2405

# NURSING STAFF DEVELOPMENT

METHODIST HOSPITAL
Memphis, Tennessee

001218

CARINI AND OWENS'
# Neurological and neurosurgical nursing

CARINI AND OWENS'

# Neurological and Neurosurgical Nursing

**BARBARA LANG CONWAY-RUTKOWSKI,** R.N., M.N.

Director, Nurse Consultation Services,
Evansville, Indiana

**EIGHTH EDITION**

with **320** illustrations and **1** color plate

## The C. V. Mosby Company

ST. LOUIS • TORONTO • LONDON    1982

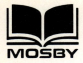

**MOSBY**

**A TRADITION OF PUBLISHING EXCELLENCE**

Editor: Pamela Swearingen
Assistant editor: Bess Arends
Manuscript editor: Carl Masthay
Design: Susan Trail
Production: Betty Duncan, Margaret B. Bridenbaugh

**EIGHTH EDITION**

The C.V. Mosby Company
11830 Westline Industrial Drive, St. Louis, Missouri 63141

**Library of Congress Cataloging in Publication Data**

Carini, Esta.
    Carini and Owens' Neurological and neurosurgical
nursing.

    Bibliography: p.
    Includes index.
    1. Neurological nursing.  I.  Owens, Guy,
1926-    .  II.  Conway-Rutkowski, Barbara Lang,
1945-    .  III.  Title.  IV.  Title: Neurological
and neurosurgical nursing.  [DNLM: 1.  Nervous
system diseases—Nursing.   WY 160 C277c]
RC350.5.C36   1982       610.73'68       81-14161
ISBN 0-8016-1035-4                       AACR2

GW/VH/VH  9  8  7  6  5  4  3  2  1     03/B/306

# CONTRIBUTORS

**MARJORIE PFAUDLER, RN, MA**
Associate Professor of Nursing, Rehabilitation
University of Rochester
Rochester, New York

**REBECCA BARNES SMITH, RN, MSN, MA**
Assistant Director of Nursing
Welborn Baptist Hospital
Evansville, Indiana

**SUSAN K. NUNCHUCK, RN, MSN**
Research Associate and Clinical Specialist
University of Texas Medical School at Houston
Houston, Texas

**JOYCE M. DUNGAN, RN, MSN**
Associate Professor
School of Nursing
University of Evansville
Evansville, Indiana

# PREFACE

The eighth edition of *Carini and Owen's Neurological and Neurosurgical Nursing* has been totally revised to include the changes that users have been requesting. Two of the most apparent changes are the reorganization of material to include more information on assessment and nursing intervention and the movement away from the medical model to a nursing model.

Neurological and neurosurgical nursing can be very challenging to teach to undergraduate students, since it encompasses such a wide variety of technical points in pathophysiology, intervention possibilities, and skills in contemporary nursing.

To make things fall into a pattern, I have begun the book with a part entitled Foundations of Neurology. The embryology facilitates better understanding of errors in formation resulting in pathophysiology. The material on anatomy and physiology has been thoroughly reorganized to facilitate the learning of normal neurophysiology. Information presented on neurotransmitters is helpful in understanding new research findings that link them with pharmacology and the neurochemistry of body functions.

Part two, Factors Affecting Neurological Outcomes, comprises seven chapters that greatly influence nursing assessment and intervention in clients with neurological problems, as described below.

Development of Perception, Integration, and Response, Chapter 5, provides the practitioner with a comprehensive environmental context of factors that underlie client performance. This chapter is particularly valuable in testing children because it gives the nurse insight into the development of performance parameters in neurological assessment.

Sexuality is considered the essence of the client's total person and as such is incorporated into the total nursing process.

In the chapter entitled Cognitive and Behavioral Impairments, approaches are suggested for working with various types of client behavior. The portion on developmental delays is totally new and incorporates important changes in living arrangements, family involvement, and potentials for nursing intervention in the intellectually impaired.

Chapter 8, Adaptive Problems in School and Learning, provides a comprehensive background on various approaches to diagnosis and remediation in learning disabilities. The reader not only learns the vocabulary essential to dealing with this common childhood problem, but also acquires the knowledge essential to nursing involvement in assessment and intervention.

In the chapter on pain, the major theories and viewpoints are detailed along with assessment, current interventions, and the neurochemical findings affecting the pain experience and pain treatment.

Impaired Consciousness, Chapter 9, includes the points in differential assessment so vital to prehospital nursing, the term used to describe care provided at the scene and in transit to the hospital. Global ischemia is reviewed in relation to barbiturates. The Glasgow Coma Scale is identified as a method for standardizing a "thumbnail" sketch on general client status. Total management for the client is also a part of the chapter.

Part three, Assessment, is composed of two chapters that detail current techniques, tests, and diagnostic studies essential to evaluate everyone across the life-span.

Part four, Disorders Affecting Functional Capacities, includes two chapters. Chapter 13, Static and Developmental Lesions, is organized in relation to Part one, Foundations of Neurology, so that disorders are discussed within a framework. Sections of nursing assessment and intervention are greatly expanded for the child with cerebral palsy and the myelodysplastic child. Chapter 14 presents a comprehensive approach to seizures, as categorized into the international classification, and to headaches — a type of pain for which nursing assessment and intervention are key ingredients to successful treatment.

Part five, Disorders Affecting Input, Integration, and Output, is a new collection of material. In giving workshops I have found that many nurses have difficulty in systematically relating disorders to interruptions in physiological functions. So I organized this section to provide a logical framework for understanding neuropathophysiology. Chapter 15 gives you everything necessary, when combined with Chapter 11, to evaluate a sensory, motor, or combined sensorimotor problem. The next four chapters divide problems into disorders arising from changes in sensibility, nutrition, and metabolism; disorders affecting motor outcomes; disorders of refined movements; and disorders arising from cranial nerves. Chapter 16 through 19 provide current comprehensive assessment and management of all major disorders in these categories, along with expected outcomes for most conditions.

Part six, Invasive Disorders, concerns the care of clients with infections and space-occupying lesions affecting the nervous system.

I am proud of Part seven, Disorders Related to Extraneurological Processes, because it includes the kind of information that prehospital and emergency room nurses need to assess clients and intervene successfully in neurological trauma. The importance of cardiopulmonary-cerebral resuscitation (CPCR) is emphasized here, as it is in coma. Another area of emphasis is hypertension, since nurses may play such an important role in prevention of severe pathophysiological outcomes associated with poorly controlled high blood pressure. Stroke is discussed in relation to the management the client and family require in both acute and long-term phases of care.

Part eight, Assistive Intervention, includes rehabilitation, surgical techniques and nursing intervention, adjunctive interventions, and medications in common use. The appendix details helpful audiovisual aids.

This book will be helpful to you both as a reference and as a means for instruction of undergraduate students in basic and advanced care of the neurological client throughout the life-span.

Special thanks goes to my parents, Lt. Col. Donald R. and Hilda M. Lang for giving me the opportunity to be where I am today; to my husband, Arthur D. Rutkowski, for his constant loving support and encouragement; to my children, Laura, Michele, and Cheryl, for their love and help; to Edna Lang, who spent a lifetime helping others; and to Granny Rathke, a shining light to many people who have weathered life's storms.

Thank you June Willis, Marjorie Pfaudler, Joyce Dungan, Becky Smith, and Susan Nunchuck for your assistance. I also appreciate the editorial assistance of Diana King.

I thank the staffs of St. Mary's Medical Center, Welborn Baptist Hospital, and Deaconess Hospital, Inc., for their encouragement and cooperation in library research.

**Barbara Lang Conway-Rutkowski**

# CONTENTS

# PART ONE

# FOUNDATIONS OF NEUROLOGY

# 1

# EMBRYOLOGY

The growth processes that characterize the formative period have far-reaching effects on the integrity and functional operations of the nervous system throughout the life cycle. Thus an understanding of neural biodynamics necessarily begins with an overview of development.

Developmental embryology is the study of the period between conception and birth, whereas developmental anatomy encompasses the entire developmental process. For the purposes of this book, let us attend to developmental embryology as a means of better understanding developmental anatomy.

## MORPHOGENESIS

The process of morphogenesis includes the fundamental components of growth, differentiation, and relative movement. In this context *growth* refers to increased size and mass resulting from protoplasmic and extracellular material synthesis rather than to the usual definition of growth as resulting from the ingestion of foodstuffs or fluids. Tissue growth is further differentiated as multiplicative, auxetic, or accretionary growth or some combination of these patterns.

*Multiplicative growth* takes place as the mitotic division of cells occurs in the zygote. It may occur once, as in the case of oocytes and neurons, or in a repetitive manner, as in the instance of epidermis and intestinal epithelium, where cellular death and regeneration are parts of a constant process. Research continues to define the precise mechanism responsible for the regulation, production, and cessation of multiplicative tissue growth.

Some general components influencing this process include genetic factors; nutritional factors; the primary organizer region; and other endocrine, thermal, photic, and mechanical determinants. Specific cell growth related to particular tissue needs and operations is probably regulated by chalones, inhibitory secretions produced by the tissue itself to regulate the mitotic cellular division.

*Auxetic growth* is the deoxyribonucleic acid (DNA)–controlled increase in cellular size. DNA present in each diploid nucleus of a cell determines the production capacities for the replacement of protein, which breaks down throughout the life cycle of the cell. Auxetic growth ceases when the cell reaches its maximum capacity to produce. Variations in growth patterns of the several cell types occur. In certain cells the nucleus divides to provide the opportunity for further growth when the limits of auxetic growth within one cell have been attained. In the granule cells of the cerebellar cortex this ongoing multiplicative growth results in a decreased cell volume in individual cells. In other cells the single diploid nucleus is aided by surrounding glial cells, which act as a functional unit with the neuron to provide additional metabolic and nuclear materials for growth. In this instance neurons may expand to a large size.

*Accretionary growth* refers to an increase in the quantity of structural intercellular material in a given tissue. Outcomes of this process include fibrous connective tissue, bone, tendon, joint capsule, cartilage, and cornea.

During the process of embryonic growth all these growth patterns—multiplicative, auxetic, and accretionary—are combined in cellular differentiation. The exact combination of these patterns depends on the specific form, size, function, age, and regenerative patterns characteristic of that

**3**

body part. Cellular death and removal are integral parts of all phases of development from embryonic life on. Through the process of death and removal of cellular components, tissue balance is maintained, and progression from rudimentary forms of growth to maturation is allowed.

## Cellular differentiation

The quest for understanding the processes that influence cells to combine into functioning tissue continues. The contemporary theory that explains cellular differentiation combines two earlier positions, namely, preformation and epigenesis. *Preformation* refers to the belief that all body parts are present in minute form in the zygote, so that growth merely implies an increase in size and development until maturity is attained. *Epigenesis* is a theory that describes organ development as the growth of new formations. The contemporary definition combines these theories and views the cytoplasmic informational content and nuclear genetic mechanisms as the ''preformation'' that is responsible for the growth and development, or ''epigenesis,'' of new body structures in the zygote (Strickberger, 1976).

Cellular differentiation is further explained in relation to protein and control complexes. Protein is the catalyst that comprises the many enzymes involved in forming the sequence of energetic and structural changes fundamental to the life process. Control complexes that regulate this elaborate process of protein synthesis include primary organization, genetic control, and an intricate system of chemical messengers that relay information within and among cells.

*Primary organization.* Two types of tissues are evident in primary organization: inductive (or self-differentiating) tissue and dependent tissue. Some tissue has an early predisposition for self-differentiation and displays an early fate. Other surrounding tissue is pluripotent, which means that it has the ability to become several different tissues in response to the specific growth of adjacent inductive tissue during the initial stages of growth.

The dorsal blastophore region exhibits powerful inductive influences on surrounding tissue and is referred to as the primary organizer region. Growth in the dorsal blastophore region results in the development of the embryonic avis and its adjacent tissue. As the organization of sequential chordate development occurs, other subordinate organizing regions become apparent.

Communication between these inductive and dependent tissues is believed to occur through undefined intracellular and intercellular chemical messengers.

*Genetic influences.* Genetic influences are the second form of powerful control that modifies cellular differentiation. Although we still understand these genetic influences only on a theoretical basis, a brief review of current thoughts on this mechanism is warranted.

The chromosome, a double strand of DNA in each cell nucleus, contains the genetic codes. This DNA comprises amino acid configurations that differ in the various genes. These genes, which are attached to each other, regulate enzyme synthesis and ultimate body metabolism through their control of ribonucleic acid (RNA).

*Chemical messengers.* The mechanism by which the foregoing elaborate, complex processes operate involves chemical messengers. DNA loci, found in functional groups called *operons,* comprise structural genes, a regulator gene, and an operant segment. The structural genes specify the polypeptides, which are the simple amino acid molecules that form either structural or enzymatic proteins. The production or inactivation of these structural genes depends on whether the operant segment is free to function or is inhibited by a repressor protein produced by its neighboring regulator gene (Fig. 1-1).

Repressor protein production from the regulator gene is controlled by chemical substances from the blastomeres and the embryonic inducers, which are discussed with the regional organizers as described under primary organization. Chalones are the substances in the local tissues that play an important role in growth processes, since they function as repressors to balance the circulating hormones and the local tissue cell genomes.

Therefore sequential growth and cellular differentiation should be viewed as an orderly process dependent on a balanced, specified pattern of operation and on inhibition of operons through the regulation of chemical interactions of inducers, circulating hormones, repressors, corepressors, and local tissue chalones. Extrachromosomal nucleic

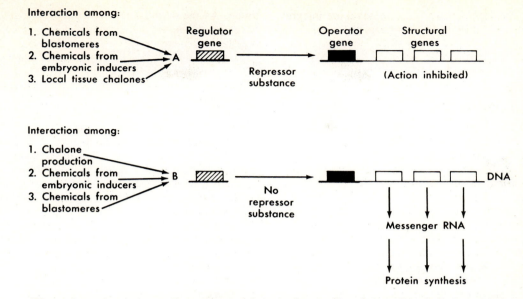

**FIG. 1-1.** Interactions among regulator, operant, and structural genes. (From Conway, B.L.: Pediatric neurologic nursing, St. Louis, 1977, The C.V. Mosby Co.)

acids may also play a role in this process, though that role is as yet undefined.

*Relative movement.* The selective interactions on tangential cellular surfaces are referred to as relative movement. Through this process, changes in the peripheral form occur so that groups of cells become sheets, balls, masses, and tubes and invaginate to make continuing embryonic development possible. Another related growth process is *contact guidance.* Some familiar examples of contact guidance are the regeneration of nerves on Schwann cell surfaces and the growth of new nerve fibers on the pathways of previous nerve fibers.

*Hereditary factors.* Factors of inheritance are key determinants of the eventual phenotype, characteristic traits in each individual, that each human possesses. Principles of inheritance are reviewed in this section, and untoward outcomes of errors during the process of embryogenesis are detailed in various portions of this text.

Meiosis and gametogenesis are the initial stages of growth. In the female 6 million primary oocytes are produced in the ovary, but only about 400 are capable of fertilization during the reproductive years. Initially these oocytes undergo the first meiotic division prenatally; this division is complete before ovulation. Then each oocyte remains dormant until ovulation, when it matures in conjunction with the ovarian follicle. Ovulation signals the beginning of the second meiotic division, which is complete by the time fertilization occurs. After the last division, one mature ovum contains 23 chromosomes and the bulk of cytoplasm, and smaller daughter cells are unable to reproduce.

Sexual maturity is attained in the male before the process of spermatogenesis occurs within the seminiferous tubules of the testes. The first and second meiotic divisions occur within 75 days. At the completion of spermatogenesis, four mature sperm cells are apparent; these have the ability to move about independently. Each mature sperm cell contains 23 chromosomes.

During the process of fertilization, the spermatozoon penetrates the ovum. The head and neck stay within the ovum, whereas the midsection and tail become detached and discarded. The head swells into a pronucleus that moves toward the center of the ovum to unite with the female pronucleus. Both nuclei duplicate their DNA material.

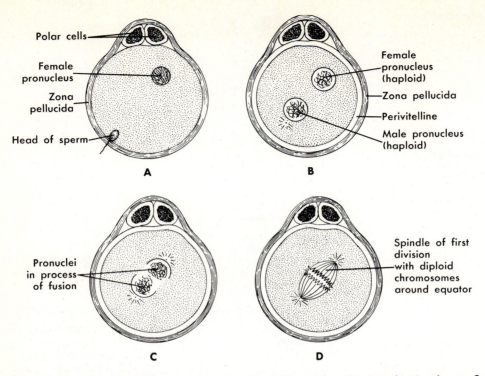

Polar cells

Female pronucleus

Zona pellucida

Head of sperm

**A**

Female pronucleus (haploid)

Zona pellucida

Perivitelline

Male pronucleus (haploid)

**B**

Pronuclei in process of fusion

**C**

Spindle of first division with diploid chromosomes around equator

**D**

**FIG. 1-2.** Process of fertilization. **A,** Sperm penetrates ovum. **B,** Pronuclei gravitate toward center of ovum. **C,** Pronuclei fuse. **D,** Appearance of two centrioles and alignment of chromosomes around equator.

Soon two centrioles are apparent (Fig. 1-2), and the chromosomes of the pronuclei align themselves on the spindle between the centrioles, where they exchange material between the two sets of 23 chromosomes. The nuclei split longitudinally, and the two sets migrate to opposite poles of the cell. A deepening groove becomes evident on the cell as the zygote progresses to the stage of cleavage or segmentation.

Inheritance is further determined by the genes in the chromosomes of all somatic cells. Each corresponding gene (allele) has a specific location on its chromosome. It is through the genes that traits from the ovum and spermatozoon are transmitted to future generations.

During fertilization each parent contributes 22 autosomes and 1 sex chromosome. Although males may provide either an X or a Y chromosome, females supply only the X chromosome. A male offspring results when the Y chromosome unites with an X chromosome, whereas a female results when two X chromosomes combine. The determination of sex in the offspring occurs when the pronuclei combine in the fertilized ovum.

Interactions of the structural and regulator genes influence cell morphology at the molecular level. The genetic traits (genotype) of an individual then become the physical characteristics of that individual (phenotype) at a more general level. The expression of an individual genotype depends on the likeness or difference of the two alleles at corresponding points in two homologous chromosomes. When one allele represents a dominant trait and one a recessive trait, the individual is heterozygous for the trait. If both alleles represent either a dominant or a recessive trait, the individual is homozygous for the trait.

The dominant trait in heterozygous individuals is expressed, whereas the recessive trait is not expressed. In the instance of homozygous expres-

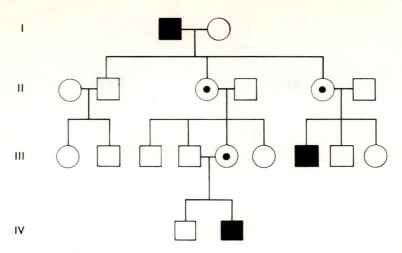

**FIG. 1-3.** Pedigree showing typical sex-linked recessive inheritance. *Dot within circle,* Females who are carriers; *black squares,* males who are affected. (From Chinn, P.L.: Child health maintenance: concepts in family-centered care, St. Louis, 1974, The C.V. Mosby Co.)

sion, both alleles carry the same trait, and expression may be either recessive or dominant, accordingly. Clinically it is difficult to distinguish a heterozygous-dominant from a homozygous-dominant trait.

Genetic linkage has a decided effect on phenotypes of individuals. Because of genetic linkage, traits from genes in proximity on the same chromosomes tend to be inherited together. Although investigation of disease-associated traits is in the initial stages, preliminary information is available. One instance of this phenomenon is apparent in sex-linked patterns of inheritance, such as that seen in hemophilia. Hemophilia, most commonly seen in males, is transmitted by females, who must be heterozygous for the trait. If a hemophiliac male mates with a female homozygous for the trait (normal), the male offspring will not have the disease, but all the female offspring will be heterozygous for the trait. Thus the disease will skip one generation and be expressed in half the male offspring produced by the affected (heterozygous) females (Fig. 1-3).

*Variable expressivity* is the phenomenon that explains why some persons inherit a trait in a differing degree from others with the same genotype. The explanation for the differences in phenotypes in individuals with the same genotypes is poorly understood.

## Critical periods of development

The chief components of the central nervous system are as follows:

| White matter | Gray matter |
| --- | --- |
| Axonal bundles | Cell bodies |
| Glial cells | Dendrites |
| Blood vessels | Axons (unmyelinated) |
| Limited extracellular matrix in contrast to other body tissue | Limited extracellular matrix in contrast to other body tissue |

These structures are susceptible to injury at various periods in neural development. In reality, a rigid timetable or an exact definition of a causative agent is not practical at this point in scientific understanding, since many defects are believed to result from the interaction of various factors. Although the causative mechanism is not clearly designated as purely environmental or inherited, resulting conditions are often described separately.

*Environmental influences.* When environmental interferences interrupt the development of the zygote during the first 2 weeks, implantation of the blastocyst is often incomplete, and spontaneous abortion or embryonic death frequently occurs. If teratogens produce mitotic nondisjunction, that is, the failure of homologous chromosomes to travel to opposite poles in the first maturational stage, some germ cells acquire 24 chromosomes, whereas others possess only 22. When the germ cell with 24 chromosomes fuses with a normal one during the process of fertilization, the resulting zygote will have 47 chromosomes *(trisomy)*. If the cell with 22 chromosomes unites with a normal germ cell, the resulting zygote will have 45 chromosomes *(monosomy)*. Monosomy of an autosome usually results in prenatal death. However, difficulties associated with a trisomy of the autosomes include common problems such as Down's syndrome (trisomy 21), whereas trisomy of the sex chromosomes occurs most often as 47XXX in females and 47XXY or 47XYY in males. Trisomy of the sex chromosomes usually is not apparent until adolescence (Figs. 1-4 to 1-6).

During the first 5 weeks of development, the nervous system is particularly susceptible to environmental interferences, since the preliminary structural formation is completed during this period. Noxious agents *(teratogens)* have great impact in this period of rapid cellular differentiation and biochemical activity that precedes morphological differentiation and structural development. Thus undesirable outcomes of these interferences may include major structural defects or embryonic death. Teratogenic factors affecting development at later points are more likely to result in less severe morphological changes or in functional disorders.

Teratogens, or substances that result in deformity more frequently than among persons not exposed, usually are associated with the following conditions: complete cranioschisis, meningoencephalocele, meningocele, cranium bifidum occultum, and congenital dermal sinuses. Further read-

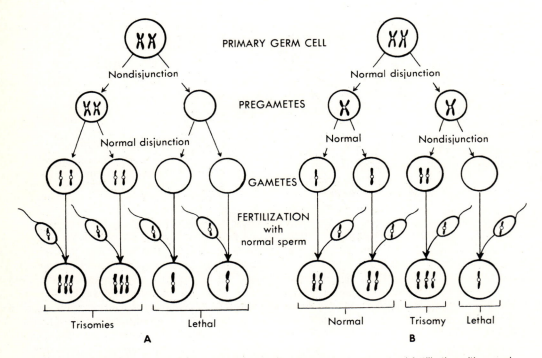

**FIG. 1-4.** Mechanisms of maldistribution of chromosomes during meiosis in ovum and fertilization with normal sperm. **A,** During first meiotic division. **B,** During second meiotic division. (From Whaley, L.F.: Understanding inherited disorders, St. Louis, 1974, The C.V. Mosby Co.)

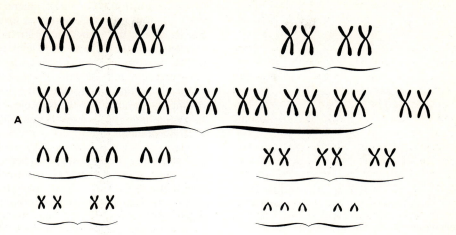

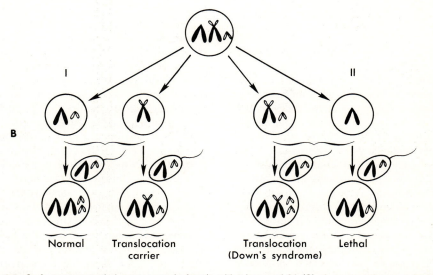

FIG. 1-5. **A,** Arrangement of chromosomes in female with trisomy of 21 (G) chromosome group, depicted as 47XX21+. **B,** Typical example of cell division in translocated chromosome. *I,* Resulting gametes receive equal amounts of hereditary material; *II,* hereditary material is unevenly distributed between gametes.

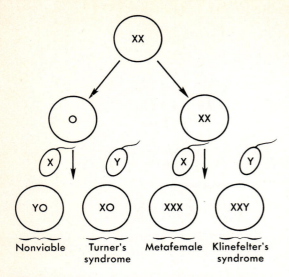

**FIG. 1-6.** Certain common sex chromosome abnormalities occur when normal sperm fertilizes ovum wherein nondisjunction of X chromosomes had occurred. (Adapted from Whaley, L.F.: Understanding inherited disorders, St. Louis, 1974, The C.V. Mosby Co.)

ing on this subject may be found among the references for this chapter.

*Genetic factors.* Other malformations may be caused by genetic factors such as mutant genes or chromosomal abnormalities. Mutant genes, which may account for up to 15% of the congenital abnormalities, become clinically apparent in accordance with mendelian laws of inheritance. Some 150 recessive and another 150 dominant autosomal disorders are known. Chromosomal abnormalities, which include problems related to abnormalities in the structure or numbers of chromosomes, account for defective development far more frequently than mutant genes. About 1 in 200 newborn infants may have a chromosomal disorder of some type. Discussion of inherited problems, many of which are apparent in childhood, is beyond the scope of this text. However, inherited problems manifested in adulthood are detailed in appropriate sections of this book (Gellis and Feingold, 1968; Gardner, 1975; Carr, 1970; Philipp et al., 1977; Holmes et al., 1972; Bergsma, 1973; Conway, 1977).

## OVERVIEW OF HUMAN DEVELOPMENT

After sexual intercourse, spermatozoa travel from the vagina through the cervical canal and uterus to the fallopian tube, where fertilization usually occurs. After the ovum is invaded by the spermatozoon, the second maturational division is complete. As the haploid pronuclei of the ovum and spermatozoon unite, the nucleus of a diploid cell *(zygote)* is formed.

As the zygote travels down the fallopian tube toward the uterus, the process of cleavage changes the zygote into blastomeres. After 3 days a sphere of 16 blastomeres *(morula)* enters the uterine cavity. Internal changes within the morula follow shortly; these cause the morula to become a blastocyst with (1) a cavity, (2) an inner cell mass that eventually gives rise to the embryo, and (3) an outer cellular layer *(trophoblast)* that encloses the cavity and the inner cell mass. By the sixth day this blastocyst has attached itself to the endometrial epithelium, and the primary germ layer of the embryo *(embryonic endoderm)* has begun its formation on the ventral aspect of the inner cell mass (Fig. 1-7).

During the second gestational week, rapid growth and cellular differentiation result in the formation of two layers: the *cytotrophoblast* and the *syncytial trophoblast (syntroblast)*. Developing lacunae soon unite into networks as the trophoblast invades maternal sinusoids to allow blood into these lacunar networks, thus establishing the early uteroplacental circulation. Primary villi are noted in the exterior aspect of the chorionic sac by this time. The process of implantation moves to completion as the bilaminar embryo becomes totally embedded in the endometrium.

Simultaneously, *extraembryonic mesoderm* arises from the inner aspect of the trophoblast, so that the original blastocystic cavity occupies less volume and is converted into the primitive yolk sac. Next the *extraembryonic coelom,* a large fluid-filled cavity bordering the amnion and yolk sac (except at the point where the amnion is connected to the trophoblast by the connecting stalk), forms from spaces in the extraembryonic mesoderm. During the development of the extraembryonic coelom the primitive yolk sac diminishes in size as a smaller secondary yolk sac forms (Fig. 1-8).

At the completion of the second week the amni-

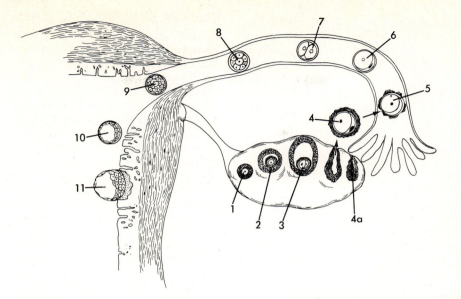

**FIG. 1-7.** Progress of zygote to implantation. *1* and *2,* Early stages; *3,* formation of polar cell; *4,* mature ovum; *4a,* corpus luteum (early stage); *5,* fertilization; *6,* segmentation of nucleus; *7,* two-cell stage; *8,* eight-cell stage; *9,* morula; *10,* blastocyst free in uterine cavity; *11,* implantation.

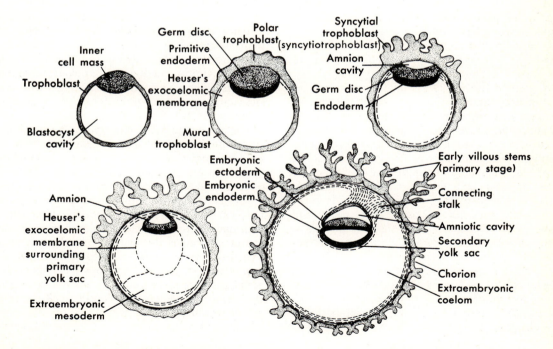

**FIG. 1-8.** Early phases of cellular differentiation. (From Conway, B.L.: Pediatric neurologic nursing, St. Louis, 1977, The C.V. Mosby Co.)

otic cavity is apparent as a narrow opening between the polar trophoblast and the inner cell mass. The inner cell mass has further differentiated into a two-layered embryonic disc where the *embryonic ectoderm* adjoins the amniotic cavity, whereas the *embryonic endoderm* is next to the blastocystic cavity. Evidence of thickening in the embryonic endoderm is termed the *prochordal plate* and forms the basis for the developing cranium and mouth.

During the third week of gestation, three primary germ layers are evident as the bilaminar embryonic disc becomes a trilaminar embryo. The primitive streak, a midline thickening of embryonic ectoderm, gives rise to mesenchymal cells that form the *intraembryonic layer* (the third germ layer located between the endoderm and the ectoderm).

The cranial thickening of the primitive streak is termed the *primitive knot*. The primitive knot gives rise to the *notochordal process,* a midline cord between the endoderm and the ectoderm, which grows until it contacts the immovable *prochordal plate*. The prochordal plate adheres solidly to the ectoderm to form the oropharyngeal membrane. Caudal to the primitive streak is the *cloacal membrane,* a round area where fused endoderm and ectoderm make the growth of the third intervening layer impossible. The only other area where the mesoderm does not intervene is in the notochord itself.

### Embryonic disc formation

The embryonic disc soon develops into a pear-shaped form as mesenchymal cells migrate away from the primitive streak. The largest part of the pearlike disc is in the cranial area, whereas caudal growth is more limited.

By the beginning of the fifth gestational week, mesenchymal cell production has greatly decreased. Gradually the primitive streak becomes a mere remnant in the sacrococcygeal area. After this remnant degenerates, it disappears in most individuals. However, when the remnant persists, it may result in a teratoma.

The next developmental event occurs as the notochord arises from the notochordal process to form the rudimentary axis of the embryo. First, the notochordal process fuses with the endoderm, and degeneration begins at the points of fusion. Soon

openings at the inferior aspect of the notochordal process are apparent. These openings allow the lumen within the notochord *(notochordal canal)* to communicate with the yolk sac. As the floor of the notochordal canal disappears, the remaining notochordal process forms the *notochordal plate,* a flattened, grooved surface (Fig. 1-9). Next, the cranial end of this notochordal plate folds over to become the *notochord*. The embryonic endoderm is then a layer anterior to the notochord.

The *neurenteric canal,* the temporary connection for the amniotic sac and the amniotic cavity, becomes obliterated when formation of the notochord is complete. At the completion of the fourth gestational week the notochord is nearly completely developed as a structure extending between the prochordal plate and the caudal primitive knot.

The next major event in neural development is the formation of the *neural tube*. As development of the notochord progresses, the embryonic ectoderm overlying the notochord and the surrounding mesoderm thicken to become the neural plate. As the neural plate continues its growth, the borders are elevated into neural folds with a longitudinal, midline separation between them, the *neural groove*. The enlargement of the neural folds, especially at the anterior aspects, and the expansion of the walls bordering the neural groove mark the first indication of brain formation. Continuing brain growth is interrupted as two transverse constrictions appear and divide the cephalic region into three areas: the *prosencephalon (forebrain),* the *mesencephalon (midbrain),* and the *rhombencephalon (hindbrain)* (Fig. 1-10).

The neural groove continues to deepen as the dorsal lips fuse to form a canal. During this process of fusion, the general body ectoderm fuses and the neural tissue fuses, and the result is the formation of the neural tube. Neural tissue fusion occurs first in the cervical, or hindbrain, area at the end of the third week of gestation and gradually continues in both directions until small openings *(neuropores)* remain at the distal ends. The function of these neuropores is to channel amniotic fluid into the neural tube and groove for purposes of bathing and possibly for nourishment. The superior neuropore closes in the middle of the fourth week, whereas the inferior neuropore is patent until the end of the fourth week. The vascular system of the neural

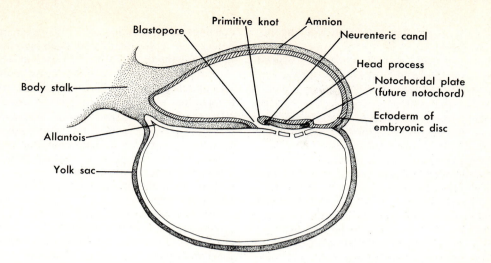

**FIG. 1-9.** Notochordal plate is precursor of notochord. (From Conway, B.L.: Pediatric neurologic nursing, St. Louis, 1977, The C.V. Mosby Co.)

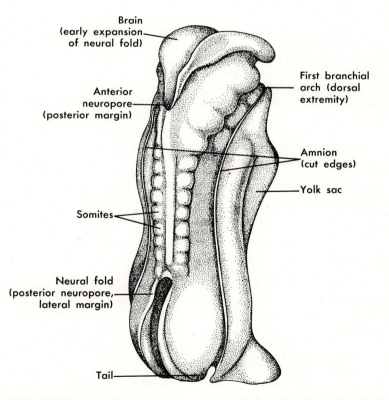

**FIG. 1-10.** Formation of neural tube occurs by end of third week of gestation. Small openings at either end (neuropores) channel amniotic fluid into neural groove and tube. (From Conway, B.L.: Pediatric neurologic nursing, St. Louis, 1977, The C.V. Mosby Co.)

tube becomes operational at the same time that the neuropores close.

Interferences with the formation of the neural tube during the third and fourth weeks of gestation account for the majority of the serious structural anomalies of the central nervous system. These interferences may include genetic disorders, environmental influences, or a combination of these. Untoward environmental influences may consist of such factors as concurrent maternal disease or metabolic disorders, effects from ingested foreign substances, infectious problems, or ionizing radiation. Most neural tube defects cannot be related to a single untoward factor and are believed to be caused by a combination of genetic and environmental problems. When the fetal involvement is severe, the defect may be incompatible with life. In other instances the problem may result in pronounced structural deformity that interferes with functional abilities (Holmes et al., 1973; Moore, 1977).

### Defective closure of midline structures

Two major groups of problems represent the outcomes of defective closure of midline structures. These defects include cerebral dysplasias with cranium bifidum and myelodysplasia with spina bifida; various other disorders are also possible. These groups contain problems that range from severe to less extensive involvement.

*Cerebral dysplasias with cranium bifidum.* Five defects make up the category of cerebral dysplasias with cranium bifidum, including the following:

  □ Complete cranioschisis
  □ Meningoencephalocele
  □ Meningocele
  □ Cranium bifidum occultum
  □ Porencephaly

*Complete cranioschisis* refers to a condition wherein the skull is lacking and the brain is defective. Three variations of this defect occur: anencephaly, hemicephalia, and exencephaly. In anencephaly the forebrain and midbrain show inadequate development, though the hindbrain may be apparent in its entirety. In hemicephalia the forebrain shows faulty development, though the midbrain may be visible as a partial or complete formation. In exencephaly the diencephalon is apparent, and parts of the hemispheres may be obvious.

The *meningoencephalocele,* the next most severe defect, corresponds to the meningomyelocele in the spinal cord. This defect is one in which the skull formation is faulty, so that a part of the brain and meninges has herniated to protrude from the exterior portion of the head. This protrusion may or may not contain portions of the ventricular system. Associated defects in brain structures are also frequently evident in this deformity.

The *meningocele* refers to an external protrusion composed of meninges without brain tissue. Abnormalities in the growth of brain tissue may also be seen with this defect.

When *cranium bifidum occultum* occurs, the bony structure is abnormal, but no saclike protrusion is seen. Overlying skin may be abnormally pigmented or evidence a "port-wine stain" (a reddish discoloration).

*Porencephaly* refers to an impairment of the cerebrum wherein cranium bifidum is associated with a cleft that opens onto the surface of the cerebral cortex. This cleft is convoluted, lined with gray matter, and connected to the ventricular system. The defect is bilateral and symmetrical.

Cranial defects of this group, collectively referred to as *encephaloceles,* occur about once in 6500 births. Anencephaly and some extreme forms of cranioschisis are not compatible with life, whereas meningoencephaloceles, meningoceles, and cranium bifidum occultum result in life characterized by a variety of functional deficiencies. Meningoencephaloceles are often accompanied by hydrocephalus. In meningoceles the bony defect is often smaller, and the external protrusion is more commonly covered by meninges and skin. Microgyria, impaired formation of the corpus callosum, and porencephaly are commonly associated with cranium bifidum. Sequestration dermoids and epidermoids are also commonly seen over the affected cranial area.

Encephaloceles are usually readily observable in the newborn. Although the size and shape of these defects may vary, they are prone to steady growth. Encephaloceles pulsate in rhythm with the body pulses. The application of pressure to these growths results in impaired consciousness, bulging fontanels, and disturbed respiration in many cases. Other cranial features in affected children include shallow eye orbits, protrusion of the eyes, receding forehead, prominent nose, and wide cheekbones.

These encephaloceles result in far-reaching health interferences, including impaired mental capacity, hydrocephalus, cerebral palsy, spina bifida, talipes equinovarus, and cleft lip and palate.

When a neural tube defect is suspected, amniocentesis may be performed. Although it is not reliable in predicting the closed types of neural tube defects (Arey, 1974; Harris et al., 1974), it has proved valuable for detection of the open forms, such as anencephaly and open spina bifida cystica. Research continues to expand the availability of this diagnostic service to individuals other than those considered at high risk for the production of neural tube defects.

In diagnosing these cranial defects, one may find the distinction between meningoceles and meningoencephaloceles difficult without the confirmation of skull films and ventricular air studies. However, the meningoencephalocele may usually be identified clinically by its tendency to be more translucent than the meningocele. Other clinical findings may also add significantly to the data needed to distinguish these two lesions. At times cranial protrusions such as abscesses, cephalhematomas, or intracranial tumors are mistakenly diagnosed as encephaloceles. Abscesses may be identified by needle aspiration yielding purulent material. Cephalhematomas may be differentiated by their tendency to grow in the parietal region rather than the midline, by their decreasing size, by the lack of pulsations, and by the evidence of new bony formation at the periphery during the first few weeks of life. Intracranial lesions such as gliomas or hemangiomas may resemble encephaloceles because of the local bony destruction they cause. However, neurodiagnostic studies allow the detection of these lesions.

When encephaloceles are extensive, death frequently occurs before the child reaches 1 year of age. Death is usually attributed in part to complications of hydrocephalus, infection, or rupture of the sac when growth of the encephalocele is rapid. Acute care is geared toward maintaining the integrity of the sac, providing supportive measures during the preoperative and postoperative period, and avoiding infection. Long-term management for surviving infants comprises a multifaceted health team approach designed to assist the child and family in coping with the many physical, social, emotional, and financial problems associated with an encephalocele. Genetic counseling and antenatal diagnosis for future pregnancies is appropriate when the family has produced one child with an encephalocele (Seller et al., 1974).

*Myelodysplasias with spina bifida.* Myelodysplasias with spina bifida may be divided into five major categories, including the following:

□ Complete rachischisis
□ Meningomyelocele
□ Meningocele
□ Spina bifida occulta
□ Congenital dermal sinuses

These defects, ranging from severe to less extensive lesions, are characterized by incomplete fusion of one or more vertebral laminae with or without impaired development of the spinal cord. Interferences, which are most likely a combination of genetic and environmental factors, probably interrupt normal developmental processes before the eleventh week of gestation, since vertebral formation from the first cervical to the fourth sacral vertebra is complete by this time.

Estimations indicate that the incidence of spina bifida occulta may be as high as 5% in the general population. However, only about 1 in 1000 infants has the accompanying protrusion of meninges and neural tissue. The meningomyelocele is the most common type of saclike protrusion and is most frequently seen in either the lumbar or lumbosacral area. After an infant has been born with a myelodysplastic defect, the incidence of the parents producing another child with a similar deformity increases to 10 times that of the general population.

*Complete rachischisis,* the most severe deformity in this category, consists of a red, exposed, flattened spinal cord within the groove formed by the bifurcated vertebral laminae. The lesion comprises poorly differentiated neural tissue in various stages of development. Although an external sac is not obvious in many cases, the lesion may appear to protrude because of the accumulation of cerebrospinal fluid beneath it. Because this lesion is often covered by meninges and skin, it may be mistaken for a meningocele. However, it may be distinguished by the concurrent evidence of paralysis in the legs and other extreme neurological symptoms. Infections commonly occur in these lesions. The prognosis is related to the extent of involvement, which may be either localized or found to include the entire spinal and cranial axis. Depending on the extent of the lesion, defects may result in severe neurological deficits or death.

The *meningomyelocele,* the next most severe lesion of the spinal cord, is a soft, rounded protrusion of the spinal cord and its roots that contains cerebrospinal fluid because of its communication with the subarachnoid space. In this defect the neural groove has closed, but paralysis below the level of the lesion as a result of adhesions or traction on the cord is consistent with the neural tissue involved.

The *meningocele* is an external protrusion that does not contain neural tissue. In these cases the cord and spinal nerve roots may be either defective or normal at the level of the lesion. Externally the defect may be covered by a thin parchment-like layer or by normal skin. Internally the meninges may be fused into a single layer or divided into the dura mater and arachnoid to form a double sac.

In *spina bifida occulta* no external protrusion exists. However, the skin overlying the defective lamina may display such abnormal markings as dimpling, unusual hair growth, or the presence of excessive fat deposits or telangiectases. The majority of these cases do not reveal any neurological abnormalities, since the neural tube has closed in this type of defect. However, faulty cord development may be associated with this defect, so that the spinal cord becomes firmly attached via a fibrous mass to the spinal column. This attachment prevents the normal ascension of the cord during the developmental process. Thus the conus of the spinal cord may be beneath the level expected in most individuals. Further information on this phenomenon is available in the sections on spinal cord development and in Chapter 2. This potential problem should be considered when a spinal tap is performed. Chapter 13 offers detailed information.

*Congenital dermal sinuses* are also included in the category of problems attributed to faulty closure of the neural tube. Although the majority of these sinuses are limited to the skin or communication with dermoid or epidermoid cysts, a few may involve the nervous system. This defect occurs when there is incomplete separation of the neuroectoderm from the epithelial ectoderm along the dorsal aspect of the embryo during the third and fifth gestational weeks. Unusual skin markings, port-wine stains, dimpling, or abnormal tufts of hair may be located on or adjacent to these sinuses. Although these sinuses may occur at any point in the axis of the central nervous system, they are most commonly found in either the posterior fossa of the head or the sacral region of the spine. When sinuses occur in the coccygeal region, they often extend only into the fascia. In these cases, termed *pilonidal sinuses,* infection is a periodic problem, but neurological deficiencies generally do not occur. Abnormalities in underlying bony structure, apparent by radiographical study, are sometimes associated.

Children with myelodysplastic problems may have associated conditions. A large number of those affected with meningomyeloceles develop hydrocephalus, which may be accompanied by Arnold-Chiari deformity. When the child has a meningocele, neurological deficiencies may be either absent or minimal. If cranium bifidum is found in association with spina bifida, the interference with the developmental process has occurred at two levels. In other cases of spina bifida occulta, progressive gliosis resulting in cavity formation in the gray matter may cause problems similar to those seen in syringomyelia.

Meningomyeloceles cause neurological problems in the myotomes innervated by involved spinal cord segments. The resulting impairment may cause any degree of involvement up to and including complete paralysis, depending on the extent and location of the lesion. Generally the most severe defects are obvious in the neonate, whereas milder impairments may not become evident until later childhood. In these latter instances early developmental progress may occur normally. However, as the abnormal saclike formation with the attached spinal cord is subjected to the stresses of spinal flexion encountered in normal activity, the lower extremities begin to develop poorly. Thus the individual eventually appears to have large shoulders in relation to a small pelvis and thin legs as development to maturity occurs. Since sudden, extreme flexion in individuals with this underlying problem may result in paralysis, consideration should be given to this possibility when children and adolescents are screened for selection in contact sports.

In individuals with congenital dermal sinuses inflammation with or without purulent drainage may be a problem. When the tract communicates with the central nervous system, recurrent meningitis and leakage of cerebrospinal fluid may be additional problems. When the tract terminates within either the spinal cord or the cranium, clinical symptoms resemble those seen when tumors occupy the same space. In cases where there is intraspinal cystic expansion of the sinus tract, neurological impairments may include disorders in the reflexes and in sensibility, problems in sphincter control, and paresis in the lower extremities. The most common location of communicating dermal tracts in the cranium is in the occipital region, where the tract leads into the posterior fossa. Resulting symptoms resemble those seen with tumors of the cerebellum or fourth ventricle and in obstructive hydrocephalus. Whenever these symptoms or those of a recurring pyogenic meningitis are evident, one should inspect the skin in the appropriate area with good lighting to ascertain the presence of a dermal sinus. Refer to other sources for information on making a definitive diagnosis among other problems and within the category of myelodysplastic problems (Ford, 1973). A variety of medical and surgical management modalities is available to individuals with these problems. Since the bulk of management for many individuals and their families occurs during childhood, further discussion of the problems of acute and long-term care is deferred to other sources (Jabbour et al., 1976; Moore, 1977; Ford, 1973; Ruhde) and to Chapter 13.

***Other disorders.*** A few other problems should be mentioned in relation to defective closure of the midline structures, including the following:

□ Diplomyelia
□ Diastematomyelia
□ Errors in cranial development

*Diplomyelia,* duplication of the spinal cord most frequently found in the midthoracic area, may be associated with normal functioning. However, when spinal cord abnormalities or congenital tumors are also present, neurological deficits may be observed. About half the individuals with diplomyelia have spina bifida. Other problems that may be associated include meningocele and various types of clubfoot.

*Diastematomyelia,* a congenital defect that occurs during gestation when deviant mesodermal cells intervene in the tissue of the neural tube rather than becoming located in their customary place at the periphery of the neural tube, results in the formation of a bony or cartilaginous spur that divides the cord into two parts. This division may extend for only one or two segments. When these dual sections of cord are evident, each cord is found to have its own sac. Associated bony defects, such as spina bifida, are frequently seen in the same area. Dermal changes, including dimples, lipomas, dermal sinus tract, nevi, unusual hair growth, and telangiectases, may also occur concurrently. Since the symptoms of this condition may not be evident at birth, practitioners who note abnormalities in sphincter control or problems in the growth or functioning of the lower extremities should consider diastematomyelia as a possibility. Common clinical findings may include atrophy, weakness, or spasticity in one or both legs; changes in the deep tendon reflexes; trophic ulceration of the feet; disturbances in gait, or difficulty in bowel and bladder control. After diagnosis is confirmed and defined through roentgenography and myelography, surgical intervention is recommended to remove the bony or fibrous septum and return both segments of cord to a single canal. Although prior damage may not be reversed, future problems are avoided because surgery eliminates the source of compression, stretching, and fixation to affected segments of the spinal cord.

The effects of several *errors in cranial development* should be considered in brief. For example, when the *corpus callosum* is missing, other formative defects—fusion of the frontal hemispheres or absence of the gyrus fornicatus or falx—may be associated. When abnormal patterns of neuronal migration occur during developmental processes, the result is a displacement in organ or tissue growth *(heterotopias).* At the histological level these abnormal migrations cause nuclear masses to accumulate in the white matter with adjacent borders of glial cells. Frequently other errors of formation are associated. *Cortical agenesis* includes several problems related to errors in the formation of different aspects of the cerebral cortex. Problems in achieving and maintaining functional integrity in cortical development and operations may also result from degenerative disease (Ford, 1973; Jabbour et al., 1976).

When the *basal ganglia* fail to develop properly because of growth interferences during the formation of the forebrain, the result may be impairments in muscular tone, often accompanied by involuntary movements.

Errors in formation of the *cranial nerve nuclei* may result in inadequate development or absence. Functions related to the involved nerves are affected accordingly. When development in the cerebellum is abnormal, the pons and olives may also reflect deviations in growth patterns.

*Special senses*—olfaction, vision, and audition—may also be affected by developmental interferences. When defective development results, the problems are usually related to the entire structure rather than to one portion of the sense mechanism.

### Histogenesis of neural tube

After the neural tube has fused, neuroectodermal cells remain at the periphery to form the neural crests of the neural tube. Neuroblasts from the neural tube and neural crest each differentiate into specific types of cells in the nervous system (Figs. 1-11 and 1-12).

Understanding the histogenesis of the neural tube, first described by Wilhelm His in 1890, is essential to orderly organization of the structure and function of portions of the nervous system.

The neural tube has three distinct layers, including (1) the *ependymal (inner) layer,* the *mantle (middle) layer,* and the *marginal (outer) layer.* Each layer is derived from a homogeneous group of pluripotent cells exhibiting appearances characteristic of the stages seen at various times in the mitotic division cycle. After the growth cycle is complete, some daughter cells remain in the ependymal layer to repeat the cycle, whereas other daughter cells differentiate into neuroblasts as they migrate to become part of the mantle layer. These neuroblasts then develop dendritic processes and are ultimately categorized as multipolar cells. Their processes extend to form the outer (marginal) layer. The marginal layer is devoid of cell bodies (Fig. 1-13).

Eventually the thickening of the lateral walls of the neural tube results in a decrease in the size of the central canal. The ependymal layer gives rise to all neurons and macroglial cells (astrocytes and oligodendrocytes) in the spinal cord. The marginal layer ultimately becomes the white matter in the spinal cord as it receives the axons from the brain,

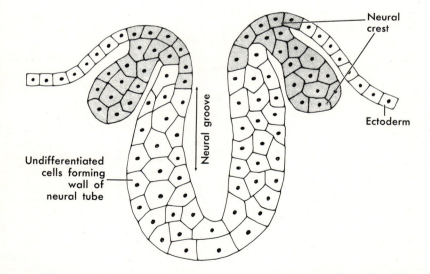

**FIG. 1-11.** Horizontal section through embryo at about 20 days of gestation. Neuroectodermal cells, *shaded areas,* remain at periphery to form neural crests after neural tube has fused. Neural crest will become neural folds and be fused at midline by twenty-fourth day of gestation.

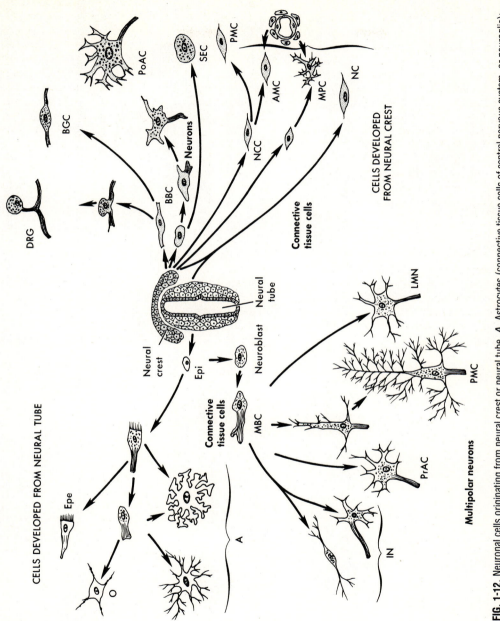

**FIG. 1-12.** Neuronal cells originating from neural crest or neural tube. *A*, Astrocytes (connective tissue cells of central nervous system, or neuroglia); *AMC*, arachnoid mater cells; *BBC*, bipolar blast cells; *BGC*, bipolar ganglion cells associated with pathways of special senses; *DRG*, dorsal root ganglion, a unipolar (single process that divides into two) neuron, and sensory neurons of cranial nerve nuclei; *Epe*, Ependymal cell; *Epi*, epithelial (lining) cell; *IN*, interneurons, association and commissural; *LMN*, lower motor neurons of anterior horn and motor nerves of cranial nuclei; *MBC*, multipolar "blast" cells of central nervous system; *MPC*, microglia phagocytic connective tissue cell; *NC* neurilemmal (Schwann) cells; *NCC*, neural crest cells; *O*, oligodendrocyte; *PMC (on right)*, pia mater cell; *PMC (on bottom)*, pyramidal motor (voluntary) cells of cerebral cortex; *PoAC*, postganglionic autonomic cells; *PrAC*, preganglionic autonomic cells; *Sec*, secreting cell of adrenal medulla.

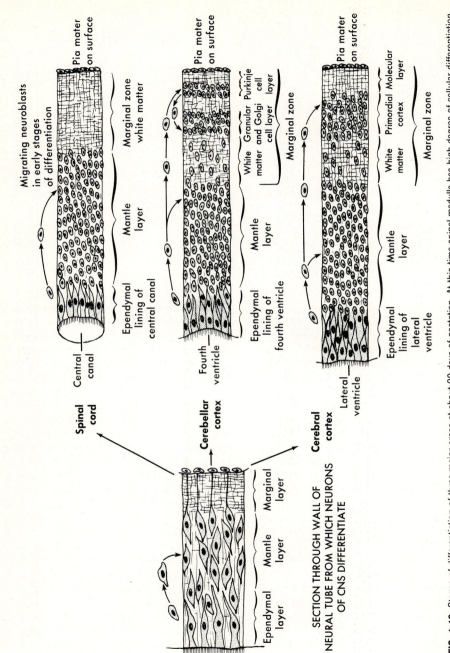

Migrating neuroblasts in early stages of differentiation

**Spinal cord**

Pia mater on surface
Marginal zone white matter
Mantle layer
Ependymal lining of central canal
Central canal

**Cerebellar cortex**

Pia mater on surface
Purkinje cell layer
Granular and Golgi cell layer
White matter
Marginal zone
Mantle layer
Ependymal lining of fourth ventricle
Fourth ventricle

**Cerebral cortex**

Pia mater on surface
Molecular layer
Primordial cortex
White matter
Marginal zone
Mantle layer
Ependymal lining of lateral ventricle
Lateral ventricle

SECTION THROUGH WALL OF NEURAL TUBE FROM WHICH NEURONS OF CNS DIFFERENTIATE

Marginal layer
Mantle layer
Ependymal layer

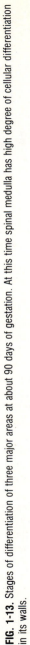

**FIG. 1-13.** Stages of differentiation of three major areas at about 90 days of gestation. At this time spinal medulla has high degree of cellular differentiation in its walls.

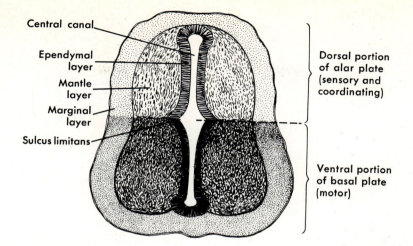

Central canal

Ependymal layer

Mantle layer

Marginal layer

Sulcus limitans

Dorsal portion of alar plate (sensory and coordinating)

Ventral portion of basal plate (motor)

FIG. 1-14. Basal and alar plates: key to functional variation. (From Conway, B.L.: Pediatric neurologic nursing, St. Louis, 1977, The C.V. Mosby Co.)

the dorsal root ganglia, and the cell bodies of the neurons in the mantle layer.

After the formation of neuroblasts is complete, the neuroepithelial cells in the ependymal layer form supportive cells of the nervous system known as *glioblasts* (spongioblasts). Some glioblasts migrate out to the mantle and marginal zones to become astroblasts and then *astrocytes*. Other cells formed in the same manner are the *oligodendroblasts*, which later become the *oligodendrocytes*. After the production of neuroblasts and glioblasts is complete, the neuroepithelial cells of the innermost layer actually form the ependymal cells that ultimately become part of the epithelial lining of the central canal in the spinal cord and ventricles of the brain.

The *microglial cells*, neuroglial cells of lesser size, are differentiated from mesenchymal cells bordering the central nervous system. They move into the spinal cord along with the blood vessels during the gestational period.

***Alar and basal plates.*** Cellular proliferation causes the lateral walls of the neural tube to thicken. The differential rate of thickening results in the development of a longitudinal groove, the *sulcus limitans,* bilaterally. The sulcus limitans divides the ependymal and mantle layers on each wall of the neural tube into two laminae, the basal (ventral) plate and the alar (dorsal) plate (Fig. 1-14).

Understanding the derivation of key components of the nervous system in relation to their origin from the alar or basal plate provides a basis for categorizing neural structures by functional variation with few exceptions. In general, neuronal cells of the alar plate become sensory and internuncial cells, whereas those of the basal plate become motor control cells.

Each area of the nervous system—the spinal medulla, the brainstem, the cerebellum, and the cerebrum—reveals some degree of development in terms of the three-layer cellular pattern and the derivation of motor cells from the basal plate and sensory cells from the alar plate. A deviation in the general growth pattern of the neural tube is evident in the development of the ventricular system and the choroid plexuses. Details on the ventricular system are presented in other sections. Because slight variations occur in the other various structures, the next few paragraphs are devoted to identifying these differences.

SPINAL MEDULLA. (Note: The term *spinal medulla* is the same as *spinal cord*.) The ependymal cells of the spinal medulla remain in a radial columnar arrangement adjacent to the central canal lumen. The gray matter of the spinal medulla, which forms an "H," is composed of the mantle zone cells. The bordering white matter surrounding this H arises from the marginal zone. The dorsal columns of the H perform sensory and coordinating functions and are derived from the alar plate, whereas the lateral and ventral gray columns are responsible for motor functions and arise from the basal plate. The white matter derived from the marginal layer is chiefly supportive in nature. However, the white matter does include the axonal bundles of neurons from the mantle layer, which combine into tracts. The discussion of specific tracts in Chapters 2 and 3 offers further detail.

BRAINSTEM. The organizational pattern in the brainstem is quite similar to that in the spinal medulla. Sensory neurons, with their dorsal location, arise from the alar portion of the mantle layer, whereas the ventral motor neurons are derived from the basal part. Neurons in the gray matter arising from the mantle zone form clusters (nuclei) according to their derivation, which dictates their ultimate operational patterns. These nuclei are flanked on all sides by the white matter of the marginal zone. The red nucleus, the pontine nuclei, and the olivary nucleus represent exceptions to the basic developmental pattern. In these three motor control nuclei, neuroblasts develop from the alar plate of the mantle layer but migrate to the basal portion of the mantle layer. Some investigators believe these variations in formation are related to the unique functions of these nuclei. Each of these nuclei is interconnected through the cerebellum or the basal nuclei (ganglia) to monitor and regulate muscular activity in relation to incoming sensory messages.

CEREBELLUM. The organization of the cerebellum represents additional changes in the basic growth model. While the dense mantle layer forms the gray matter, some of the neurons in this layer move in a peripheral direction to form a more exterior gray cortex. This gray cortex, comprising migrating neuroblasts, has two distinct layers: the inner granular and Golgi cell layers. The Purkinje cell layer covers the cortex. The cerebellar cortex is both fascinating and complex in its functions. Details of its histological structure and general operation are discussed in a later section.

CEREBRUM. During the first 3 months of gestation, the neopallial portion of the cerebral hemispheres develops in accordance with the three-layer pattern established in the neural tube. By the third month neuroblasts from the mantle layer have migrated into the marginal layer to begin the growth of the neopallial cerebral cortex. At 6 months of gestation, six distinct layers of cell bodies and their processes are obvious. The most external three layers do not complete their growth until middle childhood. It is this process of cortical refinement that distinguishes man from lower animals.

### Neuron formation

MOTOR NEURONS. Motor neurons are categorized into two major types, including (1) the *somatic motor neurons,* which innervate voluntary muscle, and (2) the *autonomic motor neurons* (preganglionic and postganglionic), which innervate glandular cells, involuntary muscle, and cardiac muscle.

SOMATIC MOTOR NEURONS. Somatic motor neurons result when the cells in the basal plate of the gray matter in the mantle layer proliferate. As this acceleration in cellular growth occurs, anterior projections on both sides of the median plane appear. These anterior projections become enlarged by the growth of anterior bundles and are responsible for causing the spinal cord to modify its growth patterns to resemble the shape it will assume at maturity. Axons of some somatic neurons migrate into the marginal zone in an anterolateral position, so that they become identified as ventral spinal nerve roots. These roots include the alpha efferent and gamma efferent fibers. Alpha efferent fibers form motor end plates on extrafusal striated muscle fibers, whereas gamma efferent fibers stimulate contractile end areas of intrafusal fibers of muscle spindles.

AUTONOMIC MOTOR NEURONS. The autonomic motor system, comprising two types of neurons (preganglionic and postganglionic), is further classified by functional divisions known as the sympathetic and parasympathetic systems.

The *sympathetic system,* the thoracolumbar system, arises from the mantle layer in the posterior region of the basal plate in the thoracic and upper lumbar areas. As development continues, it is positioned in the lateral column, where its axons combine with the ventral nerve roots to form the preganglionic fibers. These fibers continue growing until they reach the sympathetic trunk ganglia. As the preganglionic fibers mature, they become my-

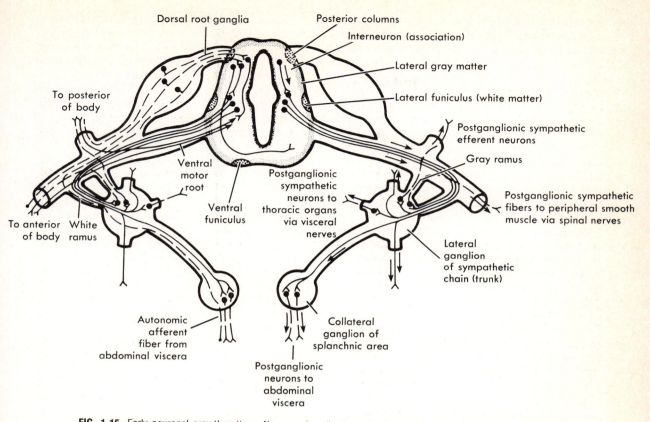

**FIG. 1-15.** Early neuronal growth pattern. Neurons described are those developing between twenty-eighth and fiftieth days of gestation. Dorsal root ganglia consist of nerve cell bodies of unipolar sensory neurons developed from neural crest. Fibers extending to anterior aspect of body join in plexuses to serve extremities. White ramus contains sympathetic preganglionic fibers. Note that autonomic afferent fiber from abdominal viscera enters spinal nerve through white ramus and then proceeds centrally and has nerve cell body in dorsal root ganglion. Lateral gray matter includes preganglionic sympathetic efferent neurons; postganglionic sympathetic efferent neurons are derived from neural crest. Gray ramus contains postganglionic sympathetic fibers en route to spinal nerves.

elinated and are termed *white rami communicantes* (Fig. 1-15).

The postganglionic fibers are those extending from autonomic ganglia in the form of axons. These axons innervate involuntary and cardiac muscle and glandular cells.

A similar pattern of growth occurs in the midsacral area. This growth results in the autonomic nerve complexes that become the *parasympathetic fibers* of the pelvic splanchnic nerves.

Investigators believe that the ganglia of the sym-

pathetic nervous system are derived either from neurons originating in the basal plate that migrate via the ventral nerve roots to become ganglia or from neurons originating in the neural crest. The ganglia of the parasympathetic system (craniosacral system) are believed to arise from the neural crest of the primitive ganglia of the oculomotor, trigeminal, facial, glossopharyngeal, and vagus nerves. The origin of the ganglia in the gastrointestinal tract has not been definitely established.

**SENSORY NEURONS.** The growth of the *dorsal col-*

umn begins as the anterior and lateral gray columns reach their final developmental stages. It is during the fourth gestational week that the dorsal column arises from the alar plate. In their earliest form the dorsal columns consist of fibers from the mantle zone and the dorsal roots of the spinal nerve ganglia, which have grown into the spinal medulla. With growth this neuronal mass appears as an oval bundle in the marginal area of the alar plate. As growth of the oval bundle continues medially, the beginning posterior funiculus is evident. This funiculus is separated into two portions by the posterior median septum, an ependymal supportive structure. At the third month of gestation, intersegmental fibers are apparent.

Sensory neurons comprise both somatic and visceral neurons. Because their development is closely associated with the formation of the spinal and cranial nerves, the following discussion includes all four of these entities.

In its beginning stages of growth the *spinal medulla (cord)* extends to the same length as the vertebral column. At this point the spinal nerves extend from the cord at 90-degree angles. By the time the embryo has reached a length of about 30 mm, vertebral growth has begun to outdistance growth of the spinal cord. Because of this phenomenon, the spinal cord, which originally had its distal point at the second coccygeal vertebra, terminates at the third lumbar vertebra. As the growth of the spinal medulla reaches the lumbar level, the external cord adheres to ectodermal tissue and is fixed in place. The medial walls encased in pia mater extend in a thread termed the *filum terminale*. If coccygeal remnants remain after birth, they may result in congenital cysts.

Every spinal nerve connects with the spinal medulla at the ventral and dorsal roots. *Ventral root fibers,* derived from mantle zone neuroblasts in the anterior and lateral positions, penetrate the marginal layer and the external membrane to gain access to the myotomes of the mesodermal somites and to form alpha and gamma efferent components of ventral nerve roots. *Dorsal root fibers,* derived from the neural crest, form ganglia that result in two particular outcomes. The ventral portion of the ganglia forms chromaffin cells, whereas other portions form symmetrical bilateral spinal ganglia equal in number to the primitive divisions, excluding the caudal area.

*Cranial nerve formation* proceeds in a fashion similar to the patterns evident in spinal nerve formation. The exception to this pattern occurs in the olfactory and optic nerves, which are categorized as brain tracts because of their origin in the forebrain. Motor axons innervating striated muscle are derived from the medial and lateral aspects of the basal plate. The medial aspect develops into the somatic efferent portion, whereas the lateral aspect forms the branchial efferent portion.

The *medial aspect,* which supplies somite-derived muscles, is characterized by its lack of ganglia and its scattered distribution of cell bodies among the motor neurons at the point where the axons exit from the brainstem. The category of somatic efferent nerves includes the oculomotor (III), the trochlear (IV), the abducens (VI), and the hypoglossal (XII) nerves (Fig. 1-16).

The *lateral aspect,* which later becomes the branchial efferent portion, comprises the accessory (XI) nerve and the motor portions of the trigeminal (V), facial (VII), glossopharyngeal (IX), and vagus (X) nerves. This category of cranial nerves innervates the striated muscle that arises from the branchial arches. These cranial nerves form both a sensory ganglion and a motor root. The accessory nerve (bulbar accessory) is considered to be part of the vagus (X) nerve, since it is enclosed with the spinal root in connective tissue. Moreover, its cranial root travels only a small distance before it rejoins the sheath of the vagus nerve.

**Myelination.** The axons of the central nervous system are ultimately totally surrounded by portions of other cells. Cell bodies are encapsulated by protoplasmic astrocytes and boutons of other neurons that are synapsing. The *neurilemmal (Schwann) cells* encase all axons of the somatic and autonomic motor neurons *only* in the peripheral nervous system. These neurilemmal cells are derived from the wall of the neural tube and the neural crest. The *satellite cells* function in a manner similar to that of neurilemmal cells because they enclose the cell bodies in the sensory ganglia of cranial and spinal nerves and the postganglionic neurons of the autonomic ganglia.

When cells are myelinated, several layers of cell membrane, oligodendrocytes or neurilemma, encase the axons. In contrast, unmyelinated axons are characterized by their coverings, which comprise only parts of cells. Most postganglionic auto-

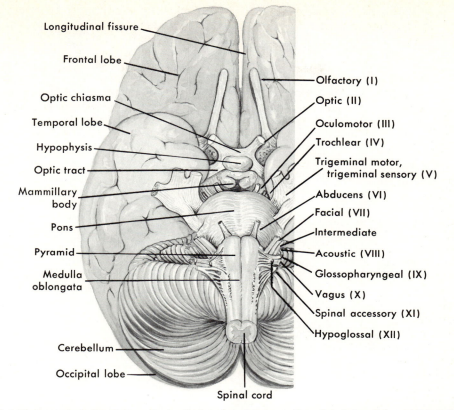

Longitudinal fissure

Frontal lobe

Optic chiasma

Temporal lobe

Hypophysis

Optic tract

Mammillary body

Pons

Pyramid

Medulla oblongata

Cerebellum

Occipital lobe

Spinal cord

Olfactory (I)

Optic (II)

Oculomotor (III)

Trochlear (IV)

Trigeminal motor, trigeminal sensory (V)

Abducens (VI)

Facial (VII)

Intermediate

Acoustic (VIII)

Glossopharyngeal (IX)

Vagus (X)

Spinal accessory (XI)

Hypoglossal (XII)

**FIG. 1-16.** Human brain from below with visualization of cranial nerves. (From Schottelius, B.A., and Schottelius, D.D.: Textbook of physiology, ed. 18, St. Louis, 1978, The C.V. Mosby Co.)

nomic neurons are not myelinated (Fig. 1-17).

Differences in the oligodendrocytes and the neurilemmal cells are also apparent. *Oligodendrocytes* form segmental sheaths for several neighboring axons, whereas *neurilemmal cells* form the myelin sheath for only one peripheral axon. Another difference between the central nervous system and the periphery is the greater distance between the nodes of Ranvier in the central nervous system.

The *myelin sheath* surrounds the axon through a spiral wrapping process whose layers eventually fuse together. The layers of these sheaths, comprising lipids and protein, appear to be a glistening white when first formed because they are composed of nearly two-thirds fatty material. As axons attain maturity, they become long tracts that form the vast part of the white matter in the nervous system. Myelinated axons are noted for their ability to fatigue slowly and react quickly after they have become fully sheathed.

Myelination of the cranial nerves in the mesencephalon and medulla oblongata begins during the third and fourth gestational months. The sheathing of these nerves facilitates functions such as sucking and swallowing in the newborn. Motor neurons are myelinated before the sensory components of the cranial nerves. For example, the optic nerve is sheathed from birth to age 2 weeks, whereas the sensory portions of the trigeminal (V) and cochlear regions of the vestibulocochlear (VIII) nerves do not form their myelin sheaths until the fifth or sixth postnatal month.

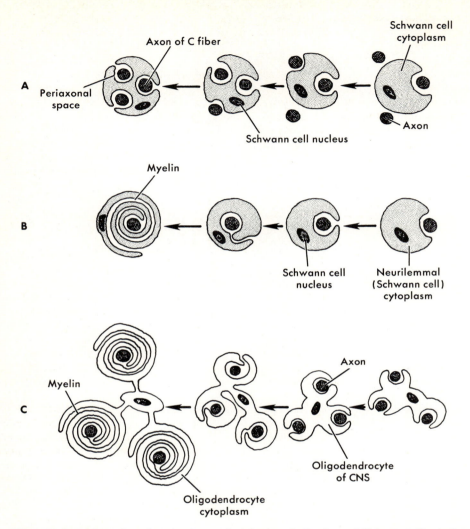

**FIG. 1-17.** Comparison of myelinated and unmyelinated axons. **A,** Neurilemmal (Schwann cell) cytoplasm un-myelinated peripheral axons in visceral or somatic motor and sensory neurons. These C fibers are being sur-rounded by neurilemma (Schwann) cell cytoplasm. Even so-called unmyelinated fibers have very thin myelin layers. **B,** Myelinated axons of somatic visceral motor and sensory neurons (A and B fibers) may be blanketed by several layers of neurilemmal (Schwann) cell membrane. The greater the diameter of the fiber, the more myelin there is in the sheath. Note that Schwann cell nucleus is developed from neural crest. **C,** Myelinated axons of central nervous system—associational, commissural, and projectional neurons—are enfolded by membrane of oligodendrocyte. Cytoplasm of oligodendrocytes surrounds unmyelinated axons in central nervous system. A fibers are heavily myelinated and form "white matter" of central nervous system. Oligodendrocytes of central nervous system, which are formed from neural tube, cannot regenerate.

At birth the neonate has sheaths around the axons of the brainstem, basal ganglia, and axons connecting the basal ganglia and cerebellum. Projectional fibers connecting the thalamus and cerebral cortex are still unmyelinated at this time. The olfactory, acoustic, and optic axons of the cerebral cortex become myelinated first. Axons of the somesthetic and motor cortices have the next priority. The projectional, commissural, and associational axons are the last ones to be sheathed. Myelination of the associational areas continues into adulthood. Some investigators link increasing maturity with myelination of the associational areas. Developmental progression in motor and sensory capacities definitely depends on myelination.

***Structures covering the nervous system.*** Chapter 2 details the function of the meninges along with the other coverings of the nervous system. The meninges, a protective covering for nervous tissue, are divided into three layers: pia mater (inner), arachnoid (middle), and dura mater (outer). The pia mater arises from neural crest cells and is ectodermal in origin. The arachnoid is derived mainly from neural crest cells but is also partially derived from mesenchymal cells. Mesenchymal cells provide the total base of origin for the dura mater. In the cranium, dura mater derived from mesenchyme is closely related to the mesenchyme that ossifies into skull. The venous sinuses distinguish the dura mater from the future skull.

The skull comprises eight bones that provide a protective covering for the brain and the other vital centers of the nervous system. Four of the eight bones—one frontal, two parietal, and one occipital—are flat and composed of two layers of compact tissue. The outer layer is thick, and the inner layer is thinner and more brittle. The base of the skull is both thicker and stronger than the roof or walls. Numerous foramina (openings) are evident at the base of the skull where the cranial nerves, blood vessels, and other vital structures travel in and out of the cranium.

Ossification of the cranial bones begins prenatally at the center and extends to include the periphery. Because this growth process is both gradual and incomplete by birth, the cranium in the newborn has membrane-filled spaces (fontanels) between the suture lines of the bones. There are six commonly mentioned fontanels, including the anterior, the posterior, two anterolateral, and two posterolateral ones (Fig. 1-18, *A*).

The diamond-shaped *anterior (bregmatic) fontanel,* found between the angles of the two parietal bones and the two sections of frontal bone, has the greatest diameter, about 25 mm (1 inch) at birth. Because of its location superior to the sagittal dural venous sinus, it pulsates. The process of involution related to bone growth, which begins at about 3 months of age, moves to completion by age 2 years in most children. Some abnormal processes may interfere with this orderly course of obliteration. For example, microcephalus may cause the fontanel to close early, whereas hydrocephalus, rickets, cretinism, and some instances of subdural hematoma may prolong closure.

The *posterior (occipital) fontanel* is a triangular space located between the occipital and the two parietal bones. This fontanel is smaller than the anterior fontanel and usually is closed within a few months after birth.

The two *anterolateral (sphenoidal) fontanels* are located at the junction of the frontal, parietal, temporal, and sphenoid bones. These anterolateral fontanels have closed by the sixth month of life.

In contrast, the two *posterolateral (mastoid) fontanels* at the junction of the parietal, occipital, and temporal bones do not become obliterated for about 2 years (Fig. 1-18).

Because the sutures and fontanels allow flexibility in the size of the head through molding or overlapping, the birth process is facilitated. The cartilage connecting the lateral and squamous aspects of the occipital bone also provides some flexibility at birth and is therefore named the *obstetric joint.*

At birth the skull is large in relation to the rest of the body, but the face is disproportionately small. As the teeth erupt, the eye orbits increase, the hard palate grows laterally, and the maxillary sinuses develop, the size and appearance of the face begin to assume more adultlike proportions.

Since brain growth is so rapid in the first 2 years of life, the bulk of expansion in head circumference is also seen at this time. At birth an average head circumference is 33 cm, but by age 2 years the head has usually grown to about 47 cm. Although practitioners should evaluate head size in relation to that seen in other members of the family, children typically have a maximum size of 50 to 55 cm. Trauma or early closure of one or more sutures may result in an unusual shape of the head. Further information on abnormal head growth is available in books listed in the references (Ford, 1973; Crelin, 1973; Seller et al., 1974).

Although the sutures do not normally fuse until adulthood, a strong fibrous tissue joint, which requires a high intracranial pressure to separate, is evident by the seventh year. After 10 years of age separation of the sutures in relation to increased intracranial pressure is unusual. This fact has application in evaluating increasing intracranial pressure at various ages.

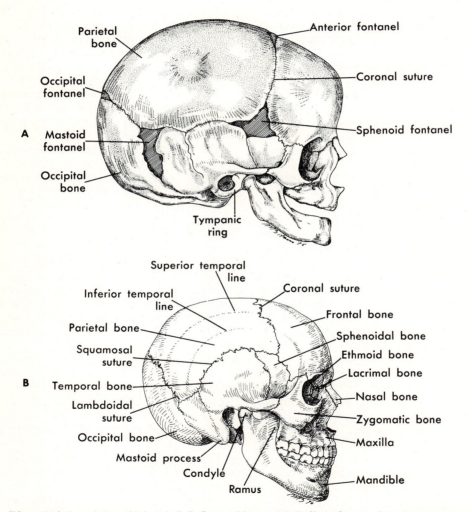

**FIG. 1-18. A,** Lateral view of infant skull. **B,** Bones of face and skull. (From Conway, B.L.: Pediatric neurologic nursing, St. Louis, 1977, The C.V. Mosby Co.)

## Brain development

Before the caudal end of the neural tube has fully evolved, the three occipital somites become further differentiated into the *prosencephalon (forebrain),* the *mesencephalon (midbrain),* and the *rhombencephalon (hindbrain).* The prosencephalon acquires lateral outgrowths, the optic vesicles. Growth continues in the optic vesicles as they branch into the optic cup and stalk, the formative structures for the optic nerve and a portion of the eyeball. The primary connection of these optic vesicles finally becomes a portion of the diencephalon, the posterior aspect of the forebrain, which is visible by the thirty-sixth day of gestation. The anterior forebrain continues its growth as it forms two telencephalic vesicles, which later mature into the cerebral hemispheres. These telencephalic vesicles are the uppermost part of the neural tube and, as such, are termed the *lamina terminalis* (Fig. 1-19).

At the same time that the optic vesicles become apparent, two curves, the *cephalic flexure* and the *cervical flexure,* are evident. The cavities of the three divisions of the brain, the prosocoele, the mesocoele, and the rhombocoele, are also formed. These cavities develop into the ventricular system in later growth.

As the forebrain subdivides, its cavity, the prosocoele, evolves into two telocoeles, the precursors for the lateral ventricles. The pocket between these lateral telocoeles is known as the median telocoele and, along with the convexity in

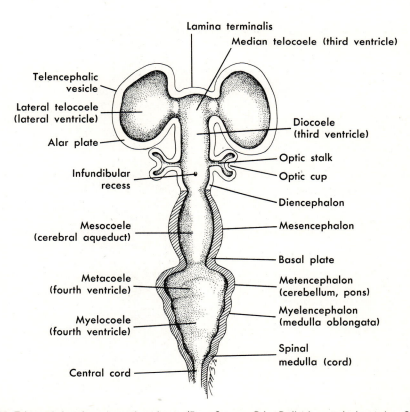

**FIG. 1-19.** Telencephalon: forerunner of cerebrum. (From Conway, B.L.: Pediatric neurologic nursing, St. Louis, 1977, The C.V. Mosby Co.)

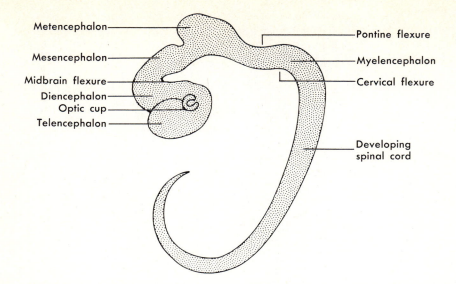

Metencephalon

Mesencephalon

Midbrain flexure

Diencephalon

Optic cup

Telencephalon

Pontine flexure

Myelencephalon

Cervical flexure

Developing spinal cord

**FIG. 1-20.** Lateral aspect of embryo at 6 weeks of gestation. Midbrain and cervical flexures delineate primary brain divisions. Pontine flexure is also obvious at this point.

the diencephalon, eventually forms the third ventricle. The pocket in the midbrain, the mesocoele, becomes the aqueduct of Sylvius. The fourth ventricle is formed by the pockets in the two divisions of the hindbrain as the rhombencephalon divides into the metencephalon (the future pons and cerebellum) and the myelencephalon (the rudimentary form of the medulla oblongata). At the same time a curve, the *pontine flexure,* occurs between the metencephalon and the myelencephalon, causing the roof of the hindbrain to become thinner (Fig. 1-20).

At 7 weeks of gestation the nervous system extends to 17 mm. Growth in the telencephalon, the ventral division of the forebrain, includes further refinements on the telencephalic vesicles as they expand into two olfactory lobes that arise from the rhinencephalon, an outgrowth of the anterior forebrain (telencephalon).

At 3 months of gestation the central nervous system is 78 mm in length. Cerebral hemispheres, formed from the telencephalic vesicles, are prominent because they have overgrown the posterior forebrain (diencephalon). The ventricles continue their growth as the connections between the lateral ventricles (one and two) and the medial ventricle (three) narrow into the interventricular foramina of Monro. The fourth ventricle develops an opening onto its roof, the foramen of Magendie, and two lateral openings, the foramina of Luschka (Fig. 1-21).

*Prosencephalon.* The forebrain has a division of the lateral walls similar to the one described for the spinal medulla. In the spinal medulla the sulcus limitans divides the walls into the alar and basal plates, whereas in the cerebrum the dividing groove is termed the *hypothalamic sulcus.* These sulci are probably related by a common origin.

The ventral roof plate of the prosencephalon, the lamina terminalis, is a thin sheet that covers the distance from the interventricular foramina to the indentation at the inferior end of the optic stalk. The floor plate and lateral walls of the forebrain rostral to the rudimentary interventricular foramina provide the space for anterior hypothalamic growth at the optic chiasma and the optic recess. The optic chiasma results from the connection and partial decussation of optic nerves located in the ventral lamina terminalis. With growth these optic tracts extend in a caudal direction, where they

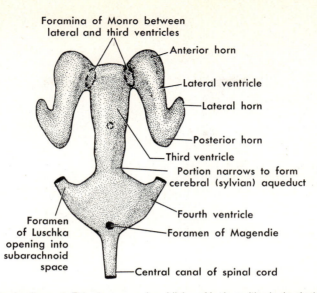

Foramina of Monro between
lateral and third ventricles

Anterior horn

Lateral ventricle

Lateral horn

Posterior horn

Third ventricle

Portion narrows to form
cerebral (sylvian) aqueduct

Fourth ventricle

Foramen
of Luschka
opening into
subarachnoid
space

Foramen of Magendie

Central canal of spinal cord

**FIG. 1-21.** Ventricular development. This shows ependymal lining of brain cavities in developing central nervous system at about 90 days of gestation.

eventually become part of the diencephalon and midbrain.

**TELENCEPHALON.** By the third month of gestation the telencephalon divides into three functionally different areas: the *rhinencephalon,* the thick basal or *striatal area,* and the *suprastriatal area.*

RHINENCEPHALON. The rhinencephalon, literally translated as the "nosebrain," is the most rudimentary portion of the telencephalon. It originates from olfactory outgrowths.

A longitudinal fissure is evident in the anteromedial portion of each ventricular floor by the fifth gestational week. A hollow sac forms from this fissure and is attached to the hemisphere by a short stalk. This sac then becomes affixed to a ganglionic mass of cells that connect with afferent axons from the sensory cells of the olfactory plate. Growth of this sac continues in an anterior direction. When the sac loses its cavity, it is a solid olfactory bulb with a lengthened stalk. Eventually this growth becomes the olfactory tract. The piriform area is the point where this tract is attached to the floor.

The rhinencephalon has a variety of functions, including olfaction, in man. The several structures

that compose the rhinencephalon are commonly known as the *limbic lobe,* with the adjective appropriately meaning "border." The limbic lobe is responsible for integrating complex olfactory and emotional data with somatic and visceral messages. At maturity the limbic lobe comprises the gyrus cinguli, the isthmus, the hippocampus, and the uncus.

The limbic lobe begins to form when the cortical area, the paleopallium, at the edge of the interventricular foramen forms a circle on the medial and inferior aspects of the hemisphere. The piriform area and the hippocampal formation both participate in this growth. As the mantle area of the cortex continues to proliferate, an elevation protruding into the medial portion of the ventricle anterior to the lamina terminalis is evident. The elevation eventually grows to connect posteriorly with the piriform area at the temporal pole of the cerebral cortex. Neurons in the marginal zone of the hippocampus form a convolution termed the *dentate gyrus,* a structure that is included as a coextension of the main structure. The ventral portion of the hippocampus is the uncus.

The hippocampal sulcus is the first groove to ap-

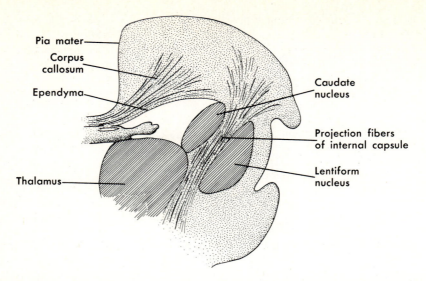

**FIG. 1-22.** Internal capsule separates caudate nucleus from lentiform nucleus. These structures compose corpus striatum, most important functional component of basal ganglia. (From Conway, B.L.: Pediatric neurologic nursing, St. Louis, 1977, The C.V. Mosby Co.)

pear on the cerebral hemispheres. It is located at the medial aspect of the hemispheric region at the hippocampal formation. By the fourth month of gestation, the calcarine sulcus traverses the area from the occipital pole to the midtemporal area. In the fifth month of gestation the sulcus cinguli begins to divide the layers of the medial portion of the hemisphere superior and anterior to the corpus callosum.

In summary, the limbic lobe comprises the medial convolution of the temporal lobe (the hippocampal gyrus), the hippocampus, the uncus, and the narrow island of cortex that connects the hippocampal gyrus with the gyrus cinguli.

STRIATAL AREA. The striatal area is better known as the *basal ganglia*. It comprises four main nuclei, which are situated deep within the cerebral hemispheres. These nuclei are the caudate nucleus, the lentiform nucleus, the amygdaloid body, and the claustrum.

The *caudate nucleus,* the *lentiform nucleus,* and the *internal capsule* dividing the two collectively form the *corpus striatum,* the most significant functional unit of the basal ganglia. The corpus striatum, closely related to the diencephalon de-

velopmentally, is an important component of the extrapyramidal system (Fig. 1-22).

The caudate nucleus first appears as elevations on the lateral aspect of the ventricular floor. Caudally the caudate nucleus forms a tail, which is the inferior horn of the ventricle and the amygdaloid complex at maturity. Ventrally the growth of the caudate nucleus extends in the direction of the thalamus, where the two structures are separated by a groove.

In the early stages of growth the lentiform and the caudate nuclei originate from the same two layers of cells. The internal capsule also begins its growth from these cells until it protrudes between the inner cellular layer, which forms the caudate nucleus, and the outer cellular layer, which forms the lentiform nucleus. The lentiform nucleus also continues to proliferate until the increase in cellular differentiation causes it to divide into the medial globus pallidus and the lateral putamen.

Thalamic growth continues until the structure joins the medial wall of the hemisphere. Thus the corpus striatum, which was once divided from the adjacent thalamus by a groove, becomes fused with the thalamus. This fusion is significant, since it provides an essential link between the diencephalon and telencephalon. Thus projectional fibers may journey between the two divisions of the forebrain.

SUPRASTRIATAL AREA. The cerebral cortex with its familiar external convolutions is termed the suprastriatal area. The neopallium is the external covering of gray matter that distinguishes man from the lower animals, whose cerebral cortex consists of only basal ganglia and olfactory brain. The convolutions in the cortex enable the neuronal area to increase without expanding the space the brain occupies.

Projectional fibers from the rapidly expanding cortex are visible by the last part of the third gestational month. These fibers extend along the pathway provided by the fusion of the thalamus and corpus striatum. The fibers further separate the caudate nucleus from the lateral lentiform nucleus. As the tract extends posteriorly and inferiorly, it reaches its caudal limit after a period of growth that spans 20 weeks and ends at the twenty-ninth week of gestation. The orderly appearance of the various reflexes can be correlated with the innervation of the various levels from this corticospinal tract.

The external appearance of the suprastriatal area begins to change by the third gestational month as the lateral (sylvian) sulcus, a minor groove anterosuperior to the temporal pole, becomes apparent. The site of this groove is in the cortex superior to the floor and lateral walls of the ventricle that encases the corpus striatum. The floor of the sulcus, termed the *insula,* is lateral to the corpus striatum. The insula grows slowly, so that the more rapid growth of the cerebral hemispheres submerges it completely. As this overgrowth of cortex occurs, significant structural changes in the olfactory areas become evident. Cortical growth also extends over the piriform area by the fifth month of gestation, so that only its inferior portion is seen at full maturity.

The shallow hippocampal and the lateral (sylvian) sulci are the only two grooves visible on the hemispheres until the end of the third month. The parieto-occipital sulcus, which appears next on the medial hemispheric surface, occurs simultaneously with the increase in fibers of the corpus callosum, the great bond of commissural fibers joining the two hemispheres. The calcarine sulcus is obvious at about the same time. Although the sulcus cinguli is apparent on the medial hemispheric surface during the fifth month, the inferior and superolateral areas show no grooves until the sixth month. During the sixth month the other major sulci become visible (Fig. 1-23).

By maturity the cerebral cortex comprises six discrete layers of cells, including the ganglionic, multiform, pyramidal, inner granular, plexiform, and outer granular layers.

One tenth of the body's weight at birth is attributed to the brain. The cerebral hemispheres account for 93% of the weight in the brain. The weight gain in these hemispheres over the first 2 years of life is about 840 gm. This rapid gain results from increased numbers of neuronal processes, greater size, and myelination, which occurs on a large scale at this time. Roughly one third of this weight gain occurs during the first 9 months; the remaining increase spans the period ending at 2 years of age (Dobbing, 1974).

Many critical factors should be considered by practitioners who attempt to provide the emotional and physical environment most conducive to optimal growth. Investigators have now linked such factors as endocrine disorders, extreme nutritional inadequacies, anoxic episodes, sensory deprivation, vascular problems, and specified viruses to interferences with the orderly process of myelination (Babson et al., 1979).

**DIENCEPHALON.** The major structures of the posterior portion of the prosencephalon, the diencephalon, include the *thalamus,* the *pineal body,* and the *hypothalamus.*

THALAMUS. The thalamus and metathalamus begin growth as the dorsal aspect of the lateral wall thickens. The structure posterior to the thalamus, the metathalamus, is more commonly referred to as the lateral and medial geniculate bodies. As the thalami continue to grow, the space between them lessens to become the cavity for the third ventricle. Medial growth results in the formation of the interthalamic adhesion, which unites the two lobes of the thalamus. As thalamic growth extends in a posterior direction, the geniculate bodies soon become situated posterior to the third ventricle. In the anterior direction the growth of the thalamus

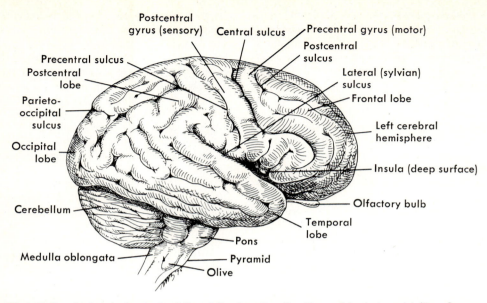

Postcentral gyrus (sensory)
Central sulcus
Precentral gyrus (motor)
Postcentral sulcus
Precentral sulcus
Postcentral lobe
Parieto-occipital sulcus
Lateral (sylvian) sulcus
Frontal lobe
Left cerebral hemisphere
Occipital lobe
Insula (deep surface)
Cerebellum
Olfactory bulb
Temporal lobe
Medulla oblongata
Pons
Pyramid
Olive

**FIG. 1-23.** Growth of cerebral cortex by ninth gestational month, with evidence of developing sulci. (From Conway, B.L.: Pediatric neurologic nursing, St. Louis, 1977, The C.V. Mosby Co.)

results in fusion with the corpus striatum of the telencephalon.

PINEAL BODY. The *epithalamus* is the collective name for the pineal body, the posterior commissure, and the trigonum habenulae. All these structures originate from the caudal roof and the lateral walls of the diencephalon. The posterior commissure consists of fibers from the pineal recesses. The nuclei habenulae are the most important component of the trigonum habenulae. The nuclei habenulae begin as a structure adjacent to the geniculate bodies but later become separated from them by distal thalamic growth. The pineal body is the most important structure of the three and is detailed more extensively in this section.

Additional investigation is needed to fully appreciate the functions of the pineal body, which Descartes once described as the seat of a man's soul. Because so little information is available, development and function are discussed together at this point. The pineal body arises as a midline evagination of the diencephalic roof and remains as two distinct sections in the rudimentary stages. However, by maturity, the anterior portion has disappeared, whereas the posterior section has become the grown pineal body. The pineal recess of the third ventricle is the only remaining indication of the presence of the anterior rudiment.

The photoreceptive quality of the pineal body in cold-blooded vertebrates explains their ability to adapt to the environment by changing skin color. The pineal body has a different function in man. In humans the pineal secretes an indole called melatonin. Melatonin inhibits gonad development and regulates estrus. The most important function of melatonin is to slow maturation. The highest concentrations of melatonin are found in the hypothalamus and midbrain, and researchers believe that melatonin has its greatest effect on the brain tissue rather than on sex organs. However, a pineal tumor may slow the process of hormone synthesis and cause precocious puberty. The question of whether melatonin is secreted into the cerebrospinal fluid or into the blood still remains to be answered.

The circadian rhythm of the pineal body is controlled primarily by the endogenous cyclic norepinephrine release. However, there is still some evidence that the pineal body is responsive to environmental lighting. Some investigators relate the earlier onset of menses in the most civilized populations of the world to the increased exposure to artificial lighting ("The pineal," 1974).

Further research in humans is necessary to understand the composition and functions of other substances produced by the pineal body.

HYPOTHALAMUS. The hypothalamus, the mammillary bodies, the tuber cinereum, and the infundibulum of the hypophysis arise from the floor of the diencephalon, whereas growth in the roof plate of the diencephalon results in the formation of the choroid plexuses.

The hypothalamus is inferior to the thalamus and superior to the pituitary gland (hypophysis). It has five major divisions, including the lateral, supraoptic, infundibular, periventricular, and mammillary areas. Major nuclei derive their names from their location in relation to these divisions. The tuber cinereum is the correct name for the medioventral area of the external hypothalamus.

The hypothalamus, an alar plate–derived structure, is regarded as the motor control center for the autonomic nervous system. The hypothalamus is also responsible for integrating and regulating autonomic-somatic behavioral responses appropriate to the source and quality of given stimuli. To accomplish these complex functions the hypothalamus has a vast network of interconnections with the thalamus, the medulla oblongata, the spinal medulla, the reticular system, the pituitary body, and the limbic system.

*Mesencephalon.* The midbrain (mesencephalon) arises from the primary cerebral vesicle. The cavity of the mesencephalon is divided from the forebrain by a constricted area and from the hindbrain by an isthmus. As the midbrain area reaches maturity, its cavity is reduced in size and is categorized as the cerebral aqueduct by adulthood. The two structures of importance in the midbrain area are the *cerebral peduncles* and the *corpora quadrigemina*.

CEREBRAL PEDUNCLES. In the anterior portion of the midbrain, cellular layers proliferate to become the cerebral peduncles. By the fourth month of gestation the cerebral peduncles have grown rapidly so that their marginal layer consists of multiple fiber tracts. These projectional fibers eventually connect the cerebral cortex with other structures in the brainstem.

The cerebral peduncles are divided into dorsal and ventral aspects. The dorsal aspect, the tegmentum, consists of the motor nuclei of the oculomotor, trigeminal, and trochlear nerves, whereas the ventral aspect contains the red nucleus (nucleus ruber). The red nucleus is an integral part of the reticular formation and is the point of origin for the rubrospinal tract of the extrapyramidal system. At the dorsal aspect the tegmentum is continuous with the pons.

The pes pedunculi is the anterior aspect of the cerebral peduncles. The pes pedunculi is located beneath the substantia nigra, an important structure in the extrapyramidal pathway.

CORPORA QUADRIGEMINA. Cells from the dorsal aspect of the alar plate proliferate and are eventually separated by a midline groove into the corpora bigemina. The transverse division that further divides these structures precedes their mature formation as the corpora quadrigemina. The final division, which results in the inferior and superior colliculi, serves an important function, since the inferior colliculi are vital components of the auditory pathway, whereas the superior colliculi are optic reflex centers. The control complex for acoustical reflexes is also located in the inferior colliculi.

*Rhombencephalon.* The three flexures in the cranial region were mentioned previously. The first flexure to appear, the midbrain flexure, causes the head to fold forward until its floor lies parallel to the floor in the rhombencephalon. The next flexure, the cervical flexure, found where the rhombencephalon joins the spinal medulla, shows rapid growth for a few weeks but becomes obliterated as the head moves into an extended position. The third curve, the pontine flexure, located in the region of the future pons, has a minimal effect on the mature shape of the head. At the time the midbrain flexure forms, the rhombencephalon occupies a greater space than both the other cranial areas combined. The pontine flexure is responsible for the thinning of the roof of the hindbrain. It also causes the hindbrain to assume a rhomboid form and results in the division of the lateral walls. These changes in the rhombencephalon influence the final growth patterns of the fourth ventricle.

At the end of the fourth week six temporary grooves are visible; the function of these grooves is poorly understood. These six transverse creases *(rhombic grooves)* are located in the basal plate of the rhombencephalon. The neural tissues between these grooves are termed *rhombomeres*. Rhombomeres are connected to the motor nuclei of the trigeminal, facial, abducens, glossopharyngeal, and vagus nerves.

The rhombencephalon is divided into two major divisions, the myelencephalon and the metencephalon. These two divisions become further refined through growth processes to form mature brain structures in the posterior aspect of the cranium.

**MYELENCEPHALON.** The posterior portion of the hindbrain encases the ninth, tenth, eleventh, and twelfth cranial nerves. It becomes the medulla oblongata at maturity.

In the area superior to the alar plate an oval bundle arises from the afferent fibers of the glossopharyngeal (IX) and vagus (X) nerves. The caudal aspect of this alar plate adjoins the roof of the rhombencephalon to become the rhombic lip. The rhombencephalon continues its lateral growth, whereas the rhombic lip folds over the neighboring area, where it becomes adjoined. Cells from the rhombic lip migrate into the marginal zone of the basal plate to form the oval bundle, the tractus solitarius, which is then encased by layers of neuronal tissue. The tractus solitarius is responsible for the reception and transmission of gustatory impulses through the facial (VII) and glossopharyngeal (IX) nerves and for the formation of the solitariospinal tract, a motor pathway that regulates respiration and vomiting.

Neuronal cells that migrate from the alar plate of the rhombic lip may also develop into the olivary and arcuate nuclei and the gray matter of the pons nuclei. Those cells that do not migrate as far as the basal plate form the nucleus of the circumolivary bundle, an oblique fold at the dorsolateral aspect of the inferior cerebellar peduncle.

The gracilis and cuneatus nuclei arise from the alar plate to occupy the caudal aspect of the myelencephalon.

By the fourth gestational month the corticospinal fibers have penetrated the anterior medulla to form the pyramids. At the caudal aspect the inferior cerebellar peduncle emerges as fibers of the spinal medulla, the olivocerebellar and parolivocerebellar fibers, the external arcuate fibers, and the bidirectional reticulocerebellar tract in combination with the vestibulocerebellar tract. Because this portion of the hindbrain is such a vital junction, it is both a control center and a link in impulse transmission to and from the higher centers of the brain.

**RETICULAR FORMATION.** The reticular formation arises from the alar and basal plates. It functions as an intermediary between the upper and lower motor neurons of the extrapyramidal system. The red nucleus of the midbrain, the cerebellar nuclei, the basal nuclei (ganglia), and the cerebral cortex each supply the reticular formation with fibers.

The motor neurons of the reticular formation are both excitatory and inhibitory. The response arising from this area is mediated by the gamma efferent fibers and includes the stretch reflexes. Thus an inhibitory stimulus on the extensor muscles facilitates the flexor motor neurons of the spinal medulla because of the inhibitory stimulus to the medial portion of the reticular system.

When stimulation is applied to the lateral anterior aspect of the reticular system, an excitatory response is induced. An excitatory response is one wherein extensor tonus is facilitated while flexion is inhibited.

Decerebrate rigidity occurs when the cerebral cortex is isolated from the reticular network by a high transection of the midbrain area. This abnormal condition results from the dominant effect of the extensor muscles and the lack of inhibition from opposing motor neurons and flexor muscles (Haymaker, 1969).

**METENCEPHALON.** The anterior region of the rhombencephalon is termed the metencephalon. It consists of two main structures, the *cerebellum* and the *pons*.

**CEREBELLUM.** The alar plate assumes a horizontal position as physical changes occur with development and as the pontine flexure forms. Concurrently, the primitive cerebellar hemispheres arise from the posterior alar plate and rhombic lip. The roof of the metencephalon separates these hemispheres at the caudal aspect. Migrating alar and basal cells travel to the roof area, and the vermis becomes visible as caudal growth continues.

The cerebellum, the largest structure in the posterior fossa, is situated inferior to the occipital and temporal lobes of the cerebrum and superior to the pons and medulla oblongata. The inferior aspect

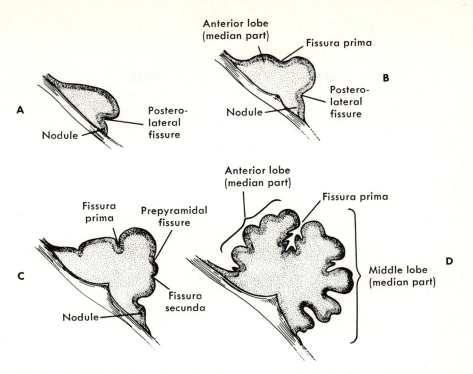

**FIG. 1-24.** By end of third gestational month, three transverse grooves appear to divide portions of cerebellum. Additional fissures form between existing ones, enabling cerebellum to have larger surface area. (From Conway, B.L.: Pediatric neurologic nursing, St. Louis, 1977, The C.V. Mosby Co.)

of the cerebellum is superior to the cranial aspect of the fourth ventricle (Fig. 1-23).

The deep fissures that eventually course the exterior of the cerebellum begin as transverse grooves on the dorsal cerebellar surface (Fig. 1-24). The posterolateral fissure, which divides the caudal portion from the rest of the cerebellum, is the first fissure to appear. In early development the flocculonodular lobes occupy the most distal region of the cerebellum. However, by maturity, growth processes in adjacent tissues have gradually pushed them forward to the anteroinferior position they occupy at adulthood.

The fissura prima is a deep transverse sulcus that forms by the third gestational month to divide the anterior cerebellum into two parts. Two other fissures appear about the same time. The fissura seconda delineates the uvula, and the prepyramidal fissure delimits the pyramids.

Since the cerebellum grows more rapidly in a caudal direction than it does at the vermis, the vermis gradually becomes located deep within a hollow termed the *vallecula*. Concurrently, a great number of parallel fissures develop between those previously described. These fissures increase the surface area of the cerebellum.

Authorities disagree on the number of major sections that compose the cerebellum. Some believe there are two, whereas others believe there are three. The following paragraphs present the portions of the cerebellum from both points of view.

The *archicerebellum (flocculonodular node)* is the oldest part of the cerebellum. Because it arises from the lateral vestibular area of the brainstem, its functions are similar to those of the vestibular system.

The *paleocerebellum (spinocerebellum)* regulates equilibrium and muscle tonus and coordinates the muscular activities involved in locomotion.

The paleocerebellum comprises the vermis of the anterior lobe, the pyramids, the uvula, and the paraflocculus. This aspect of the cerebellum receives messages through the spinocerebellar tract, particularly the ventral spinocerebellar tract, which transmits afferent messages from the stretch receptors.

The *neocerebellum,* the area of the cerebellum located in the most anterior position, is viewed by some as merely a portion of the paleocerebellum and by others as a discrete division. This division is the largest and newest region of the cerebellum from a historical viewpoint. Coordination of muscular activity in the extremities is the function of this division.

Four major pairs of nuclei are located in the cerebellum, including the *fastigial,* the *globose,* the *emboliform,* and the *dentate (lateralis) nuclei.* The most ancient of these nuclei are the fastigial or roof nuclei, which are situated near the roof of the fourth ventricle. Lateral to the fastigial nuclei are the globose and emboliform nuclei. Flanking these nuclei are the largest of all these, the dentate nuclei.

The *cerebellar peduncles* connect the cerebellum to the other parts of the central nervous system. There are three pairs of cerebellar peduncles, including the superior, middle, and inferior.

The *superior cerebellar peduncles,* the brachia conjunctiva, encase the ventral spinocerebellar afferent fibers and the dentorubral, dentothalamic, and fastigiobulbar efferent fibers. Unidirectional afferent fibers convey impulses from the spinal medulla to the cerebellar cortex, whereas efferent fibers have bidirectional pathways. Messages may exit through the red nucleus and reticular formation to the spinal medulla or through the red nucleus and the thalamus in a journey to the cerebral cortex.

The *middle cerebellar peduncles,* the brachia pontis, consist of fibers from the cerebropontocerebellar tracts. They function to convey messages from the cerebral cortex through the pons to the cerebellar cortex.

The *inferior cerebellar peduncles,* the restiform bodies, comprise the afferent fibers from the dorsal spinocerebellar, the dorsal and ventral arcuatocerebellar, the cuneocerebellar, the rubrocerebellar, the reticulocerebellar, and the vestibulocerebellar tracts. They receive efferent fibers from the cerebello-olivary, spinal, and vestibular tracts and from the fastigiobulbar fibers. The inferior peduncles are responsible for conveying impulses from afferent receptors in the spinal medulla, the medulla oblongata, and certain cranial nerves to the cerebellar cortex. They also convey efferent messages from the cerebellar nuclei to the vestibular nuclei of the medulla (Grabow et al., 1974).

PONS. The pons is literally the bridge that extends from the midbrain to the medulla oblongata. Although early growth patterns are poorly understood, investigators believe the pons develops from the three-zone pattern—ependymal, mantle, and marginal—like other portions of the neural tube. Sensory and motor nuclei of the trigeminal (V), abducens (VI), and facial (VII) nerves develop from the mantle layer. Gray matter in the reticular formation is from the basal plate, whereas that of the nuclei pontis is from the alar plate, where neuronal cells have migrated from the rhombic lip.

Fibers from the pontine and corticospinal tracts adjoin the pons by the fourth gestational month. When these fibers enter the pons, it thickens and modifies its shape to its mature form.

The isthmus rhombencephali, originally a connection between midbrain and hindbrain, experiences a number of alterations, so that it is eventually a part of the mature midbrain area. The rudimentary parts that remain are infiltrated by fibers of the cerebellar peduncles. In the early gestational period the isthmus rhombencephali encases the point where the trochlear (IV) nerves decussate. Continuing rostral growth of this area causes both the trochlear nucleus and the trigeminal nerve, which arises from this location, to become part of the midbrain.

The pontine nuclei of the pons are composed of gray matter. The corticospinal and corticobulbar tracts are the white matter of the pons. The reticular formation of the roof is a continuation of the one located in the medulla oblongata. The roof of the pons also houses the fifth, sixth, and seventh cranial nerves. The pons is essentially a point where many ascending and descending pathways are received en route to other points in the central nervous system (Fig. 1-23).

***Ventricular system.*** The ventricular system produces the fluid that bathes and cushions the central nervous system. The cerebrospinal fluid itself and implications for fluid withdrawal are considered in a later section. The development of the ventricular system and hydrocephalus are considered at this point.

DEVELOPMENT. The early development of the cavities has been discussed. As proliferation continues in the frontal, temporal, and occipital poles of the telencephalon, concurrent changes occur in the ventricular system in response to the growth process. Thus the lateral ventricles move to a more lateral position, the interventricular foramen becomes a narrow passageway, and the third ventricle becomes narrowed in the midbrain area. This narrowing is particularly noticeable in the median region, where the thalami impinge on the third ventricle before bridging it by the interthalamic adhesion. Changes of the fourth ventricle into the mature rhomboid shape in response to the pontine flexure have been discussed (Fig. 1-25).

The choroid plexus, the source of cerebrospinal fluid and the barrier between the blood and the cerebrospinal fluid, arises from the vascular pia mater and ependyma, which are devoid of nervous tissue. The vascular layers enfold into the ventricular cavity to form the fingerlike projections called villi. These villi are surrounded by epithelium from the ependymal layer. The fluid initially produced by the choroid plexus is a high protein fluid, which may nourish epithelial tissue. However, histochemical and vascular changes that occur through growth result in alterations in the constitution of this fluid.

The thin epithelial roof plate of the diencephalon located anterior to the pineal body is the first area to be invaginated by the choroid plexuses of the third ventricle. The process then includes the lower portion of the epithelial medial wall of the hemisphere, which neighbors the anterior diencephalon and the interventricular foramen. This area is ultimately the choroid plexus of the lateral ventricles. The line of invagination in the lateral ventricles is the choroid fissure, an area where neu-

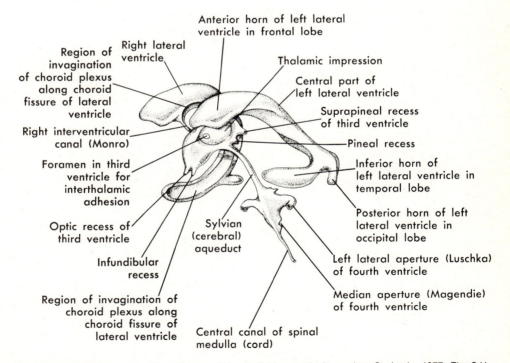

**FIG. 1-25.** Ventricular system. (From Conway, B.L.: Pediatric neurologic nursing, St. Louis, 1977, The C.V. Mosby Co.)

ronal tissue does not intervene between pia mater and ependyma. The choroid fissure of the fourth ventricle is situated at the medial aspect of the roof. This bilateral process of invagination eventually extends over the entire lateral recesses of the fourth ventricle. The choroid plexuses enter the subarachnoid space through the foramina of Luschka and Magendie.

**HYDROCEPHALUS AND OBSTRUCTIONS TO CEREBRO-SPINAL FLUID FLOW.** Interferences with cerebrospinal fluid flow may occur because of increased fluid production, obstruction within the ventricular system, or defective reabsorption of the fluid. Rarely, hypertrophy of the choroid plexus or a papilloma of the choroid plexus may cause overproduction of fluid. Obstructions of the ventricular system (internal or noncommunicating hydrocephalus) result from impaired developmental processes in ventricular structure, as inflammatory responses, or as secondary outcomes of space-occupying lesions.

When the lateral ventricle enlarges unilaterally and protrudes at the temporal area, there is faulty development at the foramen of Monro.

When interferences with cerebrospinal fluid flow occur because of atresia or stenosis in the aqueduct of Sylvius, distention of the lateral or third ventricles results. This type of hydrocephalus is the most common. When evidence of rudimentary growth is all that exists at the aqueduct of Sylvius in the form of strands of ependymal cells, blind channels, or small cysts, a normal connection between the third and fourth ventricles is not possible. Spina bifida is often concurrently associated with these developmental errors. When stenosis or total occlusion occurs, a piece of ependymal lining or glial tissue is often interfering with fluid flow by growing across the canal.

Two types of problems have been identified as the cause of noncommunicating hydrocephalus, which most frequently occurs at the foramina of Luschka and Magendie. In one type the problem is related to a thin roof and no apertures in the fourth ventricle, whereas in the other type thickened meninges and the absence of a cisterna magna result in hydrocephalus. These defects, termed the *Dandy-Walker syndrome,* account for about one third of the cases of noncommunicating hydrocephalus (Hubbert et al., 1974).

Dandy explains the obstruction at the foramina of Luschka and Magendie in terms of posterior fossa cysts resulting from developmental abnormalities or inflammatory agents. This viewpoint, formulated in 1921, was expanded by Walker in 1944; he added that this process of occlusion and cystic formation also results in interferences in union at the lateral commissures and with the closure of the posterior vermis. However, Gardner and others disagree with Dandy and Walker, theorizing the problem as one that occurs during development from genetic or teratogenic causes rather than from obstructive processes after development is complete.

When inflammatory reactions occur within the ventricular system, exudate formation results and may lead to fibrous adhesions at any of the foramina or in the subarachnoid spaces. Meningitis is a common cause of this abnormal outcome.

Causes of ventricular obstruction are further delineated in the appropriate sections on infection, cerebral hemorrhages, skull trauma, and space-occupying lesions.

*Communicating internal hydrocephalus,* an obstructive process involving either the subarachnoid space or the subarachnoid cisternae at the base of the brain, may result from adhesions secondary to an inflammatory process, congenital abnormalities in cleavage in the cerebral leptomeninges, space-occupying lesions, or interferences in absorption because of metabolic disturbances. This obstructive process impedes the flow of cerebrospinal fluid through the subarachnoid space to fill the sulci of the convex aspects of the cerebral hemispheres. This interference results in a fluid backup and ventricular distention, since the spinal subarachnoid space can assist by absorbing only one fifth of the fluid produced.

The rare condition of *external hydrocephalus* results when fluid escapes into the subdural space. Two common processes explain this abnormality. One occurs when fluid seepage results from the surgical correction of hydrocephalus, and the other occurs when the communicating internal type of hydrocephalus develops into an external form. In the second type the sulci are patent, whereas the sulci and subarachnoid spaces covering the cerebral cortex are obstructed. The fluid collection in the cisterna chiasmatis eventually causes lateral distention. This distention results in cystic extensions adjacent to the lateral hemispheres, which may result in cortical compression and distortion of the ventricles. Further increases in the pressure cause the arachnoid membrane to burst. Escaping fluid accumulates in the subdural space, where it is not reabsorbed. As fluid accumulates within the cranium, the elevation in pressure puts traction on the veins that extend from the cortex to the longitudinal sinus. Ultimately the veins may burst, so that there is bleeding in the subdural space. The increase in pressure may also compress the brain downward toward the base of the skull. Abnormal expansions in head size and increased intracranial pressure accompany this problem.

In 2% of the cases, hydrocephalus is an X-linked trait. In these cases the aqueduct is histologically normal but narrowed. When male clients without spina bifida have hydrocephalus, a careful family history should be elicited to see if other male members of the family have the same problem. In this inherited type of hydrocephalus the risk in future pregnancies is about 25% and 50% in male offspring. No specific incidence of inheritance is known when hydrocephalus is not X linked (Holmes et al., 1973).

The reader is directed to the references for details on findings in infants and children with hydrocephalus (Ford, 1973; Seller et al., 1974) and Chapter 13.

When the cerebellar tonsils and medulla oblongata are displaced downward through the foramen magnum into the cervical area of the spinal medulla, the deformity is termed an *Arnold-Chiari malformation*. In this congenital defect the lower portion of the fourth ventricle is also pulled downward toward the spinal medulla. Additionally, the foramina of Luschka and Magendie may be either patent or closed because of the compression that often occurs with the downward displacement. In extreme instances the medulla becomes twisted on the cord. Adhesions from the cerebellum to the medulla may also obliterate the cisterna magna. The upper cervical nerve roots usually travel downward toward their intervertebral exits, but the downward traction on the upper cervical nerve roots may alter their course to an upward direction. Other conditions that may be concurrent with the Arnold-Chiari deformity include myelodysplasia, internal hydrocephalus, bony defects of the upper vertebrae and base of the skull, and stenosis or forking of the aqueduct of Sylvius.

Pathogenesis is described by three popular theories, including (1) interferences with development during intrauterine life; (2) fixation of the lower region of the spinal medulla in spina bifida, which restricts the cord from ascending in fetal life and results in traction and downward displacement of the cerebellum and the medulla; and (3) descent of the hindbrain secondary to the pressure exerted by hydrocephalus. Since this problem is interesting from a developmental point of view but is primarily a pediatric complication, the reader is directed to the references for further information on diagnosis and intervention modalities (Ford, 1973; Jabbour et al., 1976).

## COMMUNICATION MODALITIES

The intricate system of receiving, integrating, and responding to stimuli is performed by *projectional, associational,* and *commissural neurons*. An explanation of development is included in this chapter, whereas details on the operations of each of these mechanisms are available in subsequent chapters.

Generally, an incoming sensory stimulus is received by the thalamus from the opposite side of the spinal medulla, except for optic sensations, which are transmitted by the same side. Activation of a small portion of the thalamus results in activation of a larger protion of corresponding neurons in the cerebral cortex. The response of the cerebral cortex is possible because of the projectional neurons adjoining the lateral thalamus and medial corpus striatum. *Projectional axons* linking the thalamus and cerebral cortex form a mass of fibers called the *internal capsule*. The internal capsule consists of the white matter that surrounds most of the* basal ganglia. Because of its location between the corpus striatum and the thalamus, it divides the caudate nuclei from the lentiform nuclei. After the sensory stimulus has reached the cerebral cortex from the corresponding side of the thalamus, it is disseminated through one hemisphere by axons of *associational neurons*. After one hemisphere receives the message it is transmitted to the other cerebral hemisphere through a connection called a *commissure*.

In the early developmental stages the telencephalon is connected by its median portion. The only place for the commissural fibers to form is the median plane in the anterior wall of the interventricular foramen (the lamina terminalis), since the roof plate becomes the area where the choroid plexuses invaginate and the floor plate is where decussating optic nerve fibers enter.

The anterior commissure is the first to form. It consists of mainly olfactory areas, including the olfactory tracts and fibers from the piriform area, prepiriform area, and amygdaloid bodies. These fibers reach the opposite hemisphere by crossing over at the lamina terminalis.

The hippocampi connect by crossing from fornix to fornix at the upper portion of the lamina terminalis. The medial aspects of the thalamus are joined through the medial commissure, which courses horizontally through the third ventricle. Other fibrous bridges form between the optic chiasma and the anterior commissure.

More commissural fibers are added to the pathways of the anterior commissure as the paleopallial cortex forms in later development. Because the numbers of fibers increase greatly in this area, the

area is referred to as the *corpus callosum*. The corpus callosum becomes the largest interconnection between the two hemispheres.

As the corpus callosum develops, it extends dorsally and superiorly to the choroid fissure. During the growth process the corpus callosum carries the commissure of the fornix on its inferior surface. Because of the affiliation of these two structures in growth, a new floor develops for the longitudinal fissure and new structures from above the epithelial roof of the third ventricle. Caudal progression of growth causes the corpus callosum to occupy the area previously occupied by the superior aspects of the hippocampal formation and the dentate gyrus, so that these structures become mere remnants as growth continues. However, the lower portions of both these structures remain intact because the brainstem becomes the obstacle that prevents further caudal proliferation by the corpus callosum (Fig. 1-26).

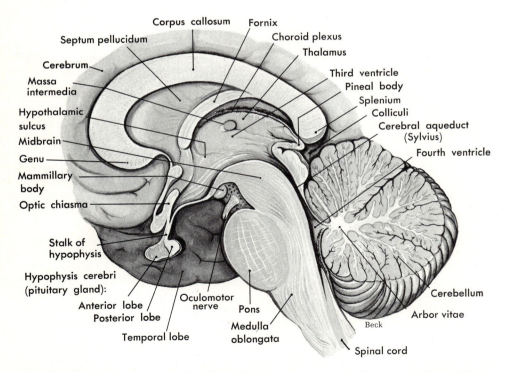

**FIG. 1-26.** Sagittal section through midline of brain showing structures around third ventricle. (From Anthony, C.P., and Kolthoff, N.J.: Textbook of anatomy and physiology, ed. 9, St. Louis, 1975, The C.V. Mosby Co.)

Impulses are transmitted to the cortex by two major pathways: the dorsal columns and the lateral spinothalamic tract. Motor responses are relayed from the cerebral cortex by the corticospinal (pyramidal) and extrapyramidal tracts. Detailed explanations on the exact formation of these tracts is beyond the scope of this book. However, discussion of general aspects of development is integrated into the sections concerning the functional operations of these pathways (Chapters 2 and 3).

## NEUROHORMONES

Neurohormones are discussed separately from the neurotransmitters that act at the point where two neurons synapse. Other sections of this book offer a complete discussion of both substances.

The neurohormones epinephrine and norepinephrine are secreted from the chromaffin cells of the medulla of the suprarenal gland. The chromaffin cells are the most primitive neuronal cells in the mature individual. These cells resemble endocrine gland cells but seem to be most closely related to the postganglionic sympathetic motor neurons, which also secrete epinephrine and norepinephrine. Both cells are derived from the neural crest. However, the two cells differ because the chromaffin cells primarily release epinephrine through the vascular system to achieve a predominance of sympathetic activity, which is sometimes referred to as Cannon's fight or flight response, whereas the postganglionic cells secrete norepinephrine at their terminal endings in the effector organ.

The supraoptic and paraventricular nuclei of the hypothalamus both have endocrine and neural functions. Each one has axonal endings in the pos-

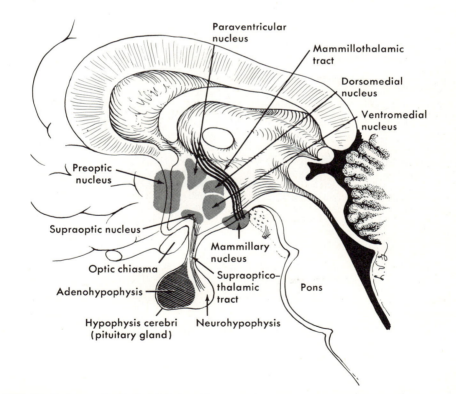

**FIG. 1-27.** Hypothalamus, showing location of nuclei and mammillary body. (From Schottelius, B.A., and Schottelius, D.D.: Textbook of physiology, ed. 18, St. Louis, 1978, The C.V. Mosby Co.)

terior lobe of the pituitary gland (hypophysis). The cytoplasm, oxytocin, and antidiuretic hormone produced in the neuron are transmitted via the axon to the hypophysis for storage. When body activity requires these hormones, the posterior lobe releases them through the vascular system to target tissues. Other hypothalamic cells secrete releasing hormones that are conveyed to the anterior lobe of the hypophysis through the hypophyseal portal system (Fig. 1-27).

The posterior lobe has its origin in primitive brain tissue, whereas the anterior lobe arises from nonneural foregut. However, the anterior lobe is interconnected with the hypothalamus to effect a profound influence on the nervous system through hormonal activity. The functional physiology of the autonomic nervous system is further detailed in Chapter 4.

## REFERENCES

Arey, L.B.: Developmental anatomy, ed. 7, Philadelphia, 1974, W.B. Saunders Co.

Babson, S.G., et al.: Diagnosis and management of the fetus and neonate at risk: a guide for team care, ed. 4, St. Louis, 1979, The C.V. Mosby Co.

Bergsma, D.: Birth defects atlas and compendium (National Foundation—Birth Defects—Original Articles Ser.), Baltimore, 1973, The Williams & Wilkins Co.

Carr, D.H.: Heredity and the embryo, Sci. J. (London) **6**:75, 1970.

Crelin, E.S.: Functional anatomy of the newborn, New Haven, Conn., 1973, Yale University Press.

Dobbing, J.: The later growth of the brain and its vulnerability, Pediatrics **53**:2, Jan. 1974.

Ford, F.R.: Diseases of the nervous system in infancy, childhood, and adolescence, ed. 6, Springfield, Ill., 1973, Charles C Thomas, Publisher.

Gardner, L.I.: Endocrine and genetic diseases of childhood, Philadelphia, 1975, W.B. Saunders Co.

Gellis, S.S., and Feingold, M.: Atlas of mental retardation syndromes, Washington, D.C., 1968, U.S. Department of Health, Education, and Welfare, Social and Rehabilitation Services Administration, Division of Mental Retardation.

Grabow, J.D., et al.: Cerebellar stimulation for the control of seizures, Mayo Clin. Proc. **49**:759, Oct. 1974.

Harris, R., et al.: Comparison of amniotic fluid and maternal serum alpha-fetoprotein levels in the early antenatal diagnosis of spina bifida and anencephaly, Lancet **1**:429, March 19, 1974.

Haymaker, W.: Bing's local diagnosis in neurological diseases, ed. 15, St. Louis, 1969, The C.V. Mosby Co.

Holmes, L.B., et al.: Mental retardation: an atlas of diseases with associated abnormalities, New York, 1972, Macmillan Publishing Co., Inc.

Holmes, L.B., et al.: X-linked aqueductal stenosis: clinical and neuropathological findings in two families, Pediatrics **51**:697, April 1973.

Hubbert, C.H., et al.: Dandy-Walker syndrome: spectrum of congenital abnormalities, South. Med. J. **67**:274, March 1974.

Jabbour, J.T., et al.: Pediatric neurology handbook, Flushing, N.Y., 1976, Medical Examination Publishing Co., Inc.

Moore, K.L.: The developing human: clinically oriented embryology, ed. 2, Philadelphia, 1977, W.B. Saunders Co.

Philipp, E.E., Barnes, J., and Newton, M., editors: Scientific foundations of obstetrics and gynecology, ed. 2, Chicago, 1977, Year Book Medical Publishers.

The pineal, Lancet **11**:1235, Nov. 23, 1974.

Ruhde, J.: Study unit on caring for the handicapped child. A project of the Wisconsin Regional Medical Program, Inc., and the Department of Nursing, Health Sciences Unit, University Extension, University of Wisconsin Press.

Seller, M.J., et al.: Maternal serum alpha-fetoprotein levels and prenatal diagnosis of neural tube defects, Lancet **1**:428, March 16, 1974.

Stevenson, R.E.: The fetus and newly born infant: influences of the prenatal environment, St. Louis, 1977, The C.V. Mosby Co.

Strickberger, M.W.: Genetics, ed. 2, New York, 1976, Macmillan Publishing Co., Inc.

Warwick, R., and Williams, P.L.: Gray's anatomy, ed. 35, Philadelphia, 1973, W.B. Saunders Co.

# 2

# FUNCTIONAL ANATOMIC CONSIDERATIONS

Neurology and neurological surgery are spheres of medicine that deal with organic disease of the nervous system. The causes of illness may vary and may be congenital, infectious, vascular, degenerative, neoplastic, or traumatic, but the fundamental clinical picture of neurological dysfunction depends on the location of the lesion and is the same regardless of cause. Therefore the first step in assessing the client is to localize the trouble. This depends on an understanding of the various parts of the nervous system and how they function.

Structurally the nervous system can be considered in subdivisions that depend on their relationships to the skull and vertebral column. The brain and spinal cord, which are contained within these bones, form the *central nervous system;* the cerebrospinal and autonomic nerves that are outside these bone cavities compose the *peripheral nervous system.* Functionally a different subdivision is used, depending on the part of the nervous system under voluntary control and the part controlled involuntarily. Most of the function of the nervous system is to receive stimuli, to interpret them at various reflex and conscious levels, and finally to transmit them for action. In this way communication is maintained between various parts of the body and the nervous system, and integration of its multiple activities is possible. The nervous system is responsible for man's perception of his internal and external environment and his reaction to it. This response may transpire on a conscious or an unconscious (reflex) level. Thus man's adjustment to life and to the environment

depends largely on the effective functioning of the nervous system (Fig. 2-1).

## NEURONS

The constituent cells of the nervous system are two, neurons and glia, and all except microglia are derived from ectoderm. The glia are comprised of *astrocytes, microglia, oligodendrocytes,* and the *ependyma.* The microglia are the phagocytes of the central nervous system and are derived from the mesoderm. The other glia cells function to support, nourish, and protect the neurons. Neurons are nerve cells, which transmit all stimuli concerned in the activity of the nervous system. They are composed of a nerve cell body (NCB), dendrites, and an axon. The cell body is a centrally located mass of granular cytoplasm encompassing a nucleus. Cellular cytoplasm contains rod-shaped bodies involved in cellular respiration (mitochondria) just as all active cells do. Neurofibrils are the fine microtubules that form the reticulum in the cell body. These neurofibrils compose most of the axon and may also be found in the dendrites. Larger dendrites and the cell body also contain chromophilic substance, which includes ribonucleic acid (Nissl substance), the basic component essential to the development of cell protoplasm. Although the fundamental structural components of neuronal cells are similar, the shape and size of various neurons vary greatly.

Neurons are classified as unipolar, bipolar, or multipolar according to the number of processes they have. The only unipolar neuron in the human

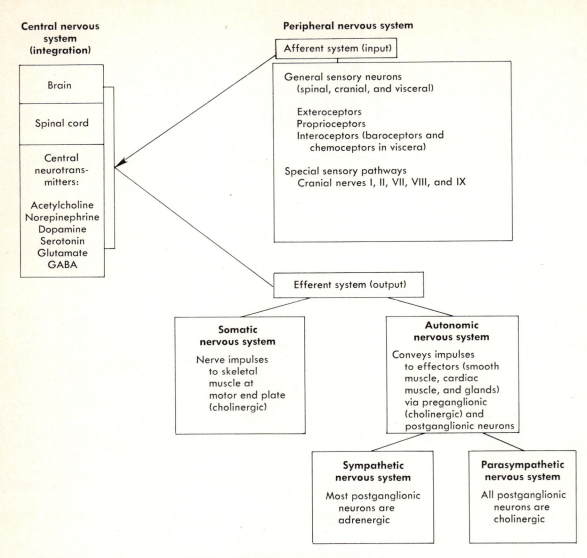

**FIG. 2-1.** Organizational pattern of nervous system.

body is the general sensory neuron (GSN), which has its nerve cell body in the dorsal root ganglion. This neuron has a single process leaving the cell body (axon) that divides shortly into a *peripheral process* (functionally a dendrite because it transmits impulses toward the nerve cell body) and a *central process*, which enters the dorsal cord.

There are bipolar neurons associated with the pathways for the special senses of hearing, taste and smell. All other neurons are multipolar (this type includes all internuncial [connecting] and motor neurons), having numerous dendrites transmitting impulses toward the nerve cell body and one process, the axon, transmitting impulses away from

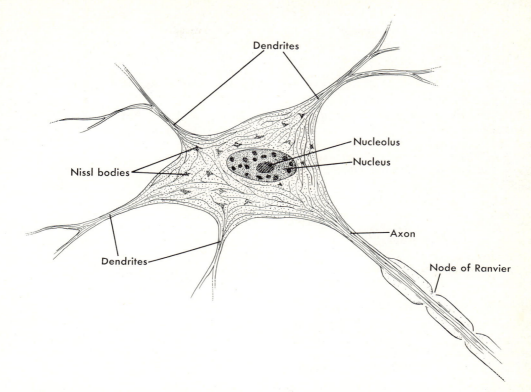

**FIG. 2-2.** Cell body of multipolar neuron. (From Conway, B.L.: Pediatric neurologic nursing, St. Louis, 1977, The C.V. Mosby Co.)

**TABLE 2-1.** Relationship between size, rate of transmission, and function of neurons

| Type of fiber | Fiber diameter in $\mu$m relative to amount of myelin | Velocity of conduction (m/sec) | Order of susceptibility to anoxia | Function (M = motor, S = sensory) |
|---|---|---|---|---|
| A | | | | |
|   Alpha | 12-20 | 70-120 | 2 | Voluntary motor—M<br>Proprioception—S |
|   Beta | 8-12 | 40-70 | 2 | Touch, pressure, kinesthesia—S |
|   Delta | 4-8 | 15-40 | 2 | Motor excitation of muscle spindle—M<br>Touch—S |
|   Gamma | 1-4 | 5-15 | 2 | Pain and temperatures—S |
| B | 1-3 | 3-15 | 1 | Autonomic preganglionic—M |
| C | 0.2-1 | 0.2-2 | 3 | Autonomic postganglionic—M<br>Pain + ?(undifferentiated)—S |

the cell center. Dendrites are short and have large points of origin and a branchlike appearance. Axons have a smooth form, decrease slightly in caliber as they extend from the cell body, and are limited to one process per cell. Axons may form one or more tiny branches termed *collaterals*. Fig. 2-2 shows an example of a multipolar neuron.

Dendrites are unmyelinated and lie with the nerve cell body in gray matter, whereas axons are myelinated and transmit impulses along pathways (white matter of the central nervous system) to another integrating center. Synapses can only occur in gray matter. Most axons are myelinated and are classified according to their diameter. The variable in this classification is the amount of myelin, which encases the axis cylinder. The significance of the myelin is related to the speed of transmission because myelinated fibers transmit impulses by saltatory transmission. The myelin sheath is broken at the nodes of Ranvier and transmission of the impulse skips from node to node (Table 2-1).

## PERIPHERAL NERVE STRUCTURE

The derivation of neurilemma and satellite cells is detailed in Chapter 1, along with information about myelinated and unmyelinated axons.

All peripheral nerve fibers are enveloped in a thin outer membrane of neurilemma. This neurilemma divides all peripheral nerve fibers from the endoneurium, the complex matrix of connective tissue surrounding each nerve fiber. Exterior to the endoneurium is the perineurium, which encloses the bundles of nerve fibers (fasciculi) with connective tissue. The outermost covering of the nerve trunk is the epineurium, a white fibrous connective tissue. Nerve trunks are composed of nerve fibers (Fig. 2-3).

Neurons may be subdivided into three functional groups: afferent, internuncial, and efferent. *Afferent neurons,* also known as sensory or receptor neurons, receive incoming stimuli. *Internuncial neurons,* also known as central, connecting, or associational cells, convey these incoming impulses to neurons of various integrating centers of the central nervous system. *Efferent neurons,* also known as motor or effector neurons, transmit impulses to effector organs such as glands and muscles.

## SPINAL CORD AND NERVES

The spinal cord and brainstem form a continuous structure (Fig. 2-4) extending from the cerebral hemispheres (brain) and serving as a connecting link between the brain and the periphery. This structure contains long conducting pathways (sensory and motor) for this purpose, as well as groups

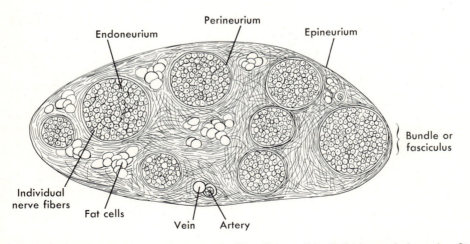

**FIG. 2-3.** Transverse section of peripheral nerve trunk. (From Conway, B.L.: Pediatric neurologic nursing, St. Louis, 1977, The C.V. Mosby Co.)

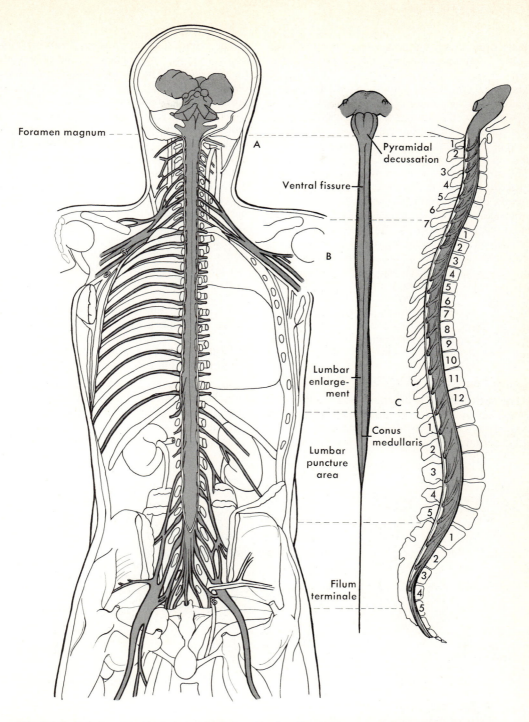

**FIG. 2-4. A,** Posterior view of brainstem and spinal cord in situ with spinal nerves and plexuses. **B,** Anterior view of brainstem and spinal cord. **C,** Lateral view, showing relationship of spinal cord to vertebrae. (From Mettler, F.A.: Neuroanatomy, ed. 2, St. Louis, 1948, The C.V. Mosby Co.)

of cells from which the nerve fibers going to the periphery originate (motor) and intersegmental fibers.

The spinal cord varies slightly in size and shape, depending on the region. The cervical region is largest in bulk; the lumbar region is next in size. These cervical and lumbar enlargements are areas of origin of the nerves to the upper and lower limbs.

The spinal cord extends from the foramen magnum at the base of the skull to the upper level of the body of the second lumbar vertebra where it terminates in a fibrous band (filum terminale) that is attached to the coccyx. (In infants the spinal cord extends to the sacral region.) The spinal cord is composed of 31 segments: 8 cervical, 12 thoracic, 5 lumbar, 5 sacral, and 1 coccygeal. Each segment has a spinal nerve for each side of the body (Fig. 2-5). The cervical and thoracic nerve roots have an almost horizontal course as they leave the spinal cord. The lumbar and sacral roots have an oblique downward course and are grouped together in such a way as to resemble a horse's tail *(cauda equina)*.

The efferent nerves consist of motor fibers that originate in the anterior horn of the gray matter of the spinal cord. The afferent nerves originate in the dorsal (posterior) root ganglia, from which one process extends into the posterior horn of the spinal cord and the other to the periphery. The motor and sensory nerve roots leave the vertebral column separately through the intervertebral foramina. Immediately outside the vertebral column the motor fibers join with the sensory fibers to form a mixed spinal nerve. To this, autonomic fibers are added, and together they constitute the peripheral nerve, which transmits sensory impulses from the skin, muscles, tendons, joints, bones, blood vessels, and viscera to the spinal cord and brain and motor impulses to the effectors. A synapse is the junction between the axon of one neuron and the dendrite or the nerve cell body of the next neuron in a pathway.

The plan of the peripheral nerve supply to the limbs is complicated by the assembly and rearrangement of the spinal nerves into plexuses. Plexuses are intricate networks of branches from the anterior division of spinal nerves. These plexuses

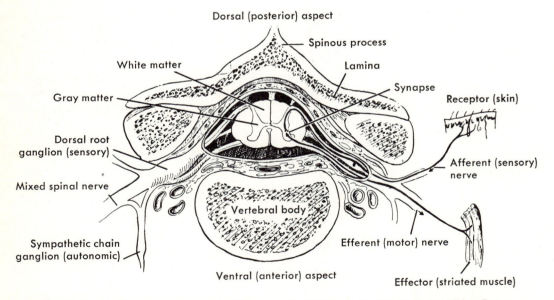

**FIG. 2-5.** Cross section of vertebral column and spinal cord. Note details of spinal cord with simple reflex arc, nerve components, dorsal root ganglion, and sympathetic chain.

have no synapses but are simply a rearrangement of fibers. After passing through the plexuses, the spinal nerves lose their individuality and emerge as peripheral nerves. These plexuses comprise the *cervical*, *brachial*, and *lumbosacral*. Branches from the thoracic area do not form a plexus but lead, instead, to the skin of the thorax and the intercostal muscles directly.

The course of these peripheral nerves and the parts supplied are outlined in Table 2-2 and Fig.

**TABLE 2-2.** Spinal nerves and peripheral branches*

| Spinal nerves | Plexuses formed from anterior rami | Spinal nerve branches from plexuses | Parts supplied |
|---|---|---|---|
| *Cervical* <br> 1 <br> 2 <br> 3 <br> 4 | Cervical plexus | Lesser occipital <br> Great auricular <br> Cutaneous nerve of neck <br> Anterior supraclavicular <br> Middle supraclavicular <br> Posterior supraclavicular <br> Branches to numerous neck muscles | Sensory to back of head, front of neck, and upper part of shoulder; motor to numerous neck muscles |
| | | *Phrenic nerve* | Diaphragm |
| *Cervical* <br> 5 <br> 6 <br> 7 <br> 8 <br><br> *Thoracic (or dorsal)* <br> 1 | Brachial plexus | Suprascapular and dorsoscapular <br> Thoracic nerves, medial and lateral anterior <br> Long thoracic nerve <br> Thoracodorsal <br> Subscapular <br> Axillary (circumflex) <br><br> Musculocutaneous <br><br><br> Ulnar | Superficial muscles† of scapula <br> Pectoralis major and minor <br><br> Serratus anterior <br> Latissimus dorsi <br> Subscapular and teres major muscles <br> Deltoid and teres minor muscles and skin over deltoid <br> Muscle of front of arm (biceps brachii, coracobrachialis, and brachialis) and skin on outer side of forearm <br> Flexor carpi ulnaris and part of flexor digitorum profundus; some of muscles of hand; sensory to medial side of hand, little finger, and medial half of fourth finger |
| 2 <br> 3 <br> 4 <br> 5 <br> 6 <br> 7 <br> 8 <br> 9 <br> 10 <br> 11 <br> 12 | No plexus formed; branches run directly to intercostal muscles and skin of thorax | Median <br><br><br> Radial <br><br><br> Medial cutaneous <br><br> Phrenic (branches from cervical nerves before formation of plexus; most of its fibers from fourth cervical nerve) | Rest of muscles of front of forearm and hand; sensory to skin of palmar surface of thumb, index, and middle fingers <br> Triceps muscle and muscles of back of forearm; sensory to skin of back of forearm and hand <br> Sensory to inner surface of arm and forearm <br> Diaphragm |

*From Anthony, C.P., and Thibodeau, G.A.: Textbook of anatomy and physiology, ed. 10, St. Louis, 1979, The C.V. Mosby Co.
†Although nerves to muscles are considered motor, they do contain some sensory fibers that transmit proprioceptive impulses.

*Continued.*

**TABLE 2-2.** Spinal nerves and peripheral branches—cont'd

| Spinal nerves | Plexuses formed from anterior rami | Spinal nerve branches from plexuses | Parts supplied |
|---|---|---|---|
| | | Iliohypogastric<br>Ilioinguinal } Sometimes fused | Sensory to anterior abdominal wall<br>Sensory to anterior abdominal wall and external genitalia; motor to muscles of abdominal wall |
| | | Genitofemoral | Sensory to skin of external genitalia and inguinal region |
| *Lumbar* | | Lateral cutaneous of thigh | Sensory to outer side of thigh |
| 1 | | Femoral | Motor to quadriceps, sartorius, and iliacus muscles; sensory to front of thigh and to medial side of lower leg (saphenous nerve) |
| 2 | | | |
| 3 | | | |
| 4 | | | |
| 5 | | Obturator | Motor to adductor muscles of thigh |
| *Sacral* | Lumbosacral plexus | Tibial‡ (medial popliteal) | Motor to muscles of calf of leg; sensory to skin of calf of leg and sole of foot |
| 1 | | | |
| 2 | | Common peroneal (lateral popliteal) | Motor to evertors and dorsiflexors of foot; sensory to lateral surface of leg and dorsal surface of foot |
| 3 | | | |
| 4 | | | |
| 5 | | Nerves to hamstring muscles | Motor to muscles to back of thigh |
| *Coccygeal* | | Gluteal nerves, superior and inferior | Motor to buttock muscles and tensor fasciae latae |
| 1 | | | |
| | | Posterior cutaneous nerve | Sensory to skin of buttocks, posterior surface of thigh, and leg |
| | | Pudendal nerve | Motor to perineal muscles; sensory to skin of perineum |

‡Sensory fibers from the tibial and peroneal nerves unite to form the *medial cutaneous* (or *sural*) *nerve* that supplies the calf of the leg and the lateral surface of the foot. In the thigh, the tibial and common peroneal nerves are usually enclosed in a single sheath to form the *sciatic nerve*, the largest nerve in the body with its width of approximately ¾ of an inch. About two thirds of the way down the posterior part of the thigh, it divides into its component parts. Branches of the sciatic nerve extend into the hamstring muscles.

2-6. However, a few observations on each plexus seem timely. One notes that the level of innervation at the spinal medulla corresponds rather closely to the area of body surface innervated by a given spinal nerve or plexus. Thus when cord functions are interrupted, practitioners performing a detailed neurological assessment are often able to define the level of interference clinically before more sophisticated diagnostic techniques are employed. Transection of the spinal cord is discussed in Chapters 17 and 23.

The phrenic nerves, which arise from the third and fourth or fourth and fifth cervical spinal nerves between the cervical and brachial plexuses, are of particular importance, since the interruption of this cord level by an infectious process such as polio-myelitis or of a higher level by trauma may halt impulses to the phrenic nerves. Such cessation of impulses results in diaphragmatic paralysis and a subsequent lack of respirations. Unless artificial means of life support are available, death may result. The brachial plexus in the shoulder area extends from the neck to the axilla. It is composed of fibers from the lower four cervical and first thoracic nerves. The nerves that emerge from this plexus innervate the hand and most of the arm. The most significant nerves in this group are the median, radial, and ulnar nerves. The median nerve is composed of fibers from the sixth, seventh, and eighth cervical and the first thoracic nerves. The radial nerve consists of fibers from the fifth, sixth, seventh, and eighth cervical and first thoracic nerves,

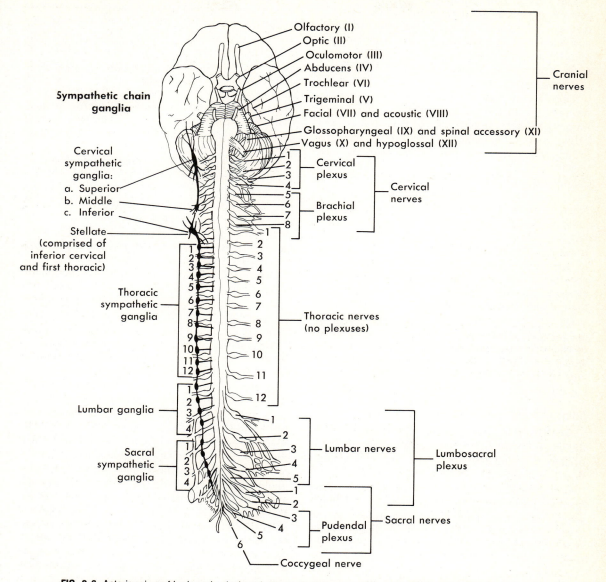

**FIG. 2-6.** Anterior view of brain and spinal cord. *Right,* Spinal nerves; *left,* sympathetic chain. Note that sympathetic chain of ganglia includes all regions even though cells of origin are only in thoracolumbar area.

whereas the ulnar nerve is derived from the seventh and eighth cervical and first thoracic nerves.

The first four lumbar nerves form the lumbar plexus, located in the lumbar area of the back in the psoas muscle. The largest nerve from this plexus is the femoral nerve, which arises from the second, third, and fourth lumbar nerves. The femoral nerve branches into other nerves to supply the lower extremity.

The sacral plexus is composed of fibers from the fourth and fifth lumbar and the first, second, and third sacral nerves. It occupies a position in the pelvic cavity on the anterior aspect of the piriform muscle. The tibial, peroneal, and sciatic nerves are the significant peripheral nerves that arise from this plexus. The tibial nerve arises from the fifth lumbar and first, second, and third sacral nerves, whereas the peroneal nerve arises from the fifth lumbar and first sacral nerves. The sciatic nerve, the largest nerve in the body, results when the tibial and peroneal nerves combine. Thus the sciatic nerve by its two branches, the tibial and peroneal nerves, innervates the posterior thigh muscles, most of the skin on the lower extremity, and the muscles in the leg and foot.

Because the spinal nerves course a considerable distance from the lumbar and sacral areas of origin to the intervertebral foramina for exit from the spinal canal, trauma or compression injuries to this area of the cord may damage several roots lying close together.

### Interrupted neuronal functions

The synthesis of protein and other substances in the cell body is vital to the functional competency of the axon and myelin sheath. When this vital flow is interrupted by disease or trauma, degeneration of the area unsupplied by this axoplasmic flow results. The early phase of degeneration is one where uniform segmental demyelination, usually reversible, occurs. When neuronal distress persists, distal areas experience wallerian degeneration.

About 7 days after injury of peripheral nerve fibers regeneration begins as new axons form along pathways already laid down by neurilemma cells. The last phase of this regrowth process is the formation of the myelin sheath. This process of re-generation does not occur in the brain and spinal cord where no neurilemma is found.

Interruption of a peripheral nerve is followed by loss of sensation and muscular activity of the part served by that nerve. The demonstrable sensory loss follows a definite pattern for each nerve (Fig. 2-7). The resulting muscular paralysis is also similar for each nerve. A muscle deprived of its peripheral nerve supply (final common pathway) does not respond either by voluntary or reflex activity. It becomes flaccid (limp), losing all normal muscle tone (a continuous state of asynchronous partial contraction that maintains the muscle in readiness for action).

Electromyography is a method of recording electrical currents produced by muscular activity and is used to confirm the presence of denervation. Atrophy, fasciculations, and fibrillations in muscles indicate a severed connection between the motor axon and the effector organ. Denervation lasting for more than 1 year results in damage, which effects an incomplete recovery.

One of the principal functions of the peripheral nerves is that of sensation. The body surface can be divided into areas supplied by each nerve. Other areas are based on a segmental plan, each skin segment corresponding to a spinal cord segment. Such a skin area is called a *dermatome*. Knowledge of the dermatomes is essential for accurate localization of spinal cord disorders. (See Chapter 3.)

In cross section the spinal cord consists of a round to oval structure formed by white matter, in the middle of which is a roughly H-shaped pattern formed by the gray matter (Fig. 2-5). The lower legs of the H are broader than the upper and correspond to the anterior horns. Herein lie the cells of origin of the fibers that form the anterior (motor) root and are essential for the voluntary and reflex activity of the muscles supplied by them. The thinner posterior (upper) horns contain central processes of general sensory neurons (GSN) entering over the posterior root, thus forming a substation in the service of sensation. In the thoracic region of the spinal cord is a projection from each side at the crossbar of the H of gray matter called the *lateral horn*. It contains the cells that give rise to the autonomic fibers of the sympathetic division. The fibers leave the spinal cord through the an-

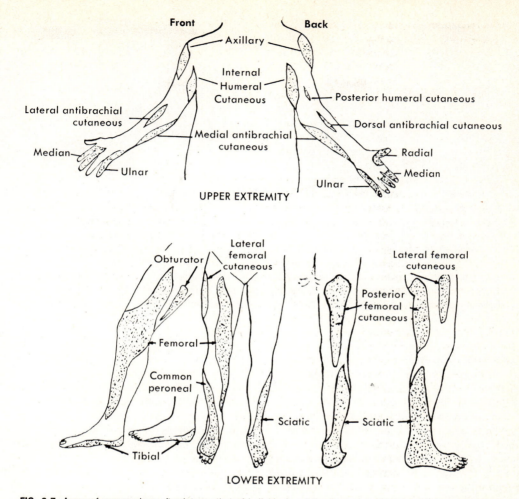

**FIG. 2-7.** Areas of sensory loss after interruption of individual peripheral nerves, which branch from plexuses.

terior roots in the thoracic and upper lumbar segments (Fig. 2-6).

## Cranial nerves

There are 12 pairs of cranial nerves (Fig. 2-6), though strictly speaking the first two pairs are tracts. They correspond to the spinal nerves serving common sensation, voluntary control of muscles, and autonomic functions in the head; in addition, they include the mechanism for the special senses of vision, hearing, smell, and taste.

1. The *olfactory nerve* is the special sense organ for smell. It consists of about two dozen nerve filaments in the mucous membrane over the upper part of the nasal septum on each side. These fibers enter the skull through the midline portion of the frontal fossa (the cribriform plate) to join cells in the olfactory bulbs. From each bulb, fibers go along the base of the brain to each side of the optic chiasma, where they enter the brain and reach the thalamus and temporal lobe in the area of the uncus.

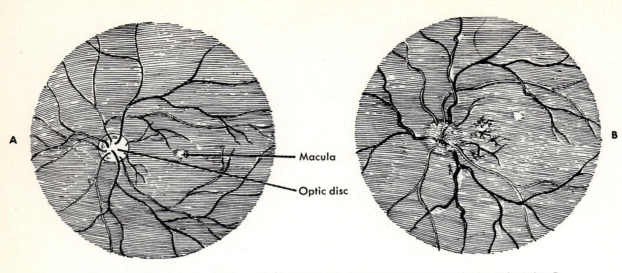

FIG. 2-8. **A,** Normal fundus showing optic nerve head with distinct outline and normal veins and arteries. **B,** Pathological fundus with papilledema (choked disc), showing optic disc with indistinct outline and swelling. Fullness and tortuosity of veins and hemorrhages in retina also are illustrated.

2. The *optic nerve* serves the special sense of vision. The sensory receptor is the retina, from which the nerve fibers run together as the optic nerve and enter the skull through the optic foramen. The optic nerve head is commonly referred to as the optic disc (Fig. 2-8, *A*). The nerve is sheathed by a prolongation of the cranial meninges. Any increase of intracranial pressure is transmitted through the cerebrospinal fluid in the subarachnoid space to the nerve head, and after a short time a swelling of the optic disc results. This can be seen on ophthalmoscopic examination of the fundus and is called *papilledema,* or choked disc (Fig. 2-8, *B*). As the optic nerve fibers pass posteriorly, approximately one half of them continue to the brain on the same side, and the other half cross to the other side of the brain. The partial crossing takes place at the *optic chiasma,* which lies directly over the pituitary body in the sella turcica. The crossed and uncrossed fibers join immediately after the partial crossing and continue as the optic tract to the lateral geniculate body of the thalamus. From this point the optic radiation courses around the tip of the temporal lobe and posteriorly to the occi-

pital cortex, the end station for vision (Fig. 2-9).

When a disturbance of the optic pathways occurs, vision can be limited in extent, though the visual acuity is normal. If one of the optic nerves were to be divided, blindness would result in that eye. If a tumor compressed the optic chiasma at its midpoint, the crossed fibers that come from the medial side of the retina would first be interrupted, and blindness would result in the temporal halves of each field of vision (bitemporal hemianopia). If the encroachment on the visual pathway were behind the chiasma, anywhere in the tract, or radiating through the temporal or occipital lobes, interference with the crossed and uncrossed fibers would occur, resulting in blindness in the same half of each field of vision (homonymous hemianopia) (Fig. 2-9).

3. The *oculomotor nerve* controls motion of the eyeball up, in, and down; raises the eyelid; and constricts the pupil. The muscles supplied are the superior, medial, and inferior recti; the inferior oblique; and the levator of the upper eyelid. The cells of origin are in the midbrain below the aqueduct. The cells for voluntary movement are grouped on each side and near the midline; the

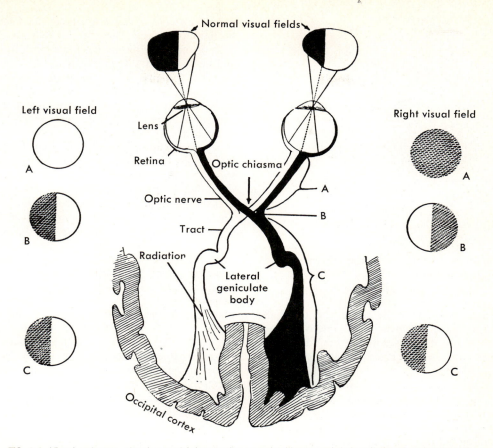

**FIG. 2-9.** Visual pathways, showing partial decussation at optic chiasma and their radiation to end station of occipital cortex. Normal visual fields show reversal of light rays, through action of lens, from nasal and temporal sides to receptors in retina. Pathological visual fields are illustrated. **A,** Loss of vision in right field resulting from complete lesion of right optic nerve; left field is normal. **B,** Loss of vision in temporal half of right and left fields caused by lesion involving optic chiasma (bitemporal hemianopia). **C,** Loss of vision in nasal field of right eye and in temporal field of left eye caused by lesion of right optic tract or radiation (homonymous hemianopia). Pathological fields are lettered corresponding to sites of causative lesions.

cells for autonomic activity form a single group lying between the paired groups and send fibers by way of each oculomotor nerve to the ciliary ganglion (parasympathetic) in the orbit, from which fibers go to the ciliary muscle and sphincter muscle of the iris. Interruption of this unit interferes with the reaction of the pupil to light, though it may still react on convergence (the Argyll Robertson pupil).

4. The *trochlear nerve* supplies the superior oblique muscle and rotates the eyeball downward

and out. The nuclei are also in the midbrain immediately posterior to the oculomotor nuclei.

5. The *trigeminal nerve* has motor and sensory components. The motor root innervates the muscles of mastication (temporalis, masseter, pterygoid, and anterior half of the digastric) and the tensor tympani and tensor veli palatini muscles. The motor nucleus is in the pons, and the motor fibers travel close to the sensory root on its medial side to the gasserian ganglion, where they join the

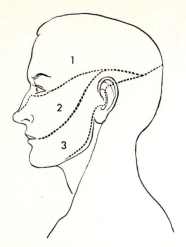

**FIG. 2-10.** Cutaneous distribution of three divisions of trigeminal nerve: *1*, ophthalmic; *2*, maxillary; *3*, mandibular.

mandibular division of the nerve and leave the skull through the foramen ovale. Interruption of the motor root interferes with chewing and opening the mouth (the lower jaw deviates toward the paralyzed side).

The sensory part of the trigeminal nerve originates in the gasserian (semilunar) ganglion, which lies in a fold of dura mater near the apex of the petrous portion of the temporal bone. The ganglion sends out three branches (Fig. 2-10): the *ophthalmic,* generally referred to as the first division, to the skin of the head, forehead, upper eyelid, and part of the nose, the cornea, conjunctiva, and the mucous membrane of the nose; the *maxillary,* second division, to the skin of the cheek, the remainder of the nose, lower eyelid, upper lip, the mucous membrane and teeth of the upper jaw, and the dura mater; and the *mandibular,* third division, to the skin of the lower lip, chin, and ear, the mucous membrane and teeth of the lower jaw, and the tongue. The posterior (sensory) root of the trigeminal nerve lies lateral to the motor root from the gasserian ganglion to the pons. The sensory trigeminal nucleus extends from the upper pons to the upper spinal cord, whereas the motor nucleus is much smaller and is located in the midpart of the pons.

6. The *abducens nerve* innervates the lateral rectus muscle, which rotates the eyeball outward. The cells of origin are in the posterior part of the pons and lie close to the facial nucleus.

7. The *facial nerve* is principally motor but also has sensory and autonomic components. It innervates the muscles of the face (forehead, eyelids, cheeks, and lips), ears, nose, and neck (platysma) through nerve fibers that originate in cells in the pons, pass into the internal acoustic meatus through the facial canal, and leave the skull by the stylomastoid foramen. The nerve then goes through the parotid gland and divides into the branches that supply the various facial muscles. The sensory component is responsible for the perception of taste on the anterior two thirds of the tongue. These fibers travel with the lingual nerve (a branch of the mandibular division of the trigeminal nerve) until they enter the facial canal in the temporal bone and join the motor elements of the facial nerve. The cells of origin of these sensory fibers are in the geniculate ganglion, the central fibers of which enter the pons and terminate in the nucleus of the tractuc solitarius. Autonomic (parasympathetic) fibers go from the superior salivatory nucleus by way of the otic ganglion to the parotid gland, by the submaxillary ganglion to the submaxillary and sublingual glands, and by the sphenopalatine ganglion to the lacrimal gland.

8. The *acoustic nerve* is purely sensory and consists of two parts: the vestibular nerve and the cochlear nerve. The cochlear nerve is concerned with hearing and originates in the spiral ganglion of the cochlea. The peripheral part ends in the special receptor mechanism, the organ of Corti, and its central fibers join with the central fibers of the vestibular portion. Together the cochlear and vestibular nerves enter the skull through the internal acoustic meatus close to the facial nerve. The vestibular nerve monitors and controls equilibrium. Its cells are in the vestibular ganglion (Scarpa), and its peripheral fibers transmit stimuli from the otolith organs of the semicircular canals. The acoustic nerve fibers enter the pons and terminate in the cochlear and vestibular neuclei. A few vestibular fibers continue uninterrupted to the cerebellum.

9. The *glossopharyngeal nerve* is small but consists of motor, sensory, and autonomic elements.

The motor fibers originate in the anterior part of the nucleus ambiguus in the medulla oblongata and innervate the constrictors of the pharynx and stylopharyngeus muscles, thus serving the act of swallowing. The sensory fibers transmit taste sensation from the same area, as well as from the soft palate, fauces, and tonsils by way of the petrous and jugular ganglia. These enter the medulla oblongata and terminate at the nucleus of the tractus solitarius. The parasympathetic fibers from the inferior salivatory nucleus reach the parotid gland by way of the otic ganglion. The autonomic sensory elements from the carotid sinus cause the blood pressure to drop and the pulse to slow. These fibers pass through the petrous ganglion to the nucleus of the tractus solitarius in the medulla oblongata.

10. The *vagus nerve* is also a mixed nerve, closely related to the glossopharyngeal in function and position. The motor fibers arise in the caudal part of the nucleus ambiguus and dorsal motor nucleus of the vagus in the medulla oblongata and leave the skull through the jugular foramen with the glossopharyngeal nerve. They control the voluntary activity of the pharynx and larynx and the involuntary activity of the esophagus, bronchi, lungs, heart, stomach, small intestines (stimulating peristalsis), liver, pancreas, and kidneys. The sensory fibers from the back of the ear and posterior wall of the external acoustic meatus originate in the jugular and nodose ganglia and enter the medulla oblongata to reach the nucleus of the tractus solitarius. There are also autonomic sensory elements from the larynx, trachea, lungs, aorta, esophagus, stomach, small intestines, and gallbladder.

11. The *accessory nerve* is motor and arises from cells in the lower medulla oblongata and upper spinal cord. The spinal cord fibers supply the sternocleidomastoid and upper part of the trapezius muscles. The cells in the nucleus ambiguus of the oblongata send a few fibers along with the vagus to the muscles of the pharynx and larynx.

12. The *hypoglossal nerve* is motor, arises in the cells of the hypoglossal nucleus of the medulla oblongata, leaves the skull by the hypoglossal canal, and supplies the muscles of the tongue.

Fig. 2-6 shows the origin of the cranial nerves on the brainstem.

## SUPPORTING STRUCTURES

Comprehension of the anatomy and physiology of the nervous system presupposes a knowledge of the associated structures that surround, support, protect, and nourish the brain and spinal cord. These structures include the bones of the skull and the vertebral column, the surrounding and supporting meninges (dura mater and pia-arachnoid), the vascular system, and the cerebrospinal fluid system.

### Bony structures

*Skull.* The skull, a rigid compartment of numerous bones fused together, protects and supports the brain and is divided into three regions: the anterior, middle, and posterior fossae. The anterior fossa contains the frontal lobes; the middle fossa contains the temporal, parietal, and occipital lobes; and the posterior fossa contains the brainstem and cerebellum. An opening at the base of the skull, the foramen magnum, is the point at which the brainstem changes structure and is identified as the spinal cord. Many smaller openings in the skull allow the cranial nerves and blood vessels to pass through. The skull is supported at its base by the atlas of the vertebral column, which forms a joint with the occipital bones.

*Vertebral column.* The vertebral column, which consists of 7 cervical, 12 thoracic, and 5 lumbar vertebrae as well as the sacrum and coccyx, supports the head and protects the spinal cord. The latter is contained in the long curved tube formed by the consecutive central canals of the vertebrae. Each vertebra has a central opening, the vertebral foramen, which is surrounded by the bony elements. In the characteristic vertebra (Fig. 2-11), these bony structures, the body of which is anterior and the spinous process posterior, are connected by a pedicle and a lamina on each side. The vertebrae are held together by a series of ligaments. Moderate motion takes place through the joints that exist between the adjacent bodies anteriorly and between the articulating facets at the junction of the pedicles and laminae posteriorly. The space between the bodies of the vertebrae is occupied by the intervertebral disc, which consists of a central cartilaginous core, the *nucleus pulposus,* surrounded by a fibrous capsule, the *anulus fibro-*

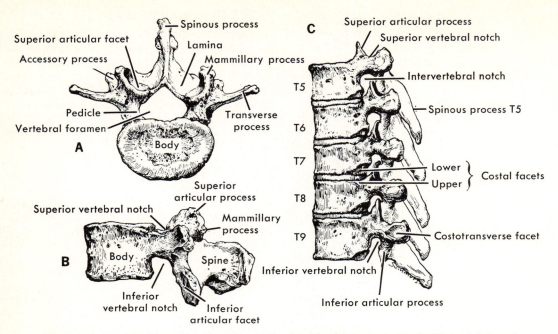

**FIG. 2-11. A,** Fourth lumbar vertebra from above. **B,** Fourth lumbar vertebra from side. **C,** Fifth to ninth thoracic vertebrae showing relationships of various parts. (From Mettler, F.A.: Neuroanatomy, ed. 2, St. Louis, 1948, The C.V. Mosby Co.)

*sus* (Fig. 2-12). Outside of this lie the longitudinal ligaments. Above and below each pedicle is an opening, the *intervertebral foramen,* through which the spinal roots pass. It is formed by a notch on the superior and inferior margins of each pedicle.

## Meninges

The meninges are the membranes between the skull and brain and the vertebral column and spinal cord. They are the dura mater, the arachnoid, and the pia mater. These membranes are fibrous connective tissue derived from the mesoderm. The dura mater within the skull differs from that within the spine in three particulars: (1) the cranial dura is firmly attached to the skull, but the spinal dura has no attachment to the vertebrae; (2) the cranial dura consists of two layers, periosteal and meningeal, whereas the spinal dura consists of one layer; and (3) the cranial dural layers separate in places and

form venous sinuses, whereas this is not possible in the one-layer spinal dura. The character of the two other membranes is the same in the cranial and spinal regions. Together they may be called the *pia-arachnoid* and may be considered as one transparent unit. The arachnoid lies next to the dura mater and has many threadlike connections with the pia mater, which is closely adherent to the brain and spinal cord (Fig. 2-13). The compartment formed by the pia mater and arachnoid is called the *subarachnoid space.* Within this space the cerebrospinal fluid circulates over the surface of the nervous system.

Folds of these membranes serve as supports for the spinal cord and brain. The spinal pia-arachnoid suspends the spinal cord by triangular extensions, which fuse with the dura mater between each cervical and thoracic segment. These are called the *denticulate ligaments.* Within the skull the dura mater folds vertically along the midsagittal line to

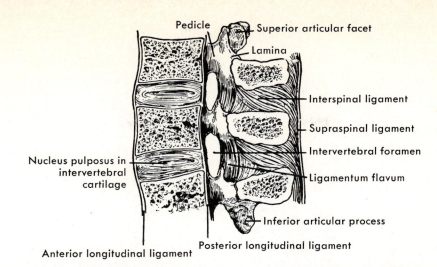

FIG. 2-12. Median section through three lumbar vertebrae showing the intervertebral discs. (From Mettler, F.A.: Neuroanatomy, ed. 2, St. Louis, 1948, The C.V. Mosby Co.)

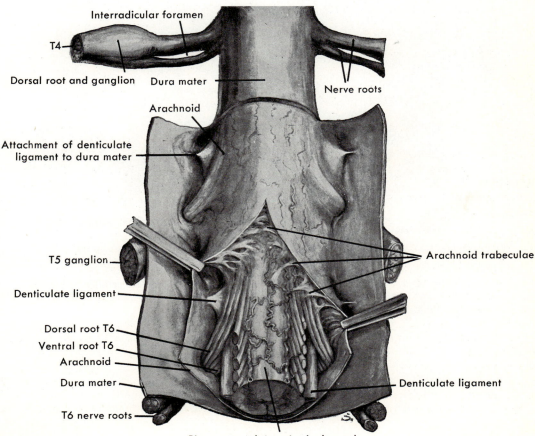

FIG. 2-13. Dorsum of midthoracic spinal cord, meninges, and roots. (From Mettler, F.A.: Neuroanatomy, ed. 2, St. Louis, 1948, The C.V. Mosby Co.)

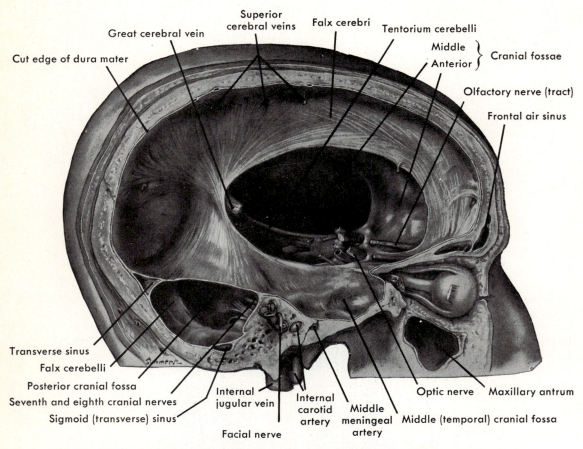

FIG. 2-14. Intracranial dura mater, showing falx cerebri and tentorium cerebelli fanning out laterally, dividing posterior cranial fossa from middle and anterior fossae. (From Mettler, F.A.: Neuroanatomy, ed. 2, St. Louis, 1948, The C.V. Mosby Co.)

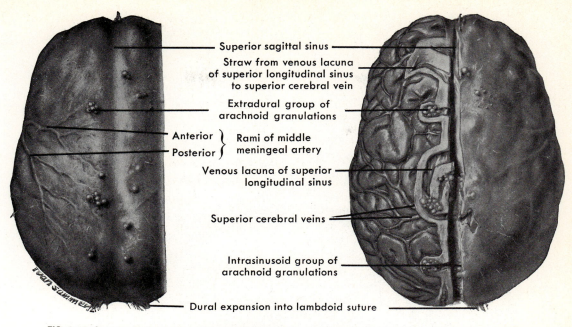

Superior sagittal sinus

Straw from venous lacuna
of superior longitudinal sinus
to superior cerebral vein

Extradural group of
arachnoid granulations

Anterior } Rami of middle
Posterior } meningeal artery

Venous lacuna of superior
longitudinal sinus

Superior cerebral veins

Intrasinusoid group of
arachnoid granulations

Dural expansion into lambdoid suture

**FIG. 2-15.** Superior surface of cranial dura with arachnoid granulations or villi. Superior longitudinal sinus, which drains veins over vertex, is shown opened. (From Mettler, F.A.: Neuroanatomy, ed. 2, St. Louis, 1948, The C.V. Mosby Co.)

form the falx cerebri, which separates the two cerebral hemispheres (Fig. 2-14). The layers of the falx cerebri separate at its superior and inferior boundaries and form the superior and inferior longitudinal sinuses. From the posterior limit of the falx cerebri the dura mater flares out laterally, forming the *tentorium cerebelli*. This supports the temporal and occipital lobes and at its periphery forms a venous channel for the lateral sinus.

The tentorium separates the posterior cranial fossa from the remainder of the cranial cavity and serves as a line of dermarcation for description when one refers to the site of operations or of lesions as *supratentorial* or *infratentorial*.

The arachnoid has wartlike formations (arachnoid or pacchionian granulations) that are found along the superior longitudinal sinus and project into the venous channel (Fig. 2-15). The arachnoid granulations push the meningeal layer of the dura mater ahead of them as they develop and perforate

this so that only a layer of endothelium of the sinus exists between these arachnoid villi and the blood, thus forming the structural mechanism for the reabsorption of the circulating cerebrospinal fluid.

The pia-arachnoid also serves as the roadbed for the vascular system of the cerebral cortex; the veins lie in the subarachnoid space, and the cortical arteries are carried with the pia mater into the cortex. The pia mater is closely adherent to the brain and even dips into the cerebral sulci, but the arachnoid spans the area without following the depressions in the surface architecture. This permits the existence of fair-sized subarachnoid spaces. At the base of the brain these spaces are large enough to be called *cisterns*. The most important of these is the *cisterna magna*, which is over the dorsum of the medulla oblongata and lies between it and the cerebellum. Other large cisterns along the base of the brain are the chiasmal, interpeduncular, and pontine (Fig. 2-16).

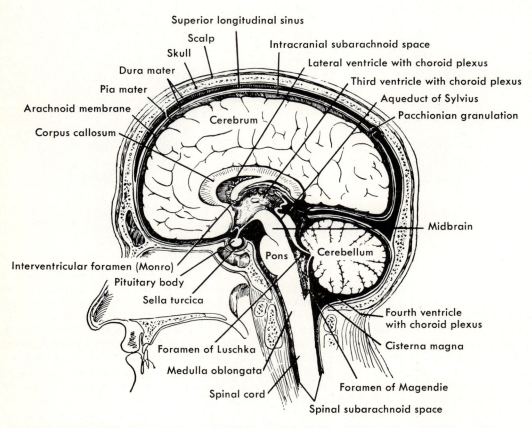

Superior longitudinal sinus
Scalp
Skull
Dura mater
Pia mater
Arachnoid membrane
Corpus callosum
Intracranial subarachnoid space
Lateral ventricle with choroid plexus
Third ventricle with choroid plexus
Aqueduct of Sylvius
Pacchionian granulation
Cerebrum
Midbrain
Interventricular foramen (Monro)
Pituitary body
Sella turcica
Pons
Cerebellum
Fourth ventricle with choroid plexus
Cisterna magna
Foramen of Luschka
Medulla oblongata
Spinal cord
Foramen of Magendie
Spinal subarachnoid space

**FIG. 2-16.** Diagram of sagittal section of head, showing cerebrospinal fluid spaces and their relationship to venous circulation and principal subdivisions of brain and its coverings.

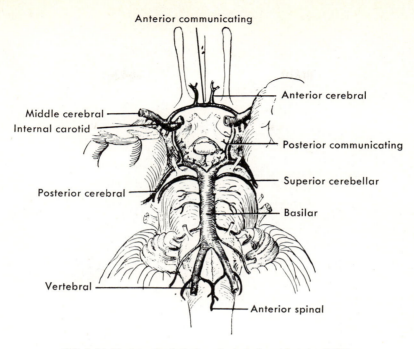

Anterior communicating

Anterior cerebral

Middle cerebral

Internal carotid

Posterior communicating

Superior cerebellar

Posterior cerebral

Basilar

Vertebral

Anterior spinal

**FIG. 2-17.** Diagram of principal cerebral arteries and circle of Willis.

## Vascular system

The arterial supply to the brain, which requires 20% more oxygen than any other organ, enters the cranium through the two internal carotid arteries anteriorly and the two vertebral arteries posteriorly. These communicate at the base of the brain through the basilar artery and the circle of Willis (Fig. 2-17), which ensures continuity of the circulation if any one of the four main channels is interrupted. The main branches for distribution of blood to each hemisphere of the brain from the internal carotid arteries are the anterior, middle, and posterior cerebral arteries. Each artery nourishes a specific area of the brain (Fig. 2-18). The anterior cerebral artery supplies the anterior two thirds of the medial surface and adjacent region over the convexity of the hemisphere, thus including about one half of the frontal and parietal lobes. The middle cerebral artery supplies most of the lateral surface of the hemisphere, including one half of the frontal, parietal, and temporal lobes. The posterior cerebral artery supplies the occipital lobe and the

remaining one half of the temporal lobe, principally on the inferior and medial surfaces. The brainstem and cerebellum are supplied by branches from the basilar and vertebral arteries.

The veins of the convexity of the brain drain principally into the superior longitudinal sinus (Fig. 2-19). This courses in the midline from the most anterior part of the dura mater to the most posterior part, where it joins the lateral sinuses. These sinuses all finally drain into the internal jugular vein to return the venous blood to the heart.

The spinal cord's arterial supply consists of the anterior spinal artery and two posterior spinal arteries, all arising from the vertebral arteries at the level of the foramen magnum. These vessels receive additional blood at each segment through the lateral spinal arteries, which, by forming a plexus around the entire spinal cord, further ensure adequate blood supply.

The spinal system of veins is extensive and is both intradural and extradural. The intradural veins follow the pattern of the arteries, whereas the ex-

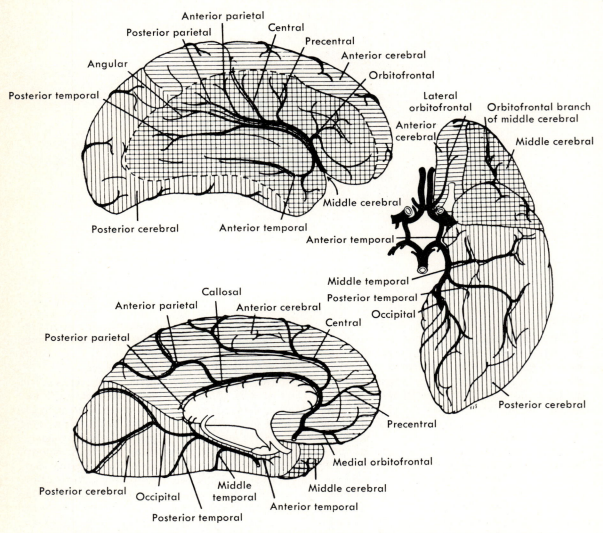

**FIG. 2-18.** Diagram of areas of distribution of anterior, middle, and posterior cerebral arteries. (From Mettler, F.A.: Neuroanatomy, ed. 2, St. Louis, 1948, The C.V. Mosby Co.)

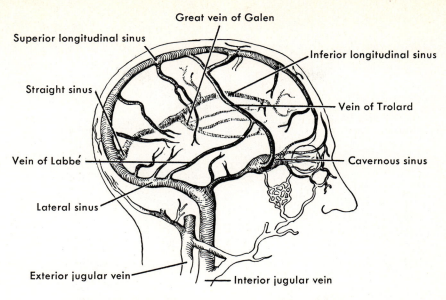

**FIG. 2-19.** Diagram of intracranial veins and drainage pathways.

tradural intravertebral veins form a plexiform network that extends from the pelvis to the cranium and has multiple communications with the veins of the abdomen, thorax, and neck.

The cranial meninges have a rich arterial supply through the anterior, middle, and posterior meningeal arteries. The most important artery is the middle meningeal (a branch of the internal maxillary artery), which enters the skull through a separate opening, the foramen spinosum. This artery is occasionally lacerated in association with fractures of the temporal bone and may lead to fatal hemorrhage if the condition is unrecognized and not treated.

### Cerebrospinal fluid system

Cerebrospinal fluid (CSF) is a clear, colorless, odorless fluid that looks like water, has a specific gravity of 1.007, and contains an occasional lymphocyte (1 to 3/mm³) and traces of the minerals and organic materials of the blood, of which the total protein is the most significant. Gravity affects the amount of protein normally found in CSF. Ventricular CSF contains 20 mg/dl, thoracic CSF 30 mg/dl, and lumbar CSF 40 mg/dl. The normal

pressure range is 60 to 180 mm CSF in the lateral recumbent position. This is frequently expressed in millimeters of water, since the specific gravity of water and that of CSF are almost the same. The total normal amount of CSF in the adult ranges from 125 to 150 ml.

CSF is formed from the blood principally through the activity of the choroid plexuses by a process of secretion and diffusion. The entire vascular bed that communicates with the subarachnoid space also acts as a source of CSF. The choroid plexuses are found in both lateral as well as the third and fourth ventricles and consist of granular tufts of capillaries and cuboidal epithelium covered by pia mater. The ventricles (Fig. 2-20) in which these plexuses lie are cavities within the brain. The parts of the lateral ventricles, one situated in each hemisphere, are the anterior horn (in the frontal lobe), the posterior horn (in the occipital lobe), the inferior horn (in the temporal lobe), and the body (in the parietal lobe). Each lateral ventricle connects through an interventricular foramen (Monro) with a central cavity, the third ventricle. This ventricle communicates posteriorly through the aqueduct of Sylvius with the fourth ventricle, a dia-

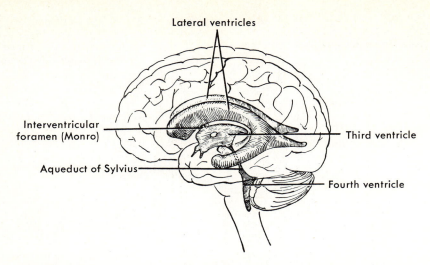

**FIG. 2-20.** Diagram of ventricular system, showing its relationship to various parts of brain.

mond-shaped space between the cerebellum posteriorly and the pons and medulla oblongata anteriorly. The structures surrounding the third and fourth ventricles are of great importance and include the nuclei of the thalamus, hypothalamus, basal ganglia, and brainstem, which form part of their supporting structure.

CSF has been referred to as the third circulation and, from its origin in the choroid plexuses, flows from the lateral ventricles through the foramen of Monro to the third ventricle and through the aqueduct of Sylvius to the fourth ventricle. It leaves the ventricular system through the medial foramen of Magendie and the lateral foramina of Luschka to enter the subarachnoid space. It circulates over the brain and down around the spinal cord and is absorbed into the venous circulation from the cranial subarachnoid space through the arachnoid granulations (or villi), which project into the large central vein, the superior longitudinal sinus (Fig. 2-15).

The function of CSF is essentially mechanical. It protects the nervous system by acting as a shock absorber, thus reducing the force of impact on the system. CSF also may carry nutrients to and waste products away from the nerve cells. The passage of CSF into the venous circulation depends on the different concentrations of these two fluids (specific gravity of blood, 1.050; of CSF, 1.007).

## BLOOD-BRAIN BARRIER

The brain differs psychologically and metabolically from other organ systems. Its metabolic requirements are such that 20% of the cardiac output flows through it, even though the adult brain is less than 1% of the weight of the total body mass. Major areas of the brain can survive total oxygen and glucose deprivation for less than 5 minutes. The accumulation of certain biochemical substances within the brain produces severe neurological disturbances. In an effort to limit these unwanted substances, a barrier to them has developed. The classic description of the blood-brain barrier is that of an absolute barrier prohibiting the entry of bloodborne solvents into the nervous system. This definition resulted from studies employing a variety of dyes that failed to stain the brain in vivo, whereas most other tissues stain deeply. Rawson and Tschirgi demonstrated that these dyes were bound predominantly to plasma proteins and that their entry into the central nervous system was actually a restriction of entry of the dye-protein complexes. Thus the classic definition became untenable. Recent electron microscopic findings have suggested that the specialized intermembranous fusions or "tight junctions" occurring between the endothelial cells of cerebral blood vessels and the lack of appreciable pinocytic activity may represent the morphological basis of the blood-brain barrier to plasma protein and other large molecules. Enhanced penetration of plasma protein and other large molecules into the brain may thus reflect an alteration in cerebrovascular permeability.

Normally, little, if any, plasma protein gains access to the central nervous system. Using a variety of experimental procedures, investigators have, in the past, been successful in modifying the entry of plasma protein into the central nervous system. Admittedly, frank damage to the central nervous system was inflicted in some cases, and entry largely represented leakage from damaged blood vessels. However, in others, increased penetration was effected without visible damage to brain tissue being produced. Experimentally induced seizures have been shown to increase the penetration of plasma protein into the brain without producing apparent damage.

The blood-brain barrier is considered to be a complex of membranes, including those comprising the capillary endothelium, pial-glial membrane, astrocytic neuroglia, ependyma, choroid plexus, and arachnoid membranes. When radioisotope techniques have been used in the study of cerebrospinal fluid formation, it has been demonstrated that the various components of this fluid are in the dynamic equilibrium from the blood into the cerebrospinal fluid across the barrier components. Materials that pass from the blood into the brain either enter from capillaries into the extracellular space of the brain or pass from the capillaries by way of the choroid plexus into the cerebrospinal fluid, from which a small amount may pass into the brain tissue. The environment of the neuron is the extracellular space, and rapid changes in the ionic components may be injurious. Thus the passage of materials into the brain is slow compared with that into other tissues, and one speaks of two barriers, the blood-brain barrier and the cerebrospinal fluid barrier, corresponding to the two routes already mentioned. If a substance passes readily into lipid material, it will pass more easily from the blood into the cerebrospinal fluid than a less lipid soluble material. This is a major property of biological membranes. Passage of soluble lipid materials across the blood-brain barrier is more rapid than across the blood–cerebrospinal fluid barrier. Certain materials are almost completely prevented

from passing across the blood-brain barrier, whereas the penetration by other substances may be rapid. The intravenous administration of deuterium (heavy water) has shown that water reaches equilibrium with all regions of the brain and the cerebrospinal fluid within 20 minutes. This factor enables the use of relatively impermeable substances such as urea or sucrose to reduce swelling of the brain. Intravenous injection of these materials in hypertonic solution causes the rapid movement of water from the ventricles to the blood, resulting in a temporarily decreased brain volume.

The barrier phenomenon has importance in drug use. Drugs do not normally accumulate in the cerebrospinal fluid because protein is unavailable for binding. Drugs exit rapidly by way of the arachnoid villi; some are actively transported out of the cerebrospinal fluid. Since the blood-brain barrier is not located at the surface of the brain cell but between the plasma and extracellular space of the brain, it can be assumed that once in contact with the cell, entry into that cell is like that into cells in any other organ. Weak electrolytes penetrate cells by simple diffusion in the nonionized form in proportion to their lipid solubility. Weak bases are concentrated slightly inside of cells, whereas weak acids are concentrated slightly less in cells than in extracellular fluids. Nonelectrolytes enter cells by diffusion and generally in proportion to their lipid solubility, but small molecules such as urea penetrate through aqueous channels in the membrane.

Lipid-insoluble drugs and inorganic and organic ions enter the brain more slowly than do lipid-soluble substances. Their rate of entrance is proportional to the size of the molecule. Large molecules like insulin or penicillin penetrate slowly, whereas small ions like chloride or small nonelectrolytes like urea penetrate more rapidly but still slowly as compared to the rate in other tissues. The choroid plexus is also slowly permeable to large lipid-insoluble substances.

The absolute nature of the barrier is as yet unproved. It has been claimed that the studies demonstrating the existence of the blood-brain barrier show only that the extracellular space of the brain is small. Thus if only a small amount of the dye injected into the blood to demonstrate the presence of the barrier enters into the extracellular space, the impression would be gained that no penetration was occurring. The amount of extracellular space is a matter of controversy. Electron microscopy of the brain done within the last several years indicates that the cells are separated by a distance of 10 to 20 nm. Calculations based on such spaces give values for the extracellular space less than 5% of the brain volume. Other studies using physiological techniques have indicated that the volume may range as high as 15%. The blood-brain barrier has permitted investigators to use this phenomenon as a means of defining normal versus abnormal parts of the brain. This has led to the development of the brain scan, which is now an important investigative tool for diagnostic purposes.

## REFERENCES

Barr, M.L.: The human nervous system, ed. 3, New York, 1973, Harper & Row, Publishers.

Bowsher, D.: Introduction to the anatomy and physiology of the nervous system, ed. 3, Philadelphia, 1975, J.B. Lippincott Co.

Carterette, E.: Handbook of perception, vol. 1-3, New York, 1973-1974, Academic Press, Inc.

Chusid, J.G., and McDonald, J.J.: Correlative neuroanatomy and functional neurology, ed. 17, Los Altos, Calif., 1979, Lange Medical Publications.

Crosby, E.C., Humphrey, T., and Lauer, E.W.: Correlative anatomy of the nervous system, New York, 1962, Macmillan Publishing Co., Inc.

Cunha-Vaz, J.G., Shakib, M., and Ashton, N.: Studies on the permeability of the blood-retinal barrier. I. On the existence, development and site of a blood-retinal barrier, Br. J. Ophthalmol. **50:**441-453, 1966.

Cutler, R.W.P., and Barlow, C.F.: The effect of hypercapnia on brain permeability to protein, Arch. Neurol. **14:**54-63, Jan. 1966.

Davison, H.: Biochemical correlates of brain structure and function, New York, 1977, Academic Press, Inc.

Dimond, S.: Neuropsychology: a textbook of systems and psychological functions of the human brain, Sevenoaks, Kent, Eng., 1980, Butterworth & Co. (Publishers) Ltd.

Dingman, J.F.: Pituitary function, N. Engl. J. Med. **285:**617-619, 1971.

Dunkerlev, G.B.: A basic atlas of the nervous system, Philadelphia, 1975, F.A. Davis Co.

Ehrlich, P.: Das Sauerstoff-Bedürfnis des Organismus, Berlin, 1885, A. Hirschwald.

Forster, F.M.: Clinical neurology, ed. 4, St. Louis, 1978, The C.V. Mosby Co.

Geldard, F.A.: The human senses, ed. 2, New York, 1972, John Wiley & Sons, Inc.

Goodman, L., and Gilman, A.: The pharmacological basis of therapeutics, ed. 5, New York, 1975, Macmillan Publishing Co., Inc.

Green, J.D., and Harris, G.W.: Neurovascular link between neurohypophysis and adenohypophysis, J. Endocrinol. **5:** 136-146, July 1947.

Guillemin, R., and Burgus, R.: The hormones of the hypothalamus, Sci. Am. **227:**24-33, Nov. 1972.

Kutt, H., et al.: The quanities of sodium diatrizoate in cerebral vessels during arteriography, J. Neurosurg. **20:**515-519, 1963.

Lending, M., Slobody, L.B., and Mestem, J.: Effect of prolonged convulsions on the blood–cerebrospinal fluid barrier, Am. J. Physiol. **197:**465-468, 1959.

Lorenzo, G.V., et al.: Temporary alteration of cerebrovascular permeability to plasma protein during drug-induced seizures, Am. J. Physiol. **223:**268-277, Aug. 1972.

Merritt, H.H., and Fremont-Smith, F.: The cerebrospinal fluid, Philadelphia, 1937, W.B. Saunders Co.

Netter, F.H.: The Ciba collection of medical illustrations, vol. 1, Nervous system, Summit, N.J., 1953, Ciba Pharmaceutical Products.

Peele, T.L.: Neuroanatomic basis for clinical neurology, New York, 1976, McGraw-Hill Book Co.

Penfield, W., and Roberts, L.: Speech and brain mechanisms, Princeton, N.J., 1959, Princeton University Press.

Perkins, W.H.: Speech pathology—an applied behavioral science, ed. 2, St. Louis, 1977, The C.V. Mosby Co.

Rawson, R.: The binding of T-1824 and structurally related diazo dyes by the plasma proteins, Am. J. Physiol. **138:**708-717, 1943.

Reese, T.S., and Karnovsky, M.J.: Fine structured localization of the blood-brain barrier to exogenous peroxidase, J. Cell Biol. **34:**207-217, July 1967.

Saffran, M., and Schally, A.V.: Release of corticotrophin by anterior pituitary tissue in vitro, Can. J. Biochem. Physiol. **33:**408-415, 1955.

Saffran, M., Schally, A.V., and Benfey, B.G.: Stimulation of release of corticotropin from adenohypophysis by neurohypophysial factor, Endocrinology **57:**439-444, 1955.

Schally, A.V., Arimura, A., and Kastin, A.J.: Hypothalamic regulatory hormones, Science **179:**341-350, 1973.

Selye, H.: The stress syndrome, Am. J. Nurs. **65:**97-99, March 1965.

Stern, L., and Gautier, R.: Recherches sur le liquide céphalorachidien. I. Les rapports entre le liquide céphalorachidien et la circulation sanguine, Arch. Intern. Physiol. **17:**138-192, Nov. 1921.

Sweet, W., and Locksley, H.: Formation, flow and reabsorption of cerebrospinal fluid in man, Proc. Soc. Exp. Biol. Med. **84:**397-404, 1953.

Tschirgi, R.D.: Protein complexes and the impermeability of the blood-brain barrier to dyes, Am. J. Physiol. **163:**756-758, 1950.

Williams, P.L., and Warwick, R.: Functional neuroanatomy of man, Philadelphia, 1975, W.B. Saunders Co.

# 3
# INPUT, INTEGRATION, AND OUTPUT

## PRINCIPLES RELATED TO NERVOUS TISSUE

Individual components of the nervous system may be described academically as distinct entities. However, the complex relationship of sensory reception, integration, and motor output is actually a process necessitating operational interdependency. The descriptions of the various disease entities throughout this book emphasize the problems that arise when any portion of this sequence is interrupted.

Sensory stimuli may be mechanical, thermal, or chemical. When any stimulus reaches adequate intensity, it causes nervous tissue to respond (excitability or irritability) and to transmit resulting nerve impulses to other cells (conductivity). Most experimental studies utilize electric current as the stimulus of choice, since the control of intensity, rate of alteration in intensity, and duration may be precisely regulated by the researcher.

Both the state of the target tissue and the intensity of the stimulus determine tissue responsiveness. The least amount of stimulus required to elicit tissue response is termed the *threshold stimulus*. When this minimal intensity is not attained, the stimulus is termed *subliminal*. Subliminal stimuli have been an issue of concern in the advertising industry for many years, since the use of subliminal input may greatly increase individual compliance with the message received at the subconscious level through the media (radio and television). Increasing intensities of a given stimulus may be applied until the tissue reaches a point of *maximal stimulus*. Any stimulus of greater intensity is *supramaximal*.

The *law of all or none* applies when a stimulus of threshold intensity or greater is experienced. Tissue response occurs at a constant amplitude within the bounds of tissue capacities. Individual action potentials of neuronal fibers are limited by the energy available in the axon at the instant of stimulation. Such factors as environment, that is, temperature changes, etc., may modify the amplitude of response. If a nerve trunk receives maximal stimulation, the tissue response represents the orchestrated effort of all involved nerve fibers.

In addition to adequate intensity, a stimulus must also last for the period of time necessary to excite the tissue. When the stimulus duration is insufficient, the tissue may fail to respond. However, when sufficient tissue capacity is combined with adequate stimulus intensity and duration, stimuli require a shorter time interval to evoke tissue response.

Nerve accommodation is another phenomenon that may be evident. In this instance a constant stimulus causes the tissue to adjust so that neuronal response noted at the time a threshold stimulus was applied becomes absent. Histologically this event is best explained by the reduction of sodium-ion concentration, which results in an increased threshold intensity with stabilization of the resting membrane potential. This universal trait of protoplasm is altered when stimulus application is either intermittent or changed sufficiently in duration or intensity.

Impulse transmission and membrane capacities in neurons are frequently likened to the conductance of electricity, though electricity travels at a speed of 300,000 meters/second, whereas neuronal impulses move at a maximum of 100 meters/second in large fibers and at a lesser rate in smaller fibers. In both instances the stimulus, the conduction pathways, and the terminal point or effector organ influence the outcome of impulse transmission. Additionally, resting nerves are similar to electrical power lines, since their long cylinders have membranes and axoplasms that resist current flow. The cellular membrane is also a capacitor, since it separates positive and negative charges.

The complex electrochemical process of nerve impulse conduction is currently theorized as a wave of depolarization changing the cell membrane's permeability to the major ions potassium and sodium. In its resting state the axonal membrane is polarized. During polarization an increased concentration of sodium ions is outside the membrane, whereas fewer sodium ions and increased numbers of potassium ions are inside the membrane. The result of this ionic arrangement during polarization is an electrically positive exterior membrane in contrast to the interior aspect.

## IMPULSE CONDUCTION

When a stimulus of at least threshold intensity is applied to a sensory receptor, a local response of slowly increasing membrane depolarization is noted. The extent of this depolarization is graded. However, no refractory period is evident, and the principle of all or none is not applicable. When the local response is sufficiently intense, sodium ions enter the axon and potassium ions move out to the exterior aspect of the axonal membrane until total membrane depolarization is achieved. This rapid sequence of events constituting the depolarization process is termed *action potential*. Action potential differs from local tissue response in the following: (1) the all-or-none principle applies, (2) the electrochemical process is brief, and (3) an absolute refractory period followed by a relative refractory period occurs.

Depolarization at one point along an axon results in a local response at the neighboring location in the direction of impulse flow. The ability of one neuronal segment to cause a local response in another area while having the energy to transmit an impulse is termed *self-propagation*. When a single stimulus is not sufficient to induce local tissue response, it may be compounded by multiple stimuli until the summation of impulses over a period of time excites neuronal tissue to propagate a nerve impulse.

After depolarization has occurred, a reversal of

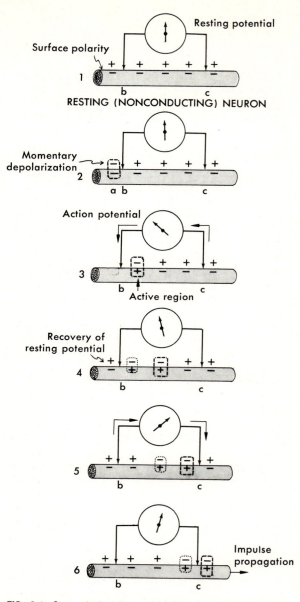

**FIG. 3-1.** Stages in impulse propagation. (From Schottelius, B.A., and Schottelius, D.D.: Textbook of physiology, ed. 18, St. Louis, 1978, The C.V. Mosby Co.)

ionic flow restores membrane polarization (Fig. 3-1). Theoretically neurons integrate excitability and inhibitory activity algebraically to polarize a nerve when the total outcome of these opposing forces is adequate to exceed the threshold intensity of a fiber.

Repolarization requires more energy than depolarization. However, neuronal tissue uses oxygen and gives off carbon dioxide according to the demands of each process. Although impulse conduction produces some heat in the energy exchange, the metabolic rate is increased 500 times less than that with maximal effort in muscle.

In heavily myelinated fibers the impulse jumps from one node of Ranvier to the next. The cell membrane is only exposed at these intervals, since it is wrapped in a myelin sheath in areas between. The influx of sodium ions is only possible at these points since it is attracted across the polarized membrane. When depolarization occurs at a node there is a great influx of sodium ions referred to as a "sodium sink." The impulse is then transmitted to the next *node*. This rapid transmission characteristic of heavily myelinated fibers is called *saltatory transmission*. The heavier the myelin sheath, the faster the rate of transmission (see Table 2-1).

## SYNAPTIC TRANSMISSION

Whereas impulse conduction along nerve fibers is an electrical process, synaptic transmission is a chemical one. The interrelationship of chemical reactions, such as adenosine triphosphate (ATP) breakdown to release energy within nerve fiber is believed by researchers to account for the constant rate of impulse speed.

The synaptic connection between one neuron and the next in a pathway occurs in gray matter. It consists of an axon bouton or knob, which contains vesicles of stored neurotransmitter, a presynaptic membrane (synaptic knob), and a postsynaptic membrane (dendrite or nerve cell body of the next neuron). There is a synaptic cleft between these two membranes and receptor sites on the postsynaptic membrane. When the impulse reaches the synaptic knob, neurotransmitter is released into the cleft and reacts with receptor sites to depolarize the next neuron in the pathway (Fig. 3-2).

Some 30 different substances are known or suspected to be transmitters in the brain, and each has a characteristic excitatory (note that "facilitory" and "excitatory" are used interchangeably) or inhibitory effect on neurons. Of these only six of the most important are discussed. Excitatory fibers are designated EPSP (excitatory postsynaptic potential) and inhibitory are termed IPSP (inhibitory postsynaptic potential). EPSP fibers, through their neurotransmitter, enhance the permeability of the postsynaptic membrane to sodium ions allowing influx and thus moving it closer to an action potential. IPSP fibers, through their inhibitory neurotransmitters, make the postsynaptic membrane less permeable to sodium ions and more permeable to negative chloride ions and thus move it farther away from an action potential.

Sherrington, in 1947, described the synapse as the point that allows flexible expression within the nervous system. This flexibility is achieved by a combination of opposing states of inhibition and excitement during the process of synaptic transmission, according to the prevailing chemical hypotheses. Eccles reported in 1957 that such integration of neuronal activities occurs at all points of the nervous system (Fig. 3-9) and that the internuncial neurons are principal links between the general sensory neurons (GSN) and the motor neurons involved in the production of human activity. Further attention to these theories has resulted in changes in the classification of neuropharmacological agents with regard to their synaptic effect as excitatory (EPSP) or inhibitory (IPSP). In other words, these agents may be categorized as either blockading or enhancing synaptic transmission.

The principal facilitatory (EPSP) neurotransmitter of the voluntary nervous system and the *parasympathetic* division of the autonomic nervous system is acetylcholine (ACh). In addition to ACh, centrally acting neurotransmitters include serotonin, dopamine, norepinephrine, glutamic acid, aspartic acid, and *gamma-aminobutyric acid* (GABA) (Fig. 3-3). Norepinephrine is the principal neurotransmitter at the postganglionic-effector junction of the sympathetic division of the autonomic nervous system and is discussed in Chapter 4. As the principle neurotransmitter of CNS cholinergic fibers, ACh is discussed in detail.

ACh controls the alteration of ions in cellular membranes that is inherent in the process of impulse initiation and propagation. The biochemical

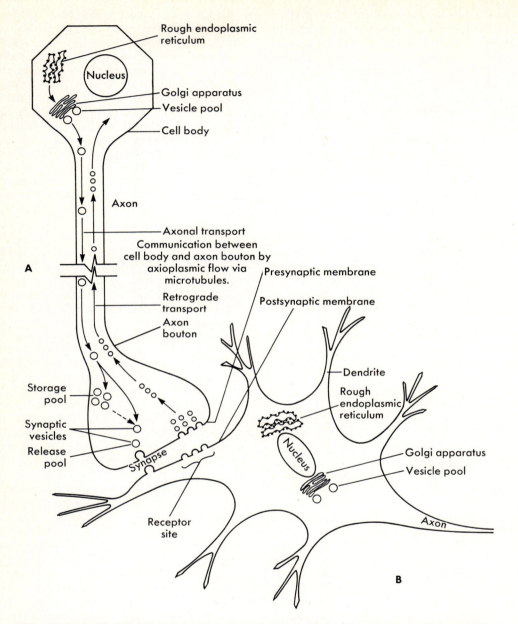

**FIG. 3-2.** Functional relationship between two neurons in pathway. Electrical impulse travels along axon of first neuron to synapse. A chemical neurotransmitter is secreted into synaptic space to depolarize membrane (dendrite or cell body) of next neuron in pathway. Cell *A* represents a unipolar cell; cell *B* represents a multipolar cell.

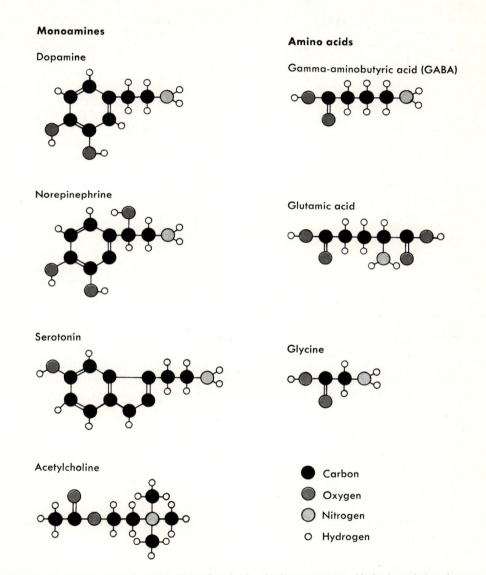

**Monoamines**

Dopamine

Norepinephrine

Serotonin

Acetylcholine

**Amino acids**

Gamma-aminobutyric acid (GABA)

Glutamic acid

Glycine

● Carbon
● Oxygen
○ Nitrogen
○ Hydrogen

**FIG. 3-3.** Transmitter chemicals tend to be small molecules that incorporate a positively charged nitrogen atom. Each has a characteristic excitatory or inhibitory effect on neurons, though some transmitters are excitatory in one part of the brain and inhibitory in another.

sequence involving ACh is as follows:

1. Stimulation is applied to the ACh complex within the cellular membrane.
2. A free ester affects the receptor protein and causes the alteration necessary to promoting membrane conductance.
3. Free ACh becomes inactivated by acetylcholinesterase (AChE), so that further ionic activity is halted.
4. ACh is resynthesized by choline acetylase.

Because this four-step sequence is completed within a few millionths of a second, in excess of 1000 impulses may travel through a nerve fiber in 1 second.

"Muscarinic" and "nicotinic" are the two terms selected to describe ACh-like activities in different body parts. Visceral activities are termed *muscarinic responses,* whereas processes involving the autonomic ganglia or neuromuscular junctions of skeletal muscles are known as *nicotinic responses*. Muscarinic responses are blocked by atropine.

Anticholinergic agents block ACh activity at the effector cells or the neuromuscular junction of smooth and cardiac muscles and glands supplied by postganglionic cholinergic nerves. These agents cause the heart to beat faster, the involuntary muscles to relax, the pupils to become dilated, and the secretions from the exocrine glands to be diminished. These agents compete for locations ACh usually occupies in the facilitation of neuronal impulse transmission and, as such, do not affect either the production or the destruction of ACh. Atropine, scopolamine, and belladonna alkaloids are well-known examples of the anticholinergic drug grouping.

Quaternary nitrogen, a synthetic substitute for atropine, may also be utilized to inhibit parasympathetic impulse propagation. Other examples of these synthetic products include methantheline (Banthine) and propantheline (Pro-Banthine), two antispasmodics utilized for relief of untoward gastrointestinal symptoms.

AChE agents are characterized by their ability to inhibit cholinesterase and to augment the activity of ACh. This category of agents may be subdivided into reversible and irreversible inhibitors. Insecticides, such as parathion, and nerve gases used in chemical warfare are included in the category of irreversible inhibitors, although atropine is known to be an effective antidote to parathion when administered immediately. This group of agents is also capable of crossing the blood-brain barrier, unlike the direct cholinergics.

The reversible AChE agents include those utilized in the treatment of myasthenia gravis. Neostigmine (Prostigmin), pyridostigmine bromide (Mestinon), and ambenonium chloride (Mytelase) are examples of these agents. The discussion of myasthenia gravis in Chapter 17 offers further information on the disease process and on current treatment regimens (DiPalma, 1974).

GABA is the prototype of the incompletely identified inhibitory neurotransmitters secreted by inhibitory central fibers most closely associated with the extrapyramidal system. GABA is an amino acid that is not incorporated into proteins and is manufactured almost exclusively in the brain and spinal cord. It is estimated that as many as one third of the synapses of the brain elaborate GABA as their neurotransmitter.

Dopamine is a monoamine precursor of epinephrine. It acts as a neurotransmitter in regions of the midbrain, especially the substantia nigra. Many dopaminergic neurons project their axons to the forebrain where they are believed to be involved in regulating emotional responses. Other dopamine-producing fibers synapse in the basal nuclei of the corpus striatum where dopamine plays a crucial role in the extrapyramidal control of complex voluntary (skeletal muscles) movement. Disease of these fibers gives rise to parkinsonian muscular rigidity.

Another monoamine transmitter, serotonin, is found in many areas of the brain and is concentrated in the brainstem. From these brainstem nuclei, fibers project to the hypothalamus and thalamus. Serotonin is believed to be involved in temperature regulation, sensory perception, and the onset of sleep.

The neurotransmitters dopamine, serotonin, and GABA are removed from the synapse by the process of *reuptake* rather than enzyme degradation. Thus they can be used through several cycles of release from the storage vesicles and reentry into the axon bouton for reuse.

Glutamic acid and aspartic acids are common amino acids that exert powerful excitatory effects on most neurons. In addition many hormones have been localized within neurons and may play a transmitter role. Again confirming the strong cooperative role of these two regulatory physiological feedback systems.

The newest and perhaps most exciting of the neuropeptides are the enkephalins and endorphins. These chemicals occur naturally within the brain and are similar to morphine in composition and effect. Receptors for these compounds are found in the region of the brain and spinal cord involved with perception and integration of pain and emotional experience. It is suggested that the use of acupuncture and electrical stimulation for relief of pain may act to release naturally occurring opiate-like substances.

There is also the experimental "substance P," which excites spinal neurons, which respond to painful stimuli from pain receptors in the periphery. Enkephalins are also found at these synapses and may act to regulate the input of painful stimuli to the brain by controlling the release of substance P at the entry point into the central nervous system. Similar inhibition of painful stimuli may take place at higher levels of the brain where concentrations of enkephalins are also found.

## INPUT

Individual perception of stimuli is both a personal and a universal phenomenon that has been extensively studied and delineated. However, research continues to reveal information on factors related to sensory mechanisms, means of enhancing desirable input, and methods of reducing or eliminating undesirable phenomena, such as pain or excessive autonomic activity. This chapter describes normal sensory mechanisms, whereas Chapters 10, 15, 16, and 25 detail problems.

Sensory input into the system is the function of general sensory neurons of the *mixed* spinal and cranial nerves and special sensory pathways associated with cranial nerves I, II, VII, and VIII (Fig. 2-1). One characteristic of sensory neurons is *divergence,* in which one neuron gives off many collaterals to synapse at various integrating levels within the central nervous system (Fig. 3-9).

### Sensory receptors

Four types of sensory apparatus are involved in the reception of incoming stimuli, including (1) special senses; (2) exteroceptors on body surfaces; (3) proprioceptors in tendons, muscles, and joints; and (4) interoceptors in the viscera.

The adaptation and response of each receptor depends on both the type of stimuli received and the threshold of stimulus intensity. For example, the tactile response to pain, pressure, and temperature is both a process of slow adaptation and one wherein increasing stimuli result in augmented response patterns. However, touch differs, since increases in stimuli do not allow similar increases in touch sensitivity beyond the stimulus threshold. Adaptation to sensory stimuli of a chronic nature occurs. After a period of time one is not generally aware of glasses on the bridge of the nose or ordinary clothing. However, changes in eyewear or seasonal changes of clothing may alert the wearer to alterations in touch stimuli.

Muscle spindles are also known to adapt gradually. Thus the afferent impulses that sustain stretch may contribute to the postural attitude of decerebrate rigidity for long periods after central nervous system insults have occurred.

When stimuli reach a threshold intensity in receptors, afferent neurons convey an impulse to some level of integration in the central nervous system (Fig. 3-9).

Several principles are important to the understanding of sensory mechanisms. First, each sensory structure complies with the *law of specific nerve energies,* which limits it to designated functions, that is, eyes see and ears hear. However, within its limits of function each sensory structure is capable of making a range of discriminations when its functional integrity is intact. For example, ears are usually able to discriminate various verbal tones, pitches, and intensities, and, with training in areas such as music, one might be able to discriminate a song in a minor key from one in a major key. Similarly, eyes are usually capable of depth perception, color discrimination, and so on. Second, the endurance of a sensory experience may be longer or shorter than its causative stimulus. Third, the functional integrity of sensory mechanisms is vital to normal functioning in humans, since localization and interpretation of sensory input are basic to adequate and appropriate responses.

*Major categories.* As mentioned, the senses are divided into four major categories, including the special senses, superficial sensations (exteroceptors), deep sensations (proprioceptors), and visceral sensations (interoceptors).

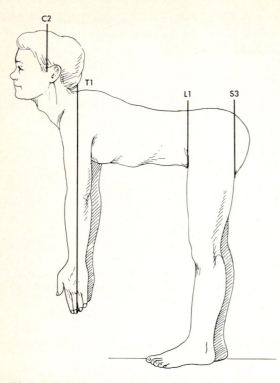

**FIG. 3-4.** Method of categorizing groups of dermatomes. (From Conway, B.L.: Pediatric neurologic nursing, St. Louis, 1977, The C.V. Mosby Co.)

Special organs of sensibility allow one to experience vision, audition, taste, olfaction, and vestibular competencies. Further discussion of the special senses is deferred to the section on assessment. Superficial sensations include touch-pressure, heat, cold, and pain-sensing capacities. Deep sensations refer to the kinesthetic sensations, pressure, and deep pain. Hunger, sexual arousal, and nausea are grouped in the category of visceral sensations received via afferent fibers of the autonomic nervous system. There is a range of stimulus intensity that evokes responses from touch to pressure; therefore these two responses lie on a continuum. When skin is displaced by unequal pressure, touch is experienced. As stimulus intensity becomes greater, the experience is perceived as pressure. The most sensitive portions of the human body are the lips and fingertips, whereas the medial portion of the back is the least sensitive area.

*Dermatomes.* The periphery is divided into areas that are innervated by neighboring spinal nerves with overlapping functions. Because of this phenomenon, the severance of a single spinal nerve may have a limited effect on sensory perception. Since the nerves in two areas pass through the brachial and lumbosacral plexuses, the resulting pattern of peripheral innervation is somewhat more complicated. The classic work describing the pattern of peripheral innervation to sensory areas by spinal nerves was done by O. Foerster (1933), whereas the dermatome arrangement in the lower extremity was greatly clarified by the work of J.J. Keegan (1943).

Two figures are available to assist the practitioner in evaluating sensory capacities in a client. Fig. 3-4 provides a rough guide to the general areas innervated by each major division of the spinal cord. Fig. 3-5 illustrates the anterior and posterior aspects of the body divided into dermatomes. Utilizing these charts, the practitioner is able to perform sensory testing to ascertain interrupted functions secondary to disease processes, trauma, or space-occupying lesions. Emerging from plexuses are peripheral nerves with very well defined surface sensory distribution (Figs. 2-7 and 3-6).

### Afferent pathways (ascending and sensory)
(Figs. 3-7 and 3-8 and Table 3-1)

*Conscious sensory pathways*
1. *Posterior columns* make up posterior funiculus (Fig. 3-7), part of the pathway of transmission for impulses of direct touch and conscious muscle sense to opposite cortex. They receive superficial impulses from the skin, including those involved in touch and touch localization, two-point discrimination, and pressure, as well as those from the deep senses (joints, tendons, and muscles). Deep sensory impulses include joint position and movement, vibration, weight appreciation, stretch excitations, postural and righting stimuli, and reflex impulses.
   a. Fasciculus gracilis—Most medial of the posterior columns; transmits impulses from lower trunk and extremities.
   b. Fasciculus cuneatus—Most lateral and wedge shaped of the posterior columns; transmits impulses from the thoracic area and upper extremity.

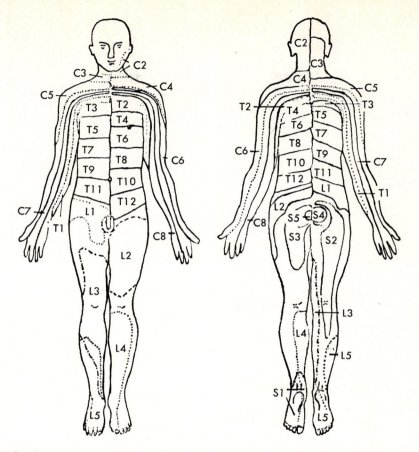

**FIG. 3-5.** Dermatomes as determined by series of transverse lesions resulting from injury of spinal cord and cauda equina.

c. Pathway composed of three neurons
   (1) Tract is formed by first-order neuron (general sensory neuron, GSN) whose axon enters posterior cord and ascends *uncrossed* to the medulla.
   (2) Second-order neuron arises in medulla oblongata and its axon crosses to opposite side of brainstem in the medial lemniscus where it ascends to the thalamus.
   (3) Third-order neuron arises in the thalamus and goes to the general sensory cortex in the postcentral gyrus of the parietal lobe areas.
2. *Anterior spinothalamic tract,* located in anterior funiculus, transmits impulses of in-

direct touch, muscle sense, tickle, itch, and sex to opposite cortex.
3. *Lateral spinothalamic tract,* located in lateral funiculus, transmit impulses of pain and temperature to opposite cortex. These pathways are composed of three neurons (both spinothalamic tracts).
   a. First-order neuron (GSN) of the pathway terminates in the posterior column of the gray matter of spinal cord where it synapses.
   b. Second-order neuron then *crosses* to the opposite side of the cord in the anterior white commissure and ascends to the thalamus.
   c. Third-order neuron of the pathway trans-

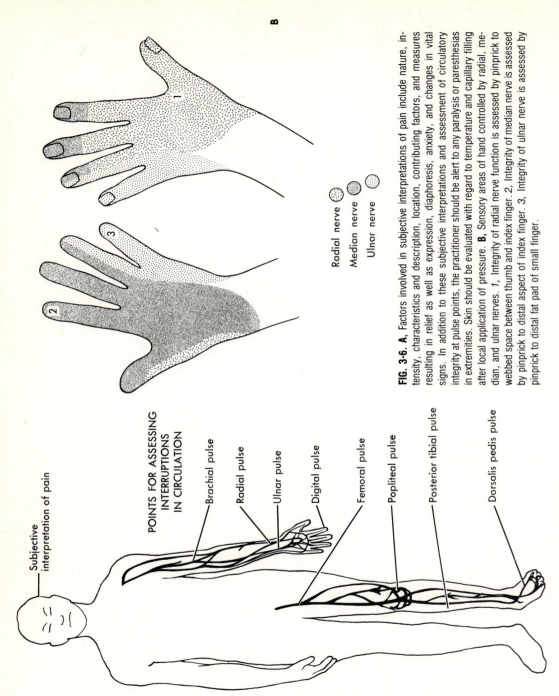

**FIG. 3-6. A.** Factors involved in subjective interpretations of pain include nature, intensity, characteristics and description, location, contributing factors, and measures resulting in relief as well as expression, diaphoresis, anxiety, and changes in vital signs. In addition to these subjective interpretations and assessment of circulatory integrity at pulse points, the practitioner should be alert to any paralysis or paresthesias in extremities. Skin should be evaluated with regard to temperature and capillary filling after local application of pressure. **B.** Sensory areas of hand controlled by radial, median, and ulnar nerves. *1,* Integrity of radial nerve function is assessed by pinprick to webbed space between thumb and index finger. *2,* Integrity of median nerve is assessed by pinprick to distal aspect of index finger. *3,* Integrity of ulnar nerve is assessed by pinprick to distal fat pad of small finger.

Radial nerve

Median nerve

Ulnar nerve

Subjective interpretation of pain

POINTS FOR ASSESSING INTERRUPTIONS IN CIRCULATION

Brachial pulse

Radial pulse

Ulnar pulse

Digital pulse

Femoral pulse

Popliteal pulse

Posterior tibial pulse

Dorsalis pedis pulse

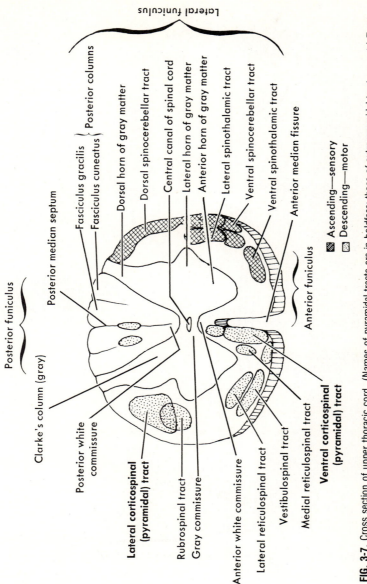

Lateral funiculus

Posterior columns

Fasciculus gracilis
Fasciculus cuneatus

Dorsal horn of gray matter

Dorsal spinocerebellar tract

Central canal of spinal cord

Lateral horn of gray matter

Anterior horn of gray matter

Lateral spinothalamic tract

Ventral spinocerebellar tract

Ventral spinothalamic tract

Anterior median fissure

Posterior median septum

Posterior funiculus

Clarke's column (gray)

Posterior white commissure

**Lateral corticospinal (pyramidal) tract**

Rubrospinal tract
Gray commissure

Anterior white commissure

Lateral reticulospinal tract

Vestibulospinal tract

Medial reticulospinal tract

**Ventral corticospinal (pyramidal) tract**

Anterior funiculus

Ascending—sensory
Descending—motor

**FIG. 3-7.** Cross section of upper thoracic cord. (Names of pyramidal tracts are in boldface; those of extrapyramidal tract are not.) Tracts and their placement will differ at different levels of cord. For instance, tectospinal tract begins in tectum of midbrain and ends in cervical cord and so does not show in this thoracic section. "Funiculus" is the term used for a large bundle of fibers. White matter, or cord, is divided into three funiculi (on each side) by H-shaped gray pattern. These are named posterior, lateral, and anterior according to their location.

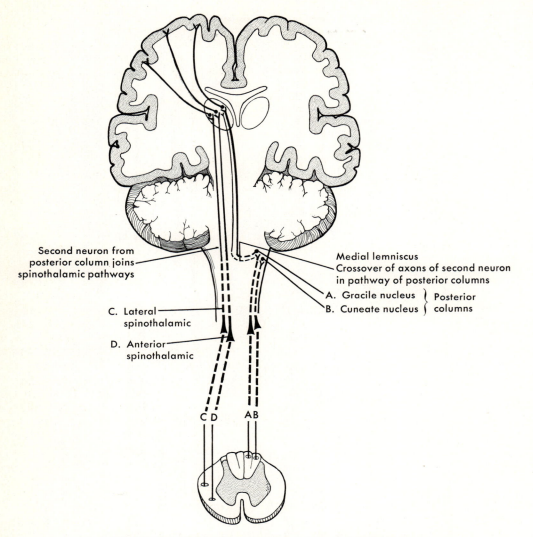

Second neuron from
posterior column joins
spinothalamic pathways

Medial lemniscus
Crossover of axons of second neuron
in pathway of posterior columns

A. Gracile nucleus } Posterior
B. Cuneate nucleus } columns

C. Lateral
spinothalamic

D. Anterior
spinothalamic

C D    A B

**FIG. 3-8.** Ascending sensory pathways to thalamus and cerebral cortex.

**TABLE 3-1.** Spinal pathways conveying afferent impulses

| Sensation | Course |
|---|---|
| Pain, thermal impulses | Short posterior root fibers terminate in substantia gelatinosa, which develops into collaterals coursing up and down one or two segments in Lissauer's tract before reaching posterior horn. Fibers of second order decussate and course upward in lateral spinothalamic tract. Medial pain pathways have different route. |
| Tactile sensations | Fibers enter ipsilateral posterior column, where a few terminate in gracile and cuneate nuclei. Most enter nucleus propius of posterior horn at point of root entry and at higher levels as they ascend in posterior column. Second-order fibers decussate and course upward through anterior spinothalamic tract. |
| Position sense and kinesthesia | Fibers course through ipsilateral posterior column and upward from there. Alternate route is Morin's tract of ipsilateral lateral column. |
| Discriminative functions | Fibers course through ipsilateral posterior column and upward from there. Alternate route is Morin's tract. |
| Vibratory stimuli | Fibers course through ipsilateral posterior column and upward. Possible alternate route is medial portion of ipsilateral lateral column. |
| Proprioception | Three ipsilateral pathways are used to convey these sensory experiences to cerebellum, including (1) pathways from nucleus dorsalis via dorsal spinocerebellar tract and into inferior cerebellar peduncle, (2) pathways from nucleus of Stilling and postcommissural nucleus through ventral spinocerebellar tract to superior cerebellar peduncle, and (3) pathways from lateral cuneate nucleus through dorsal superficial arcuate fibers and onto inferior cerebellar peduncle. |

mits the impulses from the thalamus to the sensory cortex; the thalamus is the chief subcortical relay station for conscious sensation.

The general pattern for conscious sensory pathways is as follows:

1° GSN
2° Crosses to opposite side
3° From thalamus to sensory cortex

### Unconscious sensory pathways to cerebellum

4. *Spinocerebellar tracts* transmit impulses of unconscious muscle sense, tone, and muscle coordination.
   a. Posterior (dorsal)—located in lateral funiculus.
   b. Anterior (ventral)—located in lateral funiculus.
   c. Pathway composed of two neurons.
      (1) First-order neuron synapses in nucleus dorsalis (Clark's column) in medial portion of posterior gray column.
      (2) Second-order neuron forms the tract; it ascends *uncrossed* to the cerebellum.

Interested readers may seek further detail in sources listed in the references (Cook and Browder, 1965; Haymaker, 1969).

Fig. 3-7 shows the placement of the tracts, both sensory and motor, in the white matter of the cord.

*Intersegmental tracts.* Intersegmental tracts are formed from axonal bundles arising from cell bodies at the periphery of the spinal gray matter (internuncial neurons). Axons from these cell bodies course both up and down through the white matter to link various areas of gray matter. These bundles are located in the posterolateral fasciculus of Lissauer bordering the dorsal gray column. Ascending intersegmental fibers form the cornucommissural tract, which lies posterior to the spinal gray commissure. Some of these axonal bundles *(proprius bundles)* may decussate or crop over.

*Gate control theory.* The ascending peripheral tracts arise in the somatic periphery and viscera. The cell bodies of these tracts are in the posterior root ganglia and their central processes travel into the spinal cord through the posterior spinal roots. These incoming posterior root fibers are grouped according to their length prior to synapse. Short posterior root fibers are in the lateral division (fasciculus of Lissauer), whereas intermediate and lengthy systems are in the medial division.

Incoming noxious stimuli reach the short posterior root fibers for transmission. These noxious stimuli include pain, thermal changes received from the soma that are interpreted as such by higher levels, and painful or otherwise noxious stimuli received from the viscera. These posterior root fibers transmitting incoming noxious stimuli are more numerous than the cell bodies of the lateral spinothalamic tract to which they connect. Thus these fibers become a pool for the reception of pain impulses from the periphery. Impulses received in this pool from higher levels are probably inhibitory in nature.

The gate control system is frequently mentioned as the accepted theory to understanding the phenomenon of pain. Basically the interpretation and response to pain are regulated by the interrelations of three systems: the substantia gelatinosa, the posterior column system, and the central transmission system. Incoming fine and coarse posterior root fibers terminate in the substantia gelatinosa. Coarse fibers give off collaterals that travel up the posterior columns to the gracile and cuneate nuclei. Central transmission cells (cells of the nucleus proprius) have their dendrites in the substantia gelatinosa and their axons in the contralateral spinothalamic tract. Apparently the substantia gelatinosa operates as the gate control system, since it modifies afferent input before it is received by the central transmission cells. Afferent activities in the posterior column function by eliciting appropriate brain responses, which also reinforce selected control and influence over impulse transmission. This cooperative local and cranial effort effects screening activities integral to the operation of the gate control system. Central transmission cells are then given the correct directive so that they may transmit responses that translate into the perception of and reaction to noxious stimuli (Melzack, 1973; Mountcastle, 1980).

Although the afferent fibers transmitting noxious impulses from the viscera and soma synapse with cells in the posterior horn, there are certain cells that apparently receive impulses from both the soma and the viscera. Thus the Sherrington concept of the neural pool comes into play to explain the genesis of referred pain (Haymaker, 1969).

Within the lateral spinothalamic tract, fibers of pain sensibility are located in a more ventral position than are those of temperature. A medial pain system has also been described. However, it is poorly understood in comparison to the lateral pain system just described. For further detail on the upward course of the lateral spinothalamic pathway (Table 3-1), refer to *Bing's Local Diagnosis in Neurological Diseases* (Haymaker, 1969).

***Tactile and thermal sensation.*** *Localization* and *discrimination* are the two constituents of tactile stimulation. Localization refers to awareness in the body part stimulated, whereas discrimination is the term employed to describe the capacity to detect body stimulation at two distinct points. In order for the individual to distinguish two points of stimuli, these points must be separated by a certain distance. The distance necessary varies with different body sites. For example, 8 mm must separate the two points on the palm of the hand for this discrimination to occur.

Although no particular receptors are identified, hot and cold stimuli are known to activate different nerve fibers. Both internal and external sources of temperature variation are received by dermal receptors neighboring blood vessels. Within these dermal receptors, cold receptors accelerate with decreased temperatures, whereas heat receptors respond similarly to the opposite stimuli. One exception to these responses is paradoxical cold, where extreme forms of heat have been known to activate cold fibers.

Cutaneous groupings of warm and cold receptors have been determined. These receptors tend to exhibit specific responses to the variations in temperature applied to the skin. These temperature receptors react to variations in heat and cold, as well as to the rate of temperature alteration. Once perceived, these impulses of heat and cold are transmitted largely from the skin through myelinated fibers, except in glabrous skin, which lacks myelinated fibers (Iggo, 1969).

Pain receptors (nociceptors) initiate defensive and protective reflexes whose impulses receive top priority in transmission through the nervous system.

Deep sensations include impulses from joints, muscles, and tendons (bathyesthesia), as well as those from deep pain and touch-pressure experiences. Since passive movement is effected by capsular receptors and active movement by muscle and tendon receptors, active movement is felt after passive movement is no longer perceptible. A combination of impulses from joints, muscles, tendons, and proprioceptor end-organs of muscles contribute to one's perception of position and movement of an extremity. These end organs include those of the muscle spindles (discussed later) and the Vater-Pacini and Golgi-Mazzoni corpuscles of the lamellar structure found near joints, near periosteum, and in muscle tendons. Techniques of assessing degrees of movement and motion, as experienced by the client, are reviewed in Chapters 11 and 15.

Firm pressure over superficial muscles (for example, the gastrocnemius), nerve trunks, or tendons elicits responses to deep pain. When light pressure is applied to the skin surface, investigators have noted that impulses are conveyed to the deep nerves. Thus the corpuscles of lamellar structures frequently respond to light pressure. It is interesting to note that touch-pressure sensitivity is maintained even in the absence of superficial nerve integrity. Some researchers have also noted that left-handed individuals have increased touch-pressure sensibility in the right hand (Weinstein and Sersen, 1961). However, other investigators have not discerned this variation between the lateral aspects of the body (Fennell et al., 1967). The cerebral cortex also plays a vital role in sensory discrimination, as reviewed in a subsequent discussion. Methods of testing for touch-pressure sensitivity are elaborated in Chapter 11.

Deep and superficial sensory mechanisms are involved in the perception of vibration (pallesthesia). The mechanoreceptors are probably the pacinian corpuscles in the subcutaneous tissue (most heavily located in the palms, fingertips, and soles), in the fascial planes, in the periosteum, and in the vicinity of the joints. Pacinian corpuscles must be responsive to both amplitude and frequency, since these are the two components of vibration. Thus vibration is a temporal discernment of amplitude capable of stimulating a number of fibers within the pacinian corpuscles. Testing for this sensory capacity is done when one applies a tuning fork to such bony processes as the knee, ankle, tibia, fingertip, iliac crest, malleolus, or spinous process of the vertebrae. A fork tuned to 200 to 400 Hertz (cycles/second) is perceptible by most persons (Haymaker, 1969). Men have lower thresholds for

vibratory perception than women. However, men over 45 years of age experience an increased threshold for all frequencies, whereas women of similar ages tend to be more responsive to stimuli of higher frequencies and to maintain a constant threshold of responsiveness to stimuli of lower frequencies (Calne and Pallis, 1966).

Protopathic sensation and epicritic sensation are two terms that have had various meanings since Head first utilized them in 1905 and fully described their significance in 1920 (Head, 1920). In contemporary usage the term *"protopathic sensation"* includes pressure and some types of touch, temperature, and pain, all of which are important to successful preservation of life, safety, and physical integrity. The term *"epicritic,"* or *"gnostic, sensation"* now encompasses those data that aid the individual in the acquisition of either essential or discriminatory information. Epicritic sensation includes vibration, joint position and awareness, touch, two-point discrimination, and discernment of weight, form, and texture. The following are terms commonly used in describing sensation.

### Mixed sensibilities

*epicritic sensibility*—Perception of mild temperature variations and minimal touch sensations, object identification by touch alone, and discrimination of distance between two points

*protopathic sensibility*—perception of pain and temperature extremes

*somatesthesia*—includes deep and superficial sensibility, but excludes visceral sensibility

### Movement

*bathyesthesia*—awareness of movement

*pallanesthesia*—perception only of constant sources of stimuli at bony points

*pallesthesia*—combination of deep and superficial senses to perceive vibration

*proprioception*—identification of position and occasionally movement

### Pain

*analgesia*—absence of pain

*anesthesia dolorosa*—pain and anesthesia occur at the same site

*causalgia*—burning, intense, constant pain of sudden onset after the interruption of median or sciatic nerves at the branchial plexus; sudden movement aggravates and heat and cold applications alleviate the pain

*hypalgesia*—decreased pain awareness

*hyperalgesia*—increased pain awareness

### Temperature

*hyperesthesia of head* —neuralgia and increased sensitivity to temperature extremes or pinprick after total interruption of nerve impulses; response results from ineffective inhibitory controls

*thermanesthesia* —absence of temperature sensibility

*thermohyperesthesia* —increased temperature sensibility

*thermohypesthesia* —decreased temperature sensibility

### Touch

*dysesthesia* —unusual sensation (tickling, prickling, warmth, or moist feeling) associated with peripheral nerve disturbances

*paresthesia* —uncomfortable sensations associated with touching an object, for example, wearing itchy wool clothing

*tactile anesthesia* —loss of touch sensibility

*tactile hyperesthesia* —uncomfortable state wherein discrimination is diminished and paresthesia occurs

*tactile hypesthesia* —decreased touch sensibility

Visceral afferent fibers are also an integral part of the sensory system because of their ability to relay information about the state of distention in the hollow organs, such as the bladder and stomach. Vasomotor reflexes in the carotid sinus and reflexes involved in respiration and stretch excitation of muscle tonus are conveyed by nonsensory afferents. After these impulses reach the posterior root ganglion cells, they are transmitted through a complicated matrix of ascending tracts, which are partially discussed in this text. Greater detail is available in *Bing's Local Diagnosis in Neurological Diseases* (Haymaker, 1969).

Trophic changes are discussed in Chapters 16 and 25. However, they are mentioned here to emphasize the problems a client may encounter when interference with sensory input occurs. Myelodysplastic clients are more prone to develop ulcerations on the feet because of decreased sensory input perceived by the lower extremities. Clients with traumatic cord lesions or transverse inflammatory disorders of the cord have increased potential for developing decubiti in ischemic areas because of the interruption of the normal trophic reflexes that maintain and rebuild skin integrity.

Vasomotor activities are mediated through the autonomic nervous system. Their operations are delineated in a subsequent discussion in this chapter and in Chapter 4.

**INTERRUPTED SENSORY OPERATIONS.** Although there are a number of disturbances in sensory functions associated with interrupted operations of the spinal cord, see Chapters 16 and 23 for the appropriate discussion. Other types of sensory interferences include *trauma* and *sensory deprivation*.

TRAUMA. Whenever trauma has resulted in injury to the peripheral vascular system, bone, or soft tissue, several observations are essential. A discussion of orthopedic problems related to these injuries is beyond the scope of this book (Larson and Gould, 1978; Salter, 1970). However, it is timely to mention the basic signs of interrupted peripheral functions, that is, circulation problems, pain, interrupted motor functions, skin pallor, and sensory disturbances. During the immediate evaluation, circulatory checks, including assessment of the brachial, ulnar, radial, digital, femoral, popliteal, posterior tibial, and dorsalis pedis pulses, should be made. Checks for the integrity of motor functions should accompany these circulatory assessments. Pain should also be evaluated and described in detail. In ascertaining the cause of the pain, one should look for any type of constriction in or near the area of pain. One may evaluate skin pallor by noting the color and capillary return in the extremity distal to the injury after blanching. Unusual alterations in skin temperature should be detected at the same time. Sensory disturbances might indicate either a peripheral nerve injury or problems associated with ischemia secondary to edema. A rapid method of assessing interruptions in neuronal or circulatory functions is summarized in Fig. 3-6.

**SENSORY DEPRIVATION.** Sensory deprivation is also extremely important. Although it is not a primary disturbance of the neurons, it does seriously affect an individual's total functional capacities after prolonged periods. Studies of sensory deprivation and reports of subjective experiences are largely based on controlled experimental situations and accounts from prisoners of war (Hubbell, 1976). Since most reports may not be replicated and observations are largely subjective, experimental conditions or unusual experiences are at times hard to evaluate. The use of control subjects has a number of disadvantages. Although constant testing and monitoring devices have been used to establish objective criteria for certain experiments, some investigators believe these devices alter the nature of the experience.

Some observations concerning studies clarify the problems included in examining this phenomenon. Test validity is often questionable because of directions given before the experiment, varying methods of analysis or data measurement, and procedures for selection of subjects. Other factors that may alter the outcome of a controlled situation include previous events, immediate surroundings, personal expectations, anxiety, secondary gain from the experiment, and concentration of the subject on self.

Alterations in intellectual efficiency seem to be related to the type of deprivation employed. Perceptual deprivation tends to produce more difficult problems in adjustment than does sensory deprivation. However, differences in effects from sensory and perceptual deprivation vary among studies.

Hallucinatory experiences are often reported in studies of sensory deprivation. By utilizing more sophisticated techniques of measurement and information gained through trial and error, investigators have concluded that suggestibility and expectancy may play important roles in the frequency and complexity of hallucinatory reactions. Moreover, prior exposure to an experience of isolation may contribute to this phenomenon. Studies that have tried to control these factors produce fewer reports of a hallucinatory phenomenon, and, when this phenomenon is experienced, it tends to consist of brief periods of seeing spots, light flashes, or geometric figures.

Body immobilization, even without auditory or visual restrictions, has resulted in some perceptual impairments. The explanation of this probably lies in the sensory modalities, since curtailment of kinesthetic stimuli causes the organism to utilize predominantly introspective and cognitive capacities. Unless thoughts and imaginative powers have great impact, activation levels decline sharply. Outward symptoms of this phenomenon include increased daydreaming, decreased alertness, and extended periods of sleep.

Ability to endure sensory deprivation may be a function of both the adaptive capacity of the subject and the effects of stimulus intensity as perceived by the subject. Suggestible individuals may have greater difficulty with adjustment and imagery experiences. Those who weather the experience best are probably those who rely on inner competencies and resources rather than on external sources of stimulation as predominant life patterns. Although many subjects report perceptual and sensory isolation as a boring and distasteful experience, others say the experience becomes easier to endure with practice.

In evaluating sensory deprivation the practitioner should consider both personal and situational variables. *Personal variables* include personality or character traits, level of personality integration, socioeconomic factors, family status, developmental level, psychopathological status in general, motivation, attitude, and chronological age. *Situational variables* include expectations of the deprivation experience (experimental or induced), sex, perception of the experience in relation to the individual's life, previous information about such a situation, degree and modification of sensory input, amount of tactile and kinesthetic restriction, extent of social isolation, presence of time uncertainty, satisfaction of periodic body needs, knowledge or ignorance about outcome, continuity of the isolation experience, and mechanisms of communication available.

Behavior has been described by many investigators to coincide with the various phases of adjustment experienced by individuals in isolation. In the first phase, secondary process thinking is evident as a means of reducing subjective anxiety about the situation. During this period, exaggerated response patterns tend to make the individual feel more like usual. After this initial phase, secondary process thinking gives way to thought about anything but the immediate situation. When the ability to divert thinking breaks down, anxiety is obvious. If conditions improve, one notes increased spontaneous activity, decreased focus on the self, and developing awareness of the external environment. However, if the stressor continues, the individual tends to enter the adaptive phase, where thinking is mainly confined to primary process or stimulus-bound thought. Thus all thought becomes centered on the drives and needs inherent in the immediate situation. After this period the individual enters the phase of exhaustion. In this stage the individual feels unloved and abandoned. Attempts at drawing inward and excluding external stimuli are common observations at this point. If the individual becomes too exhausted to withstand further pressure, he or she may resign him- or herself to death. The outline following provides a listing of specific symptomatic behavior that may be noted at each phase of adjustment to the deprivation (isolation) experience (further discussion of stress is available in Chapter 4):

### Phase I

Structuring the situation—thinking about personal problems, manipulating food, folding pieces of paper, thinking of situation, reciting stories, or considering plans for pursuing usual routine
Daydreaming, recalling memories
Thinking about family and friends
Appearing somnolent
Whistling, singing, counting

### Phase II

General anxiety apparent
Activation of sympathetic-adrenal response mechanism
Pain, fear, tachycardia, or slight temperature elevation
Increased perspiration and other stress responses
Irritability and restlessness
Discomfort
Panic
Tension and boredom

### Phase III

Emotional lability
Reveries of personal and emotional intensity
Impaired cognitive and intellectual functions
Impaired powers of concentration
Daydreaming
Distortions in time judgment
Blank periods
Disturbances in perception of body image
Increased hallucinatory experiences
Diffuse anger
Fears of loss of sanity
Fears of loss of control over environmental forces and self
Suspiciousness, depression, fatigue
Increased physical complaints
Feelings that others have turned against him or her
Problems in validating own thoughts
Difficulty in finding familiar objects in a known setting
Focus on body functions and processes
Loss of perspective
Attempts at self-stimulation

### Phase IV

Dazed, tense, restless appearance
Suspicious attitude

Monotony of speech inflections
Lack of spontaneity and enthusiasm
Difficulty in expressing feelings
Verbalization only when directly questioned
Paucity of emotion
Indifferent, listless attitude
Lack of initiative
Regression to self-centered needs
Feelings of abandonment and loss of love
Hostile feelings expressed with difficulty

### Aftermath

Emotional reaction to experience varying from irritation to outbursts of anger
Resolute repression of experience
Restructuring of life in pattern of usual life-style, when readjustment moves in positive direction

In making direct application of this information to nursing, one only needs to recall the variety of adjustments called for in individuals who, because of illness, are placed in a hospital. Illness in itself represents a situation where there is a loss of usual routine and where there is a need for adjustment to a strange environment and possible limitations in sociophysiological functions. The loss of familiarity and the introduction of a new situation force the person to adjust. Individual adjustment capacities to novel and often unpleasant situations may frequently be predicted through accurate assessment and diagnosis of individual problems and variables.

Some of the values that may be threatened by illness and perceptual or sensory isolation are self-perception; body image; feelings of intactness; roles in family, job, and community; adequacy and acceptability as a person and family member; success and sense of fulfillment; future socioeconomic or physical capacities; ability to relate to significant others in the usual manner; and control over events that directly affect personal welfare.

When the individual's disease process requires isolation in a separate room, the nurse should consider the alternatives that might make this experience less traumatic: isolate the client closer to the nurse's desk, visit or communicate with the client at frequent and reliable intervals, include the client in care planning, provide diversionary activity appropriate to the individual need, keep promises, provide explanations of treatment and routine, and encourage contact with significant others in the individual's life. The principle underlying this intervention is the provision of varied and constant sensory-stimulus input, which is vital to the arousal reaction generated in the reticular formation. Monotony and unchanging environmental stimulation cause reduction of arousal mechanism capacities, so that cerebral functioning patterns may be altered (Conway and McCabe, 1978; Bolin, 1974).

The reticular activating system (RAS) coordinates sensory input and modifies levels of awareness in proportion to the incoming stimuli. The RAS cooperates with the thalamocortical projection system to allow general arousal states as well as individual responses to specific stimuli. Sensory impulses reaching the cortex are subjected to stimulatory and inhibitory input through feedback systems. As this information reaches the RAS, which is both ascending and descending, appropriate integration, inhibition, excitation, or isolation of events occurs. Since the RAS may conduct these varied functions simultaneously, it is easy to see why it functions well as a screening mechanism for messages involving individual well-being and integrity. This applies particularly to the isolated or sensory-deprived person who experiences inadequate input; the subject who might be overactive and subjected to one isolated train of input to aid in control of the attention span; and the individual who experiences sensory bombardment, where input is at such an intense level that further stimuli that might otherwise be received are blocked by an intense response. Examples of individuals in the first situation were discussed previously. Those in the second situation might include hyperactive children bombarded by the treatment modalities educators employ to concentrate attention. Examples of the third situation might be busy professionals involved in a crucial, demanding project where there is an immediate time limit or assorted other projects pending or intervening.

## INTEGRATION

Integration is a function of the gray matter within the CNS (Fig. 3-9). All synapses are located within gray matter. The white matter consists of bundles of myelinated axons transmitting impulses along specific pathways between integrating centers. Bundles of fibers that transmit impulses up and down the spinal cord or to a higher level within

in the CNS central nervous system are termed *projection tracts*. Fibers that cross over from right to left and vice versa are called *commissural* fibers or tracts. Association fibers transmit impulses from anterior to posterior from one association area to another within the same hemisphere of the brain or spinal cord. The gray matter of the cord is located in the central H-shaped pattern around the central canal. The gray matter of the cerebral cortex and cerebellar cortex is arranged in convolutions at their surface. All other integrating centers at a subcortical level are islands of gray matter called nuclei. The highest level of integration is the cerebral cortex where deliberate, purposeful responses are made to conscious stimuli. All other levels of integration (subcortical) are reflex actions no matter how complex. The lowest level of integration is the simple reflex are involving only one level of the spinal cord (Fig. 2-5).

### Cerebrum (telencephalon)

The cerebrum is the largest and most important part of the nervous system. It is contained in the anterior and middle cranial fossae and is supported posteriorly by the *tentorium cerebelli,* which also separates it from the cerebellum. The cerebrum consists of two visibly similar halves called *cerebral hemispheres*. One of these hemispheres is functionally more important in the area of expressive communication using symbolic language and is called the *dominant hemisphere*. Regardless of handedness, the left hemisphere is dominant for the function of speech in 90% of the population. It is postulated that both hemispheres are equipotential at birth and that dominance evolves with the development of speech. The hemispheres are separated by the *falx cerebri* (a fold of dura mater) but are connected with each other by a broad transverse band of commissural fibers, the *corpus callosum.*

Extensive research, especially in the decade of the sixties and into the early seventies, has been done on right-sided function. Much of this work has centered on experiments and clinical studies in which communication between the hemispheres is interrupted when one either severs the corpus callosum or chemically inhibits one side. It has been determined in these studies that the right hemisphere plays an important role in intuitive and creative responses and in spatial perception. For fur-

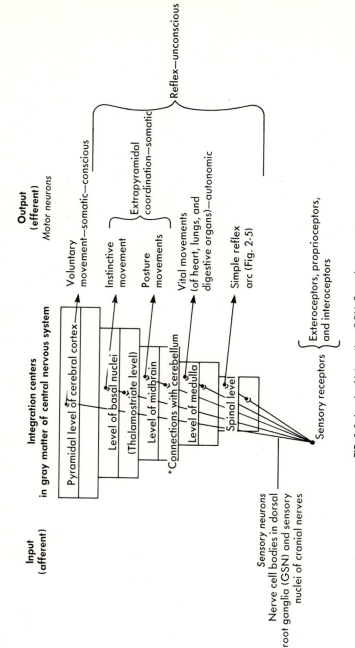

**FIG. 3-9.** Levels of integration. GSN, General sensory neurons.

ther reading in the area of split-brain research, see the references at the end of this chapter (Benton, 1972; Dimond, 1974, 1980; and Gazzaniga, 1970).

Each hemisphere can be subdivided into four lobes (frontal, parietal, temporal, and occipital) situated approximately in relation to the similarly named bones of the skull. The surface of the cerebral cortex is arranged in convolutions, or gyri (both terms are used interchangeably), to increase the surface area. These convolutions are determined by shallow fissures called *sulci*. The boundaries of the various lobes are outlined by deeper fissures: the central fissure (fissure of Rolando), which separates the frontal from the parietal lobe; the lateral fissure (fissure of Sylvius), which separates the temporal from the frontal and parietal lobes; and the parieto-occipital fissure, which separates the occipital from the parietal and temporal lobes (Fig. 3-10). The islands of Reil consist of cerebral cortex that evolves from the developing folds of the adjacent temporal and parietal lobes.

The cerebral cortex is viewed as the originating point of voluntary efferent pathways and the termination of conscious afferent pathways. The successful interpretation and transmission of impulses concerned with voluntary activity depend on intact operations of many cortical areas and pathways leading into and out of the cerebral cortex.

***Rhinencephalon.*** The rhinencephalon is the portion of the cerebral hemispheres that receives and regulates olfactory impulses. This area of the brain also plays a major role in controlling visceral activities via the hypothalamus and somatic activities via the limbic system at the level of the midbrain and medulla oblongata. The limbic system comprises the limbic lobe, the amygdaloid complex of the basal nuclei, and the fornix. (See Figs. 1-26 and 3-14.) The intricate operations of the limbic system include coded events from environmental perceptions and past experience as stored by the hippocampus as well as visceral operations from the amygdala. When this information is integrated, the individual has a basis for establishing semiautomatic responses to stimuli. These responses extend to include individual behaviors and physiological responses to such things as sex; eating; drinking; and affective, aggressive, and emotional states. Since the limbic system is also connected to the cerebral cortex through the thalamus and to the reticular formation of the brainstem, it has three other vital functions. First, the

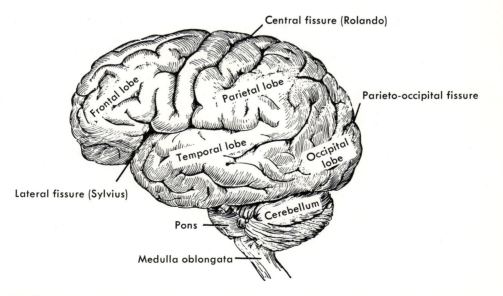

**FIG. 3-10.** Lateral view of cerebral hemisphere (showing lobes and principal fissures), cerebellum, pons, and medulla oblongata.

limbic system allows recent memories to be stored in the hippocampus, whereas distant ones are permanently retained in the neocortical area of the cerebrum (particularly in the temporal lobe). Second, the connection of the limbic system with the reticular formation provides the mechanism for the arousal-attention mechanisms vital to living. Third, the hippocampus has a tonic effect on the pituitary-adrenal axis.

*Frontal lobe.* The frontal lobe is concerned principally with personality; behavior; and the higher intellectual functions, including consciousness, learning, abstract and creative thinking, problem solving, judgment, memory, volition, and social, moral, and ethical values. The posterior limit of the frontal lobe, the precentral convolution (area 4), is the principal region for the initiation of motor function and contains the large and small pyramidal (Betz) cells. This area is subdivided into specific points (Fig. 3-11) from which movement can be elicited on electrical stimulation. These fibers are carried in the corticospinal tract to muscles on the opposite side of the body. The

specific functional areas are laid out one after the other in a definite pattern for consecutive parts of the body. One can visualize this pattern by mentally standing an individual on his head and by associating the toes and foot with the topmost part of the hemisphere and following down the precentral convolution with the leg, thigh, abdomen, thorax, shoulder, arm, hand, fingers, and face to the lowermost part of the frontal lobe, where the fissure of Rolando joins the fissure of Sylvius.

In addition to area 4 (Figs. 3-12 and 3-13), the primary motor areas (points of origin) are areas 6, 8, and 44. Just anterior to the precentral convolution is the premotor area (area 6), which is concerned with control and coordination of skilled movements of a complex nature. It has direct connections with the extrapyramidal motor nuclei and the cerebellum in carrying out these functions.

The corticobulbar tracts, which are short descending tracts to somatic motor nuclei of cranial nerves V, VII, and XII, have similar origins. Note that there is also input to the motor system from sensory areas 3, 1, 2, 5, and 7. Area 8 controls the

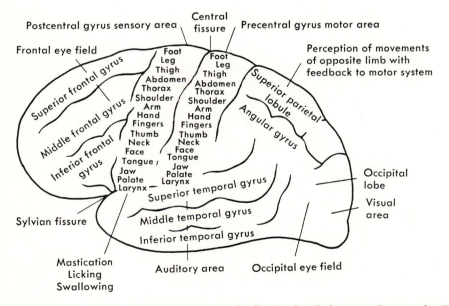

**FIG. 3-11.** Lateral view of cerebral hemisphere showing localization of cortical motor and sensory functions. (From Schottelius, B.A., and Schottelius, D.D.: Textbook of physiology, ed. 18, St. Louis, 1978, The C.V. Mosby Co.)

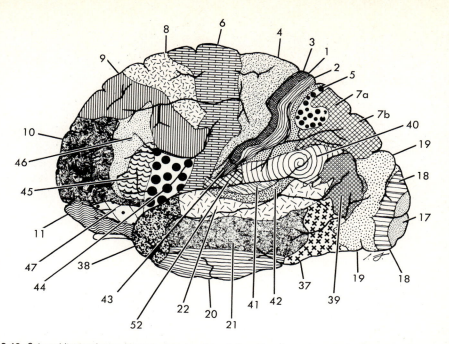

**FIG. 3-12.** Cytoarchitectural map of cerebral cortex, lateral view. Broca's motor speech area is in inferior frontal gyrus (area 44). (Based on Brodmann.)

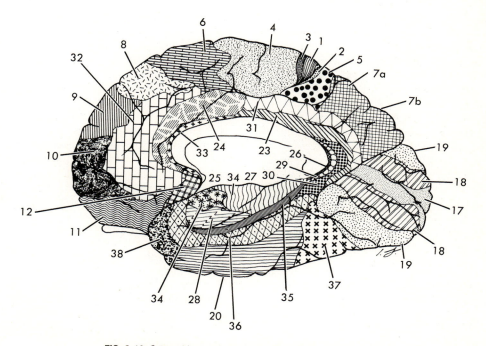

**FIG. 3-13.** Cytoarchitectural map of cerebral cortex, medial view.

frontal eye fields through its connections via the reticular substrate to the motor nuclei of cranial nerves III, IV, and VI. Area 44 (Broca's area), sometimes referred to as the speech center, is found in the inferior frontal gyrus just anterior to the motor area for control of muscles of the face, in the dominant hemisphere (Fig. 3-12). Although this area controls a major portion of the speech processes, it is actually only one point in the complex network required to produce communication. Left-sided lesions in this area result in abnormal speech production, or motor aphasia, in right-handed individuals.

The orbitofrontal lobe is composed of areas 9 through 13 on cytoarchitectural maps (Figs. 3-12 and 3-14). Although few specific activities can be assigned to this lobe, it receives an abundance of long association fibers from other lobes and is an area of integration of the personality. Recent experiments have revealed that areas 8 and 9 affect gastrointestinal movements and gastric secretions, whereas area 13 influences blood pressure and respiratory regulation. This functional association is probably made possible through the vast network of interconnections among the prefrontal lobe, thalamus, and hypothalamus.

*Parietal lobe.* The parietal lobe has a similar functional pattern for perception of general sensation in the postcentral convolution, immediately posterior to the central fissure of Rolando, as does the frontal motor area just anterior to this fissure (Fig. 3-11). This primary somesthetic area of the cortex is the terminal point of the conscious sensory (afferent) pathways (posterior columns and spinothalamic tract, Table 3-1). These pathways transmit impulses from the dermatomes of the body surface on the opposite side (except for the face). These impulses travel through synaptic connections in thalamic nuclei and terminate in areas 3, 1, and 2 of the postcentral convolution (Figs. 3-12 and 3-13). The recognition of size, shape, weight, texture, and consistency of objects and the ability to combine these to perceive three-dimensional figures (stereognosis) is a function of areas 5 and 7.

The secondary sensory area is found in the island of Reil, which begins at the base of the postcentral convolution and extends to the lower end of the Sylvian fissure. This area is the termination point of fibers from bilateral body surfaces of large cutaneous areas.

The capacities of the sensory cortex combine to allow individuals to integrate sensory input. The finished sensory experience includes related messages, past events, and emotional input from the thalamus.

*Temporal lobe.* The temporal lobe, which is inferior to the frontal and parietal lobes, receives impressions from three special senses: hearing, taste, and smell; within its substance the visual fibers of the optic radiation travel on their way to the occipital lobe. The temporal lobe of the dominant hemisphere is also important for understanding the spoken word.

Auditory fibers (see the section on the cranial nerve VIII in Chapter 2 for pathway) from the medial geniculate body of the thalamus carry impulses to the anterior transverse gyrus (Heschl, area 41), which is the primary perception area for hearing. The auditory association area occupies a part of the superior temporal gyrus (areas 42 and 22) adjacent to the primary auditory area. The supramarginal gyrus (area 40) and the angular gyrus (area 39) are important areas that interrelate somesthetic, visual, and auditory stimuli (Fig. 3-12). These association areas have the task of integrating sensory stimuli in such a way as to comprehend their meaning. This process of "knowing" encompasses comparison of sensory input with past experiences.

Olfactory sensation (cranial nerve I, Chapter 2) is carried to the olfactory gyrus at the inferior border of the island of Reil on the medial side of the temporal lobe and the periamygdaloid area, which is a small area of cortex rostral and dorsal to the amygdaloid nucleus. These areas constitute the primary olfactory cortex. The sensation of taste is closely associated with the sensation of smell, and its perception is in the same general area of the cortex. The general sensory area for the tongue is in the most inferior area of the postcentral convolution of the parietal lobe near the temporal lobe.

*Occipital lobe.* The occipital lobe of the cortex is the most dorsal apex of the cerebrum. It lies in the middle fossa separated from the cerebellum by the tentorium cerebelli. It is separated from the parietal lobe by the parieto-occipital fissure. The supramarginal and angular gyrus, described with the temporal lobe, lie at the juncture between the parietal, temporal, and occipital lobes. The calcerine fissure lies on the medial surface and is bounded on both sides by the striate area (area 17), which is the primary perception area for sight (the optic pathway is described in Chapter 2 in the discussion of cranial nerve II and in Fig. 2-9). Adjacent to area 17 are areas 18 and 19, which constitute the association cortex for visual perception and for some visual reflexes such as visual fixation (Figs. 3-12 and 3-13).

*Pain areas.* Although pain is reviewed in a later chapter, it seems appropriate at this point to discuss the cortical termination of pain reception. Nociceptors receive painful stimuli that are transmitted to postcentral convolutions by pathways described earlier in this chapter. However, when cortical influences are absent, individuals may still experience pain. Thus current investigators regard the cerebral cortex and thalamus as joint receptor bases when they use the term *"primary receptive center for pain impulses."*

*Associational areas.* Even after areas are designated with known function, large areas of the neopallium (cortex) remain for which no discrete function is known. These areas of undesignated function are also characterized by the fact that removal of large portions of or lesions to these areas may cause insignificant alterations in the functional capacities of the individual. Thus these areas, found in both hemispheres, are sometimes designated silent *"associational areas"* and are believed to provide complex connection modalities between sensory and motor areas.

In thinking about the maturation process, one realizes that the storage of information gained through experience, the retrieval of these data, and the integration of related knowledge allow the increased ability to respond to situations more maturely and appropriately. Such activity depends largely on capacities available in the associational areas.

*Factors affecting outcome.* Since cortical functions are integral events in the total organismal response, they should be viewed as part of the individual's total effort in self-preservation and self-perpetuation. When sensory impulses are received, even the most elementary response may be the result of complex interconnections between obvious sensory and motor areas and other areas of the brain that may contain relevant data. Thus complex activities often represent the integration of many points at all levels of the central nervous system (Fig. 3-9). Because coordinated response efforts depend on the collective operations of many points in the nervous system, the responses of a discrete area in laboratory experiments should not be regarded as isolated efforts in enacting activity in usual life situations.

Cortical inhibition blocks interference, so that input relevant to a situational activity may be facilitated. Thus while concentrating on learning to knit, one might not hear a dripping faucet. Anxiety and fear have varying influence on inhibiting activity. Depending on the degree to which these strong emotions affect usual behavioral patterns, individuals are categorized into groups that exhibit specific behavioral manifestations.

Since the neopallium is less developed in young children, one notes that childish behavior and rapid transitions in attention and interest are normally seen. As perceptions are recorded and cortical maturity allows molding of responses to stimuli or sets of stimuli, learning occurs. Behavior then becomes based on known patterns of performance. Predictability in behavior becomes more and more possible as more of the developmental tasks are completed. Further aspects of learning, perception, and behavior are discussed in Chapters 5 and 7.

*Basal nuclei* (often called "basal ganglia"). The basal nuclei consist of the *corpus striatum* (caudate and lenticular nuclei), the amygdaloid nucleus, and the claustrum (Fig. 3-14). These are paired structures found in each hemisphere, with the caudate nuclei forming part of the lateral walls of the lateral ventricles. They consist of groups of cells that exert a (steadying) influence on muscular activity. Disturbance of these ganglia results in tremor, muscular rigidity, and loss of the automatic movements of expression and walking (Parkinson's syndrome). These bodies have connections with the red nucleus and substantia nigra, which are cell collections in the upper midbrain, and take part in the smooth and coordinated activity of muscles. The basal nuclei are motor nuclei of the extrapyramidal system and are dis-

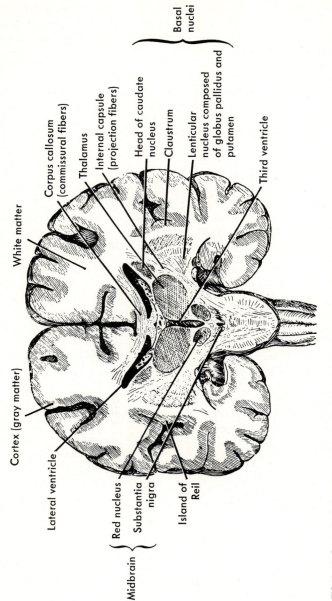

**FIG. 3-14.** Coronal section of brain showing thalamus, basal nuclei, lateral and third ventricles, and internal capsule. Note that cross section through internal capsule and basal nuclei is termed "corpus striatum."

cussed in greater detail in association with the motor output portion of this chapter.

## Diencephalon

The diencephalon is located at the distal aspect of the prosencephalon and comprises the *thalamus, epithalamus,* and *hypothalamus.* Because of its functions, the diencephalon is often referred to as the *interbrain,* or intermediary between the cerebrum and both the somatic and the autonomic nervous systems. As the interbrain, this region has a primary role in sleep, emotion, thermoregulation, autonomic activity, and endocrine control in ongoing behavioral patterns. The thalamus and hypothalamus are the only structures reviewed at this point, since the epithalamus (pineal body) was discussed in Chapter 1.

*Thalamus.* The subcortical sensory center that receives all conscious sensory stimuli, except taste, is the thalamus. After messages arrive in the thalamus, they are transmitted to the cerebral cortex. Because of its interconnections with the hypothalamus and cerebral cortex, this structure is also integrally involved in emotional activities and instinctive responses. The reticular system of the diencephalon and mesencephalon is probably partially the regulatory and distribution center for afferent impulses within the receiving areas. Because of its interconnections with the limbic area, frontal lobes, and temporoparietal cortex, the thalamus also becomes the central network for attentive processes (Figs. 3-14 and 3-15).

*Hypothalamus.* The hypothalamus (Fig. 1-27) is the group of bilateral nuclei located on the inferior surface of the brain, ventral to the thalamus, and forming the floor and part of the lateral wall of the third ventricle. It is bounded anteriorly by the optic chiasma and posteriorly by the mammil-

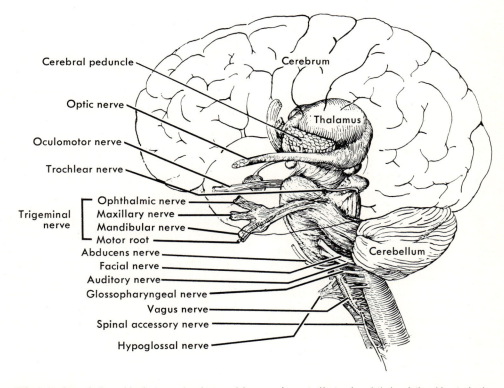

**FIG. 3-15.** Lateral view of brainstem, showing cranial nerves (except olfactory) and their relationships to brain. (See Chapter 2 for description of function of cranial nerves.)

lary bodies. The median eminence of the tuber cinereum is connected to the pituitary gland by means of a stalk, the infundibulum. The upper motor neurons of the autonomic neuron system are contained in the hypothalamus (craniosacral anteriorly and thoracolumbar posteriorly). In consort with the pituitary the autonomic nervous system and hypothalamus influence water balance, carbohydrate, and fat metabolism; growth; sexual maturity; body temperatures; pulse rate; blood pressure; and sleep.

Scarcely a single important metabolic event in the body can escape the primary or secondary effect of hormones. Most scientists agree that hormones do not initiate new events but act as regulators by their actions on enzymes and other chemical reactions. It is therefore apparent that total understanding of any disease of physiological disorder must include knowledge of the endocrine role in such states. The pituitary gland has long been called the *master gland*. If the truth of the preceding paragraph is accepted, understanding the control of this structure should offer greater insight into disease.

Since there is no direct nerve connection between the hypothalamus and the anterior pituitary, a system of blood-borne control had to be postulated. A portal system of blood vessels between the median eminence of the hypothalamus and the pituitary gland has been demonstrated. Changes in function of the endocrine glands were noted after section of the portal system. Hypothalamic nerve fibers of different types liberate hormonal substances from their nerve endings into the capillaries of the median eminence. Then by means of the pituitary portal system these ''releasing factors'' are carried to the pituitary gland where they stimulate or inhibit the release of various anterior pituitary hormones. The isolation, determination of structure, and synthesis of several hypothalamic hormones have been accomplished. Releasing factors are specific for each of the pituitary hormones controlled by this method. These events indicate that brain control of metabolic function is very important. Through the administration of synthetic hormones it is now possible to affect some control of endocrine function.

*Internal capsule.* The internal capsule lies between the thalamus medially and some of the basal nuclei laterally. It consists of the ascending and descending fiber projection tracts (white matter) as they extend from the cerebrum to form part of the midbrain. These fibers are grouped into a large bundle on each side of the mesencephalon called the *cerebral peduncles*. They form the main line for the transmission of stimuli from the cerebrum to the brainstem and spinal cord.

*Mesencephalon.* The mesencephalon (midbrain), reviewed from a developmental viewpoint in Chapter 1, is vital as a conduction pathway and a reflex control complex. The *cerebral peduncles* in the anterior aspect of the midbrain are composed of many projectional fibers extending to the cerebral cortex (Fig. 3-14). The midbrain is also integrally involved in the regulation of ocular reflexes, eye movements, and righting reflexes. The relay center for auditory and visual impulses is also located in this region.

Visceral efferent fibers that course through synaptic connections in the ciliary ganglia to innervate the smooth eye musculature originate in the Edinger-Westphal nuclei of the midbrain. *Superior colliculi* (optic reflex centers) are intricately intermeshed in reflex modification related to visual stimuli. The centers for transmission of acoustic reflexes and auditory stimuli are the *inferior colliculi*. Other key structures of the reticular formation—rubrospinal tract, substantia nigra, and tectospinal tract—have their genesis in this area.

The centers for postural and righting reflexes are also found in the midbrain region. Postural reflexes, including static and labyrinthine reflexes, are basically proprioceptive. Righting reflexes maintain the head in an upright position in accordance with the environment through the utilization of the eyes, inner ears, and neck and trunk muscles.

*Rhombencephalon.* The major regions in the rhombencephalon are the *myelencephalon,* the *metencephalon,* and the *cerebellum.* The myelencephalon is the *medulla oblongata,* and the metencephalon is the *pons,* the development, structure, and function of which are detailed in Chapter 1. The ventral part of the brainstem consists of the ascending and descending pathways.

MEDULLA OBLONGATA. The medulla oblongata, located between the foramen magnum and the pons, is anatomically complex and not usually amenable to surgery. It consists of intricate white matter pathways that are twisted around the ganglia and nuclei of the gray matter. Further information on intervention modalities and results in clients with regard to space-occupying processes is available in other sections of this text. Particular attention is paid to this problem in the discussion of tumors (Chapter 21).

Cells and nuclei in the medulla oblongata are categorized collectively as the *reticular formation*. Because the reticular formation is integrally involved in attention-arousal and consciousness, it is termed the *reticular activating system (RAS)*. Neurons of the reticular system are also integrally active in certain visceral processes, including cardiac and respiratory functions, swallowing, blood pressure control, vasomotor functions, phonation, mastication, and salivary and gastric secretions. These centers function by integrating impulses with higher centers in order to arrive at an operational outcome that suits the best interests of the individual.

**CEREBELLUM.** The cerebellum is located just below the occipital lobes, from which it is separated by the tentorium. It differs grossly from the cerebrum in that is is about one fifth as large, and its surface is formed of many thin, relatively parallel convolutions. It has two hemispheres and a central section called the *vermis* (since it is wormlike). The cerebellar peduncles (tracts) connect the hemispheres to each other and to the various parts of the brainstem as follows: the superior cerebellar peduncles (brachia conjunctiva) with the midbrain (red nucleus), the middle peduncles (brachia pontis) with the pons, and the inferior peduncles (restiform bodies) with the medulla oblongata. The cerebellum coordinates muscle tone and movement and maintains posture in space (equilibrium). To many investigators the cerebellum is the most interesting structure in the cranium because of its histological structure, functional mechanisms, adaptive capacities, and response to removal of lesions.

HISTOLOGICAL STRUCTURE AND FUNCTIONS. Ramón y Cajal of Spain in 1888 first described the neuronal circuitry of the gray matter composing the cerebellar convolutions. Although the early descriptions have been revised to reflect the state of current thinking, investigators continue to agree that the most specialized functions of the cerebellum rely on the intricate circuitry of this structure.

Seven basic types of neurons are contained in the cerebellum, including the climbing fibers, the mossy fibers, the basket cell, the stellate cell, the Golgi cell, the granule cells, and the Purkinje cell. Fig. 3-16 illustrates these various neurons. Climbing and mossy fibers conduct impulses into the cortex, whereas Purkinje cell axons are totally responsible for conveying impulses from the cortex. The remaining four types of cells are internuncial. At this point another set of afferent fibers has been identified, but since preliminary investigations continue to determine their functions, they are not discussed further at this point.

*Climbing fibers* originate in the inferior olive, a compact region of neuron cells adjacent to the medulla oblongata (Fig. 3-17). These fibers then extend into the cerebellar cortex and nuclei, where each fiber becomes permanently affixed to a single Purkinje cell. After this union has taken place, no other climbing fiber joins the involved Purkinje cell. As the Purkinje cell continues its development, its climbing fiber entwines it in a vinelike manner, touching it at some 300 synaptic junctions. Thus afferent impulses traveling through the climbing fiber result in the total excitation of that Purkinje neuron.

Unlike the climbing fiber, the *mossy fiber* has a few connections with a number of Purkinje cells because of intermediate contact with the granule cell layer, composed of interneurons beneath the Purkinje cell layer. Since each mossy fiber is connected to a number of Purkinje cells, excitation of a mossy fiber results in a more generalized response from many Purkinje cells. At the point where the mossy fiber extends beneath the Purkinje layer, it divides into a shape resembling an inverted T and is perpendicular to Purkinje cell dendrites while being parallel to other mossy fiber axons. It is this arrangement that allows each Purkinje fiber to come into contact with up to 100,000 different mossy fiber axons.

The three inhibitory interneurons in the cerebellum include the *basket cell*, the *stellate cell*, and the *Golgi cell*. Each of these interneurons affects a specific structure. The basket cell inhibits Purkinje cell soma; the stellate cell, Purkinje cell dendrites; and the Golgi cell, granule cells, so that they no longer discharge impulses to Purkinje cells. *Granule cells* number 10 times the total cells once believed to compose the entire brain. The

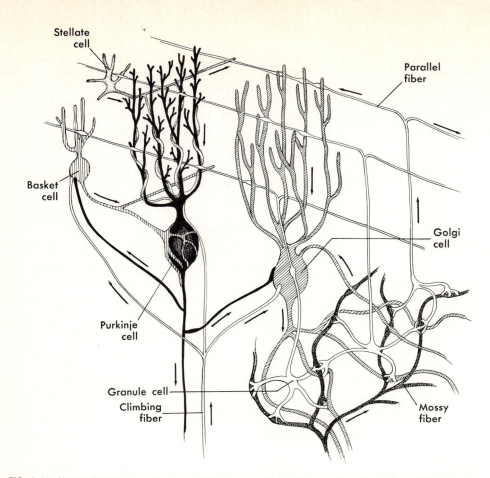

Stellate
cell

Parallel
fiber

Basket
cell

Golgi
cell

Purkinje
cell

Granule cell
Climbing
fiber

Mossy
fiber

**FIG. 3-16.** Neuronal interconnections in cerebellar cortex. (From Conway, B.L.: Pediatric neurologic nursing, St. Louis, 1977, The C.V. Mosby Co.)

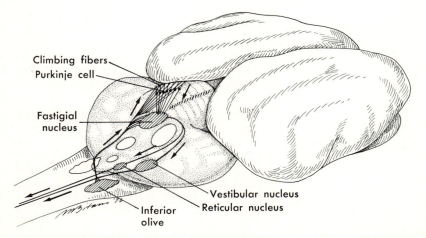

Climbing fibers
Purkinje cell

Fastigial
nucleus

Inferior
olive

Vestibular nucleus
Reticular nucleus

**FIG. 3-17.** Climbing fibers arise from inferior olive of brainstem and end in contralateral cerebellar hemisphere. (From Conway, B.L.: Pediatric neurologic nursing, St. Louis, 1977, The C.V. Mosby Co.)

functional unit of the granule cell strata is composed of Golgi cells in combination with the dendrites of the granule cells and the axons of the Golgi cells.

The *Purkinje cell,* the key component of the cerebellar neuronal network, has extensive dendrites, a bulblike body, and a long narrow axon. The cellular bodies of Purkinje cells form a dense region termed the *Purkinje cell layer.* Axons from these cells connect to the scattered areas of gray matter (nuclei) in white matter. Since the nuclei of Purkinje cells connect with climbing and mossy fibers, they become the central point for the reception of all cortical messages from the cerebrum. After these messages are received, they are further relayed either to the spinal cord or to other portions of the brain through the cerebellar network. The dendrites that initially receive these messages are conveniently located at the periphery of the cerebellar cortex, where initial contact with incoming messages occurs.

Motor responses requiring synchronized efforts from several muscle groups to effect rapid movement and abrupt termination of activity shortly after the onset of a given movement are, investigators believe, the responsibility of the climbing fiber system. On the other hand, mossy fibers are believed to activate large portions of the cerebellar cortex when necessary. The distribution of impulses toward the fiber that allows local or diffuse response is mediated through the efforts of inhibitory cells.

CEREBELLAR STIMULATOR. Through the combined efforts of all neurons, the cerebellum becomes efficient in refining or reorganizing motor activities. Its capabilities continue even when it is severed from all peripheral body input. However, in ordinary operations the cerebellum relies on the spinocerebellar tract to convey messages indicating current activities of inhibitory interneurons in the spinal cord in relation to ongoing muscular activities. Through an increased understanding of this cerebellar circuitry, investigators have developed cerebellar implants that improve motor functions for some individuals with impaired motor capacities (Grabow et al., 1974). Chapter 17 offers additional detail.

OUTCOMES OF PHYSIOLOGICAL IMPAIRMENT. When the cerebellum is damaged, the outcome depends on the portion of the structure that has sustained injury. When disequilibrium, nystagmus, or a reeling walk are apparent, the insult has affected the flocculonodular lobe. If the anterior lobe functions are interrupted, persons manifest disturbances in the postural reflexes. Posterior lobe disturbances result in such changes of voluntary movements as discrepancies in force, direction, and range of movements; lack of precision; and possible tremors in voluntary muscular activities. Interferences that interrupt functions in more than one area result in combinations of these functional disorders.

## OUTPUT

This section is limited to the voluntary (somatic) efferent system. The autonomic efferent output to the viscera is discussed in detail in Chapter 4. Both systems are capable of response to sensory input from receptors either exteroceptors, proprioceptors, or interoceptors; that is one may experience a visceral response to an external stimulus or a voluntary motor response to a visceral stimulus. There is no discrete input system for each division (Fig. 3-9). However the output system is delineated by the efferent pathways to specific effector organs. Therefore the functional division known as the somatic or voluntary nervous system controls function of skeletal muscle, whereas the autonomic division controls contraction of smooth and cardiac muscle and secretion of glands. The responding organ is termed the *effector*. All action of the human body may be described in terms of effector response. Only those actions initiated from centers of conscious response in the cerebral cortex are voluntary. All responses integrated in gray matter at a subcortical level are reflex activity. The autonomic efferent system is essentially an involuntary reflex system for the autonomic control of visceral function (Chapter 4). Much of the coordination and control of skeletal muscle contraction is also mediated at an unconscious level (extrapyramidal system).

All impulses to the skeletal muscle are transmitted by the axon of the anterior horn cell (lower motor neuron) to the motor end plate. A motor unit consists of one lower motor neuron and the skeletal muscle fibers it innervates. Each skeletal muscle is made up of numerous motor units. The neurotransmitter at the motor end plate is acetylcholine

(ACh), which exhibits a nicotinic response in this case. Numerous upper motor neurons, both pyramidal and extrapyramidal, converge upon one lower motor neuron (LMN). Pyramidal fibers are facilitory (EPSP), whereas extrapyramidal fibers are either facilitory (EPSP) or inhibitory (IPSP). The neurotransmitter for EPSP fibers is probably ACh, whereas the neurotransmitter for IPSP fibers is probably GABA or glycine. The response of the lower motor nerve is the algebraic sum of the impulses converging on it through the upper motor neurons; therefore it is called the *final common pathway* (Granit, 1970).

### Efferent pathways

*Pyramidal tracts (corticospinal tracts)* (Fig. 3-18). These tracts transmit impulses of conscious muscle contraction; they are composed of two or more neurons.

1. Upper motor neuron or Betz cell.
2. Lower motor neuron, which has its nerve cell body in the anterior horn of the gray matter of the spinal cord.
3. Lateral.
   a. Larger of the two corticospinal tracts (pyramidal).
   b. First-order neuron forms tract, which descends through internal capsule of diencephalon, cerebral peduncles of midbrain, white matter of pons, and medulla oblongata where it crosses at the *decussation of pyramids* and descends in the contralateral side of the lateral spinal cord white matter.
4. Anterior (ventral).
   a. Tract composed of first-order neuron of pathway, which descends uncrossed.
   b. Located in the anterior white matter.
   c. Many fibers cross in the anterior white commissure at the level where they synapse with lower motor neurons.

*Extrapyramidal pathways* (Fig. 3-19). These pathways modify and coordinate skeletal muscular activity.

1. Reticulospinal (lateral-anterior and medial reticulospinal in anterior funiculi); pathway begins in reticular activating system of brainstem and ends with lower motor neurons; control of *antigravity muscles*.

   a. Medial and anterior, being inhibitory—impulses from this area inhibit extensors and stimulate flexors.
   b. Lateral, being facilitatory—impulses stimulate extensors (antigravity muscles), inhibit flexors, and maintain upright position.
2. Vestibulospinal; transmits impulses that assist in maintenance of muscle tone and equilibrium.
   a. Tract is composed of first-order neuron, which has its nerve cell body in the vestibular nucleus of the medulla oblongata and descends *uncrossed*.
   b. Lower motor neuron on same side forms the second-order neuron in this pathway.
3. Rubrospinal; transmits impulses of unconscious muscle coordination.
   a. Located in the lateral white matter.
   b. Tract is composed of second-order neuron of pathway.
      (1) First-order neuron has its nerve cell body in the red nucleus of the midbrain and *crosses* to the opposite side before descending (red nucleus has connections with cerebellum).
      (2) Second-order neuron is in reticular formation of medulla oblongata (forms tract), which ends in synapse with lower motor neuron. Fig. 3-18 shows placement of both sensory and and motor tracts in the white matter of the spinal cord.

*Extrapyramidal function.* The basal nuclei are a key component of the extrapyramidal system. Their connections with the thalamus form an essential link between the diencephalon and the telencephalon. The basal nuclei are further regulated by neuronal systems arising from the cerebral cortex known as the *centrally originating extrapyramidal system* (COEPS). COEPS stems from the cerebral cortex (anterior to the central sulcus in motor areas 8, 6, and 4 and posterior to this sulcus in sensory areas 3, 1, 2, 5, and 7 and the temporal lobe). Fibers then course through the striatum, thalamus, red nucleus, reticular formation, pontile nuclei, and substantia nigra. They have numerous synaptic junctions in these areas. Activities of COEPS are constantly monitored and modified

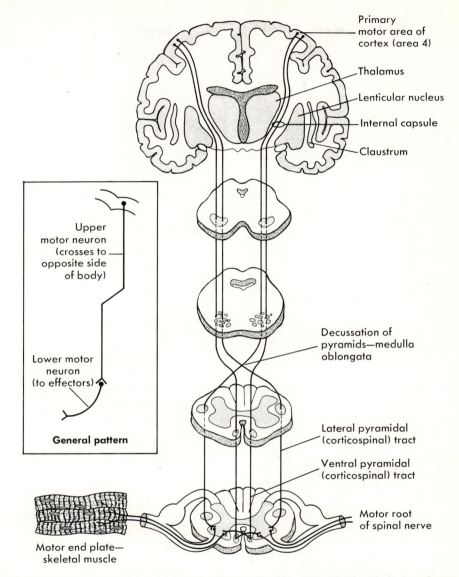

Primary
motor area of
cortex (area 4)

Thalamus

Lenticular nucleus

Internal capsule

Claustrum

Upper
motor neuron
(crosses to
opposite side
of body)

Lower motor
neuron
(to effectors)

**General pattern**

Decussation of
pyramids—medulla
oblongata

Lateral pyramidal
(corticospinal) tract

Ventral pyramidal
(corticospinal) tract

Motor root
of spinal nerve

Motor end plate—
skeletal muscle

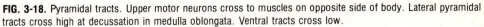

**FIG. 3-18.** Pyramidal tracts. Upper motor neurons cross to muscles on opposite side of body. Lateral pyramidal tracts cross high at decussation in medulla oblongata. Ventral tracts cross low.

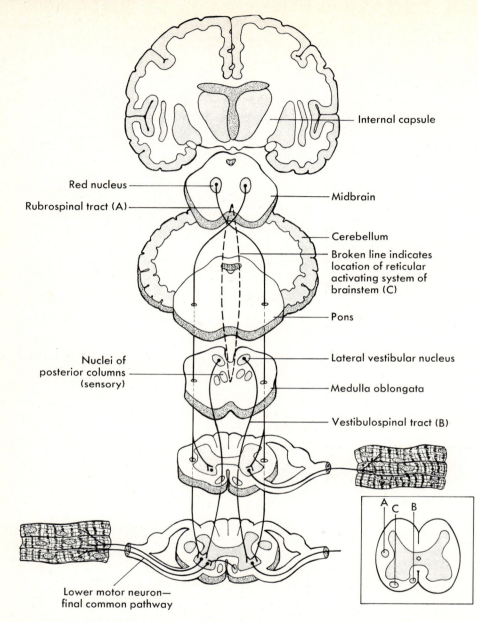

Internal capsule

Red nucleus

Rubrospinal tract (A)

Midbrain

Cerebellum

Broken line indicates location of reticular activating system of brainstem (C)

Pons

Nuclei of posterior columns (sensory)

Lateral vestibular nucleus

Medulla oblongata

Vestibulospinal tract (B)

Lower motor neuron— final common pathway

**FIG. 3-19.** Extrapyramidal descending tracts. Upper motor neurons originate below level of cortex and converge on lower motor neurons (final common pathway) along with upper motor neurons of pyramidal tracts (see Fig. 3-18). *A,* Rubrospinal tract originates in the red nucleus of the midbrain, crosses immediately, and descends contralaterally in opposite cord. *B,* Vestibulospinal tract originates in vestibular nucleus of medulla oblongata and descends ipsilaterally. *C,* Reticulospinal tracts (medial and lateral) originate from reticular activating system of brainstem and descend in general area of *C.* (These are not so well organized as others are.) Interconnections between basal nuclei, midbrain, diencephalon, and cerebellum are extensive.

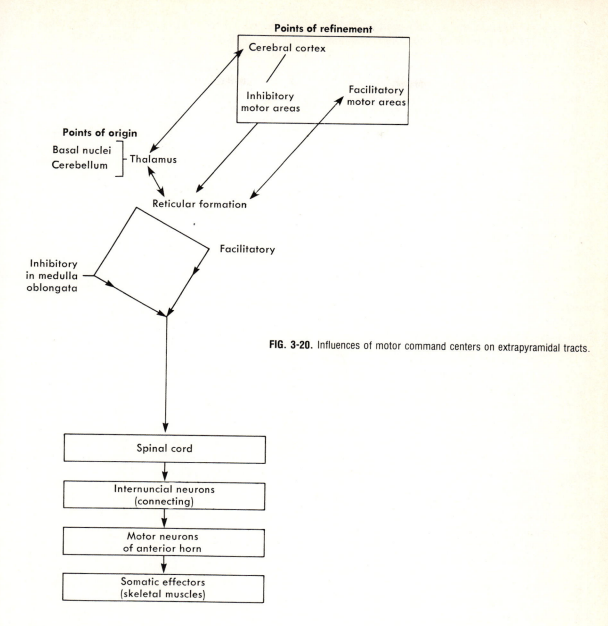

**Points of refinement**

Cerebral cortex

Inhibitory motor areas

Facilitatory motor areas

**Points of origin**

Basal nuclei
Cerebellum — Thalamus

Reticular formation

Inhibitory in medulla oblongata

Facilitatory

Spinal cord

Internuncial neurons (connecting)

Motor neurons of anterior horn

Somatic effectors (skeletal muscles)

**FIG. 3-20.** Influences of motor command centers on extrapyramidal tracts.

through feedback systems of the basal nuclei and thalamic and cortical connections (Fig. 3-20).

The basal nuclei added to the reticular nuclei and the fibers of the mesencephalon, pontile tegmentum, and cerebellum are a collective group termed the *extrapyramidal system,* from which impulses are carried to lower motor neurons by way of the extrapyramidal tracts (Fig. 3-19).

***Suprasegmental influences—summary and expansion.*** Suprasegmental influences on the local reflex act are exerted through descending motor pathways of the pyramidal and extrapyramidal tracts. Axonal processes of the pyramidal tracts, which arise from the Betz cells of the motor cortex, descend as crossed and uncrossed pyramidal tracts (corticospinal). The lateral crossed tract in the lateral funiculus terminates at every cord level near the internuncial cells of the gray matter located at the base of the anterior horn.

The uncrossed pyramidal tract in the anterior funiculus distributes fibers that course through the anterior white commissure to the contralateral horn cells at each level of the spinal cord. Although some fibers cross high and others low, the two pyramidal tracts (lateral and ventral) function to control skeletal muscle on the contralateral side of the body.

The role of the extrapyramidal tracts in affecting the anterior horn cell is far more complex than that of the pyramidal tracts. The rubrospinal tract joins the cerebellum of the same side and the contralateral portion of the pallidum with the anterior horn cells. Other connections with lower motor neurons include the vestibulospinal tract in linking the vestibular nucleus of the same side, the tectospinal tract in joining the midbrain of the opposite side, the olivospinal tract in connecting the inferior olive of the same side with the cervical cord, and of the reticulospinal tract in connecting the reticular gray matter in the brainstem with the same side. Of these extrapyramidal tracts the reticulospinal tracts are some of the more significant. The combined efforts of the extrapyramidal tracts allow an individual to perform complex, coordinated movements that may require synchronized activities on the part of several groups of muscles, automatic responses, simultaneous muscle responses, or sequences of discrete muscle movements (Oist et al., 1973). In thinking of examples of these actions, consider the act of eating, running, or swimming. More complex activities might include some sports, such as gymnastics, or some of the dance forms. Extrapyramidal tracts also regulate automatic emotional responses—grimaces or smiles—in relation to ongoing environmental and perceptual experiences (Fig. 3-20).

Before the message travels through the final common pathway, the anterior horn cell is subjected to input from a variety of sources. These sources relay both facilitory (EPSP) and inhibitory (IPSP) impulses to the anterior horn cell. The total effect of these opposing forces determines the response of the lower motor neuron. The facilitory impulses arrive at the anterior horn motor neurons through pyramidal and extrapyramidal tracts and through sensory neurons whose axons are in the posterior roots of the spinal nerves. The extrapyramidal pathways involved in facilitatory impulse transmission are the extrapyramidal facilitatory reticulospinal tracts. Impulses traveling along these pathways both facilitate lower motor neurons that innervate extensor muscles and inhibit lower motor neurons held as explanations for ways in which the higher motor centers achieve their task. In one study (Evarts, 1973) investigators credited the basal nuclei (ganglia) and cerebellum with the responsibility for being the highest motor control centers. They theorized that the basal ganglia and cerebellum transmit impulses to the thalamus for modification before reaching the cerebral cortex for ultimate transmission to the skeletal muscles. Thus the cerebral cortex is viewed as the point of refinement for muscular movement rather than the point or origin and direction for voluntary activity. The more conventional theory is opposite, since it describes the cerebral cortex as the point of origin for willed movements and the basal ganglia and cerebellum as structures responsible for refining motor output before it is transmitted to the effector organs (skeletal muscles) for implementation. At this point no one can prove conclusively which way the higher motor processes operate. Whatever the mechanism, the end result is that facilitatory impulses reaching the anterior motor neuron usually exceed inhibitory impulses, so that normal muscle tone is maintained. If impulses along inhibitory extrapyramidal pathways from basal ganglia to bulbar inhibitory centers are interrupted, facilitatory impulses dominate. The resulting increase in muscle tone is evident in the rigidity or spasticity that develops. Assessment of neurological functions after an interruption of transmission from the upper motor neurons reveals faulty impulse transmission along the axons of the pyramidal and extrapyramidal pathways. The so-called long tract, or pyramidal, signs that reflect these abnormalities are actually the result of interferences in both the pyramidal and inhibitory extrapyramidal pathways. Interruption of the pyramidal pathway results in appropriate paralysis, whereas disturbances in inhibitory extrapyramidal pathways result in spasticity and exaggerated reflexes.

Problems that may disrupt the functioning of the extrapyramidal system may be divided into the categories of metabolic and genetic disorders and static and degenerative lesions. Examples of some of these disturbances include Sydenham's chorea, cerebral palsy, Huntington's chorea, dystonia musculorum deformans, torticollis, Wilson's disease, parkinsonism, myotrophic lateral sclerosis, carbon dioxide and manganese poisoning, and effects from phenothiazines.

*Reflex characteristics.* The essential elements of the reflex arc are a receptor neuron (afferent limb) an integrating center within the central nervous system at any level below the cerebral cortex and a motor neuron (efferent limb). Theoretically, the simplest reflex arc could involve only one synapse (one cord segment) between the afferent and efferent neuron and could be termed *monosynaptic.* However in reality most reflex pathways are *multisynaptic* having one or more central connecting or internuncial neurons between the afferent and efferent limb. If the reflex act involves only one half of the body, it is termed *ipsilateral,* and if the impulse crosses over and the response is on the opposite side of the body, it is a *contralateral reflex.* The reflex time is the time that elapses between stimulus and response and is increased proportionately with the number of synapses in the pathway.

The basic purpose of all reflexes is to maintain total body integrity. However, certain responses initiated by a local reflex arc may be inhibited by powerful central states, for example, pain, fear, or acute grief, through the action of the autonomic nervous system or through the response of a cord center in a particular situation. For example, when an individual steps on a pin, a protective withdrawal of the ipsilateral aspect of the foot occurs through muscular flexion. The intensity of such a response is directly proportional to the body area stimulated and is termed a *local sign.* Most flexion reflexes are activated when noxious stimuli are experienced locally. These flexion reflexes are characterized by polysynaptic connections and the phenomenon of afterdischarge, so that the re-

action extends for a period greater than the stimulus duration. Not every application of noxious stimuli to the foot elicits the same response. For example, when pressure is applied to the plantar aspect of the foot, an extensor thrust reflex is elicited. This reflex is an important part of the locomotion act.

In continuing with the response of the pricked foot, one notes that the resulting reaction is more complex than the simple flexion and withdrawal of that extremity. The *law of reciprocal innervation* becomes involved. According to this law a particular extensor reflex may be negated and its related musculature inhibited while the opposing flexor center is positively activated. In other words, this noxious stimulus results in a flexion response while causing antagonistic muscles to remain relaxed in the involved extremity.

This example may be further extended to explain *double reciprocal extension.* Because afferent fibers in the affected leg connect with neurons of the flexors and extensors in the contralateral limb, the flexion response is accompanied by extension and flexor inhibition in the contralateral extremity. This reflex of crossed extension is part of the total movement elicited when one foot is pricked. Functionally this extension of the contralateral extremity provides the ability to support the body weight on one leg when the other leg is withdrawn in a flexor response.

Muscles that are antagonistic often work cooperatively (synergistically). Standing is an example of such cooperation, since it involves plurimuscular and synergistic muscular activity. Such smoothly coordianted muscular efforts depend on local proprioceptive reflexes in active muscle and central integration and distribution of afferent nerve impulses.

Each afferent nerve has a variety of reflex actions that may be obscured by its dominant response (*concealed reflex*). Simultaneous stimulation of two portions of the same nerve may result in two different responses. One may elicit *reflex reversal* by altering the stimulus strength, administering strychnine or chloroform, changing the original postural status, or constantly applying the same stimulus intensity to a muscle. One example of this mechanism is evident when painful plantar stimulation, such as stepping on a pin, results in flexor excitation and extensor inhibition, whereas pressure applied to the plantar surface results in extensor activation.

When an intense stimulus causes all motor units to respond to a first volley, a reflex tetanus occurs. Through the phenomenon of *afterdischarge,* muscle contractions become smoother as muscular tension is maintained between major volleys.

Through *fractionation,* usually only one portion of the motor units reacts to a stimulus even when the reflex requirement is maximal. Because of this partial response, other motor units remain available for response to subsequent incoming messages. This mechanism also facilitates *convergence*. Overlapping of reflex centers causes impulses traveling through various afferent nerves not to have arithmetical increases in muscle response through the process of *occlusion,* which is described as the ability of more powerful reflexes to occlude weaker reflexes and the possible ability of weaker reflexes to occlude certain others. Fatigue and some toxins may contribute to the process of occlusion.

*Facilitation* is the process whereby two reflexes working harmoniously result in a response greater than either one could produce singly. This augmented response occurs because of their joint ability to activate extra motor units not adequately stimulated by one set of afferent impulses. Facilitation often masks the process of occlusion or distracts from it. Strychnine promotes reflex facilitation to a detrimental degree, since it negates normal inhibitory effects and usual reciprocal innervation of antagonistic muscles. Other varied stimuli are also known to affect facilitation. The process of facilitation may be overcome by an inhibitory volley from the reflex center in the spinal cord.

Another consideration that is important in discussing the factors related to reflex activities is summation. *Summation* refers to the various central interactions of converging stimuli inherent in the functions of the reflex center. In this process the reflex center grades the extent and intensity of stimuli and relays the message to the motor units. Thus while appropriate fire frequency is achieved in the effectors, more motor units may be recruited for response from the units uninvolved in the reception of the initial threshold stimulus. Once the maximal activation level for a motor unit

is attained, a small amount of energy is required to sustain motor unit response (Grimby et al., 1974).

A *natural rhythmical sequence* is evident in most reflex activity. Therefore one reflex is frequently the stimulus for subsequent activity. Stepping and scratching reflexes are good examples of this phenomenon. Although the stepping response is possibly rhythmical, it is mediated by a central spinal reflex act so that it may be facilitated by the extensor postural state without the aid of external sensory input.

In summary, muscle tonus, stretch reflex sensitivities, excessive discharges, and coordination of muscular activity involve a complex segmental relationship of negative feedbacks and excitatory and inhibitory synaptic integration. Supraspinal structures influence this response of motor neurons by their interconnections at all levels of the spinal cord (Wilson, 1966; Merton, 1972).

REFLEX TYPES. The familiar reflex testing done as part of the neurological examination elicits *phasic stretch reflexes*. Slower stretching of the tendon results in the *static (tonic) stretch reflex*. The number of tension receptors stimulated, the degree of stretch, and the rate of discharge are determined by the rate of tendon stretch. Because of its greater intensity, the tendon jerk (phasic stretch reflex) disappears after the static stretch reflex under anesthesia. Specific reflex testing and interpretation are detailed further in Chapter 11.

When the stretch reflex is partially or completely absent because of a cumulative inhibitory effect, it is termed a *clasp-knife response*. In the clasp-knife response any amount of flexion is possible after resistance in the extensor muscles gives way. This response is evident in children with cerebral palsy.

Another response that characterizes reflexes is *Philippson's reflex*. In this instance, after a client consciously inhibits one knee extensor, the opposite knee extensor has an associated excitatory response. Static tension is developed as the individual maintains the shortened muscle in its taut position.

The fundamental unit of the stretch reflex is the fusiform capsule encasing from 2 to 10 muscle cells, or intrafusal fibers. This muscle spindle is connected to surrounding muscle spindles (extrafusal fibers) by connective tissue.

Three major nerve fibers are involved in the

functional operations of the intrafusal and extra-fusal fibers. The first two types, primary afferent fibers and gamma efferent fibers, penetrate the spindle. The third type, alpha efferent fibers, innervates extrafusal muscle (Fig. 3-21).

*Primary afferent fibers,* with a diameter of 8 to 12 $\mu$m, are distributed along the central portion of the spindle. These afferent fibers undergo degenerative changes when certain dorsal spinal roots are transected.

*Gamma efferent (fusimotor) fibers* terminate in the end plates on contractile polar areas of the spindle. These fibers are 3 to 7 $\mu$m in diameter. Other small vessels enter the spindle to innervate its vasculature.

*Alpha efferent fibers* have a large diameter and innervate extrafusal muscle fibers.

Operationally, the response mechanism is activated when the muscle is pulled down. This movement causes the central primary afferent fibers to become mobilized. From these endings, impulses are emitted to the spinal cord, which activates alpha efferent fibers and causes the extrafusal muscle fibers to contract. Contraction of extrafusal fibers reduces intrafusal tension and restores equilibrium.

When a stretch receptor is placed under a constant source of tension, there is a regular, rhythmical discharge of impulses to ensure a consistent level of tonic activity in the muscle. One example of this is the maintenance of normal mouth closure. Gravity tends to force the lower jaw to drop down, but proprioceptive impulses from the masseter and temporal muscles maintain a constant tonic state,

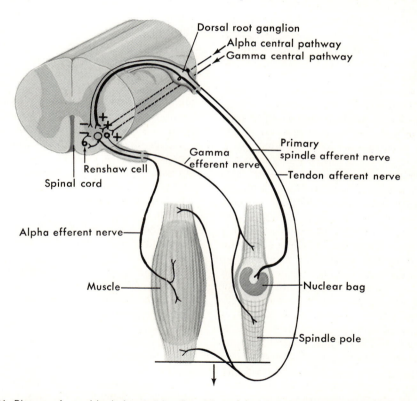

**FIG. 3-21.** Diagram of neural basis for stretch reflex. Afferent fibers from muscle spindle and tendon organs and efferent fibers to muscle and spindle (gamma fibers) are shown. Excitation is indicated by *plus signs,* inhibition by *minus signs.* Renshaw cell is interneuron that provides recurrent inhibition to active motor neuron pool. Muscle rigidly fixed at upper end and subject to stretch in direction of *arrow* at lower end. (From Schottelius, B.A., and Schottelius, D.D.: Textbook of physiology, ed. 18, St. Louis, 1978, The C.V. Mosby Co.)

so that the mouth remains closed in its position of rest. The regular firing of stretch receptors in a rhythmical pattern under tension is more accelerated during the initiation of stretch and more constant afterward to maintain a regular rate of stretch even for a prolonged period. In laboratory situations where this phenomenon is demonstrated by stimulation of a frog leg, mechanical graphs show an initial firing burst at a high frequency and a more even level of muscle activity as stretch is maintained until the demands for stretch have ended. Various muscle spindles have different thresholds of stretch stimulation, so that variable levels of discharge frequencies are required to achieve an intensity that exceeds threshold levels for a given spindle. When a given frequency and number of responsive spindles answer the call to activation, the overall result is as graded contraction of muscle in accordance with the motivating stimulus.

At the distal ends of muscles are fibrous capsules that house one or two fibers of large diameter known as *tendon afferent fibers*. These tendon afferent fibers, with their termination in fibrous capsules, are the *Golgi tendon organs* (tendon end organs) (Schoultz et al., 1974). When stretch affects a muscle, the tendon organs are displaced so that action potentials are realized in the afferent nerve. Because the Golgi tendon organs are activated when the extrafusal fibers are in operation, both passive stretch and active contraction in a muscle cause a response in tendons. One difference in tendons and muscles is that Golgi tendon organs have a threshold that may exceed that in muscle spindles by 200 to 300 times. The firing rate in the tendon increases proportionally as the intensity of stretch exceeds the threshold for a tendon. Because the tendon afferent fiber has an inhibitory effect on the alpha motor neuron in the spinal medulla where it terminates, strong muscle movements in the form of passive stretch or active contractions result in autoinhibition of a muscle's reflex stretch response. This mechanism serves as a protective feature, since it provides an avenue of tendon end-organ feedback, which regulates the amount of active muscle contraction that can be maintained.

Whenever incoming stimuli bombard the ventral root in a strong, consecutive pattern, contraction of the muscle does not diminish spindle firing. In-

stead the firing power of the spindle may increase. The gamma efferent system is partially responsible for this phenomenon. Impulses coursing through the gamma efferent system affect the polar regions of the spindle and cause them to shorten. Since the intrafusal fibers are in a stable position in relation to the extrafusal fibers, shortening in the polar areas moves in the direction opposite the nuclear bag. The subsequent stimulation of the primary endings through this distortion augments the firing rate of the receptor. However, the maximum tension level is relatively unaffected by contraction of the intrafusal fibers because they do not relay tension to their ends. Yet the gamma system has significance because it controls sensitivity of the spindle by resetting the activity level in the primary endings in relation to the extrafusal fiber length.

The capacity of the gamma efferent fibers to adjust muscles and stabilize them at new lengths is believed by some investigators to explain the plasticity of muscular responses. Central coordination of this process is achieved by tracts located at the midline of the gray matter in the spinal medulla. These tracts, composed of complex propriospinal pathways, are functionally similar to the reticular formation in the brainstem.

The gamma efferent fibers control the deep tendon reflexes, spasticity, and rigidity but not strength. A total block of the fusimotor system does not change proprioception, since this capacity is independent of muscle efferent fibers but dependent on afferent input from joints, ligaments, light touch, and vibration. When this block is effected, investigators have noted dramatic changes in pain and temperature sensibility.

Reflex patterns are also modified by the gamma system. In tracing the course of impulses in the crossed extension reflex (presented earlier in this chapter), one appreciates their role. In this instance, afferent fibers from the ipsilateral extremity are subjected to noxious stimuli and activate contralateral extensor alpha motor neurons and the gamma system in extensor muscles. The activation of the gamma system in the contralateral limb serves to reinforce the extensor response.

*Renshaw cells* complement the tendon receptors by contributing to inhibitory effects. Renshaw cells, interneurons located in the ventral horns, synapse with many alpha motor neurons. Their function is to inhibit motor neurons at the same segmental level. This negative feedback, or dampening mechanism, augments activities in proportion to the increases in motor neuron activities. This effect, known as *recurrent inhibition,* is directly related to the intensity of activity occurring in the motor neurons. Although this recurrent inhibition is poorly understood in relation to normal reflex activity, it is known to have an anticonvulsant effect.

*Tonus* may be described as resistance to passive stretch. The myotatic, or stretch, reflex is an essential part of muscle tone. The gamma efferent fiber is the specific arm controlling length and tension of the intrafusal fiber, so that the threshold of the spindle may be established. This threshold may also be termed *passive stretch*. To make essential, ongoing adjustments, gamma efferent fibers remain responsive to facilitatory stimuli from cutaneous and brainstem sources and inhibitory input from tendon receptors.

**DISTURBANCES IN REFLEX STATUS.** When an interruption of motor functions occurs, a determination of the level of disturbance (the upper or the lower motor neuron) is made. If the interruption is caused by a lesion in the central portion of the lateral column, the corticospinal fibers are affected, and the problem is identified as an upper motor neuron disturbance. When the paresis or paralysis is secondary to a disturbance in the anterior horns or roots, spinomuscular fibers are affected, and the disorder is a lower motor neuron problem. Sometimes the lesion affects both the lateral column and the anterior horns or roots.

When a local spinal cord lesion alters peripheral functions, a change in sensibility or reflexes may occur. The identification of cutaneous changes through evaluation of the dermatomes has already been presented as an assessment parameter. If the lesion interferes with the operation of a reflex arc, changes in reflex status occur in accordance with the disturbance. Table 3-2 summarizes common deep and superficial reflexes, points of stimulation, expected results, and involved segments.

Since superficial reflexes have a superimposed cortical pathway, they are of limited value in localizing the level of an upper or lower motor neuron disturbance. In contrast, the deep tendon re-

flexes are elicited by percussion of the muscle tendon or periosteum and are mediated only through the spinal arc. Deep reflexes are more valuable in localizing the level of a spinal cord lesion. When the neurological assessment reveals any abnormality, including asymmetrical, diminished, increased, or absent reflexes, findings are compared to other portions of the examination, and a specialist is informed of the disturbances (Chusid and McDonald, 1979).

A disturbance in function of the pyramidal tract results in several clinical symptoms, including spasticity, reflex changes, clonus, appearance of latent reflexes, associated movements, muscle atrophy, and chronic impairment in circulation. Spasticity is evident in affected muscles by increased tone, increased resistance at the beginning of passive movement in the flexor muscles of the arm, and increased resistance to passive range of motion in the extensor muscles of the legs. On percussion with the reflex hammer, spastic muscles respond by being more irritable than other muscles. Because of the increase in muscle tension, the deep reflexes associated with involved muscles are augmented.

In assessing the deep reflexes, the practitioner should be careful to keep the client's head in the midline, forward position and to avoid strong, sustained contractions of other muscles, since the pyramidal overflow required to sustain contractions results in a diminished pyramidal influence at the site of the reflex are being tested. Faulty positioning may cause the deep reflex at the muscle being assessed to appear increased, giving a false impression of pyramidal tract disease.

In patients in whom pyramidal tract lesions are present, crossed reflexes (described earlier in this chapter) are elicited. The presence of an obvious response in the contralateral limb during testing is abnormal after the crossed reflex of infancy has disappeared. Even though the superficial reflexes are not a definitive means of identifying a pyramidal tract lesion, disturbances in these reflexes may be apparent in the presence of a pyramidal tract lesion. Changes may indicate that the reflexes are diminished, absent, or unaffected.

The pyramidal tract is quite sensitive to pressure. Thus lesions impinging on it result in the early appearance of dorsiflexion of the great toe.

**TABLE 3-2.** Deep and superficial reflexes*

| Reflexes | | Stimulus | Normal results | Involved segment |
|---|---|---|---|---|
| **Deep** | **Superficial** | | | |
| Biceps muscle | — | Tap biceps tendon. | Forearm flexes at elbow. | C5-C6 |
| Forearm pronator muscles | — | Tap palmar side of forearm medial to styloid process of radius. | Forearm pronates. | C6 |
| Triceps muscle | — | Tap triceps tendon. | Forearm extends at elbow. | C6-C7 |
| Brachioradial muscle | — | While holding forearm in semi-pronated position, tap styloid process. | Forearm flexes at elbow. | C7-C8 |
| Finger (flexion) | — | Tap palm at tip of fingers. | Fingers flex. | C7-T1 |
| Abdominal muscles | — | Tap inferior thorax, abdominal wall, and symphysis pubis. | Abdominal wall contracts: leg adducts when symphysis pubis is tapped. | T8-T12 |
| — | Abdominal muscles | Stroke upper, middle, and lower skin on abdomen. | Abdominal muscles contract with retraction of umbilicus toward stimulated side. | T8-T12 |
| — | Cremasteric muscle | Stroke medial upper leg in adductor region. | Testicles move up. | L1-L2 |
| Adductor muscle | — | Tap medial condyle of tibia. | Leg adducts. | L2-L4 |
| Quadriceps muscle (knee jerk) | — | Tap tendon of quadriceps femoris muscle. | Lower leg extends. | L2-L4 |
| Triceps surae muscle (ankle jerk) | — | Tap Achilles tendon. | Plantar flexion of foot occurs. | L5-S2 |
| — | Plantar area | Stroke lateral side on sole of foot. | Plantar flexion of toes occurs. | S1-S2 |

*From Conway, B.L.: Pediatric neurologic nursing, St. Louis, 1977, The C.V. Mosby Co.

Since dorsiflexion of the great toe depends on the extensor hallucis longus, innervated by L4 and L5, disturbances beneath this level of the spinal medulla do not result in the presence of the extensor toe response. The extensor toe response, or *Babinski toe sign,* often occurs simultaneously with the flexion withdrawal reflex of the lower limb (described earlier in this chapter). Dorsiflexion of the great toe may be elicited by the application of a stimulus in the traditional way, that is, by applying a firm stroke to the lateral aspect of the plantar surface of the foot, by wide extension of the little toe, or by squeezing pressure applied to the Achilles tendon. A positive Babinski sign in clients more than 2 years of age consists of responsive dorsiflexion of the great toe with or without associated movements or fanning of the other toes on the ipsilateral foot.

When hyperreflexia exists, clonus may often be demonstrated. *Clonus* is elicited as the practitioner rapidly dorsiflexes the foot to maintain pressure and added tension to the gastrocnemius muscle. The result is a rhythmic seesaw motion of the foot being stimulated.

Several latent reflexes may be demonstrated when a lesion of the pyramidal tract is present. These reflexes are significant only if they are quite exaggerated or if they are evident on only one side. They include Wartenberg's sign, Hoffmann's sign, Mendel-Bekhterev's reflex, Rossolimo's reflex, and the snout reflex.

*Wartenberg's sign* is elicited as the practitioner places the index finger across the client's supinated, lightly flexed four fingers and taps the client's fingers lightly with a reflex hammer. When a pathological condition exists, the response is flexion of the four fingers and of the distal segment of the patient's thumb.

*Hoffmann's sign* is elicited by percussion of the distal end of the radius with a reflex hammer; clients with neurological disturbances respond by flexing the fingers and thumb.

To elicit *Mendel-Bekhterev's reflex* the examiner percusses the lateral area of the dorsum of the patient's foot and notes the pathological toe flexor response. This sign is a latent deep plantar muscle reflex.

*Rossolimo's reflex* is elicited as the examiner percusses the pulps of the client's toes. A resulting response of turned-up toes with subsequent stretching of the toe flexors and flexion of the toes is positive for this sign.

The *snout reflex* is elicited by light tapping of the closed lips in the midline. When a disturbance in the pyramidal innervation of the facial muscles exists, the individual responds by pursing the lips.

All voluntary movements have concomitant associated movements. For example, when a person makes a fist with the hand, dorsiflexion of the hand also occurs. When pathological changes exist in the pyramidal tract, certain associated movements have been identified as signs accompanying these problems. The major associated movements include the tibialis sign of Strumpell, trunk-thigh sign of Babinski, Wartenberg's sign, and interosseous phenomenon of Souques.

To elicit the *tibialis sign of Strümpell* the practitioner asks the person to lie in a supine position with legs extended. The examiner places a hand on the person's knee and applies resistance as the person lifts the leg. In normal individuals the foot assumes a position of plantar flexion, but in individuals with pathological conditions the foot appears dorsiflexed and supinated during this test. The anterior titialis muscles also appear prominent.

To elicit the *trunk-thigh sign of Babinski,* one asks the person to lie in a supine position with legs extended and abducted and arms folded across the chest. Without the use of the arms, the person is asked to pull up to a sitting position. This sitting-up exercise should be accomplished without the aid of associated movements in the arms and legs. In persons with pathological conditions of the pyramidal tract the attempts to rise to a sitting position are accompanied by flexion of the affected thigh and trunk and involuntary elevation of the leg and heel. When the lesion involves both sides of the pyramidal tract, both legs rise as this test is being performed.

Another method for eliciting this sign occurs as the examiner assesses the presence of *Wartenberg's sign* by asking the person to bend the four fingers of the hand to counter the resistance offered as the examiner pulls the fingers in the opposite direction. In normal individuals the thumb remains in abduction and extension during this exercise. In persons with pathological conditions the thumb adducts, flexes, and opposes the fingers.

The *interosseous phenomenon of Souques* is evaluated as the patient elevates and extends the involved upper extremity. When a neurological disturbance exists, the fingers simultaneously hyperextend and spread involuntarily. In normal individuals this response is not evident.

Some muscle atrophy from disuse of muscles may also be evident when spasticity is present as a result of a pyramidal tract lesion.

Disturbances in circulatory function or impaired pilomotor activities should be noted with the time of onset and the extent of involvement. Generally lesions at the level of the spinal medulla result in vasomotor impairments more frequently than lesions in other portions of the central nervous system.

**Pyramidal tract disorders.** Several conditions have been identified as disorders that predominantly affect normal functions of the pyramidal tract. A prolapsed intervertebral disc may also interfere with pyramidal tract operations by exerting traction on the lateral portion of the cord through stretching of the related dentate ligaments. When multiple sclerosis affects only the pyramidal tract, the client may have an early complaint of stiffness in the limbs. The spastic syndrome may also occur when primary lateral sclerosis interferes with pyramidal tract operations bilaterally unless amyotrophic lateral sclerosis also develops. The cortical tract may also be selectively impaired by Strümpell-Lorrain's familial spastic paraplegia.

**Disturbed operations of the anterior horn.** When paralysis of the muscles results from an anterior horn lesion, the initial paralysis is complete. However, after a period of time some degree of function returns in those muscles supplied by fibers from anterior horn cells that did not suffer direct impairment. In most cases a lesion in the anterior horn does not affect all the muscles in an extremity. The reasons for this are twofold. First, the anterior horn cells at a given level are located in groups covering a wide area, so that each cell grouping innervates different muscles. No lesion is generally expansive enough to interfere with all these cell groups. Second, even when a lesion has a large diameter, it is seldom large enough longitudinally to affect the cell groups, which may be spaced a few centimeters apart.

Some disease entities—notably hereditary spinal muscular atrophy (Werdnig-Hoffmann disease), Japanese B encephalitis, and poliomyelitis—are clear-cut examples of conditions causing peripheral paralysis. In these examples the anterior horn is impaired, whereas the adjacent pyramidal tracts remain uncompromised.

When flaccid paralysis exists, there is a deficiency in voluntary movement because of the decreased availability of motor units for response. The affected muscles lack tone, since their nerve supply, essential to muscle tension, is inadequate. This lack of tone may be noted by the practitioner as absence of normal irritability in response to direct mechanical stimulation. Other signs that confirm the presence of muscle atonia include laxity of joint movement from lack of muscle support, facility of joint hyperextension by passive maneuvers, diminished resistance to passive movement, and ability to place extremities in abnormal postures.

Because of the interference with impulses in the centrifugal limb of the spinal reflex arc, there is a cessation of reflexes. Anterior horn lesions are also noted for their ability to leave the pyramidal tract reflexes undisturbed. For example, reflexes such as the Babinski (mentioned in the previous section) do not seem abnormal when tested. There is also a lack of the pathological associated movements accompanying lesions of the pyramidal tract, since these movements are possible only when the lower motor neuron is intact. Unlike lesions of the pyramidal tract, lesions in the anterior horn have a profound effect on vasomotor responses. The rationale for this vasomotor disturbance is that sympathetic cells regulating vasomotor functions are more densely congregated in the gray matter of the cord than in the lateral column.

After the muscle weakness in paralysis secondary to interrupted functions of the anterior horn cells, there is a somewhat immediate response in the form of muscle atrophy, fasciculation, and degeneration reactions.

In some disorders both the pyramidal tract and the anterior horn cells are affected. An example of this type of disturbance is amyotrophic lateral sclerosis.

## EVALUATION OF MOTOR SYSTEM

Although a detailed comparison of upper and lower motor neurons is presented in Chapters 15 and 17, it seems timely to mention the importance of motor functions of this point, since their functional integrity is vital to normal motor output.

The components that are important in assessment of the motor system include muscle size, tone, and strength and the presence or absence of involuntary movements.

Muscle size may be evaluated accurately by comparison of both arms, calves, and thighs with a tape measure. Observation for missing muscles, estimations of muscle bulk, and determination of nutritional status may be made concurrently.

Muscle tone is assessed as the practitioner notes posture and adequacy of movement during normal activity and relates these observations to appropriate capacities for both developmental and chronological age. Additional information may be gleaned as the practitioner observes the client in such motor activities as walking, running, and hopping. Observations that should be made during these activities include notations about excessive arm swing, asymmetrical characteristics, clumsiness, and the use of muscles not ordinarily required by the activity.

Muscle strength is assessed as the practitioner moves all joints through the full range of motion with and without resistance. Muscle weakness or asymmetrical muscle power in corresponding muscles requires referral to a specialist for further evaluation.

Because the condition of some clients makes them unable to cooperate in neurological assessment, special techniques are necessary to estimate the degree of muscle strength. Muscle power may be evaluated as the client is observed in manipulating everyday objects or objects the examiner has deliberately handed to the client. One may assess the strength of the shoulder girdle by asking the client to resist force placed on the shoulder through pushing the shoulders upward. The muscles of the pelvic girdle and proximal lower extremities may be evaluated as the practitioner observes the client climbing steps or rising to a stance from a supine position. In step climbing a rotary motion of the legs indicates muscle weakness. Undue assistance in using objects for support or in rising by climbing up the legs with the hands may also indicate muscle weakness.

Involuntary movements such as dystonic twistings; jerky, irregular movements; muscle contractions; tics; and tremors should be noted. In describing such movements as tremors one should notice whether rest or intentional activity aggravates the tremor. Wasting and fasciculations should also be noted because they indicate the possibility of a lower motor neuron problem and the need for additional neurological assessment.

## RELATED FACTORS

Since no part of the neurological system operates as a discrete entity, one should be careful to consider all components of the neurological assessment, as outlined in Chapters 11 and 15, before making a definitive conclusion as to the nature or source of a problem. Although certain interferences with motor functions might well be local problems, the involved structures are subjected to influences from higher levels as well. At times an individual may seem to be physiologically intact but still unable to function normally because of environmental or psychosocial factors. In assessing the total functional capacity of the individual one should be aware of all the resources and limitations in the perceptual world of that client. Not only do these factors have bearing on immediate functional capacities, but also they may influence the outcome of efforts geared toward the prevention of problems or rehabilitation efforts after acute disturbances.

## REFERENCES

Anthony, C.P., and Kolthoff, N.J.: Textbook of anatomy and physiology, ed. 9, St. Louis, 1978, The C.V. Mosby Co.

Benton, A.L.: The 'minor' hemisphere, J. of Hist. Med., **27:**5, 1972.

Bolin, R.H.: Sensory deprivation: an overview, Nurs. Forum **13**(3):240, 1974.

Cain, D.P.: Kindling in sensory systems: thalamus, Exp. Neurol. **66:**319, 1979.

Calne, D.B., and Pallis, C.A.: Vibratory sense: a critical review, Brain **89:**723, 1966.

Chusid, J.G., and McDonald, J.J.: Correlative and functional neurology, ed. 17, Los Altos, Calif., 1979, Lange Medical Publications.

Conway, B.L., and McCabe, S.: Isolation: an historic critique. Unpublished paper, 1968.

Cook, A.W., and Browder, E.J.: Functions of the posterior columns in man, Arch. Neurol. **12:**72, 1965.

Dimond, S.: Neuropsychology: a textbook of the human brain, Sevenoaks, Kent, Eng., 1980, Butterworth & Co. (Publishers), Ltd.

Dimond, S.J., and Beaumont, J.G., editors: Hemisphere function in the human brain, New York, 1974, John Wiley & Sons, Inc.

DiPalma, J.R.: Drug therapy today: cholinergic and anticholinergic drugs, RN **37:**83, May 1974.

Eccles, J.C.: The physiology of nerve cells, Baltimore, 1957, The Johns Hopkins University Press.

Evarts, E.V.: Brain mechanisms in movement, Sci. Am. **209:**96, July 1973.

Fennell, E., Satz, P., and Wise, R.: Laterality differences in the perception of pressure, J. Neurol. Neurosurg. Psychiatry **30:**337, 1967.

Foerster, O.: The dermatomes in man, Brain **56:**1, 1933.

Fortuyn, J.D.: On the neurology of perception, Clin. Neurol. Neurosurg. **82**(2):97, 1979.

Gazzaniga, M.S.: The bisected brain, New York, 1970, Appleton-Century-Crofts.

Gilman, S., and Denny-Brown, D.: Disorders of movement and behavior following dorsal column lesions, Brain **89:**397, 1966.

Glencross, D.J., and Koreman, M.M.: The processing of proprioceptive signals, Neuropsychologia **17:**683, 1979.

Goodman, L.S., and Gilman, A.: The pharmacological basis of therapeutics, ed. 6, New York, 1980, Macmillan Publishing Co., Inc.

Grabow, J.D., et al.: Cerebellar stimulation for the control of seizures, Mayo Clin. Proc. **49:**759, Oct. 1974.

Granit, R.: The basis of motor control, New York, 1970, Academic Press, Inc.

Grimby, L., et al.: Differences in recruitment order and discharge pattern of motor units in the early and late flexion reflex components in man, Acta Physiol. Scand. **90:**555, March 1974.

Hamberger, A., et al.: Glutamate as a CNS transmitter. I. Evaluation of glucose and glutamine as precursors for the synthesis of preferentially released glutamate, Brain Res. **168:**513, 1979.

Hamberger, A., et al.: Glutamate as a CNS transmitter. II. Regulation of synthesis in the releasable pool, Brain Res. **168:**531, 1979.

Haymaker, W.: Bing's local diagnosis in neurological diseases, St. Louis, 1969, The C.V. Mosby Co.

Head, H.: Studies in neurology, vol. 2, Oxford, 1920, Oxford University Press.

Hubbell, J.G.: P.O.W.: the American prisoner-of-war experience in Vietnam, Reader's Digest **650:**195, June 1976.

Iggo, A.: Cutaneous thermoreceptors in primates and subprimates, J. Physiol. (Lond.) **200:**403, 1969.

Iversen, L.L.: The chemistry of the brain, Sci. Am. **241:**134, Sept. 1979.

Keegan, J.J.: Dermatome hyperalgesia associated with herniation of intervertebral disc, Arch. Neurol. Psychiatry **50:**67, 1943.

Larson, C.B., and Gould, M.: Orthopaedic nursing, ed. 9, St. Louis, 1978, The C.V. Mosby Co.

Llinas, R.R.: The cortex of the cerebellum, Sci. Am. **232:**56, Jan. 1975.

McGeer, E.G., and Singh, E.A.: Inhibition of angiotensin converting enzyme by substance P, Neuroscience Letters **14:**105, 1979.

Melzack, R.: The puzzle of pain: revolution in theory and treatment, New York, 1973, Basic Books, Inc.

Merton, P.A.: How we control the contraction of our muscles, Sci. Am. **226:**30, May 1972.

Mountcastle, V.B., editor: Medical physiology, ed. 14, St. Louis, 1980, The C.V. Mosby Co.

Oist, C., et al.: The learning process for fine neuromuscular controls in skeletal muscles in man. VI. The relationship between the ability to control random and fine neuromuscular activity, Electromyogr. Clin. Neurophysiol. **13:**505, 1973.

Plaitakis, A., et al.: Thiamine deficiency: selective impairment of the cerebellar serotonergic system, Neurology **28:**691, July 1978.

Robertson, L.T., et al.: Morphological changes associated with chronic cerebellar stimulation in the human, J. Neurosurg. **51:**510, 1979.

Salter, R.B.: Textbook of disorders and injuries of the musculoskeletal system, Baltimore, 1970, The Williams & Wilkins Co.

Schottelius, B.A., and Schottelius, D.D.: Textbook of physiology, ed. 18, St. Louis, 1978, The C.V. Mosby Co.

Schoultz, T.W., et al.: Ultrastructural organization of the sensory fibers innervating the Golgi tendon organ, Anat. Rec. **179:**147, June 1974.

Sherrington, C.S.: The integrative action of the nervous system, ed. 2, New Haven, Conn., 1947, Yale University Press.

Sibley, W.A.: Polyneuritis, Med. Clin. North Am. **56:**1299, Nov. 1972.

Weinstein, S., and Sersen, E.A.: Tactile sensitivity as a function of handedness and laterality, J. Comp. Physiol. Psychol. **54:**665, 1961.

Wilson, V.J.: Inhibition in the central nervous system, Sci. Am. **214:**102, May 1966.

Willis, S.G., et al.: Cerebral processing of spatial and verbal-analytic tasks: an EEG study, Neuropsychologia **17:**473, 1978.

# 4

# AUTONOMIC NERVOUS SYSTEM— A SPECIAL CASE OF OUTPUT

The autonomic nervous system (visceral, involuntary) consists of the efferent neurons to smooth muscle, cardiac muscle, and glands of the viscera (effectors). Visceral responses are primarily on an involuntary, reflex, unconscious level. However, through the phenomenon of biofeedback (Chapter 10), experimental studies are showing that conscious control of visceral function is possible. Two major differences separate the autonomic and voluntary nervous systems. First, despite advances in biofeedback, the autonomic nervous system functions remain largely beyond volitional control in normal activity. Second, interference with a peripheral motor neuron of the somatic system results in impaired function, whereas severance of an autonomic nerve may not cause permanent functional impairment or atrophy of the involved organ. There are numerous connections between association cortex (especially areas 9 to 13 of the frontal lobe) and the thalamus and hypothalamus by which visceral reactions are elicited in response to emotions related to cultural, moral, and ethical values. Fear, rage, humiliation, love, ecstasy, hate, and other strong emotions certainly do cause a visceral response, and it is through these thalamocortical radiations that this influence is exerted on the hypothalamus and by way of the hypothalamus to the autonomic nervous system. Visceral reactions can occur in response to input (from exteroceptors and proprioceptors) over general sensory fibers of the cranial and spinal nerves and in response to special sensory impulses from cranial nerves I, II, VIII, VII, and IX, as well as to stimuli from baroceptors and chemoceptors in the viscera. There are no discrete input systems for the somatic and autonomic divisions of the nervous system. That is the reason why the autonomic nervous system is often considered an efferent system. From the central nervous system to the effector (smooth muscle, cardiac muscle, or gland) there are two neurons in the pathway so the second neuron must have its nerve cell body in a ganglion outside the central nervous system.

There are two divisions of the autonomic nervous system that may be contrasted according to function, neurotransmitter secreted by postganglionic fibers at the effector junctions, and anatomical placement of preganglionic neurons and ganglia. Most effector organs (except the sweat glands, arrector pili muscles of each hair follicle, most blood vessels, and the adrenal medulla) are innervated by both sympathetic and parasympathetic fibers. In the organs served through double innervation one fiber is inhibitory and the other facilitatory to achieve the balance required in that organ. Other structures may benefit from dual innervation as fibers of each category work to supply antagonistic muscles that complement each other to achieve functional integrity, for example, the filling and evacuation of the rectum. The autonomic nervous system also acts in a synchronous way with structures of the somatic system to adjust and support voluntary activity. The hypothalamus contains the upper motor neurons for both divisions of the autonomic nervous system. The nuclei for the integration of sympathic (thoracolumbar) output is in the posterior of the hypothalamus, and the nuclei for the parasympathetic (craniosacral) division output is in the anterior part. The sympathetic division has the nerve cell bodies of its preganglionic neurons in the lateral horns of the gray matter of the thoracic and upper lumbar segments of the spinal cord (therefore named "thoracolumbar"). Its postganglionic fibers have their nerve cell bodies in a chain of each 18 vertebral or lateral ganglia just lateral to the vertebral column (Figs. 2-5 and 2-6), or in three pairs of collateral ganglia in the abdominal cavity—the coelic, superior mesenteric, and inferior mesenteric. Only one preganglionic fiber of the sympathetic division does not synapse in a ganglion but goes directly to its effector, which is the adrenal medulla. This is an important link between nervous and endocrine function just as is the control of the pituitary gland by the hypothalamus. The neurotransmitter secreted by the sympathetic *post*ganglionic fibers at their effector junctions is *norepinephrine;* therefore they are said to be adrenergic.

By contrast the parasympathetic division has nerve cell bodies in the motor nuclei of cranial nerves III, VII, IX, X, and perhaps XI (with the greatest parasympathetic control coming over the vagus nerve to thoracic and upper abdominal viscera) as well as the lateral gray of some sacral segments of the spinal cord. The ganglia of the parasympathetic division of the autonomic nervous system lie near the viscera they innervate or actually within their walls. These postganglionic fibers secrete acetylcholine at their effector junctions and so are termed *"cholinergic" (muscarinic action)*. Remember that cholinergic fibers are widespread in the somatic nervous system as well. Acetylcholine is also the neurotransmitter in the *ganglia of both divisions* of the autonomic nervous system. Its effect at the somatic motor end plate and autonomic ganglia is termed *nicotinic action*.

## SYMPATHETIC GANGLION CONNECTIONS

Recall that autonomic preganglionic fibers are myelinated B fibers whereas postganglionic fibers are relatively unmyelinated C fibers or gray fibers (Table 2-1). Each spinal nerve in the thoracolumbar area is connected to its corresponding sympathetic ganglion by a white ramus. Although there are three cervical sympathetic ganglia, a superior, a middle, and an inferior (the inferior forms a large ganglion in union with the first thoracic and is called the *stellate* ganglion), and one or two sacral ganglia in the lateral (vertebral) sympathetic chain, they do not communicate directly to the cord because there are preganglionic cells only in the thoracic and lumbar segments (Fig. 2-6). Only these segments (thoracolumbar) have *white rami communicantes* formed by preganglionic fibers. Communication up and down the chain is possible through branching and connecting neurons. Post-

**TABLE 4-1.** Functions of the autonomic nervous system

| Organ | Sympathetic | Parasympathetic |
|---|---|---|
| Heart | Accelerates | Retards |
| Iris | Dilates pupils | Constricts pupils |
| Bronchi | Dilates | Constricts |
| Gastrointestinal peristalsis | Inhibits | Stimulates |
| Gastrointestinal secretion | Inhibits | Stimulates |
| Bladder emptying | Inhibits | Stimulates |
| Internal urinary sphincter | Constricts | Relaxes |
| Gastrointestinal sphincters | Constricts | Relaxes |
| Salivary secretion | Causes viscid flow | Causes watery flow |
| Suprarenal secretion | Stimulates | Inhibits |
| Coronary arteries | Dilates passively | Little effect |
| Helicine arteries | Constricts | Dilates |
| All other arteries | Constricts | Little or no effect |
| Sweat glands | Stimulates | No supply |
| Pilomotor and dartos muscles | Stimulates | No supply |

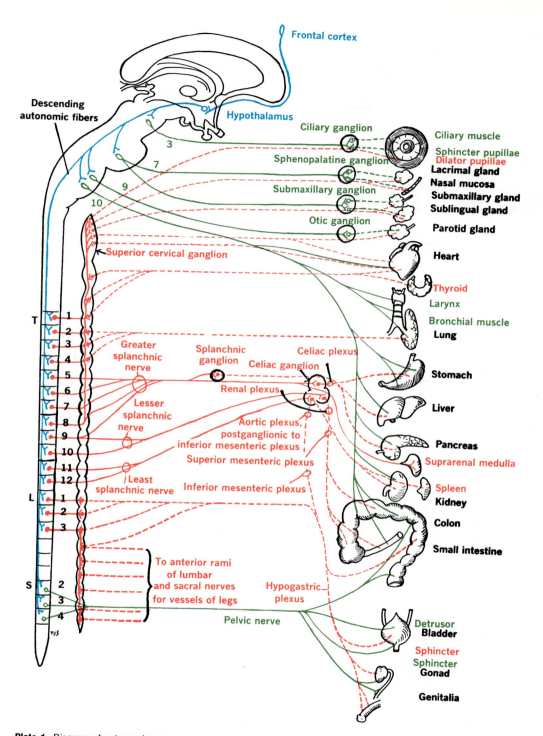

**Plate 1.** Diagram of autonomic nervous system. *Continuous lines,* Preganglionic fibers; *broken lines,* post-ganglionic fibers; *red,* sympathetic components; *green,* parasympathetic; *blue,* central connections. (After A. Brazier Howell; from Mettler, F.A.: Neuroanatomy, ed. 2, St. Louis, 1948, The C.V. Mosby Co.)

ganglionic fibers to the smooth muscle structures at the surface of the body (sweat glands, blood vessels, and arrector pili muscles) are distributed by the spinal nerve branches. Therefore each of the 31 pairs of spinal nerves receive *gray rami communicantes* (unmyelinated C fibers) from the sympathetic chain. Structurally, preganglionic fibers of the sympathetic division are short (from cord to chain—white rami), and postganglionic fibers are relatively long (from chain to viscera). Since there are only three sympathetic cervical ganglia and eight cervical spinal nerves, several gray rami branch from each cervical ganglion to the cervical spinal nerves. This is also true in the sacral region. In the lower thoracic area preganglionic fibers course through the chain without synapse and form the splanchnic visceral nerves, which travel to the collateral ganglia in the abdomen (coeliac, superior mesenteric, and inferior mesenteric). Postganglionic neurons then branch to abdominal viscera through corresponding plexuses. Only the preganglionic neuron to the adrenal medulla does not synapse along the way as already described.

It is through the interconnections made possible by the chain that the sympathetic system is able to effect such a diffuse response during times of threat, to prepare the body to meet an emergency. At such times the normal functioning mediated through the discrete homeostatic feedback loops of the parasympathetic division of the autonomic nervous system are overridden. The unique anatomical feature of the direct connection of the sympathetic preganglionic fiber to the adrenal medulla causing secretion of the hormone epinephrine into the bloodstream augments and prolongs the sympathetic response.

## PARASYMPATHETIC GANGLIA

In contrast to sympathetic ganglia, parasympathetic ganglia have long preganglionic fibers and short postganglionic fibers that are located on or adjacent to the organs innervated. The parasympathetic, or craniosacral, division derives its name from its cells of origin in the brainstem and sacral segments of the spinal cord. Unlike the postganglionic fibers of the sympathetic system, the parasympathetic postganglionic fibers course only a short distance to innervate a single or-

gan. Thus impulses through the parasympathetic division of the nervous system effect a local response.

A detailed discussion of the pharmacological action of acetylcholine, the neurotransmitter of cholinergic fibers, is contained in Chapter 3. A detailed account of norepinephrine, the neurotransmitter of postganglionic sympathetic adrenergic fibers is presented in the following discussion of stress. In addition, some of the drugs that specifically stimulate the sympathetic division are epinephrine, amphetamine sulfate, cocaine, ephedrine, and phenylephrine; ergonovine in large doses depresses it. Those that stimulate the parasympathetic division are acetylcholine, methacholine, neostigmine, physostigmine, and pilocarpine; atropine and its derivatives depress it.

Plate 1 (p. 118) contrasts the anatomical and pharmacological differences. Table 4-1 contrasts functional differences between the two divisions of the autonomic nervous system.

## STRESS

Physical and psychological responses to stress may not have a definitive sequential correlation. For example, when an individual fractures a femur in an automobile accident, the stages of psychological stress may not correspond to the physical processes of catabolism and anabolism. Thus although bony callus is successfully laid down and anabolism is occurring, the individual may still be experiencing extreme psychic stress that seems unrelated phasically to the positive physical changes.

Stress is in the eye of the beholder. Thus an event that results in extreme stress for one individual may not elicit the stress response in another person. Such individual differences are assigned to the personal variations in perceptual worlds. Events are perceived in the context of self in relation to past and current experiences and future expectations.

Living implies some stress. The volitional obligations of living necessitate some stress for the learning of behavioral patterns inherent in coping with the complexity of life.

Stimulus novelty affects response. The first time you speed in a race car you might experience extreme stress. As you become more familiar with the feeling of speed, the dangers, and the skills essential to safety, varying degrees of pituitary-adrenal response are noted.

Stress manifestations differ among individuals. The perception of the stressor and one's interpretation of stress affect the disruption in homeostasis that an event may have on an individual. Sociocultural and family styles may cause the individual's response to stress to vary. Individual differences may also result in variances of autonomic activity in different parts of the system. Thus stress in some individuals may cause ulcers or headaches, whereas others may experience diarrhea.

Because of the wide range in individual responses to stress, the practitioner needs to base therapeutic intervention on a thorough history and assessment of personal characteristics and capacities, developmental patterns, age-related needs and concerns, and familial-sociocultural influences. Moreover the practitioner needs to realize that therapeutic intervention, that is, electrolyte stabilization, intravenous fluid therapy, and administration of pharmacological agents, alters the manifestation of autonomic activity.

Selye's investigations of the pituitary-adrenal stress mechanism form the foundation for continuing study in stress. However, his original work is more currently viewed as dealing with an integral response involving psychological as well as physiological stressors. The operational mechanics of the adrenal-pituitary axis are shown in Fig. 4-1. The last step of the process, wherein adrenocorticotropic levels regulate corticotropin-releasing factor production, provides a cyclic biofeedback mechanism.

*Local response.* Local effector organs—smooth vascular muscle, fatty tissue, liver, heart, and brain—are affected in daily operations by the catecholamine norepinephrine. Understanding the mechanism affecting this local response is fundamental to understanding autonomic activity and the actions of many pharmacological agents.

Scientists have utilized advanced fluoroscopic techniques and electron microscopy to reveal outpouchings on a branched axon that look like varicosities and house neurotransmitters. These outpouchings (storage vesicles) measure about 50 nm in diameter and are believed to release their contents through cell membranes when chemical stimulation causes membrane depolarization. This process is similar to that affecting neurotransmitters at all synapses.

To understand the process of norepinephrine activity at the local level, it is important to review the process from production to reuptake. The following enzymatic reactions occur in the production of norepinephrine:

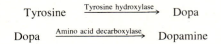

These reactions occur in the cytoplasm, but after dopamine is formed, it enters the storage vesicles to combine with the enzyme dopamine $\beta$-hydroxylase and become norepinephrine.

The same process occurs in the adrenal medulla. However, the adrenal medulla is the only structure capable of taking the process one step further so that the enzyme phenylethanolamine-$N$-methyltransferase acts on norepinephrine to form epinephrine.

Returning to norepinephrine distribution, after norepinephrine is discharged into the synapse from its storage vesicle either in the brain or the peripheral nervous system, it may be distributed in three major ways: (1) entry into the circulation to reach the liver, where it is metabolized through the activity of the enzymes catechol-$O$-methyltransferase (COMT) and monoamine oxidase (MAO); (2) metabolism in the effector organs by the same enzymes (COMT and MAO); and (3) release and reuptake by the storage vesicle. By far the greatest amount of norepinephrine is retrieved through the rapid and effective process known as reuptake. Through reuptake, catecholamine reserves are maintained, and amine-induced reactions are halted. Because the storage vesicle confuses like substances, it may fill with related endogenous (epinephrine, dopamine) or exogenous (amphetamines, metaraminol) substances. When filled, the storage vesicle disallows further reuptake, so that effects from circulating biogenic amines are potentiated. For the effects of these and other drugs in the cycle of catecholamines, refer to Table 4-2.

Detection of circulating catecholamines has also proved valuable in the diagnosis of such conditions as neuroblastoma, since this tumor elevates the urinary output of vanillylmandelic acid. The assessment of blood levels of circulating catechol-

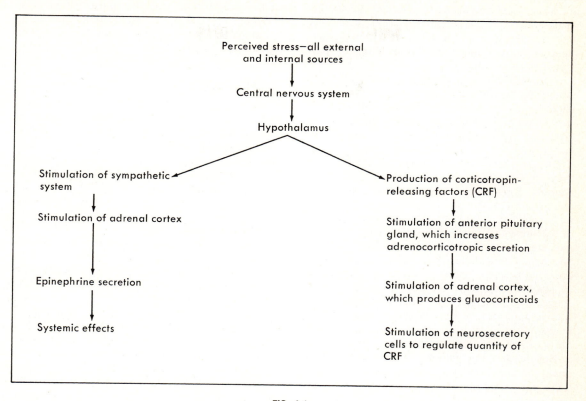

**FIG. 4-1**

**TABLE 4-2.** Adrenergic drugs*

| Drug | Effect | Resulting action | Therapeutic use |
|------|--------|------------------|-----------------|
| α-Methyl-p-tyrosine | Inhibits tyrosine from conversion to dopa | Decreases norepinephrine in tissues | Hypertension associated with pheochromocytoma |
| α-Methyldopa | Replaces norepinephrine in storage container | Works through central adrenergic processes | Hypertension |
| Disulfiram (Antabuse) | Inhibits dopamine-β-hydroxylase | Depletes tissue norepinephrine | Alcoholism |
| Cocaine | Prevents reuptake | Potentiates tissue norepinephrine effects | Local anesthetic |
| Imipramine, amphetamine, tricyclic antidepressants | Prevents reuptake | Potentiates effects of circulating biogenic amines | Psychological disorders |

*From Conway, B.L.: Pediatric neurologic nursing, St. Louis, 1977, The C.V. Mosby Co.

amines requires sophisticated technological assay methods. Unmetabolized amines may also be detected in the urine. Vanillylmandelic acid and 3-methoxy-4-hydroxyphenylglycol are metabolites of norepinephrine, whereas homovanillic acid and methoxytyramine are metabolites of dopamine. Research into the diagnostic implications of these metabolites continues.

***Catecholamine activity in the brain.*** The process of production, distribution, and reuptake, apparent in the peripheral nervous system, also occurs in the brain. However, because of the blood-brain barrier, catecholamines in the periphery are not utilized in the brain and vice versa.

Biogenic amines in the brain are contained in three types of neurons: (1) the noradrenergic neurons, found mainly in the pons and medulla oblongata; (2) the serotonergic neurons of the raphe nuclei; and (3) the dopaminergic neurons of the substantia nigra. Biogenic amine activity is indicated in assays of cerebrospinal fluid that contain vanillylmandelic, homovanillic, and 5-hydroxyindoleacetic acids. Therapeutic application of synthetic biogenic amines is in the pioneer stages. The door was opened as investigators utilized L-dopa to treat Parkinson's disease. Experiments continue as investigators attempt to excite the reticular activating system with products such as Sinemet (a combination of carbidopa and levodopa) in clients who are comatose and beyond treatment with conventional modalities. Other investigators are exploring the use of biogenic amines in the treatment of other conditions, including depression. The section on Parkinson's disease and Chapter 18 offer more data on the biogenic amines.

In reviewing the homeostatic cycle one notes that a stressor results in increased sympathetic nervous system activity, causing tyrosine to be converted to norepinephrine and epinephrine. When the stressor is overcome and sympathetic response is not required, the catecholamines are stockpiled in storage vesicles. The production of further catecholamines is self-regulated, since catecholamines have an inhibitory effect in proportion to available quantity of the enzyme tyrosine hydroxylase, which results in a proportional decrease in the synthesis of dopa from tyrosine. The activation or cessation of the generalized sympathetic response is controlled by adrenocorticotropin and other corticoids. The enzyme phenylethanolamine-*N*-methyltransferase is responsible for the conversion of norepinephrine to epinephrine. In contrast, peripheral conversion of tyrosine to norepinephrine is a dynamic, ongoing process integral to normal organ functions and is induced by stimulation of the sympathetic postganglionic nerves.

## VISCERAL FUNCTIONS

Several visceral functions—vasoconstriction and vasodilatation, sweat secretion, pilomotor response, pupillary response, urination, defecation, male sexual functions, and respiration—are regulated by autonomic control centers in the cord. Information on autonomic innervation of the heart is available in sources listed in the references. The relationships between the higher control centers of the brain and the hypothalamus have been documented in Chapters 2 and 3.

***Vasoconstriction and vasodilatation.*** Specific cells in the central and lateral anterior horn in the thoracic and upper lumbar region within the sympathetic nervous system regulate vasoconstriction through postganglionic fibers that connect with spinal nerves to influence activity in the blood vessels. When an interruption in vasomotor function occurs, as in the instance of spinal shock associated with acute cord transection, capacities for vasoconstriction are lost in large areas. Subsequently, a transient drop in blood pressure may become evident because of lack of tonic vasomotor impulses coursing from the medulla to the thoracolumbar cord, on to the sympathetic cells from T1 to L2, and then to the vasoconstrictor fibers, which leave the spinal cord through the anterior roots. Stabilization in blood pressure resumes when spinal sympathetic cells regain their capacities for independent functioning, causing smooth muscle in blood vessels to contract. Externally the practitioner notes that skin is at first red and warm and then cold and cyanotic because of the circulatory embarrassment resulting from disturbances in voluntary muscle contractions.

In the rehabilitation phase of management of paraplegics with lesions between T5 or T6 and L2, flushing may be used to determine bladder distention and to guide the patient in sexual functions. Bladder distention in these clients results in vasoconstriction in the lower limbs and adaptive vaso-dilatation above the level of the lesion, particularly in the fingers. A detailed account of assisting the paraplegic client with sexual functions is available in Chapter 6.

*Sweat secretion.* Sweat secretion, also termed *sudorific* or *diaphoretic function,* is influenced by cholinergic activity. However, sweat secretion is considered an independent function, as apparent in the paleness and clammy skin seen in fear. Vasodilatation increases sweat secretion, whereas vasoconstriction diminishes it. Five types of sweat secretion are commonly seen as outcomes of diaphoretic functions, including thermoregulatory sweating, emotional sweating, gustatory sweating, drug sweating, and spinal reflex sweating.

When an individual ingests hot liquids or salicylates, generalized *thermoregulatory sweating* may occur as a result of hypothalamic activity. Central processes affect sweating primarily of the face, hands, and feet in highly stimulating *emotional* situations. When individuals ingest spicy foods, a parasympathetic reflex of the face results in *gustatory sweating*. When sweating is related to pharmacological agents, the reaction is caused by either central or cholinergic nerve activity in accordance with involved *drug* action. Sweating that follows the pathway of sympathetic cholinergic fibers is termed *spinal reflex sweating*.

At times unusual sweat patterns have been correlated with underlying pathological conditions. However, the value of localizing pathological conditions by sweat patterns is much more limited than the use of sensory level determinations.

*Pilomotor response.* In thinking of superficial responses one often recalls the pilomotor reaction termed *gooseflesh*. This response represents an ipsilateral reflex to cold originating from the sympathetic cells of the thoracic region. Pilomotor fibers in the facial region travel the same pathway as the trigeminal nerve. The diagnostic value of the pilomotor response is somewhat limited in localizing a lesion.

*Pupillary response.* The corticomesencephalic area regulates pupil dilatation via descending fibers that course through the brainstem to the intermediolateral horns of the sympathetic nervous system at the C8 to T1 levels. Because of this mechanism, local or remote stimuli may result in pupil-lary dilatation. Secretion of the catecholamine epinephrine may also induce pupil dilatation in states of anxiety and pain.

The oculosensory and the ciliospinal are two important reflexes related to pupillary dilatation. Painful stimulation applied to the eye or its adnexa activates the oculosensory reflex, which consists of either pupillary constriction or dilatation, followed by constriction. The ciliospinal reflex is used to assess the functional integrity from the level of the brainstem to that of the mesencephalon. The assessment consists of pinching the skin on the neck to cause ipsilateral pupillary dilatation. This response is explained by the inhibition of the constrictor tonus mediated by parasympathetic fibers present in the third cranial nerve. The ciliospinal reflex is especially useful because it is not regulated by the sympathetic nervous system.

Whenever sympathetic innervation of the eye and neighboring areas is disrupted, Horner's syndrome is apparent. In this entity the sizes of the pupils are unequal, the affected pupil being the smallest; the eyelid droops slightly (ptosis); and sometimes the eyeball appears sunken into the orbit (enophthalmos).

*Urination.* Clients with neurological problems frequently have disturbances in urinary functions. A review of physiology is helpful in understanding how these interruptions occur. The process of urination requires parasympathetic impulses for involuntary control and input from the cerebrospinopudendal pathway for voluntary regulation. The sympathetic nervous system has a minimal effect on urination, but researchers continue to investigate possible influences on urethral functioning. The level of interrupted neuronal activity determines the type of disturbance in urinary function, which may include uninhibited neurogenic bladder, reflex (automatic) bladder, or autonomous neurogenic bladder. Also included are problems related to lesions in the cauda equina and posterior lumbar roots.

*Uninhibited neurogenic bladder* is seen in two groups of clients: the elderly and those with disease processes that interrupt suprasegmental impulses to a vital segment. This problem is evidenced by reduced bladder capacity, increased residual urine, and sudden premature emptying of the bladder.

When lesions interrupt cord functions above the sacral level, a *reflex (automatic) bladder* results. In instances of complete transection, bladder activity depends on the spinal reflex arc. Thus the mechanism for urination is stimulated when retention causes overflow incontinence and subsequent automatic, incomplete emptying of the bladder without dribbling. Bladder evacuation may then be completed by stimulation of the perineum, rectum, abdomen, or plantar aspect of the foot, because the reflex bladder functions as part of the mass reflex, which includes priapism and withdrawal of the foot on stimulation. When space-occupying lesions impinge on the cord above the sacral level, their presence may often be detected in early stages by interferences in bladder functions.

When lesions involve the cord at the sacral level, the urinary disorder is an *autonomous neurogenic bladder*. Since these lesions interrupt connections with the spinal cord, retention and overflow do not result in spontaneous emptying of the bladder. Paralysis or incontinence occurs. As a result, there is hypertrophy of the bladder wall and lack of the reflex emptying usually associated with the mass reflex.

Outcomes of *lesions in the cauda equina* include incontinence and possibly sciatica and weakness and numbness in the lower extremities. When the lesion interrupts motor connections but leaves sensory nerves intact, the result is sensory awareness of bladder filling or emptying, but paralysis of the detrusor muscle.

*Lesions in the posterior lumbar roots* are apparent in impaired afferent functions, resulting in the absence of the micturition reflex. Since the client is unaware of bladder status, dribbling incontinence, overdistended bladder walls, and stress incontinence may result. Urinary tract infections and renal calculi are particular problems for these patients; practitioners should be cognizant of these difficulties so that early preventive treatment may be initiated as necessary.

Urinary disturbances may be caused by a number of problems, including spinal cord trauma and space-occupying lesions. A common cause of such an interruption in children is meningomyelocele. Some 60% of the children affected with this myelodysplastic problem have some type of interference with urinary function, though the level and extent of the disturbance remains individual.

***Defecation.*** The sympathetic nervous system regulates rectal filling in the process of defecation. This mechanism operates as afferent impulses relay messages to the cerebrum to indicate filling. After the rectum is filled the cerebrum relays impulses through the lateral columns to signal anterior horn cells from T6 to T12 to contract abdominal musculature. Abdominal muscle activity greatly influences the effect on the rectum. Defecation moves to completion as the parasympathetic cells in segments S3 through S5 cause sigmoidal and rectal muscles to contract and the internal sphincter to relax.

When lesions impinge on the spinal cord above the sacral level, there is a loss of voluntary regulation of the anal sphincter and the feeling of associated fullness with subsequent fecal retention. This usually results in reflexive and spastic anal constriction. The practitioner may verify this spasticity by inserting a lubricated finger into the rectum. In cases of complete cord transection there is usually a total absence of reflex sphincter contraction. Involuntary defecation that occurs at widely spaced intervals is known as *reflex intermittent defecation*. When defecation control is interrupted by a nonneoplastic lesion of the hypothalamus, the reflex to defecate occurs only when high intrarectal pressure is attained. The effect on the defecation reflex is reversed when the lesion involves the tuber cinereum.

Lesions of the sacral cord result in permanent paralysis of the anal sphincter. In these instances the client has fecal incontinence even though retaining hard masses of feces. The degree of paralysis is related to the elasticity of the anal sphincter.

***Male sexual functions.*** For an overview of sexuality the reader is referred to Chapter 6. However, an explanation of the physiology of male sex functions at this point is of value as the practitioner reviews theoretical considerations basic to counseling. Acts of erection and ejaculation are regulated by the sympathetic and parasympathetic cord centers, with suprasegmental influences from the cerebrum and vasomotor centers of the medulla oblongata through the lateral columns. When cord transections occur above the sacral level, normal erections are still possible, even when suprasegmental impulses are blocked. If the problem in-

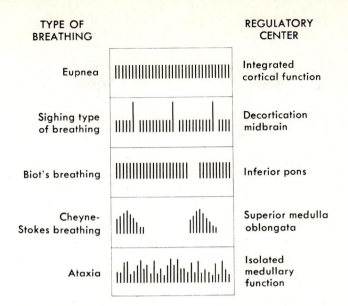

| TYPE OF BREATHING | | REGULATORY CENTER |
|---|---|---|
| Eupnea | | Integrated cortical function |
| Sighing type of breathing | | Decortication midbrain |
| Biot's breathing | | Inferior pons |
| Cheyne-Stokes breathing | | Superior medulla oblongata |
| Ataxia | | Isolated medullary function |

**FIG. 4-2.** Analysis of origin of periodic respiration. Several intermediary stages of periodic respiration characterized by slow rhythm of all-or-nothing type of breathing separate fully integrated respiration, in which all higher coordination centers participate, and nonintegrated, atactic respiration on medullary level. (From Koos, W.T., and Miller, M.H.: Intracranial tumors of infants and children, St. Louis, 1971, The C.V. Mosby Co.)

cludes suprasegmental lesions that partially interrupt cord functions or partial transections, a painful engorgement in the penis, termed *priapism,* results. Priapism may result from the slightest stimulation, since it is part of the mass reflex. Local stimulation may provoke the muscles into ejaculation or clonic contractures.

*Respiration.* Respiratory functions are influenced cranially by respiratory centers in the orbitofrontal cortex, hypothalamus, and midbrain tegmentum. Contemporary investigators believe the rhythmical breathing mechanism is regulated reciprocally through associated inspiratory and expiratory neurons in the brainstem. Two centers greatly affect this mechanism: the pneumotaxic and the apneustic centers. The *pneumotaxic center,* located in the tegmentum of the lateral pons, is the inhibiting center for respiration, whereas the *apneustic center,* found in the median and distal aspects of the pontile tegmentum, is the area exerting tonic influence on bulbar inspiration.

Interference with breathing patterns depends on the location of the lesion in the nervous system. Some common disorders in respiratory function are shown in Fig. 4-2. When the upper cervical pathways are interrupted, temporary losses of pulmonary tidal volume greater than 50% occur, with recovery in a few minutes. Other respiratory interferences are caused primarily by abnormal innervation of the diaphragm, intercostal muscles, or other muscles of respiration. Lesions possibly responsible for such interruptions include ascending myelitis, poliomyelitis, and syringomyelia.

**REFERENCES**

Appenzeller, C.: The autonomic nervous system, ed. 2, Amsterdam, 1976, North Holland Publishing Co.

Axlerod, J.: Neurotransmitters, Sci. Am. **230:**59, June 1974.

Axlerod, J., and Weinshilboum, R.: Catecholamines, N. Engl. J. Med. **287:**237, 1972.

Bannister, R.: Brain's clinical neurology, ed. 5, Oxford, 1978, Oxford University Press, Inc.

Bannister, R.: Degeneration of the autonomic nervous system, Lancet **2:**175, 1971.

Braunwald, E.: Regulation of the circulation, pt. 1, N. Engl. J. Med. **290:**1124, May 16, 1974.

Braunwald, E.: Regulation of the circulation, pt. 2, N. Engl. J. Med. **290:**1420, June 20, 1974.

Dicara, L.V.: Learning in the autonomic nervous system, Sci. Am. **222:**30, 1970.

Ferguson, M.: The brain revolution, New York, 1973, Taplinger Publishing Co., Inc.

Forster, F.M.: Clinical neurology, ed. 4, St. Louis, 1978, The C.V. Mosby Co.

Hee, L., editor: Neurotransmitters, vol. 2, Sixth International Congress of Pharmacology, Helsinski, New York, 1976, Pergamon Press, Inc.

Iverson, L.L.: Uptake and storage of noradrenaline in sympathetic nerves, Cambridge, 1967, Cambridge University Press.

Knowles, F., and Vollrath, L.: Neurosecretion—the final neuroendocrine pathway, Proceedings of the Sixth International Symposium on Neurosecretion, London, New York, 1973, Springer-Verlag New York, Inc.

Levine, S.: Stress and behavior, Sci. Am. **224:**26, Jan. 1971.

Mason, J.W.: The integrative approach in medicine—implications of neuroendocrine mechanisms, Perspect. Biol. Med. **17:**333, Spring, 1974.

Mountcastle, V.B., editor: Medical physiology, ed. 14, St. Louis, 1980, The C.V. Mosby Co.

Pick, J.: The autonomic nervous system, New York, 1970, J.B. Lippincott Co.

Pitts, F.W., Jr.: The biochemistry of anxiety, Sci. Am. Feb. 1969.

Research News: New information about the development of the autonomic nervous system, Science **206:**434, Oct. 1979.

Selye, H.: The stress syndrome, Am. J. Nurs. **65:**97, March 1965.

Selye, H.: The stress of life, New York, 1956, McGraw-Hill Book Co.

Selye, H.: Stress without distress, Philadelphia, 1974, J.B. Lippincott Co.

Spielberger, C.D., and Sarason, I.G.: Stress and anxiety (4 vol.), New York, vol. I, 1975, vol. II, 1975, vol. III, 1976, vol. IV, 1977, Halsted Press.

Trotter, R.J.: Listen to your head, Sci. News **100:**314, Nov. 1971.

Warwick, R., and Williams, P.L.: Gray's anatomy, ed. 35, Philadelphia, 1973, W.B. Saunders Co.

Weiss, J.M.: The psychological factors in stress and disease, Sci. Am. **226:**104, June 1972.

Yagi, K.: Structure and function of biomembranes, Forest Grove, Oregon, 1979, International Scholarly Book Service.

# PART TWO

# FACTORS AFFECTING
# NEUROLOGICAL OUTCOMES

# 5

# DEVELOPMENT OF PERCEPTION, INTEGRATION, AND RESPONSE

Nurses make a unique contribution to the health team in screening populations for neurological problems and in redefining the status of a problem where a known impairment exists. This assessment depends on their diverse exposure to basic behavioral and biological sciences and on the application of these sciences to activities of daily living in all phases of health and disease. The goal of these efforts is to minimize or prevent health impairments when possible, maintain acceptable biopsychosocial patterns for clients during illness, and assist individuals in returning to their highest level of well-being in convalescence.

To achieve these goals, nurses may find it useful to apply principles of systems engineering, so that they view human beings in terms of their internal structures as well as in the context of the total environment. Thus human operations become subject to analysis for system-design problems. Some state that systems have been the major method of studying humans for a long time and that the approach represents nothing new. However, the difference is that contemporary science no longer views functions within a system as discrete occurrences but as events working in conjunction with other systems that receive input from a multiplicity of sources.

The human body presents some challenges that are not apparent to engineers that deal in modalities other than living systems. Unpredictability and incomplete information on all aspects of human functioning cause many experimental situations to result in mostly descriptive, qualitative, and empirical data rather than the concrete data that char-

acterize areas concerned with man-made systems. Moreover, isolated investigations of physiological operations may result in phenomena that differ from those experienced in the context of ordinary functioning. For this reason, man must be considered in the context of life experiences, which encompass four basic principles: (1) consideration to simple stimulus-response patterns, consisting of inflow and outflow of matter and energy with subsequent reactions; (2) attention toward the many mechanisms in the body geared toward preserving or restoring homeokinesis in dynamic, constant body operations; (3) human functioning as a complex process that utilizes many different mechanisms to provide order, consistency, and continuity in living; and (4) the person as a being continually engaged in active interchange with the environment.

The first chapters have been concerned primarily with the specific components of operations related to the first two principles. Physiological mechanisms geared toward the provision of consistency and continuity in living have also been presented. This chapter reviews psychosocial parameters of influence as they relate to the third and fourth principles of dynamic environmental interchange and orderly processes of living. It is the addition of these variables that allows practitioners to assess neurological problems within the gestalt of total human experience.

## SOCIETAL INFLUENCES

The United States and Canada primarily comprise immigrants and their descendants. Because of this fact, nurses encounter a wide variety of subcultural practices and beliefs, depending on the geographic locality and persons in their patient population. Familiarity with characteristic group patterns is essential to effective functioning in the planning and accomplishment of health care objectives.

In addition to these local patterns, several general trends have emerged about the dominant sector in contemporary western society. The key aspects of these trends may be summarized as follows:

1. In comparison to other countries, North Americans enjoy a higher standard of living.
2. North America is characterized by rapid strides in scientific technology and industrialization.
3. Large, impersonal organizations and conglomerates are in operation to provide goods, services, or human processing on a massive production scale.
4. Extended family groups are being rapidly replaced by mobile nuclear family units that have futuristic orientations.
5. Socioeconomic positions are increasingly related to employment ranking and consumption patterns rather than to family origins.
6. Rapid change causes families to establish more temporary goals and more superficial, transient relationships.
7. The mass media have promoted fads and trends that bear great similiarities even at geographically distant points.
8. Traditional male and female roles are in flux.

### Family—the central unit

*Nuclear family.* As a result of the societal pressures just mentioned, more and more young families consist solely of the biological parents and their offspring. This unit, known as a nuclear family, a "launching platform" (Margaret Mead) or a "launching-pad" family (Carol Taylor), is the product of the rapid movement and constant flux readily apparent in contemporary Western society. Dissolution of this unit occurs when the marriage breaks up.

The nuclear family units are less efficient than those of extended families, which utilize all members to perform vital services and provide information related to young family life, child-rearing, and activities of daily living. With more experienced family members often living some distance away from the young family, many questions and problems arise concerning normal child care and management in family living that the young couple may be unable to handle financially, emotionally, or practically. Additionally, the public sector of society is not prepared to assume all the functions that the extended family once provided. Thus the modern family is often caught in an ambiguous position at times of crisis. As a result, many nurse practitioners are redirecting their focus to overcome these deficiencies and provide the assistance required by this life-style.

*Matrifocal family.* In contrast to the nuclear family, the matrifocal family comprises the mother and her children. Biological fathers have a temporary place in this young family unit but a more permanent position in their original families. These males may contribute to child support, engage in adult male-female relationships, and provide a male model for the young, but are unable to become part of a stable family unit because of their lack of consistent economic support. Common characteristics of this type of family structure include the following:

1. Economic means are at subsistence levels and therefore the family is oriented toward the present and its basic needs.
2. Males have unreliable and frequently inadequate employment and vocational preparation.
3. Elderly females, less qualified for employment, rear the children while the biological mother seeks employment to support the family unit.
4. As family members become employable, they are urged to seek gainful employment.

This family structure is frequently frowned on by persons socialized in the nuclear family structure. Since many professional persons have their origin in a nuclear family, they may need to identify sources of potential biases and misconceptions, so that they may function more effectively in therapeutic health management and in the formulation of realistic health care objectives for clients and their families who belong to this type of family group.

*Single parents.* Another group in family living is composed of the single parent and offspring.

Circumstances resulting in this situation may include primary single parenting where no marriage existed or war, desertion, divorce, or death as the main causes for the loss of a spouse. Such a group has a multitude of psychologic and socioeconomic problems that are beyond the scope of this book; other sources may be helpful in approaching some problems encountered by the single parent.

According to the U.S. Census Bureau: (1) 19% of U.S. families with children were maintained by a single parent in 1979, (2) one half of the black families with children were maintained by one parent, and (3) 31% of families maintained by a single female lived below the poverty level in 1978.

***Kinship model.*** A third type of family group is centered around nuclear families who have maintained close ties with the extended family structure. In this arrangement, family policy is frequently formulated by a mother-daughter axis. In these instances the maternal grandmother is not only the most significant figure in child-rearing, but is also the person who makes decisions for the young family unit. Often such arrangements are frustrating when poorly understood by health care professionals, because young parents who seem to comprehend and agree with a therapeutic plan may be unable to follow through with appropriate action because of interference from a maternal grandmother, whose ideas may differ. Such family units are characterized by four main points:

1. Maternal grandmother dominance
2. Clearly delineated sex roles
3. Resistance to change
4. Child-rearing by the maternal grandmother

Another cultural model that bears great similarity to the mother-daughter axis is the father-son kinship model. In this model, paternal grandfathers dominate in family and community affairs. In southeastern mountain areas families are frequently organized in this manner.

***Group living.*** Some young persons seek group living as a means of escaping materialism and lifestyles that incorporate competitive living patterns. Within these groups they hope to find meaning, identity, and humanism through an introspective search of self, which differs from the superficial orientation that their parents seem to represent. In searching, these individuals may exhibit hostility toward their family and dominant social groups, as they join others with similiar problems. They may communicate in a different language, engage in sexual promiscuity, wear odd clothing, and become involved in other demonstrations of deviance from the established societal norms. The use of psychedelic drugs may also accompany this behavioral pattern. Characteristics exhibited by persons attracted to these groups include the following:

1. Rejection of some social norms and values, especially those associated with materialism
2. Orientation to living in the present, with resultant short-term goals and immediate plans often taking priority
3. Short-term planning to effect social change
4. Emotional problems and dissatisfactions
5. Past history of material rewards for competitive achievements
6. Lack of warm, loving relationship with parents
7. Rejection of symbolic items generally used by dominant social groups
8. Engaging in social causes and philosophic discussions in a chronic quest for meaning and purpose in living

Conformity to this group subculture causes individuals to try to justify its existence and their own needs for belonging. As they become more deeply involved, these individuals may lose the ties that bound them to the dominant sector of society and may develop a perspective that differs from the perspective shared by the majority of persons. If they are unable to adjust to the group-living process, these persons may appear confused and psychologic disturbances may surface. With adequate guidance, reentry into the dominant sector of society on a more mutually satisfying basis is possible.

With regard to children born within the group-living structure, a great deal of supportive assistance in terms of growth and health promotion and prevention of health interferences may be necessary to stimulate normal developmental patterns.

## Life-styles

Within these family configurations are many behavioral patterns that are dependent on cultural habits, beliefs, and values; individual personalities; family systems; and community standards.[24,25] Effective health care delivery depends on the practitioner's ability to make objective assessments and take definitive action in the context of individual situations and groups.

Dominant religious and political beliefs, social structures, influences of power figures, customs, characteristic ways of spending time, socioeconomic conditions, and related data provide basic information about the client's style of living and frame of reference within the community. Such information may be gleaned from the family itself, professionals specializing in psychosocial studies, and community agencies serving a specified locality.

Benefits from studies by extrafamily agencies are evident in the following situation. A community in a rural area bordering a highway about 10 miles from small towns in either direction composed the target population. The population was termed a "bedroom community," because the only businesses were a grocery store, a service station, and a church, and employed community members commuted to one of the two nearby towns to work. Economically the group was a homogeneous population living at subsistence levels. In the area of health care, many deficiencies existed in the prevention, identification, and treatment of interferences with well-being. Socially the community revolved around the local church, and the people regarded the preacher as the most respected and influential group member. Thus when the community needed immunizations, a teaching program and clinic were set up outside the church after Sunday services to include the cooperation of the preacher, who received the first injection to ensure program success, as predicted by prior evidence from situational study and information from extrafamily agencies.

Similar methodologies were utilized in another situation to elicit meanings of local verbal expressions. Term clarification proved valuable in the assessment of various paroxysmal disorders in a group of epileptics. When queried, families did not understand the term "seizure." "Convulsion," "fit," "big spell," or "falling-out spell" were synonyms commonly used to describe a major motor episode. However, none of these words were selected by these families to describe minor motor seizures, which were characterized by these families as a problem of lesser magnitude.

Knowledge of this semantic gap caused the practitioner to identify seizure patterns carefully before reporting treatment outcomes or making recommendations to the neurologist.

## FOUNDATIONS OF DEVELOPMENT

In this section the processes of socialization, growth potentials, and parent-child interactions are briefly reviewed, and theories concerning developmental patterns and cognitive growth and concept formation are highlighted. Refer to other references for detailed coverage of these topics.

### Socialization

When infants are born, they are immediately subjected to significant others in the environment who manifest behaviors that the infants learn and internalize for eventual use in functioning as integral members of particular families, subcultures, and societies. This process is called socialization and is characterized by the following principles:

1. The group to which the child belongs existed before the child was born.
2. The addition of each member cannot be viewed as gaining one person, because it converts the entire group into a new organization with more than one new potential relationship.
3. Socialization negates individual differences, and it stresses likenesses that facilitate the learning and implementation of behavioral patterns congruent with the group.
4. The primary focus of the group does not revolve around individual perceptions and subsequent need-satisfaction patterns. Instead it is based on the person as one who is capable of learning and behaving in accordance with group norms.
5. Social contact is the means of transmitting and reinforcing acceptable behavioral and attitudinal patterns.
6. According to group norms, certain positions are assigned to members (status) that require a given set of behaviors (roles) to meet the standards of conformity.
7. Individuals learn responses, attitudes, and motivations appropriate to their assigned group status.
8. When appropriate patterns are learned and

acceptable behaviors are exhibited, they are reinforced by positive movement and emotion from significant others.

9. The repetition of behaviors results in the internalization of system values and beliefs.

10. Language is a symbolic device that incorporates jargon and gestures and tends to unite the group and identify individuals as members.

As children grow, their developing behavioral competencies and future objectives must be viewed by their group as appropriate if the group is to consider them well-adjusted members. Because of local variations, acceptable patterns (belching to show gustatory pleasure) in one portion of the world or country may be totally unacceptable in other geographic localities.

Children are challenged with the problem of growing in two different directions simultaneously as they seek individual identity while striving to mesh with their cultural group. This may create cognitive dissonance, so that individual behaviors inconsistent with group expectations result in activities that either move children toward or away from the group as a means of restoring psychologic equilibrium.

Children socialized in minority cultures and societies frequently experience disadvantages in opportunities, health maintenance and care, and socioeconomic progression, since many of these items are based on an individual's ability to comply with the dominant social sector's group standards in growth, achievement, behavior, and performance. Recognizing this fact, nurses must increase their sensitivity toward particular variants characteristic of a subcultural group, so that health care planning and implementation and developmental opportunities proceed in accordance with family and child capacities, resources, and aspirations. However, when such family patterns result in negative outcomes, appropriate nursing intervention may be activated.

## Growth potentials

Within the context of society, the family unit is charged with the responsibility for rearing children. This function is dependent on a child's biologic capacities coupled with patterns related to environmental events, learning opportunities, and health and ecologic considerations, as illustrated in the boxed material on p. 134. By considering these factors the nurse may formulate a fairly comprehensive picture of the child within the family and environmental structures. Based on these gross observations, plans for definitive assessments and appropriate actions could be activated.

## Parent-child interactions

Viewing an individual from embryonic formation through birth and the ensuing developmental sequences is best accomplished in a professional context when one utilizes the previously mentioned principles of systems engineering, which define the individual in the context of the total external and internal environments, with the designation of departures from acceptable patterns as system design problems. A dominant component that recurs in system design analysis related to humans is the impact of the parent-child relationship throughout life. Describing this interaction as a complex interplay of biologic, psychologic, and environmental forces is the only accurate way to depict these influences that evade exact quantification.

In the first few days of life, infants perceive all objects and persons as being coexistent with them and belonging to them. The world revolves around immediate needs as each activity becomes all absorbing to the exclusion of others. Need-gratification and tension-reducing movements by significant others probably appear as unorganized sensory experiences, which provide the initial matrix for emerging personality and role processes. With time the infants learn to identify mother from self and begin the lengthy sequences of growth interactions that move them from initial dependence to independent functioning and repetition of the cycle with their own infants.

Early contact with parents establishes a framework of reciprocal expectations and patterns for future role exchanges. These patterns develop as learning proceeds through imitation, identification, projection, and transference in individual development.

Through these learning processes, parents play a major role in providing the security, safety, guidance, and orientation necessary for acceptable growth and mature identity as the infant develops

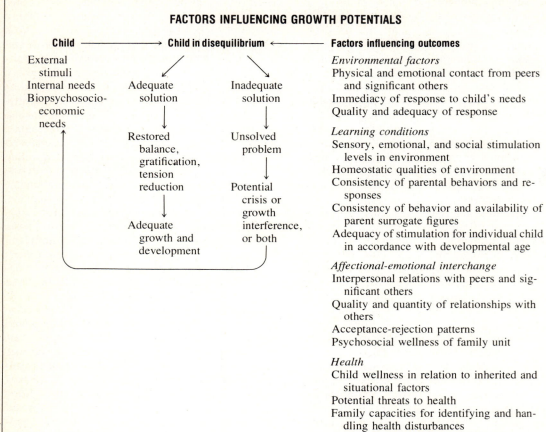

**FACTORS INFLUENCING GROWTH POTENTIALS**

Child ⟶ Child in disequilibrium ⟵ Factors influencing outcomes

External stimuli
Internal needs
Biopsychosocio-economic needs

Adequate solution

Inadequate solution

Restored balance, gratification, tension reduction

Unsolved problem

Adequate growth and development

Potential crisis or growth interference, or both

*Environmental factors*
Physical and emotional contact from peers and significant others
Immediacy of response to child's needs
Quality and adequacy of response

*Learning conditions*
Sensory, emotional, and social stimulation levels in environment
Homeostatic qualities of environment
Consistency of parental behaviors and responses
Consistency of behavior and availability of parent surrogate figures
Adequacy of stimulation for individual child in accordance with developmental age

*Affectional-emotional interchange*
Interpersonal relations with peers and significant others
Quality and quantity of relationships with others
Acceptance-rejection patterns
Psychosocial wellness of family unit

*Health*
Child wellness in relation to inherited and situational factors
Potential threats to health
Family capacities for identifying and handling health disturbances
Activities of daily living related to health maintenance
Perceptions and values related to health

*Ecological considerations*
Quality of environmental air, water, sanitation, living quarters and facilities, and recreation
Adequacy of nutrition
Freedom from infectious processes
Positive and negative components of life space

the cortical association areas that allow spontaneous, creative, present-oriented infants to gradually profit from past experiences and anticipate future objectives.

Early parent-infant relationships have become the focus of increasing attention as their importance continues to be revealed. Emphasis has shifted from the view of the infant as a passive recipient of tension-reducing movements to the infant as an active, selective respondent of biopsychosocial stimuli who progresses from simplistic to complex learning with practice.

Initial maternal-neonatal interactions seem to be instrumental in formulating and indicating future interactions. Research into the sensitive period of the first few days of extrauterine life have caused concern over traditional hospital practices as impediments to natural maternal-neonatal contacts. Further study is needed to investigate the potential impact that prolonged separation may have on premature and low birth weight infants in relation to later learning and development. Possibilities for early hospital discharge for these infants also need exploration.

In one agency, a study was conducted on the problem of early separation in a nonfamily-oriented, traditional hospital setting, where the care involved in subspecialties physically isolates new mothers and fathers from neonates requiring special care. Unnecessary separation has been avoided in this setting because of the changes recommended by this study, which caused maternity and pediatric nurses to unite in utilizing an integrated staffing pattern in the special care unit for neonates. In this milieu the family unit has become the key focus in caring for neonates with special needs, as positive parenting behaviors are fostered and early crisis intervention and anticipatory guidance earmark the total health care delivery approach (McFadden and Kopf).

Dr. Klaus of Case Western Reserve University has explored the differences in later mothering patterns in two groups of primiparas, where one had limited contact while the other group had 15 additional contact hours with their neonates during the first 3 days of life. Observations in a controlled setting when the infants were 1 month of age demonstrated greater maternal responsiveness and attention by the group who spent the most time with their infants during the critical period. Another study of early adaptive patterns and their predictive value in successful maternal-neonatal adjustment centers around feeding patterns as a primary and significant interaction between mother and neonate.

Another aspect of shifting emphasis is that of extending the total childbearing process to incorporate considerations other than the physical gestation and the relationship of the mother and the infant. Current concepts in maternity nursing approach changing individual needs in terms of various family configurations and view the birth process in the context of the entire family unit. Moreover, added emphasis on family involvement and renewed interest in family participation has given impetus to breast feeding, prepared childbirth classes with labor and delivery involvement for fathers, and more liberal visiting and neonatal contact for fathers (and even siblings in some hospitals) during the critical period in many settings.

### Developmental patterns

As the neonate continues to mature, progression through the various developmental stages suggested by various theoreticians ensues. Although no theory seems complete in its ability to unlock all the mysteries and complexities inherent in development, each opinion adds perspective to the data needed by practitioners in their assessment of the total child. A broad discussion of prevailing theories at each stage of personality development and social growth is beyond the space limitations of this book. Therefore this text is necessarily based on the assumption that the reader has a thorough understanding of growth and development. An informative, current review of the topic is available in *Child Health Maintenance*. The bibliographies contained in the aforementioned book are divided by age group and offer opportunities for seeking additional knowledge.

### Cognitive growth and concept formation

Maturity of the neurological system and the advent of learning and cognitive development are interdependent entities. Consideration is therefore given to all known aspects of learning and cognitive development in thorough evaluations of an individual's neurological status.

The learning capacities of infants have received increasing attention, as previously mentioned. Thus significant parent figures and early environmental influences have become paramount factors in affecting not only total development, but also in establishing the boundaries of learning capacities. The impact of varying biopsychosocial stimulation levels on cognitive growth and functioning in infants in relation to later intellectual development has been explored by a number of researchers. One classical study by Spitz of infants in a foundling home relates stimulus deprivation and the lack of mothering to growth interferences and maldevelopment in all areas of growth. Other studies have added evidence to the argument that early stimulation has profound effects on later intellectual capabilities. Such findings form the basis for establishing primary intervention programs, as discussed later in this chapter.

In 1949 Hebb proposed a significant theory that compares brain input-output mechanisms, storage, and associational interconnections to a computer network. Thus early patterns of learning stored in permanent networks have long-range effects on future learning, intellect, and behavioral responses.

Probably one of the greatest contributions to the understanding of developing cognition in childhood is provided by Jean Piaget. The basic development of his ideas is presented here, but the reader is referred to his works and the many interpretations by others for explicit details of each developmental stage.

In Piaget's theory, intellectual behavior is composed of function and structure. Function is a constant throughout the life cycle and is subdivided into organization and adaptation. Organization is the process that provides meaningful patterns and consistency to all activity. Active, ongoing commerce with the environment is termed adaptation. Adaptation is further subdivided into two functional categories, assimilation and accommodation. First, an individual identifies, uses, and incorporates an element from the surroundings (assimilation). This process may involve physiologic ingestion of food or perception and integration of an event or object. Each time this process occurs, the act is viewed from former experience, and the current act adds data to the perception of future events. Interesting research on the laws governing perceptual experiences, especially in sensory illusions, is presented in the works of Dember and Hochberg.

As current acts add to and alter the internal patterns, modification occurs and affects behaviors in similiar future situations (accommodation). When an infant receives an initial bath, for example, it may seem to be a relaxing or, at times, an irritating experience. As repeated experiences in bathing occur and the infant matures in locomotion capabilities, the joint processes of assimilation and accommodation may result in the infant's perception of the bath as a playtime filled with splashing, fun, and toys. Warm water may still seem relaxing, but being washed may remain an irritating departure from play. Thus adaptation may be viewed as an interplay between assimilation and accommodation in an attempt to achieve equilibrium.

The second major premise of Piaget's theory consists of structural units (schemata), mental frameworks composing each developmental stage that fit the barrage of perceptual experiences of living and offer meaning and organization to all events. Although these stages and schemata occur sequentially, the chronologic age of their appearance may vary among individuals in accordance with different growth rates in children, past experience, and environmental factors.

## MOTIVATION

The structural and functional patterns of infants and children at various developmental ages within the context of their individual family units does not totally account for behavior. An intervening, unobservable variable termed motivation is also a significant factor inferred from behavior. In this section cursory attention is given to the principles underlying the theory and application of motivation as a therapeutic technique.

### Concepts

Several researchers have added depth and varying opinions to the definition of motivation. Freud, Miller, Hill, and Dollard regard motives as deficit tension states designed to activate an organism to attempt to regain homeostasis and obtain relief. Hebb disagrees with this definition, believing that organisms are already in a state of dynamic activity and that motives are needed merely to direct energies. McClelland views motivation as an activity that links past experience with behaviors geared toward anticipated goal achievement of specific ends or emotional states. Malamud adds a further shade of meaning to these definitions, regarding motivation as a basic process that channels behavior and experience through the interaction of conscious and unconscious components, though such movement may or may not be goal directed. Suffice it to say that motivation is a fundamental force that is continually active and in flux within each organism as that organism engages in lifelong commerce with its environment.

## Behavioral studies

The element of motivation is apparent in the discussion on stimulus input in Chapter 3. As previously mentioned, behavioral scientists are able to place animal subjects in a relatively controlled situation, to consider most of the variables in the situation, to apply some kind of stimulus as the changing variable, and then to observe the response pattern. From numerous experiments they can compile data to predict responses that occur under specified conditions. In essence they are able to demonstrate a simple stimulus-object-response pattern, which is a fundamental form of motivation.

Perceptual psychologists are also gathering data about basic stimulus-response patterns in human beings. For example, these investigators have explored the responses given when minimal visual or auditory information (threshold stimulus) is introduced. In this type of experiment the human subject indicates the first detection of the stimulus. By computing the response patterns for subjects in several given sets of conditions, the researchers are able to draw a probability curve, where response probability is an increasing function of stimulus intensity (Fig. 5-1).

After completion of the experiment and computation of the mathematical data, the following statements may be made: (1) Perceptual tasks may be categorized by the quantity of data needed for completion. (2) Informational thresholds may vary from person to person, as well as within the same person at various times.

These attempts to measure thresholds are significant because they represent efforts to correlate

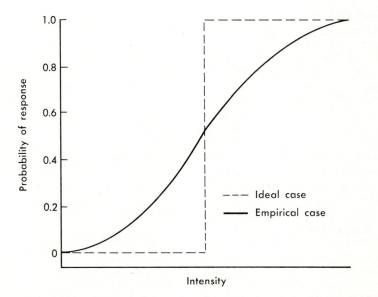

FIG. 5-1. Responses to stimulus intensity. (From Conway, B.L.: Pediatric neurologic nursing, St. Louis, 1977, The C.V. Mosby Co.)

input with output. From these studies, scientists propose to formulate principles that have global implications when specified conditions exist. Practically, such information is applied to matters such as subliminal advertising, wherein the success of subliminal input has shown a direct relationship to purchases of the product presented.

### Nursing implications

A descriptive study was done to identify possible motives for client behavior. When client movement did not result in predetermined objective completion, the nurse reassessed and modified the approach in relation to behavioral cues from the patient or family. Based on continuing reassessment, success often resulted in positive movement toward the goal. Such continuing reassessment necessarily included consideration of habits, inhibitions, sociopsychobiologic phenomena, self-concept, past experience, perceptions, conscious and unconscious factors, needs, emotions, health status, and developmental age within the family context. Since all behavior has meaning and may provide insight for further efforts, practitioners should utilize all data gained from client behavior.

### DEVELOPING POTENTIALS

Several components compose the child's ability to function adequately. In addition to factors previously discussed, consideration should be given to learning theory, memory, language skill acquisition, perceptual-motor development, and transcultural phenomena related to early successes, failures, and growth processes as well as deprivation and enrichment experiences. Ascertaining such information is essential in planning a cooperative team approach aimed at prevention, health maintenance, and primary intervention in processes interfering with growth and well-being.

### Learning theory

Cognition and intellectual development have been previously discussed. In this section, learning is viewed as an isolated factor in an attempt to provide perspective on various points of view needed in the evaluation of teaching-learning encounters. At one pole lies the specific empirical definition of learning as an observable stimulus-response sequence. However, the other, more general definition at the opposite pole refers to learning as an internal process dependent on certain experiential input that results in the production of behavior and potential behavioral changes. Practitioners benefit from a combination of these definitions, since they acknowledge the elusive qualities of the teaching-learning situation while being in the practical position of generating positive activity toward specified objectives. Such objective completion necessitates the calculation and management of environmental factors, the application of behavioral reinforcement techniques, the progression in learning at the level of the child within the family context, and the documentation of goal-directed movement.

### Memory

Discussions of learning, motivation, and related topics are incomplete without consideration of the phenomenon of memory. Memory is described as an intervening variable, since it is an inferred, unobservable operational process dependent on the reunification of disjointed mnemonic events. Some have likened the mnemonic process to a hologram, a photographic plate devoid of meaning until appropriate lighting illuminates the image.

Functionally the association areas in the cerebral cortex probably work in conjunction with incoming messages in the brainstem to effect memory by rejoining distributed bits of information. However, pragmatically the only significant aspect of memory is the child's ability to organize, code, and decode messages in a manner appropriate to the developmental level. An example of one association methodology that simplifies the process includes the "hill and valley" approach to figuring the number of days in a month by the use of the knuckles on the hand, because this process adds meaning and context to the calculations.

### Language skill acquisition

Language is a dynamic, complex vehicle that includes interchanges to convey thoughts, feelings, or questions experienced by another person. Functionally it is the mechanism that allows individuals to communicate messages of value to others. Language is significant because of its influence on learning potentials and attitudes and because of its unique function in assisting individuals to become part of a social system.

In children, language is learned through processes of imitation and trial and error. Because of a child's reliance on others in the immediate environment as models for language acquisition, communication skills necessarily incorporate the vocabulary, usage, pronunciations, and variety practiced by available resource persons.

Because of the modes of language skill acquisition, powers, functions, and meanings are assigned to communication symbols that may have deeply personal significance, frequently evading logic or literal interpretation.

*Maternal influences.* Investigation is needed to establish the effects of various teaching modalities (television, books, rhymes, educational toys, songs, discussions, and stories with and without tangible examples), of various milieus, of possible outcomes for varying capacities in children, and of unique mother-child interactions specific to every relationship. By consideration of all these factors, developmental trends that encompass situational variability might be formulated.

Currently, three general phases in language skill development emphasize the mother-child relationship as one of the most important factors in influencing language skill acquisition. In the first stage the mother expends effort to interpret her performance, discuss and respond to infant sounds and movements, state her perceptions about the surroundings, including available resources and events, and translate concrete objects and pictures into verbal descriptions. In the second stage she tests the success of encoding and responds positively, neutrally, or negatively to the infant's ability to react appropriately to cues. Interactions characteristic of this phase begin with maternal who-where-why-what verbalization. The infant progresses toward the ability to provide acceptable verbal feedback to these questions. In the third phase the mother reinforces the description or tries to alter the response through her reaction. The third stage of response is evident when the child is capable of spontaneous verbalization without props

or encouragement. Naturally this final stage of verbal ability and interpretation progresses to a more sophisticated level as cognitive growth and environmental conditions allow.

*Physical structures.* In addition to the psychosocial influences in language development, the practitioner should carefully assess physical factors related to perceptual capacities, for example, hearing, sight, and sensory organs and endings; intelligence; structures essential to communication (tongue, lips, jaws, palate, and muscles); and behavioral competencies. Assessment techniques are further described in Chapters 8 and 11 and in the sources given in the references.

## Perceptual-motor development

A discussion of developing perceptual-motor abilities in children is timely at this point, since it represents an important part of the neurologic evaluation, especially when impaired abilities interfere with these basic skills. This section emphasizes abilities that are evident from birth through middle childhood, theoretical viewpoints on aiding perceptual-motor development, visual perception patterns, development of manual dexterity, and the maturational sequence involved in graphic skills.

### Birth through middle childhood

BEGINNING ABILITIES. Although motor movements are evident in utero, specific perceptual-motor functions are not generally assessed or are not conspicuous unless absent until birth. Early neonatal examinations depend heavily on the status and presence of certain reflexes, which are primarily essential to normal functioning and life. Precise descriptions of early reflexes, methods for eliciting these reflexes, and the significance of the various reflexes are detailed in Chapter 11.

INCREASING INDEPENDENCE. As neural growth and maturation proceed in a cephalocaudal direction, a proximal to distal pattern, and a manner where large muscles and gross movements occur before the mastery of finer movements, increasing voluntary and independent functions are commanded by the growing infant. Prior to walking and lower limb coordination, head, arm, and neck coordination are more refined, as is evident in the creeping movements that are precursors for crawling and sliding in many infants. Appearance and patterns in prewalking activities are highly individualistic and may show great variation among infants.

As the infant gains the ability to move around in an upright position at about 1 year of age, movement and independent activity capacities increase greatly. At first, walking is characterized by a wide-based stance, an irregular rhythm, and a distinct preference to continue crawling when destination is important. With practice the gait becomes more rhythmic, and the base of support is narrowed. Outward direction of the toes is replaced by a more mature toddlelike movement, which is more and more easily utilized as maturity progresses. Later additions to the maturing gait include appropriate arm swing, increasing muscle strength in the legs, and the ability to lock the knees for added support in the extremities. Emphasis on the locomotion process and visual inspection of gait and obstructions in the pathway require less attention as they become more integrated into multiple simultaneous activities with advancement around 3 years of age. As walking is mastered, the 2-year-old child may walk sideways and backward or travel on tiptoe. In the third year the child may enjoy turning in circles to become dizzy.

Skill in running progresses on a continuum beginning at about 18 months of age, when the child appears to run but is unable to allow both feet to leave the ground together. With use, leg muscles become strong and the child exhibits true running ability between the ages of 2 and 3 years. However, practice continues as the child masters the ability to start and stop suddenly. By 5 years of age, most children run at a fair velocity with coordinated movements of the arms and feet.

At about 18 months of age the child begins to step off low objects as a preliminary activity to jumping. By 2 years of age the jump involves both feet, and leaping over low objects closely follows this ability. Most children are skillful at jumping by 3 years of age.

Hopping one to three times in place on the preferred foot is a task that most children 3½ years of age accomplish easily. By 5 years of age, 8 to 10 unilateral hops are common, and children easily hop about 50 feet forward. Girls seem to perform this task more easily than boys. Girls also show a greater ability to hop on either foot, whereas boys

have difficulty alternating the hopping movements. Both sexes still have problems alternating from foot to foot in a rhythmic manner at 5 years of age.

Skipping and galloping are complex refinements of the hopping movement. Although beginning efforts at skipping may be evident by 4 or 5 years of age, most children do not show proficiency in these skills until they reach 6½ years of age. Girls tend to prefer skipping, whereas boys may gallop better.

Integrated functioning in righting reflexes and visual control mechanisms is assessed at several points in the neurological examination. One measure of this neurological competency is balance. By about 3½ years of age, many children can walk for a distance of about 10 feet in a straight line. However, the ability to walk on a circular line is not mastered until almost 4 years of age. Average 5-year-olds are also able to balance on one foot without extending their arms for a few seconds. However, studies on the ability to maintain the Romberg position—eyes closed, hands on hips, and feet in a heel-to-toe position—indicate variance among the ages reported in the different investigations.

Climbing is a more complicated activity that involves arm-leg coordination as well as such emotional factors as adventure, courage, and independency patterns of individual behavior. Early crawling movements up stairs may be seen in infants before walking is mastered. After walking ability is attained, many toddlers move readily up the steps with the assistance of another person or a rail for support by 17 months of age. By 3½ years of age, the child moves up the steps by alternating feet. Sometime around 5 years of age, children may attempt to descend a staircase, if their past experience has prepared them sufficiently.

Other coordination skills such as toe tapping and hand clapping in rhythm are frequently employed to establish neurological status. Girls 5 years of age accomplish such tasks more readily than boys. However, more difficult rhythms are not easily achieved by either sex.

Another complex skill that the preschool child becomes adept at is throwing and catching a ball, in that order. Whereas first attempts at throwing are underhanded motions, later efforts reflect a variety of styles that gradually utilize body weight and movement to advantage. By about 5 or 6 years of age, children shift their weight by taking a step forward during the throwing movement. Children seem to throw small balls more readily than large one, and individual proficiency seems to be related to family and cultural values, as well as to practice.

Catching balls is a more difficult task to master. Children younger than about 3½ years of age tend to hold their arms stiffly in front of them, but by 4 years of age, many extend their hands in anticipation of the ball. By the middle of the fifth year, many children show arm flexibility and even lateral positioning of the arms to increase versatility in catching. At all ages, larger balls are caught more easily than small balls. However, the perception of ball trajectories that are not self-initiated are still hard to predict by 5 years of age.

LATERALITY. Over the past few years evaluations of preferred extremity and eye use have been considered important in assessment of perceptual-motor problems in children. Current investigation reveals that although preferences in eye, hand, and foot usage seem to be inherited, they probably are somewhat modified by sociocultural forces that are largely geared toward right-sideness. By 6 years of age, most children show a fairly consistent pattern of dominant hand use, which stabilizes at age 10 years. However, children may continue to utilize one hand for one task and the contralateral hand for another activity. Preferential patterns in hand use are individual, and the degree of dominance or cross dominance is on a continuum in different children. Additionally, about one half the number of normal children use one hand and the contralateral eye predominately, whereas the others use the ipsilateral eye and hand most often. These patterns of eye-hand use have received attention by some investigators because of their alleged connection with cognitive-motor impairment and subsequent interferences with education. Preferred dominant leg use is more likely to be correlated with the hand rather than the eye used predominately. However, all investigations that link laterality with perceptual-motor impairment or cognitive disturbances should be carefully scrutinized with regard to the testing techniques uti-

lized. Practitioners will also want to learn updated information in the exciting research about laterality in relation to control of artistic and humanistic qualities versus cognitive and logical functions.

MIDDLE CHILDHOOD. During the elementary years, children continue to grow in their ability to perform and coordinate perceptual-motor tasks. Boys tend to show the greatest ability in achieving physical tasks, since their muscles are frequently more developed in the hip and shoulder region, whereas girls perform tasks requiring agility and rhythm best, such as skipping and hopscotch. Assessment of skills in these years is discussed further in Chapter 8.

*Theoretical viewpoints.* Motor activities have become the focus of theoreticians, who strive to improve children's performance in all spheres of activity by the use of prescribed programs. Although competent motor functioning is vital in keeping pace with peers, in gaining peer acceptance and inclusion, and as a prerequisite in the successful accomplishment of a variety of skills, programs emphasizing perceptual-motor activities may not remedy existing problems in all children. However, enthusiastic parents and educators who make many sacrifices to participate fully in a program for the child who has limited treatment alternatives may experience bitter disappointment and guilt when the program fails to result in demonstrable improvements in the child's performance. Furthermore, questions regarding progress related to maturation versus program success have not been satisfactorily answered.

Even though other aspects of learning disability and motor impairment are discussed fully in Chapter 8, the three major theories of perceptual-motor training are reviewed here.

Kephart offers one theory of child development that is based on increasingly complicated levels of general performance in the child. This theory relies heavily on the successful completion of previous levels of general perceptual-motor skills. All learning is said to be dependent on the expanding motor potentials in the growing child. When these motor capacities do not develop in an acceptable manner, free exploration is impaired, as the child focuses on inabilities rather than freedom in space and the dynamic relationship with environmental objects. Also, Kephart emphasizes the importance of the child's sense of orientation of the body and its parts in relation to space occupancy and gravity as a prerequisite in accurately perceiving and evaluating other spatial relationships. Adequate body image is also related to laterality, which is the basic coordinate in the orientation of objects to the body. A third premise is termed perceptual-motor matching. In this instance the child must receive sensory input and correlate it accurately with motor abilities and object manipulation. The inability to achieve this function causes impairments in identifying appropriate directionality in spatial relationships outside the body. Such problems are often said to result in reading and form reproduction reversals. Since these stages of development rely on previous levels, this theory relates the problem of spatial directionality to the previous stage of body laterality.

Other, later, generalized stages include form perception and finally conceptualization. A concept, the highest form of generalization, is the extraction of components from one set of circumstances and their subsequent application to a novel situation. In the remedial program Kephart emphasizes the need to begin at the level of the most elementary faulty generalization, since further development requires a sound foundation. To date, other investigators have revealed a variety of findings that do not always support Kephart's theories, but that point to the need for further study and validation of some of his ideas.

Another popular theory, the Delacato method, has received sharp criticism from many health professionals. This method is based on the premise that specific areas of the brain have particular control over given perceptual-cognitive-motor functions and that a program can be developed to affect certain brain layers. As explained in Chapter 3, current thought emphasizes complex locomotor and perceptual activities as regulated at several points in the nervous sytem rather than at one single point. Central aspects of the Delacato theory include the use of a variety of specific tasks designed to result in hemispheric dominance, the use of the ipsilateral eye and hand, and subsequently improved sensory and speech functions. Music, supposedly controlled by the nondominant cerebral hemisphere, is said to interfere with the operation of the dominant hemisphere, and thus musical ex-

periences are not allowed. Furthermore, patterning activities to allow the child to experience the creeping and crawling activity are done according to a specific routine despite socioemotional considerations involving the family or the child's desires or life-style. Naturally this rigid aspect of the program has been criticized for the potential harm it may do to the child with respect to psychosocial realms.

However, in observing the program in operation, some positive points are obvious. First, an entire detailed evaluation and program is prepared for each child. This program contains careful, detailed instructions that are conveyed to the parents so that the child has one centrally integrated format to follow that is understood by the parents. This consistency of approach, involvement of parents, and central planning as well as the regular sensory stimuli through all avenues of perceptual input are points that could be modified and integrated into other types of programs. Such planning and periodic follow-up might make children with perceptual-motor problems and their families feel less splintered by specialists and subspecialists who often function autonomously with limited interspecialty communication.

Another theory describing motor control and coordination as the basis for intellectual functions is proposed by Getman. This program emphasizes the development of muscle efficiency and movement as well as visual-perceptual processes. Learning abilities are correlated with the adequacy of visual-perceptual development and organization. However, studies by other experts on his methods conclude that although near-point fusion and ocular functions may be significant factors, they should not be the only points emphasized. Cognitive capacities and adequate functioning of the higher centers in the central nervous system also play a vital role in learning and reading skills. In summary, although blanket application of this theory seems unwise, further investigation may reveal some merit in the ideas proposed by Getman.

*Visual perception patterns.* Although the area of visual perception is complex and includes many questions about the relative contribution of such factors as visual apparatus, perceptual response patterns, functional intellectual levels, cognitive capacities, and environmental and experiential opportunities, some widely accepted ideas currently prevail. First, ocular activity in neonates has received renewed attention, since a relationship between environmental and novel stimuli and tracking and visual regard patterns has been noted. Additionally, by observing binocular fixations of the eyes and changes in head movements as infants visualize objects, investigators now believe that infants 2 months of age experience figure and size constancy. Second, early perception and integration of directionality of lines occur first with the organization of horizontal and vertical lines and then oblique lines. Third, perception and integration occur in a maturational sequence that begins with gross object awareness and continues until complex, intricate refinement of the perceptual and motor experience occurs. This maturational process is interdependent with the concurrent development of neurologic pathways. Fourth, experience is a significant factor in causing a variety of perceptual characteristics to be assigned to objects and events. By the time a child is 5 years of age, many of the existing visual perceptions experienced are similiar to those perceived in adulthood.

***Development of manual dexterity.*** Infants begin the long course toward physical control and manipulation of certain environmental objects with an intense interest in their own hands sometime between 1½ and 2 months of age. An enriched level of environmental stimulation may delay this hand-regard phase for about 1 week, whereas an environment with diminished visual stimuli and physical contact may cause infants to focus on their hands sooner.

Between 2 and 4 months of age, infants attempt to make physical contact with environmental objects by utilizing a sweeping or encircling arm movement toward an object. In times of generalized excitement, infants may strive for contact by vertical arm movements involving either one or both upper extremities. By 4 months of age, experience teaches infants to approach objects more deliberately. Thus infants may be observed as they shift their eyes from hand to object until contact with the object is made. Often hand preferences are indicated at this time.

In general the period from 2 to 6 months of age is characterized by progression from the palmar grasp of objects to the use of a pincer movement. Activity centers on banging, shaking, stacking, and throwing objects in countless novel ways to produce noise and on many creative uses for objects. Since novel objects attract attention more readily than familiar objects, Solokov has proposed a motor-copy theory to explain this phenomenon. Apparently, when cortical neurons do not have previous data stored on a particular object, they stimulate other portions of the brain to extend exploration activities. After object familiarity is attained, feedback inhibition causes the infant to shift this focus to other stimuli.

Another significant accomplishment of this early period of environmental-infant interaction is the acquisition of information on object-distance relationships, which the infant acquires through play with objects and visual inspection of object placement. Through these basic hand-eye movements, data is accumulated that contributes greatly to the growing infant's perception of the world. Since infants are exploring objects, it is wise to present them with a variety of sizes, textures, shapes, consistencies, and colors to enrich their exploratory experiences.

Beginning at 6 months of age, the infant utilizes more cognitive and social operations as a part of object manipulation. Uzgiris classifies these operations as schemata that range from simple banging and object movement to a stage of intense object examination and then to throwing and dropping items that enable the infant to integrate auditory and visual activity. By 11 months of age, the infant uses object exchange with others as a simple type of social interaction. Sometime between 18 and 22 months of age, the infant links verbal ability with other perceptual data, as the naming and identification of objects becomes possible.

In later years, as dexterity continues to improve, it is utilized as one parameter to assess neurological functioning. One test that is frequently employed to evaluate such capacities is the rapid thumb-finger contact, which includes an orderly approximation of the thumb with each finger in succession. At 5 years of age a child performs the test deliberately and visualizes the fingers carefully to avoid errors. Small movements are often noted in the uninvolved hand as the child focuses on the hand in motion. By age 7 years, slightly more than half the number of normal children can touch each finger to the thumb without breaking the sequence in less than 5 seconds. This ability improves to include nearly all children by 8 years of age. In general girls perform this task better than boys.

There are many other forms of definitive testing techniques available to evaluate perceptual-motor competencies. These methods are discussed further in Chapter 8.

*Graphic skills.* Many children who require definitive neurological examinations also need an assessment of their ability to draw, reproduce figures, and print numbers and letters as a partial measure of their developmental patterns. Whereas the manipulation of drawing and writing objects is heavily influenced by practice, availability to materials, and values placed on such skills by significant others, specified developmental capabilities are consistently seen at certain ages.

Graphic skills appear between about 12 and 16 months of age for most children, starting with spontaneous scribbling. Practice with drawing instruments results in bold, repetitive marks in several directions (Fig. 5-2). If a small square is present on the page, the child may scribble through it or draw in another area of the page to offset the preexisting form. If the existing square is larger, the child may attempt to scribble within the margins.

With increasing visual-motor maturation and coordination, the child 2 years of age begins to make lines that ultimately result in the ability to encircle a space. Concurrently, the child frequently discovers the ability to draw wavy lines. These wavy lines precede the ability to form series of loops, which the child may enjoy drawing from one end of the page to the other (Fig. 5-3). Next the child frequently discovers the ability to make a spiral and gradually a larger central area with multiple boundaries. By 3 to 4 years of age, the child is able to complete a primitive circle spontaneously. The ability to copy a circle is evident sooner. About 75% of all children master the ability to copy a circle by 3 years of age.

By late in the third year of life, the child usually attempts to draw a cross and sometimes figures of multiple intersecting vertical and horizontal lines. The emergence of squares seems to be somewhat individualistic, since some children leave

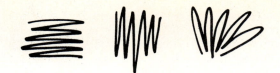

**FIG. 5-2.** Early scribbling patterns. (From Conway, B.L.: Pediatric neurologic nursing, St. Louis, 1977, The C.V. Mosby Co.)

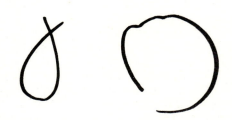

**FIG. 5-3.** Steps in drawing a circle. (From Conway, B.L.: Pediatric neurologic nursing, St. Louis, 1977, The C.V. Mosby Co.)

larger central areas between the vertical and horizontal lines, whereas others follow the form of the page or draw circles in a square manner.

The production and copying of geometric figures has become an important measure of perceptual-motor integration and is frequently included as a part of the neurological examination. In general children are able to reproduce certain figures by given chronologic ages. However, practitioners may learn as much about children by observing behaviors, verbalizations, parent-child interactions, and techniques employed in completing the task as from assessment of the figure.

General age guidelines for figure completion are noted in Fig. 5-4. Some characteristics of the production process seem worthy of enumeration, as follows:

1. Circle formation begins at a superior point after 5½ years of age, and many children in this age group, if right-handed, complete the figure in one counterclockwise motion.

2. Although cross formation is attempted by 4-year-olds, the finished product is not well drawn until 6½ or 7 years of age and is not flawlessly

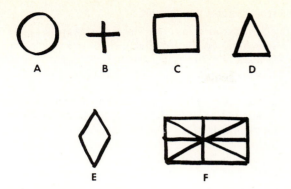

**FIG. 5-4.** Average abilities in figure reproduction. **A,** Circle, a skill achieved at 3 years of age. **B,** Cross, one of simple and complex patterns achieved at 3½ and 6½ years of age, respectively. **C,** Square, an achievement at 4 years of age. **D,** Triangle, accomplished at 6½ years of age. **E,** Diamond, a figure completed at 7 years of age. **F,** British flag, an accomplishment of children 8 to 9 years of age. (From Conway, B.L.: Pediatric neurologic nursing, St. Louis, 1977, The C.V. Mosby Co.)

mastered until 9 years of age. By age 5 years, right-handed children draw the vertical line by beginning at the top and the intersecting line commencing with the left side.

3. Before 5 years of age a square is often drawn as two parallel horizontal lines that are then linked by two vertical lines. By 5 years of age, many right-handed children are able to complete the figure in one counterclockwise sweep, beginning in the upper left-hand corner, whereas left-handed children draw in the opposite direction, from the upper right-hand aspect.

4. Whereas children 5 years of age may make an imperfect attempt to complete a triangle, this form is reproduced flawlessly by 7 years of age using a motion that begins at the top and proceeds in a counterclockwise manner. Diamond production is similiar to triangle production.

5. The figure resembling the British flag (Fig. 5-4, *F* ) is reproduced beginning with the rectangle and filling in of the internal figure with eight lines drawn from the center to the periphery. Problems in forming this figure occur as late as 10 years of age.

6. Whereas children under 5 years of age make most drawings large, older children often reproduce difficult figures in a smaller size.

7. Children often turn the paper so that the line being constructed is near them and does not have to be produced by a horizontal mark on the page.

In neurologic assessments the Bender test is frequently administered to evaluate the child's ability to combine more than one geometric figure in a contiguous arrangement. Such definitive testing should be done only by a person thoroughly trained in the technique. However, practitioners may elect to have a child reproduce one or more figures to gather added initial data on a child. Accuracy in copying such complex figures is not mastered until about 7½ years of age.

Children identify and label primitive efforts at drawing according to their perception of the surrounding environment. Additionally, the majority of children approaching 5 years of age are able to draw a human figure with three parts. By 5½ years of age, most children construct the human figure with six parts. This ability to reproduce the human figure proceeds in the following sequence. First, the child draws marks in a circle that remotely resemble a face. Second, the child extends a stick-like body directly from a circle (Fig. 5-5, *A*). Third, the child extends the central line to form a trunk and draws fingers and feet at the ends of the extremities (Fig. 5-5, *B*). Fourth, refinement of body parts becomes the focus (Fig. 5-5, *C*). Finally, the extremities assume some breadth (Fig. 5-5, *D*). Psychosocial aspects of these drawings are beyond the scope of this book, but the practitioner may wish to refer to the *Mental Measurements Yearbook* for a description of the various tools available (Buros).

**LETTERS AND NUMBERS.** In neurological evaluations the ability to reproduce letters and numbers is frequently evaluated. During testing it is helpful to ask the child to print these figures, since printing reveals more trends than script.

By 4 years of age, the child may print letters, but these letters have no linear organization on the page and may often be faced in the wrong direction. Many children 5 years of age print their given name, but it is not until 6 years of age that the last name, the alphabet, and the numbers through 10 can be produced. During the sixth and seventh years of life children demonstrate a better ability to place their figures in horizontal lines and to make figures that are not so large. However, uni-

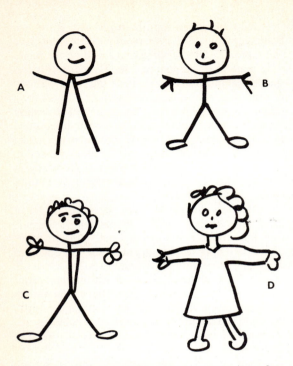

**FIG. 5-5.** Emergence of drawing of a human body. (From Conway, B.L.: Pediatric neurologic nursing, St. Louis, 1977, The C.V. Mosby Co.)

formity in distances between the figures is not achieved until after 7 years of age.

In observing the production of numbers, children are frequently noted to make the numbers 3, 4, and 5 in one continuous pencil motion, while utilizing two distinct movements to form the numbers 7, 8, and 9.

Letter and number reversals have received great attention in recent years. Five- and six-year-old children are frequently noted to make 30 into 03 or merely to form the 0 prior to the 3, while attaining a correct end product. Letter reversals are also quite common until the age of 7 years. However, only about 12% of all children continue these reversals beyond 7 years of age.

Three-dimensional figures present a much more difficult challenge. Most children do not master the ability to draw cubes and cylinders until they reach about 10 years of age.

## Transcultural phenomena

*Success and failure.* Since education is highly valued in the United States, it is not acceptable to learn at a pace that does not meet peer norms. However, various subcultural pockets have standards for success and failure that differ from those of the dominant sector of society. Unfortunately, most children compete in a school situation where the standards of the dominant social sector prevail. Such standards include all behavioral parameters as well as learning skill–acquisition trends. According to many educators, the motivation to perform in a certain manner is heavily influenced by past experience, expectations about the event, self-concept, and the value of the immediate incentive.

In one study by Deutsch, middle-class parents were found to consistently encourage and reward academic achievement at an early age. Thus the aura of success was often associated with task completion rather than with extraneous rewards. This factor was frequently found to be missing in lower socioeconomic groups and tended to have a pronounced effect on scholastic goals and achievements.

*Deprivation of stimulating experiences.* Restrictions to maximal accomplishment in each of the aforementioned phases of language development may be imposed on a child by the deprivation of stimulating experiences. Frequently this stimulus impoverishment is accompanied by limited vocabularies for expression and a predominance of negative social and emotional responses along with more physical means of stating emotions and feelings.

McCarthy's investigations show that children who come from an environment of diminished opportunity are slow in all areas of development, with the greatest area of impaired growth occurring in language development. This environmental restriction not only limits the number of words used, the ability to construct mature sentences, and the interpretation of another's comments, but also retards the progress of the child in school. This happens because children pattern themselves after those in their immediate environment. Therefore the amount of information available to the child in the form of mental stimulation, language aptitude, and experiences determines the quantity and quality of thought, verbal ability, and idea production.

The culturally impoverished environment has been well described in the literature, but at this point it seems important to review some of its characteristics. In many cases, parent figures left school at an early age. Thus they often lack the vocabulary necessary to communicate extensively and correctly by dominant social sector standards. Additionally, these adults often produce large families, a situation that causes them to work long hours to support the family group. Such long working hours may result in limited adult-child contact. Limited monetary means may result in older children caring for younger siblings until the older children are employed. As a result, directions and verbal contacts with parents may be limited to gestures or a few words, since time does not permit lengthy, relaxed interactions. Thus the children learn most of their language on the streets and where they play. This language usage is quite limited, since play is often physical and conversation remains at a minimum. Additionally, such language usage is often unsuitable for classroom settings, since it is frequently a form of unacceptable or inadequate expression. In summary, opportunity-deprived children may have great difficulty in competing with children from enriched environments, who probably use about 8000 words, comprehend concepts, and utilize simple, compound, and complex sentences by the time they enter school.

The practitioner should not overlook other groups that may contain opportunity-deprived children. Working parents with inadequate socioeconomic means may be compelled to place their young children in a crowded private care setting where positive learning experiences and adequate mothering are insufficient. Additionally, there are those situations wherein parents or parent surrogates are unable to provide acceptable environments for their children because of existing emotional disorders that they may have or because they lack the necessary information about rearing children. At times these situations may be unrelated to inadequate socioeconomic means. When detected, such situations may improve greatly with appropriate therapeutic intervention or intensive counseling in parent-child interactions and stimulus re-

quirements of the various developmental ages.

One revealing clinical experience that assists the practitioner in becoming acquainted with a preschooler's perceptual framework involves presenting a list of common words and asking for meanings from the child in a gamelike fashion. Naturally such investigation should be done only with the consent of the appropriate adults. A pilot investigation of this type was conducted in a nursery school setting for low-income families. The child's definitions, mannerisms, and other characteristics were correlated with known data about the child's background. It was interesting to note that there was great consistency between what the child revealed and the subculture and personal situation in which he or she lived. Tools such as this are valuable because of the limited means available to evaluate the perceptual world of the preschool child.

***Environmental enrichment.*** Since many investigators view infants and young children as active, selective respondents to learning within their immediate environmental contexts, programs that emphasize the enrichment of the family as the primary unit affecting growth and developmental outcomes in children have been developed. However, other programs also attempt to augment this primary unit with an enriched preschool program.

The program goals in many preschool centers designed to assist the opportunity-deprived child in gaining the skills to compete successfully have a twofold purpose. First, they assist the child in gaining experiences, including those of investigation, experimentation, imagination, creative abilities, problem solving, and peer socialization by aiming to meet the following objectives: (1) increased capacities for independent action through bolstering the child's self-confidence and feelings of security in a variety of situations; (2) broadened understanding of self, family, and others; (3) expanded appreciation of self-expression through art, music, and rhythm; (4) expanded horizons beyond the immediate environment to include the community, the state, the country, and the world; and (5) improved hygienic practices, nutritional habits, health practices, and social patterns. Second, they allow a self-determined pace for learning and exploring in a "safe" environment, with constant interpretation of individual and age-related needs to parents. These centers also may serve as a central place for child health maintenance and intervention in health impairments, since they may set up a referral network connected to many members of the health delivery system. Finally, the center may serve as a resource or primary referral center designed to assist families who are experiencing acute crisis or chronic stress.

Several preschool programs have been evaluated. Two of the most promising are GOAL, a small-group game approach to the development of standard school curriculum readiness, and the Bereiter-Englemann program, where basic academics are taught in structured drills. These programs have the following qualities: (1) sound theoretical base, (2) daily reassessment of program effectiveness, and (3) emphasis on development in the total range of cognition, psychosocial patterns, and motor skills.

Several programs have been conducted with children in the early childhood years, wherein paraprofessionals assist the mother in improving her activities and communications in relation to her child and others in the home. One of the most outstanding programs of this type is the Milwaukee project, which was conducted by Heber and Garber. This program was a 3-year stimulation program involving inner-city youngsters. When compared with a control group of peers, the study participants showed an increase of 33 IQ points on tests.

The nurse practitioner based in one of these centers may have impact in five major areas: (1) family instruction in routine health maintenance, opportunities in the community that would benefit this family unit, nutrition and household management, first aid, and community health resources; (2) prenatal preparation and infant care, including maternal care, instruction on fetal growth and child development, practical suggestions about infant care, stimulation, and communication; (3) preschool readiness, including constant communication with parents about preschool goals and ways that the home may assist the child in gaining more experience in preparation for school; (4) school readiness, involving health maintenance and motivation of the family to enroll the child in a program that utilizes a cognitive approach in conjunction with other learning activities; and (5) continuing emphasis on the parent as the primary factor in influencing the child's academic and social success. Nurses may make these contacts in a variety of ways, including office visits, home visits, clinic visits, involvement in school and community programs, and through formal courses offered in appropriate neighborhoods.

*Teaching techniques.* Because of the orientation of lower socioeconomic persons, nurses may find it necessary to employ several specific principles in reaching their audience effectively. First, physical and visual methods of demonstration about topics that are immediately relevant are received best. Second, the use of introspection and abstraction should be minimized, while the use of externally oriented material and problem-centered approaches is emphasized. Third, spatial material and inductive methods are more successful than temporal materials and deductive methods. Fourth, meaningful examples and one-track thinking, as well as action-oriented words, are utilized to fuller effect. Finally, the discussion should be geared to the present and to complete or partial goal accomplishment where gratification is immediate. Follow-up sessions and methods to reinforce initial teaching and parent endeavors are also helpful.

## REFERENCES

Affel, H.: System engineering, Int. Sci. Technol., p. 18, Nov. 1964.

Aguilera, D.C., and Messick, J.M.: Crisis intervention—theory and methodology, ed. 3, St. Louis, 1978, The C.V. Mosby Co.

Allport, G.: The open system in personality theory, J. Abnorm. Psychol. **61:**301, 1960.

American Academy of Pediatrics: Policy statement on day care, Pediatrics **51:**947, 1973.

Anthony, E.J., and Benedek, T., editors: Parenthood: its psychology and psychopathology, Boston, 1970, Little, Brown & Co.

American Baby **36:**entire issue, Feb. 1974.

Ayres, J.A.: Patterns of perceptual-motor dysfunction in children: a factor analytic study, Percept. Mot. Skills Monogr. Suppl. I-V20, 1965.

Bayley, N.: Behavioral correlates of mental growth: birth to Thirty-six years, Am. Psychol. **5:**1, 1968.

Bellugi, U., and Brown, R., editors: The acquisition of language, Chicago, 1972, The University of Chicago Press.

Bender, L.: Psychological principles of the visual motor gestalt test, Trans. N.Y. Acad. Sci. **II:**164, 1949.

Bernard, H.W.: Human development in western culture, ed. 5, Boston, 1978, Allyn & Bacon, Inc.

Bijou, S.W.: Helping children develop their full potential, Pediatr. Clin. North Am. **20:**579, 1973.

Billingsley, A.: Family functioning in the low income black community, Soc. Casework **50:**563, 1969.

Bower, T.G.: The visual world of infants, Sci. Am. **215:**80, 1966.

Bower, T.G.R.: The object in the world of the infant, Sci. Am. **225:**30, 1971.

Bowlby, D.: Attachment, Attachment and Loss ser., vol. 2, New York, 1973, Basic Books, Inc., Publishers.

Browder, J.A., and Mershom, P.M.: Speech and language development: the physician's role, Postgrad. Med. **56:**151, 1974.

Brown, R.: The development of wh questions in child speech, J. Verbal Learning Verbal Behav. **7:**279, 1968.

Brown, R.C.: The effects of a perceptual-motor education program on perceptual-motor skills and reading readiness, Paper presented to the Research Section of the American Association for Health, Physical Education and Recreation, St. Louis, April 1, 1968.

Buros, O.K.: The seventh mental measurements yearbook, Highland Park, Ill., 1972, The Gryphon Press.

Caldwell, B., and Ricciuti, H.N., editors: Child development research: child development and social policy, vol. 3, Chicago, 1976, The University of Chicago Press.

Cazden, C.: The situation: a neglected source in social class differences in language use, J. Soc. Issues **26:**35, 1970.

Chapman, A.H.: Management of emotional problems of children and adolescents, Philadelphia, 1974, J.B. Lippincott Co.

Chinn, P.L.: Child health maintenance, ed. 2, St. Louis, 1979, The C.V. Mosby Co.

Clausen, J.P., et al., editors: Maternity nursing today, ed. 2, New York, 1976, McGraw-Hill Book Co.

Combs, A.W., et al.: Perceptual psychology: approach to the study of persons, New York, 1976, Harper & Row, Publishers.

Combs, A.W., et al.: Helping relationships: basic concepts for the helping professions, ed. 2, Boston, 1978, Allyn & Bacon, Inc.

Committee on Government Operations: Background papers prepared for the 1970-1971 White House Conference on Children and Growth, Washington, D.C., 1971, U.S. Government Printing Office.

Conway, B.L.: The effect of using a word list to ascertain the perceptual world of a four year old in a low socioeconomic category, Unpublished data.

Conway-Rutkowski, B.: Divorce, potential for growth in common problems in primary care, St. Louis, 1982, The C.V. Mosby Co.

Cratty, B.J.: Perceptual and motor development in infants and young children, ed. 2, New York, 1979, Prentice-Hall, Inc.

Cutright, P.: Incomes and family events: marital stability, J. Marriage Family **33:**2, 1971.

Delacato, C.H.: Neurological organization and reading, Springfield, Ill., 1973, Charles C Thomas, Publisher.

Delacato, C.H.: The diagnosis and treatment of speech and reading problems, Springfield, Ill., 1974, Charles C Thomas, Publisher.

Dember, W.N.: The psychology of perception, ed. 2, New York, 1979, Holt, Rinehart, & Winston, Inc.

Despert, J.L.: Children of divorce, Garden City, N.J., 1962, Dolphin Books.

Elkin, F.: The child and society, ed. 3, New York, 1978, Random House, Inc.

Extended neonate contact makes for better mother, Ob. Gyn. News **6:**1, 1971.

Farley, R., and Hermalin, A.J.: Family stability: a comparison of trends between black and white, Am. Sociol. Rey. **36:**1, 1900.

Festinger, L.: Cognitive dissonance, Sci. Am. **207:**27, 1962.

Fleishman, E.A., et al.: The dimensions of physical fitness: a factor analysis of speed, flexibility, balance and coordination tests, Tech. Rep. 3, The Office of Naval Research, New Haven, Conn., 1961, Yale University Department of Psychology.

Flick, G.L.: Sinistrality revisited: a perceptual-motor approach, Child Dev. **37:**613, 1966.

Folta, J.R., and Deck, E.S.: A sociological framework for patient care, ed. 2, New York, 1979, John Wiley & Sons, Inc.

Freed, D.J., and Foster, H.H.: Divorce American style, Ann. Am. Acad. **38:**71, 1969.

Friedenberg, E.Z.: The vanishing adolescent, New York, 1972, Dell Publishing Co., Inc.

Gallagher, J.J.: Preventive intervention, Pediatr. Clin. North Am. **20:**681, 1973.

Gehrke, S., and Kirschenbaum, M.: Survival patterns in family conjoint therapy, Family Process **6:**no. 1, 1967.

Gesell, A., and Ames, L.B.: The development of handedness, J. Genet. Psychol. **70:**155, 1947.

Gesell, A., et al.: Vision: its development in infant and child, New York, 1967, Hafner Publishing Co., Inc.

Getman, G.N.: How to develop your child's intelligence, a research publication, Luverne, Minn., 1952, published privately.

Getman, G.N.: The physiology of readiness experiment, Minneapolis, 1963, Programs to Accelerate School Success, Inc. (P.A.S.S., Inc.)

Glass, G.V.: A critique of experiments on the role of neurological organization in reading performance, Urbana, Ill., 1967, University of Illinois Center for Instructional Research and Curriculum Evaluation.

Glidewell, J.C., editor: The social context of learning and development, New York, 1977, Halsted Press (John Wiley & Sons, Inc.)

Goldfarb, W.: Effects of psychological depreciation in infancy and subsequent stimulation, Am. J. Psychol. **102:**18, 1945.

Greene, H.A., et al.: Developing language skills in the elementary schools, ed. 5, Boston, 1975, Allyn & Bacon, Inc.

Guillaume, P.: Imitation in children, Chicago, 1973, The University of Chicago Press.

Haith, M.M.: The response of the human newborn to visual movement, J. Exp. Child. Psychol. **3:**235, 1966.

Harlow, H.F.: Love in infant monkeys, Sci. Am. **200:**68, 1959.

Harris, A.J.: Diagnosis and remedial instruction in reading. In innovation and change in reading, 67th Yearbook, pt. II, of the National Society for the Study of Education, Chicago, 1968, The University of Chicago Press.

Hebb, D.O.: The organization of behavior, New York, 1949, John Wiley & Sons, Inc.

Hecaen, H., and Albert, M.L.: Human neuropsychology, New York, 1978, John Wiley and Sons, Inc.

Hershenson, M.: Visual discrimination in the human newborn, J. Comp. Physiol. Psychol. **58:**270, 1964.

Hochberg, J.E.: Perception, ed. 2, Englewood Cliffs, N.J., 1978, Prentice-Hall, Inc.

Ilg, F.L., and Ames, L.B.: School readiness: behavior tests used at the Gesell Institute, New York, Harper & Row, Publishers.

Joint Commission on Mental Health of Children: Mental health from infancy through adolescence, New York, 1973, Harper & Row, Publishers.

Karr, S.D., and Dent, O.B.: In search of meaning: the generalized rebellion of the hippie, Adolescence **5:**187, 1970.

Keller, F.S.: Learning: reinforcement theory, ed. 2, New York, 1969, Random House, Inc.

Keogh, J.F.: Analysis of individual tasks on the Stott Test of Motor Impairment, Tech. Rep. 2-68, USPHS Grant HD 01059, Los Angeles, 1968, University of California, Department of Physical Education.

Keogh, J.F.: Rhythmical hopping tasks as an assessment of motor deficiency, Paper presented at the International Congress of Sports Psychology, Washington, D.C., 1968.

Kephart, N.C.: Perceptual-motor correlates of learning, Conference on Children with Minimal Brain Impairment, Chicago, June 1963, National Society for Crippled Children and Adults.

Kessen, W., and Kuhlman, C., editors: Thought in the young child, Chicago, 1971, The University of Chicago Press.

LaPray, M., and Ross, R.: Auditory and visual perceptual training. In Figurel, J.A., editor: Vistas in reading, Int. Reading Assoc. Conf. Proc. **9:**530, 1966.

Learning to see, American Baby **36:**41, 1974.

Maslow, A.H.: Motivation and personality, ed. 2, New York, 1970, Harper & Row, Publishers.

May, R.: The meaning of anxiety, New York, 1979, Pocket Books, Inc.

McClelland, D.C.: The achievement motive, New York, 1976, Prentice-Hall, Inc.

McFadden, E., and Kopf, R.: Integrated staffing for a special care unit, Supervisor Nurse **6:**26, 1975.

Middleton, N.: When family failed, London, 1971, Victor Gollancz, Ltd.

Moerk, E.: Changes in verbal child-mother interactions with increasing language skills of the child, J. Psycholinguist. Res. **3:**101, 1974.

Monaco, J.T., and Conway, B.L.: Motivation: by whom and toward what, Am. J. Nurs. **69:**1719, 1969.

Montagu, A.: Touching: the human significance of the skin, New York, 1971, Columbia University Press.

Motard, R.: Systems engineering: engineering comes of age, Engineering Educ. **56:**198, 1966.

Moustakas, C.E.: Psychotherapy with children: the living relationship, New York, 1979, Harper & Row, Publishers.

O'Grady, R.S.: Feeding behavior in infants, Am. J. Nurs. **71:** 736, 1971.

Parad, H.J., editor: Crisis intervention, New York, 1973, Family Service Association of New York.

Piaget, J., and Inhelder, B.: The psychology of the child, New York, 1969, Basic Books, Inc., Publishers.

Phillips, J.L., Jr.: The origins of intellect: Piaget's theory, ed. 2, San Francisco, 1975, W.H. Freeman & Co., Publishers.

Piaget, J.: The theory of stages in cognitive development, New York, 1969, McGraw-Hill Book Co.

Piaget, J.: The child's conception of movement and speed, New York, 1970, Ballantine Books, Inc.

Policy statement: The Doman-Delacato treatment of neurologically handicapped children, Neurology **18:**1214, 1968.

Pribram, K.H.: The neurophysiology of remembering, Sci. Am. **220:**73, 1969.

Purkey, W.W.: Inviting school success, Belmont, Calif., 1978, Wadsworth Pub. Co., Inc.

Robbins, M.P., and Glass, G.V.: The Doman-Delacato rationale: a critical analysis. In Hellmuth, J., editor: Educational therapy, vol. 2, Seattle, 1968, Special Child Publications, Inc.

Rutherford, W.L.: Perceptual-motor training and readiness. In Figurel, J.A., editor: Reading and inquiry, Int. Reading Assoc. Conf. Proc. **10:**194, 1965.

Satire, V.: Conjoint family therapy, Palo Alto, Calif., 1967, Science & Behavior Books, Inc.

Smith, O.W.: Developmental studies of spatial judgments by children and adults, Percept. Mot. Skills **22:**3, 1966.

Smith, O.W.: Spatial perceptions and play activities of nursery school children, Percept. Mot. Skills **21:**260, 1965.

Spitz, R.: Hospitalism, Psychoanalytic Study of the Child ser., vol. 1, New York, 1945, International Universities Press.

Spitz, R.: Hospitalism: a follow-up report, Psychoanalytic Study of the Child ser., vol. 2, New York, 1946, International Universities Press.

Stein, R.L.: The economic status of families headed by women, Mon. Labor Rev. **93:**3, 1970.

Strickland, R.G.: The language arts in the elementary school, ed. 3, Lexington, Mass., 1969, D.C. Heath & Co.

Sussman, M.: The isolated nuclear family: fact or fiction? Soc. Probl. **11:**Spring, 1959.

Taylor, C.: In horizontal orbit, New York, 1970, Holt, Rinehart, & Winston, Inc.

Ten Houten, W.D.: The black family: myth and reality, Psychiatry **33:**145, 1970.

Thant, U.: Report on trends in the social situation of children, New York, Jan. 8, 1970, United Nations Economic and Social Council.

Toffler, A.: Future shock, New York, 1970, Random House, Inc.

Travers, R.: The essentials of learning, ed. 4, New York, 1977, MacMillan Publishing Co., Inc.

U.S. Department of Health, Education, and Welfare, Social and Rehabilitation Service: Suggested guidelines for evaluation of the nutritional status of preschool children, Washington, D.C., 1967, U.S. Government Printing Office.

U.S. Department of Labor: The Negro family: the case for national action (the Moynihan report), Washington, D.C., 1965, U.S. Government Printing Office.

U.S. White House Conference on Children: Profiles of children, Washington, D.C., 1970, U.S. Government Printing Office.

Van Hattum, R.J.: Communication disorders in children: a guide for detection and referral, Nursing75 **5:**12, 1975.

Vernon, M.D.: The nature of perception and the fundamental

stages in the process of perceiving. In Uhr, L., editor: Pattern recognition, learning and thought: Computer-programmed models of higher mental processes, New York, 1973, Prentice-Hall, Inc.

von Bertalanffy, L.: Robots, men, and minds, New York, 1967, George Braziller, Inc.

Warren, S.A.: Adult expectations and learning disorders, Pediatr. Clin. North Am. **53:**705, 1973.

Whitsell, L.J.: Delacato's neurological organization: a medical appraisal, Calif. School Health **3:**1, 1967.

WIC Currents: News of women, infants, and children programs, Ross Timesaver, vol. 1, no. 2, March-April 1975.

Widdowson, E.M., and McCance, R.A.: A review: new thoughts on growth, Pediatr. Res. **9:**154, 1975.

Wright, J.C., and Kagan, J., editors: Basic cognitive processes in children, Chicago, 1973, The University of Chicago Press.

Zaner, A.R.: Differential diagnosis of hearing impairments in children: developmental approaches to clinical assessment, J. Commun. Disord. **7:**17, 1974.

# 6
# SEXUAL FUNCTION AND DYSFUNCTION

In contemporary health literature, sexuality has become an increasingly popular topic for development as a discrete entity. It is discussed in this text in a separate chapter to emphasize the importance of sexuality in relation to disease processes and individual adaptations to living. Although the chapter presents an overview of the topic of sexuality, it does not contain sufficient detail to arm the practitioner with an in-depth coverage of physiology and psychosocial considerations for intense counseling purposes. Other sources are devoted entirely to these ends. This chapter should serve as an introduction to traditional sexual norms, alternative considerations, and specific problems that some neurological clients may encounter. Interested individuals may apply general principles but should seek more comprehensive sources when they counsel intensively.

Sexuality should not be viewed merely as a life force that distinguishes men from women but rather as an integral component of the total individual on a continuum from birth to death. It represents the summation of one's behavioral competencies and feelings in terms of total personality, as well as the unique qualities that identify one as male or female in processes such as growth, development, life space, and communication capacities. Moreover, sexuality as a life force necessarily operates within the context of sociocultural and emotional realms to incorporate social patterns of learning along with bodily drives. Thus practitioners identifying competencies in sexuality need to review the process in the broadest context to elicit the gamut of comprehensive significance sexuality may have for the individual. Moreover, careful assessment of the client reveals the personal meanings, ideas, and values that affect the individual's concept of sexuality in terms of self. Given a thorough understanding of the client's background, viewpoint, and feelings, contemporary practitioners are able to counsel and assist clients in electing or exploring styles, patterns, and standards that improve their quality of life.

## PREMISES OF INTERVENTION

Nurses, like many other practitioners, have their own set of beliefs and values that govern individual behaviors and attitudes in sexuality. For some clients, these nurse-held values may be ideal, whereas for others such individual values may hamper meaningful communication and realistic guidance. To be effective in counseling a client on sexuality, the nurse needs sufficient education and experience in factual information and counseling techniques. Moreover, the nurse should have specific assistance in recognizing personal values and attitudes that might render the nurse unacceptable in interviewing and in counseling certain clients on general or specific aspects of sexuality.

Societal attitudes about sexuality are in flux. The roles of men and women are changing rapidly. Many believe that the next generations will rear their children with a number of different ideas on what men and women ''are'' and on what roles and behaviors are normative.

On more specific sexual behaviors, a number of things have changed. Public media convey programs and advertisements on specific sexual activities and products related to reproductive functions during times when children view television. Classes in school are more explicit. Publications reveal more in pictures and words than was possible even a few years ago. Adults become concerned sooner about the implications of adolescent boy-girl relationships.

Other changes are also afoot. In reading publications on sexuality released recently, one will find that attitudes conveyed in the health care literature are changing dramatically. For example, homosexuality is no longer an illness according to the American Psychological Association.

The health practitioner needs to remain informed about individual values and sexual behavior in relation to contemporary trends and interim and long-term outcomes. By doing so the practitioner is best able to present realistic options, discuss current social pressures, and work jointly with the client to arrive at the decision most appropriate to the individual. Client decisions, at best, in these times, are those wherein informed choice emerges above conformity to include options that are selected with complete awareness of interim and terminal outcomes. After decisions are made about one's own sexual behavior and patterns, the client may benefit by further follow-up wherein satisfaction and actual outcomes may be evaluated and modified as necessary. When the ramifications of sexual behavior become complicated or the assistance approaches the intensive therapy level, the practitioner may wish to refer the case to another professional better equipped to provide the needed intervention. The nurse may remain involved in other areas of care and may participate as a co-therapist or liaison in sexual issues as well.

The following nursing care standards are suggested as guidelines for working with the client who has a neurological problem. Consistent with these guidelines, the client may expect:

1. An identification of personal values, pleasure-giving stimuli, and sexual patterns when the client desires this type of assistance.
2. A tactful, thorough assessment of the specific neurological problem in relation to its effect on role performance, vocational and educational productivity, total functional ability, and self-concept.
3. A discussion of specific information on sexual functions and behavior and alterations arising from illness and aspects of the health care process.
4. The assurance of respectful handling of all personal data and strict confidentiality to include only appropriate professionals and mutually identified significant others.
5. Competent, professional management of any problem related to personal beliefs, relationships, and behaviors.
6. Therapeutic intervention that offers factual information and apparent outcomes in a milieu of realistic, nonjudgmental guidance and behavioral support.
7. Physical privacy and personalization of care to make institutional management as humanistic and client-centered as possible.

## CONTEMPORARY RESEARCH

Great attention has been focused on the human sexual response since Masters and Johnson's classic work was made available in 1966. Since that time the literature has abounded with information and studies that have dispelled widely held misconceptions.

The biological significance of sexuality is not necessarily more important or vital in shaping total development than are other essential biological activities. Instead, sexuality as a force is complexly interrelated with a number of other biological and emotional phenomena that operate together to produce the total range of psychosocial competencies within an individual. Most theorists agree that one's foundations in sexual behavior are established during the first 5 years as the child incorporates the nonverbal behaviors of significant others in the environment. Moreover, current investigators and members of women's liberation efforts have explored the fact that sexual drives, desires, and expressions of women may be less passive, submissive, and subordinate than previously thought, even if such behaviors have previously been accepted through sociocultural learning patterns and values. Finally, sexuality is both an individual and a life-long expression that is variously expressed but nevertheless formulates an integral part of comprehensive health, development, and biopsychosocial well-being.

In infants, sexual responses that distinguish males and females are variously ascribed by investigators to innate, learned, or combinations of nature-nurture forces. However, Stone and Church (1979) raise the point that one of the first questions settled at the birth of an infant is the sex of the child, and from that point verbal and nonverbal behaviors from the parents and significant others begin to mold behaviors in the child, including appropriate vocalization, and object selection and manipulation. Within the context of sociocultural forces, then, the major task of the child from the beginning is largely related to incorporation of the gender role. The gender role is greatly affected by the total response of significant others and expectations of the child, so that somewhere between 18 months and 4 years the child knows his or her gender. Moreover, the child has learned to build a set of values and emotions related to the continuum of acceptance for his or her body and its biological processes by incorporating the messages relayed verbally and nonverbally by significant others. In-depth discussion of developmental tasks and concerns that require successful completion to result in the highest level of biopsychosocial health may be gleaned from sources on growth and development. The works of Freud and Erikson (1963) are also important to a basic understanding of psychosocial development.

In looking at the childhood era, from roughly age 2 to 12 years, or pubescence, one notes vast changes in growth and development that are too extensive to review in this text. Thus some of the major trends and tasks are merely reviewed in the broadest sense to add continuity to this discussion.

Many agree that anal awareness is followed in preschool years by sexual awareness characterized by Freud as the Electra and Oedipus complexes. As these fantasized relationships between the child and parent of the opposite sex subside, the child enters the grade-school years, where latency of biological drives is upstaged by the conflict of industry versus inferiority, according to Erikson. By the time latency has occurred, the child should have developed a sense of morality from the resolution of the Electra-Oedipus complex. During the school years where latency prevails, the child tackles and accomplishes problems of the world in general that prepare him or her for moving into ever-widening circles away from the family.

During the early school years a differential level of school performance is evident between boys and girls; this may be ascribed to individual competencies (Maccoby, 1972) or to socialization by the school (Bardwick, 1972).

In terms of sexual identity the child 2 or 3 years of age can identify the two sexes and assign him- or herself to one category. Prior to this stage the foundation for successful sexuality and life relationships is being formed in a basic, broad way as the child learns and feels a sense of nurturing, love, oral gratification, and trust (as opposed to mistrust) during infancy. From the age of 2 or 3 years the child begins to learn and imitate behaviors compatible with the socially defined concept of gender and to learn values for actions that imply logic, intellect, physical prowess, sensuality, emotion, aggression, love, and so on. All these, including perception, interpretation, and response, are then incorporated into his or her real and ideal sexual role identity. During latency, children become curious about many processes related to bodily functions and sexuality and need accurate and healthy responses to their inquiries.

Principles that underlie the preadolescent period in relation to healthy resolution of sexuality include behaviors that relate to the attitudes and expectations of the sexual role as learned by the child from the parents. To effect this healthy resolution the parent of the same sex needs to present an image that is not weak or punitive so that sexual identification is possible. The parent of the opposite sex needs to avoid seductive activity and emotional instability that might cause the child to distrust or develop negative feelings toward the opposite sex. Together parents need to present acceptance of biological functions and feelings inherent in sexuality so that sexual identity and realistic sexual standards may be incorporated as a part of the total makeup of the child. When the basic foundations of love, trust, and sexual identification and exploration proceed in an abnormal manner, alternative patterns of sexual behavior may result. When children are reared in family groups that deviate from the traditional family pattern, a parent needs to provide healthy contact with members of the opposite sex. An example of such a model is the single-parent family. Interested readers should consult the references for readings in alternate family styles and sexual relationships.

Adolescence may roughly be divided into three stages, including the early, middle, and late periods. During the *early* period the adolescent is confronted with the physical changes heralding puberty, changes that necessitate an alteration in body image and self-concept. At this early point the adolescent tapers off his or her dependence on parents, moves out of the hobbies of middle childhood, and gravitates toward peer groups. By *middle* adolescence more rebellion and experimentation are apparent as the adolescent continues movement away from parents and toward strong peer alliances. Heterosexual interest becomes important as the adolescent is intermeshed in a life-style and value system that define personal worth and identity as being contingent on peer acceptance and group involvement. Selective peer activities predominate as the sexual drives apparent in the preschool age reemerge. Family confrontations are common as the adolescent relies on the love, trust, and support that parents optimally provide for successful resolution of sexual identity and establishment of a moral code. Where interpersonal problems and a lack of support prevail in parent-adolescent interactions, adolescents turn to less desirable modes of acceptance or expression through rebellious acts, which may include the use of drugs or sexual promiscuity. By *late* adolescence the well-adjusted individual has attained consolidation of identity, social integration, and an orientation toward the future. For many this is a time when they leave home to obtain employment or seek further education or training. Testing and switching of life and vocational objectives are common. Friends become limited to fewer peers, and dating becomes more exclusive and intimate as the adolescent strives to attain close, loving intimacy with a member of the opposite sex. Basically the entirety of the adolescent period may be characterized as the bridge between childhood and maturity.

North American culture provides constraints on the physically mature adolescent, barring adult rights, privileges, and responsibilities for several years after biological maturity. These restraints may add to the pressures and insecurities the adolescent feels while emerging toward mature identity. During the adolescent period, individuals are confronted not only with sexuality as a total image and conceptual framework but also with discrete concerns and events that are more specifically identified with sexuality. Healthy assistance in the acceptance of menstruation, masturbation, sexual autonomy, transient homosexual encounters, and questions related to premarital sex are some of the major requirements of the adolescent. When parents are unable to supply needed information or advice and treatment in contraception and venereal disease control, health team practitioners need to be available and accepting so that needy individuals are provided essential therapeutic intervention.

As the individual matures into adulthood, movement beyond the egocentric concerns of adolescence is evident. The external restrictions of adolescence are lifted, and the individual is confronted with a wide range of choice about sexuality in general and the expression of sexual activity. Since scientists have made such great strides in contraception, procreation as the overriding objective of sex is being reevaluated in the minds of many individuals in general society. Contemporary young persons seem to be approaching sexuality in marriage and adulthood in a more open manner than individuals of previous generations. Even with this increasing societal openness to issues of sexuality, health practitioners need to be integrally involved so that wide dissemination of factual information is available for individuals engaged in personal decisions about sexuality.

For many the period of adulthood is earmarked by marital union and parenting. However, methods of population control now allow consenting adults to remain childless. Moreover, young persons are remaining single for longer periods or returning to single life in increasing numbers through divorce. However, according to Erickson the key question of this period remains one of generative existence versus stagnation or self-absorption. Although increased freedoms for women and alternative sexual styles or diversity in living arrangements continue to be widely discussed in contemporary literature and through the media, the traditional family still seems to be the most widely accepted, stable relationship for heterosexual fulfillment, child-bearing, and general life productivity.

Even after all the psychosocial problems and concerns of biological integrity are resolved, situations remain that have the potential for altering an individual's sexual image. These factors include pregnancy, trauma, illness that interrupts usual sexual patterns, and disfiguring traumatic or surgical events. Responses to such interruptions are dealt with later in this chapter, after the discussion of sexuality and age is complete.

As age increases and manifests itself in visible physical changes, the couple approaches the interim period wherein children leave home, but retirement has not occurred. This age range is from about 50 through 65 years. It is earmarked by the task of resolving feelings of self-esteem versus those of despair. Key issues individuals face at this time include severing dependent ties with adolescents, coping with peak career and social demands, solving problems and interacting with aging parents, renewing the one-to-one relationship with a spouse, and facing the preparation for future years. Evaluating one's life success and coping with illness or death of a spouse may be additional issues at this point. Simultaneously, individuals are faced with physiological changes compatible with aging. Feelings about general sexuality are both personal and related to concerns and processes inherent in aging. Interest in sexual expression continues to be an integral need of this age group.

In later years establishing a retirement income that provides for physical comforts and needs, as well as psychosocial and emotional needs, seems important. Problems in health and possible loss of a spouse may cause the aged individual to realign life patterns to find new meanings in life. Little is done in our society to assist aging individuals in accepting physiological aging, death, and questions of sexuality. Studies on aging individuals reveal that these persons remain sexually active when the appropriate partner is available and when their health status is adequate. Certainly placement in segregated nursing home facilities may be one issue health practitioners might address as they consider the needs of aging individuals in the light of contemporary research.

## NORMAL PHYSIOLOGY

Vasocongestion and myotonia are the two major physiological processes that make up the human sexual cycle. Several portions of the nervous system are involved in sexual functions, including the cerebral cortex, the limbic lobe, the hypothalamus, the reticular activating system, the somatic pathways, the autonomic pathways, the reflex centers, and the peripheral nerves.

The first phase of sexual arousal is termed the *excitement phase,* wherein descending corticomotor or ascending sensory pathways relay impulses arising from psychic or physical stimuli.

The glans penis and the clitoris are the two primary neural areas of tactile stimulation and are both heavily populated with peripheral nerve endings. When either the external genitalia are stimulated or tension and pressure build up in the pelvic organs, impulses course to the pelvic or pudendal nerves through afferent fibers. From these nerves, impulses reach the sacral cord to synapse with parasympathetic efferent nerves of the pelvis, causing a possible reflex erection. In men, erection becomes possible as the parasympathetic nervous system transmits impulses from the sacral spinal cord through the nervi splanchnici pelvini to the penis. The resulting erection comprises arterial dilatation, some venous constriction, and subsequent vasocongestion of the cavernous sinuses of the penis.

Although psychogenic stimuli may influence reflex centers of the brain to trigger an erection, erections may also occur even when a total disruption exists in sacral cord functions through centers in the thoracolumbar area of the cord. Genital stimulation is still effective in causing ejaculation even when pathways relaying psychic stimuli from central structures have been completely severed.

In women, sexual excitement is an outcome of both local and psychic stimuli. When stimulation occurs at the local level, the pudendal nerve and sacral plexus transmit impulses to the lumbar and sacral areas of the cord. Sexual excitement of the erectile tissue in the female pelvis is regulated by parasympathetic impulses from the sacral plexus coursing through the nervi splanchnici pelvini to the genitalia. The modus operandi of the parasympathetic innervation is similar to that seen in men, wherein arteries of the orgasmic platform dilate and some venous congestion occurs, subsequently resulting in vasocongestion and vaginal lubrication.

After the excitement phase, a *plateau* ensues, wherein sexual tension mounts. At this point parasympathetic impulses in men result in mucus secretion from bulbourethral glands at the two sides of the urethra near the prostate gland.

Orgasm is an intense sexual state wherein rhythmic sympathetic impulses course to the penis from reflex centers in the cord. Reflex centers in the thoracolumbar cord regulate emission through the sympathetic nerves, resulting in propulsive contractions to move sperm to the penile urethra.

As emission occurs, the prostatic membranous urethra conveys afferent impulses through the pudendal and possibly pelvic nerves to the sacral cord, where they synapse with somatic efferent fibers of the pudendal nerve. The sexual act is made intense as the ischiocavernous and bulbocavernous muscles experience clonic contractions. During ejaculation the bladder neck is occluded to avoid entry of semen by synergistic neuronal activity at the sacral and thoracolumbar levels.

Ejaculation occurs as sympathetic pathways emit afferent impulses, which synapse with efferent fibers of the hypogastric nerves to stimulate the bladder neck, vas deferens, smooth muscles in the prostate, and spermatic vessels into peristalsis. Reflex centers regulating ejaculation are probably located in the sacral area of the spinal cord.

In women the neuronal stimuli and control through pathways are like those of men. However, the result in women is contraction of the perineal musculature and subsequent orgasm.

Several of the central structures may be responsible for sexual arousal as somesthetic, auditory, visual, and olfactory stimuli activate the hypothalamus, temporal lobe, and portions of the limbic system. As these higher centers are stimulated, somatic and visceral efferent fibers relay these impulses down to centers in the spinal cord.

## EFFECTS OF HOSPITALIZATION AND ILLNESS

The very character of the hospitalization process indicates both depersonalization and failure to individualize routines to the needs of each client. At a time when illness or disability may already threaten a client's image, bureaucratic hospital procedures compound the insult by confronting him or her with questions that result in the assessment of life and career successes and assets. Next the person is separated from valuables that link him or her to societal and personal identities and is dressed and treated in the manner of large institutional routine. All these verbal and nonverbal gestures serve to insult one's concept of sexuality and promote the feeling of being neuter sexually.

When illness interferes with functional capacities in a man, his partner may need to assume new roles and responsibilities in the home setting. Such role adjustment may be threatening to the man and may open new vistas for the woman, altering the relationship and functional roles of both partners from that point forward.

As a part of diagnosis and treatment, the client is further subjected to a role that banishes privacy and necessitates intrusion into psychosocial realms, privacy, and bodily parts as a matter of routine. The adult, used to control of his or her body and environment to a large extent, becomes helpless, dependent, and passive as a recipient of those services designed to stabilize the physical condition and return him or her to the highest functional level.

Too often the person's own feelings about illness, hospitalization, and role in relation to developmental tasks have not been adequately explored. Thus expectations and guidance related to separation from loved ones, disturbance of sexual functions, and lack of privacy may remain unconsidered in the total plan of care.

Neurological conditions frequently necessitate hospital admission either on a long- or a short-term basis. The nature of the illness—temporary, progressive, or chronic—has much to do with individual adjustment. When the illness results in problems or concerns that limit the individual from engaging in activities characterizing the preillness state, changes in self-image and life-style are often necessary. One such adjustment in life patterns is detailed in Chapter 10, where individuals afflicted with chronic pain begin to gear total responses to anticipation, coping behaviors, and preventive aspects to avoid discomfort. In several other chronic neurological diseases the practitioner is struck by the grief patterns that typify the client and family experiencing crisis and loss of former capacities and life patterns. Consider some of the mental and emotional changes that may occur with cerebrovascular accidents and that cause the client to be a far different person from what he was in the preillness state. Still other neurological problems have periods of exacerbation and remission, so that the grief process and adjustment patterns inherent in one's total concept of sexuality appear to wax and wane in relation to the immediacy of the symptoms. Individual responses to crisis in terms of life-style and body image compose a whole area of study for the practitioner who wishes to pursue the subject. Parad (1973) has edited a book on crisis intervention that provides a good basis for understanding this situation.

## Illness cycle

In individuals affected by illness, Lederer (1965) has identified three rather discrete stages of illness that influence the client in relation to sexuality in the broadest sense and that lend themselves to consideration by health practitioners planning comprehensive health care. These stages should be applied as the reader continues to review the neurological disorders described later in this text.

The first phase is one of *transition,* wherein the individual is confronted with the fact that illness has precluded participation in the mainstream of life. Responses at this point run the gamut from denial to aggression and seem to be heavily laden with personal interpretation of the meaning of this illness in the individual's total context. Does it make one feel aged or less sensuous and attractive as an individual? Are illness and inactivity signs that one is unmasculine, incapable, or unproductive? Does it threaten one's ability to hold a position in a vocation, academic role, or social group?

In transition, fantasy about real or imagined changes in body image related to sexual or physical attractiveness may cause the individual to worry about guilt, shame, and rejection. In this youth-oriented culture, disfiguring problems may cause one to fear loss of the ability to compete, to retain loved ones, or to face the usual life-style and friends.

Illness and submission to the care of others may be quite difficult for the controlling personality, who may deny illness or the need for assistance until no alternative is possible. In others, illness may represent secondary gains, that is, opportunities for attention, dependency, and escape from life's responsibilities. Either of these responses indicates a problem in accepting the self and in coping with one's own image.

As illness becomes a statement of fact to the client, transitory behaviors give way to responses identified with acceptance of the illness. At this point some persons seem aggressive and obnoxious, whereas other regress to less mature styles of operation. Other coping patterns emerge on the continuum between these two extremes. In North America, where achievement and goal orientation are values, illness and its states of dependency may make the individual feel weak and inadequate. As the individual gropes with acceptance, the practitioner notes increased egocentric concerns in daily activities and communications, as in the great detail the patient assigns to descriptions of pain, bowels, or food. Many jokes are generated in society about the sexual adjustments of this period, for example, the masculine client chasing the voluptuous nurse about the bed theme. All these jokes necessarily center about the key issues that pervade this period, for there is a bit of truth in every jest. For the client the following questions become quite significant: Am I still sexually attractive? Do I have the capacity to control my life? Will I overcome this passive, impotent phase, or is my former capacity gone forever? Verbally the client may lash out at personnel or facilities as a way of expressing dissatisfaction with the current status in life. One of the best books I have read on the anthropological events that affect both staff and patients in the hospital setting is Carol Taylor's *In Horizontal Orbit*. Ms. Taylor's wonderful British humor keeps the reader absorbed as one finds many points of personal identification with the deep issues that concern all hospital professionals in providing care for the hospitalized client.

In the convalescence phase the staff assists the client in regaining the total competencies for returning to a normal pattern of living. Dependency patterns are replaced by increasing client initiative and independence. Communication for the client returns to levels that include concerns beyond the self. Concerns increase as the client faces the problems of realigning body image and coping with his or her identity in relation to his or her real or desired life-style. Clients may become upset as the staff withdraws attention and support and centers these efforts on other clients with more acute needs.

During hospitalization a client may act out sexually to test his or her own sexuality and attractiveness to others. Such situations require tact and insight on the part of the staff, since they may result in embarrassing encounters and, at times, legal problems. Consider the woman who parades down the unit in a sheer negligee, the man who makes a pass at the female nurses, or the woman who accuses an orderly, male nurse, or physician of physical aggression.

Three major steps may be taken to avoid increased problems with one's sexual image. First, psychological and physical privacy should be provided for the client. Acknowledgment of feelings and explanation of procedures are warranted when intrusive procedures and exposure of private body parts are necessitated. Second, provision should be made to hold individual disclosures in confidence and to provide privacy for the client to act out emotional and sexual behaviors during hospitalization. Third, after assessment of the client's sexual needs, time, privacy, and arrangements should be allowed within the restrictions of illness and institutional routine.

## Sexual functions in patients with spinal cord injury

The most blatant confrontation with sexuality occurs for some clients and nurses when paralysis is involved after spinal cord impairment. At this time the client is faced with the fact that in addition to restrictions in mobility and its problems and needs for assistance in toileting and other functions of daily living, the possibility of sexual functioning may be gone forever. Fears about sexual ineptness in relation to body image and conduct of total life patterns may adversely color the client's total will to become rehabilitated.

Thus the issue of sexuality must be confronted early. To effectively encounter and assist the client who is concerned about sexual functions, the nurse needs to be personally comfortable with perspectives on the topic. In addition, the nurse needs to be equipped with factual information on sexual functions in the client with spinal cord injury. As the nurse encounters the client in a discussion of sexuality, the client may relate moral standards or practices that differ from those of the nurse. Self-understanding allows the nurse to be open and nonjudgmental as the best alternatives are explored for the individual client. As open communication proceeds, confidentiality about client disclosures beyond therapeutic professionals is a must. As the nurse interviews the client with regard to sexuality, it is important to gain information on preillness

concepts of sexual functions per se and sexuality as a whole, and it is imperative to discern what alterations in communication, sexual patterns, and other forms of affection are necessary to effect harmony between client and partner. Continuing support is necessary as the client and partner continue to explore alterations in their behavioral patterns. Other issues arise when a sexual partner is unavailable.

## Sexual functions in paralyzed patients

Increasingly since World War II, studies of male paraplegics have appeared to provide practitioners with essential statistics for rehabilitation counseling in sexual functions. A study of note was done by Bors and Comarr in 1960 as they interviewed 529 men with spinal cord injuries. Table 6-1 summarizes the findings of this study, which includes three important phenomena: (1) complete disruption of upper motor neurons of the cervical region results in only reflexogenic erections, (2) incomplete lesions result in both reflexogenic and psychogenic erections, and (3) complete lower motor neuron lesions result in only psychogenic erections.

The level and type of cord interruption profoundly affect sexual experience. Psychogenic erections are possible only in clients in whom complete or incomplete transection occurs beneath the level of T12. In either complete or incomplete transections of the cord at upper motor neuronal levels, sexual activity in the sacral region was found to have an inhibitory effect on ejaculation in some clients.

The orgasmic experience is widely variant in individuals who have experienced spinal cord injury and may range from a normal experience to anesthesia. In clients with upper motor neuron impairments, ejaculation may be preceded and accompanied by extreme flexor and extensor spasticity, followed by total relaxation in skeletal muscles. Some men with upper motor neuron lesions also report rousing sensations in the skin on the back superior to the lesion.

Clients with complete sacral cord transections state that sexual excitement is accompanied by sensual arousal in the inner thighs, groin, and lower abdomen.

In general, paraplegics relate successful experi-

**TABLE 6-1.** Type of spinal cord lesion and associated components of sexual function*

| Type of lesion | Erection | Ejaculation | Orgasm |
|---|---|---|---|
| Upper motor neuron | | | |
| Complete | Frequent (93%) Reflexogenic only | Rare | Absent |
| Incomplete | Most frequent (99%) Reflexogenic (80%) Reflexogenic and psychogenic (19%) | Less infrequent (32%) After reflexogenic erection, 74% After psychogenic erection, 26% | Present if ejaculation occurs |
| Lower motor neuron | | | |
| Complete | Infrequent (26%) Psychogenic only | Infrequent (18%) | Present if emission occurs |
| Incomplete | Frequent (90%) Psychogenic and reflexogenic | Frequent (70%) After psychogenic and reflexogenic erections | Present if ejaculation occurs |

*From Woods, N.F.: Human sexuality in health and illness, St. Louis, 1975, The C.V. Mosby Co.; based on the findings of Bors, E., and Comarr, A.E.: Urol. Surv. **10**:191-222, Oct. 1960.

ence and satisfaction in coitus to pleasure in satisfying the partner simultaneously.

In contrast to male paraplegics, few studies have involved female paraplegics. However, some observations have been made. For example, women with spinal cord injuries are believed to experience varying levels of libido in relation to age and psychodynamic factors. The same pathways referenced in the discussion of men are probably affected by the various levels of lesions. However, women have a more passive role sexually when sensory impairment accompanies the injury.

After the question of sexual functions is addressed, clients may raise questions related to fertility. In studies of complete and incomplete spinal cord transections sperm count remained essentially unaffected, except in clients with lumbosacral and cauda equina lesions, wherein the count was somewhat diminished. However, when microscopic examinations were performed in testicular biopsies, tubular atrophy was found, whereas Leydig's cells remained normal.

When sterility is a problem, it may be the result of hormonal disturbances or autonomic denervation, which alters temperature regulation. It may also be related to a mechanical problem wherein reflex emission lacks sufficient projectile power for impregnation. In these instances, electroejaculation may be utilized to gain semen for artificial insemination in the wives of paralyzed men.

In women the level and extent of the spinal cord interruption seems to be unrelated to fertility. Although some women have some interruption in menses, most resume menstrual periods within 6 months of the onset of paralysis. Menstruation frequently fails to resume in women who are near or into menopause.

Spinal cord transections do not seem to interfere with pregnancy, normal vaginal deliveries, or breast feeding. If lesions are above the level of T10, labors are painless, although in one small sample there was an increased incidence of effacement and dilatation of the cervix before the thirty-fourth week of gestation.

In lesions below the level of T10, normal sensory experience is retained during uterine contractions. However, spastic paraplegics may experience increased muscle spasms and ankle clonus during labor.

Complications during labor in paraplegic women result from autonomic dysreflexia, a cardiovascular phenomenon resulting in bradycardia, headaches in the last stages of labor, and hypertension.

**Common concerns**

As previously mentioned, psychosocial concerns need resolution, especially when the paraplegic is the head of a household. Economic problems and ego-related issues may become paramount in families with limited incomes as the man has varying successes in returning to employment and the woman has to assume breadwinning functions. Individual concerns from these arenas of problems deserve personal attention and calculated individual planning.

Another concern may center around the return of sexual function. For many clients the permanent level of sexual function will be apparent 6 months after spinal cord disruption. A complete neurological assessment is indicated at this time, with particular attention to the evaluation of the segments from S2 through S4, which innervate the bladder and sexual organs. When rectal tone is present and the bulbocavernous reflex can be elicited, the interference is at the upper motor neuron level. When these reflexes are absent, the problem is located in the lower motor neuron.

In upper motor neurons the retention of pinprick sensation in sacral segments is far more indicative of successful erection and ejaculation than is intact function in pelvic floor muscles or light touch perception. Other physiological problems that may interfere with successful coitus include incontinence, decreased muscle strength, and lack of ability to support body weight. Flexion spasticity may either induce an erection or interfere with coitus. This resumption of erection capacities in men is coincidental to recovery from spinal shock and reestablishment of sexual autonomic reflexes.

Another concern may revolve around coping with incontinence. Catheters may be left in place during coitus in both men and women, though the traction on the catheter may be problematic for the man. To avoid involuntary bladder evacuation, clients following intermittent catheter programs or with condoms should drain the bladder before coitus. Since chronic bladder infections in the paraplegic may be a source of infection for the partner, the preventive measures of bladder evacuation and thorough cleansing of the penis provide means of reducing the risk.

For clients unable to participate in normal coitus, alternative modes of sexual stimulation and positions should be explored.

## SUMMARY

Timing is everything. The practitioner who introduces sexual matters at a time when the client is occupied with toileting may receive a poor response. However, one should not wait too long after injury to introduce the subject lest the client assume silence is an affirmation of his or her loss of sexual functions. Realistic goal establishment and attainment depend on an open, trusting, ongoing series of encounters between the spouse and partner and the practitioner. Confidentiality, tact, and patience are essential ingredients of this process.

## REFERENCES

Aguiler, D.C., and Messick, J.M.: Crisis intervention: theory and methodology, ed. 3, St. Louis, 1978, The C.V. Mosby Co.

Anstice, E.: Helping the motherless family, Nurs. Times **69:** 432, April 5, 1973.

Athearn, L.M.: What every formerly married woman should know, New York, 1973, David McKay Co., Inc.

Atkin, E.: Part-time father: a guide for the divorced father, New York, 1976, Vanguard Press, Inc.

Ballivet, J., et al.: Aspects of hypersexuality observed in parkinsonian patients treated by L-dopa, Ann. Med. Psychol. (Paris) **2:**515, Nov. 1973.

Bardwick, J., editor: Readings on the psychology of women, New York, 1972, Harper & Row, Publishers.

Bardwick, J.: In transition: how feminism, sexual liberation and the search for self-fulfillment have altered America, New York, 1978, Holt, Rinehart & Winston, Inc.

Berezin, M.A.: Psychodynamic considerations of aging and the aged: an overview, Am. J. Psychiatry **128:**1483, 1972.

Berlin, H.: Effect of human sexuality on well-being from birth to aging, Med. Aspects Hum. Sexuality, July 1976.

Bors, E.: Sexual function in patients with spinal cord injury, proceedings of a symposium on spinal injuries, Royal College of Surgeons of Edinburgh, June 1963.

Bors, E., and Comarr, A.E.: Neurological disturbances of sexual function with special reference to 529 patients with spinal cord injury, Urol. Surv. **10:**191-222, Oct. 1960.

Bors, E., et al.: Fertility in paraplegic males, a preliminary report of endocrine studies, J. Clin. Endocrinol. Metab. **10:**381, 1950.

Braversman, S.: Homosexuality, Am. J. Nurs. **73:**652, 1973.

Comarr, A.E.: Observations on menstruation and pregnancy among female spinal cord injury patients, Paraplegia **3**(4): 263, 1966.

Comfort, R.L., and Kappy, M.: Pediatrician and social worker as a counseling team, Soc. Work **19:**486, July 1974.

Curtis, J.: Working mothers, New York, 1976, Doubleday & Co., Inc.

Despert, L.: Children of divorce, New York, 1962, Doubleday & Co., Inc.

Downey, G.W.: Sexuality in a healthcare setting, Mod. Health Care **5:**20-23, 25-27, May 1976.

Duncan, B., and Duncan, O.D.: Sex typing and social roles: a research report, New York, 1978, Academic Press, Inc.

Eiduson, B.T.: Looking at children in emergent family styles, Child. Today **3**:2, July-Aug. 1974.

Erikson, E.H.: Childhood and society, ed. 2, New York, 1963, W.W. Norton & Co., Inc.

Fisher, P.: The gay mystique: the myth and reality of male homosexuality, New York, 1972, Stein & Day Publishers.

Fisher, S.: The female orgasm, New York, 1973, Basic Books, Inc., Publishers.

Frommer, E.A.: Families at risk, Nurs. Times **69**:1408, Oct. 25, 1973.

Gadpaille, W.J.: Adolescent sexuality and the struggle over authority, J. School Health **40**:479, Nov. 1970.

Gardner, R.A.: Boys and girls book about divorce, New York, 1970, Bantam Books, Inc.

Gearhart, S., and Johnson, W.: Loving women/loving men: gay liberation and the church, San Francisco, 1974, Glide Publications.

Goode, W., and Price, S.: The second time single man's survival handbook, New York, 1974, Praeger Publishers, Inc.

Grollman, E.A.: Talking about divorce: a dialogue between parent and child, Boston, 1975, Beacon Press.

Hanion, K.: Maintaining sexuality after spinal cord injury, Nursing75 **5**:58, May 1975.

Henry, G.W.: Sex variants: a study of homosexual patterns, New York, 1979, AMS Press.

Hite, S.: Sexual honesty: by women for women, New York, 1974, Warner Paperback Library.

Jackson, R.W.: Sexual rehabilitation after cord injury, Paraplegia **10**(1):50, 1972.

Jaco, G.E., editor: Patients, physicians and illness, ed. 3, New York, 1979, The Free Press.

Kadushkin, A.: Single-parent adoptions: an overview and some relevant research, Soc. Serv. Rev. **44**:263, Sept. 1976.

Karr, S.D., and Dent, C.B.: In search of meaning, the generalized rebellion of the hippie, Adolescence **5**:187, 1970.

Katchadourian, H., and Lunde, D.: Fundamentals of human sexuality, ed. 2, New York, 1975, Holt, Rinehart & Winston, Inc.

Kinsey, A.C., Pomeroy, W.B., and Martin, C.E.: Sexual behavior in the human male, Philadelphia, 1948, W.B. Saunders Co.

Kinsey, A.C., et al.: Sexual behaviors in the human female, Philadelphia, 1953, W.B. Saunders Co.

Klein, C.: The single parent experience, New York, 1978, Avon Books.

Krantzler, M.: Creative divorce: a new opportunity for personal growth, New York, 1974, J.B. Lippincott Co.

Krantzler, M.: Learning to love again: beyond creative divorce, New York, 1979, Bantam Books.

Krell, R.: Problems of the single-parent family unit, Can. Med. Assoc. J. **107**:867, Nov. 1972.

Lederer, H.D.: How the sick view their world. In Skipper, J., and Leonard, R.C., editors: Social interaction and patient care, Philadelphia, 1965, J.B. Lippincott Co.

Long, R.C.: Common sexual problems and their management, J. Ky. Med. Assoc. **72**:273, May 1974.

Lorenz, N.: Sex after sixty-five, Public Affairs Pamphlet No. 519, New York, 1975.

Lowenthal, M.F., and Chiriboga, D.: Transition to the empty nest: crisis, challenge, or relief, Arch. Gen. Psychiatry **26**: 8, 1972.

Masters, W.H., and Johnson, V.E.: Human sexual response, Boston, 1966, Little, Brown & Co.

Masters, W., and Johnson, V.: Homosexuality in perspective, Boston, 1979, Little, Brown & Co.

McCary, J.: Human sexuality, ed. 3, New York, 1978, Van Nostrand Reinhold Co.

Maccoby, E.E.: Sex differences in intellectual functioning. In Bardwick, J.M., editor: Readings on the psychology of women, New York, 1972, Harper & Row, Publishers.

McFadden, M.: Bachelor fatherhood, New York, 1978, Ace Books.

*Medical Aspects of Human Sexuality,* a monthly journal available from Hospital Publications, Inc., 609 Fifth Ave., New York, New York 10017.

Money, J., and Ehrhardt, A.A.: Man and woman, boy and girl: the differentiation and dimorphism of gender identity from conception to maturity, Baltimore, 1973, The Johns Hopkins University Press.

Montague, A.: Touching: the human significance of the skin, New York, 1971, Harper & Row, Publishers.

One-parent families, Lancet **2**:92, July 13, 1974.

Parad, H.J., editor: Crisis intervention, New York, 1973, Family Service Association of America.

Pfeiffer, E., and Davis, G.C.: Determinants of sexual behavior in middle and old age, J. Am. Geriatr. Soc. **20**:151, April 1972.

Pfeiffer, E., et al.: Sexual behavior in middle life, Am. J. Psychiatry **128**:1262, 1972.

Roberts, A.R.: Childhood deprivation, Springfield, Ill., 1974, Charles C Thomas, Publisher.

Robertson, D.N.S., and Guttman, L.: The paraplegic patient in pregnancy and labour, Proc. R. Soc. Med. **56**:381, 1963.

Rosenfeld, J.M., and Rosenstein, E.: Towards a conceptual framework for the study of parent-absent families, J. Marriage Family **35**:131, Feb. 1973.

Satir, V.: Changing with families, Palo Alto, Calif., 1976, Science & Behavior Books, Inc.

Schwartz, L.H., and Schwartz, J.L.: The psychodynamics of patient care, Englewood Cliffs, N.J., 1972, Prentice-Hall, Inc.

Schaffer, K.F.: Sex-role issues in mental health, Reading, Mass., 1980, Addison-Wesley Publishing Co., Inc.

Skolnick, A., and Skolnick, J.H.: Family in transition: rethinking marriage, sexuality, child-rearing, and family organization, ed. 2, Boston, 1977, Little, Brown & Co.

Start, C.: When you're a widow, St. Louis, 1968, Concordia Publishing House.

Stone, J., and Church, J.: Childhood and adolescence, ed. 4, New York, 1979, Random House, Inc.

Sutterley, D.C., and Donnelly, G.F.: Perspectives in human development, Philadelphia, 1973, J.B. Lippincott Co.

Taylor, C.: In horizontal orbit: hospitals and the cult of efficiency, New York, 1970, Holt, Rinehart & Winston, Inc.

Toffler, A.: Future shock, New York, 1970, Random House, Inc.

Weber, D.K., and Weissman, H.C.: A review of spinal cord trauma, Phys. Ther. **51**:290, 1971.

Weinberg, G.: Society and the healthy homosexual, New York, 1973, Doubleday & Co., Inc.

Whaley, L., and Wong, D.: Nursing care of infants and children, St. Louis, 1979, The C.V. Mosby Co.

Wilbur, C., and Aug, R.: Sex education, Am. J. Nurs. **73:**88, 1973.

Wilson, D.: Counselling the person with spinal cord injury on sex and sexuality, Canadian Paraplegic Association, March 1973.

Women in transition: a feminist handbook on separation and divorce, New York, 1975, Charles Scribner's Sons.

Woods, N.F.: Human sexuality in health and illness, ed. 2, St. Louis, 1979, The C.V. Mosby Co.

# 7

# COGNITIVE AND BEHAVIORAL IMPAIRMENT

This chapter is intended to serve as a guide to the nurse who is confronted with the mental, emotional, and behavioral problems of neurological and neurosurgical clients. It can scarcely be called an orientation in psychiatric nursing, but it is hoped that the reader will be stimulated to increase the scope of his or her knowledge by referring to some of the books on psychology, psychosomatic medicine, psychiatry, and psychiatric nursing. An understanding of the underlying mechanisms motivating human behavior is an essential requisite of all nurses.

Major physical illness that requires hospitalization and a variety of medical or surgical treatments generally is accompanied by emotional reactions. Some clients freely express their fears and anxieties; others try to control or deny them; still others react by demonstrating great changes in mood and behavior. The observant, perceptive nurse can help the clients by providing opportunities to discuss the illness and the problems associated with it and by accepting expressions of anxiety.

Some clients whose emotional and physical needs are not met may react by being hostile and demanding. Generally these clients have difficulty in accepting the limitations imposed by illness and in adjusting to depending on others. The staff tends to perceive these clients as uncooperative and unappreciative. They are labeled as being difficult, problem clients and usually are rejected and treated summarily by the staff. Because the dynamics underlying their behavior are not understood, the staff cannot meet the special needs of these clients. Consequently, the negative expectations of

the staff reinforce and perpetuate the client's maladaptive behavior.

Although one may assume that most clients confronted with a serious illness experience some fear and anxiety, it is important to recognize that each client handles these emotions differently. The individual's reactions will be determined and influenced by learned habits of response; by constitutional and psychological makeup; and by racial, cultural, educational, religious, social, and vocational background.

Fear may be expressed indirectly in many ways; the aggressively demanding client, the client who puts the call light on frequently for seemingly trivial requests, and the client who is irritable or uncooperative and resistive may each be trying to overcome fear and may be communicating a need for the supportive presence of someone who understands and can help.

Generally the person who has difficulty in adjusting to depending on others or who is overdependent while in the hospital has had problems in this regard before. Whether or not the hospital experience is a strengthening one depends to a large extent on the staff.

Regardless of the mood, behavior, or mental status of a client, the registered nurse is responsible for providing the standard of nursing care that will maximize safety within the hospital. The nurse is responsible for monitoring physical and psychological environments and for alerting the physician and administration when a change in the client's condition requires modification. In planning the assignments of nursing personnel, one must know the level of knowledge and competency of each member of the staff to delegate only those functions and components of nursing care that can be performed safely and efficiently.

The clinical specialists, head nurses, team leaders, or primary care nurses, through personal attitudes, verbal and nonverbal communication, and behavior, create the climate in which nursing is administered and to a great extent determine its quality. If they respect the dignity and individuality of each client, so will their staff. If they express interest in and concern about the clients, so will their staff. If they attach high priority to using problem-solving techniques, so will their staff. If they are sensitive to the total needs of the client and intervene to prevent crisis situations and complications, the client's welfare, comfort, and safety are assured.

## OVERACTIVITY

Any client who has periods of elation out of proportion to the actual situation; who is seemingly tireless, physically overactive, mentally overproductive, and emotionally unstable; and who manifests extreme self-confidence may be considered overactive. These expressions of overactivity may vary considerably in degree. The overactive (manic) client may have flights of ideas, a short attention span, and little awareness of his or her behavior and its effect on others. This person may be manipulative, domineering, and disruptive. The attitude of superiority may alienate and irritate both clients and staff. If the client who is admitted to the neurological service presents any of these symptoms, one cannot ignore them when planning medical and nursing care. Clients with the following diseases most frequently present these manifestations to some degree; alcoholism, arteriosclerosis, brain tumor, acute and chronic encephalitis, epilepsy, head injury, general paresis, and senility.

### Nursing intervention

The responsibility of the nurse is reality centered and based on supportive, protective, and sedative therapies that are essential in the care of overactive clients. When an organic disease coexists, treatment and nursing care are planned to meet the client's needs, physical and psychological.

*Objectives.* Regardless of whether these symptoms are superimposed on a well-delineated organic disease or are the fundamental reason for the client's admission to the hospital, the nursing care is directed toward achieving the same objectives: (1) Observing the client carefully and accurately and recording pertinent conversation and behavior in exact detail; (2) protecting the client from injuring self or others; (3) preventing exhaustion and collapse; (4) increasing comfort and the therapeutic effect of the procedures and treatments administered; (5) understanding the etiology of the behavior and reacting objectively to the client; (6) planning total care in response to the physical, mental, and emotional needs of the individual client; (7) maintaining an adequate fluid and food intake; (8) providing safe outlets for physical energy; and (9) developing an effective interpersonal relationship.

*Approach.* The nurse's approach to the overactive client is most important in achieving these objectives. Understanding why he or she behaves in this manner allows one to react objectively with a minimal display of emotion. Do not show amusement, irritation, repulsion, or confusion about the behavior. Be firm, kind, nonjudgmental, and considerate in contacts with the client, and make every attempt to understand the reasons for the deviant conversation and activity. Recognizing that the erratic behavior and mood swings are symptoms of an illness, maintain the environment most suited to the client's needs and the amelioration of the condition. However, avoid indulgence and permissiveness; these attitudes may reinforce and increase the ''acting-out'' behavior. Set limits, and, if the client cannot exercise self-control, establish external controls to protect him or her and others. When an overactive client demonstrates aggressive tendencies toward another client or member of the staff, intervene promptly. Crisis situations frequently can be avoided when one removes the disturbed client from the group, accompanies him or her to a private room, remains with him or her, and talks quietly. Sustained personal contact can be supportive to the client and can help in developing self-control.

Effective, frequent communication among members of the staff is necessary for planning the care of the overactive client. The health team should be consistent in their approaches to the client and should create positive expectations so that he or she will develop more appropriate behavior and conform to certain standards of social interaction.

*Aspects of nursing care.* (1) Maintenance of nutrition by supervision of meals to ensure adequate intake. (2) Development of regular habits of elimination with supervision of visits to the toilet. (3) Supervision of hygiene with emphasis on the client's personal appearance. (4) Administration of sedatives, ataractic drugs, or prolonged neutral baths to ensure adequate rest and sleep. (5) Provision for participation in physical, recreational, and occupational therapy in view of needs, interests, and capacity. (6) Supervision of the client to prevent injury to self or others. (7) Control of the external environment with removal of harmful objects and reduction of external stimulation as necessary. (8) Assistance with diagnostic tests and therapeutic procedures. (9) Keeping of accurate records of all data pertaining to the client's behavior, attitudes, cooperation, coordination, and individual and group activity. (10) Treatment of the client as an ill adult and not as an individual who must be dictated to, corrected, and disciplined. (11) Development of a relationship so that psychological and social needs will be fulfilled. (12) Involvement of significant members of the family for the achievement of treatment goals.

## UNDERACTIVITY

Any client whose actions are retarded, appears sad and dejected, shows signs of inferiority, or expresses feelings of guilt or self-accusation may be called underactive. Some of these manifestations are the logical result of certain traumatizing experiences, but generally they should recede progressively. Any depressed, inactive client must be considered potentially suicidal. This assumption influences planning. These symptoms may be demonstrated in the following conditions: arteriosclerosis, epilepsy, senility, spinal cord injuries, and toxic states.

The disabled, chronically ill client, before accepting and adjusting to disability, may go through a period during which the symptoms just listed are manifested to a certain degree. Any assurance given by such a client that he or she would never harm him- or herself should serve to make the nurse more vigilant rather than provide a feeling of false security. This client may deliberately try to disarm the nurse by this approach in order to commit suicide at the first opportunity. If anything, he or she is more of a suicidal risk than the client with a psychosis, who is so retarded mentally and physically as to be unable to plan and attempt suicide.

## Nursing intervention

Many of these clients ultimately recover their emotional equilibrium. By accepting the basis of his or her reaction to disability and the change in self-concept, one can show interest and concern and can help the client adjust to and accept the limitations imposed by illness. Communicate belief in the client's worth and ability to cope with the problems that now seem overwhelming and without solution; express willingness to help and create opportunities to express feelings, fears, and anxieties; and help develop whatever intellectual and physical resources he or she has to compensate for any impairment of essential function. Increase independence and decrease dependence on the staff. As the client's condition improves, short- and long-term goals should be developed with the help of the client and family.

*Objectives.* The objectives outlined earlier for overactive clients apply to the care of underactive clients as well.

*Approach.* The approach to the underactive client differs in that concentration on using the right suggestions, techniques, and devices to stimulate and interest him or her must be emphasized. Cultivate patience, understanding, and perseverance. The development of rapport with a depressed, underactive client is a slow, tedious, and frequently discouraging process. Days, weeks, or even months may elapse before the client begins to respond by showing interest in surroundings and life. If he or she expresses delusional ideas, the staff should not try to reason or argue but should point out that they do not share these beliefs and attempt to redirect attention to other topics or engage in another activity.

Despite this client's seeming disinterest in what goes on, he or she is generally aware of and well oriented to the surroundings. A careless individual can further increase the state of depression by making thoughtless comments to co-workers within the client's hearing. An understanding professional will take every opportunity directly or indirectly to give positive assurance, show interest in the client's welfare, and offer encouragement despite apathy and lack of response. The recognition that nursing personnel tend to avoid the depressed, withdrawn client should encourage the perceptive nurse to spend time with him or her and give the emotional support this person needs so much.

*Aspects of nursing care.* (1) Prevention of self-injury by close, constant supervision. This should be done openly so that the client is aware of your concern and interest. A client may react negatively to constant supervision, be frustrated by the thwarting of plans, and resent the lack of privacy. Because of these feelings, he or she may begin to direct anger and hostility toward the staff member who is literally ''dogging his footsteps.'' This in itself may be therapeutic. (2) Maintenance of a pleasant, therapeutic milieu to stimulate interest. (3) Maintenance of nutrition by supervising the client's meals, making trays attractive, and encouraging eating. At times, it may be necessary to tube-feed these clients. (4) Maintenance of regular habits of elimination. The client should be taken to the toilet at specified times; output should be measured; retention of urine and severe constipation should be prevented. (5) Administration of stimulants or antidepressants, with observation of the client's reactions. (6) Supervision of the client's hygiene and personal appearance. Despite his or her lack of interest, assist the client in achieving a good cosmetic effect. Shaving under supervision is as important for male clients as applying cosmetics and dressing the hair becomingly are for female clients.

Plan a daily routine to occupy the client. This should include activities that can be achieved through suggestion without coercion. Mild exercises, walking, and simple occupational therapy may prove a point of departure and are essential if muscular tone is to be maintained and circulatory and psychological complications prevented. As the client convalesces, the schedule should be varied and activities progressively increased. At first the practitioner will have to initiate all activity and encourage the client to participate even in a passive way. As he or she convalesces, the client should become increasingly independent and should be guided to make plans and decisions. The ambulatory or wheelchair client should also be encouraged to engage in group activities with other clients.

## MALADJUSTMENT

Any client is maladjusted who has difficulty in adapting to the environment and who manifests to an abnormal degree any of the following symptoms: nervousness, palpitation, insomnia, asthenia, anxiety, irritability, inability to concentrate, vague somatic complaints without demonstrable organic causes, gastrointestinal disturbances, fatigue, anorexia, or fear. These manifestations of neurotic or maladjusted personalities may be present concomitantly with or follow an organic illness. They may be precipitated by injuries, infections, operations, or chronic disease. Approximately 65% of all clients seen in private medical practice manifest some of these symptoms and are suffering from a form of ''psychoneurosis.'' Some of these clients, unable to adapt to the stresses and strains of life, unconsciously transfer their emotional conflicts into physical symptoms and thus make an inferior form of adjustment that serves temporarily to ease the conflict. This is called *conversion hysteria* and is characterized usually by loss of sensory or motor function in some part of the body.

The scope of this chapter does not permit discussion of psychosomatic medicine, which has directed attention to the emotional factors involved in many organic diseases. It emphasizes the importance of treating every client as an individual, a complete personality, rather than the symptoms and signs of physical disease alone.

### Nursing intervention

*Approach and treatment.* The clients who have developed disabling symptoms that keep them from living up to their capacities and potentialities depend on those in authority and need considerable guidance and support. Understand the meaning of the symptoms and the dynamics underlying behavior. Only through knowledge and understanding of these problems can the client be assisted toward good health. Many of these clients unconsciously cling to their symptoms because they are unable to give up the security the hospital situation affords them. Treatment is directed so that clients will develop insight and will ultimately reorganize their personalities so that they may function effectively in personal relationships within the community.

Never imply disbelief in the client's illness. Guard against making the easy judgment that because there is no organic cause for illness, the client is not ill and does not deserve any time, patience, understanding, or care. Less effective practitioners may even be so intolerant of this type of client that they reject and neglect him or her. Some go as far as to inform the client that there is nothing wrong and that he or she should stop acting like a baby or a sissy and get back on his or her feet. Denial of the client's illness only causes loss of confidence in the staff and develops even more symptoms in an unconscious effort to gain the sympathy and help needed.

Establish good rapport with the client in an effort to gain confidence, recalling that he or she is ill, psychologically helpless, and frequently dependent on you.

The adult client should never be treated like a child. A friendly, matter-of-fact relationship should be established from the beginning. Do not encourage the client in unconscious, but frequently persistent, efforts to remain childlike, making exorbitant demands for attention and affection.

Recognize the fact that the client will improve and be able progressively to do things he or she is now unable to do. Suggestions, reassurance, and encouragement are important techniques used in the care of these clients. The nurse, guided by the physicians, can contribute a great deal in these areas during contacts with the client. Avoid criticizing or blaming the client for being unable to perform a certain task; on the other hand, give praise whenever possible. These clients are generally emotionally unstable and respond very readily to suggestion. Strive to be optimistic without displaying inappropriate and insincere behavior. The projection of positive expectations frequently produces positive reactions.

Important observations may be made on the client's behavior when he or she is alone or in a group. A program of activities (occupational therapy, physical and recreational therapy, and outdoor exercise) should be planned for the client to reestablish interests and to distract from ailments.

Supervised group activity should be directed toward building up self-confidence and facilitating the development of social and personal relationships.

Psychotherapy is given to the client not only to free him or her of symptoms but also to aid in the development of insight into the causes of illness and to guide in reorganizing personality so that he or she can function as a respected, useful, and happy member of the community.

To become well-adjusted, the client must be able to face reality, to adjust to its demands without developing any symptoms, and to react to stress and strain without security being threatened. Adjustment may be facilitated when the home environment is modified as necessary.

Bed rest, because of its psychological implications, should be restricted to a minimum throughout hospitalization. Action absorbs anxiety, and this maxim should be a basic consideration when one is making the plan for treatment. If the client also has an organic disease, treatment and nursing care should proceed hand in hand with the principles previously outlined. Only such diagnostic study as is necessary to rule out organic disease should be done. Too often the client's attention is further fixed on symptoms by unnecessarily elaborate diagnostic measures.

## AGE

Any older client who has cerebral alterations that result in changes in intellectual activity, responsiveness to stimuli, and the capacity for adaptation to the environment may be considered aged. Some clients are victims of the aging process before they are 60 years old; others who are 70 years of age are still able to function and to react to and cope with the realities and stresses of life. Reaction to increasing years varies with the individual. However, inevitably certain physiological changes take place that influence one's self-concept, functioning, mood, and behavior.

The progressive alteration of body structure and function results in certain pathological manifestations that characterize the aging process: changes in equilibrium and coordination, slowed reflexes and responses to stimuli, impaired sensory perceptions (hearing, vision, smell, taste, pain, and temperature), impaired intellectual functions (memory for recent events; orientation to time, person, and place; confusion at intervals, especially at night; misinterpretation of stimuli) and emotional reactions, diminished central nervous system response to postural changes (orthostatic hypotension), and less efficient detoxification of drugs.

The aged client may manifest some or all of these characteristics in varying degrees. Depending on the severity and number of physiological changes, he or she may become increasingly anxious and fearful about the ability to be independent and to take care of him- or herself. If hearing is impaired, the client tends to withdraw and to become unduly suspicious. If vision is impaired the client has poor tolerance of strong lighting and glare and may be unable to read, look at television, or pursue usual interests and hobbies. If the sense of smell is impaired, the client may be unable to taste food, may lose appetite, and may become undernourished. If intellectual perception of pain and heat is impaired, disease processes may not be recognized or burns may result. Because the central nervous system reacts less readily to the effect of gravity in the erect position, heart rate is not increased, and the small arteries and veins constrict more slowly, with pooling of blood in the abdomen and lower extremities. As a result, when the client assumes an erect position after bed rest, the blood pressure may fall, and he or she may complain of dizziness or faintness. If equilibrium is poor, the client may have a tendency to fall. In the case of forgetfulness, confusion, or disorientation the client may compensate with stereotyped behavior to avoid the risk of failure. The aged client is less able to tolerate and deal with stress and changes in the environment. He or she may not be able to control physiological functions. This person may feel worthless and be depressed.

Since the detoxification of drugs by the liver and their excretion by the kidneys are less efficient, the client is more likely to react adversely to certain drugs. Central nervous system reactions to the bromides and barbiturates are more easily precipitated and more prolonged. Daily doses of these drugs, though small, may increase mental confusion. Since the cough reflex generally is weakened and ciliary activity diminished, codeine may induce clogging of the bronchial tubes and cause atelectasis. Since secretions are not expectorated, these clients are especially susceptible to pneumonia.

The physiological and psychological reactions to the aging process may be intensified when the elderly client is removed from home to the hospital. Fears of dying and of being deserted, alone, unloved, and unwanted are reinforced by the separation from family and friends. Self-esteem may change to feelings of worthlessness and hopelessness. When the natural consequences of the aging process are considered and are superimposed on a primary illness, the special needs of these clients for understanding, support, and encouragement are better appreciated.

## Nursing intervention

The care of the aged client is facilitated if a climate of understanding and acceptance is created that focuses on the client as a person with strengths and abilities as well as limitations and problems.

*Objectives.* The care of the aged client is directed toward achievement of the following objectives: (1) helping the client adjust to the hospital environment, (2) helping the client function as independently as possible, (3) helping the client participate in the activities of daily living, (4) involving the client in daily planning and decision making, (5) providing experiences through which the client can achieve feelings of worth, (6) promoting the client's self-esteem, (7) helping the client develop control over body functions, (8) providing active and passive activities as deterrents to regression and deterioration, (9) helping the client socialize within capabilities, (10) promoting the client's physical and emotional well-being, (11) maintaining optimal intake of food and fluid, (12) recording and reporting accurately reactions to drugs, (13) helping the client express feelings and communicate effectively with others, and (14) preventing physiological and psychological complications.

*Approach.* The approach to the aged client is most important for the achievement of the objectives just listed. All attitudes and approaches are based on respect for the client as a person of dignity and worth. This approach will enhance self-esteem, mobilize strengths, and prevent further deterioration, regression, or depression. The elderly client should not be hurried; he or she needs more time to react and to follow hospital routine. Establish, with his or her help, a schedule of daily activities that will facilitate adjustment. Frequent reference to the time of day, the day of the week, and the sequence of meals and other activities will help to orient the client and diminish confusion and feelings of insecurity. Careful explanation of any change in routine or of any new procedure is most important in the prevention of unnecessary frustration, anxiety, or stress. Providing the client with opportunities to be as independent as possible and to achieve a feeling of accomplishment will contribute to feelings of worth and individual identity.

In some instances when an elderly client has a prolonged hospitalization, he or she may become the "pet" of the ward, be treated like a child, and be addressed in an informal, familiar manner. Even though this behavior by the staff may be motivated by their positive and kindly attitudes toward the client, it should not be condoned or tolerated. At all times the elderly client, like any other mature individual, should be treated as an adult. The client, even though his or her behavior is childish, should be addressed formally as Mr. _____, Mrs. _____, or Miss _____. This helps to create a climate in which the client is accepted as a person and expected to function at optimal level. It increases personal identity and prevents further regression or deterioration.

The staff who has positive expectations of the client and helps him or her to do what is possible at the right time and place, no more and no less, is creating opportunities for the client to utilize and maintain skills. The assignment of the same staff to care for the client also will facilitate adjustment. The number of different staff members caring for the client should be as few as possible. Not only is the client less threatened and confused, but also the staff develops more understanding of the client's needs as well as skill in meeting them.

Close observation of the client and reactions to drugs, treatment, and nursing care and planned interactions provide the data needed to evaluate progress and to revise and modify the nursing care plan. Involvement of the family in care and sustaining their interest and support will alleviate some of the client's fears of isolation and desertion.

*Aspects of nursing care.* (1) Maintenance of nutrition and fluid balance by supervision of meals and by providing of interval feedings to ensure optimal food and fluid intake. (2) Development of regular habits of elimination with scheduled, supervised use of facilities. (3) Encouragement of self-care, personal grooming, and interest in appearance. (4) Fostering as much independent activity as possible. (5) Provision of a schedule of meals and daily activities with opportunities for the client to make choices about participating in certain activities. (6) Creation of a climate of acceptance in which the client is treated as an adult and respected as a person of worth. (7) Provision of experiences that will enhance self-esteem. (8) The understanding of verbal and nonverbal communication; interpretation and sharing with other staff members assigned to the client's care. (9) Development of a meaningful relationship so that emotional, intellectual, and social needs are met. (10) Encouragement of the family to visit and bring the client small personal possessions that will contribute to security. (11) Placement of a large clock and calendar where they can be seen by the client as aids to orientation. (12) Controlling and modifying the environment to ensure adequate rest and sleep (a small light at night is recommended). (13) Administration of medications as ordered; observation of therapeutic and toxic effects; recording and reporting reactions. (14) Appreciation of physical limitations and sensory impairments and development of a nursing care plan in light of accumulated data. (15) Recognition that bed rest and immobility may exaggerate physical and emotional problems and that activity and socialization may diminish these problems. (16) Avoidance of any hurried, unexplained change of position to wheelchair or stretcher that might cause the client to become disoriented and fearful of losing control of time and space. (17) Supervision of client in any change of position from bed to standing. (18) Prevention of physiological and psychological complications should be emphasized.

Some hospitals have a policy that elderly, infirm, or confused clients must have side rails on the bed at all times. Every effort should be made to explain the reasons for this policy to the client. If he or she is bedridden, a member of the family, a friend, or a volunteer may stay with the client and the side rails may be lowered or removed. Restraints should be used with extreme caution and only as a last resort. The client may interpret this procedure as punishment; confusion and disorientation may increase; feelings of worthlessness may be reinforced; and he or she may waste valuable strength fighting the restraints. Enforced immobilization increases the possibility of skin breakdown, problems of elimination, and respiratory and thromboembolic complications, as well as undesirable emotional reactions.

If the nursing and medical staff really understand and appreciate the nature of the aging process and its impact on the individual, they will accept the aged client as a person who presents a challenge to them and who merits the collaborative use of their knowledge and skill.

## DEVELOPMENTAL DELAY

One of the disadvantages of diagnosing a mentally impaired individual as "retarded" is the label that follows that person from that point. The label "mental retardation" has some negative connotations that may result in undesirable outcomes and the receipt of stereotyped behavioral responses from a variety of individuals and agencies.

To avoid this problem, professionals are beginning to term those whose cognitive and behavioral levels are inappropriate to chronologic age as developmentally delayed individuals. In reality, developmental delay is a catch-all term that can include the mentally retarded, the learning disabled, and those impoverished by inadequate social, environmental, or emotional deprivation. At times, it is difficult to distinguish which factor or factors apply to a given individual. In other cases, practitioners promptly arrive at a definitive conclusion. Even when a diagnostic category is reached, practitioners may retain the label of developmental delay with explicit descriptions of individual client characteristics, since this general label offers more flexibility and may have less stigma attached. However, some agencies do not accept the developmental delay term. Health care specialists continue to debate issues on the use and abuse of the

term "developmental delay." For further insights, refer to Chapter 5 and to the remaining problems discussed in Chapter 8.

## Mental retardation

When one considers the range of problems that interfere with cognitive and behavioral functions, the area of mental retardation frequently comes to mind. Although many entities resulting in retardation are outcomes of childhood problems, medical advances have enabled retarded citizens to live well into adulthood in many instances. In the United States about 13.59% of the retarded citizens have borderline intelligence, 2.6% fall into the educable range, 0.3% are trainable, and another 0.1% are grouped in the category requiring custodial care.

Methods of categorizing the mentally retarded include groups usually related to etiology or severity.

### *Definitions*

ETIOLOGY. The etiological definition and classification of mental retardation that have received the widest acceptance were proposed by the American Association on Mental Deficiency (AAMD). In this statement, mental retardation is defined as "subaverage general intellectual functioning" that results in impairments in adaptive behavior. Mentally retarded individuals include those who fall more than 1 standard deviation below the mean on intelligence tests. However, an important point of consideration is that placement within a category of intelligence may not be permanent. Instead, through adequate professional intervention or environmental enrichment, the possibility exists for the person to improve intelligence scores even to the point of normal intellectual functioning.

Mental retardation is further defined by the AAMD in relation to the following eight major causes:

1. Mental retardation resulting from infection, which occurs during two periods: prenatal and postnatal. Prenatal infections that cause neuronal damage leading to mental retardation include those of viral (herpes simplex, rubella, cytomegalic inclusion disease), protozoal (toxoplasmosis), and bacterial (syphilis, *Haemophilus influenzae* infection) origin. Sequelae from infections such as bac-

terial meningitis or encephalopathies account for the neuronal damage that results in mental retardation in the postnatal period.

2. Mental retardation may be caused by intoxication from exogenous or endogenous sources. In the prenatal period, maternal ingestion of medications such as opiates, reserpine, or quinine; toxemia; and Rh incompatibility leading to bilirubin encephalopathy are some causes of mental retardation. In the postnatal period such factors as lead poisoning, hyperbilirubinemia from large doses of vitamin K, and postimmunization encephalopathies are implicated as some causes of mental retardation.

3. Mechanical agents or physical injury may result in mental retardation. In the prenatal period such factors as hemorrhage, threatened abortion, or irradiation may be causative events. In the postnatal period, particularly at the time of delivery, such problems as mechanical injuries during delivery, intracranial hemorrhage, anoxic episodes, extended use of anesthesia, and cesarean section may result in mental retardation. Such agents as automobile accidents may also result in impaired mental capacities throughout the life cycle.

4. Mental retardation may result from disturbances in growth, metabolism, or nutrition. Rh and ABO incompatibilities with their resulting sequelae also belong in this category. Hormonal imbalances in either the prenatal or postnatal period resulting in impaired growth and mental retardation are also included in this category.

5. Mental retardation may result from new growths. Conditions in this category include intracranial neoplasms, neurofibromatosis, tuberous sclerosis, and Sturge-Weber syndrome.

6. Unidentified factors may result in mental retardation, particularly in relation to abnormalities in the embryonic period. Some of these entities include certain chromosomal disorders, anencephaly, and encephalopathies associated with cranial malformations such as microcephaly, hydrocephalus, cranium bifidum, and craniostenosis.

7. Mental retardation may result from undefined factors associated with impaired functioning of the central nervous system. Cerebral sclerosis is an example of this type of encephalopathy.

8. Mental retardation may also result from un-

defined disorders that result in impaired behavioral or functional categories. This category includes cultural-familial factors, psychogenic or psychosocial influences (sociocultural deprivation, emotional disturbances), and major alterations in personality (autism, childhood schizophrenia).

SEVERITY. Mental retardation may be ranked with reference to *severity*. Three categories compose this ranking system, including educable, wherein the intelligence quotient (IQ) is from 50 to 70 points; trainable, wherein the IQ is from 30 to 49 points; and custodial, wherein the total is less than 30 points. These three categories are based on a child's adaptability to academic and behavioral competencies necessary for adequate school performance.

The categorization based on severity fails to include a significant number of children whose scores lie somewhere in the range between normal and educable. For these children competition in the normal classroom situation is impossible without special assistance from the teacher. They may also have the added problem of possessing an IQ too high for candidacy in special education programs in some states.

Educational instruction of the slow learner is aimed at enhancing the child's ability to construct meaningful learning strategies and systems for data collection, comprehension, storage, utilization, and subsequent recall, particularly within the realms of concepts, abstractions, and relationships of objects. Techniques designed to facilitate these educational objectives and create intrinsic motivation have resulted in increases of as much as 20 points on intelligence tests.

Some learners are not only slow, but also difficult to arouse so that meaningful learning and communication may take place. One of the newer treatments for causing lethargic, slow learners to "come alive" for maximal benefit in special learning centers is stimulation to the reticular activating system. This method is termed "sensory integrated processing therapy." The child is suspended in a net from a free-hanging, sturdy rope, and spun around rapidly to the point of dizziness. The response is dramatic in increasing behavioral and intellectual output and total activity. The arousal and awareness levels are also noticeably increased.

When successful, this method is utilized at the beginning of a productive learning session and is often done as a daily routine.

Individuals categorized in the educable range may master academic material at the maximum level of the fifth grade. Assessments of development frequently reveal significant delays, even though many of these children appear normal outwardly. School programs practicing contemporary philosophies vary in approaches to include such innovations as individualized curriculums that allow for mainstreaming (remaining within the regular class) and entry into a well-staffed resource room as the situation requires. When possible, integration with normal children is preferred over the self-contained classroom setting wherein retarded children are constantly grouped together because it gives the child normal role models to identify with. Modifications of the individual curriculum allow this integration to occur with a minimum of negative feedback from inability to compete.

Vocational counseling and direction in concerns of daily living are imperative with advancing age to enhance the individual's opportunities for achieving independence and functioning within the range of jobs available to the intellectually limited. Gainful employment and independence in activities of daily living in adult years are important objectives.

When school programs do not allow for the needs of the retarded citizen, parents may need to seek the assistance of one of the state or federally supported programs that provide a broad range of services to the retarded individual and the family. Some of these reach down to meet the needs of infants and up to include the needs of adults who have experienced mental retardation throughout life or have experienced some type of trauma or disease process that has left residual cognitive impairments. More alternatives to life management and concerns inherent in mental retardation are becoming available for affected citizens of all ages as society and professionals continue to explore ways of integrating these individuals into the mainstream of living. In coming years investigators will strive to identify more causes of mental retardation and concurrent preventive measures for avoiding cognitive impairments.

In trainable mentally retarded children the goals are mainly related to independence in social skills and self-care. Vocational opportunities are frequently restricted to supervised situations, and intervention is often necessary for the management of personal affairs. Phenotypically, trainable individuals may exhibit outward evidence of specific syndromes or may have perceptual defects.

Frequently the only course open to the most retarded group, the custodial mentally retarded, has been home care throughout life or institutionalization. Either decision is very difficult for the involved family, and both situations have advantages and disadvantages. Because placement in an institution results in so much guilt and turmoil for parents, they need intensive guidance and support as they confront the decision and resolve the situation to conform to their individual life pattern. Where facilities exist, some families are able to reach a happy medium as they find a care setting wherein the retarded citizen may go for day care or care through the week, while being able to be at home other times.

### New developments

The retarded citizen may now look forward to the growth of the community residential housing program, wherein institutions are returning their clients to supervised apartment living in their own local communities. Progress in this trend, as well as other current trends and laws may be monitored by reading the *P.C.M.R. Newsbreak,* a periodical published by the President's Committee on Mental Retardation, Department of Health, Education, and Welfare, Washington D.C. 20201. For current information on accreditation standards applying to this group, write to the Accreditation Council for Services for Mentally Retarded and Other Developmentally Disabled Persons, Joint Commission on Accreditation for Hospitals, 875 Michigan Avenue, Chicago, IL 60611.

Awareness of laws and facilities within the community and state is an important prerequisite to effective counseling. Two of the most significant laws currently are PL 94-142, a law that mandates individually appropriate special education for all school-aged children who have any type of physical, intellectual, or emotional handicap, and PL

93-112, a massive law of rehabilitation acts passed in 1973, which include nondiscrimination in all respects for handicapped individuals. Examples of nondiscrimination extend to include such things as architectural barriers, employment, and education.

Careful assessment of the client-family dynamics and the total cultural, psychosocial, and economic climate will provide the practitioner with the data necessary for counseling and intervention.

### Involving families

To effectively change the total milieu of the client, the home setting must be altered as positive growth and improved functional capacities result from the therapeutic treatment setting. Parents are a valuable resource and may be involved in a variety of meaningful ways as in groups designed to facilitate personal and family growth and acceptance; in a number of volunteer activities, which may involve direct contact with clients or indirect services to benefit public relations, administration of services, or fund raising for an agency; in support to parents of a newly diagnosed client; or in home training programs for self or others. There are a number of reasons why parents fail to become involved. The agency may indicate a lack of interest for what may be a threat to their exclusive control of educational processes, threatening behavior from staff members, or what they may view as inappropriate parent behavior, attitudes, or accessibility. To avoid poor first contacts with parents and significant others, the nurse may be the one who makes the first approach. A home visit is often a good idea because it allows the nurse to increase the data base on the child's total environment and life space. A few conditions, beyond harmony and willingness for a family outreach at the agency, must exist. These include (1) the necessity for the nurse to thoroughly assess the child and family and to individualize the approach for each situation, (2) a thorough working knowledge of agency and community resources, (3) a time for the initial contact that is mutually convenient for both the nurse and the family, and (4) an attitude that conveys positive feelings about the client and the proposed intervention and one that does not heighten parental feelings about guilt, blame, and frustrations of pursuing the problem without adequate support systems.

### Nursing intervention

Nurses may be involved in a limited way with the retarded citizen or in a manner wherein they have more total responsibility for the individual. The following objectives may be utilized as they apply:

1. Maintain a therapeutic environment wherein a positive self-concept is emphasized and wherein expectations and protocols are geared to individual capacities.

2. Remain informed about the issues in management of the mentally retarded client in the community, the state, and the nation. Work to change laws, practices, public opinions, and misconceptions that disadvantage the retarded citizen.

3. Plan care to include physical, behavioral, cognitive, and sociocultural needs within the framework of realistically available resources.

4. Assess the abilities, disabilities, and potential capacities of the client with other professionals in the health care and educational delivery systems so that a total plan emerges for augmenting individual abilities and talents.

5. Participate in family/client assessment and education and in implementing methods of stimulating sensory, motor, and cognitive functions.

6. Write exact behavioral objectives for each individual client with other members of the helping team. Evaluate these daily, and rewrite them whenever they are necessary to the progress of the individual.

7. To maintain objectivity, observe the client carefully and record all pertinent conversation and behavior to document the progress of the individual in relation to individual objectives.

8. Learn about the specific condition that underlies the mental retardation, and include appropriate items in acute and chronic care as it pertains to the individual.

9. Monitor the general health, growth, and development of the client, including such things as immunizations, so that the total well-being of the individual may be assured.

10. Involve family members and significant others in the total plan of care. Utilize opportunities to include them in programs for families, and in working on projects that give them a sense of "helping" and some insights into others with similiar problems.

11. Work as a liaison between the client with significant others and the agencies that provide health care, education, and vocational services, so that efforts benefit the client maximally.

## Helpful resources in mental retardation

- International Council for Exceptional Children, National Education Association, 1201 16th St. N.W., Washington, D.C. 20036. Provides reading lists on request, publishes the *Exceptional Child* periodical, and has local chapters in the United States.
- National Association for Retarded Citizens, P. O. Box 6109, Arlington, Texas. Provides reading lists on request, offers some free reading materials. This is the national organization for children and parents. Information on local chapters is available.
- *Residential Schools and Homes for the Mentally Deficient: A Directory.* Published by the American Association on Mental Deficiency. Lists public and private residential schools by state with a limited description of each facility.
- *Directory for Exceptional Children,* E. Nelson Hayes, editor, 11 Beacon St., Boston, Massachusetts 02108. A comprehensive guide of day, state, and residential schools for the mentally retarded, blind, deaf, and psychologically disturbed. The source lists clinics as well and provides a fairly adequate description of facility capacities and limitations (3,000 facilities; 1304 pp.).
- *Mental Retardation,* American Association on Mental Deficiency, Box 96, Willimantic, Connecticut 06226. A bimonthly, nontechnical publication that emphasizes treatment techniques and training programs.
- *Training School Bulletin,* Training School, Vineland, New Jersey 08360. Prints human-interest, technical, and nontechnical material on mental retardation.
- Children's Bureau, U.S. Dept. H.E.W., Social Security Administration, Washington, D.C. 20402. Ask for directories and current reading materials on the mentally retarded.
- Berkman, Gloria: *Training parents as members of the educational team,* ED 122 570 and EC 182 948 ERIC. Paper presented at the annual international convention, The Council for Exceptional Children, April 1976. Self-paced modules to assist parents in working more effectively with their child. A total approach included.
- Reisinger, James John: *Educating parents as primary service providers,* ED 122 568 and EC 082 946 ERIC. Paper presented at the Annual International Convention, The Council for Exceptional Children, April 1976.
- Markel, Geraldine, and others: *Assertiveness training for parents of exceptional children,* ED 122 569 and EC 082 947 ERIC. Paper presented at the annual international convention, The Council for Exceptional Children, April 1976.
- Donaldson, Joy: *Working with parents: a values clarification approach,* ED 122 567 and EC 082 945 ERIC. Paper presented at the annual international convention, The Council for Exceptional Children, April 1976.

## REFERENCES

Aguilera, D.C.: Review of psychiatric nursing, St. Louis, 1977, The C. V. Mosby Co.

Baroff, G.S.: Mental retardation: nature, cause and management, New York, 1975, Halsted Press.

Begab, M.J., and Richardson, S.A.: Mentally retarded and society: a social science perspective, Baltimore, 1975, University Park Press.

Blake, K.: Mentally retarded: an educational psychology, Englewood Cliffs, N.J., 1976, Prentice-Hall, Inc.

Burnside, I.M.: Clocks and calendars, Am. J. Nurs. **70:**117-119, Jan. 1970.

Burnside, I.M.: Loss: a constant theme in group work with the aged, Hosp. Community Psychiatry **21:**173-176, June 1970.

Burnside, I.M., editor: Psychosocial nursing: caring throughout the life-span, New York, 1979, McGraw-Hill Book Co.

Burton, G.: Interpersonal relations: a guide for nurses, ed. 4, New York, 1977, Springer Publishing Co., Inc.

Campbell, M.E.: Study of the attitudes of nursing personnel toward the geriatric patient, Nurs. Res. **20:**147-151, March-April 1971.

Carlson, C.E., editor: Behavioral concepts and nursing intervention, Philadelphia, 1970, J.B. Lippincott Co.

Chappelle, M.L.: The language of food, Am. J. Nurs. **72:**1294-1295, 1972.

Chinn, P.C., Drew, C.J., and Logan, D.R.: Mental retardation: a life cycle approach, ed. 2, St. Louis, 1979, The C.V. Mosby Co.

Chodil, J., and Williams, B.: The concept of sensory deprivation, Nurs. Clin. North Am. **5:**453-465, 1970.

Comstock, R., Mayers, R., and Folsom, J.: Simple physical activities for the elderly, Hosp. Community Psychiatry **20:**377-380, 1969.

Conover, M., and Cober, J.: Understanding and caring for the hearing-impaired, Nurs. Clin. North Am. **5:**497-506, 1970.

Crary, W., and Crary, G.: Depression, Am. J. Nurs. **73:**472-475, 1973.

Curtin, S.R.: Nobody ever died of old age, Boston, 1973, Little, Brown & Co.

Davidites, R.M.: A social systems approach to deviant behavior, Am. J. Nurs. **71:**1588-1589, 1971.

Davis, R.W.: Psychologic aspects of geriatric nursing, Am. J. Nurs. **68:**802-804, 1968.

Deutsch, E.B.: A stereotype—or an individual? Nurs. Outlook **19:**106-108, Feb. 1971.

Eckelberry, G.: The nurse as a patient, Nurs. Outlook **12:**20-23, Dec. 1964.

Elms, R., and Diers, D.: The patient comes to the hospital, Nurs. Forum **2**(3):89-97, 1963.

Faas, L.A.: Learning disabilities: a competency based approach, Boston, 1976, Houghton Mifflin Co.

Fallon, B.: And certain thoughts go through my head . . ., Am. J. Nurs. **72:**1257-1259, 1972.

Fowler, R.S., and Fordyce, W.: Adapting care for the brain-damaged patient, Am. J. Nurs. **72:**2056-2059, 1972.

Francis, G.M., and Munjas, B.A.: Manual of sociopsychologic assessment, New York, 1976, Appleton-Century-Crofts.

Freedman, A., and Kaplan, H.I.: Modern synopsis of comprehensive textbook of psychiatry, ed. 2, Baltimore, 1975, The Williams & Wilkins Co.

George, J.A.: Teaching the young about the old, Nurs. Outlook **20:**405-407, 1972.

Gerdes, L.: The confused or delirious patient, Am. J. Nurs. **68:**1228-1233, 1968.

Glaser, K.: Learning difficulties; causes and psychological implications: a guide for professionals, Springfield, Ill., 1974, Charles C Thomas, Publisher.

Goldsborough, J.: Involvement, Am. J. Nurs. **69:**66-68, Jan. 1969.

Gould, G.T., editor: Symposium on compassion and communication in nursing, Nurs. Clin. North Am. **4:**651-729, 1969.

Hagerman, Z.: Teaching beginners to cope with extreme behavior, Am. J. Nurs. **68:**1927-1929, 1968.

Hansell, N.: The person in distress: on the biosocial dynamics of adaptation, New York, 1976, Behavioral Publications, Inc.

Hershey, N.: Safety of the difficult patient, Am. J. Nurs. **71:**1766-1767, 1971.

Hewitt, H., and Pesznecker, B.: Blocks to communicating with patients, Am. J. Nurs. **64:**101-103, July 1964.

Hulicka, I.M.: Fostering self-respect in aged patients, Am. J. Nurs. **64:**84-89, March 1964.

Johnson, J., Dumas, R., and Johnson, B.: Interpersonal relations: the essence of nursing care, Nurs. Forum **6**(3):325-334, 1967.

Jordan, T.E.: Mentally retarded, ed. 4, Columbus, Ohio, 1976, Charles E. Merrill Publishing Co.

Kalkman, M.E.: Recognizing emotional problems, Am. J. Nurs. **68:**536-539, 1968.

Kindred, M., et al.: Mentally retarded citizen and the law, The President's Committee on Mental Retardation, New York, 1976, The Free Press.

Koncelik, J., and Snyder, L.: The role of design in behavior manipulation within long-term care facilities, Nurs. Homes **20:**6, 20-23, Dec. 1971.

Kraegel, J., et al.: A system of patient care based on patient's needs, Nurs. Outlook **20:**257-264, April 1972.

Kyes, J.J., and Hofling, C.: Basic psychiatric concepts in nursing, ed. 3, Philadelphia, 1974, J.B. Lippincott Co.

Langlois, P., and Teramoto, V.: Helping patients cope with hospitalizations, Nurs, Outlook **19:**334-336, May 1971.

Leland, H., and Smith, D.: Mental retardation: present and future perspectives, Worthington, Ohio, 1974, Charles A. Jones Publishing Co.

Levine, M.E.: Adaptation and assessment, a rationale for nursing intervention, Am. J. Nurs. **66:**2450-2453, 1966.

Levine, M.E.: The pursuit of wholeness, Am. J. Nurs. **69:**93-98, Jan. 1969.

Levine, M.E.: The intransigent patient, Am. J. Nurs. **70:**2106-2111, 1970.

Linden, M.: The emotional problems of aging, Nurs. Outlook **12:**47-50, Nov. 1964.

Lindenberg, R.E.: The need for crisis intervention in hospitals, Hospitals **46:**52-55, 110, Jan. 1, 1972.

MacGregor, F.C.: Uncooperative patients: some cultural interpretations, Am. J. Nurs. **67:**88-91, Jan. 1967.

Matheson, W.E., et al.: Control of screaming behavior using aversive conditioning and time-out, J. Psychiatr. Nurs. **14:**27, Sept. 1, 1976.

Mead, M.: The right to die, Nurs. Outlook **16:**20-21, Oct. 1968.

Mereness, D.A., and Taylor, C.M.: Essentials of psychiatric nursing, ed. 10, St. Louis, 1978, The C.V. Mosby Co.

Metropolitan Life: Number of elders growing nationwide, Statistical Bull. **54:**4-8, Jan. 1973.

Miller, W.H.: Systematic parent training: procedures, cases and issues, Champaign, Ill., 1975, Research Press.

Moore, B.C., et al.: Mental retardation: causes and prevention, Columbus, Ohio, 1977, Charles E. Merrill Publishing Co. (Text, instructor's manual, and six 20-minute filmstrips.)

Morris, M., and Rhodes, M.: Guidelines for the care of confused patients, Am. J. Nurs. **72:**1630-1633, 1972.

Moss, B.B.: The aging process, Nurs. Homes **20:**23-24, 48, March 1971.

Niemeier, D.F., and Allison, T.S.: Nurses can be effective behavior modifiers, J. Psychiatr. Nurs. **14:**18, Jan. 1976.

Orlando, I.J.: The dynamic nurse-patient relationship: function, process and principles, New York, 1961, G.P. Putnam's Sons.

Patrick, M.: Care of the confused elderly patient, Am. J. Nurs. **67:**2536-2539, 1967.

Peplau, H.E.: Interpersonal relationships in nursing, New York, 1952, G.P. Putnam's Sons.

Peplau, H.E.: Psychiatric nursing skills and the general hospital patient, Nurs. Forum **3**(2):28-37, 1964.

Peterson, D.I.: Developing the difficult patient, Am. J. Nurs. **67:**522-525, 1967.

Petrillo, M.: Preventing hospital trauma in pediatric patients, Am. J. Nurs. **68:**1469-1473, 1968.

Powers, M., and Storlie, F.: The apprehensive patient, Am. J. Nurs. **67:**58-63, Jan. 1967.

Preston, T.: Meeting the needs of nursing home residents, Nurs. Outlook **12:**44-46, Dec. 1964.

Reorganization study of human services programs. Interim report written mid-1978. Write to President's Reorganization Project, Human Resources Division, Office of Management and Budget, New Executive Office Building, Room 3206, Washington, D.C. 20503.

Robinson, L.: Psychological aspects of the care of hospitalized patients, ed. 3, Philadelphia, 1976, F.A. Davis Co.

Rodstein, M.: Health problems of the aged, RN **35:**39-43, Aug. 1972.

Rossier, M., and Steiger, T.: Teaching attendants to cope with stressful patient situations, Am. J. Nurs. **69:**305-309, 1969.

Rossman, I., editor: Clinical geriatrics, ed. 2, Philadelphia, 1979, J.B. Lippincott Co.

Rubin, R.: Body image and self-esteem, Nurs. Outlook **16:**20-23, June 1968.

Schwab, Sister M.: Caring for the aged, Am. J. Nurs. **73:**2049-2053, 1973.

Schwartzman, S.T.: Anxiety and depression in the stroke patient: a nursing challenge, J. Psychiatr. Nurs. **14:**13, July 1976.

Scott, M.L.: To learn to work with the elderly, Am. J. Nurs. **73:**662-665, 1973.

Sharp, C.: First or last name? Am. J. Nurs. **71:**958-959, 1971.

Shurley, J., and Pokorny, A.: Handling the psychiatric emergency, Med. Clin. North Am. **46:**417-426, 1962.

Sorenson, K., and Amis, D.: Understanding the world of the chronically ill, Am. J. Nurs. **67:**811-817, 1967.

Spitzer, S.P., and Volk, B.A.: Altercasting the difficult patient, Am. J. Nurs. **71:**732-735, 1971.

Stafford, L.: Depression and self-destructive behavior, J. Psychiatr. Nurs. **14:**37, Aug. 1976.

Steinberg, F.U., editor: Cowdry's the care of the geriatric patient, ed. 5, St. Louis, 1976, The C.V. Mosby Co.

Stephens, L., compilator: Reality orientation, a technique to rehabilitate elderly and brain-damaged patients with a moderate to severe degree of disorientation, Washington, D.C., 1969, American Psychiatric Association, The Hospital and Community Service.

Sullivan, H.S.: The interpersonal theory of psychiatry, New York, 1968, W.W. Norton & Co., Inc.

Todhunter, E.N.: Meanings of food to the consumer, Nurs. Homes **22:**22-24, March 1973.

Topalis, M., and Aguilera, D.C.: Psychiatric nursing, ed. 7, St. Louis, 1978, The C.V. Mosby Co.

Tuck, B.R.: The geriatric nurse, pioneer of a new specialty, RN **35:**38, Aug. 1972.

Ushely, G.B.: What is realistic emotional support? Am. J. Nurs. **68:**758-762, 1968.

Velasquez, J.M.: Alienation, Am. J. Nurs. **69:**301-304, 1969.

Walsh, J.: A specialized activity program for acutely disturbed patients, J. Psychiatr. Nurs. **14:**12, April 1976.

Wedell, K.: Learning and perceptuo-motor disabilities in children, New York, 1973, John Wiley & Sons, Inc.

Weymouth, L.T.: Nursing care of the so-called confused patient, Nurs. Clin. North Am. **3:**709-715, 1968.

Wingquist, D.: Of life's span the final stages, Nurs. Homes **22:**32-34, March 1973.

Wortis, J., editor: Mental retardation and developmental disabilities, vol. 11 (an annual review), New York, 1979, Brunner/Mazel, Inc.

# 8
# ADAPTIVE PROBLEMS IN SCHOOL AND LEARNING

Although statistics vary, some experts have predicted that as many as 10% to 30% of all school-aged children experience problems in adapting to their appropriate grade level in school. These problems may be evident in perceptual-motor impairments, learning difficulties, unacceptable social relationships, or behavioral disorders.

Early efforts toward identification and intervention in these impairments represent not only a savings in human potential, but also an opportunity to correct initial or possible problems before they become increasingly complex and more difficult to remediate. This early approach in prevention and primary intervention should be geared to incorporate the principles and considerations developed in Chapter 5. By including these factors, practitioners may approach children in toto rather than segmentally and avoid treating dominant problems to the exclusion of other needs. Moreover, as the practitioner regards the value system of the subcultural group wherein the child has membership, appropriate therapeutic responses may be evaluated in view of desired outcomes within the child's individual situation. For example, in some groups proficiency in manual skills outweighs the acquisition of language skills and creative art abilities. Such emphasis would probably be quite acceptable if the child socialized within that particular system did not have to compete with children from the dominant sector of society, who have opposite values. Thus, when the child socialized in the minority group faces the competition with peers that occurs naturally in the school setting, the child tends to consistently demonstrate an apparent in-

ability to succeed in one or more activities, shows an increasingly negative self-concept, and exhibits problems in adaptive behaviors involving peers, school, and other facets of living. These problems along with those categorized as specific learning disabilities, mental retardation, emotional disorders, abnormal physical development, seizures, malignancies, and opportunity deprivation constitute the essential factors in diagnosing impaired functioning in school and learning situations.

## DEVELOPMENT OF INVOLVED AGENCIES

Since the 1960s learning disabilities have been identified as a specialized area in education. The disciplines of psychology and medicine have also demonstrated an interest in assisting the child who has impaired learning capabilities. However, each of these disciplines utilizes a different model in approaching the child with learning problems: these models include different terminology and treatment modalities often not commonly used by the other disciplines. To overcome these differences, a conference was held in 1963 with the combined cooperation of the National Society of Crippled Children and Adults and the Neurological and Sensory Disease Control Program of the Division of Chronic Diseases, United States Public Health Service, who jointly concluded that some agreement was necessary in deciding on necessary research, services, terminology, and identification of problems inherent in the management of children with learning impairments. Since these initial efforts in coordination and interdisciplinary cooperation, many other agencies have become involved. Additionally, funding from PL 88-164, passed in 1963, provided support for initial research and training within a framework that encompassed programs related to learning disabilities.

By 1964 the Association for Children with Learning Disabilities (ACLD), a group closely aligned with the educational model, became organized. Their major objective is to enhance the learning and overall status of children with normal intelligence who have perceptual, motor, or conceptual impairments in learning, frequently accompanied by behavioral problems. In considering their use of the term ''learning disabilities'' to encompass the scope of the problem, one readily realizes that the organizational goals emphasize remediation and treatment rather than etiologic factors. Currently the group remains extremely active on national, state, and local levels in their influence on legislation, funding, and interdisciplinary communication.

By 1966 funding was allocated for learning disabilities as a separate entity within the Division of Training Programs, Bureau of Education for the Handicapped, United States Office of Education. This resulted in the creation of 11 university training programs and the establishment of another conference to resolve problems of terminology and definitions within the scope of learning disabilities.

Kass and Myklebust published a classic paper on the educational definition of learning disabilities and techniques in remediation combining the efforts of 15 special educators attending an advanced study institute at Northwestern University. Later the National Advisory Committee to the Bureau of Education for the Handicapped drafted the following definition, which has been utilized in formulating subsequent federal and state legislation:

Children with special learning disabilties exhibit a disorder in one or more of the basic psychological processes involved in understanding or in using spoken or written language. These may be manifested in disorders of listening, thinking, reading, writing, spelling, or arithmetic. They include conditions which have been referred to as perceptual handicaps, brain injury, minimal brain dysfunction, dyslexia, developmental aphasia, etc. They do not include learning problems which are due primarily to visual, hearing, or motor handicaps,
to mental retardation, emotional disturbance, or to environmental disadvantage.*

As the area of learning disabilities continued to gain momentum, several more institutes for special education were convened by the Bureau for Education of the Handicapped, Office of Education. Furthermore, those needs that remained unmet by the ACLD were met by the Division for Children with Learning Disabilities (DCLD), a group formed under the auspices of the Council for Exceptional Children (CEC) and especially credited with the establishment of learning disabilities as a distinct type of exceptionality.

When the Learning Disabilities Act of 1969 was passed as Title VI-G of the Elementary and Secondary Education Act of 1970, funds became available for providing direct services to children with learning disabilities and for offering supportive services to various related projects throughout the nation.

PL 94-142 and PL 93-112 also apply to these children. Refer to section on mental retardation, Chapter 7.

## APPROACHES TO SPECIFIC LEARNING DISABILITIES

The recognition of learning disabilities has been documented since the seventeenth century. Although the exact causes of this problem are not well understood, the functional outcome clearly demonstrates impaired learning of adaptation requiring individualized programs of remediation.

### Treatment philosophies

Although the educational focus has been primarily geared toward the assessment of current individual capacities as a base line for establishing intervention modalities for remediation, medical emphasis has remained on diagnosing underlying causes that respond to preventive or curative techniques within the realm of medicine. The disagreement between the medical approach and the educational approach centers on medicine's tendency to study persons with impairments as a ho-

*From National Advisory Committee on Handicapped Children: Special education for the handicapped children, the first annual report of the National Advisory Committee on Handicapped Children, Washington, D.C., 1968, Office of Education, Department of Health, Education, and Welfare.

mogeneous category to ascertain common approaches that could benefit all members of that group. Unfortunately, medical findings have offered little help to these children, except in ruling out other health problems or providing supportive counseling and medication, as required, since the broad category of learning disabilities represents a diverse collection of symptoms that vary among children and within the same child from time to time.

However, as medical research continues into specific subdivisions of behavioral and functional capacities, more information may become available on etiological factors and relationships of treatment modalities to symptom changes. With increasing communication between health professionals and educators, future clients with learning disabilities may have the joint benefit of a thorough background investigation with subsequent medical follow-up coupled with a highly specialized program of remediation for current problems that includes multidisciplinary contributions (Conway, 1970).

*Recent advances.* Medical research has produced a new wealth of information on prenatal, perinatal, and postnatal factors and their relationship to later learning, growth, and development. Because of this information, the health team is better able to avoid problems related to hypoxia, nutritional deficiencies, maternal complications during pregnancy, hereditary conditions, and disorders acquired in utero. Moreover, research has identified many growth interferences and problems of childhood related to the socioenvironmental factors presented in Chapter 5 and to developmental, physical, or intellectual limitations in potential capacities. In these instances, management is geared toward the alleviation of immediate problems, early assessment of the entire situation, correction and counseling in long-term events, and intervention in behalf of future children.

## TREATMENT SETTINGS

In reviewing the available literature and current community practices and in formulating a philosophy for treating children with learning disabilities, nurse practitioners may encounter a wide variety of treatment settings and approaches incorporating education, medical management, behavior modification, and pharmacology. A thorough review of each major type of setting and method is essential to the nurse practitioner who becomes involved in the specialized area of learning disabilities.

EDUCATIONAL SETTINGS. There are several educational settings wherein intervention occurs on behalf of the child with learning disabilities. Some are included in special programs within the public school system, and others are part of a private or remedial school.

A comprehensive review of the public school philosophy is presented in the film *Learning Disabilities: Invisible Learning Handicaps,* a public television film, and in *You're Not Listening* (1976, available from the Ciba Pharmaceutical Company) as three main concepts aimed at the assessment and remediation of individual impairments. First, there is the self-contained classroom, a traditional approach of segregating learning disabled children from their peers. Although some educational systems make this separation total, others attempt to integrate these children into the normal school routine whenever possible. Because of pragamatic problems and limited funds, special programs for learning disabled children have often been compelled to include mentally retarded children. This grouping plus the isolation from normal classes has tended to reinforce the negative self-concept and intensify some problems of the learning disabled child who has normal intelligence.

Second, a compromise between this self-contained classroom and the total integration into the normal classroom has been the resource room. When the concept of resource rooms is employed, the child remains with the class as much as possible but leaves to attend special sessions designed to improve performance in those areas wherein functional abilities are not at peer level. Resource rooms emphasize a higher teacher-to-pupil ratio, unique teaching methods, and selected skills training tailored to the needs of each individual child. In terms of self-concept this method tends to be less disruptive to children, since they are spared from classroom participation when their weakest skills are taught and are moved to the resource room, just as other pupils move to participate in classes taught by a variety of teachers.

"Mainstreaming" is the third approach and individualizes curriculum planning for all children, including those with learning disabilities. In this approach the classroom teacher utilizes the consultative services of a special educator to identify appropriate skills, equipment, and techniques for managing the child with specific learning disabilities within the normal classroom setting. Many educators favor this model, because of the continuing education potential built into the system, the regular opportunity for the classroom teacher to converse with educational specialists about classroom problems, the tendency to develop teaching techniques that utilize a prescriptive approach for all children, and the opportunity for children with learning problems to associate with and model themselves after normal peers.

Private school settings offer a wide variety of philosophies and approaches for children requiring special assistance in learning and adaptation to school. A comprehensive list of names and addresses of these programs may be obtained by writing:

**Closer Look**
Box 1492
Washington, D.C. 20013

In the evaluation of each program it is helpful to recognize the philosophy and methods utilized.

MEDICAL SETTINGS. Frequently the first professional assistance to be sought when behavioral and learning disorders are evident is from the nurse, the family physician, a pediatrician, a neurologist, a psychologist, or a diagnostic clinic. The person offering this professional assistance often becomes a key individual in organizing and implementing the diagnosis, management modalities, and referral systems for the case. Typically one begins the evaluation by performing a physical examination, doing a neurologic assessment, and taking a history. Depending on the impairments noted, physicians may seek evaluation and consultation from other professionals, especially neurologists, psychologists, educators, or an outpatient facility specializing in the team diagnosis of learning disabled children. Final recommendations may come from the original professional or the consultants, or both, involved in the assessment process. However, the appropriateness and success of the treatment regimen is directly related to professional awareness of current educational management and community resources.

*Nursing role.* Interdisciplinary referrals and communications vary greatly from setting to setting throughout the country. Naturally the contributions that each discipline may offer remain extremely important to the thorough assessment and prescriptive treatment for each learning disabled child. However, vigorous involvement by several disciplines at the same time may fragment efforts and result in the lack of a coordinated approach.

Nursing can play a vital role in ensuring an acceptable outcome for the child in two important ways. First, the unique background of nurses allows them to function in a variety of settings, with the primary base of operation being a school; a community health facility or agency; a hospital, with diverse possibilities for extended roles; a private practice; or a clinic. Thus they are in a natural position to be liaison persons between all specialists involved in the management of the learning disabled child. Second, nurses have a perspective in assessment that incorporates not only physical or functional findings, but also patterns of daily living that focus on the individual child within the gestalt of the routine life-style. Thus nurses with these particular assets may be the members of the team of helping professionals best suited to coordinate a comprehensive intervention program with the total needs of the child within the family context as the primary consideration.

In one setting the clinical nursing specialist in pediatric neurology participated in a total team approach in diagnosing children with specific learning disabilities. This nurse specialist formed a one-to-one relationship with each child and family at the beginning of the assessment process, so that testing and care plans could be individualized throughout the evaluation. Several short encounters with family and child throughout the 2-day stay allowed them to verbalize problems, voice feelings, and obtain assistance in understanding the child's situation and planning their future course. The final summary and therapeutic regimen, derived from a round-table discussion by involved multidisciplinary professionals, were presented to each family by the neurologist and the nurse specialist. Family reactions and needs were handled accordingly, and appropriate recommendations were forwarded to the referring physician after thorough interpretation to the child and family. If these families had not lived in scattered areas throughout the state, more direct follow-up through community resources could have been possible. (See Conway, 1970).

## EDUCATIONAL PRESCRIPTIVE METHOD

The educational prescriptive method is based on the evaluation of children through various test batteries and the application of these findings in the educational process. Testing is divided into initial screening to identify learning disabilities and assessment testing to verify and specify individual strengths and weaknesses.

Any health care team professional involved in specific learning disabilities may conduct the initial assessment to detect the presence of a learning problem. When a learning disability is suspected to exist, more definitive evaluation techniques are employed, as discussed later in this chapter. Additionally, after a learning disability is confirmed in a child, referrals to specialists for further testing and treatment are appropriate.

Referrals for remediation of a learning disability may be made to a public or private program. Some of the better known approaches emphasizing language and academic training are briefly reviewed here.

*Language models.* Two of the leading models emphasizing impaired language skill correction as a means of improving general academic performance include programs by Johnson, Myklebust, Kirk, and Kirk (see references).

The program by Johnson and Myklebust defines psychoneurological learning disorders as neurological problems that may be caused by developmental impairments, disease, or accidents and that exclude impairments related to low intelligence level, sensory disorders, or psychological difficulties. Although the identification of diagnostic problems frequently remains an elusive complexity, these authors have found that disturbances in auditory integration have a more profound impact on general orientation and functioning than disorders in visual integration. Moreover, written language is the highest form of verbalization, and as would be expected, children with impaired learning capacities, speech disorders, social problems, and reading disabilities also tend to have difficulty with written language.

The theory proposed by Johnson and Myklebust is based first on a sequence of auditory input, integration, and output in the form of speech or auditory language. Second, this auditory language is essential in learning visual language, better known as reading. The final output of written language depends on the input of visual language through reading. Thus the teacher practicing this method gears remedial efforts toward overcoming problems identified with particular functional levels. A thorough acquaintance with the intelligence quotient and the sociopsychological events inherent in each situation is stressed. Ongoing objective testing and continuous behavioral observations also typify this method. This philosophy is practiced in the Meeting Street School in Rhode Island.

In the model formulated by Kirk and Kirk, children with a learning disability have at least one impairment in speech, language, reading, spelling, writing, or arithmetic that may be caused by cerebral disorders or psychogenic problems. This definition excludes such causative factors as mental retardation, lack of cultural and stimulating opportunities, and unacceptable educational methods. Testing for deficiencies is accomplished by using a revision of the Illinois Test of Psycholinguistic Abilities (ITPA), which measures three dimensions of linguistic ability: (1) communication channels, including auditory or visual input and vocal or motor output; (2) organizational levels, including the automatic-sequential level and the representational or meaning level; and (3) psycholinguistic abilities, including receptive language ability (decoding), internal manipulation of linguistic symbols (association), and expressive capacities in words or gestures (encoding). The first dimension is the reception of visual or auditory input and its translation into appropriate action. The second is best explained by considering the child's use of the word ''bye-bye.'' Children functioning at the automatic-sequential level utilize memory and imitation to say bye-bye. When children associate bye-bye with the activity of leaving and express the word at the appropriate time, they are operating at the representational level. The third dimension may be correlated with medical terminology, since decoding problems are synonymous with sensory aphasia and visual agnosia, whereas encoding impairments are termed "motor aphasia" or "apraxia."

When testing with the ITPA is completed, the child is categorized according to the learning problems that are apparent, such as (1) academic (reading, writing, arithmetic), (2) nonsymbolic (perceptual-expressive), or (3) symbolic (linguistic difficulty in reception or idea expression). These problems are treated on an individual basis by the use of traditional teaching methods aimed at correcting individual weaknesses.

*Academic models.* Strict academic models analyze student abilities in basic subjects—reading, writing, and arithmetic—and construct drills as a means of correcting weaknesses. Such methods generally ignore the cause of problems and focus only on the task at hand. Currently only one of these approaches, the Fernald method, has applicability. The Fernald method attempts to integrate visual and auditory abilities by developing the kinesthetic sense through exercises such as manual tracing over large letters.

*Developmental models.* In Chapter 5 the theories of Getman, Kephart, and Delacato are reviewed. Two other major professionals who stress the developmental model are Cruickshank and Frostig. The work of Cruickshank, based on the classic efforts of Werner and those of Strauss, stresses the use of minimal selective stimuli and a one-to-one teacher-to-pupil ratio in a controlled environment to facilitate learning in hyperactive children. To minimize environmental stimuli, isolation booths are employed as part of this method. Emphasis in this approach is also placed on increasing developmental capacities, especially in fine muscle activity, eye-hand coordination, figure-ground discriminations, concepts in laterality, and incorporation of acceptable behavioral patterns into the matrix of the entire educational processes (Hallahan and Cruickshank, 1973, and Cruickshank, 1975).

The Frostig program is an extremely popular method of treating children with learning disabilities based on serial assessments, including obser-

vations, interviews, and testing; detailed analysis of individual strengths and weaknesses; and the tailoring and application of any combination of three training methods, including (1) the single approach to remediate a particular impairment; (2) the comprehensive ability training program, which integrates skill and developmental ability training with appropriate subject matter; and (3) the usual methods of academic instruction geared to the level of learner ability.

Four stages of developmental abilities are stressed by Frostig in her method of evaluation and remediation. The sensorimotor stage occurs in the first 18 months of life. For most infants and toddlers this period is one wherein all the perceptual modalities are integrated with motor activities to allow environmental exploration. Children later diagnosed as having impaired learning capacities may demonstrate basic problems in individual awareness, movement, and manipulative abilities that stem from problems related to this initial stage. Remediation is geared toward exercises in movement designed to enhance the perception of self and others and the orientation in time and space. Communication abilities may improve as better perspective is gained in these other realms.

The second stage is entered during the second year of life when language skills are highlighted. The Frostig program tests the outcome of these abilities and disabilities in language development by utilizing the ITPA.

The third phase lasts from about 3½ to 7 years of age, the time when most children experience the development of auditory and visual perceptual capacities. During this phase, object recognition should become so automatic that the child is able to identify an object without hesitation or the use of movement as an aid. Two tests are utilized to assess the acquisition of these abilities: the Developmental Test of Visual Perception and the Auditory Discrimination Test.

The final stage of concrete operations begins at about 6½ years of age and is characterized by the ability to relate present situations to those stored in the memory and to associate future consequences with past events. After 5 years of age these cognitive skills are tested by the Wechsler Intelligence Scale for Children (WISC-R), which has tended to be a useful tool in preventing learning problems and in guiding remediation efforts because of its expression of final scores as 12 subtests plus verbal and performance evaluations.

Other popular intelligence tests are the Wechsler Preschool and Primary Scale of Intelligence (WPPSI), which may be utilized at 4 years of age, and the McCarthy Scales of Children's Ability, which is administered as early as 2 years of age. In infancy the Bayley Scales of Infant Development (BSID) tend to be the most accurate determination of development.

In summary, although these intelligence tests are available, one must regard results as mere guidelines, since testing in young children necessarily reflects the transitional nature of development with its integration of mature and immature patterns. Thus periodic retesting with these tools is appropriate in the reassessment of changing abilities and educational needs.

*Behavioral models.* The behavioral models in education are based on the principles of operant conditioning as spelled out by Skinner. Basically, operant conditioning differs from the pavlovian reflexive conditioning in one major way. In operant conditioning the behavior occurs first and is reinforced by a stimulus, whereas in reflexive conditioning the stimulus precedes the response. Thus in operant conditioning, stimulus presentations are designed to reinforce or increase the frequency and probability of a given preceding response or to extinguish certain previous behaviors. In this approach only the overt, observable human responses are acknowledged, whereas internal explanations of forces, such as perception, will, instinct, drive, or neurophysiology, are not considered in the evaluation of responses.

Two educational methods have evolved from skinnerian behavioral engineering techniques; these are precision teaching and contingency management.

In the *precision teaching* method developed by Lindsley, frequent charts are made to establish the continuous effect and adequacy of individualized student curricula on learning in each child. Approaches and techniques that do not result in movement toward identified objectives are modified. Precision teaching allows evaluation of the need for modification when the movement cycle and the changes in behavioral rates are considered.

The movement cycle is defined as a repetitive behavioral unit observable in a child. Changes in behavioral rates refer to the number of movement cycles counted within a specified time period. For example, an overactive child may leave his seat 20 times in 1 hour. This activity may be identified as one that interferes with academic learning. Thus the educator may plan a favorite game to encourage the child to leave the seat fewer times within the hour. Daily charts on this activity would indicate the effectiveness of the approach and any need for modification.

*Contingency management* is an effective system of reinforcing behavior that is characterized by offering a reward when a specific behavior is observed. Rewards may be social or may consist of tangible items. Each act of acceptable behavior may be acknowledged consistently, or rewards may be intermittent. Setting limited goals that are easily achieved by the child seems to be the most successful way to encourage children to gradually modify academic efforts or behavioral patterns. One important principle in this method is to acknowledge a positive behavior rapidly and to interpret the reinforcing action clearly to the involved child. In addition, behaviors may be extinguished when one ignores the occurrence of the undesired activity.

## Classroom observation

When nurses visit classroom settings to observe a learning disabled child or to confer with an educator, they may notice that no educational method is strictly enforced. Instead many educators combine the most effective techniques from several methods in accordance with their own personal philosophy. The important point is to identify and understand prevailing plans within the setting so that effective counseling may occur with the child and family as they return to the nurse or physician for continuing health maintenance, correction of health problems, and assistance in psychosocial and developmental areas.

## MEDICAL EVALUATION SYSTEM

The role of medical professionals is primarily one of identifying a learning problem, excluding the possibility of a pathological condition, referring the child for psychoeducational diagnosis and treatment, and continuing child health maintenance within the context of the individual situation. This program of total evaluation and management may be performed by the nurse or the physician, or both, depending on the situation.

## Pathophysiology

The physical findings in the child with a learning disability vary greatly from child to child and within the same child at different times. To cloud the issue further, medical professionals have selected terminology to describe specific learning disabilities that implies etiology, for example, the medical term used to describe a child with specific learning disabilities is minimal brain dysfunction, which is defined as follows:

This term as a diagnostic and descriptive category refers to children of near average, average or above average intellectual capacity with certain learning and/or behavioral disabilities ranging from mild to severe, which are associated with deviations of function of the central nervous system. These deviations may manifest themselves by various combinations of impairment in perception, conceptualization, language, memory, and control of attention, impulse or motor function. These aberrations may arise from genetic variations, biochemical irregularities, perinatal brain insults, or other illnesses or injuries sustained during the years critical for the development and maturation of the central nervous system. . . .*

The outcome of minimal brain dysfunction is a specific learning disability, which is the descriptive term for the resulting impairment in functional abilities. This impairment may be one of three types: (1) a pure learning disability, (2) a pure mixture of symptoms known as the hyperkinetic syndrome, or (3), as is usually the case, a combination of both hyperkinesis and learning disabilities.

Characteristics of a pure learning disability might include *dyslexia* (problems in reading), *dysgraphia* (writing impairments), or *dysorthographia* (spelling problems), or all three. Although these impairments are frequently accompanied by problems in right-left orientation, they are not general-

*From Clements, S.D., project director: National project on minimal brain dysfunction in children: terminology and identification, monograph No. 3, Public Health Service Publication No. 1415, Washington, D.C., 1966, Superintendent of Documents, U.S. Government Printing Office.

ly associated with the symptoms of hyperkinesis. Instead these children are often strikingly underactive in comparison with their normal peers.

The hyperkinetic syndrome represents the other end of the continuum. Its appearance as a separate entity is rare. The management of this overactivity is discussed in the last section of this chapter.

Since most children have a combination of hyperkinesis and specific learning disabilities, these conditions are combined in the following review of components in assessment.

## Symptoms

Symptoms of unusual behavior are frequently reported by parents of children with minimal brain damage even before 2 years of age as impaired sleeping or feeding patterns, poor health in infancy, and even delayed speech acquisition or coordination problems. The family history often reveals a father who was a difficult child to manage behaviorally, who had problems in adapting to school, and who may be impatient, short-tempered, and restless as an adult. The hyperactive syndrome is six times more prevalent in boys than girls. Moreover, interviews with 45 mothers of adolescents who had been diagnosed as being hyperactive about 5 years previously revealed that these adolescents continued to display tendencies such as restlessness, excessive talking, impaired concentration, poor ability to complete tasks, inadequate self-conceptualization, and problems in behavioral and disciplinary areas (Stewart, 1970).

Other symptoms reported by various authors are described by such terms as hyperactivity, impulsivity, distractibility, and short attention span. Since these symptoms are most frequently seen in concentration, poor ability to complete tasks, inadequate self-conceptualization, and problems in behavioral and disciplinary areas (Stewart, 1970).

## Initial screening

The first indication of either hyperactivity or specific learning disabilities may not be evident until the child is given preschool tests or performance is noted in early school years. At this time parents or teachers, or both, may refer the child to the family physician or clinic for further evaluation.

In the early school years, tests are administered by nurses or educators to assess school readiness and detect potential learning disabilities. Two examples of the types of tests that may be administered include the Preschool Readiness Experimental Screening Scale (PRESS) and the Meeting Street School Screening Test (MSSST).

The PRESS is a screening tool that detects developmental interferences and impairments that might result in maladjustments in social contacts or academic functioning. This tool does not estimate intellectual capacities. Most children 5 years of age should be able to complete the test without difficulty.

Areas tested include knowledge of colors, numbers, general knowledge, drawing, coordination, comprehension and performance during testing, and personal-social maturity. Scoring is simply measured on a 10-point system that includes three divisions to indicate school readiness, borderline school readiness, or inadequate school readiness.

The MSSST is an individually administered test that requires about 20 minutes to complete. It is designed to detect impaired functioning in language or in visual-perceptual-motor control that interferes with normal school adaptation in kindergarten or first-grade children. The test is divided into three categories, including motor patterning, visual-perceptual-motor integration, and language. These areas are further subdivided to incorporate a wide variety of skill testing. Directions for use and complete information on clinical implications and test evaluation are available by writing:

**The Meeting Street School**
Crippled Children and Adults of Rhode Island Inc.
Rhode Island

Other sources of referral include educators or parents. If the adaptive or learning problem remains undetected until the child is attending school, first indications of the disorder may be manifested as a dislike for or reluctance to attend school, poor grades, complaints about performance or academic skills from the teacher, problems in peer relationships, and a poor self-concept. Hopefully, the problem becomes identified before these negative qualities become deeply rooted in the child.

Another source of referral is by parents or parent surrogates who notice abnormal behaviors and performance capacities in their child and seek medical expertise to solve the problem.

## Differential diagnosis

Examination of the child who has been referred for evaluation of minimal brain dysfunction, behavioral problems, specific learning disabilities, devleopmental lags, impaired academic performance, or inability to keep pace with peers should begin with a complete assessment and a neurologic evaluation, as described in Chapter 11. Naturally such testing should include complete ophthalmological and otological testing.

Next, a detailed family and child history is elicited, with particular attention being given to the child's disorder from the family's and child's perceptual viewpoints; the family's life-style, collectively and individually; and all other psychosocial and economic factors relevant to the situation. Additional important details include antenatal, perinatal, and postnatal events; medical or surgical conditions; accidents or incidents, especially those related to the central nervous system; psychological disorders; convulsions; inherited familial disorders; and the history of progression through developmental milestones. Eliciting this information is fundamental in ruling out such potential causes of learning disability as mental retardation, emotional disorders, abnormal development, seizures, malignancies, endocrine impairments, and opportunity deprivation.

*Mental retardation.* Refer to Chapter 7 for a discussion on mental retardation.

*Emotional disturbances.* One important determination in the comprehensive assessment of the child with behavioral disturbances or problems in adapting to school is a careful assessment of the emotional states of both child and family. Although an emotional disorder can certainly cause problems in school adaptation, social adjustment, and general performance, the evidence of psychologic disturbances should not prevent the practitioner from continuing the evaluation into an underlying specific learning disorder, since undetected learning impairments in children with normal intelligence may cause them to receive undue pressure to achieve when such performance is not possible without remedial help.

This discussion continues with the typical findings in the history of the child with minimal brain dysfunction. It contrasts this clinical picture with two important differential diagnoses: social or reactive patterns and primary psychogenic problems.

**CLINICAL FINDINGS OF MINIMAL BRAIN DYSFUNCTION.** Although each child presents a different mosaic of symptoms, many children tend to exhibit similar behavioral and performance patterns. Mothers of children who have minimal brain dysfunction may recall that the infant or toddler seemed restless and hard to satisfy and remained in constant motion after mastering locomotor skills, preferring to run rather than walk. These children also tend to be great explorers and are reported as being into everything. During preschool years these children may be unable to stay at the dinner table or remain interested in television programs. When they enter school, teachers frequently report that these children cannot sit still for long periods of time and that while sitting at the desk, their feet and hands are in perpetual motion. However, when teachers relate to these children on an individual basis outside the highly stimulating classroom setting, behavioral responses may be entirely within normal limits. In summary, many of the symptoms discussed are directly linked to impairments in attention span. Although some researchers report that problems in attention disappear by adolescence, it is more commonly assumed that the problems continue to persist in a more subtle form.

As children reach the age of group activity, parents frequently report that the child with minimal brain dysfunction is excluded from team play by peers. This exclusion from play is caused by the child's clumsiness and lack of coordination, which is usually apparent in earlier developmental task mastery as well. For example, fine motor coordination may have been delayed, as evidenced by the child's slowness in fastening shoes and clothing, in coloring, or in learning to write. Moreover, impaired eye-hand coordination is often detected by playmates, who, for example, master the various tasks required in a ball game at a much faster rate. Finally, practitioners should inquire about gross motor patterns by asking when the child mastered the tricycle, bicycle, or roller skates. In the gross motor history, one should carefully rule out the lack of these skills because of limited family finances, lack of sidewalks, paren-

tal overprotectiveness, or other situational circumstances. (See Fig. 8-1).

Since underachievement in school, poor grades, or the inability to compete with peers may be the first sign or signs of a learning disorder, the practitioner should evaluate school progress thoroughly as a part of the family history.

In the area of pyschosocial behaviors, several problems are often observed. In peer relationships, children with minimal brain dysfunction are often found to be bossy, aggressive, and unable to comply with group norms. Thus peers reject them as friends. Parents report that these children, unlike their siblings, tend to be difficult to discipline and socialize. Deviant behavior often persists even when parents do a reasonable job of being consistent and firm in setting limits. Parents may also describe this child as being impulsive and into all sorts of trouble in school, including stealing, lying, pranks, and truancy. Problems tend to become more serious with increasing age and may even require intervention from law enforcement agencies at some points. Since these deviant behaviors are common initial complaints, practitioners should seriously regard poor insight into consequences and inadequate social adjustments as potential symptoms of minimal brain dysfunction. Mood lability is also frequently noted in these children. Additionally, they find little satisfaction in goal attainment, exhibit high frustration levels, and seem short-tempered. Outward aggression is often a mask for inadequacy and a poor self-concept. Another characteristic of children with these behaviors is the tendency to cause marital and sibling discord, especially when the problem is poorly understood, and blame and guilt are continually accepted in patterns compatible with individual family personalities. In speaking to the parents of a child with minimal brain dysfunction, one finds that they often have great difficulty in thinking of positive attributes of the child. However, in one study on parent interviews (Graham and Rutter, 1968), more than half of the parents failed to report negative behavioral patterns in their children, such as lying, stealing, school truancy, and disciplinary problems. Such information seemed sensitive and could only be elicited indirectly by skillful interviewing about broader, less emotionally charged symptoms, such as attention span, temperament, peer relations, disciplinary patterns, or cognitive-

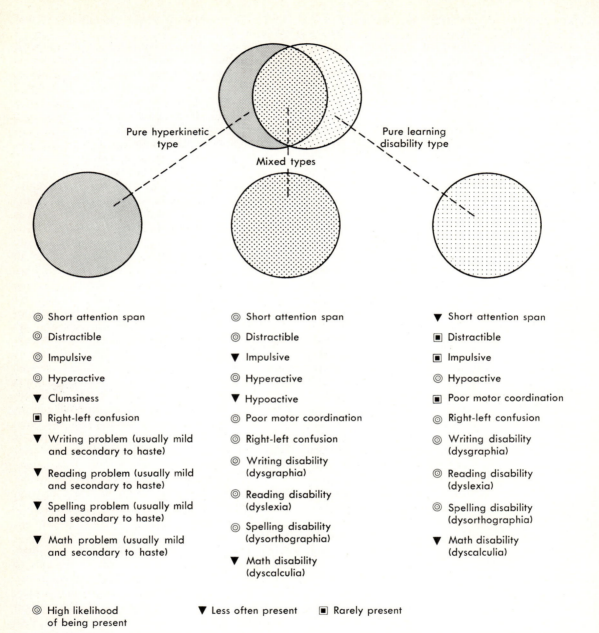

**FIG. 8-1.** Minimal brain damage: overlapping and discrete characteristics. (From Peters, J.E., et al.: Physician's handbook for screening for minimal brain dysfunction, Chicago, 1973, Ciba Medical Horizons.)

motor skills. To supplement data from the parental history, the practitioner should utilize the classroom teacher's observations as a valuable additional source of information.

**REACTIVE PATTERNS.** In contrast to minimal brain dysfunction as a cause of behavioral disorders are the reactive problems that are environmentally induced. Precipitating factors may be evident in the history as psychosocial or economic difficulties, for example, alcoholism, divorce, or any situation perceived by the family or child as an acute crisis or chronic problem.

In other situations there are normal children without learning disorders who exhibit a variety of symptoms, such as "stomachaches," headaches, or behavioral changes, to avoid school or who attend school but are characterized as underachievers. These children may be having difficulty coping with unrealistic parental demands to achieve, excel, compete, and produce beyond their capacities. Often nurses may elicit the presence of such pressure and tension as parents mention homework routines, grades, future career expectations for the child, or their estimation of current abilities. Counseling is often effective in educating, offering insight, and assisting these parents in seeking more acceptable plans of alternative action.

A third type of reactive problem is sometimes termed "school phobia." This phobia is a neurotic anxiety of the child that most frequently stems from conflicts in the mother-child relationship and is manifested as syncope, fatigue, vomiting, headache, or other vague symptoms that occur on school days and prevent attendance. When the possibility of school attendance has passed, the symptoms vanish. It is important for the practitioner to look beyond the superficial problems that precipitate the school avoidance behavior, such as the birth of a sibling, divorce, fear of failure in school testing or classroom presentations, or humiliation over a teacher's comment. Closer investigation may reveal basic conflicts in the mother-child relationship. For example, tense home situations or insecure feelings about child rearing may result in a "double message" when the time approaches for the child to attend school. On the one hand, the mother encourages the child to make major steps toward separation and independency, yet she is unable to release the child from dependency on her.

When the child develops symptoms to avoid school, the mother may be unable to give the encouragement required to foster school attendance. Thus detection of this problem by the nurse practitioner requires two main types of intervention: counseling with the parent and child to resolve the conflict and prompt return of the child to school with the cooperation of the teacher, as necessary.

**PRIMARY PSYCHOGENIC PROBLEMS.** Another major differential diagnosis that should be considered as a possible cause of impaired interpersonal relations is childhood schizophrenia. In these cases the history tends to reveal the child as a person who is anxious and withdrawn and who has a clinging dependency on the mother or mother surrogate, but shares no warm spontaneous relationships with anyone.

*Abnormal physical development.* In physical functioning, one of the first obvious difficulties demonstrated is usually a developmental lag and an inability to perform at a level compatible with chronological age. As the nurse assesses the child, careful evaluation of perceptual-motor-cognitive capacities is essential, since defective hearing, speech, sight, touch, or proprioception are often remediable causes of school maladaptation. Other children may have noticeable physical handicaps, such as missing or impaired limb use, that require early evaluation and treatment and a flexible program of habilitation. Early detection of handicapping physical conditions, such as cerebral palsy, is important in preventing or diminishing the incidence of secondary problems. For further information on cerebral palsy refer to Chapter 13.

*Other factors.* Seizure disorders are discussed in Chapter 14. In referring to this section, the reader will note that abnormal brain-wave activity may interfere with consciousness, and thus attention, or may cause the child to exhibit unusual behaviors, particularly when a temporal lobe focus is evident.

Malignancy in the central nervous system is certainly a consideration when an acute onset of unusual behavior, weight loss, signs of increased intracranial pressure, or other "hard" neurological signs appear.

Finally, the practitioner has to evaluate the child in the context of individual "life space." Chapter 5 reviews factors related to growth, environment, and opportunity.

## Components in evaluation

The examination of the child begins with a thorough physical assessment. If screening tools such as the DDST, PRESS, MSSST, or Denver Articulation Screening Examination (DASE) are utilized, cautions on interpretations of these devices should be heeded, as discussed in connection with the DDST in Chapter 11.

A variety of conditions may interfere with normal growth and development. In the physical examination, unusual findings may indicate static or progressive processes that dictate the need for specific laboratory and radiological follow-up, referral to appropriate specialists, and therapeutic intervention, as discussed in instances throughout this book.

Evaluation of sensory modalities may elicit problems in perceiving various stimuli. Although impaired proprioceptive and tactile input may result in problems in motor abilites, such limitations are not nearly so severe as those imposed by defective auditory or visual input. Of the latter two impairments, auditory disturbances result in more profound developmental impairments than visual handicaps.

## SYSTEMATIC NEUROLOGICAL EXAMINATION

The neurological examination begins with the traditional assessment techniques, as detailed in Chapter 11. Further studies and tests are dictated by the findings. In evaluating events that have physiological significance for the central nervous system, many investigators have reported that children who manifest symptoms of minimal brain dysfunction frequently were subjected to prematurity, complications during pregnancy, or hypoxic episodes during the perinatal period. Lead poisoning and especially lead encephalopathies also seem to be connected to later learning disabilities. Other investigators have attempted to correlate learning impairment with inadequate nutrition, postencephalitic states resulting from viral infections, prenatal ingestion of medication, and environmental pollution. Further research is needed to identify the significance of these findings.

Children with minimal brain dysfunction are often described as having "soft" neurological signs. These soft signs are sometimes used to designate perceptual or cognitive behaviors that are evident beyond the usual chronological age in development. One example is the persistence of problems in distinguishing left and right until the late age of 9 years. Another meaning for soft signs is in the description of nonspecific entities, such as clumsiness, that are subject to interobserver variability. Although the appearance of these signs is common in children with minimal brain dysfunction, the absence of the signs does not exclude the possibility of minimal brain dysfunction. Investigators agree that the maturity of the central nervous system is probably delayed in children with minimal brain dysfunction (Dykman et al., 1973). Thus the documentation of soft signs is an important initial measurement that may be used as a base line for comparison in the evaluation of clinical changes resulting from the effects of increasing age and remedial intervention.

Common findings in the clinical assessment of the child with minimal brain dysfunction include few or no abnormalities, numerous soft neurological signs, reflex asymmetry, minimal speech and hearing impairments, mixed laterality, increased general activity, short attention span, clumsiness, impaired fine perceptual-motor coordination, and problems in reading, writing, spelling, and arithmetic.

The following sections describe the tests that are frequently added to the conventional neurological examination to reveal the range of problems that may be apparent in the child with minimal brain dysfunction. These are presented in the order recommended for their administration, with due regard for the child's ability to perform for a limited period of time before becoming bored or fatigued. The practitioner should evaluate each child individually and tailor the procedures to the child's needs. Hyperactive children should perform confining activities first because these children may be difficult to handle once active testing situations are introduced; other children may require a break after a few confining tasks, and active and confined tests may be interspersed for these children.

## Perceptual-motor function

One difficult task for many children with a learning disability is to perceive a stimulus and to make the appropriate motor response, particularly in basic academic skills.

***Visual-motor abilities.*** Visual-motor abilities may be observed when one asks the child to reproduce the geometric figures detailed in Chapter 5 (see Fig. 5-4). Normative values for reproduction are listed in the legend for Fig. 5-4.

Careful observation of the child's behavior and efforts in figure production are as significant as the accuracy of the end product. When one is evaluating visual-motor abilities, the following functional abilities in the child should be considered: eye-hand coordination, spatial and directional organization, and visual-motor coordination. Many children with minimal brain dysfunction have problems in drawing the figure in a smooth motion; in turning corners, especially at right angles; in changing directions; and in accurately reproducing the figure in the perspective presented. These require the child to make frequent erasures.

TESTING PROCEDURE. To conduct the test, the examiner gives the child a piece of white, unruled paper, a pencil, and a separate picture of each geometric design. The exercise is explained to the child, and erasures are discouraged. When the child wants to correct an error, the correction should be merely produced again on paper. In this way a permanent record of the child's efforts may be maintained. After the child copies the designs the nurse should record observations as to the manner in which the child reproduced the figures and any other significant points. These notes may be utilized to compare present capacities with results of the test given at some time in the future.

***Auditory-motor functions.*** Children with minimal brain dysfunction frequently have difficulty with the perception of a verbal command and its subsequent translation into motor activity essential to academic functioning, general adaptation, and concept formation.

One test of the integration of auditory and motor functions involves giving verbal directions that must be reproduced in writing.

TESTING PROCEDURE. The selected procedures are those that tend to cause the child with minimal brain dysfunction the most difficulty. They are dictated in simple phrases or sentences for the child to reproduce with a pencil on unruled paper.

Again, erasures are discouraged. Examples of items that may be used include the following: (1) A boy had a dog. (2) A dog saw a bird. (3) My name is _____. (4) I am _____ years old. (5) Write the numbers from 1 to 10. (6) Write the alphabet.

In administering this test, the nurse may find that the child tries to avoid the task by such maneuvers as needing to go to the bathroom, changing the subject, or becoming thirsty. After the nurse has encouraged the child to print these letters, figures, and words, observations are recorded as to the child's production and organization of symbols, the behaviors and effort exerted during the production process, the spacing, and only disjunction of letters (if writing is used). Erasures, spelling errors in relation to age and school grade, and haste or poor task accomplishment are also noted. The finished product should be evaluated for letter reversals or inversions and word reversals.

Frequent problems are noted with the letters *d/b, y/h,* and *d/g*. Often a *d* is drawn for a *b;* an *h* for a *y,* or a *d* for a *g*. Words such as "was" become "saw," and "dog" becomes "god."

Although one or two letter reversals are common in the 6- or 7-year-old child, reversals should be infrequent by 8 years of age. Additionally, the child 6 years of age should be able to print the first and last names, the numbers from 1 to 10, and the alphabet. These figures should be in a horizontal line and should become more evenly spaced by 7 years of age. Chapter 5 offers more details.

***Concept formation.*** To test the child's thought processes and concept formation, the nurse practitioner should become familiar with the usual fund of knowledge possessed by children at each grade level within the community. After establishing a basis for comparison, the nurse may ask the child to answer a variety of questions or to perform various tasks, such as the following: Who is the President of the United States? Count as far as you can. What state (city) do you live in? Additionally, the nurse practitioner may utilize a book such as Scarry's *Best Word Book Ever* as a basis for facilitating conversation or as a means of assessing the child's ability to identify objects and discuss their relationship to each other. At this point the nurse may also summarize the child's memory, quality, and continuity of thought, as demonstrated throughout the assessment process.

*Motor ability.* Before the testing of speech and reading skills the child might appreciate a break and some motor activity to release the tension that may build as a result of attempting various confining academic skills.

Some motor skills are detailed in Chapter 5 according to the usual capabilities of various age groups. However, specific testing beyond that detailed in the neurological assessment in Chapters 5 and 11 is suggested to elicit the neurological soft signs frequently associated with minimal brain dysfunction.

Practitioners should realize that children less than 7 years of age are often unable to complete these tasks without errors or some difficulty.

TESTING PROCEDURE. The child is instructed to lie down in a supine position. (It is abnormal to assume the fetal position after the age of 2 years.) Then the child is asked to stand. Posture, head tilting, and position of the hands, legs, and toes as well as the degree of straightness in the spinal column are noted. Next, the child is asked to walk the distance of about 30 steps forward and backward. The gait should then be assessed for exaggerated or asymmetric arm swinging, clumsiness, or problems in balance.

The child is requested to walk about 25 steps on alternating heels. This task should be accomplished after 5 years of age without difficulty in maintaining balance.

The ability to stand on one foot to hop and skill in skipping and galloping are easily demonstrated by many children before 7 years of age, as discussed in Chapter 5. The inability to complete these skills by 8 years of age is abnormal.

Even though there is some disagreement on the significance of the Romberg test for young children, it is generally included in the assessment. In this test the child closes both eyes, stands with both feet together, projects the tongue, and extends both upper extremities with the fingers spread apart. This position is maintained for about 45 seconds. The practitioner should document any choreiform movements in the fingers, as well as the child's ability to follow directions.

Coordination and fine motor skills are tested by use of the following exercises. The smoothness and symmetry of eye movements are tested when one swings a disc through the full visual range while instructing the child to fixate the head and follow the object with both eyes. Other than the rhythmic eye jerks that guide eye movements, the eyes should move in a smooth, coordinated manner bilaterally. Any deviation from usual eye movements should be carefully documented.

Fine motor functioning and coordination in the extremities may be assessed by use of the following tests: First, the child is asked to imitate simple activities, such as touching the nose with the left hand while touching the right ear with the right hand. Next the child touches the nose with the left hand and the left ear with the right hand. As the child repeats this exercise, any tremors, unusual effort, deviations in fine motor movements, or right-left confusion should be noted.

The second exercise involves asking the child to touch the index finger to his nose and then to the index finger on the examiner's hand. This procedure should be done repeatedly, using one hand at a time. The child should be asked to move as rapidly as possible while maintaining accuracy in touching both targets.

Third, the child is asked to imitate the examiner, who taps the upper and lower extremities first unilaterally and then bilaterally at the same rhythmic pace.

Fourth, the child is requested to perform repetitive movements. To begin this sequence, the child is asked to touch and then separate the index finger and the thumb on one hand as rapidly as possible. After the exercise is done several times on one hand, it is repeated with the opposite hand. Next, the child is asked to pronate and supinate each hand separately in rapid succession. Finally, the child is asked to touch each finger to the thumb in rapid succession on one hand and then on the other hand. During these exercises the examiner notices the child's ability to follow directions and perform the tasks. The amount of effort exerted including difficulty with or behavioral responses to the tests, and limb symmetry and smoothness of movements are important. However, nurses should realize that young children may normally exhibit overflow movements in joints or extremities not actively engaged in the exercise.

*Tactile perception.* The perception of tactile

stimuli is the next area that is included in the assessment. Several simple tests are utilized to test tactile input after the child has had an adequate trial of practice. With the eyes closed, the child is asked to move the same finger on the left hand that the examiner is touching on the right hand, and vice versa. Next, the examiner touches the child at two different points simultaneously (chin and right hand, nose and left hand, and so on) and asks the child, whose eyes are closed, to identify the points of tactile contact. Then the examiner may place an object in the hand of the child and ask the child to identify the object without looking at it. Objects used in this test should be familiar items, such as a comb, coin, safety pin, or button.

As a part of tactile sensations, the child should be able to discriminate heat, cold, smoothness, pain, or roughness without viewing the stimulus. Additionally, the intact sensation of all body areas should be established along with an adequate ability to feel two simultaneous points of tactile stimulation.

*Academic abilities.* At this point the nurse has spent sufficient time with the child to have a relaxed interaction with both the child and the parent. Thus it is a good time to summarize the patterns of communication that the child demonstrates, both by history and in the testing situation. Such items as the child's ability to stick with the topic at hand, the speed of speech, the adequacy of word usage, the tone of voice, and the presence of any prevailing themes in spontaneous conversation should be recorded. The manner in which the child becomes involved in communication, that is, spontaneous speech, responses after parental encouragement, constant silliness or interruptions, responses limited to answering of direct questions only, or inability to answer questions because of parent interference, should also be noted.

At some point in the examination the practitioner may utilize the DASE if the child is between the ages of 2½ and 6 years. Further assessment of speech and language development is discussed in Chapter 11.

As a part of the academic assessment, the practitioner should utilize excerpts from a standardized reading test to evaluate the reading level and comprehension capacity. Additionally, the nurse may utilize a school-administered test on comprehen-

sive achievement to assess arithmetic, word recognition, and spelling. To test memory, the nurse practitioner may ask the child to repeat five digits. By the age of 7 years, the child should be able to recall all five digits accurately.

*Social capacities.* A summary of the total ability of the child in social realms may be included at this point. It should include data from the history, observations on parent-child interactions, impressions derived from the child's response to the nurse practitioner and the assessment situation, and data from other sources, such as schoolteachers.

*Attention and concentration.* In those children with specific learning disabilities who also have impaired attention spans, nurses should attempt to document the base-line behavior during the initial assessment. Thus later progress may be measured. It may be helpful to describe the behavior and the situations that improve attention or make it worse. Additionally, it may be helpful to time the attention span during periods of free activity, stress, concentration, and conversation both in a stimulating situation and in the quiet examining room after the child has become thoroughly acquainted with the room and the nurse practitioner.

### Hyperkinesis

The child who is hyperkinetic has a variety of problems. Basically the child has a great difficulty in concentrating on static tasks and finds attention to active movements far easier to achieve. Thus parents may report that the child operates better in the free-play setting than in the confined academic role. Additionally, the child is easily distracted from the current activity by usual environmental stimuli. Pattern perception may also be distorted, so that responses to various types of input are inappropriate or clumsy. Perseverance is another problem in these children. For example, the child may show impaired ability to identify a course of action, define logical priorities, and follow activities that result in goal completion. Thus the child who plans to go into the bedroom to dress for school may be found looking out the window and thinking about model airplanes moments later. Momentary observation also reveals the constant, excessive quality of movement and conversation in the hyperactive child. Moreover, in addition to the excessive motion patterns, the quality of movement is poor because of the continuous, nonselective responses to assorted, unrelated environmental stimuli. Impulsiveness and spontaneous, unplanned actions are also characteristic of these children. Emotions are labile, and hyperkinetic children are prone to mood swings, impatience, inappropriate responses, and outbursts.

*Medical management.* Although the exact etiology of hyperkinesis has not been determined, physicians attempting to diagnose this problem generally utilize the differential diagnoses mentioned earlier in this chapter along with assessments of hypoglycemia and current classroom situations to decide whether hyperkinesis is the problem. Certainly one should know if the classroom is noisy, crowded, poorly staffed, or unacceptable in terms of the child's needs before categorizing the child as the source of the problem.

After the diagnosis of hyperkinesis is established by the procedures summarized in the boxed material on pp. 195 and 196, most nurses believe that a comprehensive treatment plan that includes all aspects of support to the child and family, as well as a progressive plan for remediation, should be drafted. In addition to emotional support and appropriate referrals, many nurse practitioners believe that the child should be given medications or a special diet.

Two of the medications that have been most widely used in the control of hyperkinesis are dextroamphetamine and methylphenidate (Ritalin). Whereas dextroamphetamine is available in liquid or capsule form and has the advantage of having been on the market for a longer period of time, methylphenidate is said to have less effect on growth suppression (Safer et al., 1973). In one study, investigators worked with a group of children for a period of 5 years to determine the impact of treating children with methylphenidate, chlorpromazine, or no medication. Although children taking methylphenidate were more manageable in school and at home, none of the groups showed statistical differences in long-range improvements as measured by standardized tests for emotional adjustment, motor skills, intelligence, or academic performance (Weiss et al., 1975). However, many practitioners still agree that the use of stimulant drugs is appropriate for improvement in target behaviors, such as school participation. Some prac-

titioners prescribe a dosage for use during school only, some use a medication schedule that spans the clock, and some discontinue medications during vacations or school breaks, since use is primarily aimed at assisting the child to learn in the confined academic environment.

Although the effect of central nervous system stimulants on the learning process is not well understood, it is generally believed that action is related to the metabolism of catecholamines, as described in Chapter 4. Thus the displacement of catecholamines from the sympathetic nerve terminals by stimulants probably affects the reticular activating system.

Over the past several years there has been an increase in interest in the orthomolecular concept and the food-additive question in relation to behavior and learning.

The orthomolecular theory gained much of its current impetus from the works of Pauling, who expounded the importance of having certain substances available within the body to ensure optimal functioning. This type of thinking underlies the reasons for megavitamin therapy. Wender and Wender have also contributed to this area with a discussion of biochemical abnormalities and their connection to behavior. Weiss and Kaufman added another dimension by introducing the connection between hyperkinesis and food allergies. Another popular method of treating hyperkinesis is by the use of the dietary management program proposed by Feingold, this program eliminates artificial food colors, flavors, and the salicylates that occur normally in certain foods.

In summary, these methods continue to be investigated. The significance of nutritional metabolic, and biochemical factors in learning and behavior is only beginning to be realized. More research in these areas is needed.

### Nursing intervention

Most clients and families have a backlog of negative experiences and feelings when they arrive at the health care facility for problem assessment. After the nurse does a comprehensive assessment, and identifies individual areas of actual functioning and possible developmentally appropriate potentials for increasing functional capacities, the client and family need a thorough explanation of

## ASSESSMENT SUMMARY FOR SPECIFIC LEARNING DISABILITIES

I. History
   A. Previous growth and development
   B. Current growth and development (Denver Developmental Screening Test until child is 6 years of age)
   C. Prenatal and perinatal events
   D. Physical problems, accidents, surgeries, hospitalizations, and so on
   E. Inherited disorders, especially related to central nervous system
   F. Behavioral history
II. Adaptation to school
   A. Teachers' report
   B. Results of readiness tests (Preschool Readiness Experimental Screening Scale and Meeting Street School Screening Test)
   C. Grades
   D. Parents' comments
   E. Child's perception of school
III. Physical assessment
   A. Review of systems
   B. Emphasis on otological and ophthalmological tests
   C. Speech screening (Denver Articulation Screening Examination)
   D. Body measurements
   E. Nutritional status
   F. Immunizations and childhood disease history
   G. General health status and practices
IV. Neurological examination
   A. Cranial nerves
   B. Reflexes
   C. Muscle strength and tone
   D. Visual motor abilities
      1. Geometric figures
   E. Auditory motor functions
      1. Writing from dictation
   F. Concept formation
      1. Fund of knowledge
      2. Memory
      3. Quality and continuity of thought

G. Motor ability
   1. Supine position
   2. Stationary stance
   3. Gait
   4. Heel walking
   5. Skip, hop, and gallop
   6. Romberg test
   7. Fine motor skills
      a. Eyes
      b. Extremities
      c. Right-left confusion
H. Tactile perception
   1. Contact
   2. Object identification
   3. Sensory discrimination
   4. Two-point discrimination
I. Academic abilities
   1. Communication and speech patterns
   2. Reading level and comprehension
   3. Arithmetic, word recognition, and spelling
   4. Digit recall
J. Social capacities
   1. Summary of data from parent history and teachers' reports
   2. Observations during assessment
K. Attention and concentration
   1. Behavioral description
   2. Timed attention-span sequences
   3. Response to various levels of environmental stimulation
L. Hyperkinesis (if present)
   1. Distractibility
   2. Response patterns
   3. Perseverance
   4. Priority setting and goal completion
   5. Impulsivity
   6. Emotional lability
   7. Insight into consequences

## BEHAVIORAL RATING SCALE FOR CHILDREN WITH SPECIFIC LEARNING DISABILITIES*

Date: _____

Teacher: _____ Physician: _____

Name: _____ Age: _____ yr _____ mo  Sex: _____  Grade: _____

Current medications (include name, dosage, frequency, length of time taking medication, side effects, etc.):

    1. _____

    2. _____

    3. _____

Diet:

Height: _____ feet _____ inches _____ percentile for age   Weight: _____ pounds _____ percentile for age

Vital signs: Blood pressure: _____ Respirations: _____ Temperature: _____ Pulse: _____

System review:

Teacher's observations:

Date of last laboratory tests: _____

### Rating behavioral observations

| Behavior | 0 | 1 | 2 | 3 |
|---|---|---|---|---|
| 1. Restless or overactive | | | | |
| 2. Excitable or impulsive, or both | | | | |
| 3. Disturbs other children | | | | |
| 4. Fails to finish things started; short attention span | | | | |
| 5. Constantly fidgeting | | | | |
| 6. Inattentive; easily distracted | | | | |
| 7. Demands must be met immediately; easily frustrated | | | | |
| 8. Cries often and easily | | | | |
| 9. Sudden, radical mood swings | | | | |
| 10. Unpredictable behavior; explosive emotional outbursts | | | | |

**KEY TO RATING SYSTEM:**
**0** Does not show this behavior    **2** Shows this behavior 50% of the time
**1** Shows this behavior 25% of the time    **3** Shows this behavior 75% or more of the time

*Modified from Conners' Abbreviated Teacher Rating Scale in Sprague, R.L., and Sleator, E.K.: Pediatr. Clin. North Am. **20**:726, 1973.

the testing and treatment goals of the health team. Assist the family of focusing on positive behaviors and ways that they can work together to improve the client's functional abilities and self-concept. Provide a therapeutic climate for supportive counseling as the client and family discuss problems encountered in living with a child who competes inadequately with peers. Modify stimulus-response patterns that result in negative outcomes by applying techniques of behavior modification so that the client may be managed more successfully at home and at school. Acquaint the family with specific resources and approaches for handling specific problems of the child. Coordinate educational and health care interventions, so that services are not fragmented and all needs of the client and family are considered in acute and long-term interventions.

Regardless of the comprehensive treatment approach selected, the nurse has a role in evaluating the effectiveness of the problem-specific therapy for the individual child. After the initial assessment is summarized, along with specific interventions that have been prescribed by the nurse, the physician, or other involved professionals, the nurse may utilize a modified form of the Conners' Abbreviated Teacher Rating Scale, as shown in the boxed material on p. 196, to evaluate periodically behavioral progress in the child. As mentioned previously, the child may exhibit different behaviors in various settings. When improvement is not apparent in the individual child, the plan of intervention should be reevaluated and modified accordingly.

At the present time no universal scale for measuring the effect of medication on behavior in children with specific learning disabilities is available. However, the Conners' Abbreviated Teacher Rating Scale has repeatedly shown a sensitivity to the effects of central nervous system stimulants in children with specific learning disabilities. Since it is a tool that is rapidly administered, it has gained wide acceptance. However, its reliance on subjective evaluations should be taken into account when one evaluates the results of testing.

Sprague and Sleator recommend that their tool be utilized on a monthly basis to measure the effectiveness of central nervous system stimulants on school behavior and performance. The tool that appears in the boxed material is adapted from their tool. If offers more data that are specifically needed by the nurse. However, at the time of each observation by the nurse, the teacher should also complete the portion detailing behavioral observations and add comments about the child's overall progress. In this manner the interobserver objectivity may be increased.

## REFERENCES

Baldessarini, R.J.: Pharmacology of the amphetamines, Pediatrics **49:**694, 1972.

Brown, R.T., and Sleator, E.K.: Methylphenidate in hyperkinetic children: differences in dose effects on impulsive behavior, Pediatrics **64:**408-411, 1979.

Buros, O.K., editor: The seventh mental measurements yearbook, N.J., 1972, Gryphon Press.

Charles, L., et al.: Effects of methylphenidate on hyperactive children's ability to sustain attention, Pediatrics **64:**412-418, 1979.

Conway, B.L.: The role of the teacher-practitioner in pediatric neurology, 1970 (unpublished paper).

Cruickshank, W.M., and Johnson, G.O., editors: Education of exceptional children and youth, 1975, Englewood Cliffs, N.J., 1975, Prentice-Hall, Inc.

Dykman, R.A., Peters, J.E., and Ackerman, P.T.: Experimental approaches to the study of minimal brain dysfunction: a follow-up study, Ann. N.Y. Acad. Sci. **205:**93, 1973.

Eisenberg, L.: The clinical use of stimulant drugs in children, Pediatrics **49:**709, 1972.

Feingold, B.F.: Hyperkinesis and learning disabilities linked to artificial food flavors and colors, Am. J. Nurs. **74:**797, 1975.

Fernald, G.: Remedial techniques in basic school subjects, New York, 1943, McGraw-Hill Book Co.

Frostig, M.: Move-grow-learn, Chicago, 1969, Follett Publishing Co.

Frostig, M.: Testing as a basis for educational therapy, J. Spec. Educ. **2:**1, 1967.

Frostig, M., et al.: The Marianne Frostig Developmental Test of Visual Perception, ed. 3, Palo Alto, Calif., 1964, Consulting Psychologists Press.

Graham, P., and Rutter, M.: The reliability and validity of the psychiatric assessment of the child. II. Interview with the parent, Br. J. Psychiatr. **114:**581, 1968.

Hallahan, D.P., and Cruickshank, W.M.: Psychoeducational foundations of learning disabilities, Englewood Cliffs, N.J., 1973, Prentice-Hall, Inc.

Johnson, D., and Myklebust, H.R.: Learning disabilities: educational principles and practices, New York, 1967, Grune & Stratton, Inc.

Kass, C.E., and Myklebust, H.R.: Learning disability: an educational definition, J. Learn. Disabil. **2:**38, 1969.

Kirk, S.A.: A behavioral approach to learning disabilities, Conference on Children with Minimal Brain Impairment, Chicago, 1963.

Kirk, S.A., McCarthy, J.J., and Kirk, W.D.: The Illinois Test of Psycholinguistic Abilities, rev. ed., Urbana, Ill. 1968, University of Illinois Press.

Kirk, S.A., and Kirk, W.D.: Psycholinguistic learning disabilities: diagnosis and remediation, Urbana, Ill., 1971, University of Illinois Press.

Lindsley, O.R.: Direct measurement and prosthesis of retarded behavior, J. Educ. **147:**62, 1964.

McCarthy, D.: McCarthy Scales of Children's Ability, New York, 1972, The Psychological Corporation.

Meeting Street School Screening Test, Providence, R.I., 1969, Crippled Children and Adults of Rhode Island.

Myklebust, H.R.: Psychoneurological learning disorders in children, Conference on Children with Minimal Brain Impairment, Chicago, 1963.

Pauling, L.: Orthomolecular psychiatry, Science **160:**265, 1968.

Rogers, W.B., Jr., and Rogers, R.A.: A new simplified Preschool Readiness Experimental Screening Scale (the PRESS), Clin. Pediat. **11:**10, 1972.

Rogers, W.B., Jr., and Rogers, R.A.: A new simplified Preschool Readiness Experimental Screening Scale (the PRESS): a preliminary report, Clin. Pediatr. **11:**558, 1972.

Rosenberg, L.A.: Psychological examination of the handicapped child, Pediatr. Clin. North Am. **20:**66, 1973.

Safer, D.J., et al.: Factors influencing the suppressant effects of two stimulant drugs on the growth of hyperactive children, Pediatrics **51:**660, 1973.

Scarry, R.: Best word book ever, ed. 16, New York, 1974, Golden Press.

Skinner, B.F.: Beyond freedom and dignity, New York, 1971, Vintage Books.

Sprague, R.L., and Sleator, E.K.: Effects of psychopharmacologic agents on learning disorders, Pediatr. Clin. North Am. **20:**719, 1973.

Stewart, M.A.: Hyperactive children, Sci. Am. **224:**94, 1970.

Strauss, A., and Lehtinen, L.: Psychopathology and education of the brain-injured child, vol. 1, New York, 1947, Grune & Stratton, Inc.

Strauss, A., and Kephart, N.C.: Psychopathology and education of the brain-injured child, vol. 2, New York, 1955, Grune & Stratton, Inc.

Wechsler, D.: Wechsler Preschool and Primary Scale of Intelligence, New York, 1967, The Psychological Corporation.

Weiss, G., et al.: Long-term treatment of hyperactive children with methylphenidate, Can. Med. Assoc. J. **112:**159, 1975.

Weiss, J., and Kaufman, H.S.: Subtle organic component in some cases of mental illness, Arch. Gen. Psychiatr. **24:**25, 1971.

Wender, P.H., and Wender, E.H.: The hyperactive child and the learning disabled child, New York, 1978, Crown Pubs., Inc., New York, 1971.

Wepman, J.M.: Wepman Auditory Discrimination Test, Chicago, 1958, Language Research Associates.

# 9

# IMPAIRED CONSCIOUSNESS

## DEFINING IMPAIRED CONSCIOUSNESS

Unconsciousness is the outcome of an underlying problem; thus each case varies significantly in onset, duration, depth, and other characteristics in accordance with the specific etiology. Because consciousness implies individual awareness and response to stimuli related to self and environment, lack of consciousness necessarily refers to loss of these capacities or to a state that may be described as unarousable unresponsiveness.

Unconsciousness is a state of depressed cerebral function in which the appreciation of stimuli is lost and the response to such, if present at all, is on a reflex level. The depth of unconsciousness may vary from stupor to coma. In the former a client may respond to noxious stimuli by withdrawal, grimacing, or making unintelligible sounds; in the latter there is no observable response.

There are several conditions that may be mistaken for coma. A client may have *acute global aphasia* so as to be totally unable to communicate information successfully perceived. *Akinetic mutism (coma vigil)* is a state wherein the client experiences sleep-wake cycles while appearing silent, immobile, and alert but with no indication of functional higher brain processes. A similar condition, termed the *apallic state,* may resemble akinetic mutism or cause the immobile client to be rigid or spastic, but it specifically refers to the generalized damage and degeneration that occurs in patients who have encephalitis, head injuries, or anoxic episodes. *Locked-in syndrome* is a condition wherein the patient suffers paralysis of the lower cranial nerves and all four extremities. The state of consciousness may or may not remain intact. When it does remain intact, the only means of communication available to the client involves vertical eye movements and blinking. These limited responses might be missed by the unskilled eye.

## CONFUSED STATES

Some individuals experience an alteration in *content level* rather than in their *awareness* or *arousal level.* These clients are termed *confused.* Examples include those who perceive stimuli in a distorted manner, in a manner that misinterprets stimuli or in response to the lack of stimuli. Confusion is a frequent problem of elderly clients and those with psychosocial disturbances. These two groups should be considered separately. Refer to Chapter 7 for additional detail.

## STAGING PROCESS

As an individual begins to experience an impairment in the level of consciousness (LOC) the problem of measurement becomes important. Most frequently, parameters of measurement are based on motor activity, particularly speech and the pattern of somatic and eye movements. The correlation of consciousness and motor behavior is presented in the following schema:

| Normal consciousness | 1. Spontaneous (voluntary) speech at a normal rate |
|---|---|
| *See next page.* | Normal voluntary and reflex somatic motor activity |
| | Eyes open; normal oculomotor activity |

**199**

Lethargy

Stupor

Coma

2. Spontaneous sentences, spoken slowly
   Decreased speed of voluntary motor activity
   Eyes open; decreased oculomotor activity
3. Spontaneous words, spoken infrequently
   Decreased speed and coordination of voluntary motor activity
   Eyes open or closed; decreased oculomotor activity
4. Vocalization only to stimuli that cause pain
   Greatly decreased spontaneous motor activity
   Eyes generally closed; some spontaneous eye movements
5. No vocalization
   Appropriate defensive movements, generally flexor, to stimuli that cause pain
   Eyes generally closed
6. No vocalization
   Mass movements to stimuli that cause pain
   Eyes closed; decreased spontaneous conjugate eye movements
7. No vocalization
   Decerebrate posturing to stimuli that cause pain, or no response
   Eyes closed; absent spontaneous eye movements

When individuals experience progressive brain lesions such as expanding hematoma, the neurological capacities often seem to deteriorate in steps, as those just outlined, as they progress to coma. Similarly, as individuals regain their capacities, the capacities seem to progress in a steplike fashion upward to higher levels of consciousness. This mode of progression suggests the interrelationship of various structures of the brain in maintaining consciousness. (See Fig. 3-9.)

Another system of organization is a four-stage grading process, as follows:

*Stage I: Stupor*—Means the client is arousable for brief periods and able to exercise simple motor and verbal responses. This stage sometimes occurs alternately with delirium, a state wherein motor excitement and mental confusion predominate.

*Stage II: Light coma*—Painful stimuli results in semi-

purposeful acts of avoidance and moaning without arousal.

*Stage III: Deep coma*—No meaningful response is apparent with painful stimuli that often evoke extension and pronation of the arms (decerebrate posturing).

*Stage IV: Client is apneic and flaccid*—The individual has no brainstem functions and is breathing by artificial ventilation. Some spinal reflexes may still be evident. This phase is termed *brain death,* wherein (1) two electroencephalographic tracings taken 24 hours apart reveal complete absence of brain waves; (2) all cerebral functions, including pupillary and spontaneous breathing capacities, are lacking for at least 24 hours, even if local spinal reflexes remain; and (3) expert opinions confirm that the absence of brain activity is not secondary to hypothermia or drug intoxication.

## ROSTRAL-CAUDAL PROGRESSION OF COMA

Another set of terms that interface with the preceding two descriptions includes grouping according to the portion of the brain involved in the progression of coma. This type of classification is broadly termed the *rostral-caudal progression* of coma. Symptoms relate to interference at the diencephalic, midbrain, lower pontine, or medullary areas.

### Diencephalon

Interferences at the diencephalic level result in a depressed state of consciousness, Cheyne-Stokes respiration, slightly responsive pupils that react briskly, roving eye movements, and evidence of the full range of eye movements only with the use of the doll's head maneuver or the calorics technique. The doll's head maneuver is demonstrated as rapid turning of the head results in conjugate deviation of the eyes in the direction away from the head movement when the brainstem centers for eye movements remain intact. The calorics techniques are detailed in Chapter 27. The contralateral side of the body is most commonly affected when the individual has a diencephalic lesion, unless the lesion is a lateral expanding mass in the supratentorial area, wherein herniation of the uncus through the supratentorial notch causes the oculomotor (third) nerve to be compressed, with subsequent dilatation of the pupil on the affected side.

Early in the course of lesions affecting this area,

aversive movements of the face and limbs are evident in response to painful stimuli. However, as the lesion progresses, the client becomes immobile and evidences decorticate posturing. *Decorticate posturing* refers to the state wherein there is adduction to the shoulders; flexion at the elbows, wrists, and fingers; and extension and adduction in the lower extremities.

If the space-occupying lesion is in a position in the lateral hemisphere, assessment of the client reveals tonic deviation of the eyes away from the side of the body affected by hemiplegia. Since problems in the diencephalon do not involve the brainstem centers for eye movement, this eye deviation may be demonstrated by the doll's head maneuver or calorics technique. The response is usually most dramatic with the calorics technique, since it is the stronger stimulus. The practitioner should realize that this tonic deviation of the eyes may not be apparent for 8 to 12 hours after the onset of hemiplegia. After this period, if these techniques do not reverse the eyes, the problem may be an acute pontine lesion.

### Midbrain

As disrupted functioning affects the midbrain area, decorticate posturing becomes *decerebrate posturing* and Cheyne-Stokes respirations change to neurogenic hyperventilation. Although decerebrate posturing may not be observed, the response may be stimulated by knuckle pressure to the sternum. To best observe decerebrate posturing, one should place the client's arms in a semiflexed position across the abdomen and apply knuckle pressure to the sternum. The response includes internal rotation of the forearm away from the painful point of stimulation. Additional symptoms of midbrain involvement include fixed pupils and extension of both the upper and lower extremities.

### Lower pontine area

When involvement progresses to the lower pontine area, findings include flaccid quadriplegia; absence of eye movements in responses to the calorics technique and doll's head maneuver; fixed, nonreactive pupils located in the medial position; and a breathing pattern wherein normal breathing is interrupted by pauses at the peak of the inspiratory cycle.

### Medulla

As the medulla becomes involved, respirations become arrhythmical and assume a gasping pattern. Blood pressure begins to fall. Death frequently results with medulla involvement.

## DIAGNOSIS

Causative mechanisms for coma may roughly be divided into four categories, including metabolic encephalopathy, supratentorial space-occupying lesions, infratentorial space-occupying lesions, and psychogenic coma. The first objective when one evaluates the client is to ascertain which of these categories is involved so that interventions may be implemented for the specific problem.

When unconsciousness results from a *metabolic encephalopathy,* the metabolism of the cerebral cortex and brainstem is disrupted. Agents affecting this disruption include such conditions as drug overdosage, hypoglycemia, and situations resulting in anoxic episodes. When coma is caused by metabolic encephalopathy, abnormal motor movements are symmetrical bilaterally. Pupils are small and reactive and reveal conjugate eye movements in response to calorics testing. Some clients who have ingested overdoses of drugs will present a different picture. If the drug was an opiate, pupils will be pinpoint sized but reactive. In atropine and scopolamine overdosage the pupils are dilated and fixed. Pupils are fixed in the midline in glutethimide overdosage. In barbiturate poisoning the pupils are variable; skin is usually cyanotic; muscle twitching may be evident; reflexes are sluggish or abolished; and respirations assume a shallow, slow pattern.

When related to a *supratentorial space-occupying lesion* (abscess, tumor, hemorrhagic accumulation), coma occurs as the mass distorts and compresses the brainstem reticular formation. Supratentorial lesions frequently include the following symptoms: hemiplegia, small reactive pupils, conjugate ocular deviation away from the hemiplegic side, and Cheyne-Stokes respirations. These lesions continue to progress in the rostral-caudal pattern previously described until pupils become fixed in the midline, respirations become rapid and deep, and decerebrate rigidity occurs.

In *infratentorial space-occupying lesions* (cerebellar hemorrhage, infarcts from basilar artery oc-

TABLE 9-1. The characteristics of organic and functional coma

| Organic | Functional |
|---|---|
| No response to noxious stimuli | Response to noxious stimuli with manifestations such as withdrawal and grimacing |
| Loss of sphincter control | No loss of sphincter control |
| All reflexes are absent (pupils fixed, corneal reflexes absent, swallowing impossible) | Reflexes are present |
| Skin may be abnormal in color, texture, temperature, and moisture, depending on specific disease | Skin has normal characteristics |
| If a convulsion occurs and the client falls, invariably injury is sustained, and generally tongue biting is evident | No injury with falling; generally before an audience; no tongue biting |
| Eyelids may be elevated without difficulty; pupils are visible | Pronounced resistance to elevation of eyelids; eyeballs generally rotated upward; pupils not visible |
| May be pathological changes in blood pressure, pulse, respiration, and temperature | Pulse and respiration may be accelerated; temperature usually unremarkable |
| Paralysis of one or more extremities may be present | No true muscular paralysis |

clusion), coma results from direct pressure or destruction of the brainstem reticular formation. Symptoms include hemiplegia, disconjugate or conjugate ocular deviation toward the hemiplegic side, and several possible abnormal pupil responses—pinpoint, fixed, or fixed at midposition. These symptoms are observable in the early stages of coma.

At times coma may have a *psychogenic origin*. In these cases the client is unresponsive to the environment, even though physiologically intact. Examinations of neurological status reveal findings within normal limits. When ice-water calorics testing is performed, normal rapid-phase nystagmus occurs toward the opposite side. See Table 9-1 for distinctions between organic and functional coma.

## COMMON CAUSATIVE PROBLEMS

Acute alcoholism is frequently a cause of coma. In such cases the level of coma is not deep, and the client reacts to painful stimuli. The temperature may be normal or decreased. Other symptoms include involvement of the conjunctiva, hyperemia of the face, equal but moderately dilated pupils, and deep, noisy respirations. When blood alcohol levels are measured, a concentration greater than 200 mg/dl is often revealed.

In cerebrovascular accidents the client usually reveals a history of either hypertension or cardiovascular disease. The age of the client is usually greater than 40 years. Symptoms in these cases include sudden onset; asymmetrically flushed or cyanotic face; variable findings in the vital signs, usually elevated blood pressure; unequal, unreactive pupils; and frequent paralysis. When a lumbar puncture is performed, the cerebrospinal fluid is under increased pressure and may appear bloody or xanthochromic. Chapter 24 gives further details on cerebrovascular disease.

Sometimes clients are in the postictal phase of a grand mal seizure when they appear to be in "coma." In these cases a relative may report previous seizures, or an identification tag on the client may indicate epilepsy. Symptoms include sudden onset; normal vital signs, unless multiple seizures have resulted in elevation; incontinence; and possible injury from biting the tongue or, often, portions of the mouth.

If the coma is related to syncope, it is superficial and transient. The episode is sudden, and emotional problems are frequently noted as precipitating events. These clients appear pale and often have pulse rates that are initially slow but become rapid and weak.

When coma is related to hypoglycemia, many warning signs usually precede the attack, including diaphoresis, nausea, pallor, palpitation, vomiting, hunger, abdominal pain, and light-headedness. However, the episode may be acute and is, at times, accompanied by seizures. Findings during the episode include hypoglycemia, exaggerated

---

## COMMON CAUSES OF COMA

Vascular diseases—ruptured intracranial aneurysm, cerebral thrombosis, embolus, hemorrhage

Space-occupying lesions—tumor, abscess, chronic subdural hematoma

Head injury—severe concussion, contusion, laceration of the brain, extradural hemorrhage, subdural hematoma, penetrating wound

Toxic problems—uremia, diabetes, hypoglycemia, alcoholism, drug overdose, lead poisoning

Infectious processes—encephalitis, meningitis

Seizures—postictal phase, status epilepticus

Psychogenic disorders

---

deep tendon reflexes, moist, pale skin, and a positive Babinski sign.

Some symptoms related to coma caused by drug overdose are mentioned in the discussion of metabolic encephalopathies.

When cranial trauma is the cause of coma, the incident may have occurred within the past few hours so that the bleeding is superficial and arterial in origin, or it may have occurred up to 2 weeks before, so that the hemorrhage is probably deeper in the cranium and of a venous origin. In either case there is a history of cranial insult, and, in some cases, the point of injury is observable. The onset of coma is variable, depending on the nature of the lesion. The temperature may be normal or elevated. Bleeding may be apparent from the cranial orifices: nose, ear, or throat. Pupils are often unequal and unreactive. Respirations vary among individuals but are frequently slow or irregular. Pulse rates may also fluctuate but are often rapid at first and then slow. Alterations in blood pressure may or may not be eivdent. Reflexes are frequently abnormal. Incontinence and paralysis may occur. When a lumbar puncture is performed, the cerebrospinal fluid is often bloody and under increased pressure. Radiographic films of the skull may show a fracture. Carotid arteriography and computerized axial tomographic (CAT) scanning are frequently required to make a definite diagnosis and localize the lesion.

It is noteworthy to mention alcoholics in the context of cranial trauma, since they frequently sustain unrecalled injury during a stuporous state. They are frequently known to have chronic subdural hematomas because of repeated cranial trauma. Thus even when the state seems to be one of alcoholic overdose, the judicious practitioner should look further to eliminate the possibility of concurrent problems.

## DATA COLLECTION

Because the client is unable to relate a history, it is imperative that the practitioner utilize any other informed individuals available. Such persons may include witnesses to the problem, the police, relatives, or friends. Questions of these persons are geared toward attaining the following information: (1) pattern of onset or injury, (2) infections, (3) previous seizures, (4) concurrent problems (psychogenic disturbances, diabetes mellitus, nephritis, hypertension, cardiovascular disease), and (5) presence of a headache. An immediate problem is to decide if the client has ingested any type of toxic substances, such as alcohol or drugs. Containers in the vicinity of the incident should be retained for testing so that identification of a toxic substance may proceed when ingestion is a possibility. The client should be rapidly assessed for signs of cranial trauma, hemorrhage, or incontinence. Identification of the client or a tag or bracelet signaling a medical problem may add valuable information or may assist in allowing the medical team to contact a close friend or relative.

To further define the nature of the problem and evaluate the depth of coma, the practitioner may apply pressure adequate to evoke a painful response.

The physical assessment continues as the practitioner attempts to make pertinent observations in several areas. Vital signs are measured. The temperature is taken rectally or at the axillary site to avoid injury to the client. The skin is examined carefully for irregularities, that is, petechiae, rashes, injection sites, trauma, and changes in color. The scalp is carefully inspected for any evidence of trauma or laceration that may have occurred. The eyes are examined carefully for pupillary response, corneal reflex, and ocular palsy, and funduscopic assessment is performed. The cranial orifices are examined for the presence of blood drainage. The mouth is examined for lacerations or old scars. The underside of the tongue is inspected for needle tract marks, since drug addicts may use this concealed site for injections. Respiratory rate, volume, and patterns are noted. The practitioner also attempts to detect any odors on the breath because they may provide clues in diagnosis. In cyanide poisoning the breath smells like bitter almonds.

The examination continues with elevation of the cardiovascular system. First, the apical and radial pulses are measured. Quality, rhythm, rate, and volume are noted. Asymmetry in these pulses and other major pulses is noted as the pulses are compared bilaterally. Blood pressures are measured and compared in both arms. Efforts are made to document any apparent sclerosis in peripheral vessels or cardiac insufficiency. The abdomen is assessed for rigidity and spasms. Clubbing, cyanosis, and paresis are noted in the periphery, including the extremities. Significant neurological findings may include seizures, asymmetric deep tendon reflexes, a positive Babinski sign, muscular twitchings, hemiplegia, or signs of meningeal irritation, for example, Kernig's sign.

If a space-occupying lesion is suspected, a skull radiograph is often taken unless the client is in shock. A neurosurgical consultation is initiated, and cerebroangiography and computerized axial tomographic (CAT) scanning are commonly done to further delineate the problem. When it does not compromise the client, a lumbar puncture is frequently indicated to provide further data.

If the possibility of a metabolic encephalopathy exists, a urine specimen is obtained by catheter for evaluation of the presence of glucose, albumin, and acetone. Blood samples are tested for glucose, blood urea nitrogen, and hemoglobin and are subjected to spectroscopy, wherein abnormal blood pigmentation, indicating the presence of sulfhemoglobin and methemoglobin, is apparent. In suspected overdoses or poisonings, gastric lavage is performed for diagnostic and therapeutic reasons.

## BRAIN RESUSCITATION THERAPY

The new emphasis has shifted from the well-known CPR to CPCR (cardiopulmonary *cerebral* resuscitation). Because of experiments in reflow-promoting measures and barbiturate loading after global ischemia (such as cardiac arrest results), the theory of irreversible brain damage after cessation of blood flow for 4 to 6 minutes has been challenged. Although barbiturates are not a panacea, findings resulting from these experiments have caused experts to believe that neuron-saving and neurotransmitter-related advances will continue to relate to pharmacological and physiological measures. The relevance of these efforts are their attempt to avoid current outcomes; that is, about 20% of survivors of cardiac arrest or brain trauma have long-term deficits ranging from minimal dysfunction to extended coma or permanent vegetative existence. As research continues, new criteria will emerge regarding predictions about irreversible coma and the degree of extensive brain damage. New optimism about client outcomes is evident because of these new vistas in cerebral resuscitation that are becoming well integrated into critical care.

Because of spatial limitations, key points, which the reader may wish to explore further in the references, are outlined below:

### Factors to consider in brain resuscitation

Types
  Global ischemia—cardiac arrest
  Focal ischemia—stroke
Mechanism causing damage, such as
  Trauma
  Metabolic cause
Protective measures—before, during and after, such as
  Hypothermia before elective surgery
  Hypothermia during traumatic event, such as cold-water drowning
  Resuscitation after event
Importance of early resuscitation, including prehospital treatment
Key points to research
  Hyperventilation to keep $Pco_2$ between 25 and 28 mm Hg and $Po_2$ above 100 mm Hg
  Pros and cons of early steroid use
  Barbiturate loading
  Mannitol use to decrease increasing intracranial pressure (see also Chapters 21 and 23)
  Prevention of hypertension while ensuring adequate arterial perfusion
  Importance of establishing base-line data and doing Glasgow Coma Scale initially and serially
  Adequate basic life and brain support (Safar, Nemoto, Smith, Bleyaert)

## VITAL INTERVENTIONS

The immediate goal in the care of the unconscious client is to *sustain the highest level of well-being possible, to maintain life, and to avoid permanent damage*. Thus several problems receive priority attention even while the underlying cause of the coma remains elusive. Naturally, as these life preserving measures are enacted, a concurrent goal is to identify the underlying problem so that definite action that is designed to solve the problem may ensue.

The client must have a *patent airway*. Endotracheal suctioning may be the only assistance necessary in providing a patent airway. In deep coma a cuffed endotracheal tube may be necessary, and ventilation maintenance may require a respirator. Arterial blood should be drawn for assessment of the oxygen saturation level, and supplemental oxygen may then be administered in accordance with the findings. In clients with a metabolic encephalopathy the head is placed beneath the rest of the body, whereas the prone patient is turned from side to side to facilitate drainage from the respiratory tract. The head *should not* be lowered in patients with intracranial lesions.

The *circulation* needs to be adequately maintained. After blood is obtained for laboratory analysis, an intravenous infusion line is kept in place to maintain adequate fluid levels, to treat clients who may be hemorrhaging or in shock, and to administer medications. A *cardiac monitor* may be attached to the client whose condition is unstable or who has ingested a toxic substance.

*Glucose in a 50% concentration is administered immediately to the comatose client*. If the coma is caused by hypoglycemia, glucose administration will avoid brain damage while providing evidence to support the diagnosis. It has no adverse effects on brain tissue in individuals who are not hypoglycemic.

If *intracranial pressure* is increased, the client receives treatment to decrease the pressure. Chapters 21 and 27 detail these procedures.

*Seizure activity* is halted by the use of diazepam. Ventilatory assistance should be available, since large doses of diazepam may result in respiratory depression. Once the seizures are controlled, phenytoin sodium is utilized to maintain seizure control. Chapter 14 offers further detail on seizures.

If the client has a *nervous system infection,* a lumbar puncture is performed, and cerebrospinal fluid is analyzed as described in Chapter 20. In emergencies, lumbar punctures are done only when infection is suspected, since they may compromise the condition of the client with an intracranial space-occupying lesion or increased pressure.

*Acid-base imbalances* need to be regulated to avoid further depression of respiratory status and the possibility of cardiovascular problems.

*Body temperature* should be carefully monitored, since temperature extremes may have adverse effects on the client. Clients are placed on a hypothermia blanket so that they may maintain a temperature no lower than 96° F. Chapter 27 gives more information on hypothermia.

The administration of substances to the comatose client is carefully controlled. Depressants such as morphine are contraindicated. Stimulants are reserved for those instances when toxic states require reversal procedures or when heart block occurs, as in Adams-Stokes syndrome.

In the past few years there have been a large number of comatose clients who have ingested one or more narcotics, hallucinogenic agents, tranquilizers, or other substances. Although these clients need the symptomatic support as outlined, they may also require an agent that can reverse effects such as respiratory depression. Naloxone (Narcan) is a drug often given to combat narcotic overdose. However, because its duration is limited, it may need to be given again to counteract the effects of longer acting substances for those individuals who have been overdosed. Care is taken in giving Narcan to a drug addict, since it may precipitate the acute symptoms of drug withdrawal, which necessitate additional treatment, or temporary arousal and refusal of further treatment.

## MONITORING LEVEL OF CONSCIOUSNESS

The Glasgow Coma Scale (GCS) is becoming the standardized model for assessing the level of consciousness (LOC). The scale allows one to evaluate eye opening, verbal response, and best motor response and is sensitive and rapid for evaluation of deteriorating consciousness. However, it

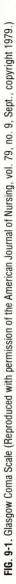

**FIG. 9-1.** Glasgow Coma Scale (Reproduced with permission of the American Journal of Nursing, vol. 79, no. 9, Sept., copyright 1979.)

is only intended to supplement the complete neurological assessment process.

The GCS is objective because is equates these three areas of measurement to numerical values. The normal individual score is 14; one is in coma at 7 or less; and a value of 3 is often evident in brain death. The GCS score alerts health professionals to client needs and care acuity. See Fig. 9-1.

## NURSING INTERVENTION

Caring for the comatose client and his or her significant others is one of the greatest challenges in nursing. The quality of care that the client receives directly affects the future quality of the individual's life. The nurse has an important role in maintaining life at the highest possible level, while recognizing developing problems and preventing complications through appropriate intervention. The principles of nursing care are essentially the same, no matter what the cause of coma. Educational and behavioral support systems provided for significant others may influence their emotional resolution of the event and their subsequent general well-being. To provide the most favorable nursing care climate, the nurse may follow these standards for nursing intervention.

1. Adhere to the applicable standards outlined on p. 248.
2. Provide physical privacy and respect for the client as an individual.
3. Speak around and to the client as if every word were appropriately comprehended.
4. Document the base-line status of all biopsychosocial capacities and complete a thorough assessment of the preillness state.
5. Conduct, document, and communicate findings from thorough, systematic assessments performed at appropriate intervals.
6. Use the GCS at defined intervals for rapid, objective, general-status determinations.
7. Utilize the nursing process to define client needs, specify measures for maintaining and improving functional capacities, determine interim and terminal deadlines, and assess effectiveness of interventions in accord with predefined outcome criteria. Alter nursing interventions in response to these periodic evaluations and new plans. In-

crease the frequency and completeness of client care to compensate to what the client would require or self-monitor if he or she were alert and aware.
8. Plan nursing interventions to support biopsychosocial functions, while minimizing additional injury or complications arising from inappropriate functional capacities.
9. Observe the client for biopsychosocial findings that may enhance the discovery of the underlying causative mechanism. Document findings and convey them to appropriate health professionals.
10. Involve significant others as historians during the assessment process; as those needing thorough explanations, understanding, and special consideration during the client's illness; and as participants in active client care. Involvement and education in care problems and interventions allow significant others to provide valuable assistance, while resolving personal issues and preparing for possible long-term management of the client.

*Observations.* At times the physician may have difficulty in making a diagnosis; the nurse's observation of the client while administering nursing care frequently can help. The nurse can contribute to the client's welfare by making detailed observations.

The following observations should be charted on the nurse's notes in detail, and any change should be reported to the physician in charge:

Any change in the level of consciousness as manifested by the client's spontaneous behavior, resistance to care, or response to noxious stimulation

Voluntary motion of the extremities and any change in muscular tone or position of the body or head

Equality, size, and reaction to light of pupils

Changes in the color of the face, lips, extremities, and trunk

Changes in texture, temperature, and moisture of the skin; early evidence of pressure areas

Quality and rate of pulse and respiration (taken at frequent intervals as ordered)

Rectal temperature every 2 to 4 hours, depending on the need of the individual client

Blood pressure (taken as ordered or determined by the nurse according to the condition of the individual client)

Accurate measure and record of fluid intake and output

Accurate and complete description of focal or generalized convulsions

Early signs of periocular or facial edema, especially after head injury or cranial surgery

Signs of meningeal irritation, stiffness of neck, and so on

After intracranial operations, dressings checked frequently for bloody drainage or leakage of cerebrospinal fluid.

Adequacy of ventilation

Status of blood gases and other laboratory data

Monitoring device values

Symptoms related to an underlying problem

*Environment.* Many unconscious clients are 60 or more years of age. Persons in this age group are more sensitive to atmospheric changes and are highly susceptible to respiratory complications; therefore it is most important to provide the environment best suited to the individual client's well-being and comfort. An unconscious client cannot express preferences; therefore provision for adequate warmth should be made routinely. The room should be well ventilated and free from odors. If hyperthermia is a complicating factor, body temperature should be reduced.

The nurse is responsible for the safety of the client and for providing protection from injury. Side rails are raised unless someone is staying with the patient.

*Hygiene.* Because the care of the client with regard to hygiene is so important in the prevention of complications, the skin and mucous membranes of the body demand special attention.

SKIN. The blood supply to the skin may be poor, and, in the aged, tissue changes are characterized chiefly by signs of wasting and insufficient or inappropriate repair. It is essential to cleanse the skin of infectious agents that may be present from bowel, bladder, or respiratory tract contamination. The number of microorganisms on the surface of the body can be reduced by meticulous bathing with warm, soapy water. If the skin is dry, a superfatted soap (castile, lanolin, or cold cream) is used to prevent further irritation and dryness. Cotton-seed oil is applied daily on the hands and feet to prevent a deficiency of cutaneous oils. Frequent rubs over all pressure areas and the back with baby lotion, Keri lotion, or another lubricating preparation are indicated to stimulate the circulation and to prevent decubitus formation. Bed linen should be kept dry, taut, and without wrinkles. Hot-water bags should not be applied to unconscious clients or to clients with impaired sensation because of the danger of burns.

EYES. When unconsciousness has an organic cause, the corneal reflexes are absent, and the cornea is likely to become irritated by being scratched on the pillow or by dust particles. There is also excessive dryness because of diminished secretions and incomplete closure of the eye; this requires treatment as well as adequate protection. The eyes should be examined frequently and carefully for early signs of irritation or inflammation, cleansed with suitable solutions, and lubricated with mineral oil at frequent intervals. At times it may be necessary to cover the eyes with shields made of radiographic film or to close them with a butterfly dressing or gauze and collodion to prevent complications. Neglect can lead to corneal ulcerations, keratitis, and even blindness. Be certain to remove and appropriately store contact lenses in comatose clients.

NOSE. Frequently the nares become occluded by crust formation. To facilitate breathing, one should keep these passages open by gentle cleansing and lubricating. After a head injury, if bleeding is present, the nostrils are cleansed only on the physician's order. Sterile cotton is placed gently in the nares, changed when soiled, and examined carefully for any indication that rhinorrhea exists as a complication. Cerebrospinal fluid drainage from the nose is a serious complication. If it is suspected, the nurse should report immediately to the physician.

MOUTH. Dentures, if present, are removed and placed in a proper receptacle until the client becomes conscious. Frequently the unconscious client is a mouth breather. The mouth becomes excessively dry or thickly coated with mucus. Brush the teeth at least three times a day, and cleanse the mucous membrane with normal saline or aromatic alkaline mouthwash, which keeps the tissue well lubricated.

Coat the lips with cold cream or rub them with Chap Stick to prevent cracking and fever blisters. An alternate method for cleansing the client's mouth and maintaining the tone of the tissues is to use Gly-Oxide, an oral lavage solution. A piece of gauze is saturated with the solution, and all surfaces of the teeth and soft tissues of the mouth are rubbed thoroughly.

The airway must be kept open and suction used as necessary. A soft rubber catheter, whistle tip No. 20 or 22, is usually most effective for this purpose and least likely to cause trauma. If unconsciousness is prolonged, a tracheostomy may be indicated to maintain adequate ventilation of the lungs and to ensure an open airway.

HAIR. The hair is kept neatly combed and, if long, plaited in braids for comfort. Unless contraindicated because the client is critically ill, a shampoo is given every 10 to 14 days. As the female client convalesces, having her hair styled in an attractive way will sometimes stimulate her interest in getting well.

For black individuals, cleanse hair with a warmed 1:4 mixture of alcohol to mineral oil. Apply additional warmed baby oil or petroleum jelly to the scalp and hair. Towel the excess oil away. Arrange short hair with a wide-toothed comb in a loose style; braid longer hair.

EARS. After a head injury, if there is bleeding from the ears, sterile cotton should be placed loosely in the external ear and changed whenever necessary to prevent contamination. Cleanse only as ordered by the physician. Cerebrospinal fluid discharge from the ears should be noted and reported.

*Nutrition.* During the initial 24 to 48 hours in the hospital the fluid balance is usually maintained by intravenous infusion or hypodermoclysis. If the state of coma continues or if, because of poor veins or frequent change of position, these methods are not feasible, a nasogastric tube is inserted through the nostril into the stomach, and feedings are given every 2 to 3 hours in 100 to 300 ml amounts, depending on the needs and tolerance of the client. If the general condition of the client is good and especially if he or she is unconscious because of a head injury or a sudden illness, nutritional needs may be met and normal stomach function and capacity maintained when the ingredients of three meals of a regular diet are mixed in an electric blender and given to the client by tube three times a day. Otherwise the number of calories and the contents of the tube feeding are specified by the physician for each client. If not contraindicated, a high-vitamin, high-protein feeding with 2500 to 3000 calories in about 2500 to 3000 ml of fluid each 24 hours is recommended for an adult. Its protein content helps prevent the formation of decubitus ulcers by maintaining the skin in good nutrition. Supplementary vitamins or other medications may also be given as necessary through the tube.

The nasal tube generally is not left in the same nostril longer than 5 days and should be kept lubricated at the orifice to prevent the formation of crusts. Each feeding is followed by 30 ml of water to clear the tube and prevent blocking. Avoid overfilling the stomach, since regurgitation or vomiting may occur. In the unconscious client aspiration of vomitus is a real danger, since the airway may be obstructed or pulmonary complications may ensue.

After the client begins to respond and the ability to swallow has been tested, start small, palatable, liquid oral feedings given at frequent intervals. Increase the amount until the nasal feedings can be stopped. The client then gradually progresses to a soft diet. Some clients may require a different regimen of feedings. The client with facial paralysis is postured with the affected side up before feeding is attempted. The convalescent client with residual facial paralysis is encouraged to take food and fluids into the unaffected side of the mouth to lessen drooling and facilitate chewing.

*Elimination.* Unconscious clients are generally incontinent of urine. This increases their susceptibility to decubitus ulcers. A retention catheter (male Foley No. 16 to 22) is inserted into the bladder to keep the client dry, and, if possible, a closed system of drainage is established. If the client is a man, external condom drainage may be used instead of a catheter to reduce local irritation and infection. (The high incidence of urinary tract infection with an indwelling catheter requires frequent monitoring of the client. Chemotherapy or antibiotics may be indicated.) Consult your infection control nurse for a current protocol.

Give a mild cathartic every second or third

night, followed the next morning by a colon lavage to prevent fecal impactions, constipation, and involuntary stools. If signs of increased intracranial pressure exist, use saline cathartics for the dehydrating effect. If the client develops an impaction, hydrogen peroxide retention enemas may be given with good results.

As soon as the client is conscious and able to cooperate, initiate a regimen of bowel training, and discontinue the cathartics and lavages. The regular intake of fluids up to 3000 ml, 1 to 3 ounces of prune juice each morning, Dulcolax suppositories, and regular toileting are effective in achieving regular bowel movements for most clients.

*Safety and mobility.* Accident precautions should be included in the care standards for the unconscious client. Clients with decreased awareness are unable to avoid burns from hot objects, falls from unsecured positions, or constructions of circulation from inappropriately placed clothing or unsupervised use of restraining devices. Any equipment used on the client should be periodically evaluated for adequate functional integrity and safety.

*Posture and exercise.* The client is postured at all times in the optimal position in good alignment to prevent the complications of deformities, contractures, footdrop and wristdrop, muscle strain, and decubitus ulcers (Fig. 9-2).

Place a turning sheet (a large sheet folded lengthwise and then in half) under the client from above the shoulders to below the buttocks to facilitate change of position with minimal strain and fatigue on the part of the nurses in attendance. Turn unconscious clients every 1 to 2 hours, and keep them postured on either side. They should not lie on their backs except for short periods of time when receiving necessary treatments. Lying on the side facilitates the circulation of oxygen through

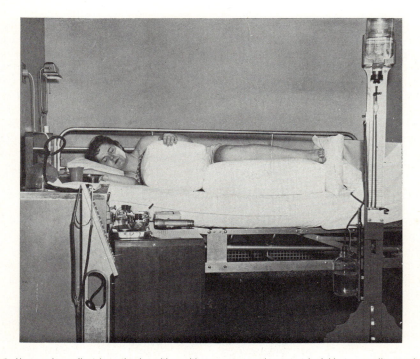

**FIG. 9-2.** Unconscious client in optimal position with necessary equipment at bedside to expedite nursing care. (One side rail has been removed temporarily.)

the lungs and lessens the danger of aspiration or obstruction of the airway by the tongue. This positioning reduces the incidence of atelectasis and other respiratory complications. Frequent turning of the client not only helps prevent pressure sores but also facilitates drainage of oral secretions.

**POSITIONING CLIENT ON SIDE.** Place a small, firm pillow under the client's head, which is elevated 10 degrees; support the upper extremity on a square bolster or a large, firm, doubled pillow. Support the upper leg, flexed at the knee at a right angle to the hip, from the knee to the foot on two firm, rubber-covered pillows, bolsters, or crib mattresses; keep the foot in firm dorsiflexion with an adequate bolster and sandbags. The client's lower leg is slightly hyperextended and flat on the bed with the foot supported with a sandbag at a right angle to the leg; the lower arm is flexed at the elbow, placed flat on the bed with the hand parallel with the head; the buttock, if well pulled out, will anchor the client in place. If the back is straight

and the weight evenly distributed on the shoulder, side, and hip, a back pillow is superfluous and contraindicated. If the client is in the right position, he or she will remain as postured (Fig. 9-3). Place a cradle over the foot of the bed to prevent pressure of the bedclothes over the feet. If a footboard is used, this will serve to elevate the bedclothes, and the cradle may be omitted; consequently, there is less possibility of drafts and chilling. If the cradle is used, it should be covered with extra blankets during cold weather to afford adequate warmth.

**POSITIONING CLIENT ON BACK (INDICATED ONLY WITH FAVORABLE CONVALESCENCE).** A low to medium head Gatch bed is used as indicated by the client's condition. Place the client's body in correct alignment with a small bolster under the knees for slight flexion (10 degrees) to prevent muscle strain and contractures of the knees. A flat bolster about 4 inches thick, extending from the knee bolster to 1 inch above the heels, supports the calves and elevates the heels from the bed to avoid pres-

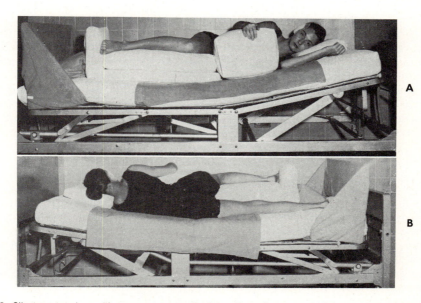

**FIG. 9-3.** Client postured on side to prevent complications. Note alignment of back, position of extremities, use of supportive devices, small head pillow, and position of turning sheet, which extends above shoulders and below buttocks. **A,** Anterior view. **B,** Posterior view. Note that no pillow is used to support back. This is not only unnecessary but also contraindicated.

sure; the feet are supported in firm dorsiflexion at right angles to the body by a footboard, bolsters, or sandbags. A paralyzed upper extremity can be supported on a pillow or across the chest in a sling to avoid muscular strain and prevent wristdrop.

Splints and casts are rarely employed. Massage with active and passive exercises to all extremities will help stimulate circulation and maintain muscular tone and normal range of motion of the joints. This is done at least daily and more frequently unless contraindicated. Consult a physical therapist for an individualized plan.

POSITIONING CLIENT IN CHAIR. The client under consideration may be unconscious, hemiplegic, paraplegic, or quadriplegic. To help in the prevention of complications place the individual in a large sturdy armchair once or twice a day. When transporting the client from bed to chair, a mechanical lift or a large sheet folded in half lengthwise may be used. It is important to support the entire body during the process of transferring from bed to chair. After the client is in the chair, place two 4-inch shock blocks under the front legs of the chair. Place the chair against the wall to prevent it from tipping over backward. The client's legs are postured on a firm leg pillow or on a knee roll and foot bolster on the seat of a second chair. If the legs are not elevated, place the feet on a foot stool. The upper extremities are supported in a relaxed, comfortable position at a right angle to the trunk on a flat traylike board. Place a firm pillow behind the client's head. If necessary, a Posey bolero or a stitched cotton strap, 4 inches wide, may be used behind the client's neck and under the armpits and tied to the back of the chair to maintain a good anatomical position.

## PREVENTION OF DECUBITUS ULCERS

Change the client's position every hour (posture as just described). Never use doughnuts (cotton or otherwise); these merely serve to transfer pressure from the bony prominences to the area of contact. Keep the client dry. During the period of unconsciousness prevent involuntary defecations by the regular use of colon lavages about every third day. Use a sponge rubber or air mattress to ensure optimal distribution of body weight, thus preventing excessive pressure on vulnerable bony prominences. Keep linen taut, smooth, and free from crumbs. Substitute Pliofilm, or semitransparent plastic sheeting, for protective rubber sheeting (perspiration is reduced; easier to maintain free of coarse wrinkles). Administer scrupulous skin hygiene and frequent rubs, with special attention to all vulnerable areas (heels, ankles, pelvic crests, sacrum, scapulae, elbows, ears, and head). Do not use powder, since it may cake and cause welts. If the skin is very fragile, sheepskin may be used as an added deterrent to breakdown. Maintain adequate nutrition with a high-vitamin, high-protein, high-caloric diet. Maintain adequate fluid intake. Give massage and exercises to stimulate circulation. Chapter 25 gives further details.

## DEATH

In a significant number of neurological conditions, death lies at the end of either an acute or a chronic disease course. As a result, the practitioner caring for neurological clients frequently confronts the multidimensional concerns of client, family, and staff when the last stage of life approaches.

Because there are a great many issues that arise in association with assisting a client and family through the experience of death, it is beyond the scope of this text to deal with these concerns in the depth required. Readers are referred to the bibliography and to the many seminars and workshops devoted to this topic. In learning how to assist others in coping with the experience of their own death, the writings and seminars presented by Elizabeth Kubler-Ross are among the most valuable works.

In reviewing the issues of death, one should particularly consider personal philosophies and needs, family and client needs, concerns and patterns of response, and legal aspects inherent in the entire area. Some issues include the acceptance of the living will,* the definition of neurological death, the point at which heroic measures may be withheld, and the health care delivery system and trends of society in general with regard to these areas.

*Guidelines and forms for a living will are available from the Society for the Right to Die, 250 West 57th St., New York, N.Y. 10019.

## SUMMARY

The comatose client depends completely on nursing personnel for the fulfillment of physiological needs. As he or she becomes increasingly alert, the nurse must help the client become progressively independent in order to move away from the role as a client and assume a healthy social role.

It is especially important for the elderly client recovering from the acute phase of illness to be actively involved in the activities of daily living and to reestablish identity as a responsible individual. In short, the objective is to help this person function as effectively as possible within the limitations imposed by physical residuals or the aging process.

As the client convalesces, definite periods of rest are provided to avoid fatigue. If there are residual disabilities such as hemiplegia, aphasia, memory, or visual difficulties, the client's wants and needs should be anticipated to prevent unnecessary emotional trauma and to conserve strength. It is most important that these clients have emotional and physical security during this period of convalescence. The nurse can do much, by approach and interest and by doing little things to reassure the client, to stimulate the desire to get well. As soon as possible, the client is encouraged to do things and, if he or she has residual handicaps, taught how to make the most of remaining abilities. If facilities are available, reeducation and rehabilitation should be carried out according to the needs of the individual client.

Throughout the hospitalization period, the family of the client receives special consideration. When the client is critically ill and unconscious, the nurse must be sensitive to the family's emotional needs and provide opportunities for them to talk and, if possible, be involved in the care of the patient. During periods of crisis brought about by changes in the client's condition, the family is helped by the attitude of the nurse, expressions of concern, the time spent with the client, and little acts of kindness, such as frequently stopping by the visitor's room to inform them of the status of the client, listening, and trying to make them comfortable during their vigil.

Inevitably some clients die. The nurse is then responsible for discussing the death with the staff and helping the family to cope with their grief. Some hospitals that provide special programs for the terminally ill have established bereavement clinics and hospices to aid families after the death of the patient. Physicians, nurses, psychiatrists, and sociologist participate in providing supportive counseling services to the family.

### REFERENCES

Adam, N.R.: Prolonged coma: your care makes all the difference, Nursing77 **7**:21-27, 1977.

Anthony, C.: Fluid imbalances, formidable foes to survival, Am. J. Nurs. **63**:75-77, Dec. 1963.

Beresford, H.R.: Who should decide to withhold care in chronic coma, Arch. Neurol. **33**:371, May 1976.

Bleyaert, A., et al.: Effect of postcirculatory-arrest life-support on neurological recovery in monkeys, Crit. Care Med. **8**:153-156, March 1980.

Bower, P., and Hicks, D.: Maintaining muscle function in patients on bed rest, Am. J. Nurs. **72**:1250-1253, 1972.

Brooks, H.L.: The golden rule for the unconscious patient, Nurs. Forum **4**(3):12-18, 1965.

Brownlowe, M., Cohen, F., and Happich, W.: New washable woolskins, Am. J. Nurs. **70**:2368-2370, 1970.

Bunch, B., and Zahra, D.: Dealing with death: the unlearned role, Am. J. Nurs. **76**:1486, Sept. 1976.

Burton, C.: Families in crisis, Nursing75 **5**:36-43, Dec. 1975.

Carlson, C.E., coordinator: Behavioral concepts and nursing intervention, Philadelphia, 1970, J.B. Lippincott Co.

Chamo, L.: Psychotherapy with comatose patients, Psychother. Psychosom. **25**:7, 1975.

Davenport, R.: Tube feeding for long-term patients, Am. J. Nurs. **64**:121-123, Jan. 1964.

Engel, G.L.: Grief and grieving, Am. J. Nurs. **64**:93, Sept. 1964.

Feldman, M.H.: Physiological observations in a chronic case of locked-in syndrome, Neurology **21**:459, 1971.

Foss, G.: Postural drainage, Am. J. Nurs. **73**:666-669, 1973.

Fry, E.N.: Levels of consciousness in comatose patients, Lancet **1**:422, Feb. 21, 1976.

Gakley, D.E., et al.: Glycerol and hyperosmolar nonketotic coma, Am. J. Ophthalmol. **81**:469, April 1976.

Gaul, A., Thompson, R., and Hart, G.: Hyperbaric oxygen therapy, Am. J. Nurs. **72**:892-986, 1972.

Gibbs, G.E.: Perineal care of the incapacitated patient, Am. J. Nurs. **69**:124-125, Jan. 1969.

Gould, H.: How to remove contact lenses from comatose patients, Am. J. Nurs. **76**:1483-1485, 1976.

Grant, M., and Kubo, W.: Assessing a patient's hydration status, Am. J. Nurs. **75**:1306-1311, 1975.

Grier, M.: Hair care for the black patient, Am. J. Nurs. **76**:1781, 1976.

Gyulay, J.: The forgotton grievers, Am. J. Nurs. **75**:147, Sept. 1975.

Hägerdal, M., et al.: The protective effects of a combination of hypothermia and barbiturates in cerebral hypoxia in the rat, Anesthesiology **49**(3):165, Sept. 1978.

Hitchcock, E.R.: Management of the unconscious patient, Philadelphia, 1970, J.B. Lippincott Co.

Jackson, P.L.: Chronic grief, Am. J. Nurs. **74:**1239, July 1974.

Jennett, B., et al.: Prognosis in coma (letter), Lancet **1:**100, Jan. 11, 1975.

Jones, C.: Glasgow Coma Scale, Am. J. Nurs. **79:**1551-1553, 1979.

Keegan, L.: Fecal incontinence bag, Nurs. Homes **20:**40-41, March 1971.

Kirklin, J.K., et al.: Treatment of hydrazine-induced coma with pyridoxine, N. Engl. J. Med. **294:**938, April 22, 1976.

Kirilloff, L., and Maszkiewicz, R.: Guide to respiratory care in critically ill adults, Am. J. Nurs. **79:**2005-2012, Nov. 1979.

Kottke, F., and Blanchard, R.: Bedrest begets bedrest, Nurs. Forum. **3**(3):56-72, 1964.

Kubler-Ross, E.: Death: the final stage of growth, Englewood Cliffs, N.J., 1975, Prentice-Hall, Inc.

Langford, T.L.: Nursing problem: bacteriuria and the indwelling catheter, Am. J. Nurs. **72:**113-115, Jan. 1972.

Lindemann, E.: Symptomatology and management of acute grief, Am. J. Psychiatry **101:**141, 1944.

Ludwig, A.M.: Hysteria, a neurobiological theory, Arch. Gen. Psychiatry **27:**771-777, 1972.

McCaffrey, C.: Performance checklists: an effective method of teaching, learning and evaluation, Nurse Educator, pp. 11-13, Jan.-Feb. 1978.

Muller, E.A.: Influence of training and of inactivity on muscle strength, Arch. Phys. Med. Rehabil. **51:**449-462, 1970.

Nemoto, E.M.: Pathogenesis of cerebral ischemia-anoxia, Crit. Care Med. **6:**203-214, July-Aug. 1978.

Olson, E.V.: The hazards of immobility, Am. J. Nurs. **67:**779-797, 1967.

Perlmutter, I.: The comatose patient (letter), J.A.M.A. **234:**1321, Dec. 29, 1975.

Plum, F., and Posner, J.B.: The diagnosis of stupor and coma, ed. 2, Philadelphia, 1972, F.A. Davis Co.

Posner, J.B.: The comatose patient, J.A.M.A. **233:**1313, Sept. 22, 1975.

Reitz, M., and Pope, W.: Mouth care, Am. J. Nurs. **73:**1728-1730, 1973.

Rudy, E.: Early omens of cerebral disaster, Nursing77 **7:**59-62, 1977.

Safar, P.: Amelioration of postischemic brain damage with barbiturates, Curr. Conc. Cerebrovasc. Dis.—Stroke **15:**1-5, Jan.-Feb. 1980.

Safar, P., et al.: Resuscitation after global brain ischemia-anoxia, Crit. Care Med. **6:**215-227, July-Aug. 1978.

Salibi, B.S.: Positioning and turning comatose patients in mass casualties, Wis. Med. J. **74:**512, Jan. 1975.

Schwab, M.: Caring for the aged, Am. J. Nurs. **73:**2049-2053, 1973.

Schoenberg, B., et al., editors: Bereavement: its psychosocial aspects, New York, 1975, Columbia University Press.

Smith, A.L.: Barbiturate protection in cerebral hypoxia, Anesthesiology **47:**285-293, 1977.

Sonstegard, L., et al.: The grieving nurse, Am. J. Nurs. **76:**1490, Sept. 1976.

Sparagana, M., et al.: Clinicopathologic conference: hypothermia and lethargy, Postgrad. Med. **58:**156, Oct. 1975.

Stanley, P.E.: Electric shock hazards—2, Hospitals **45:**78-80, Jan. 16, 1971.

Stover, S.I., et al.: Head injury in children and teenagers: functional recovery correlated with duration of coma, Arch. Phys. Med. Rehabil. **57:**201, May 1976.

Swift, N.: Head injury: essentials in excellent care, Nursing74 **4:**926-933, Sept. 1974.

Teasdale, G., and Jennett, B.: Assessment of coma and impaired consciousness: a practical scale, Lancet **2:**81-84, 1974.

Teasdale, G., et al.: Observer variability in assessing impaired consciousness and coma, J. Neurol. Neurosurg. Psychiat. **41:**603-610, July 1978.

Vijayan, N.: Eye deviation in coma, N. Engl. J. Med. **291:**106, 1974.

Walker, A.E., et al.: The neuropathologic findings in irreversible coma: a critique of the respirator, J. Neuropathol. Exp. Neurol. **34:**295, July 1975.

Wentzel, K.B.: The dying are the living, Am. J. Nurs. **76:**956, June 1976.

Westmoreland, B.F., et al.: Alpha-coma: electroencephalographic, clinical, pathologic, and etiologic correlations, Arch. Neurol. **32:**713, Nov. 1975.

Williams, A.: A study of factors contributing to skin breakdown, Nurs. Res. **21:**238-243, May-June 1972.

Willis, W.D., and Grossman, R.G.: Medical neurobiology: neuroanatomical and neurophysiological principles basic to clinical neuroscience, ed. 2, St. Louis, 1977, The C.V. Mosby Co.

Works, R.F.: Hints on lifting and pulling, Am. J. Nurs. **72:**260-261, Feb. 1972.

# 10
# PAIN EXPERIENCE

Pain, a scientific issue and human malady that has evaded explanation by researchers since the beginning of time, has received increasing attention in experimental settings in the past decade. For a moment, consider this powerful and complex physiological puzzle that necessarily involves a vast overlay of emotional, affective, cultural, social, and cognitive factors. Not only does the objective picture seem intricate, but the personal perception also has interesting qualities. Healthy individuals, free from the trappings of pain, may deal with issues beyond the confines of bodily limits. However, when the pain experience begins, the individual draws in to various degrees to focus on the subjective discomfort. When moderate to severe pain persists, the individual has difficulty in recalling its onset, in dealing with issues beyond the self, and in believing that the pain will ease. After the pain has gone, the individual often has great difficulty in recalling the subjective experiences present during the pain experience.

This chapter reviews the definition of pain, current theories of pain, assessment of pain, clinical situations relating to specific disease entities, referred pain, and treatment modalities.

## DEFINITION

Pain, from the purely physiological viewpoint, is defined as actual or potential tissue damage from causative stimuli and the measurable responses indicating its presence. Causative stimuli capable of evoking pain include *mechanical factors* (pressure), *thermal factors* (radiant heat), *chemical factors* (presence of the substance bradykinin), and *electrical factors* (shock). As the individual perceives pain, there may be verbal expressions of discomfort, changes in usual behavioral patterns, and physiological responses (Fig. 10-1). In measuring physiological response, researchers have constructed highly refined methods of quantifying stimuli and recording subsequent output from the affected individual. Moreover, clinicians have the advantage of knowing about the dermatomes, a map of surface areas of sensibility, in tracing confirmed neural pathways (see Fig. 3-7, p. 81). However, this approach to the study of pain is incomplete, since interruption of the involved sensory pathway is not the total answer to elimination of pain. In fact, response to pain may not only be disproportionate to actual or potential tissue damage but may also be totally caused by psychogenic phenomena. Additionally, one might note differences in children who experience the same injuries or trauma an adult encounters. In children the lack of previous experience or information regarding expectations may cause them to require little or no pain medication, when the adult in a like situation requires narcotics. Beecher (1946, 1956) studied wounded soldiers utilizing injury as a means to leave the battlefront in comparison to civilians undergoing surgery. The personal meaning of the soldiers' injuries resulted in 25% requesting narcotics, whereas postoperatively the civilians, focusing on the gravity of the situation rather than its potential for freedom from a situation, requested narcotics 80% of the time.

Other features of pain further confound the issue. For example, in causalgia, burning pain associated with displacement of nerves by high-velocity missiles such as bullets, the pain experience

215

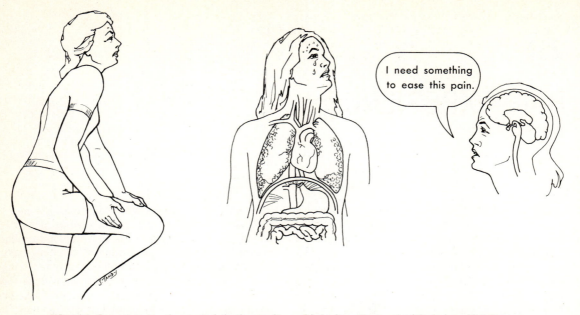

**FIG. 10-1.** Responses to pain may include changes in usual behavior patterns, physiological manifestations, or verbal expressions.

may still be evident for several months after the tissue has healed. Another example of a pain experience, solved through clinical research, is that of phantom pain after the amputation of an extremity. The experience of a phantom limb occurs in most amputees, whereas severe pain at the surgical site is evident in 10% or less of these clients. This pain may be activated by slight stimuli but is frequently eliminated forever through the injection of a local anesthetic that supposedly has an effect for only a few hours (Melzack and Bromage, 1973).

Since studies of the past decade have revealed a multiplicity of factors in all domains, many researchers are now viewing pain in relation to psychosocial and cultural phenomena in addition to physiological factors. As part of this effort, central processes are credited with a greater role in pain perception (Melzack, 1973), and interpretations of pain allow for human responses and attempts at communication about the meaning of pain with the affected individual (Plainfield and Adler, 1962; Zborowski, 1969).

## CURRENT THEORIES OF PAIN
### Psychophysiological theories

Pain, at first consideration, is usually thought of in terms of a physiological response to physical danger. Although such pain is described later in this chapter, it seems more appropriate to begin with theories explaining psychological pain, since pain from psychogenic sources is common in daily living and is often a compounding factor to identified sources of physiological pain.

Headaches are frequently the result of psychological problems. Pain of various types is also a chief complaint commonly seen in individuals with psychological problems (Devine and Mersky, 1965). However, response to noxious stimuli differs among individuals. As beauty is in the eye of the beholder, pain also takes on ramifications that may be complexly related to the perceptual world and experiences of the affected individual. Thus whether or not an obvious cause is ascertained, pain is still a real phenomenon to the person having the experience and as such should not be lightly dismissed. It signals the need for attention, assessment, and remediation. Aside from an experience that results in bodily discomfort, one must also consider the entire range of problems capable of producing mental pain or anguish, including grief and loss.

Mental pain or anguish may also be evident in bodily symptoms caused by three major mechanisms: conversion hysteria, pain related to muscle tension, and pain arising from psychological disorders.

Classic examples of *conversion hysteria* include the headache that prevents one from going to a distasteful event, the numbness in the arm of a pianist about to perform in a concert, and the labor pains in the expectant father during the time when his wife is giving birth. In some children, abdominal pain may be observed on school days when they cannot cope with the pressures of school. On weekends and holidays, such pain is not apparent. Other cases of this type may be more subtle. Thus close observations, a detailed history, and correlation of pain with possible disease entities and life patterns are essential for detection of the problem. Once detected, the pain, which is quite real to the affected individual, should be skillfully handled so that one may both eradicate it and reach the source of the problem without offering undue secondary gain to the affected individual.

Anxiety and stress causing *muscle tension* through persistent muscular contractions are also credited with causing much physical discomfort. So-called tension headaches may also be included in this category of problems, which respond well to heat applications, sedatives, relaxation techniques, and reassurance.

*Psychological disorders* may cause pain. Pain may be an outcome of a hallucinogenic experience in some depressed and psychotic individuals who believe that a body part is being altered or destroyed. In one example an individual thought that her stomach was being consumed by worms and constantly doubled up in pain. Although this type of pain is rare, pain from neurotic states of anxiety, tension, and depression is quite commonly seen by all health professionals. This pain may include conversion reactions, discomforts related to muscle tension, or exaggerated responses to pain, which may actually be detected in relation to physiological causes. It is important to emphasize the

fact that such pain may be only chronically apparent in a mild degree and not necessarily overwhelming or disabling.

Individuals who seem eager to frequent the physician and seem more than happy to accept elective surgery and medical treatment with evidence of long drawn-out elaboration of symptoms and treatments need further assessment for underlying motives after a thorough clinical investigation has eliminated the sources of serious pathological conditions. Often, these persons insist on treatment, become known for their lengthy elaboration of problems and frequent calls to the physician, and even "physician-shop" when a practitioner fails to prescribe treatment in concert with their expectations. In studies of such individuals, themes of anger, guilt, unhappiness, and masochistic tendencies seem to be recurring traits (Menninger, 1938; Mersky and Spear, 1967).

Three theories are utilized to explain psychogenic pain. Szasz (1957) contends that pain is the outcome of perceived threats to body integrity. In this theory the works of Freud are drawn on heavily to explain how the ego perceives emotional and objective threats to self. Threat (psychogenic or objective) must then be determined by the practitioner, who assesses it in relation to reality.

Although the other two theories overlap to some degree, they are still somewhat discrete. The second theory, endorsed by Weiss, Eisenbud, and most recently Engel (1956), speaks of pain as an outcome of hostility. The third theory discusses pain in relation to rather defined personality types, where the pain experience becomes an important mode of communication (Engel, 1958, 1959).

Perhaps practically the clinician should incorporate all these theories, since the assessments of the client, history, individual styles of pain description, and purposes the pain serves combine to give the practitioner the total meaning of the pain experience to the individual. In considering cases where pain is either severe or of paramount concern to the affected individual, one notes that attention to the pain and detailed, elaborate descriptions about the pain experience are quite common. Although the absence of a clear-cut causative factor in pain may be an indication for some to conclude that there is a psychogenic cause, one might do well to continue the data collection while treating the problem empirically. Whereas pain from psychogenic causes may be manifested in a variety of ways, it seems that this type of pain does not disturb the sleeping client, even though it may be a continuing problem during the waking hours and over a prolonged period of time (Mersky and Spear, 1967). Although psychogenic pain may involve more than one body part, it frequently includes bilateral, symmetrical headaches or bouts of acute abdominal pain.

**Personal perceptions.** Perhaps the reason scientists have had such difficulty in pinpointing the elusive qualities of the subjective pain experience is that the total gestalt of pain has a personal quality hard for the uninvolved individual to grasp. Pain is a lonely experience, though researchers have identified common factors in relation to age, sex, and ethnic origin that seem to have general implications within the subjective interpretation of the pain experience. Still the subject may believe he or she is the only one having such an experience; in some ways this is true, since the acuteness or chronicity of the pain problem has a distinct outcome and impact on each isolated life and varies from situation to situation.

The universal aspect of the pain experience involves the degree of noxious stimulation and the extent of real or perceived damage or danger to tissues or to the organism itself. The response to this universal phenomenon may be proportional or seemingly out of proportion to the degree of stimuli. The variability in response among individuals related to differences in past experience and psychosocial-cultural factors probably accounts in part for some of the difficulty in making objective, quantitative determinations about the pain experience. These factors might be categorized for descriptive purposes into cognitive and affective domains influencing the pain experience.

In the cognitive domain, researchers have found that the anticipation of pain, that is, when pain is discussed as an event associated with an upcoming laboratory experiment, and the lack of control, that is, the inability to stop the pain stimulus or know when incoming stimuli will cease, have great impact on the subjective response to pain (Murray, 1971).

In the affective domain, it seems that pain and subsequent measures utilized to relieve pain can and often do operate independently from usual patterns of expectation related to quality and quantity of stimuli and type and amount of analgesic administered. Thus one quickly enters the area where the power of suggestion with or without a placebo may have strong effects in pain reduction. Placebos, substances that are organically inactive but active through psychological mechanisms to effect a therapeutic outcome, are believed to achieve the desired response because the client believes he or she has been treated and has interpreted this treatment as being effective. Similarly, it is helpful for the same psychological feelings to accompany a physiologically active analgesic for maximum benefit to occur.

In considering the affective domain, one might assume a *theoretical summary*. In a physiological context a stimulus is the mechanism that evokes an involuntary, unpleasant response. However, from a psychological point of view the stimulus-effect pattern may be less significant or equally important to the outcomes, secondary gains, or purposes the pain serves.

**Group variations.** In attempts to gather data that shed light on the variability of the subjective pain experience, researchers have evaluated such factors as age, sex, differences in perception at various points on the body, family size, race, and athletic involvement. However, the relationship of these factors is often hard to evaluate by comparison of these studies, since researchers have utilized different types of noxious stimuli in these studies. Moreover, some evaluate perceptible pain thresholds, whereas others measure the point of pain tolerance. Another complicating factor involves the circumstantial variables. For example, if a woman were told that this study was a test to find out whether women have abilities to tolerate pain superior to those of men, she might be motivated to experience more or less pain then she might in a situation where this factor or others such as ethnic origin were not issues either through background or reinforcement of certain stereotypes. Finally, as the following experimental findings are discussed, one should carefully evaluate the difficulties in controlling variables inherent in quantifying this subjective data, in evaluating sample size and subject selection, in formulating testing modalities, and in arriving at stated outcomes.

In relation to age throughout the life cycle, one might hypothesize certain reactions to stressful situations, such as pain, by considering the issues, tasks, and developmental competencies inherent in the age group. For instance, a great deal is known about needs, fears, perceptions, and points of self-development at various ages in childhood. By knowing these factors within the context of North American culture and even within subcultural groups, normative attitudes and responses may be predicted. At other points on the continuum, such as in senior age groups, awareness of age-related problems might cause the individual to associate pain with such problems as debility or loss of independence or to view it as a disturbance that threatens functional integrity and independence (Whipple, 1966; Sutterly and Donnelly, 1973). At any rate, practitioners who have a thorough understanding of growth and development, of holistic theory, and of human interactions at each point with the environment and others have valuable data to construct intervention modalities, since these considerations are valuable in comprehending each individual's perceptual framework.

Sex is frequently cited as a factor that influences responses to pain. Although studies do not establish any significant variation in pain perception between male and female subjects, studies indicate that males tolerate more pain than females (Kennard, 1952; Petrovich, 1958; Petrie, 1960). However, significant variability among subjects of both sexes indicates that factors related to personality and past experience are also important determinants in responses noted at various points of pain tolerance.

A number of studies have been done on responses to dermal stimuli. Investigators have done studies wherein hands and feet were submerged in water baths at approximately 32° C in an effort to detect correlations between hand preference (dextral or sinistral) and sensitivity of extremities. Studies to date (Murray and Hagen, 1973) have utilized small samples, and results should be viewed in that light. The findings from these studies indicate that in both sinistral (left-handed) and dextral (right-handed) individuals there is a greater level of sensitivity in the left hand and foot, though the left hand is more sensitive than the left foot. It is thought that the feet have higher pressure thresh-

olds, greater concentrations of warm and cold spots, and more pain points than the hands and that the pain threshold is probably higher in the feet than in the hands (Geldard, 1972). Preferred hand use as an explanation for the diminished pain sensitivity in the right hand did not seem to be validated as the cause of this phenomenon, since some sinistral subjects had even less sensitivity in their hands than did dextral subjects. Further research is needed at this point, but even this initial data might be utilized by the practitioner in electing the right hand for an intravenous infusion rather than the left when problems related to pain outweigh the disadvantages of immobilizing the preferred hand for functioning.

Family size has been studied as a factor in response to pain. However, many variables other than birth order and family size seem to be operating. Thus data supporting differences in individuals are inconclusive at this point (Sweeney and Fine, 1970).

Another aspect of response related to pain tolerance has been investigated in relation to athletic participation. In these investigations, subjects are usually separated into two categories, depending on whether the athletic event is a contact or a noncontact sport. It has been hypothesized that although the initial choice of sport may reflect differences in pain threshold among individuals, factors influencing pain tolerance may be psychosocial in nature, that is, desire to remain on the team, to be accepted by the peer group, to please the family, and so on. Moreover, with a given psychological set (football is rough and injury is inevitable—take it like a man!) the individual may be willing to accept the discomforts inherent in the sport. Yet in another setting the "brave" football player may show a great reaction to a lesser stimulus, such as the administration of an injection by a nurse. The other hypothesis is that repeated experience with pain that is usually acute and not debilitating may cause the football player to adjust expectations to cope with temporary discomforts as a part of the total picture. Individuals with less experience in contact sports are probably less certain of the outcomes, more apprehensive of potential injury, and less tolerant. Petrie and associates (1967) have hypothesized from their studies that extroverted individuals tend to minimize incoming noxious perceptual experiences and have diminished responses to pain. Similarly, they tolerate experiments in sensory deprivation more poorly because of their outer-directed nature. This hypothesis may suggest why individuals who enjoy activity and contact are often more outgoing and may select contact sports in the first place. Obviously, inferences about pain tolerance in relation to athletics is at a beginning stage, and much more research is necessary before definitive conclusions may be reached.

In a large study of 41,119 individuals of various descriptions in relation to age, race, and sex, measurable amounts of pressure were applied to the Achilles tendon to elicit pain tolerance responses to deep pain. However, these researchers were careful to state that an experimental study on healthy individuals is not comparable to the physiological and psychological problems inherent in endogenous pain, wherein control and limitations inherent in the experimental situations are not possible. With regard to problems involved in quantifying subjective experience, several findings in this study are both interesting and may offer useful insights for practitioners. In consideration of responses to pain with advancing age, superficial pain such as that associated with applications of radiant heat is tolerated more successfully, whereas deep pain, for example, pressure applied to the Achilles tendon, results in a diminished level of tolerance. This study further reported that although male and female subjects do not differ consistently in pain threshold, males definitely exhibit a greater tolerance for pain than do females. In terms of ethnic origin, this study revealed that whites were able to tolerate the most pain, blacks tolerated an intermediate amount, and Orientals tolerated the least, even after such factors as education and socioeconomic status were considered (Woodrow et al., 1972).

**Cultural factors.** In consideration of responses to the pain experience, testing in a variety of cultural and ethnic groups reveals no consistent differences in pain perception but rather significant variability in pain tolerance among groups. These intergroup differences are ascribed by most experts to products of socialization and sociocultural expectations. In other words, as one grows, he or she experiences noxious stimuli and looks to signifi-

cant others for attitudes and acceptable behaviors in relation to the stimuli. In experimental settings of all types, one should also consider the motivation for the subject (money, grades, and so on) and the possibility that sexual, racial, or personality issues between the examiner and the examinee may influence outcomes. In one study where differences among ethnic groups were evident, researchers followed the experiment by using electrical shock as a stimulus, with a questionnaire where subjects were asked to rank the intensity of several stimuli with a standard shock. Even though this same group demonstrated differences in pain threshold, they showed no ethnic differences in ranking the stimulus (Zborowski, 1969; Weisenberg et al., 1975). Problems that arise in data collection in this aspect of pain experience include the facts that those approaching the problem from the physiological framework frequently omit data that might relate to significant cultural aspects, and those approaching sociocultural phenomena may not detail physiological parameters of measurement in sufficient detail to identify significant factors.

**Experimental situations.** In controlled settings the attempt is made to vary and control the input of noxious stimuli in an effort to relate causative factors to behavioral outcomes. Because a human with a wide range of behavioral and experiential potential is between the calculated input and the outcome, there is still an uncontrolled factor that may cause the outcome to vary from hypothesized expectations even in the laboratory setting. However, it is this very cause-effect relationship that needs closer scrutiny through research to provide valuable data for practitioners in clinical settings. Obviously, certain factors exist in the behavioristic laboratory setting that differ sharply from problems and variables inherent in the clinical setting. Considering these aspects is helpful in practice, as pragmatic individuals attempt to apply principles and findings to real-life situations.

Modeling is one phenomenon that alters the response to experimental settings. Either through perceived or stated directions or because of repeated trials with the experimental setting, individuals change their patterns of responsiveness, so that they react more or less to a constant stimulus. This phenomenon of modeling is apparent in real-life situations as individuals model their behavior to respond in accordance with sociocultural or peer norms. (Recall the behaviors discussed in relation to contact sports.) Such behaviors may be evident even in novel situations because of both formal and informal anticipatory guidance an individual has received. However, such behavior and attitudes are most definitely reinforced by the trial and error inherent in repetitive experience.

The so-called rehearsal for a pain experience may have a positive or a negative effect. Consider the young child sitting in a physician's office who observes several children entering an examining room and from behind the closed door hears crying and protest. When the child takes his or her turn, he or she is somewhat anxious and even anticipates what might happen to make him or her cry. Turning the situation around, an informed parent or practitioner may take the time to explain and orient the child to the situation and even use play to help the child achieve mastery and knowledge about coming events both objectively and perceptually, so that extraneous anxiety and fear of the unknown may be diminished (Conway et al., 1970).

Preoperative teaching and similar therapeutic interventions also provide an individual with control and data about a situation that may reduce the ominous and threatening qualities of the situation. Similarly, lack of intervention at appropriate times may cause persons to arrive at faulty conclusions by dwelling on incorrect data (Blitz and Dinnerstein, 1968).

In the context of rehearsal, personality style is certainly a consideration, since some personality types accent input whereas others diminish the significance of the input in relation to their responses to pain. Certainly, any attempts to allow the subject to control or predict as many situational factors as possible increase one's capacities to handle unpleasant situations more effectively (Staub, 1968). For example, it may seem less painful to pull off your own bandage or remove a splinter from your finger than it would if someone else performed these operations. Allowing *realistic* choice when there are alternative ways to approach an uncomfortable procedure may also assist the individual in handling the situational anxiety more constructively. (You may squeeze my hand during this procedure, or how may I remove these ban-

dages so it makes you less uncomfortable?)

Another factor inherent in the pain experience is attention. Much can be done to allow anxiety to rise to a point of incapacitation or to remain at a level where the powers of perception are keen and protective in nature. One example of pain control through technqiues of relaxation and concentration involves the various methods taught as part of prepared childbirth classes.

When attention to the pain serves to magnify the problem, the affected individual might cope more effectively when presented with diversionary stimuli.

One last factor that should definitely be mentioned is that experimental subjects have chosen to be in the elective setting, whereas those experiencing pain in the clinical situation have not. Thus the pain experience for these two groups probably differs greatly in personal significance. For these reasons, determination of outcomes related to placebos may differ because of the variables inherent in the clinical context, which may be either absent or purposefully superimposed on the experimental situation.

*Measurement.* Quantification of sensory experiences such as sight and audition have been possible because the introduction of a stimulus may be controlled and carefully correlated with subjective responses. Although pain is also a sensory phenomenon, the control of stimuli and the subsequent response patterns have evaded attempts at precision control. Early attempts at quantification of pain in terms of the dol, a unit giving pain a relative unit of comparison, failed to stand the test of replication (Beecher, 1950). This problem is possibly related to the difficulty in comparing and grading different stimuli, in evaluating differences between clinical and laboratory settings, and in identifying the different subjective responses to the pain experience. In other words the pain phenomenon is not a simple stimulus-object-response pattern. Nor can the laboratory setting truly replicate the subjective meaning that similar pain might have in states of disease and trauma. Double-blind studies are helpful in pointing out some of the paradoxical and little-understood problems in the pain experience, which may include such factors as emotion, the significance of the problem to the individual in relation to suffering, the role of active medication and placebos, and the degree to which psychological interpretation of the experience accounts for perception and response to the noxious event. In summary, work to date has been largely descriptive, and exact correlations between pain sensation, processing, and the many variables have not been possible. Work continues in the attempt to delineate and quantify the various factors in operation in the pain experience. We hope that such research will continue to make predictions about pain more reliable and valid.

### Physiological theories

This section necessarily summarizes the findings of many researchers who have evolved theories of pain from earliest times, since further discussion goes beyond the intent of this text. Readers seeking more detailed information should consult "The Gate-Control Theory of Pain: a Critical Review" (Nathan, 1976).

One problem in identifying theories of pain is that the theoretical conceptual frameworks postulated have been difficult to prove because scientists have not been able to completely identify the mechanism underlying the pain experience. Three major theories represent most viewpoints in describing conceptual frameworks of pain: the specificity theory, the pattern theory, and the gate control theory.

*Specificity theory.* The specificity theory is a rather simplistic concept that identifies distinct pain receptors in body tissue. These pain receptors, in the form of free nerve endings, transmit pain impulses through A-delta and C fibers in peripheral nerves and through the lateral spinothalamic tract of the spinal medulla to a terminal pain center in the thalamus. The implication in this theory is that these peripheral receptors are responsive only to a specific type of sensory input and, in fact, are pain receptors. Although it is true that some receptors are specialized, it does not follow that such receptors have a direct, constant channel to the brain, so that each impulse is automatically interpreted as pain and only as pain by the brain. In fact the processing of that pain impulse, which includes psychosocial factors, may alter the final perception and individual response to the noxious stimuli. Thus the specificity theory has validity in relation to physiological reception in peripheral tissue but

is inadequate to identify why stimulation of specific fibers does not always elicit the subjective pain response.

To further clarify the problems that this theory poses, it is helpful to consider further research. Researchers have continued to look at the functionally specialized fibers and sensory receptors in the skin in an attempt to find fibers that respond only to pain. Burgess and Perl (1967) identified a specialized group of A-delta, myelinated fibers of a small circumference that have a slow conduction velocity. They are connected to specific nociceptors, which convey impulses only when tissue damage has occurred. Thus these A-delta fibers carry impulses related to pain, but they are not the only avenue for the transmission of impulses that may be eventually interpreted as pain. There are several other cutaneous experiences and interrelationships between stimulus and response that also contribute to the perception of painful experiences caused by cutaneous sources. Consider such noxious stimuli as the chemical bradykinin or extremes of heat and cold; these do not excite the A-delta fibers. Additionally, note the pain experiences of clients with neuralgia, where stimuli are not adequate to reach the threshold of these fibers. Finally, A-delta fibers have two additional properties—rapid powers of adaptation and the lack of afterdischarge—that also limit their capacities to transmit some noxious stimuli and thus identify them as the exclusive modality for the reception of cutaneous pain impulses.

A more plausible explanation is that all cutaneous fibers are on a continuum in relation to threshold. These A-delta fibers merely have a high threshold and are fired when stimulation is extreme. However, the activation of A-delta fibers does not automatically result in pain. In reviewing Chapter 3, one notes that the response of any sensory receptor is governed by many situational variables, including receptor response to the type of stimulus (mechanical, temperature, chemical, or electrical); alteration of receptor threshold by physiological conditions or chemical, mechanical, or temperature factors; adequacy and endurance of stimulus intensity; adaptation of specific fibers; and the phenomenon of afterdischarge. It is such factors that control and alter response to stimulation and limit the notion that a given receptor may consistently react in a cause-effect relationship regardless of intervening variables.

C fibers have also received attention by researchers. In these experiments, C fibers are specifically blocked by the use of pharmacological agents, with a subsequent client response of sensory loss. These experiments still do not show C fibers as a specific pain modality, since many scientists believe that C fibers have a high threshold and are activated when an incoming stimulus exceeds the threshold of all fibers. Thus the results of selectively blocking C fibers do not necessarily point to these fibers as a pain-specific modality but rather indicates that the total interrelated response of fibers has been interrupted.

In looking at the lateral spinothalamic tract as a pain-specific conduction modality, researchers have found that surgical interruption in the thalamus or spinothalamic tract may terminate pain caused by disease states. Although this tract does carry pain impulses, it may not be a specialized pain modality because the surgical interruption results in more complex outcomes than may be apparent initially. Specifically, such an interference limits the number of neurons available for response, alters interrelationships among all ascending tracts, and modifies the descending feedback system, changing impulse transmission from the periphery to the involved cells of the dorsal column. This complex account is further substantiated by the fact that pain often returns after a successful chordotomy.

In summary, researchers believe that cutaneous fibers evidence a high degree of physiological specialization. However, it does not necessarily follow that specific fibers consistently transmit pain impulses when stimulated. The variability in response is related to principles about stimulus-receptor relationships and the intricate matrix of psychosocial factors that affect the individual pain experience.

*Pattern theory.* In response to the weaknesses noted in the specificity pattern, some researchers proposed theories that are collectively grouped in the category termed "pattern theory." In 1894 Goldschneider identified stimulus intensity and central summation as the most significant factors influencing pain. Livingston (1943) was the first investigator to identify a theory of neuronal cir-

cuitry to account for this phenomenon. This theory is as follows: Extreme stimuli result in reverberating circuits in spinal internuncial pools, which may then be further stimulated by nonnoxious stimuli because of the existing state of hypersensitivity. Abnormal volleys thus generated may be interpreted centrally as pain.

Other theorists have added information to support theories of central summation by stating that the response described by Livingston is evident only when there is an interference with the input control system that normally prevents the central barrage or overload state seen in some diseases. In these theories the fiber system characterized by rapid conduction (also known as epicritic, fast, new, and myelinated fiber systems) inhibits impulse transmission in the fiber system, which conducts more slowly and conveys impulses indicating pain. This slow system is also known by a variety of names: protopathic, slow, old, and unmyelinated fiber systems. When disease states interfere with the balance between the two systems so that impulses in the slow system predominate, the outcome is described as *hyperalgesia, diffuse burning pain, protopathic sensation,* or *slow pain.*

In contrasting pattern theories with theories of specificity, one notes that these theories dissociate pain from psychosocial factors and, instead, relate pain perceptions to alterations in the relationship of the two fiber systems involved. These theories of central summation and input regulation have added greatly to the explanation of the pain experience, but they all leave many questions unanswered. It is, however, well accepted that temporal and spatial patterns of neuronal impulses are basic to a contemporary understanding of the nervous system.

*Gate control theory.* Although the pattern theory and the theory of specificity offer valuable information about the questions of stimulation, processing, and response to pain, many points still remain vague and unanswered. Thus the gate control theory has been proposed to answer some of these concerns.

In this theory the individual perceives pain because the output of the central transmission system in the dorsal horn (T cells) reaches threshold or suprathreshold limits. In other words, through temporal summation of incoming impulses in central cells the critical level is attained and surpassed, and pain is experienced.

Since the gate control theory was proposed by Melzack and Wall in 1965, additional data have been added that necessitate revisions in this theory. These revisions are presented here, but certain limitations of contemporary data should be considered while one is reading this information.

It seems that substantia gelatinosa cells are extremely difficult to stain and study, so that gaps in data remain about interconnections, synapses, destiny of axons, and ability of these cells to generate nerve impulses. Another problem is that the power of descending impulses and variables initiating this central output to affect the dorsal horn cells is poorly understood. An additional factor that strikes the reader making a critical analysis of this theory is the paucity of information provided about the interrelationship of the gate control mechanism with such systems as the endocrine and nervous systems. It would seem that even further revision of the theory is needed to include the biochemical and neuroendocrine processes and their interrelationships with regard to normal functions, anxiety, and stress as these factors relate to pain perception and response. Since such a compilation of data is not currently available, the remaining discussion on gate control theory will be confined to the expanded area of information that has become known since the theory was first proposed.

One major finding responsible for expanding the knowledge of the gate control theory is the increased understanding of the laminar organization of the dorsal horns.

Anatomically the cutaneous afferent fibers terminate in the posterior two thirds of the dorsal horns on cells organized into five laminae. Lamina 1 is composed of a sparse layer of marginal cells whose operations evade explanation. Lamina 2 is the substantia gelatinosa, consisting of three elements: terminals of afferent fibers, dendrites of deeper cells, and small cells with their interconnections. The delicate afferent fibers in lamina 2 travel directly into dorsal gray matter from the dorsal roots through the medial aspect of the Lissauer tract. Dendrites of the large cells from deeper laminae become large formations in a rostro-caudal pattern that separates the lamina into component parts. Small cells in this lamina interconnect through short axons and through the long axons that compose the Lissauer tract. Lamina 2 also contains many axons that are probably peripheral afferent fibers that interconnect with each other and probably with some small cells in lamina 3. Lamina 3 has the same composition as lamina 2. However, the afferent fibers in lamina 3 are from large, myelinated, cutaneous afferent fibers and are interconnected with dendrites of cells from deeper laminae. Small cells in this layer receive primary afferent fibers and send their axons out to lamina 2. Lamina 4 has large cell bodies whose dendrites extend into laminae 2 and 3 and whose axons may travel through the ipsilateral dorsolateral tract, in part. Lamina 5, composed of afferent fibers, extends its axons into dorsolateral white matter of the ipsilateral side and possibly to undefined regions of the brain, such as the thalamus, through the ventral crossed spinothalamic tract. Each of these five laminae connect with descending fibers from the brain through tracts that also include input from the pyramidal tract.

Physiologically the mechanism of the gate control theory remains somewhat elusive. However, it is known that membrane potential of the terminals is regulated both by a central mechanism and by opposing effects of small and large afferent fibers, particularly in laminae 2 and 3. Moreover, the control of incoming impulses is assumed to be connected to presynaptic membrane potential control and possibly to some concurrent alteration in the presynaptic membrane.

From the data collected about the five laminae, several points have been theorized. First, all five laminae are recipients of cutaneous afferent fibers. Lamina 1, with its sparse cell population, is a point of reception and multiple convergence from skin and muscle but is not thought to transmit impulses to contralateral ventral white matter. Although the actual physiology of laminae 2 and 3 is inadequately described, they are believed to modify the afferent impulses to larger cells. Lamina 4 has limited fibers for cutaneous reception extending to lamina 5 cells and to ipsilateral white matter. Lamina 4 cells show response to light pressure and to A-beta afferent volleys but not to A-delta or C volleys. Lamina 5 has larger receptive fields that respond not only to all types of cutaneous stimuli but also to messages from deep and visceral structures. Through the organization at lamina 5, inhibition is produced by large fibers and facilitation by small fibers, possibly through the involvement of cells in laminae 2 and 3 and through presynaptic and postsynaptic changes. Facilitatory mechanisms are inhibited by barbiturate anesthesia, which results in strong tonic descending impulses of an inhibitory nature from the brainstem. Small afferent fibers in lamina 5 arise from three places: cutaneous delta afferent, small muscle afferent, and small visceral afferent fibers. All cells are activated through the small afferent fibers from any of these three origins and dampened by the large afferent fibers from cutaneous sources. When the total effect of facilitatory impulses exceeds a preset level, the pain response is triggered.

The activity of the dorsal horn is probably only the initial screening, interaction, and modification of the total input of incoming sensory impulses. Similar activity and interrelationships of cells involved in the transmission of noxious impulses extends up to include the brain, though the nature of functional operations, relays, and interconnections at these higher levels is still debatable.

It is believed that the aspect of sensory discrimination involved in pain is modulated through the neospinothalamic tract. The drive that motivates the individual to respond to noxious stimuli is determined by the messages received in the reticular and limbic structures through the paramedial ascending system. Further refinements of motivation and discrimination in individual response patterns are regulated by neocortical areas that store data valuable for the assessment of particular input in light of previous experience. The interaction of these systems is believed to provide the individual with accurate perceptions of pain with respect to site, intensity, and spatiotemporal characteristics as well as subsequent cognition of all aspects, so that the strategy for response may be formulated.

Many researchers now believe that the reticular and limbic systems are responsible for the aversive drive and behavioral response noted when individuals have been subjected to noxious stimuli. The mechanism for these responses is as follows: The

reticular and limbic systems, known as the central intensity monitor, become activated when the total output of the T cell in the dorsal horn exceeds a critical intensity after the modulating forces of the gate control system have been exerted. Activation of this central intensity monitor leads to negative affect, aversive drive, and appropriate activation of motor cells, so that the total message received through interactions of sensory and cognitive processes might receive appropriate response.

In further evaluation of central processes the central trigger mechanism is theorized. This theory revolves around the concept that a mechanism in the central nervous system excites specific, selected portions of the brain, which in turn have regulatory power over sensory input. Perhaps descending messages from this mechanism travel through the dorsal column–medial lemniscal and dorsolateral systems, systems noted for their capacities to transmit impulses rapidly. It is assumed that the rapid flow of impulses through these systems not only affects neurons of the cerebral cortex in such a manner as to prepare them for subsequent afferent volleys but also affects the gate control system in the dorsal columns. Thus such a system allows brain processes to become ready for additional messages traveling upward through slower conduction pathways. The addition of this theoretical mechanism further offers an explanation for ways in which emotion, attention, chemical and biological substances, and past experience play roles in the perception of incoming noxious stimuli. It is well known that powerful emotional states such as fear or anxiety may block or open the gate for all sensory input at any body location, whereas other central activities may operate in a more specific, localized way on the gate control mechanism. Thus any signals that may potentially be interpreted as pain are screened through several processes, including past experience and physiological and psychosocial inhibition, before they are perceived in relation to location and individual significance as pain.

## ASSESSMENT

Pain remains a personal experience felt only by the individual. As previously mentioned, it originates from a disease state, trauma, or other condition sufficient to excite receptors through electrical, thermal, chemical, or mechanical stimuli. From there, impulses are relayed to the central nervous system, including the thalamus, where pain is perceived as a conscious, undesirable sensory phenomenon. After interpretation in the cerebral cortex the physiological responses occur through the skeletal muscles and autonomic nervous system. Table 10-1 summarizes the outcomes after a body system is activated in response to a painful stimulus.

Next, what can be done to assess the problem as accurately as possible, even though absolute quantification and predictions about the pain experience may elude the scientist? Clinically the practitioner organizes data in the attempt to comprehend the client's experiences, to define the causative agent or problem, and to learn about the factors that influence the pain. The practitioner should also identify the significance and effect this pain experience has on the individual. To glean such information the following data should be elicited from the history, physical assessment, and clinical observation:

1. Brief but thorough review of past history and previous experience with pain
2. Clinical description of personality and subjective and clinical evaluation of methods used in coping with pain of various intensities
3. Brief, thorough discussion of pain location
4. Mode of onset
5. Detailed description of how pain evolved
6. Quality and characteristics of pain (dull, aching, shooting, and so on)
7. Duration, intensity, and severity of pain
8. Changes in pain since it was first perceived
9. Precipitating or associated factors
10. Measures that relieve pain
11. Associated symptoms such as autonomic reactions
12. Meaning of pain experience to the individual
13. Clinical observation and validation of collected data

The client's descriptions of pain may often be more exact when the individual can compare sensations with a written list of words. The boxed material on p. 227 lists the 39 pairs of words utilized in the University of Washington Pain Clinic during the process of diagnosis. In further evaluation of pain the practitioner might benefit from the use of a pain reaction rating scale such as the one found in the programmed instruction on pain from the *American Journal of Nursing* (p. 228).

**TABLE 10-1.** Functions of body systems after activation by a pain stimulus

| Clinical observation | Purpose | Outcome |
|---|---|---|
| **Autonomic response** | | |
| Rise in blood pressure | More blood available to brain and muscles | Increased perception, which aids in detecting threat |
| Increased heart rate | More blood available to brain and muscles | |
| Rapid, irregular respirations | More oxygen available to brain and muscles | Narrowed perspective to focus on painful stimulus |
| Augmented perspiration | Mechanism for removal of excess body heat | Control of body temperature |
| Dilatation of pupil | Allows more light to enter eye | Improved vision to view threats to integrity |
| **Musculoskeletal response** | | |
| Muscle tension or activity is increased | Increases power of response in nerves and muscle | Preparation for rapid motor activities |
| **Psychological manifestations** | | |
| State of expectation, anxiety, irritability | Augment powers of perception and response | Keen power of perception for rapid processing of potential threat |
| Perception narrowed to focus on painful stimulus | | Musculoskeletal readiness for instantaneous response |
| Communication of pain | Tension-releasing problem-solving act | Expression of discomfort and effort to seek assistance from others |

## HOW PATIENTS DESCRIBE THEIR PAIN*

The left and right columns below form 39 pairs of opposite descriptions of pain used in diagnosis at the University of Washington Pain Clinic. Patients are told to make one choice from each pair and indicate it with an **X** on one of seven spaces between each pair. They mark a space close to the word if the description applies closely or a space toward the middle if the description is not so close. Choosing the middle space shows that both descriptions apply equally or that neither applies.

|  | |  |
|---|---|---|
| Cold | | Hot |
| Nonlocalized | | Localized |
| Real | | Phantom |
| Steady | | Throbbing |
| Flattening | | Pinching |
| Still | | Moving |
| Severe | | Mild |
| Steady | | Pulsating |
| Soft | | Hard |
| Sensitive | | Numb |
| Evening | | Morning |
| Heavy | | Light |
| Contracting | | Expanding |
| Frosty | | Burning |
| Always | | Sometimes |
| Pointed | | Blunt |
| Working | | Relaxing |
| Casual | | Intense |
| Stable | | Fleeting |
| Deep | | Shallow |
| Tingling | | Numb |
| Varying | | Constant |
| Dull | | Sharp |
| Shrinking | | Growing |
| Lifting | | Pressing |
| Short | | Long |
| Straight | | Twisting |
| Reclining | | Upright |
| Not bothersome | | Bothersome |
| Nighttime | | Daytime |
| General | | Specific |
| Pulling out | | Knifing in |
| Seldom | | Often |
| Loose | | Tight |
| Fixed | | Spreading |
| Unbearable | | Bearable |
| Irregular | | Regular |
| Squeezing | | Tearing |
| Limp | | Stretched |

*Copyright Jan. 1975, RN Magazine; reproduced with permission.

## PAIN REACTION RATING SCALE*

| | | | |
|---|---|---|---|
| 1. Attention | Almost complete attention to pain—very difficult to distract | Some attention to pain—some to distraction | No attention to pain—easy to distract |
| 2. Anxiety | Extreme tension, irritability, or worry | Some tension, irritability, or worry | No tension, irritability, or worry |
| 3. Verbal | Severe pain | Some pain | No pain |
| 4. Skeletal muscle response | Very restless or very tense | Slightly restless or slightly tense | Quiet or relaxed |
| 5. Respiration | Very irregular | Slightly irregular | Regular |
| 6. Perspiration | Profuse perspiration | Some perspiration | Normal perspiration |

*Adapted from *A Study of Nurse Action in Relief of Pain,* by Mildred E. Newton and others. Columbus, Ohio, Ohio State University Research Foundation, 1964, p. 44, Fig. 4. Copyright May, 1966, The American Journal of Nursing Company. Reproduced with permission from the American Journal of Nursing.

**TABLE 10-2.** Classic peripheral and central pain syndromes

| Pain | Description | Pain | Description |
|---|---|---|---|
| **Peripheral type** | | **Brainstem pain syndromes** | |
| Trigeminal neuralgia (tic douloureux) | Common problem whereby brief, paroxysmal, extreme pain is evident, usually along one division of trigeminal nerve | Disease processes—direct stimulation | Stimulates sensory pathways to convey message that results in pain responses |
| Nerve root compression syndromes | Intermittent, radicular, stabbing pain along one or more nerve roots. Any activity that stretches nerve intensifies pain | **Diencephalon pain syndromes** | |
| | | Thalamic syndrome | When infarction affects ventroposterior lateral nucleus, extreme dysesthetic and hyperpathic symptoms occur in contralateral extremities |
| Causalgia | Extreme, continuous burning or tearing sensation often after acute, incomplete nerve injury | **Cerebral pain syndromes** | |
| **Central pain syndromes** | | Pain of cortical origin | Inadequately understood by researchers; causes disturbed sensations on contralateral side of body; difficult to discriminate this central type of pain from nerve root pain |
| Spinal cord | | | |
| Tabetic crises | Involves sensory fibers entering spinal cord; dysesthetic, paresthetic, poorly localized sensations | General headache | Variable pain focus and symptoms; symptoms, treatment regimen, and outcomes depend on underlying cause |
| Multiple sclerosis | Involves interference with ascending sensory pathways; dysesthetic, poorly localized sensations | | |
| Trauma | Involves interferences with ascending sensory pathways; dysesthetic, poorly localized sensations | | |
| Low back pain | Complex problem where symptom outcomes are related to underlying cause and available treatment | | |

## CLINICAL SITUATIONS RELATING TO SPECIFIC DISEASE ENTITIES

The gate control theory offers plausible explanations for several types of pain. In alcoholic or diabetic neuropathies, selective damage to large peripheral nerve fibers occurs, leaving small fibers mainly unaffected. Therefore impulses through small fibers pass into the dorsal laminae unopposed and provide the explanation of the severe, pathological pain that ensues. The delay in pathological pain experiences by such individuals is further explained by the reduction in functional peripheral fibers that results in a greater time interval between the point of stimulation and the transmission of sufficient impulses to excite T cells to the level where pain is triggered. A similar mechanism is offered as an explanation for the pain of trigeminal neuralgia. In lesions of the brain, those augmenting descending inhibitory impulses cause the gate to close, whereas those interfering with descending inhibitory impulses result in facilitation of sensory impulses at the level of the gate control system.

The gate control system suggests the following three plausible explanations for pain experiences resulting from interferences within the autonomic nervous system: (1) There is an alteration of sensitivity at afferent nerve endings through the release of neurohormones by autonomic efferent activity. (2) The presence of bradykinin, a pain-causative substance found at points of tissue breakdown, is regulated by local circulation and autonomic nervous system activity. (3) Somatic afferent fibers course through the sympathetic ganglia. Thus the process of summation and facilitation of impulses through input from the autonomic nervous system may be the result of either direct or indirect activity at either the receptor fiber or the central cell level.

Several classic peripheral and central pain syndromes have been identified, as found in Table 10-2.

## COMMON DISORDERS RESULTING IN PAIN

*Backache.* There is nothing like a backache to reduce its sufferer to approaching the simplest tasks with monumental effort, pain, and apprehension. Yet, it is a common malady because of the architecture of the spine and the posture and habits of modern individuals. Refer to Chapter 23 for further detail.

*Headache.* Headache is another common disorder that most of us endure at some time. Chapter 14 details this common type of pain.

*Cervical spine syndrome.* The cervical spine syndrome is also a common painful disorder. About 90% of these injuries result from automobile accidents. Injury is usually caused by hyperextension and prolongation of the neck, a very mobile part of the spinal column. Symptoms vary in different individuals, depending on the nature and location of the injury. Usual symptoms may include neck pain, headache, and loss of range of motion in the neck. Shoulder weakness, pain, stiffness; arm pain; changes in sensory capacities in the upper extremities; and even loss of hand grip may occur. Whatever the symptoms, clients are usually unable to continue their routine functions, and they become focused on ridding themselves of pain and regaining lost functional capacities. Muscle weakness, atrophy, and sensory changes should be promptly reported to the physician, since they may signal the need for prompt intervention to avoid such problems as paralysis caused by potential compression.

As clients undergo radiographic studies, tomography, electroencephalograms, and similar studies, findings may be minimally abnormal, if at all, compared to the actual symptoms that the client reports. Thus these clients are too often dismissed as "a pain in the neck," crocks, or neurotics.

Great patience and understanding is needed to restore functional capacities. A thorough assessment is important. When evidence does not support the existence of protrusion of the intervertebral disc or spondylosis caused by cervical osteoarthritis, appropriate treatment may consist of moist heat applications, ultrasound treatments, traction, medications, immobilization, relaxation techniques, and exercise to maintain function and prevent disuse atrophy. Through all of this the important *client outcomes* are to inform the client so that he or she can (1) discuss the problem and treatment plan in detail, (2) identify underlying principles in treatment, (3) demonstrate his or her conviction to cooperate with the treatment plan, and (4) utilize medications for pain, depression, and relaxation judiciously.

The use of pain medication may also deaden the warning mechanism that protects the individual from reinjury of the affected area. When use continues over a long period, there is also the chance that the user will become medication dependent. Practitioners must work closely with the client so that the right medicine usage is established. For some individuals minimal use of medications may be warranted, so that pain operates as the control for indicating individual activity limits.

## REFERRED PAIN

The concept of referred pain is one that has evaded explanation by one theory throughout the twentieth century. In situations of referred pain the peripheral or visceral site of stimulation is not the body area where the pain is felt; instead the pain is referred to a remote area.

When pain occurs in the viscera or muscles, it may be projected to the dermatomes (Fig. 3-5, p. 79). However, such referred pain is not necessarily limited to the segments of innervation or to a fixed anatomical location. Three mechanisms are commonly utilized to describe this phenomenon: (1) convergence-facilitation, (2) convergence-projection, and (3) set-point view.

*Convergence-facilitation* is a phenomenon by which impulses generated in the viscera result in an irritating focus at the segment where they course into the cord. Thus there is a concurrent intensification of cutaneous afferent impulses, and the client perceives pain in the corresponding radicular cutaneous area. Therefore impulses of a visceral origin facilitate somatic pain (MacKenzie, 1918).

*Convergence-projection* occurs as both visceral afferent and cutaneous afferent fibers converge on the same neurons at spinal, thalamic, or cortical levels. Because of previous experience the brain interprets the source of this input as cutaneous impulses. This view is based on the neuron pool concept proposed by Sherrington (Ruch, 1965).

The *set-point view* revolves around the premise that pain occurs when the total result of afferent impulses is greater than the preset level of a presynaptic filter. This presynaptic filter is affected by input from supraspinal structures or responses, or both, from the afferent barrage preceding sensation (Melzack and Wall, 1965; Wall, 1970).

Although disease states involving viscera result in localized and referred pain from the somatic and visceral afferent fibers serving these structures, referred pain is the only type of pain considered at this point in the text. Somatic afferent fibers arising in the lining of the visceral structures result in the referral of pain to the locations outlined in Table 10-3. Referred pain from visceral afferent fibers to various points is summarized in Table 10-4. Visceral afferent fibers carrying pain impulses travel into the central nervous system through specific routes of the cranial parasympathetic, sympathetic, and sacral parasympathetic systems.

In some instances, pain of cutaneous origin may

**TABLE 10-3.** Somatic afferent fibers from visceral structures and sites of pain projection*

| Structure | Nerves carrying pain impulses to central nervous system | Radicular segments involved in pain protection | Site(s) of referred pain |
|---|---|---|---|
| Central zone of diaphgram (pleural and peritoneal sides) Portions of pericardium Biliary tract | Phrenic nerve | C3-C4 | Region of junction of neck and shoulder |
| Borders of diaphragm | Intercostal nerves | T6-T12 | Anterior abdominal wall laterally; occasionally to back |
| Parietal pleura Parietal peritoneum Roots of mesentery | Thoracic and upper lumbar nerves | T1-L2 | Anterior thorax and abdomen; occasionally to posterior thorax |

*Partly from Ruch and associates, 1965; from Haymaker, W.: Bing's local diagnosis in neurological diseases, ed. 15, St. Louis, 1969, The C.V. Mosby Co.

**TABLE 10-4.** Sources of visceral afferent fibers and sites of referred pain*

| Structure | Nerves carrying afferent pain impulses | Radicular segments involved in pain protection | Site(s) to which pain is referred |
|---|---|---|---|
| **Cranial parasympathetic system** | | | |
| Larynx | Tenth | — | No referred pain; pain felt in superior or inferior laryngeal area |
| Upper esophagus, trachea, bronchi | Tenth | — | Midline, lowermost neck, and xiphoid |
| **Sympathetic system** | | | |
| Apical pleura | Brachial plexus | | — |
| Heart | Cardiac | T1-T5 | Right shoulder and neck |
| Ascending aortic arch (aneurysm) | Cardiac | T1, T2 | Thorax and inner upper arm |
| Gallbladder | Right splanchnic | T7-T9 | Above umbilicus on right side |
| Pancreas | Splanchnic | T7-T9 | Anterior upper abdomen, occasionally through to back |
| Lower esophagus, gastric cardia, duodenal cap | Splanchnic | T7 | Region of xiphoid |
| Duodenum | Splanchnic | T7-T10 | Midline and deep, from xiphoid to umbilicus |
| Jejunum, ileum | Splanchnic | T10 | Region of umbilicus |
| Appendix | Splanchnic | T11, T12 | Right lower quadrant of abdomen (second-stage pain) |
| Upper colon | Splanchnic | T11-L1 | Side of abdomen below umbilicus |
| Kidney pelvis | Lower splanchnic | T10-L1 | Region of costovertebral angle, occasionally to glans penis |
| Ureter | Renal, spermatic, and hypogastric plexus | T11-L1 | Lateral border of rectus muscle, suprapubic region up to umbilicus, groin, down leg, occasionally to glans penis |
| Bladder fundus | Hypogastric | T11-L1 | Suprapubic region |
| Testis | Spermatic plexus | T10 | Groin |
| Uterine fundus | Superior hypogastric plexus | T11-L1 | Lower lateral quadrants of abdomen |
| Ovary, fallopian tube | Along ovarian arteries | T10 | Small of back, also lateral to and below umbilicus |
| **Sacral parasympathetic system** | | | |
| Lower colon, rectum | Pelvic | S2-S4 | Lower midabdomen |
| Prostate | Pelvic | S2-S4 | Glans penis, lumbar region |
| Bladder neck | Pelvic | S2-S4 | Hard to define zone; maximal pain in region of buttock; may radiate from sacral region, around ilium, to lower abdomen |
| Seminal vesicles | Pelvic | S2-S4 | Lumbar region |
| Uterine cervix, upper vagina | Pelvic | S2-S4 | Lumbar region |

*From Behan (1914), Capps and Coleman (1932), Jones (1938, 1943), McLellan and Goodell (1943), Ray and Neill (1947), White (1943), and White and Sweet (1955); from Haymaker, W.: Bing's local diagnosis in neurological diseases, ed. 15, St. Louis, 1969, The C.V. Mosby Co.

be projected to deep structures. Herpes zoster provides an example of this phenomenon, since it may result in pain in the heart area, and the erroneous diagnosis of angina may be made until additional data appear in the form of cutaneous vesicles.

## INTERVENTION MODALITIES

In treating pain the importance of *accurate and ongoing assessment coupled with a sincere effort on the part of the practitioner to solve or alleviate the problem cannot be overemphasized (Fig. 10-2). Certainly the establishment of effective rapport with clients is one major step in assuring them that their pain is significant and that they may rely on the expertise and human comfort the practitioner lends.* Too often, acute care settings augment the client's anxieties of the unknown through hurried encounters, deal minimally with the psychosocial realm, and give the client a feeling of depersonalization—all of which intensify personal discomfort, tension, and pain. Although

such outcomes are not intentional but often the result of pressures related to time, stress, and routine in the situation, failure to lay this basic groundwork can actually result in a greater time expenditure for the practitioner and more pain, uncertainty and medication for the client in the long run. The adage about a stitch in time saving nine applies here.

Personality is certainly a factor in the pain experience, as previously mentioned; therefore *care should be individualized to cope with the problems of individuals on the continuum between those who augment and those who reduce the pain experience. Attention to client needs during the absence of pain, explanations about individual diagnosis, treatment, and the reason for the pain with hints at control, that is, relaxation techniques or methods of avoiding precipitating factors, may aid individuals in experiencing less pain or less frequent episodes as they participate actively to decrease the incidence or severity of their pain.*

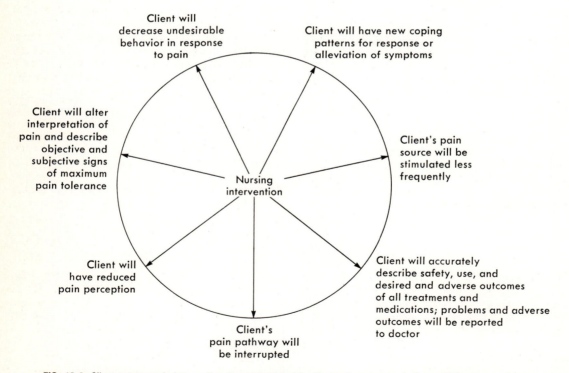

**FIG. 10-2.** Client outcomes in intervention for pain relief. After thorough assessment, the practitioner may elect to alleviate pain by intervening to achieve one or more items.

Certainly, *medication is a valuable adjunct to the services of the practitioner and should be given promptly and as often as needed.* However, it cannot replace nor should it be a substitute for an open relationship, physical presence of the practitioner when comfort is needed, touching, and provision of the nurturing necessary when the client is overwhelmed with personal discomfort, fears, or anxiety. Nor should medication replace the need to voice concerns an have them answered in accordance with the significance they have for the client. *Individuals should be allowed to express emotion in pain and feel supported in a nonjudgmental manner as they do so.*

*Chronic pain* presents problems different from those of acute pain. In chronic pain there is often a causative factor or disease state that cannot be removed. The pain response that signals harm or threat to integrity may have even more significance for the chronically ill client who worries about the threat to life and functional integrity when pain cannot be eradicated. Unable to remove the underlying source of pain, such a client may feel particularly anxious and frustrated. If these feelings are coupled with lack of acceptance from practitioners because of the client's physical condition or limitations, appearance, odor, isolation, or terminal illness, the problems for the client may be even further augmented. *Whatever the client's situation, each request for pain assistance should be personally considered and treated in accordance with the severity of that particular episode.* For example, a client with a terminal illness may have a narcotic ordered for some type of severe, recurring pain but may need a less powerful medication to treat an ordinary headache. *When disease states are chronic and even terminal, pain serves as a reminder to the individual that something is wrong and may cause a number of emotions:* guilt, anger, fear, aloneness, and so on. Clients may even believe that pain is a personal punishment for some act they have performed. *Particular support and understanding is needed to assist both client and family in handling unsettling experiences. Understanding the facts about the client's situation also aids the practitioner in lending appropriate and realistic support without offering false hope and assurance.*

Practitioners not only tend to avoid clients in chronic pain because of personal difficulty in dealing with the problem but may actually withhold necessary pain medication for fear of addicting the client. *Client care conferences and understanding of situational objectives may assist practitioners in utilizing all therapeutic means, including medications, within the context of individual client needs.* Professionals who work extensively with pain control in terminal cancer have found pain control regimens to be most effective when the client participates in decisions about what medications and dosages should be used. In these instances, small doses are given at specified intervals to eliminate the client-staff bargaining that occurs with an "as-needed" schedule. An excellent article on these issues is "The Patient in Pain: New Concepts" (Benoliel and Crowley). Refer also to the Symposium on Client Compliance to be published by *Nursing Clinics of North America* in September 1982.

## Pharmacological control of pain

Pharmacological agents are known to act at three levels of the nervous system: the receptor level, the dorsal horn, and higher levels such as the brainstem. Some drugs act at one or more of these levels. At the receptor level, analgesics presumably act to limit specific receptor activity so that tissue breakdown, edema formation, vasodilatation, and pain are decreased. Further research is needed to establish the exact process of tissue and serum breakdown as it relates to the pain experience. At this point, aspirin and phenylbutazone are known to interfere with the action of bradykinin, though the precise mechanism of this antagonistic process is yet to be determined.

The action of pharmacological agents at the level of the dorsal horn is explained in terms of the gate control theory. Although three ways have been suggested for the operation of these agents at the dorsal horn level, these ways are not necessarily exclusive operational modes. Instead, they may function in harmony. The three suggested ways analgesics operate at the level of the dorsal horn include decreasing excitation caused by separate impulses, increasing inhibitory effects on individual impulses, and disorganizing the usual volleys of spatial and temporal impulses.

Nitrous oxide at analgesic levels and barbiturates have been documented as decreasing the amplitude of potentials emitted by the midbrain reticular formation. Some researchers believe that action at this level is at least partially attributed to interference with the summation of sensory input necessary for the critical level to be attained before the pain reaction.

## Placebos

Placebos continue to occupy an important position in modern medicine but should be used judiciously. Recent information reveals that placebos result in both psychological and physiological changes. Administration of placebos probably results in the activation of the mechanism that releases endorphins. Thus clients who believe that they are receiving medication may experience side effects related to the placebo effect. Older beliefs about placebos working only in the imagination of the client or mainly in ''neurotic'' clients should be discarded. Emphasis should once again be placed on the importance of the physician and nurse relationships with the client, since research shows that medication effectiveness is related to the faith in the cure that health professionals transfer to the client (Perry and Heidrich, 1981).

## Pain clinics

When pain becomes chronic, it affects the entire quality of an individual's life. Patterns of life begin to revolve around pain, and drastic changes in personality may become apparent. In the effort to eradicate pain the individual may visit a series of physicians, become dependent on powerful pain medications, and undergo numerous surgical procedures in the attempt to correct the problem. Dr. John Bonica, chairman of the Department of Anesthesiology and Anesthesia Research Center of the University of Washington School of Medicine in Seattle, became aware of this problem and formed a multidisciplinary team of specialists to tackle this complex area. Underlying their approach are principles of operant conditioning and the systematic commitment to assist clients in unlearning pain and the undesirable behaviors they have formulated to cope with chronic pain. Although the waiting list is lengthy and represented by persons from all over the nation, clients with pain from terminal cancer are admitted immediately.

After intensive multidisciplinary screening; review of a diary of the individual's pain and details of treatment; a workup, which may include laboratory evaluation, diagnostic nerve blocks, percutaneous stimulation, hypnosis, placebo trials, and test batteries such as the Minnesota Multiphasic Personality Inventory; and weekly staff conferences, the client is assigned to a treatment regimen. Unless the client is drug dependent, he or she is treated as an outpatient. If drug dependent, he or she is admitted to the inpatient facility for detoxification before continuing in the program. During this period the client receives intense emotional support and ''pain cocktails'' at regular intervals as he or she enters the difficult processes of unlearning the behaviors related to the pain experience and of withdrawing from drug dependency. As drug-related symptoms disappear, the client may be more accurately diagnosed. If symptoms are psychological and drug related, the combination of detoxification and physical therapy may effect a cure.

Some other clients in the program are placed in a program of operant conditioning that attempts to decrease responses related to learned pain and increase physical ability through positive reinforcement. Through this program, deficiencies related to inactivity and negative patterns of living are reversed.

In summary, these programs have met with such success that the University of Washington Pain Clinic and other like facilities are vital and common in chronic pain treatment.

## Hypnosis

At some point in the practitioner's career, hypnotic techniques are used either knowingly or unknowingly. Placebos, back rubs, attempts to make the atmosphere of the room quiet and tranquil, soft statements and hand holding aimed at relaxing the client, and other such methods designed to reduce anxiety, relax muscles, and decrease pain awareness are all examples of such techniques. Although not previously mentioned, most practitioners recognize the therapeutic value of suggestion and quiet reassurance as invaluable tools for treatment.

Hypnosis as a valid medical technique first became approved by the American Medical Association in 1958. Today the American Society for Clinical Hypnosis has a membership of some 2600 physicians, dentists, and others holding doctoral degrees, whereas the Society for Clinical and Experimental Hypnosis has a membership of about 300 physicians and 350 other professionals. A discussion on techniques employed in hypnosis is available in an article by Barrins (1975). It is beyond the scope of this text to identify these steps at this point.

Theoretical differences exist as to what constitutes hypnosis, how it affects the individual, and how hypnotics operate. Hilgard (1973) has defined hypnosis in relation to levels of consciousness. He believes that although the painful stimulus is still perceived at a lower level of consciousness in hypnotized clients, the hypnotic state is effective because it allows the client to keep pain perception from a distressing level of conscious awareness. Hilgard's article presents a most informative critique of various theories on hypnosis.

Barber et al. (1975) have conducted a number of laboratory experiments and have demonstrated that under certain conditions unhypnotized and highly motivated clients perform the same as hypnotized persons in situations involving pain. Barber et al. do not believe that hypnosis creates a state different from what is apparent in the waking individual. Instead, they believe that a variety of techniques utilized in hypnosis may be effective in assisting individuals in coping with surgical pain. These techniques include diminishing levels of pain and anxiety and creating positive expectations, attitudes, and motivations toward the experience. Other techniques include distraction, the power of suggestion for analgesia and decreased pain experience, and cognitive strategies, including imagination and though processes, to desensitize a body part. This work further places surgical pain into perspective by reviewing the fact that most body tissues and organs are not pain-sensitive structures, so that the use of a local anesthetic for numbing the pain-sensitive structure of the skin during initial opening of the surgical wound is sufficient when the client is prepared psychologically to cope with awareness during the remaining procedure. In summary, these authors contend that psychosocial factors, including motivation and a client's capacity to be open to suggestion, are powers that most practitioners utilize in creating a therapeutic situation even when hypnosis is not used. Basically, all these techniques work in an advantageous manner when a trusting relationship exists between practitioner and client.

Not all researchers are in agreement with the findings of Barber et al. Although these findings have added greatly to the subject by placing hypnosis into a scientific perspective, others still contend that hypnosis alters the waking state in the individual. Hilgard (1973) agrees that no physiological changes occur strictly as an outcome of hypnosis but notes that some physiological changes may be induced when certain suggestions and conditions are imposed on the client. The type of stimulus used, that is, ice water or ischemia, to induce pain seems to influence the client's response.

On the other hand, Thompson defends the effectiveness of utilizing relaxation as a means of lessening pain, whereas Hilgard (1973) believes that relaxation has little effect on pain reduction. Thompson has a video presentation of hypnosis and pain control during dermabrasion that effectively shows the operation of hypnosis in pain relief. Theorists such as Sarcedote (1970) present data supporting the use of hypnosis as a valid and valuable technique to alleviate pain.

In summary, there remains much debate about the operational mechanics and effects of the techniques that make up the method known as hypnosis. The reader is encouraged to read the works of the various aforementioned theorists to gain further insights.

## Acupuncture

Over the last decades, acupuncture techniques have gained increasingly wide acceptance in China and worldwide as a means of combating such problems as neuralgia, phantom limb pain, and pain related to surgical procedures. One of the most intriguing aspects of acupuncture involves the sites selected for insertion of the stainless steel needles, which in anesthesia are connected to phasic direct current of minimal voltage, that is, 6 volts at 150 cpm. If voltage is not utilized to maintain stimulation at the sites of acupuncture needles, the needles are often turned to stimulate tissue or heated through moxibustion of herbs. In essence, acupuncture depends on ongoing intense stimulation at the site of the acupuncture needles to be effective. When the acupuncture technique is utilized, a period of time lapses between stimulation of the acupuncture needles and the onset of analgesia. Once induced the analgesia may extend beyond the period when actual needle stimulation is occurring. If a local anesthetic is injected at the acupuncture site, it interferes with the neuronal impulses traveling to block pain at the identified remote site.

Several questions remain about the mechanism of effective analgesia in acupuncture. Who elects acupuncture and why? What consistent methods are utilized to evaluate the individual effectiveness of acupuncture? Of those receiving acupuncture, how many effects are related to acupuncture and how many are outcomes of the analgesic agents that are often administered simultaneously? One final point is that individuals electing acupuncture are convinced that this technique is an effective method of analgesia. How would skepticism interfere with the effectiveness of acupuncture?

Acupuncture involves three major factors that have been substantiated through research. First, there is a rather intense stimulus at the acupuncture site that effects analgesia at a remote site, even though the pharmacological mechanism underlying this phenomenon evades explanation. Second, the selection of cutaneous sites for the insertion of acupuncture needles does not seem to have an established anatomical connection to the remote body portion that experiences analgesia. Third, the pain-relieving capacities of this method extend beyond the period when stimulation is applied to the acupuncture needles. It may help to elaborate on these factors individually.

First, stimulus at a nonpainful site resolves pain at a remote point. Although the underlying rationale here seems to be suggestion, distraction, and counterirritation, these factors do not seem to adequately explain the phenomenon of acupuncture. Perhaps one explanation for this phenomenon is that pain of short duration at one site alters the basic threshold for pain occurring simultaneously in other body parts. Experimental validation of this point has included situations such as injection of hypertonic saline solution into back tissues to alleviate phantom limb pain or intense cold applications to the chin to diminish the pain threshold for teeth subjected to electrical stimulation.

The second factor refers to the interrelationships of remote body sites. Such an interrelationship may be explained according to the discussion of referred pain presented earlier in this chapter. Because of the phenomenon of referred pain, intense stimuli through extreme cold application, repeated needling of an area, or injection of a trigger point often result in pain relief at the involved remote area.

In relation to the third factor, scientists have found no appropriate explanation of why a local anesthetic injection into a stump can permanently cure the pain resulting from the amputation of a limb or why stimuli of a short-lived nature result in pain relief for hours beyond stimulation. Obviously the answer does not lie in a discrete, simplistic, cause-effect relationship.

Three major theories are utilized to explain how intense stimuli at a remote site affect pain, why certain sites affect remote points, and the nature of temporal qualities related to stimuli and degree of analgesia: the Chinese theory, Kroger's (1973) and other workers, and Melzack's gate control theory.

According to the *Chinese theory,* two great universal forces are expressed at the human level in the spirit *(yin)* and the blood *(yang)*. Yin and yang are transmitted along different avenues (meridians). The acupuncture points visualized in Chinese illustrations are either along these meridians or at the interconnections of meridians. This theory revolves around the belief that disease and pain are outcomes of disharmony between yin and yang. Thus intervention at certain sites through acupuncture needles allows yin and yang to return to harmony. Although the origin of acupuncture sites in relation to meridians remains obscure, the choice of these sites has definitely included reliance on empirical observation. There is suggestive data to support the idea that resistance to electrical flow at acupuncture sites is different from that at other cutaneous sites, but much more research is necessary to substantiate these data.

Some practitioners, such as Kroger (1973), believe that acupuncture is quite similar to hypnosis and that similar phenomena may be seen while the client is hypnotized during surgical procedures. Although the significance of psychosocial influences and positive motivation by the individual certainly have a bearing on the outcomes of acupuncture, these factors do not totally explain the underlying mechanics of acupuncture. In hypnosis, specific client education and induction must occur before the hypnotic state, but in acupuncture, previous introduction to the technique is not necessary. About 20% of the population may be hypnotized to the extent of an anesthetic response for surgical procedures, whereas some 90% are able to undergo surgery with the acupuncture technique. No change in either the conscious state or the subjective behavior is evident during acupuncture, whereas hypnotized subjects require directions to move and speak. A final remark of interest is that some animal species undergo surgery successfully with acupuncture when hypnotic techniques prove to be ineffective.

Of all explanations of acupuncture the *gate control theory* offers the most plausible and widely accepted explanation. Some believe that the suitability of the gate control theory to acupuncture is one of its strongest applications. The gate control theory is a mechanism by which the dynamically active nervous system modifies and modulates input and output related to pain in a flexible manner. In relation to pain modulation, stimulation of acupuncture needles activates more large than small fibers and thus has the effect of closing the gate. (Refer to the explanation of the gate control theory earlier in this chapter.) To explain the position of acupuncture needles in relation to pain in remote organs, theorists believe that neuronal input from acupuncture needles travels to the brainstem, which in turn has a strong inhibitory effect both on other portions of the brain and on the gate control related to the area experiencing pain.

Psychological processes—fear, shock, pain, and anxiety—all have profound effects on the pain experience. These pain-augmenting experiences are alleviated to an amazing degree because the history of acupuncture suggests effectiveness, and the environment in which acupuncture is performed contains positive expressions of assurance.

## Shiatsu

Shiatsu (Japanese for 'finger pressure' and pronounced shee-aht-soo) is the use of finger pressure over a pressure point to allow the client to have self-power and -control.

## Acupressure

Acupressure is compression of a bleeding vessel by insertion of needles into adjacent tissue.

## Biofeedback

The alteration of functions involving autonomic system activity has been possible through biofeedback in recent years. Biofeedback is founded on the principles of operant conditioning, whereby the stimulus reaches the client, and the client then alters visceral response as a result of learning.

At the Menninger Foundation in Topeka, Kansas, clients with histories of migraine headaches engaged in a biofeedback program and learned to shunt blood from their heads to their hands. Ninety percent of the subjects involved were able to control their migraine headaches in this manner, since migraine headaches begin with a distention of the cranial blood vessels (Ferguson, 1973).

A great deal of work is currently being done in utilizing galvanic skin response (GSR) to assist individuals in tuning into and gaining control of their psychological and emotional realms as these factors influence the quality of life.

Kamiya, at the University of Chicago, has also experimented with the control of brain waves, as evidenced on electroencephalographic recordings during relaxation, and has demonstrated that alpha waves may be consciously eliminated or increased in frequency through subjective control after the individual has an indication of their presence through a connection to a sound or blinking light in the laboratory setting (Speeth and Tosti, 1973).

Biofeedback offers many exciting uses in the control of man's internal states. Since these states are inextricably interwoven into the pain experience, recognition and control of these states should continue to have bearing on the issue of pain prevention and remediation as research continues (Danskin and Walters, 1973).

## Relaxation

Mastery of relaxation techniques is important to the nurse who may successfully decrease subjective pain and the use of pharmacological agents through skilled implementation of these methods.

In addition to acupressure, practitioners may utilize a wide variety of techniques in assisting the client to gain control over such pain augmenters as anxiety and increased muscle tension.

Galvanic skin response equipment is utilized in biofeedback to give the client data on the success of relaxation, as well as of autonomic control.

Breathing exercises, wherein the client takes rhythmic large breaths through the nose and then exhales through the mouth in a stimulus-diminished environment, work well when the practitioner or a well-instructed significant other stay with the client to provide a soft, monotone voice in coaching and supportive care. This method often helps the client drift into sleep.

Meditation involves special techniques and exercises to relax specific body parts. Such control is also valuable in reducing pain perception.

Depending on the type of pain, individually tailored exercise may be beneficial in pain control.

### Electrical stimulation

The transcutaneous stimulator for the relief of intractable pain has received widespread attention and has been quite successful in alleviating certain types of pain since about 1967 when it gained wide usage. Its use is based on the gate control theory, so that electrical stimulation to the dorsal columns of the spinal cord activates the large sensory fiber system and thus reduces the excessive activity in the small fiber system. To employ this technique, the client is provided with a pocket-sized transmitter that he or she controls to send radio-frequency impulses to the receiver implanted in the chest wall. The receiver is then connected to electrodes surgically inserted in the medulla or specified brain nuclei. When the client wishes to supersede an undesirable sensory experience, he or she merely manipulates the external transmitter. Details about the transcutaneous stimulator are available in an article by Galvan and Burzaco (1976).

In another article on peripheral neurostimulators the authors disagree with the gate control theory as the underlying explanation and hypothesize the effectiveness of the technique on the basis of altered neuronal activity before the first synapse in the spinal cord (Ignelzi and Nyquist, 1976).

### Surgical relief of pain

Because of the vague and subjective criteria for evaluating the nature and extent of an individual's pain experience, the neurosurgeon is often confronted with the difficult decision of suggesting or negating surgical intervention as a relief modality. When speaking of the surgical procedures utilized to relieve pain, many contemporary writers refer to Shurmann's categorization of these techniques in terms of the first, second, and third neurons (Fig. 10-3).

The *first neuron* refers to surgical intervention in the region of the receptor apparatus of the peripheral afferent nerves and ganglia and at the afferent spinal nerve roots. Such procedures are termed ''radicotomies'' or ''posterior rhizotomies.'' Operative procedures at the level of the first neuron are both successful and commonly done. One type of pain amenable to resection at this level is the local neuroma pain associated with the irritative focus at the stump in amputation. Although resection of the sensorimotor nerve is an uncomplicated measure resulting in relief, regeneration of the neuroma may occur as the central nerve stump revitalizes and regenerates. Thus to prevent such regeneration from central activity, the surgeon must perform endoneural alcohol injection or endoneural destruction with a needle electrode and interrupt the course of axon cylinders that might proliferate from the central nerve section. However, even after all these surgical measures are employed, results from surgical intervention are far from encouraging, particularly when a delay between the onset of pain and surgery has occurred. When simple surgical intervention at the local source of stimulation fails to relieve pain, one realizes that the substantia gelatinosa in the dorsal horn cells of the spinal medulla has begun to respond to the spontaneous neuronal discharges from the neuroma.

When the problem has extended to the level of the dorsal horns, surgical intervention at the posterior roots is no longer helpful. Instead, the problem, if surgically corrected, requires resection at the level of the second neuron in the form of a chordotomy of the spinothalamic tract. Other indications for surgical intervention at the level of the first neuron include problems originating from herpes zoster, neuralgias, and pain from deep-lying organs. Facial pain is most commonly treated with medication rather than surgery. In some conditions at this level, surgical resection to solve the

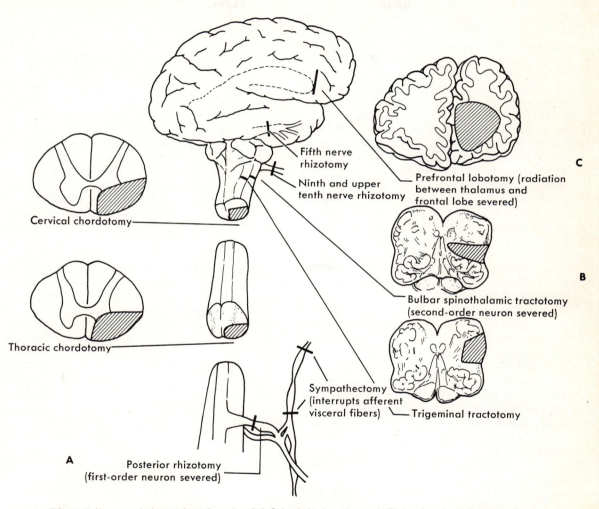

Cervical chordotomy

Thoracic chordotomy

Fifth nerve
rhizotomy

Ninth and upper
tenth nerve rhizotomy

Prefrontal lobotomy (radiation
between thalamus and
frontal lobe severed)

**C**

**B**

Bulbar spinothalamic tractotomy
(second-order neuron severed)

Sympathectomy
(interrupts afferent
visceral fibers)

Trigeminal tractotomy

**A**

Posterior rhizotomy
(first-order neuron severed)

**FIG. 10-3.** Neurosurgical procedures for pain relief. Spinothalamic pathway. *A,* First-order neuron from receptor transmits impulse to cord. Neural cell body is dorsal root ganglion. *B,* Second-order neuron. Neural cell body is dorsal gray matter of cord. This crosses to opposite side and ascends as spinothalamic tract. *C,* Third-order neuron. Neural cell body in thalamus ends in sensory cortex.

pain problem adds increasing difficulty because the nerves severed in the surgical resection contain both sensory and motor components.

The surgical procedure known as posterior rhizotomy involves intradural interruption of the first neuron at a point proximal to the spinal ganglion but distal to the posterior horn cells. This surgical procedure is of particular assistance to clients affected with traumatic or degenerative disorders wherein resulting partial spinal cord lesions have caused painful paraspastic contractions because the posterior rhizotomy diminishes the increased irritability in both the posterior and anterior horns of the spinal medulla (Fig. 10-3).

The explanation underlying the effectiveness of posterior rhizotomy is as follows: When a lesion impinges on the thoracic or cervical cord, forces of extrapyramidal inhibition usually affecting the anterior horn cell operations are rendered ineffective. As a result, striated muscle evidences augmented tone. Concurrently, afferent impulses pass through the spinal reflex arc to the anterior horn cell without the modification normally present from inhibitory forces. The strength of the outgoing motor response is further augmented as intramedullary synaptic neurons transmit the stimulus from one posterior nerve root concurrently to several anterior nerve roots. The resulting neuronal impulse therefore becomes communicated to several segments. For the client, this uninhibited flow of neuronal impulses results in the production of extreme flexion reflexes from slight cutaneous irritation, such as the bed linens resting on the skin. As the surgical intervention interrupts neuronal flow through involved posterior nerve roots, the extreme contractions and pain are alleviated.

Posterior rhizotomy may also be justified for relief of intractable pain, neuralgia caused by herpes zoster, and pain from deep structures. When the procedure is utilized for intractable pain, it should include the nerve roots of all the involved segments to be successful. When posterior rhizotomy is utilized to combat pain from herpes zoster, it may meet with limited success, because this virus may invade nerve processes both in the periphery and in the posterior horn. In such an instance the surgical procedure known as chordotomy of the spinothalamic tract would have preference over the posterior rhizotomy. A posterior rhizotomy may also be unsuccessful when the operative site is not so extensive as necessary. Since sensitivity may extend through overlap into neighboring segments, an adequate operative site for posterior rhizotomy includes the two or three segments on each side of the area involved. A resection of the posterior roots for relief of referred pain from deeper structures meets with success in some clients when surgical resection includes all segments involved in pain production and in other clients is only successful when performed concurrently with a sympathectomy.

The *second neuron* includes intramedullary chordotomies and tractotomies of the spinothalamic tract at different segmental levels of the mesencephalon, medulla oblongata, and cervical or thoracic areas. A disappointing response for permanent pain relief has been reported in relation to surgical intervention at this point. When a chordotomy is performed to alleviate intractable pain in a client with a terminal malignancy who survives less than 18 months, the procedure is deemed a success. However, beyond 18 months there is often renewed pain sensation in the area, as adjacent neuronal tissue assumes the functions for the inactivated neuronal tissue originally responsible for the transmission of pain impulses. Noordenbos (1972) has noted this phenomenon particularly in the anterolateral quadrant of the spinal cord, which is known to contain multiple synapses and fibers. Thus surgery effective in alleviating pain for the longest period should be performed over the largest possible area of the spinal cord. However, the disadvantage of more extensive surgery is that it increases the possibility of interference with other functions of the spinal cord. In considering the point of surgical intervention, one notes that higher points of pain origin require both higher points of surgical intervention and more extensive surgical resections. Pain located in the lower limbs and abdomen may be alleviated by high thoracic chordotomy, whereas pain in the arm and chest is relieved by chordotomies in the cervical region. Since central autonomic pathways are interspersed throughout the medial portion of the spinothalamic tract, a bilateral division of the tract in the thoracic area may result in incontinence in a large number of clients. Because these pathways are more discrete in the cervical area, chordotomies in this region are associated far less frequently with incontinence. When a cervical chordotomy is done, an inadequate division of the nerve fibers may not affect pain relief, whereas a procedure that is too vigorous may cause paralysis of the leg on the opposite side.

Bilateral resection of the cervical or medullary cord should not be performed simultaneously because of the complications arising from the cord edema that might ensue when both sides are involved. However, high bilateral thoracic thoracotomies have proved to be most valuable in interrupting the spinothalamic tracts conveying pain impulses from deep structures and organs. For the most part, mesencephalic tractotomy is not so effective as chordotomies because it does not relieve pain so consistently and because it is associated with severe side effects such as visual and auditory disturbances and severely painful dysethesias that even negate the advantages of a successful surgical procedure.

One additional factor to weigh in considering the merits of chordotomies in individual cases is that less extensive surgical intervention may only compromise pain and thermal sensory modalities, leaving the modalities of touch and position unaffected. If sensory modalities are affected in this manner, the total operations of the individual are not seriously hampered because diminished pain and thermal sensibility in the trunk are not vital components of human functioning. However, when posterior rhizotomies are extensive, the sensory modalities of touch and positional orientation are often compromised. Since positional orientation is significant for human functioning, the loss of such a sensory modality in the trunk may represent a serious infraction interfering with overall mobility.

Surgical relief of pain in the area of the *third neuron* involves stereotactic thalamotomies, which include division of cord fibers between the thalamus and the cortex and corticectomies.

In stereotactic thalamotomies, destruction of adjacent structures may be an outcome of the surgical procedure, and thalamic pain syndromes of an intense nature may occur. Because of the associated problems, thalamotomies should be reserved as a final solution for intractable pain, probably in those with cancer when the malignant invasion is one involving the cranium and facial structures. Even when the impinging thalamic lesion is precisely detected preoperatively by electrophysical means, these complications remain as a detriment to the choice of thalamotomy as a surgical procedure. Once this procedure is elected, leading neurosurgeons believe that the occurrence of the central pain syndrome is less probable when the thalamotomy is extensive enough to include the destruction of both the caudal ventral and the dorsomedian nucleus.

The highest level of interruption for fibers causing pain is the *frontal lobotomy*. The affective response to pain seems to be mediated especially in the bundle of medial white matter known as the cingulum. A lobotomy does not alter the pain threshold but alters the affective response to pain. Thus when questioned, the client reports pain awareness but states that it does not bother him or her even when narcotics are withheld. The problem with frontal lobotomies involves the concurrent changes in personality, that is, loss of finer individual characteristics, apathy, lack of consideration for others, socially unacceptable behavior, aggression, or incontinence. If surgery is unilateral, pain responses are modified, but relief may last for only a few months. Bilateral destruction of these pathways effects permanent changes. A newer technique that involves freezing the involved area may reduce the damage ordinarily related to larger areas included in a resection.

Another intervention for the relief of pain is the use of resections of the sympathetic trunk (sympathectomies). *Sympathectomies* are often indicated for causalgia because of the genesis of pain, wherein excited sympathetic fibers emit impulses to partially damaged nerve fibers. However, even in causalgia, permanent cures are not usually effected by sympathectomy because of the powers of regeneration and the intricate network of pathways through which stimuli may course in the sympathetic system.

Disappointing long-term results have also been noted in sympathectomies for the treatment of chronic and intractable pain, since the sympathetic pathways are utilized by interoceptive pain fibers

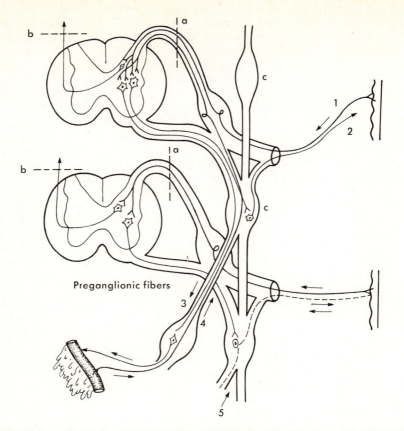

**FIG. 10-4.** Conduction pathways for painful stimuli from visceral organs. The following surgical intervention may occur: *a,* posterior root resection; *b,* chordotomy of spinothalamic tract; or *c,* sympathectomy. *1,* Afferent peripheral impulse transmission; *2,* efferent peripheral impulse transmission; *3,* efferent visceral impulse transmission; *4,* afferent visceral impulse transmission.

of the peripheral nervous system merely as an avenue. Thus sympathectomy often results in less complete resolution of the pain problem than does posterior rhizotomy, unless extensive denervation of a specific organ is accomplished. Still, the problem of pain becoming rerouted over alternate pathways and the regenerative capacities of the sympathetic network make the prospect for long-range success bleak (Fig. 10-4).

## NEW VISTAS

For clients with intractable pain, removal of the pituitary or destruction of it has recently been utilized as a method of controlling generalized pain, such as that occurring in terminal cancer. The pituitary connection is probably attributable to the opiate-like I peptides known as endorphins in the pituitary and hypothalamus. The relationship of hypophysectomy and endorphins is not clear. Other methods of pain control include the introduction of a probe into the sella turcica for electrocoagulation and injection of alcohol. Stereotactic brain lesions in the hypothalamus or the pituitary, or both, might also prove to be useful.

Experiments wherein electrodes are implanted to allow client control of endorphin release for pain regulation will provide important information in the next few years. Some researchers are conducting experiments on endorphin release to better understand psychogenic factors accompanying placebo administration. Others are studying a variety of other stimuli that might effect endorphin release, as well as the results of this phenomenon. Look for a profusion of papers on endorphins in the next few years.

## THE HOSPICE

The word "hospice" goes way back in time. Its derivation from the Latin word *hospitium,* meaning 'hospitality and lodging,' was known to early pilgrims who sought lodging as they traveled. The term later was used to indicate a place where the dying could seek refuge and needed care. Since St. Christopher's Hospice was established in London, England, a few years ago, there has been renewed interest in incorporating the hospice concept as a means of providing comprehensive care for the dying. The hospice approach includes an interdisciplinary effort to care for all needs of the dying client. Trained volunteers are also an important aspect of this movement. The hospice not only meets the needs of the client, but also provides the significant others with essential concrete solutions to problems and emotional support. Some hospices are extending their programs to include home services for those clients that have made the decision to die at home. This effort at encouraging death at home may have psychosocial as well as economic advantages for the client and involved significant others.

An important aspect of the hospice effort is in coping with pain that may be a part of some terminal conditions, such as cancer. Medications are quite often scheduled to avoid the problem of nurse-client bargaining. Bromptom's cocktail is quite often effective in the control of pain, but may need to be combined with other treatments to be totally effective. Phenothiazines and marijuana are used for the control of nausea and vomiting. The use of marijuana, though apparently effective, is still the topic of continuing control and controversy.

## REFERENCES

Barber, T.X., Spanos, N.P., and Chaves, J.F.: Hypnosis, imagination, and human potentialities, Elmsford, N.Y., 1974, Pergamon Press, Inc.

Barrins, P.C.: What nurses need to know about hypnosis, RN **38**:37, Jan. 1975.

Beecher, H.K.: Pain in men wounded in battle, Ann. Surg. **123**:96, 1946.

Beecher, H.K.: Relationship of significance of wound to the pain experienced, J.A.M.A. **161**:1609, 1956.

Beecher, H.K.: Increased stress and effectiveness of placebos and "active" drugs, Science **132**:91, 1960.

Benoliel, J.Q., and Crowley, D.M.: The patient in pain: new concepts, American Cancer Society, Professional Educators Publications, Inc. (Reprinted from Proceedings of the National Conference on Cancer Nursing.)

Black, P.: Management of cancer pain: an overview, Neurosurgery **5**(4):507-517, 1979.

Blitz, B., and Dinnerstein, A.: Effects of different types of instructions on pain paramenters, J. Abnorm. Psychol. **73**:276, 1968.

Breeden, S.A., and Kondo, C.: Using biofeedback to reduce tension, Am. J. Nurs. **75**:2010-2012, Nov. 1975.

Burgess, P.R., and Perl, E.R.: Myelinated afferent fibers responding specifically to noxious stimulation of the skin, J. Physiol. (Lond.) **190**:541, 1967.

Carlen, P.L., et al.: Phantom limbs and related phenomena in recent traumatic amputations, Neurology **28**:211-217, March 1978.

Conway, B., et al.: The seventh right, Am. J. Nurs. **70**:1040-1043, April 1970.

Conway-Rutkowski, B., guest editor: Patient compliance, Nurs. Clin. North Am., March 1983.

Danskin, D.G., and Walters, E.D.: Biofeedback and voluntary self-regulation, Nurs. Digest **1**:9, Sept. 1973.

Devine, R., and Mersky, H.: The description of pain in psychiatric and general medical patients, J. Psychosom. Res. **9**:311, 1965.

Diamond, B.I., and Borison, R.L.: Enkephalins and nigrostriatal function, Neurology **28**:1085-1088, Nov. 1978.

DiBlasi, M., and Washburn, C.J.: Using analgesics effectively, Am. J. Nurs. **79**:74-78, Jan. 1979.

Engel, G.L.: Studies of ulcerative colitis. IV. The significance of headaches, Psychosom. Med. **18**:334, 1956.

Engel, G.L.: Psychogenic pain, Med. Clin. North Am. **42**:1481, 1958.

Engel, G.L.: Psychogenic pain and the pain prone patient, Am. J. Med. **26**:899, 1959.

Ferguson, M.: The brain revolution, New York, 1973, Taplinger Publishing Co., Inc.

Fuller, G.D.: Current status of biofeedback in clinical practice, Am. Psychol. **33**:39-48, Jan. 1978.

Galvan, J., and Burzaco, J.A.: A new transcutaneous stimulator for the nervous system, Med. Biol. Eng. **14**:215, March 1976.

Geldard, F.A.: The human senses, ed. 2, New York, 1972, John Wiley & Sons, Inc.

Gramse, C.A.: For control of severe pain: dorsal column stimulation, Am. J. Nurs. **78**:1022-1025, June 1978.

Hilgard, E.R.: A neodissociation interpretation of pain reduction in hypnosis, Psychol. Rev. **80**:396, 1973.

Hogan, L., and Beland, I.: Cervical spine syndrome, Am. J. Nurs. **76**:1104-1107, July 1976.

Ignelzi, R.J., and Nyquist, J.K.: Direct effect of electrical stimulation on peripheral nerve evoked activity. Implications in pain relief, J. Neurosurg. **45:**159, Aug. 1976.

Isler, C.: New approach to intractable pain, RN **38:**17, Jan. 1975.

Jacox, A.K.: Assessing pain, Am. J. Nurs. **79:**895-900, May 1979.

Janecki, C.J., Jr., and Lipke, J.M.: Whiplash syndrome, Am. Fam. Physician **17:**144-151, April 1978.

Kennard, M.A.: Responses to painful stimuli of patients with severe chronic painful conditions, J. Clin. Invest. **31:**245, 1952.

Kroger, W.S.: Acupunctural analgesia: its explanation by conditioning theory, autogenic training and hypnosis, Am. J. Psychiatry **130:**855, 1973.

Livingston, W.K.: Pain mechanisms, New York, 1943, Macmillan Publishing Co., Inc.

MacKenzie, J.: Symptoms and their interpretations, ed. 3, London, 1918, Oxford University Press.

Melzack, R.: The puzzle of pain, New York, 1973, Basic Books, Inc., Publishers.

Melzack, R., and Bromage, P.R.: Experimental phantom limbs, Exp. Neurol. **39:**261, 1973.

Melzack, R., and Wall, P.D.: Pain mechanisms: a new theory, Science **150:**971, 1965.

Menninger, K.A.: Man against himself, New York, 1938, Harcourt Brace Jovanovich, Inc.

Merskey, H., and Spear, F.G.: Pain: psychological and psychiatric aspects, London, 1967, Baillière Tindall.

Morley, S.: Partial reinforcement in human biofeedback learning, Biofeedback Self-Regul. **4:**221-227, 1979.

Murray, F.S., and Hagan, B.C.: Pain threshold and tolerance of hands and feet, J. Comp. Physiol. Psychol. **84:**639, 1973.

Murray, J.B.: Psychology of the pain experience, J. Psychol. **78:**193, 1971.

Nathan, P.W.: The gate-control theory of pain: a critical review, Brain **99:**123, 1976.

Noordenbos, W.: Causes of failure of surgical treatment in pain: basic principles, pharmacology, therapy, Stuttgart, 1972, Georg Thieme Verlag KG.

Perry, S.W., and Heidrich, G.: Placebo response: myth and matter, Am. J. Nurs. **81:**720, April 1981.

Petrie, A.: Some psychological aspects of pain on the relief of suffering, Am. N.Y. Acad. Sci. **86:**13, 1960.

Petrie, A.: Individuality in pain and suffering, Chicago, 1967, The University of Chicago Press.

Petrovich, D.V.: The pain apperception test: psychological correlates of pain preception, J. Clin. Psychol. **14:**367, 1958.

Plainfield, S., and Adler, N.: The meaning of pain, Dent. Clin. North Am. **6:**659, 1962.

Putt, A.M.: A biofeedback service by nurses, Am. J. Nurs. **79:**88-89, Jan. 1979.

Ruch, T.C.: Somatic sensation: pathophysiology of pain. In Ruch, T.C., et al., editors: Neurophysiology, ed. 2, Philadelphia, 1965, W.B. Saunders Co.

Sacerdote, P.: Theory and practice of pain control in malignancy and other protracted or recurring painful illness, Int. J. Clin. Exp. Hypnosis **18:**160, 1970.

Saunders, C.: The management of terminal illness, Chicago, 1978, Year Book Medical Publishers, Inc.

Silman, J.: Reference guide to analgesics, Am. J. Nurs. **79:** 74-78, Jan. 1979.

Speeth, K., and Boorstein, S., editors: Explorations in transpersonal psychotherapy, Palo Alto, Calif., 1981, Science and Behavior Books.

Staub, E.: Reduction of a specific fear by information combined with exposure to a feared stimulus. Proceedings of the 76th Annual Convention of the American Psychological Association **3:**525, 1968.

Sterman, L.T.: Clinical biofeedback, Am. J. Nurs. **75:**2006-2009, Nov. 1975.

Sutterly, D.C., and Donnelly, G.F.: Perspectives in human development, Philadelphia, 1973, J.B. Lippincott Co.

Sweeney, D.R., and Fine, B.J.: Note on pain reactivity and family size, Percept. Mot. Skills **31:**25, 1970.

Szasz, T.S.: Pain and pleasure: a study of bodily feelings, London, New York, 1975, Basic Books, Inc., Publishers.

Thompson, K.F.: Hypnosis in dental practice: clinical views in control of pain. In Weisenberg, M., editor: Pain: clinical and experimental perspectives, St. Louis, 1975, The C.V. Mosby Co.

Wall, P.D.: The sensory and motor role of impulses travelling in the dorsal columns towards cerebral cortex, Brain **93:** 505, 1970.

Weisenberg, M., et al.: Pain: anxiety and attitudes in black, white and Puerto Rican patients, Psychosom. Med. **37:**123, 1975.

Whipple, D.: Dynamics of development: euthenic pediatrics, New York, 1966, McGraw-Hill Book Co.

Woodrow, K.M., et al.: Pain tolerance: differences according to age, sex, and race, Psychosom. Med. **34:**548, 1972.

Wolff, B.B.: Perceptions of pain, The Sciences **20:**10-13, 28-29, July-Aug. 1980.

Zborowski, M.: People in pain, San Francisco, 1969, Jossey-Bass Inc., Publishers.

# PART THREE

# ASSESSMENT

# 11

# NEUROLOGICAL ASSESSMENT

As researchers study the frontiers of the nervous system, the resulting knowledge is a constant reminder about the significance of neurophysiology to life as we know it. When the functional integrity of the nervous system is impaired, interruptions may occur in behavioral, cognitive, perceptive, and neuromotor capacities.

Nurses are involved in examining the neurological status as part of the total physical assessment of the client in two situations. In the first situation the client is a member of the normal population with no previously identified neurological problem. Examination may confirm normal neurological functioning, or it may reveal an interruption of neurological capacities that deserves more definitive assessment. In the second situation the individual has a neurological disorder that requires definition for purposes of diagnosis and treatment.

Before reading this chapter on neurologic assessment, nurses may find it helpful to review the first four chapters. A thorough acquaintance with normal embryology, neuroanatomy, and neurophysiology is essential before the nurse may identify potential and actual neurological abnormalities, or prior dormant processes. Additionally, the nurse needs a background in normal growth and development at all ages in the life cycle before completing a client assessment.

In this chapter, the emphasis is placed on a neurological assessment as an isolated phenomenon, when in practice it is integrated into a total examination. However, in spotlighting the neurological assessment, the nurse gains the kind of detail needed when thorough evaluation of the nervous system is required.

When the individual has an interruption in neurological functions, the assessment process needs to be ordered in such a way as to place the problem first within a broad category and then through specific testing into a definitive entity. One of the key components in initiating such categorization is a complete and detailed history. As data are uncovered, they may point to a specific category of diseases such as extrapyramidal problems and cerebrovascular problems. Explicit questions are necessary to confirm the problem as a member of the specific group.

The physical assessment and the findings from laboratory, radiological, and specific neurodiagnostic testing are valuable in confirming impressions formed during the history. As abnormal functional capacities appear, the nurse may review the applicable general chapters on behavioral considerations, sleeping disorders, motor disorders, or sensory disturbances, along with specific chapters on infection, degenerative disorders, space-occupying processes, cerebrovascular disturbances, paroxysmal disorders, and developmental, traumatic, or inherited disorders. A review of specific entities within the identified category assists the nurse in formulating definitive questions or determining tests applicable in the individual situation.

When a neurological problem is found, the meticulous process of defining the disturbance is a time-consuming matter that should be done thoroughly. As the physician, nurse, and other health team members uncover the problem, their goals are twofold: First, to offer appropriate assistance to the client and, second, to consider the implications for other family members. For example, if the client has an inherited single-gene disorder (Wilson's disease, Huntington's chorea), remaining family members should be encouraged to have thorough genetic evaluations, especially during pregnancy, to determine whether offspring will have the problem. Because of this objective, there is an increasingly popular trend to take individuals who have been institutionalized for unknown types of mental retardation and completely evaluate their problems in the light of contemporary findings. Although the retarded individual does not always benefit, the findings may assist other family members in choosing childbearing practices or in seeking early intervention, if there is an identified treatment for the problem.

## STANDARDS OF CARE

Assessment is the first step of the nursing process, wherein the next three are planning, implementation, and evaluation. Throughout the application of the nursing process, every attempt should be made to provide quality nursing care. One may get a better idea of the defined standards; activities that measure structure, process, and outcome; and increasing demands for accountability by reading materials such as the 12 volumes of the *Nurse Planning Information Series* available from the National Technical Information Service (5285 Port Royal Road, Springfield, Virginia 22161), the *Accreditation Manual for Hospitals* available from the Joint Commission on Accreditation of Hospitals (875 North Michigan Avenue, Chicago, Illinois 60611), the *Code for Nurses* published by the American Nurses Association, and the *Standards of Nursing Practice* available from the American Nurses' Association (2420 Pershing Road, Kansas City, Missouri 64108). Other materials from the American Nurses Association include specialty-related standards, *Issues in Evaluation Research* (1976), *Standards of Nursing Practice* (1973), and *Plan for Implementation of the Standards of Nursing Practice* (1975). A publication that would be of particular interest to nurses working with the neurological patient would be *Standards of Neurological and Neurosurgical Nursing* (1977), also available from the American Nurses' Association. For a current discussion on particular issues and events in quality assurance, the reader is referred to nursing journals publishing articles on management, which often include this information, and specifically to the *Quality Assur-*

*ance Bulletin,* a monthly publication devoted to the topic.

Some general guidelines for providing quality nursing care to clients throughout their contact with the health care delivery system include the following:

1. Behavior consistent with the ANA Code for Nurses.
2. The use of the nursing process wherein
   a. Data is collected and documented systematically and continuously on client health care status.
   b. Intervention objectives and plans are jointly planned, implemented, and evaluated by the caretaker, client, and nurse, as feasible.
   c. Continual reassessment and revision of written and actual care planning and intervention based on accomplishing preset client outcomes within prescribed interim and terminal deadlines.
3. Follow-up care in prevention, health promotion, or restoration beyond the agency walls. When an abnormality needs to be monitored or treatment plans are prescribed, the client should have written and verbal instructions on self-care or care administered outside of the agency. A method should be developed in each agency to provide structure for a postdischarge contact with the client or others providing care, after the client has been on the treatment program for an appropriately defined period.
4. A complete level-appropriate explanation from a qualified professional of the assessment process, any specific testing that is required, and any findings—normal or abnormal—complete with the significance of said event or problem(s). The nurse may be this individual for parts of this educational process, as appropriate from the educational and experiential background and practice opportunities within the bounds of agency and state governance.
5. The integration of the total individual within his or her perceptual world into the health care delivery system in such a way that the life-style, need systems, and behaviors are preserved within the boundaries of the situa-

tional circumstances, with the nurse functioning as a client advocate.

6. Utilization of appropriate resources and expert others within the health care delivery system to maximize quality care of the client.
7. Coordination of various health care services to maximize benefits for the client and his or her family.

## EQUIPMENT

Before proceeding with the assessment, the practitioner assembles the equipment required for the physical assessment.

An ophthalmoscope with good batteries, so that light is adequate for visualization, is essential. The practitioner also needs a flashlight with a rubber extender so that the skull may be illuminated. A stethoscope and a watch with a second hand in good working order are essential for evaluation of vital signs and bruits. A sphygmomanometer is required to take the blood pressure. A penlight flashlight is valuable because it emits a bright beam for assessing pupillary response. A percussion hammer is needed to evaluate reflexes. In selecting the sharp objects (pins) to be used to test response to pain, one should probably choose sterile needles or safety pins and discard them after use on one individual, since hepatitis may be transmitted by repeated use of the same needles. To assess the visual field the practitioner may purchase from a yard-goods store 1 yard of 2- or 3-inch trim with a repetitive pattern of characters. This fabric is moved steadily and rapidly in a horizontal direction through the visual plane as a means of detecting abnormal eye movements. Some individuals utilize a blunt two-point discriminator or esthesiometer as equipment for one of the sensory tests. A tuning fork and an otoscope are essential for evaluation of auditory integrity, vibration, and hearing. A Snellen eye chart is needed for evaluation of visual acuity. Salt, sugar, vinegar, and quinine are used in the assessment of taste. Stoppered vials of oil of cloves, peppermint, coffee, and soap are often utilized to evaluate the sense of smell. Vials of cold and hot water are used to determine temperature sensibility. Common objects—paper clips, coins, safety pins, and cotton—are needed for a portion of the sensory discrimination. A cotton applicator with the cotton twisted

out over the end is useful in the evaluation of corneal reflexes. A tongue depressor is useful in testing of reflexes and cranial nerves and in assessment of some aspects of sensibility. A diagram of dermatomes (Figs. 3-4 and 3-5) is useful in the evaluation of sensory capacities. Interruptions in sensory capacities may result from disease processes, trauma, space-occupying lesions, or emotional problems. A clean piece of paper and a pencil should also be available if the practitioner believes a writing sample, the production of geometric figures, or a projective drawing test would augment the findings. The practitioner may wish to make a notebook of reading samples at various grade levels for use in the assessment of reading language and comprehension, as well as the educational and cognitive levels. A measuring tape might be quite handy if the disease process has altered body size, as in hypertrophy of calves in muscular dystrophy, wasting of an extremity in paralysis, or increasing head size.

A developmental history is important in many neurological conditions. A number of tools are available, some of which require specialized training to administer, such as standardized psychological or intellectual testing. Others, such as school readiness tests, the Denver Developmental Screening Test, or the Denver Articulation Screening Examination may be readily administered by the nurse. However, the choice of testing tools is often limited by age. Improvisation may be necessary for older individuals. In compiling data samples, the practitioner should base questions and norms for answers on well-accepted information.

Two other instruments may be helpful in assisting the practitioner with a thorough assessment. A dynamometer measures grip strength, whereas a goniometer measures joint motion, like a protractor measures angles in mathematics.

While gathering equipment, the practitioner should pay attention to the environment wherein the history and physical examination will occur. The area should be esthetically as pleasing as possible. The arrangement of furniture should allow for facilitation of relaxed discussion. Equipment for testing should be arranged so that it is organized for orderly use.

For the history the client should be comfortably positioned in a chair; for most of the physical assessment he or she should be placed on an examining table in drapes. For the parts of the examination where client participation is required the client should be allowed to dress comfortably in such a manner as to provide an unobstructed view of the body part under study. Age-appropriate modifications are made as applicable.

## HISTORY

After the equipment has been assembled and the practitioner has attempted to make the client comfortable, the history is taken. Quite often the history is most important in identification of the nature of the problem. Although the physical assessment is also valuable in providing adjunctive preliminary data, it may often be used to validate a presumptive diagnosis gleaned from the history.

Since the nervous system is often affected by problems arising from other systems (diabetes, pernicious anemia, cancer, infections, hypertension) or manifests symptoms of disturbed functions in organs outside the nervous system, that is, bowel, bladder, and sexual disturbances, the history and physical examination should be comprehensive enough to identify these abnormalities.

When the nurse asks the series of questions to clarify the problem and the events preceding it, it is important to be certain that words the client uses in description have the same meaning to the nurse. For example, in describing a convulsion, many lay persons define the episode as a grand mal event only and may think of other types of seizures as spells. Accurate term clarification avoids the possibility of the nurse counting a number of episodes different from what the client has experienced.

The practitioner should carefully detail the client's perception of the problem and the events leading up to the disturbance. Where possible, the client's words for a symptom or problem should be indicated in parentheses, especially when they represent unusual usage. In identifying a point of difficulty—numbness, pain, or anesthesia, one should elicit exacting details with specific adjectives about the character of the problem, the mode of onset, the length of endurance, the frequency of episodes, the precipitating factors, or associated events. The client should point to the area involved so that it may be delineated in precise anatomical terms. Such vague descriptions as

''I have pain in my hand'' or ''my arm just feels funny'' should be discouraged.

Because so many neurological entities have distinct modes of onset, it is extremely important to clearly define the characteristics and progression of those symptoms. It is important to note abrupt versus gradual onsets and waxing and waning versus consistent symptoms. The sequence of progression should be in chronological order so that any reader can understand the logical history of the problem.

When a client explains symptoms that could fit into more than one disease entity, it is important to ask questions that rule out the possibility of other symptoms. By recording the lack of some symptoms, the practitioner may eliminate some of the diagnostic possibilities.

Identify the pathological condition in the family tree over the past three generations (pedigree). List all significant medical conditions, surgical interventions, and hospitalizations over the client's lifetime. In recording this section one needs to be concise but accurate.

The practitioner needs to know about any allergies or adverse reactions to drugs or other substances. If the client takes any medication, it is detailed. Often when this question is posed, individuals quickly describe prescriptive medications but fail to mention regular use of aspirin, laxatives, or other self-prescribed medications. Oral contraceptives cause a number of symptoms, and the practitioner needs to verify their use in a discreet manner.

Ask the client what his or her expectations are in relation to the problem, treatment modalities, and outcomes. One should also elicit information about how to make the situation as agreeable as possible in terms of maintaining client comfort, safety, protection, and security in such a manner that the client feels cared for.

After speaking to the client, the practitioner utilizes available opportunities to speak to relatives, especially when the client's problem hampers a comprehensive view of the situation. Items the client may have problems relating include alterations in behavior and personality, particularly when such changes are gradual. The family may also be able to relate further data about incidents the client cannot recall—events of a stroke, concussion, or paroxysmal disorder. If the client seems to be an unreliable historian for any reason, interviews with a relative may give a more accurate history. The family may also relate a detail about the individual's psychological or economic status that sheds new light on the problem.

## Client interview

The interview begins as the nurse obtains enough information to get a overview of the situation. Thus any immediate needs may be met. When the client is able to continue, the remaining history may be taken. If the client has problems that interfere with the history-taking process, the practitioner may need to elicit information from an appropriate significant other.

The sociocultural data and the vital statistics frequently alert the nurse to a presumptive diagnosis on a statistically probable basis. Many disorders of the nervous system are related to factors such as age, sex, environmental conditions, trauma, activity level or safety, inheritance, opportunities in life, or a behavioral phenomenon.

Many practitioners can identify characteristics of the local community in relation to belief systems, language usage, or ethnocultural affiliations that directly affect coping behaviors, emotional support systems, nutritional and health care practices, and other key behaviors. The practitioner should particularly seek information about the relationship of these factors to health maintenance practices. Continue questioning to learn about the type, quality, specific professional or professionals, and frequency of any health-maintenance activities.

Individual adjustment capacities have a great impact on the provision of health care, individual response patterns, and comprehensive outcomes to the health care process. Obtain the information suggested in the following outline to acquire a framework for better understanding of the client.

## CLIENT HISTORY
### Summary of health care status

*Name, age, sex, race, marital status*
*Description of client* —Height, weight, phenotype, obvious physical or behavioral health care problems.
*Previous health history* —Major illnesses, childhood communicable diseases, hospitalizations, surgery.

*Immunization status* —Prescriptive and nonprescriptive.
*Current medications* —Medications, alcohol, tobacco, socially related substances.
*Allergies* —Ingestive and environmental
*Immediate needs* —Stop the interview to provide essentials for the client such as insulin, suction, oxygen, positioning, food, rest-room break, significant other needs.

### General sociocultural data

*Educational level* —Note response and performance level.
*Developmental milestones*
*Personality and psychosocial development* —Utilize the Eight Stages of Man according to Erickson to evaluate this.
*Members of living group* —Age, relationship, school level or vocation.
*Client role and performance level in living group, community vocation, or school* —Include income figures and insurance coverage.
*Pedigree*
*Environmental evaluation*
  Description of housing.
  Infection and pollution control.
  Work and living environment.
  Architectural barriers (if applicable).
  Alterations needed to improve client health care.
*Community resources*
  Ethnocultural affiliations that may affect coping behaviors, emotional support systems, nutritional and health care practices, and so on.
*Health maintenance practices*
  Note type, by whom, professional title, frequency.

### Individual adjustment capacities

Identification of significant others and the relationship.
Personal and family response to current problem or illness, if any.
Interaction patterns between significant others and client.
Effect illness or problem has on livelihood, life goals, and daily living.
Spiritual resources or religious affiliation (determine beliefs that affect nutrition, health practices, prescribed treatments, and views on life and death).
Avocational interests, hobbies, pasttimes.
Typical daily schedule in usual health and with current problem, if any.
Ideal versus real roles and performance expectations within the family, community and work or school environments.
Special needs related to age or inappropriate adjustment.

### Dependency, independency, and coping patterns

What is the level of independence in ADL (activities of daily living—areas of need, use of significant others, and use or need of community resources)?

What makes client afraid? What helps?

What makes the client sad? What helps?

What makes the client happy?

What are the major changes or crises that have occurred in the past year?

What are the client's three worst problems right now?

What are the client's three greatest strengths?

When the client has problems, how does he or she solve them?

Is there anyone or anything that the client turns to for hope and strength?

Is that resource currently available?

Does the client have special needs related to inappropriate behavior or age?

How does the client cope in relation to others in his or her opinion?

What would help the client cope more effectively?

What can we do during this visit or hospital stay to make matters and routines better for the client?

Would the client like a significant other or others to be included in health care or education?

What are the client's expectations related to possible needs or problems, treatment, professional care, outcomes for self and significant others?

Describe previous experience with illness or hospitalization and need for education or orientation.

Give explanation regarding possible client and nurse planning and review of nursing care.

### Behavioral response patterns

General mood, verbal and nonverbal expression.

Incidence of involuntary behaviors or sounds.

Response to varying levels and types of environmental stimuli.

Discomforts that may inhibit observation of typical behaviors.

General activity level.

Attention and concentration.

Ability to follow directions.

Priority setting and goal completion.

Insight into consequences.

Emotional stability.

Input from significant others, reports from school or work, or other professional evaluations.

### Routine activity patterns

#### Rejuvenation

Past or current problems with sleep, rest, or relaxation.

Rest and sleep patterns (times, wakeful periods, insomnia, and so on).

Does rest routine cause client to feel adequately rested?

What measures or aids facilitate sleep?

#### Nutritional patterns and related factors

Past or current problems with eating or digestion.

Evaluate adequacy and intake of basic four foods.

Quantity of daily fluid intake.

Preferences and dislikes.

Pattern of meals and snacks.

Change in food habits in illness.

Assistance and aids required in eating.

Problems in chewing and swallowing.

Oral-hygiene routine or care of cleanliness of oral cavity prosthesis.

Condition of teeth and gums.

Evaluate possible problems related to appropriate appetite, thirst, weight maintenance, and digestive disturbances (include assessment of abdominal feeling after eating: pain, discomfort, nausea, vomiting, and excessive gas production).

Special needs related to disease or age.

#### Elimination patterns and related factors

Bowels

Past or current disorders.

Time and frequency of bowel movements.

Description of stool (color, consistency, amount, presence or absence of blood).

Hemorrhoids.

Pain (location, relationship to defecation; see the pain rating scale, p. 228).

Medications and habits that interfere with bowel functioning.

Medicinal aids and routines that facilitate adequate bowel habits.

Special needs related to disease or age.

Urinary system

Past or current problems with the urinary tract.

Daily fluid intake.

Nature of urinary output (frequency during day and night, bedwetting—especially after toilet training is complete or usual—loss of sphincter control, dysuria, amount, color, odor, specific gravity from urinalysis, if available).

Special needs related to disease or age.

Edema.

### Sensation

Pain assessment (refer to Chapter 10).

Past or current problems with smell, taste, sight, hearing, spatial orientation, touch, temperature, pain, pressure, speed of response, equilibrium.

Use and care of prosthetic devices.

Unusual sensory experiences.

### Musculoskeletal functions

*Past or present problems* with muscle strength, tone, reflexes, range of motion, motility, muscle control, or physical endurance.

*Perceptual-motor problems*—"soft signs" such as clumsiness, impaired fine motor coordination, increased or decreased general activity or level of minimal brain dysfunction, hyperkinesis, learning disability. Refer to Chapter 8 for more detail.

*Activity level*

Aids.

Safety factors related to age or impaired mobility.

Assistance required in activities of daily living.

Description of current muscular impairment or limitation in range of motion.

Current medication that interferes with or enhances muscular functions.

Special needs related to age or impaired functions.

### Nervous system

Past or current problems with intellectual functions, sensation, movement, or pain.

Past or present problem that was inherited or in other family members.

Problems with "nerves," that is, behavioral capacities.

Mental retardation in client or family.

Seizure disorders or "spells" in client or family.

Fainting spells, dizzy spells, or lapses in awareness or consciousness (see Chapter 14).

Tics and involuntary movements.

Headaches, back problems, or whiplash.

Malignancy.

Accidents that involve damage to head, spinal area or peripheral nerves.

Ability to learn new skills, perform them, and remember new information.

Communication and speech patterns.

Current medication usage that inhibits or enhances nervous system activities.

Special needs related to age or disease process.

### Integument

Past or current conditions of the skin, scalp, and nails.

Description of skin (color, temperature, turgor, circulatory impairment, and texture).

Lesions (note appearance, size, and precise location).

Skin care routine (hair, bathing, nails, special aids or treatments).

Sensitivity to pollens, insect bites, contact poisons, sun, and other substances resulting in an allergic response).

### Endocrine functions

Growth patterns.

Conditions related to underfunctioning or overfunctioning of the endocrine system.

General stress level.

Use of steroids within the past year.

Medication usage that facilitates or inhibits endocrine functions.

Disorders that require special assistance.

Family history of undergrowth, overgrowth, diabetes, or reproductive problems.

### Sexual functions

*History of sexual activity, infections, and disorders of reproductive system*

*Birth history* (gestation, labor, delivery, Apgar score, and perinatal period, if client remembers)

*Reproductive facts*

Number of pregnancies.

Outcome—sex and health of each offspring

Menstrual pattern, problems with menses, and menopause.

Family planning—philosophy, methods.

Gynecological problems.

Health routines.

Breast self-examination.

Vaginal examination and Pap smear.

Attitudes toward sexuality (refer to Chapter 6).

*Medication that affects the reproductive system*

### Cardiovascular system

Past or present disease of the cardiovascular system.

Presence of hypertension, high cholesterol levels, any unusual spell, edema, chest pain, or "little strokes."

Activity endurance or fatigability.

Subjective temperature differences in varying body parts.

Tingling or burning sensation in extremities.

Medications used that enhance or inhibit cardiovascular functions.

### Respiratory functions

Past or current respiratory problems.

History of allergies, asthma, frequent infections, orthopnea, or hemoptysis.

Cough (note frequency, type, and duration; describe sputum, if cough is productive).

Last test for tuberculosis (type, date, and reaction).

Shortness of breath (precipitating factors, frequency, measures that relieve symptoms, and effect on activities of daily living).

Smoking (type, frequency, duration, and success at eliminating the habit).

Environmental pollutants affecting respiration.
Medications that enhance or inhibit respiratory functions.

*Summary*

1. Note behaviors, symptoms, and historical findings support, and also those that seem inconsistent with, the practitioner's impressions.
2. Identify areas that require further investigation during the physical assessment, through specialized evaluations and through diagnostic testing.
3. Consult the appropriate physician about findings that may influence the medical or general management. Plan client objectives, interventions, and evaluation at least jointly, if not with additional health professionals, so that all health care is well coordinated.
4. Continue the assessment process with the physical evaluation.

Health care and the state of wellness in an individual has the potential for bringing out both the best and the worst in individuals as their patterns of dependency-independency and coping are bared to the practitioner. A thorough review of these patterns during the history may equip the practitioner with essential information for planning further care and in anticipating an individual's responses. A closely related area of importance is that of behavioral response patterns. Knowledge in these areas may make the difference between what works and what does not for neurological clients who may face a multiplicity of physical, behavioral, or cognitive problems.

Making nursing decisions is also contingent on a thorough investigation of a client's routine activity patterns and biologic rhythms and on an understanding of specific operations of bodily functions and systems. After the history-taking process is over, the practitioner should do the following: (1) Identify areas that require further investigation through further verbal questioning or physical assessment, (2) consult a neurologist or the appropriate physician about findings that may influence medical or general case management, (3) continue the assessment with the physical evaluation, and (4) involve the client and his or her significant others, as indicated, in the care-planning process. From this point onward, the practitioner may continue the health care delivery process appropriately when following guidelines suggested in the section on Standards of Care.

Refer to the preceding outline of significant points when taking a client history, as follows.

## FACTORS IN PRENATAL AND INFANT ASSESSMENTS

Adequate provisions for programs of assessment and health maintenance from conception to maturation occur in a variety of settings. For the midwife the assessment and subsequent treatment of the mother and the unborn child begin during pregnancy and continue through the first few weeks of neonatal life. Practitioners specializing in labor, delivery, and hospital nursery settings also have increasing responsibilities in the prenatal and perinatal periods for the early detection of congenital anomalies or functional impairments in the neonate. These observations become extremely critical, since the practitioner's most intensive period of contact with the mother and neonate has been reduced by shortened hospital stays and early discharges for both mother and neonate.

In Desmond's study the importance of serial observations during the first 6 hours after birth were stressed, since the neonate experiences many changes in physical reorganization during this period. Abnormal events may occur at this time even when the prenatal progress and delivery seemed unremarkable.

After discharge the practitioner in the community setting has a growing responsibility to detect impairments in growth and development, incorporating the latest information in diagnostics and case management.

### Problem definition

A great deal of emphasis has been placed on the detection of impaired functions in infancy. However, periodic assessments throughout life are also important in spotting abnormalities, which may not be manifested immediately; impairments resulting from disease; or trauma occurring after birth.

Early recognition and precise definition of impaired neurological functioning or maturation are paramount, affording the opportunity for early referral to appropriate health team members for intervention and potential avoidance of secondary problems.

The assessment guide detailed in this chapter is

divided into age-related characteristics and is usually only utilized in its entirety when a suspicion of neurological problems exists. Even though the neurological evaluation may be performed by age groups, a comprehensive history frequently is the key component when one determines the basic neurological problem at all ages.

In neurological assessments where a potential impairment exists the practitioner should consider the outcome of the assessment in terms of the general groupings presented throughout this book, which include (1) static lesions in prenatal, perinatal, and postnatal development; (2) abnormalities in metabolism; (3) progressive degenerative or demyelinating diseases; (4) inherited disorders; (5) muscle defects; (6) nerve root, central, or peripheral nerve problems; (7) autonomic nervous system dysfunctions; (8) paroxysmal disorders; (9) trauma or space-occupying lesions in the nervous system; (10) infections and invasive disorders; and (11) problems related to specific learning disabilities or functional capacities.

After deciding which category of nervous disorders best characterizes a client's problems, the practitioner should continue testing to obtain a more definitive picture of the problem within the given disease group. The specification of neurological problems through complete clinical examinations is important in providing adequate treatment, in ensuring adequate diagnostic testing, and in defining the problem sufficiently so that the appropriate specialists may be utilized. Moreover, a thorough understanding of the components of the various categories allows practitioners to play a major role in guidance and long-term management of neurological disturbances, which may have a prolonged effect on health outcomes and usual living patterns.

The assessment process begins with an inquiry into the paternal and maternal history, the growth patterns of other siblings, prenatal course, emotional factors, and socioeconomic influences.

## Paternal life patterns

To better comprehend the life context that the newborn enters, the practitioner should elicit details on the father's background and current status. First, it is helpful to discern the axis of organization that characterizes this family. (See Chapter 5 to review common models.) Next, the practitioner should become acquainted with the cultural system and the groups in which the family holds membership. Such information leads naturally to a view of family values and expectations.

The practitioner attempts to summarize key events in the father's growth and development. Included in this synopsis are items such as inherited disorders in the family lineage, significant illnesses, maturational delays, and other medical or surgical events. Careful interviewing is required at this point to be certain that all neurological impairments in relatives, such as mental retardation, seizures, degenerative illnesses, complications in pregnancy in the paternal grandmother, or death in siblings, have been explained. It should be pointed out that neurological problems that occurred many years ago may have evaded modern clinical description. For example, a pathological condition in the family lineage in one instance was recalled as the father casually mentioned an uncle who had always lived with the paternal grandparents and did things that made everyone laugh. In fact, in detailing the memory, the father said, "Something must have been wrong with him, but no one ever discussed it. . . . I don't know what ever happened to him."

Current health status, age, occupation, and learning capacities are evaluated next. In discussing learning capacities, the father should be asked what was the last grade he completed in school. The practitioner should also be alert to a history of any specific learning disabilities, as discussed in Chapter 8.

## Maternal life patterns

A similar line of interviewing is appropriate to elicit details on inherited disorders in the mother's family lineage, pattern of growth and development, significant illnesses, impairments, and medicosurgical events. Learning capacities of the mother are also an important area to explore, since they are related to the child's values with respect to learning and language acquisition, as detailed in Chapter 5. It is also helpful to know the mother's current health status, age, blood type, level of education, occupation, and her plans concerning employment and child-rearing.

*Age and parity.* The extremes of age in childbearing, that is, under age 16 years or over age 36 years for the primipara and over age 40 years for the multipara, tend to be associated with a higher number of problematic fetal outcomes. Increased risk is also evident in women who have had five or more children or who produced their children in rapid succession. Maternal age is apparently a causative factor in disorders, such as Down's syndrome, since chromosomal material changes with advancing age. Multiple or closely spaced pregnancies present a problem, since they strain the biological abilities of the body to support the demands of fetal growth. Further investigation is necessary to delineate the exact factors interacting in extremes of age and parity as they relate to increased fetal risk.

## Siblings

At this point the practitioner should elicit detailed information on the health and well-being, age, growth sequences, learning capacities, sex, and any untoward events related to siblings of the fetus. In listening to the sibling history, the practitioner should be alert to any psychosocial or physiological factors that might have a bearing on the status of the fetus or child.

## Prenatal course

The history of the prenatal course should begin with information as to the mother's initiation of menses, typical menstrual cycles, past pregnancies, and associated complications. Any miscarriages, congenital anomalies, or other problems noted in reproduction should be noted. Some examples of other problems might be prematurity, cervical incompetence, stillbirth, ectopic pregnancy, placenta previa, or any fetal or neonatal deaths.

Finally, attention is focused on the current pregnancy. One of the first areas of exploration comprises the beliefs, attitudes, and subsequent health practices that the expectant mother utilizes. Knowledge of superstitious beliefs or cultural and personal practices that may damage the unborn child are essential to the practitioner, who is trying to establish a realistic approach to prenatal care and instruction. When a mother refuses to heed a necessary health practice after apparent understanding and acceptance of the matter, the practi-

tioner should take a closer look at the family organization to determine the possible influence of a strong family member who may encourage the mother to disregard the advice.

## Emotional factors

In most cases the birth of a child is a happy, long-awaited event. However, in situations where the family income is inadequate, the child is born out of wedlock, the pregnancy is unwanted, the parents are poorly educated or mentally retarded, or the mother or father is afflicted by a problem such as mental illness, alcoholism, or drug addiction, the birth of the infant may not be well received. Practitioners should be alert to instances wherein a pregnant woman fails to have prenatal care, to attend clinic or doctor's office appointments regularly, or to make provisions for the hospitalization. The practitioner should also be alert to the woman who exhibits excessive stress or anxiety and who may have inadequate psychic reserves for coping with pregnancy. Such an individual needs careful follow-up and possibly referral for psychotherapy to avoid behaviors that may potentially harm the fetus or child.

## Socioeconomic factors

In recent years socioeconomic factors have received increasing attention because of their profound effect on the health, well-being, and nutritional status of the expectant mother and her unborn child. Investigators are beginning to associate poor health care and nutrition with low birth weights, inadequate intrauterine environments, prematurity, and growth interferences. Severe dietary deficiencies have also been related to impaired neuronal growth in the brain. However, because of limitations in measurement techniques, attention has been focused on defective glial multiplication and myelination mainly in animals.

In addition to those environmental factors that are observable and potentially within practical individual control are those potentially hazardous elements in the environment that may be beyond the awareness or direct control of the average expectant mother and father. Examples of such hazards include air and water pollution levels, irradiation in the surrounding atmosphere, and increasing amounts of psychological and physiological stress associated with the accelerated pace of modern living.

## Intrauterine environment

A multiplicity of factors interact to produce an adequate intrauterine environment. Thus even when the practitioner elicits a deviation from the normal prenatal course, it is often difficult to predict the exact effect that the factor has on fetal outcome, except in instances where definitive testing is available.

## Placenta

One of the first considerations in evaluating the fetal environment is the efficient functioning of the placenta, the interconnection between the mother and the fetus that provides vital products of life and waste removal. After birth it is wise to keep the placenta until it may be thoroughly examined by a specialist to determine any physiological deviations, particularly in cases where the neonate has problems.

In assessing maternal requirements and fetal outcomes in relation to medications, it is safest for the practitioner to assume that all medications cross the placental barrier. Thus consultation with appropriate specialists and current research is imperative when any unusual material is being given to the mother or when the mother is known to have ingested such material, since the teratogenic effects of many materials are difficult to evaluate and may even vary at different points of pregnancy within the same individual.

Placental inadequacy during pregnancy is also a consideration when the height of the fundus is not compatible with the gestational age or when there is a history of preeclampsia, toxemia, prolonged gestation, or vaginal bleeding.

## Maternal conditions associated with fetal outcomes

A number of concurrent medical problems in the mother are assumed to have an effect on fetal development. Included in the metabolic category are diabetes mellitus and malnutrition. Diabetes mellitus in the mother increases the fetal risk for prematurity, hyaline membrane disease, hyperbilirubinemia, macrosomatia, hypocalcemia, renal vein thrombosis, polyhydramnios, and congenital mal-

formations. Additionally, as the fetus of a diabetic mother develops, the maternal stimulation of hyperglycemia causes the fetal pancreas to overproduce insulin. Thus at birth the neonate is large and has a peach-colored appearance and an overabundance of fatty tissue.

Malnutrition in the mother not only constitutes a socioeconomic problem, but also prevents acceptable fetal metabolism, because of the inadequate supply of the essential materials for growth. Such inadequate resources result in intrauterine growth retardation with the sequelae mentioned earlier in this chapter.

Maternal endocrine disorders such as Addison's disease may result in prematurity and intrauterine growth retardation, whereas hypothyroidism is associated with abnormalities of the central nervous system and hypothyroidism in the neonate.

Certain cardiovascular problems in the mother are associated with placental insufficiency in the developing fetus and potential prematurity, delayed growth, and asphyxia.

Pulmonary interferences, such as intractable asthma with hypoxemia and hypercapnia or status epilepticus, may result in hypoxia or asphyxia in the fetus.

Two of the hematological problems that cause concern are blood incompatibilities and anemias. The major problems of incompatibility associated with the Rh factor or the major blood groups between fetal and maternal circulation are manifested in hyperbilirubinemia and erythroblastosis fetalis.

In the case of Rh-factor incompatibilities, maternal antibodies are developed against the Rh-positive blood cells in the fetus. These antibodies then cross placental barriers, where they have a destructive effect on cells in the fetal circulation. Since the D antigen is involved in about 93% of these cases, with rarer Rh antigens composing the remaining percentage, the availability of anti-D globulin has resulted in successful outcomes for many individuals affected by Rh isoimmunization. Since a little as 0.5 ml of fetomaternal bleeding has been known to cause maternal sensitization, practitioners should consider Rh isoimmunization in maternity patients who have undergone cesarean section, prolonged labor, forceps delivery, manually removed placenta, or early abortion or who have received oxytocin. Early abortions are known to sensitize affected women, since the Rh antigen is present by the sixth week of pregnancy. Moreover, practitioners should recognize that the effects of Rh isoimmunization on previous siblings is not indicative of the current fetal status. However, Liley's method of evaluating the bilirubin level in the fetus provides data necessary to the physician, who must decide if an intrauterine transfusion or an early delivery is warranted.

Anemias occur in several forms, such as megaloblastic, sickle-cell, or iron-deficiency anemias. Megaloblastic anemia is associated with abruptio placentae, sickle-cell anemia with a low birth weight, and iron-deficiency anemia with a low birth weight and prematurity. These anemias are not always responsive to adequate dietary measures and may cause fetal insufficiencies as a result of their effect on maternal hemoglobin levels and the decreased concentration of red blood cells in the maternal circulatory system.

Another category of diseases that interferes with fetal growth and normal functioning includes viral, protozoan, and bacterial infections. Sepsis in the newborn may be associated with maternal infections transmitted in either the prenatal or the perinatal period.

Rubella, one of the best-known viruses that crosses the placental barrier, causes devastating effects, such as cataracts, congenital heart disease, deafness, mental retardation, and microcephaly, especially when the infection occurs during the first month of gestation. Other invasive agents associated with undesirable fetal outcomes are *Toxoplasma gondii,* cytomegalovirus, and herpesvirus hominis; these are further detailed in Chapter 13.

## PRENATAL ASSESSMENT

For pregnant women receiving prenatal care, practitioners usually assess the adequacy of fetal growth by making serial evaluations of fundus height in relation to the last menstrual period and current gestational age. Auscultation and palpation of uterine contents reveal fetal heart sounds, movement, and position as the pregnancy progresses. Viewing the cervix and vagina in early pregnancy provides the practitioner with information on the pelvic structure. To accompany this external view, pelvic bone measurements are re-

corded during an early visit. Thus pelvic dimensions may be gauged in relation to adequacy for delivery.

Throughout pregnancy the mother is monitored for general health and specifically for body functions that may interfere with a normal gestational period. At frequent intervals, weight, urine, blood, and blood pressure are evaluated to ascertain functional adequacy. Serological tests for veneral disease and vaginal smears, as indicated, for other infections result in early intervention and treatment of potentially harmful conditions. Special tests or treatments may be indicated in accordance with the individual history or disease problems prevalent in certain geographic locales or populations.

### Special techniques

When the usual methods of monitoring the fetus are inadequate in evaluating the gestational age and well-being of the fetus, several biochemical and electronic testing devices are available for the practitioner's use. Understanding the principles and indications involved in the utilization of each of these parameters of measurement is essential to the practitioner.

The major testing procedures utilized include radiological examination, ultrasonic cephalometry, amniocentesis, and assessment of maternal urine.

*Radiological examination.* Radiological studies of bone growth centers, especially in the long bones and skull, during the later part of pregnancy are utilized to assess fetal maturity. However, this method does not reveal inadequate intrauterine growth.

*Ultrasonic cephalometry.* Ultrasonic cephalometry, a newer, less hazardous method of gauging fetal growth by monitoring the deflection of ultrasonic waves from the fetal skull on an oscilloscope, reveals the three-dimensional measurements of the skull. This measurement may be accurately correlated with gestational age.

*Amniocentesis.* Amniocentesis, a method of removing amniotic fluid from the uterus for assay during pregnancy, is used in estimating fetal growth and well-being, maternal conditions, and inherited disorders. The first two reasons for amniocentesis are reviewed here. Studies on cultured cells of amniotic fluid may be done on clients where inherited disorders are a problem. The resulting findings may assist the client in deciding about elective abortion.

As the fetus matures, chemical and cellular changes in the amniotic fluid have an important diagnostic value. By the fourteenth week of gestation, the amniotic fluid contains fetal urine. When fetal kidneys function normally, the levels of creatinine and urea increase, whereas osmolality decreases in the amniotic fluid as the fetus matures. As the hepatic system matures in fetal life, levels of bilirubin in the amniotic fluid vary. Unconjugated bilirubin levels increase until the thirteenth week of gestation and decrease sharply at term.

Changes in the fat content of various fetal cells that are apparent in amniotic fluid are also utilized as determinants of gestational age. Of the lipid measurements, the lecithin-sphingomyelin (L-S) ratio is one of the most significant determinations. In this measurement the changing level of the phospholipid lecithin is compared to sphingomyelin, a stable substance in amniotic fluid. When lecithin in the amniotic fluid occurs in a 2:1 ratio to sphingomyelin, adequate lung surfactant is generally present to allow the lungs to inflate and function properly after birth. Inadequate quantities of surfactant result in respiratory distress syndrome (formerly called "hyaline membrane disease").

Gestational age may also be determined by the use of special staining techniques to show the presence of two types of desquamated fetal cells, basal and precornified, which appear in varying quantities and form, according to the stage of fetal maturity.

*Assessment of maternal urine.* Maternal urine may also be monitored for estriol concentrations. Estriol is a substance synthesized by the fetus that is eventually excreted through maternal urine. Thus adequate estriol concentrations are associated with acceptable placental functioning and fetal well-being. When serial estriol levels reveal low concentrations, intrauterine growth retardation is indicated. Decreasing estriol levels are associated with impending fetal death, and thus immediate delivery is warranted when possible.

## PERINATAL ASSESSMENT

In monitoring the process of labor and delivery, the practitioner should carefully describe and re-

port the following symptoms to the obstetrician: (1) changes in fetal activity or fetal heart rate; (2) presence of meconium during or after membranes rupture, since the passage of meconium is probably the result of increased peristalsis and relaxation of the fetal and sphincter in response to anoxia; and (3) bradycardia or tachycardia persisting after contractions. These occurrences are correlated with maternal events. Thus all activity, changes, vital signs, details on medications, status of membranes, bleeding, and progress in labor should be noted with the time of the event.

### Fetal monitoring

Traditionally the fetal heart rate has been monitored periodically throughout labor by the use of stethoscopic auscultation. However, newer methods are widely available that allow for more complete and consistent monitoring. Such sophisticated monitoring mechanisms provide valuable information essential to fetal heart rate interpretation for all labors and deliveries. However, such data are especially crucial to the fetus and mother subject to increased risk. Although techniques in fetal electrocardiography are generally available, two other types of monitoring are in more common use, namely, ultrasonic and electronic monitoring. An additional method involves the use of pH determinations.

*Ultrasonic monitoring.* Ultrasonic monitoring utilizes the Doppler high-frequency sound waves to monitor both uterine contractions and fetal heart rate transabdominally. The apparatus is best understood through the description and explanation given in the manufacturer's instructions.

*Electronic monitoring.* Electronic monitoring is a direct method wherein an electrode is attached to the presenting portion of the fetus and a catheter electrode is introduced into the uterus after the maternal membranes have ruptured.

*pH determinations.* Another method of monitoring the fetus is by conduction of blood gas and pH determinations of fetal scalp capillary samples. These determinations provide valuable adjunctive data to ultrasonic and electronic monitoring.

Basically the fetal scalp capillary pH decreases from a range of between 7.32 and 7.35 to between 7.25 and 7.28 as labor progresses; this is a result of the concurrent drop in maternal bicarbonate and pH levels. Levels below 7.25 indicate hypoxia and excessive acidosis in the fetus.

The acid-base determinations obtained from fetal scalp samples correlate highly with the 1-minute Apgar scores (see subsequent discussion of Apgar score), which reflect the degree of birth asphyxia and the subsequent need for resuscitation. However, the 5-minute scores more accurately predict morbidity and long-term survival. In fact, the collaborative study done by the National Institute of Neurological Diseases and Stroke in Bethesda, Maryland, from 1957 to 1970 on cerebral palsy, mental retardation, and other neurological and sensory problems in infancy and childhood revealed that neonates with an Apgar score of 0 to 3 at age 5 minutes have three times the number of neurological impairments as those with Apgar scores of 7 or more. Moreover, those with a birth weight of 1,001 to 2,000 gm have six times the number of neurological problems as those weighing 2,500 gm or more. Thus every effort should be made to provide the highest level of care prenatally and during labor and delivery, so that the flow of fetal nutritional supplies and waste removal processes operate as efficiently as possible. When impediments in this process occur, the newborn may evidence distress in the form of flaccidity, apnea, cyanosis, low heart rate, seizures, or metabolic imbalances.

## The fetus at risk

This section reviews abnormal perinatal progress that may indicate fetal problems. Common signs of impaired fetal functioning are identified, along with methods of assessing the level of fetal and neonatal well-being. For a discussion of care during normal labor and delivery and of nursing care for the mother and the neonate, the reader is referred to other sources.

In considering concurrent maternal conditions that may affect the fetus, the practitioner should consider clients who have diabetes, cyanotic heart disease, hypertension, chronic renal disease, preeclampsia, or other diminished pulmonary capacities, such as those related to pneumonia, asthma, or aspiration, that may interfere with maternal oxygen levels in arterial blood and thus fetal supply. Other high-risk situations include those where the membranes have been ruptured for

an extended period, where the fetus is postmature, and where the fetus exhibits problems, such as infection or congenital anomalies. Problems such as diminished vital supplies caused by impaired placental functioning, inadequate growth or maturity, cerebral edema, traumatic intracranial hemorrhage, or stillbirths are also included in the high-risk category.

During the process of labor and delivery, several factors may increase the risk of fetal impairment or death. These factors include (1) labor that extends beyond 8 hours in the multipara or 18 hours in the primipara; (2) the occurrences of uncontrolled or precipitous deliveries, where frequent, forceful contractions occur in the first or second stage of labor and where delivery occurs less than 3 hours after labor begins; (3) abnormal fetal presentations with difficulty in delivery of the head; (4) tetany or cessation of uterine contractions; (5) extensive use of or high or middle application of forceps; (6) version of extraction of the fetus; (7) anesthetic or pharmacological depression; (8) cesarean sections; (9) prolapsed or compressed cord; and (10) infection and subsequent temperature elevations in the mother.

Mechanical problems may also diminish the necessary blood flow to the fetus during labor. When the mother is lying in a supine position, the weight of the uterus may compress the inferior vena cava, causing a diminished blood flow to be available to the uterus. The ensuing hypoxia is reflected in the fetal heart rate. However, the problem may be alleviated by frequent repositioning of the maternity client and avoidance of prolonged dorsal recumbency.

## Oxygen levels

Any condition that causes a decrease in the arterial oxygen level of maternal blood also results in a diminished oxygen supply to the fetus. Examples of conditions that result in a decreased oxygen supply include maternal health problems and diseases, abnormalities in pregnancy such as abruptio placentae or placenta previa, or difficulties in labor that compromise the fetus by reducing the available oxygen supply.

A decreased oxygen supply forces the fetus to obtain oxygen by utilizing anaerobic metabolic pathways. Chemically this causes the following reaction:

H lactate + NaHCO$_3$ → H$_2$CO$_3$ + Na + Lactate

In short, this chemical reaction results in fetal acidosis because of the buildup of carbon dioxide and the decreased quantity of serum bicarbonate. Additionally, the problem that causes the decreased perfusion of oxygen also results in interferences with the removal of carbon dioxide.

## Status of the newborn

When one is evaluating the status of the newborn, the following measurements are particularly valuable: the Apgar score, the relationship of birth weight to gestational age, and the estimation of gestational age.

*Apgar score.* The Apgar scoring system is a widely accepted evaluation of the neonate's general condition. It not only represents the neonate's current heart rate, respiratory status, muscle tone, reflex irritability, and color, but also reflects long-term adaptation and neurological intactness.

Scoring is routinely done at 1 and 5 minutes of age. Each of the five signs may receive 0 to 2 points, and the maximum score is 10 (Table 11-1).

The score for heart rate is assigned after stethoscopic auscultation is done. A score of 100 or more beats each minute is scored as 2 points, a rate under 100 beats receives 1 point, and the absence of a heartbeat is graded as 0. In evaluating the heartbeat, the practitioner should consider a heart rate of 160 or more beats each minute as a symptom of moderate asphyxia of recent occurrence. When bradycardia is evident, a more prolonged and severe type of depression has occurred, and therapeutic intervention may be warranted. If the newborn does not have a favorable cardiac response to resuscitation, it is considered a poor prognostic sign.

Respiratory status is second in importance to acceptable cardiac functioning and is scored as follows: Apnea receives 0, ineffective or arrhythmic respirations are scored as 1, and vigorous, effective respirations that result in a good ventilatory exchange are assigned 2 points.

Muscle tone is the next parameter of measurement. Vigorous, spontaneous movements of flexion and extension in the extremities are awarded 2 points. More limited movement in the arms and legs, accompanied by the inability to resist passive extension, receives 1 point. The flaccid, limp infant is given a score of 0.

Reflex irritability represents the neonate's reaction to stimuli. Such stimuli may include nasopharyngeal suctioning or a brisk slap on the sole of the feet by the practitioner's open hand. If the neonate cries in response, a score of 2 points is assigned, a grimace receives 1 point, and no response is graded with a 0.

Color is determined by general observation of the neonate. A blue or extremely pale neonate is rated 0. If the hands and feet are dusky or cyanotic, the score is 1 point. When the entire body is a healthy pink, the neonate receives 2 points.

## Birth weight

After the birth weight is recorded, it is evaluated in relation to gestational age (Fig. 11-1).

On a chart the horizontal axis is divided into weeks of gestation, and the vertical axis represents birth weight in grams. Infants who are between the 10th and 90th percentiles are considered appropriate for gestational age (AGA), those falling beneath the 10th percentile are small for

**TABLE 11-1.** Apgar scoring method

| Sign | Score | | |
|---|---|---|---|
| | 0 | 1 | 2 |
| Heart rate | Absent | Less than 100 beats/min | More than 100 beats/min |
| Respiratory rate | Absent | Hypoventilation, weak cry | Strong cry |
| Muscle tone | Limp, flaccid | Some flexion in extremities | Well-flexed extremities, spontaneous motion |
| Reflex irritability | No response | Some motion | Cry |
| Color | Blue, pale | Body pink, hands and feet blue | Entirely pink |

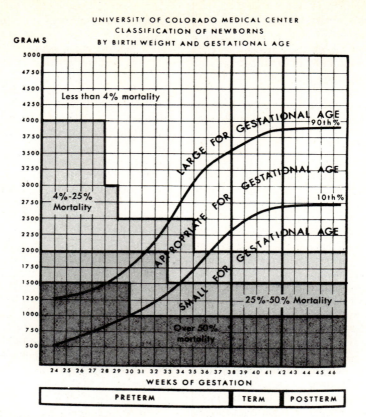

UNIVERSITY OF COLORADO MEDICAL CENTER
CLASSIFICATION OF NEWBORNS
BY BIRTH WEIGHT AND GESTATIONAL AGE

**FIG. 11-1.** Birth weight and mortality related to gestational age. (From Conway, B.L.: Pediatric neurologic nursing, St. Louis, 1977, The C.V. Mosby Co.)

gestational age (SGA), and those scoring above the 90th percentile are large for gestational age (LGA). These categories of weight are coupled with determinations of gestational age, including the following: (1) prematurity, consisting of 38 weeks of gestation or less, (2) term, comprises 38 to 42 weeks of gestation, and (3) postmaturity, which is 42 or more weeks of gestation.

Thus the neonate is assigned to one of nine groups as the three periods of gestation are combined with the adequacy of birth weight for gestational age (Battaglia and Lubchenco).

After these determinations are made the practitioner compares the results with the history. When the neonate has a weight that is inappropriate for gestational age or when the neonate is not the product of a full-term pregnancy, potential causative factors may be evident in the history. For example, inadequate intrauterine growth may be related to such factors as a concurrent metabolic problem in the pregnant woman, malnutrition, infection, or placental malfunctions. Thus the placental integrity should be carefully examined after delivery.

Growth interferences may result in untoward problems for the neonate, such as failure to thrive, hypoglycemia, hypocalcemia, or apnea, with the possibility of seizures as a result of the imbalance. At the other end of the continuum is the neonate who is classified as LGA. One usual cause for this is maternal diabetes. Thus practitioners should encourage evaluation of the mother when the condition has not been previously suspected, as it may be an undiagnosed problem.

Other determinations that should be made at this time include length, chest, and head circumference measurements. These should be plotted according to percentiles, so that all dimensions of the newborn may be compared for proportion and baseline measurement for future use.

## Gestational age

Since it is not always possible to rely on the mother's estimation of gestational age or the size and weight of the neonate as the primary factors in judging development and maturity, the practitioner needs a tool that is simple to administer and interpret. Ballard et al. have designed a tool that is currently available (Fig. 11-2).

*Test administration.* Ballard's test to assess gestational age is a tool that requires less than 5 minutes to complete after some practice with the testing procedure. The test should be administered during the first 48 hours of the infant's life.

The practitioner begins by completing the data shown in Fig. 11-2. After the information is recorded, the physical assessment is started. Each description within a category has a point value. When the neonate's response or characteristic has been observed, it is compared with the appropriate description and given a point value. At the completion of testing the combined score of neuromuscular and physical maturity is totaled on the maturity rating scale, since each score corresponds to a gestational age for the neonate expressed in weeks.

NEUROMUSCULAR MATURITY. The techniques for administering each category under neuromuscular maturity are as follows:

1. *Posture.* The neonate is placed in a supine position and observed for the degree of flexion present in the upper and lower extremities. At 28 weeks of gestational age the neonate is totally hypotonic. By 32 weeks of gestational age the lower limbs are flexed, and at gestational age 36 weeks flexion of the upper and lower limbs is evident. From this point the amount of hypertonicity increases in all limbs until term.

2. *Square window (wrist).* The wrist is flexed on the forearm until the point of resistance is reached. The angle is measured and a score as-signed. It should be noticed that the angle at the wrist becomes more acute with increasing maturity.

3. *Arm recoil.* With the neonate in a supine position, the forearm is held in extension for 30 seconds and then released. After the arm recoils the angle at the elbow is measured and points are assigned. Until gestational age 34 weeks the arms are extended and hypotonic. By the thirty-fourth gestational week a tendency to flex the forearms is apparent. At 36 weeks of gestational age there is a strong recoil that is inhibited when the forearm is held in extension for 30 seconds. By 38 weeks of gestation, even after the forearm is maintained in extension for 30 seconds, spontaneous recoil of the forearm occurs.

4. *Popliteal angle.* With the pelvis flat on a hard surface, the thigh is flexed at the hip until the knee-chest position has been attained. With the thigh against the chest, the lower leg is extended along the thigh to the point of resistance. The angle at the popliteal space is measured and points assigned. It should be noted that the popliteal angle becomes more acute with maturity.

5. *Scarf sign.* The neonate's hand is drawn across the chest and as far over the opposite shoulder as it will go, as a scarf would encircle the neck. Before 32 weeks of gestational age the elbow may be moved across the chest to be parallel with the opposite shoulder without resistance. However, maturity of muscle tone usually prevents the elbow from crossing the midline by gestational age 40 weeks.

6. *Heel to ear.* With the neonate in a supine position and the pelvis flat on a hard surface, the lower limb is rotated at the hip in an attempt to touch the feet to their respective sides. The distance between the foot and the ear when resistance prevents further approximation is compared. It should be noted that the distance between the feet and the ears is greater as muscle tone increases.

PHYSICAL MATURITY. Physical maturity is ascertained by observation and inspection and comparison of the neonate to the descriptive material, as follows:

1. *Skin.* The texture is visualized by examination of a fold of abdominal skin between the examiner's finger and thumb.

2. *Lanugo.* In a well-illuminated area the neo-

# A SIMPLIFIED SCORE FOR ASSESSMENT OF FETAL MATURATION OF NEWLY BORN INFANTS

## NEUROMUSCULAR MATURITY

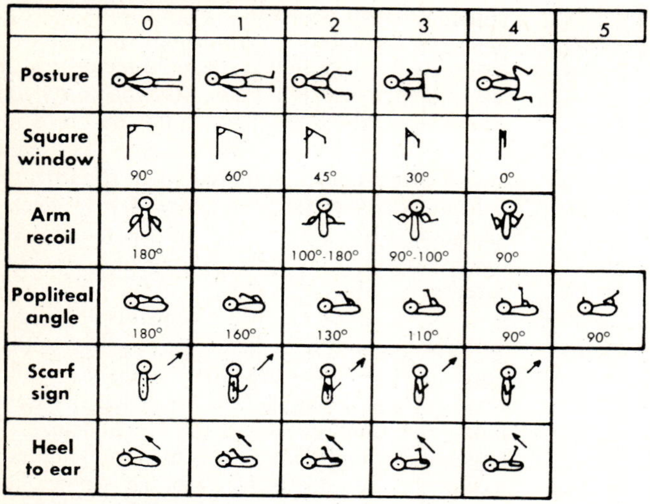

| | 0 | 1 | 2 | 3 | 4 | 5 |
|---|---|---|---|---|---|---|
| Posture | | | | | | |
| Square window | 90° | 60° | 45° | 30° | 0° | |
| Arm recoil | 180° | | 100°-180° | 90°-100° | 90° | |
| Popliteal angle | 180° | 160° | 130° | 110° | 90° | 90° |
| Scarf sign | | | | | | |
| Heel to ear | | | | | | |

Apgar _____ 1 min _____ 5 min

Age at exam _____ hr

Race _____ Sex _____

BD _____

LMP _____

EDC _____

Gestational age by dates _____ wk

Gestational age by exam _____ wk

Body weight _____ gm ____ percentile

Length _____ cm ____ percentile

Head circumference ____ cm ____ percentile

Clinical disturbances ____ None ____ Mild ___

Moderate ____ Severe

## PHYSICAL MATURITY

| | | | | | | |
|---|---|---|---|---|---|---|
| Skin | Gelatinous red, transparent | Smooth pink, visible veins | Superficial peeling and/or rash, few veins | Superficial cracking, pale area, rare veins | Parchmentlike cracking, no vessels | Leathery, cracked, wrinkled |
| Lanugo | None | Abundant | Thinning | Bald areas | Mostly bald | |
| Plantar creases | No crease | Faint red marks | Anterior transverse crease | Creases cover anterior two-thirds | Creases cover entire sole | |
| Breast | Barely perceptible | Flat areola, no bud | Stippled areola, 1-2 mm bud | Raised areola, 3-4 mm bud | Full areola, 5-10 mm bud | |
| Ear | Pinna flat, stays folded | Slightly curved pinna; soft with slow recoil | Well-curved pinna; soft, ready recoil | Formed, firm, instant recoil | Thick cartilage, ear stiff | |
| Genitals ♂ | Scrotum empty, no rugae | | Testes descended, few rugae | Testes down, good rugae | Testes pendulous, deep rugae | |
| Genitals ♀ | Prominent clitoris, and labia minora | | Labia majora and minora equally prominent | Labia majora large; minora small | Clitoris and labia minora completely covered | |

### MATURITY RATING

| Score | Wk |
|---|---|
| 5 | 26 |
| 10 | 28 |
| 15 | 30 |
| 20 | 32 |
| 25 | 34 |
| 30 | 36 |
| 35 | 38 |
| 40 | 40 |
| 45 | 42 |
| 50 | 44 |

**FIG. 11-2.** Assessment of gestational age. (From Ballard, J.L., et al.: J. Pediatr. **95**:770, Nov. 1979.)

nate's back is examined, and the findings are compared to the descriptive material.

3. *Plantar creases.* The skin on the soles of the feet is stretched from the toes to the heel and the creases that remain compared with the descriptive data.

4. *Breast.* By inspection, palpation, and measurement of breast tissue diameter, the development of breast size and nipple formation may be determined.

5. *Ear.* The ear is palpated to determine the extent of cartilage formation, and the upper pinna is folded over gently between the examiner's finger and thumb. The response of the ear when released and the status of cartilage formation is compared to the descriptive material.

6. *Male genitalia.* The neonate is placed in a supine position, so that the scrotum may be visualized and palpated. Findings are compared to the descriptive material in the test.

7. *Female genitalia.* The characteristics of the female genitalia are easily determined when the neonate is placed in a supine position and the area is observed.

**Neurological development.** It is significant to realize that neurological development occurs in an orderly, sequential manner that is unaffected by premature deliveries. For example, a newborn who was delivered at 32 weeks of gestational age but has lived in an incubator for 4 additional weeks has the same degree of neurological maturity as one remaining in utero for the 36-week period, excluding impairments in either of the two.

The estimation of gestational age is an important measurement in caring for the neonate, since low birth weights are not necessarily indicative of prematurity, and birth weights of 2500 gm or more are not always associated with term pregnancies. However, clinical progress in the fetus is closely allied to the level of maturity.

Because of the birth shock, the neurological examination done within 48 hours of delivery is valuable mainly in the estimation of gestational age. Neonates with possibly abnormal conditions should be serially monitored and treated in accordance with their individual needs. However, further evaluations for all neonates are necessary after 48 hours to confirm problems.

Basically the examination during the first 48 hours reveals the neonate's reflexes, reactions, and muscle tone. At 28 weeks of gestation the neonate is flaccid. With maturity the muscle tone increases in a cephalocaudal direction, beginning with the distal segments. At term, flexor hypertonicity is apparent in all extremities. One may make an objective evaluation of the degree of passive tone present by measuring the various limb angles, as described in Ballard's test. These angles decrease as muscle tone increases with maturity.

In addition to neuromuscular status, certain physical characteristics in the neonate are valuable in estimating fetal age, since they develop independently from functional capacities or growth failures during the last month. These features include creases in the sole of the foot, breast nodule diameter, lanugo, earlobe development, appearance of the skin, and external features of the genitalia, described previously.

In general, infants of less than 36 weeks of gestational age have smooth skin covering the plantar aspect of the foot, small or absent breast nodules, fine bristly hair on the head, and flexible earlobes that lack cartilage. Males have partially descended testicles that are not in the scrotum, whereas females have protruding labia minora not covered by the labia majora.

By 38 weeks of gestational age the plantar aspects of the feet are well demarcated, the breasts are prominent, the scalp is covered with straight, silky strands of hair, and the earlobes are well supported by cartilage. In females the labia majora cover the labia minora, and in males at least one testis is palpable in the scrotum.

Between 36 and 38 weeks of gestational age the features are in various stages of transition.

## NEONATAL EXAMINATION

After completion of the evaluation of the initial vital signs, measurements, and determination of gestational age, the neonate is examined more generally. In addition to the usual examination, observations should include a description of the neonate's overall appearance, including the following: (1) skin marks, rashes, turgor, consistency, and condition; (2) skin and nail bed color during rest, feeding, and crying and inspection for neonatal jaundice; (3) body posture at rest, as well as symmetry and adequacy of spontaneous movement; (4) intactness of body structures and documented functioning of appropriate orifices; (5) infection; and (6) behavior, especially excessive irritability, dissatisfaction even after feedings or after solutions for physical discomfort are enacted, or twitching.

## NEUROMUSCULAR ASSESSMENT

The neuromuscular assessment begins with the detailed description of facial symmetry, skull molding, and individual features that characterize the neonate. The ears should be checked to determine their alignment with the outer canthus of the eye. Facial movements should be observed to detect transient paralysis caused by birth trauma and compression of neurological tracts.

Temporary types of cranial characteristics are detected at this time. Caput succedaneum, generalized swelling under the scalp, occurs soon after delivery, but resolves in a few days. Cephalhematoma is an excessive accumulation of fluid beneath the suture lines. In cephalhematoma, swelling beginning after delivery may continue until the head appears misshapen. Reabsorption of this fluid may require 3 months. Other characteristics of importance include the degree of molding or separation of cranial sutures; the presence, size, and fullness of fontanels; and the comparison of head circumference to both the established norms and the neonate's chest circumference as measured at the nipple line.

Next, infant responses in relation to alertness, eye functions, and hearing are assessed. The neonate is generally observed for movement and response to environmental stimuli. In addition to newborn instillation of silver nitrate, the eyes are observed to detect the color of the sclera, lacrimal functioning, and freedom from infection. After having opened the infant's eyes through upright positioning of the infant, dimming the light source, and placing a nipple in the infant's mouth, one assesses the eyes for pupillary reaction to light, ability to fixate, and coordination of movements. Regard for the human face and the ability to track movements to the midline may be observed in the newborn. Hearing is checked as the infant shows movement and blinking in response to a sudden loud noise, such as a whistle or a ringing bell.

Neuromuscular capacities are further evaluated after 48 hours of age through exercise of the complete range of motion for all movable parts, observation of hand posturing, evaluation of active tone, response to primary reflex testing, and transillumination of the skull.

### Active tone

To reliably evaluate the neonate's active tone and reflex status, the practitioner should wait until the second day of life and select a time when the neonate is comfortable and not reacting to excessive stimulation or fatigue. Midway between feedings is often a time when acceptable conditions exist and when the neonate is neither too full nor hungry.

One evaluates active tone by assessing the neonate's posture and the righting responses of the head and extremities. When the neonate is placed in the supine position, there is external rotation of the shoulders and hips and flexion at the elbows, knees, fingers, and thumbs. The tonic neck reflex slightly alters this position, whereas the Moro reflex greatly alters this position.

The righting reaction of the trunk and lower extremities may be tested when the neonate is placed in a supported, standing position. By term the newborn has a proprioceptive supporting reaction that allows support of the body weight for a few seconds. This response results in the movement of the trunk, neck, and lower extremities into a brief opisthotonic posture.

Since differences in the neck flexors and extensors are not so great by term, when the infant is required to right the head on the trunk, the head may follow the trunk without falling backward for a few seconds.

Neck extensors at the dorsal aspect of the neck may be tested when the neonate is placed in a sitting position with the head tilted forward on the chest and the neonate's trunk is moved backward slowly. At 36 weeks of gestation the neonate may right the neck, but cannot maintain the position. By 38 weeks of gestation the neonate may keep the head in line with the trunk for a few seconds. At a gestational age of 40 weeks the head stays aligned with the trunk for more than a few seconds.

Neck flexors may be tested when one places the

neonate in a supine position and pulls the neonate gently to a sitting position by grasping the hands, or supporting the shoulders in a small premature infant. The relationship of the head to the trunk is observed during this maneuver. Before 32 weeks of gestation the head remains in a pendulous position. By 32 weeks of gestation the effort of muscle contraction is apparent but ineffective in aiding head control. By 36 weeks of gestation the head hangs back and then quickly moves forward to a pendulous position on the chest. At term the head should follow the trunk and lag less than 45 degress behind the trunk as the neonate is pulled to a sitting position.

## Primary reflexes

The reflexes that are generally assessed in the neonate and infant include the Moro reflex, traction response, grasp response, plantar response, Babinski reflex, rooting and sucking reflexes, supraciliary tap, automatic walking response, trunk elevation response, crossed extension reflex, dorsolumbar incurvation, ventral suspension, asymmetric tonic neck response, and pupillary response (included in the subsequent discussion of cranial nerve functions).

*Moro's reflex.* In eliciting the Moro reflex, the infant is gently lifted a few centimeters off the bed by the hands and is suddenly released back to the bed. The normal reaction is rapid neck extension resulting in symmetric extension and abduction of the arms, extension and fanning of the fingers, and the formation of a C by the thumb and index finger. By 24 weeks of gestation this reflex is barely obvious. At a gestational age of 28 weeks the reflex is apparent, but easily exhausted. After 28 weeks of gestation the reflex should be apparent in all healthy infants. Before the age of 8 weeks after birth asymmetry in the Moro reflex indicates possible injury or paralysis, such as a brachial plexus palsy, whereas absence suggests a severe neurological problem. Between 8 and 18 weeks after birth, the response may be limited to a body jerk. The reflex is absent after 6 months of age.

*Traction response.* Along with the early automatic grasp of the neonate the traction response occurs (Fig. 11-3, *B*). The traction response may be elicited as the practitioner pulls gently on the neonate's arm to stretch the shoulder adductor muscles. This effort results in a strong synergistic flexed position at all joints. As the grasp reflex develops, the traction response is lost.

*Grasp response.* The grasp response is elicited as the examiner places a finger across the palmar aspect of the neonate's palm, and the neonate closes the fingers around the examiner's finger (Fig. 11-3). However, the true grasp reflex is not developed until 2 to 4 months of age, and the initial grasping patterns are actually avoidance patterns. When the true grasp reflex has developed, stimuli applied to the medial part of the hand will produce flexion and adduction of the fingers, a position that is sustained when the fingers are pulled on (Fig. 11-3, *C*). Between the ages of 5 and 10 months the infant begins to utilize this crude grasp to reach for objects (Fig. 11-3, *D*). Next, the infant acquires the ability to move digits singly without causing all the other digits to flex simultaneously. When such fractional hand movement is readily possible, the ability to oppose the thumb and index finger in the pincer grasp is evident (Fig. 11-3, *E*). At this point, true voluntary prehension has begun.

*Plantar response.* The plantar response may be elicited when the examiner's finger is placed firmly across the base of the toes. The toes should curl downward (Fig. 11-4). This response should be symmetric and is less intense by 8 months of age.

Four different reactions compose the plantar response, including the flexor reflex, the avoidance response, the proprioceptive positive supporting reaction, and the grasp reflex of the foot. Thus the movement of the toes in a plantar or dorsal direction is heavily dependent on the type of stimulus—painful or proprioceptive—and the portion of the foot stimulated. For example, stimuli applied to the lateral border of an infant's foot cause dorsiflexion, whereas stimuli applied to the medial side of the foot result in plantar flexion.

*Babinski's reflex.* In infants, when the lateral portion of the foot is stroked from the heel upward and across the ball of the foot, hyperextension or fanning of the toes occurs. As myelination of the pyramidal tract is completed, the normal response becomes flexion of all the toes, whereas hyperextension of the great toe becomes the pathological sign. This sign, known as Babinski's reflex, is the most significant clinical sign in ascer-

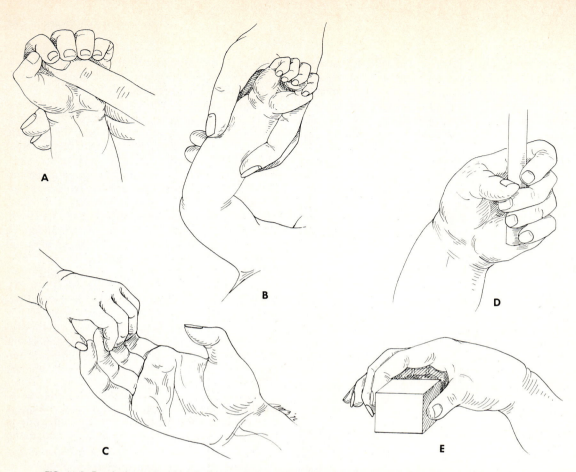

**FIG. 11-3.** Developing prehension. **A,** Grasp or palmar response. **B,** Traction response at birth. **C,** True grasp reflex, present at 2 to 4 months of age. **D,** Instinctive grasp reaction, present at 5 to 10 months of age, used for active reach. **E,** Pincer grasp. (From Conway, B.L.: Pediatric neurologic nursing, St. Louis, 1977, The C.V. Mosby Co.)

**FIG. 11-4.** Plantar response. (From Conway, B.L.: Pediatric neurologic nursing, St. Louis, 1977, The C.V. Mosby Co.)

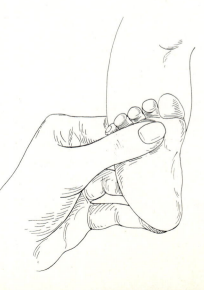

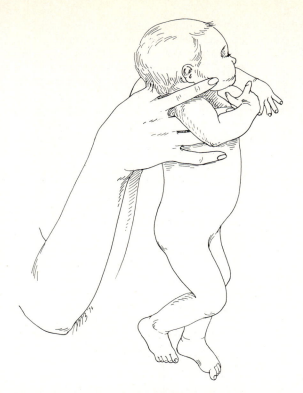

**FIG. 11-5.** Automatic walking, involving supporting reaction and stepping. (From Conway, B.L.: Pediatric neurologic nursing, St. Louis, 1977, The C.V. Mosby Co.)

taining the presence of a pyramidal tract lesion after a child is 2 years of age. When it is observed, a specialist should be consulted to consider it in relation to other clinical findings.

*Rooting and sucking reflexes.* The response of cardinal points, or the rooting reflex, is obtained as the tactile stimulus in the perioral area causes the neonate's head to turn toward the stimulus. This reflex is first noted at 24 weeks of gestation and is well established by 32 weeks of gestation.

Along with the rooting reflex the sucking reflex develops. At 24 weeks of gestation the sucking reflex is first seen. By 32 weeks of gestation the sucking response is well developed, and by 34 weeks of gestation it is coordinated with swallowing.

When a nipple touches the perioral area of the hungry neonate's face, the rooting and sucking responses are elicited. Absence or exhaustibility of these reflexes usually indicates a young gestational age. When absence of these reflexes occurs in term infants, the practitioner should suspect central nervous system depression from maternal medication or anesthesia during delivery, hypoxia, or congenital abnormalities. When sucking and rooting reflexes are not adequate to allow the infant to feed sufficiently, the practitioner may assist the mother by applying such techniques as chin traction, utilizing a high-calorie formula or a thickened feeding when swallowing is a problem, selecting an appropriate nipple and schedule, flexing the spastic or rigid infant to facilitate swallowing, burping the infant well, and using a semi-Fowler's position after eating. Before the practitioner assists the mother in learning to feed the infant, the professional may elect to feed the infant first to become familiar with the individual problems. In the immature premature infant, oral feedings may need to be supplemented with nasogastric feeding to avoid excessive fatigue and expenditure of calories.

*Supraciliary tap.* The supraciliary tap (Mc-Carthy's reflex), similar to the corneal reflex, is a trigeminal afferent–facial efferent reflex. It is elicited by gentle percussion directly above the eyebrows (supraorbital ridge) and results in closure of the ipsilateral eyelid. This reflex is evident after 32 weeks of gestation.

*Automatic walking.* Automatic walking is achieved when the infant is held by the trunk and tilted slightly forward with the feet in firm contact with a solid surface (Fig. 11-5). Early efforts to step may reveal excessive flexion of the hips and knees with overextension at the ankles. The additional feature of overadducted legs may cause the neonate to have a scissorslike gait.

Automatic walking is first observed as momentary tiptoeing and righting efforts at 32 weeks of gestation. By 38 weeks of gestation the neonate walks on tiptoe with great facility. By 40 weeks of gestation the premature infant walks either in a pattern of toe-heel placement or on tiptoe, whereas the full-term neonate walks in a heel-toe pattern and utilizes the entire sole of the foot.

During the first 4 months of life the tendency to crouch while being supported in a standing position gradually disappears as the infant increases in ability to support some body weight. In most infants the ability to support the bulk of the body weight is apparent by 10 months of age.

After 4 months of age, occasional scissoring of the legs and standing on tiptoe may be observed. However, persistent tendencies to scissor the legs or stand on tiptoes after 4 months of age should alert the practitioner to seek further evaluation from a specialist. While the neonate is in the supported standing position, the practitioner should notice any deformities of the hip, knee, and foot.

After 6 months of age the supporting reaction is less clearly demonstrated as the infant matures toward the ability to stand voluntarily. Maturity also causes the crude partial placing responses to give way to elaborate contact-placing reactions. For example, the older infant makes immediate adjustments in the foot and steps up onto the tabletop whenever any aspect of the foot is lightly touched by the table edge. Such adeptness in foot reactions is a necessary precursor to the later activity of standing and to various forms of mobility.

**Trunk elevation response.** The trunk elevation response is seen when the infant is held against the examiner's body with the trunk horizontal and the legs vertical while the soles of the feet are stimulated. At 37 weeks of gestation the trunk straightens on the hips, and at 40 weeks of gestation the head also extends.

**Crossed extension reflex.** The response of crossed extension is normally seen in infancy. It is elicited when one rubs the sole of one foot while the leg is maintained in extension and movement is noted in the opposite leg. The complete response of the contralateral leg is developed by 36 weeks of gestation and is a three-part movement consisting of rapid flexion and then extension of the leg, adduction of the leg and foot, and fanning of the toes. After the pyramidal tract has become myelinated, the presence of the crossed extension response may indicate pyramidal tract or frontal lobe lesions.

**Dorsolumbar incurvation.** Dorsolumbar incurvation of the trunk is elicited with the infant in the prone position and the examiner moving a finger down the paravertebral portion of the spine, first on one side and then on the other. The response should be a movement of the pelvis toward the side of stimulation. After 4 weeks of age the response cannot be elicited in most infants.

**Ventral suspension.** Two reflexes are commonly associated with positions of ventral suspension: the Landau reflex and the parachute reflex.

To obtain *Landau's reflex* the infant is suspended carefully over a bed or table with the trunk or abdomen supported. The newborn should respond by flexing the legs and assuming a slightly convex position with the head a little below the horizontal line of the body. If the newborn collapses into a limp concave posture, it is an abnormal sign. By 3 months of age the head should be slightly above the horizontal plane, and by 10 months of age the infant should assume a position wherein the spine is concave and the head is above the horizontal plane. The absence of these postural responses is abnormal and should be reported to a specialist.

The *parachute reflex* should be done carefully to avoid injury by accidental dropping of the infant. Positioned over a table or bed, the infant is held in an upright form of suspension and then is quickly plunged forward with the arms moving over the head (Fig. 11-6). The infant should respond by extension of the arms and fingers, as if to break the fall. Although this response may be seen in some infants as early as 3 months of age, other infants may not manifest the sign until 9 months of age or later. Asymmetry or absence of the response after 9 months of age should be called to the attention of a specialist.

**Asymmetric tonic neck response.** The asymmetric tonic neck response is inconstant during the first 3 months of life and as such as dubious neurological significance. By about 3 months of age the reflex may be elicited in most infants. With the infant in a supine position, the head is passively rotated to one side. The arm and leg on the ipsilateral side extend, whereas the arm and leg on the contralateral side exhibit diminished tone (Fig. 11-7). When the response is either persistent after 7 months of age or extremely strong on one side, the practitioner should examine the infant further to see if torticollis or cerebral palsy is a problem.

The disappearance of the asymmetric tonic neck response is generally replaced by the neckrighting reflex, wherein passive or active rotation of the head laterally results in the infant moving the

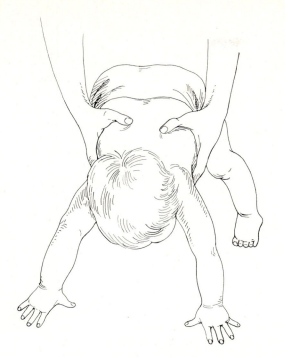

**FIG. 11-6.** Parachute reflex. (From Conway, B.L.: Pediatric neurologic nursing, St. Louis, 1977, The C.V. Mosby Co.)

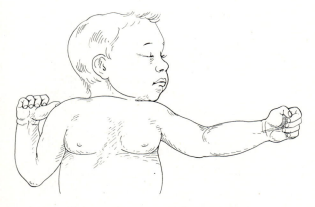

**FIG. 11-7.** Asymmetric tonic neck reflex.

shoulders, trunk, and hips in the same direction after a momentary delay. Movement should be readily observed as the practitioner turns the head in either direction. When the infant persists in holding the head to one side or has difficulty in turning readily to one side, the practitioner should examine the infant more closely to rule out the possibility of cerebral palsy. The disappearance of this reflex is hard to pinpoint; an extension of the response may be seen in the two-step procedure involved as the young child turns over to assume a sitting position before rising upward to a stance.

## NECK AND BACK

Since the neck and shoulders are often subjected to trauma during birth, it is important to palpate the neck for masses, asymmetric features, and injury. After the intactness of the clavicles has been ascertained, the head should be rotated passively in all directions to evaluate the adequacy of the range of motion.

At this point it is usually convenient to place the infant in a prone position to inspect and palpate the spinal column for abnormalities. Any dimpling superior to the gluteal fold should be documented, as it may indicate spinal column irregularities caused by the late embryonic closure of the spinal column, as described in Chapters 1 and 13.

The arms should be rotated through the full range of motion to observe any defects or limitations of movement in the muscles of the shoulders or back.

## EXTREMITIES

The hands should be inspected to note the position that the neonate usually assumes. Normally neonates hold their hands in a closed fist. Overlapping of fingers or extension of the thumb should be noted, as either may indicate a chromosomal disorder. Creases in the palmar aspect of the hand are also significant.

Presence, symmetry, and functioning of all muscles should be noted as each body joint is passively moved through its usual range. Limitations of movement or dislocations are noted.

## CRANIAL ASSESSMENT

Chapter 2 contains a discussion of the assessment of the skull, fontanels, and skull dimensions.

In addition, Fig. 1-18 may be helpful in visualizing important features.

When the chest is auscultated in the course of the general examination, the practitioner should also listen to the skull with the stethoscope to detect possible bruits. The best location for *auscultation* is either the temporal region or the area of the anterior fontanel. In infants younger than 4 years of age, symmetric, soft bruits are normal. When bruits are loud or localized, further investigation is warranted. Some causes of unusual bruits include arteriovenous malformations in the middle cerebral artery or the vein of Galen, cardiac murmurs that are transmitted to the skull area, extreme anemia, and increased intracranial pressure.

*Transillumination* of the skull is a simple screening device that is valuable in revealing defects in the central nervous system, such as cysts, deviations, or absences of vital central structures. To perform the procedure, the practitioner takes the infant into a darkened room and places a flashlight with a flexible rubber attachment directly on the infant's scalp. The illumination in the frontal area should not be visible under the scalp for more than a 1 to 2 cm circumference beyond the area of the flashlight. The parietal and temporal regions should reveal even less transillumination of the scalp beyond the periphery of the flashlight, and the occipital area should show the least of all. When transillumination of the scalp exceeds these general guidelines, further follow-up by a specialist is warranted.

As part of the cranial examination, the practitioner should make an *observation* of dimples, clefts, or asymmetric features of the face. In addition, the practitioner should note close spacing (hypotelorism) or wide spacing (hypertelorism) between the eyes. The relationship of the top pinna of the ear to the outer canthus is also significant. A small or recessive chin is also an important finding, since it is associated with some syndromes as well as problems of obstruction, wherein the tongue falls backward to obstruct the nasopharynx. All these findings are considered in relation to the remainder of the examination and may provide clues in diagnosis when the child has problems.

When the practitioner suspects hyperirritability, hyperventilation, or tetany from irritation to a lower motor neuron, causing facial muscle spasms or contractions, the cheek may be tapped in front of the ear. The resulting reflexive grimace or cramp-like contraction on the same side is termed *Chvostek's sign.*

Two other phenomena may occur when one is examining the skull, namely, craniotabes and Macewen's sign. *Craniotabes,* or softening of the exterior skull layer, is a normal finding in infants up to 3 months of age. However, it is also associated with such abnormal conditions as prematurity, rickets, syphilis, hypervitaminosis A, and hydrocephalus. It may be elicited by firm compression of the temporoparietal suture area above and behind the ears. When present, the practitioner notices a snapping sensation that has been likened to an indented table tennis ball returning to its former shape.

*Macewen's sign,* popularly termed the cracked pot sound, is the increased resonance associated with increased intracranial pressure that results on percussion of the skull. The sound is normal in infants with open fontanels but is an abnormal finding after the fontanels close.

## EVALUATION OF DEVELOPMENT

During the first 2 years of life the brain attains about 90% of its adult growth, and myelination of the corticospinal tract is completed in the cephalocaudal and proximodistal directions. Thus the infant exhibits control over body parts in the following order: head, trunk, arms, hands, pelvis, and eventually legs. After 2 years of age the child can accomplish most movements associated with maturity, though speed, strength, fine activity, and coordination are not refined for several more years, as discussed in Chapter 5.

Growth patterns and developmental sequences depend heavily on the stimulation level to which the infant is exposed. When stimulus opportunities are limited, growth patterns tend to reflect impoverished experiences and deprivation. Chapters 5 and 8 discuss several theoretical viewpoints that emphasize the importance of previous operations and experiences as fundamental components of adequate functional capacities in later life.

## RESPONSE TO STIMULI

When an infant is first born, the response to environmental stimuli seems to be grossly generalized and undifferentiated, so that noxious stimuli, temperature extremes, and other forms of physiological discomfort result in generalized body movement and crying. With maturity, responses to stimuli become more selective and specific. These more differentiated responses are probably partially the result of the increasing myelination of the cerebral cortex and the corticospinal tracts.

Since myelination in the cortical pathways is incomplete, the infant is unable to make voluntary, appropriate responses when presented with olfactory or gustatory stimuli. However, the infant will respond to a noxious odor by crying or exhibiting generalized body movement. It is interesting to note that the receptors for taste and smell are fully developed at the time of birth.

At birth the receptor apparatus for hearing is fully developed but does not attain full function for several years because of the incomplete myelination and functioning of the cortical auditory pathways. The newborn responds to types of sounds in a generalized way. For example, loud noises may cause agitation, whereas soft sounds may calm and comfort the infant. At 2 to 3 months of age the infant has developed some ability to localize sounds and is able to turn the head toward the origin of a sound. However, the integration of auditory capacities into complex, meaningful communication patterns requires several years.

## SPEECH

From the first cry of the infant after birth, the practitioner is atuned to the quality, type, pitch, frequency, and intensity of the infant's cry. As a matter of fact, along with the feeding patterns of the infant, crying often provides the first clue that the child may have a problem. For example, a weak cry and a poor sucking reflex may be identified with a premature infant, a critically ill infant, or an infant with central nervous system damage. High-pitched cries and feeble feline cries are also associated with central nervous system deficits.

Acceptable speech patterns are heavily dependent on the intactness and appropriate functioning of the auditory apparatus. Hearing impairments are fully covered in the subsequent discussion of auditory capacities. While considering the ears, the external ear should be inspected for deformity, asymmetry, unusual slant or placement, or protrusion. The area anterior to the ear should be examined for any pinhole-sized openings because these may be dermal sinuses that penetrate deeply into the cranial tissues, offering a portal to infection. Ear tags should also be noted, since they may have significance in relation to other findings in the examination. The presence of a cleft lip and palate or a bilirubin concentration of more than 20 mg/dl during the first week of life increases the risk of an auditory problem and therefore indicates the need for complete audiometric testing.

Generally in early infancy some vocalization and cooing are common before 4 months of age. The infant should also turn toward the source of the sound by 4 months of age. Speechlike sounds are often heard between 6 and 9 months of age. Many toddlers say one to four meaningful words between 12 and 18 months of age, know 10 to 20 words by 15 to 25 months of age, and use two words in rapid succession by 2 years of age. After 2 years of age, there is rapid vocabulary expansion. However, there is great interchild variability in the rate of language acquisition because of differences in environment, intelligence, and perceptual experiences. Suspicion of an auditory problem should exist if the infant begins to babble, but quits by 6 months of age, shows no response to name or commands between 6 and 9 months of age; seems unresponsive to environmental noise changes; is not startled by loud, sudden noises during the first year; or does not blink in response to loud noises in the neonatal period.

Inspection of the mouth and nose for anomalies is important, since deformities in these areas may interfere with speech.

## VISUAL DEVELOPMENT

At birth the eye is not fully developed and does not possess the capacities that are present after further maturity of the eye structures and neural pathways. Hyperoptic acuity is normal in the infant, since the shape of the eyeball is less spheric than in adults. Although the pupils respond to changes in light intensity at birth, accommodation to near and distant objects by the lens is not possible for several months. It is not until the second or third month that the lacrimal ducts are functional.

One of the first abilities that the infant demonstrates to indicate visual integrity is the ability to fixate on and follow objects. Because of the incomplete myelination of the cerebral neural pathways, convergence may not be possible for about 3 months. Although voluntary control of eye muscles is not possible until about 3 months of age, the practitioner should be alert to disconjugate, constantly roving eye motions as a clue to blindness and to a fixed position in one eye that does not allow symmetric movement in accordance with movements in the other eye.

Whereas peripheral vision is fully developed because of complete maturity in the peripheral areas of the retina at birth, the central area surrounding the optic disc, the macula, is poorly developed. As this central area matures, the infant begins to experience sharp, clear images and light contrasts. By 8 months of age the combination of myelination of cortical pathways and maturity of the macula allows infants to differentiate colors. At 9 months of age the long process of integrating the images received by the macula of each eye begins. Simultaneously, cerebral maturity (which is complete by the first year) and further coordination of the eye muscles continue. These two processes are vital to the infant in integrating two separate visual images into one perceptual experience.

As part of the eye examination, the practitioner should also be alert to indications of concurrent pathological conditions. The setting-sun sign, that is, downward displacement of the eye bulbs as a result of depression of the roof of the orbit or sixth-nerve palsy, may indicate increased intracranial pressure and is often associated with hydrocephalus. When one cornea is larger than the other, the practitioner should examine the infant further to rule out congenital glaucoma. Opacity or clouding of the lens or its capsule in infancy may cause the practitioner to question the possibility of congenital cataracts associated with rubella. Later, cataracts may indicate metabolic disease, trauma, or poisoning of certain types. In all nonoriental infants the practitioner should inspect the inner aspect of the eye for an extra fold (epicanthic fold) of skin superior to the eye, since this extra fold of skin may be associated with Down's syndrome.

Other minor deviations of the eye should also be noted, since further examination of the infant for a major problem is warranted when three or more minor defects are noted. Noteworthy items include hypotelorism, hypertelorism, wide, bushy brows that meet in the middle of the nose, peculiar placement of the eyes, or striking differences in the size of the two eyes.

## NEUROMUSCULAR DEVELOPMENT

Most practitioners are well acquainted with the sequence of neuromuscular events that compose increasing developmental maturity and physical mastery of the environment. One of the most popular screening tools for detecting developmental disorders is the Denver Developmental Screening Test (DDST) (Fig. 11-8). However, care must be taken to utilize the DDST only as a screening device rather than as a diagnostic determinant. When problems in any of the four areas of gross motor, language, fine motor–adaptive, or personal-social development are detected, more definitive methods of testing are warranted. Through this additional testing a functional analysis or profile of strengths and weaknesses may be detailed to provide the basis for appropriate intervention.

## CONTINUING DEVELOPMENT

As auditory abilities, communication skills, and visual capacities become more mature, they are amenable to more reliable methods of assessment.

### Auditory abilities

Testing the young child for auditory abilities offers the practitioner a challenge, since test results are heavily dependent on one's ability to gain full cooperation and attention from the child. Particular difficulty may be experienced when the child is either young or afflicted with multiple handicaps. Some simple techniques for measuring hearing ability may be employed, including playing games with the child that involve whispered directions given to the child while the examiner's lips are out of the child's visual range or varying the volume on a record player or radio and asking the child to identify the first time that sound is heard.

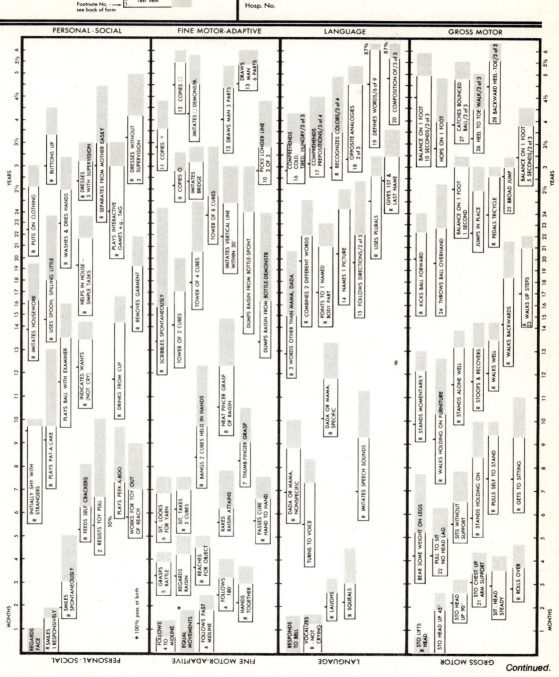

**FIG. 11-8.** Denver Developmental Screening Test (DDST). (From Conway, B.L.: Pediatric neurologic nursing, St. Louis, 1977, The C.V. Mosby Co.)

1. Try to get child to smile by smiling, talking or waving to him. Do not touch him.
2. When child is playing with toy, pull it away from him. Pass if he resists.
3. Child does not have to be able to tie shoes or button in the back.
4. Move yarn slowly in an arc from one side to the other, about 6" above child's face. Pass if eyes follow 90° to midline. (Past midline; 180°)
5. Pass if child grasps rattle when it is touched to the backs or tips of fingers.
6. Pass if child continues to look where yarn disappeared or tries to see where it went. Yarn should be dropped quickly from sight from tester's hand without arm movement.
7. Pass if child picks up raisin with any part of thumb and a finger.
8. Pass if child picks up raisin with the ends of thumb and index finger using an over hand approach.

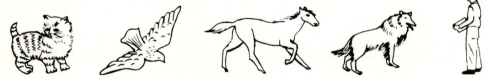

9. Pass any enclosed form. Fail continuous round motions.
10. Which line is longer? (Not bigger.) Turn paper upside down and repeat. (3/3 or 5/6)
11. Pass any crossing lines.
12. Have child copy first. If failed, demonstrate

When giving items 9, 11 and 12, do not name the forms. Do not demonstrate 9 and 11.

13. When scoring, each pair (2 arms, 2 legs, etc.) counts as one part.
14. Point to picture and have child name it. (No credit is given for sounds only.)

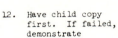

15. Tell child to: Give block to Mommie; put block on table; put block on floor. Pass 2 of 3. (Do not help child by pointing, moving head or eyes.)
16. Ask child: What do you do when you are cold? ..hungry? ..tired? Pass 2 of 3.
17. Tell child to: Put block on table; under table; in front of chair, behind chair. Pass 3 of 4. (Do not help child by pointing, moving head or eyes.)
18. Ask child: If fire is hot, ice is ?; Mother is a woman, Dad is a ?; a horse is big, a mouse is ?. Pass 2 of 3.
19. Ask child: What is a ball? ..lake? ..desk? ..house? ..banana? ..curtain? ..ceiling? ..hedge? ..pavement? Pass if defined in terms of use, shape, what it is made of or general category (such as banana is fruit, not just yellow). Pass 6 of 9.
20. Ask child: What is a spoon made of? ..a shoe made of? ..a door made of? (No other objects may be substituted.) Pass 3 of 3.
21. When placed on stomach, child lifts chest off table with support of forearms and/or hands.
22. When child is on back, grasp his hands and pull him to sitting. Pass if head does not hang back.
23. Child may use wall or rail only, not person. May not crawl.
24. Child must throw ball overhand 3 feet to within arm's reach of tester.
25. Child must perform standing broad jump over width of test sheet. (8-1/2 inches)
26. Tell child to walk forward,  ⬭⬭⬭➤  heel within 1 inch of toe. Tester may demonstrate. Child must walk 4 consecutive steps, 2 out of 3 trials.
27. Bounce ball to child who should stand 3 feet away from tester. Child must catch ball with hands, not arms, 2 out of 3 trials.
28. Tell child to walk backward,  ◀⬭⬭⬭  toe within 1 inch of heel. Tester may demonstrate. Child must walk 4 consecutive steps, 2 out of 3 trials.

DATE AND BEHAVIORAL OBSERVATIONS (how child feels at time of test, relation to tester, attention span, verbal behavior, self-confidence, etc,):

**FIG. 11-8, cont'd.** For legend see p. 275.

**TABLE 11-2.** Appraising hearing*

| Age (months) | Method | Response |
|---|---|---|
| 4 | Attract infant's attention by using silent toy in motion while making sound with another object—bell, shoe on floor, toy—outside of visual field. Perform tests on both sides. | Infant suspends active attention toward silent toy, as shown by widening of eyes, minimal turning toward origin of sound, or cessation of motion with apparent listening. |
| 6 | | Infant turns head in direction of sound, though exact localization of sound may not be possible. |
| 8 | | Infant turns head as much as 45 degrees to origin of sound and localization of sound above or below the body possible. |
| More than 18 | Test high-frequency sound sensitivity by rubbing fingers together by each ear. | Infant identifies rubbing of fingers by appropriate ear. |
| More than 18 | Place ticking watch next to each ear. | Infant identifies ticking sound. |
| More than 18 | Strike tuning fork and place it in center of forehead, asking child to indicate where sound is heard (Weber's test). | Sound should be heard equally on both sides. |
| More than 18 | Strike tuning fork and place it first on mastoid process and then next to external ear. Child should indicate when sound is gone in each position (Rinne test). | Infant should be able to hear sounds in each location bilaterally. Sounds through bone conduction at mastoid process should not be heard as long as sounds at external ear measuring air conduction. |

*Refer all clients with abnormal findings for complete audiometric evaluation.

The use of a tuning fork for measuring bone and air conduction is also valuable in arriving at an impression about auditory abilities. Additional techniques are outlined in Table 11-2.

When problems with auditory capacities are first suspected, they may be manifested in impaired speech and language development. In making the differential diagnosis, the practitioner should attempt to determine if the hearing loss results from lack of cooperation in the testing situation, if speech delays are related to abnormal intelligence or emotional disorders, if organic impairments exist in receptive or integrative apparatus, or if impaired muscle coordination is evident in the structural apparatus required for expression—a common problem in cerebral palsy.

In evaluating the family history, the practitioner should be alert to conditions that might be associated with hearing defects. Such factors as congenital rubella, anoxic episodes any time after 16 weeks of gestational age, when the cochleae have formed, the administration of ototoxic drugs, prematurity, birth trauma, meningitis, low birth weight, extended hospitalization at birth, or family history of deafness place the child in a high-risk category and suggest the need for complete audiometric testing.

In evaluating the child's history, the practitioner should question the parent or test the infant to detect the lack of response to slight noises, the consistent appearance of behavior that is inappropriate to environmental activity and often unrelated, and any paucity of babbling or abnormal speech rhythms. In the young child, emotional problems or hearing disabilities may be evident in delayed speech or speech deterioration, constant requests to have conversation repeated, cupping of the hand to the ear or cocking of the head toward the sound source, lack of attention to conversation or environmental noise, emotional lability, poor expressive inflection, and frequency of articulation errors.

If the hearing loss is in the range of high-pitched tones, the child may have great difficulty in hearing /sh/, /ch/, /th/, /s/, /f/, /v/, and /t/, since these sounds all occur in the high-frequency range. The examiner may also notice that the child utilizes excessive gesturing to express thoughts.

When any of these unusual findings is noted in the physical examination, referral to an audiologist and continued definition of the underlying problems by other specialists is appropriate.

## Communication skills

Receptive and expressive language comprises three important components: phonology, semantics, and syntax. *Phonology* consists of the 35 individual sounds, or phonemes, that compose the English language. Receptive phonology involves the conversion of speech sounds into neural impulses at the cochlear level and the further transmission of these impulses to the temporal lobe for organization into the correct sound sequence. In contrast, *semantics* involve the cortical relation of word and meaning. Since one word is often inadequate to express a thought or activity, several words in a given order or words in varied forms, such as tense or plurality, are utilized in communication. This process of word variation and sequence is known as *syntax*. Obviously semantics and syntax in receptive language are closely related and probably are interpreted together by the neurological apparatus. In expressive language the cortical area supplies words to correspond to the intent of the incoming message in expressive semantics and syntax. Expressive phonology is involved with the transmission of appropriate speech sounds through neural pathways to the structures and muscles of speech production, that is, the organs of phonation: the jaw, the tongue, the soft palate, and the pharynx. Further investigation is necessary to understand more specific brain functions related to the reception, association, integration, and expression of language.

Since there is wide variability in the rate of language acquisition in children and in the number and types of problems that may occur, early detection and referral of all speech defects to specialists remains imperative.

The Denver Articulation Screening Examination (DASE) is a valuable screening tool designed for use in children 2½ to 6 years of age (Fig. 11-9) that readily identifies articulation skills in the English-speaking child. Children who have problems as identified by this screening test should be referred for further evaluation. Further information on communication disorders and remedial measures is available in other sources.

## Visual capacities

Both the Denver Eye Screening Test and the Snellen Screening Test may be utilized as asessing visual problems. The Denver Eye Screening Test has the advantage of being geared to the preschool group and has proved valuable in detecting such eye problems as refractive errors, strabismus, and amblyopia. The Snellen Screening Test reliably estimates visual acuity, but is dependent on the child's ability to cooperate and identify the correct direction of the **E.** Since color discriminations are significant in the accurate perception of the environment, it is important to identify color blindness early. Although complete testing for color blindness involves the use of a test such as the Ishihara test, the practitioner may detect the existence of a potential problem in color identification by asking the child to describe items in the immediate environment.

When visual acuity is 20/20 but the child seems to have difficulty in translating visual perceptions into coordinated activity, several simple measures may be used to further delineate the nature of the problem. To assess eye movement, one may hold a pencil about 13 to 16 inches from the child's nose and ask the child to follow the object with the eyes only in all planes. Slow, awkward, or arrhythmic movements should be noted. Additionally, nystagmus and the use of associated head movements to visualize the object should be noticed. Sometimes persistence in the use of head movements to follow an object constitutes the inability to follow directions because of a limited attention span, as further described in Chapter 8.

Near-point convergence of the eyes may be estimated when an object is moved toward the nose while the child is asked to continue watching the object. When the object is very near the nose, one eye will turn outward. At this point the direction of the object should be reversed. When the object has been moved outward to about 7 inches from the nose, the child should have realigned the eyes.

Distant fixation may be tested when the child is asked to fixate on an object no more than 20 feet away and then one eye is covered. The uncovered eye should not require readjustment to remain fixed on the distant object. Alternate covering of each eye in a successive pattern is also valuable

### Denver articulation screening examination*

For children 2½ to 6 years of age

INSTRUCTIONS: Have child repeat each word after you. Circle the underlined sounds that he pronounces correctly. Total correct sounds is the raw score. Use charts.

Name:

Hosp. No.:

Address:

Date:_____Child's age:_____ Examiner:_____ Raw score:_____

Percentile:_____ Intelligibility:_____ Results:_____

| | | | |
|---|---|---|---|
| 1. table | 6. zipper | 11. sock | 16. wagon | 21. leaf |
| 2. shirt | 7. grapes | 12. vacuum | 17. gum | 22. carrot |
| 3. door | 8. flag | 13. yarn | 18. house | |
| 4. trunk | 9. thumb | 14. mother | 19. pencil | |
| 5. jumping | 10. Toothbrush | 15. twinkle | 20. fish | |

Intelligibility: (circle one)

1. Easy to understand
2. Understandable half the time
3. Not understandable
4. Cannot evaluate

Comments:

To score intelligibility:

| | NORMAL | ABNORMAL |
|---|---|---|
| 2½ years | Understandable half the time or "easy" | Not understandable |
| 3 years and older | Easy to understand | Understandable half time Not understandable |

Test result:
1. *Normal* on DASE and intelligibility = *normal*
2. *Abnormal* on DASE and/or intelligibility = *abnormal*
   If abnormal on initial screening, rescreen within 2 weeks. If abnormal again, child should be referred for complete speech evaluation.

*By Amelia B. Drumwright, University of Colorado Medical Center, 1971.

*Continued.*

**FIG. 11-9.** Denver Articulation Screening Examination.

To score DASE words: Note raw score for child's performance. Match raw score line (extreme left of chart) with column representing child's age (to the closest *previous* age group). Where raw score line and age column meet, number in that square denotes percentile rank of child's performance when compared to other children that age. Percentiles above heavy line are *abnormal* percentiles and below heavy line are *normal*.

PERCENTILE RANK

| Raw score | 2.5 yr | 3.0 yr | 3.5 yr | 5.0 yr | 4.5 yr | 5.0 yr | 5.5 yr | 6 yr |
|---|---|---|---|---|---|---|---|---|
| 2 | 1 | | | | | | | |
| 3 | 2 | | | | | | | |
| 4 | 5 | | | | | | | |
| 5 | 9 | | | | | | | |
| 6 | 16 | | | | | | | |
| 7 | 23 | | | | | | | |
| 8 | 31 | 2 | | | | | | |
| 9 | 37 | 4 | 1 | | | | | |
| 10 | 42 | 6 | 2 | | | | | |
| 11 | 48 | 7 | 4 | | | | | |
| 12 | 54 | 9 | 6 | 1 | 1 | | | |
| 13 | 58 | 12 | 9 | 2 | 3 | 1 | 1 | |
| 14 | 62 | 17 | 11 | 5 | 4 | 2 | 2 | |
| 15 | 68 | 23 | 15 | 9 | 5 | 3 | 2 | |
| 16 | 75 | 31 | 19 | 12 | 5 | 4 | 3 | |
| 17 | 79 | 38 | 25 | 15 | 6 | 6 | 4 | |
| 18 | 83 | 46 | 31 | 19 | 8 | 7 | 4 | |
| 19 | 86 | 51 | 38 | 24 | 10 | 9 | 5 | 1 |
| 20 | 89 | 58 | 45 | 30 | 12 | 11 | 7 | 3 |
| 21 | 92 | 65 | 52 | 36 | 15 | 15 | 9 | 4 |
| 22 | 94 | 72 | 58 | 43 | 18 | 19 | 12 | 5 |
| 23 | 96 | 77 | 63 | 50 | 22 | 24 | 15 | 7 |
| 24 | 97 | 82 | 70 | 58 | 29 | 29 | 20 | 15 |
| 25 | 99 | 87 | 78 | 66 | 36 | 34 | 26 | 17 |
| 26 | 99 | 91 | 84 | 75 | 46 | 43 | 34 | 24 |
| 27 | | 94 | 89 | 82 | 57 | 54 | 44 | 34 |
| 28 | | 96 | 94 | 88 | 70 | 68 | 59 | 47 |
| 29 | | 98 | 98 | 94 | 84 | 84 | 77 | 68 |
| 30 | | 100 | 100 | 100 | 100 | 100 | 100 | 100 |

**FIG. 11-9, cont'd.** For legend see p. 279.

in detecting difficulty in realigning an eye fixed on a distant object. Problems in perceptual-motor integration and coordination are detailed in Chapters 5 and 8.

## CONSIDERATIONS IN ASSESSING NEUROLOGICAL CAPACITIES IN YOUNG CHILDREN

In the strict sense of interpretation, all body functions are related to neurological processes. However, practically, problems in the neurological functions are divided into categories. Evaluation of acceptable neurological functioning involves a comprehensive description of behavior; learning capacities; patterns of adaptability to living; orientation to time, person, and place; perceptual-motor capacities; proprioceptive integrity; and competency of various physiological structures routinely tested in a neurological examination. Since the subjects of perceptual-motor integration and behaviors related to such factors as mental retardation, hyperkinesis, learning disabilities, as well as normal skills required for adaptation to school, learning, and life patterns are developed in Chapters 5 and 8, they are not discussed further at this point.

### Cerebral functions

By the time the practitioner is required to summarize the cerebral functions, which include such factors as general mental status, thought processes, emotions and behaviors, state of consciousness and orientation, memory, appropriateness of intellectual capacities in relation to developmental age, and language usage, the examiner has had the opportunity to take a history, to observe the parent and the child during the office visit, and to administer screening tests appropriate to the child's age and development. The summary of maturity and general cerebral capacities is a written statement based on the data obtained. If a perceptual, motor, or learning disability is suspected, the practitioner may desire to evaluate the child in more detail.

### Cranial nerve functions

The ability to evaluate the cranial nerves adequately is dependent on the child's ability to cooperate and respond to each portion of the examination. When such cooperation is not possible, estimations of function should be attempted by modification of the testing approach. There are 12 cranial nerves, which are tested in the following order: olfactory (I); optic (II); oculomotor (III), trochlear (IV), and abducens (VI); trigeminal (V); facial (VII); auditory (VIII); glossopharyngeal (IX); vagus (X); accessory (XI); and hypoglossal (XII).

Discussion of the details on physical assessment continue under the following heading: Physical Examination of Older Child and Adult.

## PHYSICAL EXAMINATION OF OLDER CHILD AND ADULT

The physical examination should be thorough, with emphasis on neurological assessment in light of a problem. The examination begins with an evaluation of behavioral and cognitive capacities. Although the initial impression of mental capacities is established at this point, it is validated continually throughout the contact period with the client.

### GENERAL BEHAVIOR

The first consideration is general behavior. Much data may be gleaned on this point by observation of the appearance, posture, dress, and manner of the client. In opening comments continue this assessment by noting responses, behaviors, and body language in relation to the conversational topics. Also form a general impression as to the patient's capacity for cooperation. The ability to cooperate may be influenced by emotional states that range on the continuum from temporary status to frank psychosis or from impairments in sensory capacities, that is, hearing or visual disturbances, to problems like receptive dysphasia. Assuming that the receptive apparatus is intact, continually evaluate the behavioral and emotional status of the client with particular reference to body tension; personality traits; affect; mood; appropriateness; and the relationship and responses to, and comments about, the situation at hand. Extremes of emotion may indicate a neurological problem. Spontaneous, inappropriate crying or laughing is a common behavior in clients with pseudobulbar palsy. Inappropriate behavior may also be obvious in clients who have head injuries, brain damage, or frontal lobe disease. Temporal lobe lesions result in hallucinatory experiences that may be mistaken for psychiatric disturbance. Evidence of progressive behavioral or cognitive deterioration may indicate the presence of organic cerebral disease.

## INTELLECTUAL CAPACITIES AND MEMORY

Along with the behavioral evaluation, assess intellectual capacities, including memory. Intellectual performance is grossly estimated in the adult as one considers vocabulary range, the fund of knowledge revealed in the total assessment process, and the combination of socioeconomic status, life achievements, and educational preparation. More definitive tests are available when the gross estimation seems inadequate.

Memory is tested for recent and past events. Past memory is assessed as the client provides the history. Logic, sequence of events, and capacity for remembering personal data are evident. Recent events may be evaluated when the client is asked to recite a few facts and perform some simple exercises, such as the following:

1. Ask what events happened today.
2. Ask what the client was doing last Monday.
3. Ask the client for the name of the building you are in.
4. Give the client a name and address to remember and in about 5 minutes ask him or her to recall this information.
5. State a series of seven or eight digits and ask the client to repeat them.
6. Recite a series of five digits and ask the client to repeat them in reverse order.

In using series of digits write them out in advance so as to avoid replication of a character.

Calculations are assessed when the client is asked to add, subtract, multiply, and divide two digits. Another popular exercise is to ask the client to count backward from 100 by 7's — 100, 93, 86, 79. . . .

In evaluating the outcome of this intellectual performance, consider powers of concentration and attention versus problems related to organic disorders.

Orientation to time, person, and place is an important factor that may be altered by some organic disorders. To assess orientation, ask the client about common facts in his or her environment: name, age, city of residence, where he or she is, name of spouse or family member, name of the president of the United States of America, date, and time of day. Abstract reasoning may be assessed when the client is asked to identify the meaning of a famous adage such as "A stitch in time saves nine."

## REVIEW OF GENERAL OBSERVATIONS

At this point you have gained a vast amount of data that may require further elaboration and exploration. It is a good time to reflect on this preliminary data in light of subtle behaviors that may reveal a great deal about the client and serve to overcome the unnatural situation inherent in the formal process of examination. First, note the client's level of comfort with the office situation: Does the client seem to feel strange and nervous or does he or she act as if visiting a medical situation is a customary practice? Is the client punctual, late, or extremely early for the appointment? Why? In listening to and observing the client approach the examining room, do you note if there is an obvious postural or gait deformity, or do the feet meet the ground with an unusual slap, dragging motion, or shuffle (Table 11-3)? Is the client relaxed and self-confident or does he or she look at the ground and seem overly conscious of his or her appearance to others?

When the face is observed, does it seem to have expression? Does the client seem to be able to gauge direction by looking forward or does he or she have to turn the head to see because of a defect in the visual field, such as hemianopia? Is the base of support normal or wide during walking? Are any signs of ataxia or unusual associated movements obvious? Does the client have any peculiar mannerisms or tics?

Other general observations about the stance include size, body proportions, obesity, evidence of wasting, and striking deformities (kyphosis, scoliosis, torticollis). Observe the head to see if it is abnormally large or small in relation to the body. Does the client seem to be abnormally weak? Are auxiliary muscles used in walking or sitting, or does the client seem to have difficulty in correct-

**TABLE 11-3.** Common gait disorders

| Condition | Characteristics |
|---|---|
| Hemiplegia | Dragging one foot when walking |
| Spastic paraplegia | Legs dragged through bilaterally |
| Tabes dorsalis | Short, irregular, unstable, double sound related to profound postural disturbance |
| Drop foot | Double "ker-lump" |
| Parkinson's disease | Short, variable shuffle with accelerating sound; fixed expression; flexed trunk, arms, and hands |
| Arteriosclerosis | Marche à petits pas—even, short, constant shuffle |
| Phenytoin (Dilantin) toxicity | Wide-based gait |
| Advanced disseminated sclerosis | Reeling, broad-based gait with cane, which is moved in an exaggerated manner forward and sideways; explosive speech; exaggerated smile |
| Cerebellar ataxia | Reeling gait with capacity to compensate and regain balance |
| Cerebellopontine angle tumor | Ataxia with head turned toward side of the face that is paralyzed |
| Extremely swollen legs | Legs probably dependent for extended period; evaluate circulation |

ing a drooping neck? As the client sits down, notice the hands and legs. Multiple injuries or burns may suggest impaired sensory perception, which occurs in such conditions as syringomyelia. Do the joints seem misshapen or painful and limited in movement? If so, consider arthritis.

Observe the face carefully. Is it fat and hairy, as in Cushing's syndrome, or smooth, round, and yellow, as in hypopituitarism? Do the eyes bulge (exophthalmos) while the lids remain retracted as in those individuals with hyperthyroidism? Do the eyelids droop? If so, describe the drooping lids carefully because they may indicate several problems: variable bilateral droop of myasthenia gravis, wrinkled forehead and fixed unilateral droop of ocular myopathy, or fixed unilateral droop of paralysis of the third cranial nerve. A face drawn down in combination with muscular atrophy, baldness, and cataracts possibly indicates dystrophia myotonica. Does the client blink bilaterally? If

not, are the cranial nerves intact or does the client possibly have parkinsonism? If the eyes turn upward without the lids closing, the client may have lower motor neuron facial paralysis. Is the client cachectic and drawn, as in malignancy? Note scars and tremors in the facial muscles.

In evaluating the voice, reflect on the volume, quality, clarity of words, content, and organization of thoughts. Inappropriate emotional outbursts may reveal primary brainstem lesions or pseudobulbar palsy.

After clarifying initial data, evaluate impressions and subjective complaints for continuity. For example, if the client relates unbearable pain but shows no signs of discomfort or if he or she speaks about impaired use of an extremity that appears operational, clarify the nature of the complaint. It may either be an ill-defined organic problem, wherein more data are needed, or a psychogenic problem.

## CEREBRAL FUNCTIONS

Specific testing is required for assessment of the functional integrity of the various cortical areas. In general these tests are divided into three categories of cortical functions: (1) sensory integration, (2) motor integration, and (3) language.

### Sensory integration

Specific areas of the cerebral cortex are responsible for sensory integration at the cortical level as object recognition occurs through feeling, vision, and audition. When one is unable to effect sensory integration at this level through the special senses, the problem is termed *agnosia*. Visual agnosia occurs when there is a disturbance in the occipital lobe. Interference with the lateral and superior aspects of the temporal lobe results in auditory impairments. Disrupted functions in the parietal lobe result in disturbed tactile capacities. Interferences in the posteroinferior areas of the parietal lobe result in disturbances in identifying the relationships of body parts.

### Motor integration

Various portions of the neurological examination require the client to execute motor functions in response to specific directions. In the absence of motor impairments or diminished strength the

**TABLE 11-4.** Assessment of agnosia, apraxia, and aphasia

| Behavior/task | Testing procedure |
|---|---|
| **Sensory interpretation** | |
| Sound identification | Instruct client to close eyes and state recognition of familiar noises. |
| Auditory-verbal integration | Direct client to both answer a question and follow instructions. |
| Identification of body parts and sidedness | Point to body parts and ask client to identify them. Test client for discrimination between right and left sides. |
| **Motor interpretation** | |
| Skilled motor activities | Direct client to retract point of ballpoint pen, close safety pin, drink from cup, snap fingers, and so on, after receiving your verbal directions. |
| **Language capacities** | |
| Visual object recognition | Present familiar objects to client and ask to name. |
| Visual-verbal integration | Ask client to read passage from book or newspaper aloud; if client cannot verbalize, ask to indicate comprehension of printed instructions. |
| Motor qualities of speech | Ask client to repeat sounds ''ba-ba,'' ''ti-ti,'' and phrases of progressive difficulty. Listen carefully for unusual verbalization during this test and in other conversations. |
| Automatic speech | Ask client to name days of week and months of year. |
| Volitional verbalization | Determine if answers are appropriate to questions posed. |
| Written communication | Ask client to close eyes and write a word and his or her name. Have client open eyes and copy words you name. |

inability to perform specified tasks is termed *apraxia*.

## Language

The term ''language capacities'' is a broad designation referring to the total process of reception, integration, and response in written, verbal, or body language form. Gestures, inflections, and other subtleties may significantly alter the meaning of a given communication. When language functions are disrupted, the individual is said to be *aphasic*. There are several types of aphasia, each one dependent on the region of brain where the disturbance has occurred. Auditory-receptive problems are caused by temporal lobe disturbances, expressive writing disabilities by posterior frontal cortex lesions, expressive writing disabilities by posterior frontal cortex disturbances, and visual-receptive problems by parieto-occipital cortex disorders. Although this discrete division is valuable for an academic separation of types of aphasia, clinical situations infrequently point to one discrete type of aphasia; instead more than one language deficiency is seen. Mild aphasic problems are frequently not indicative of the location of a lesion, since they are often the result of generalized

brain damage, residua from more complete aphasia, or characteristic of early evidence of a progressive lesion.

The assessment of agnosia, apraxia, and aphasia is summarized in Table 11-4.

## EVALUATION OF SPECIFIC PHYSICAL FEATURES
## Head

Begin the examination with a general evaluation of the head. An overall impression of position, shape, and size is important. Data about the head are gained through inspection and measurement, palpation, percussion, and auscultation.

Through *inspection and measurement* of the head, the appropriateness of head size is determined. If the head is too large, assess cranial symmetry, since hydrocephalic heads appear as inverted triangles, whereas macrocephalic heads are large and symmetrical. If the head is small, consider microcephaly and craniostenosis. In microcephaly the head rises to a point and looks like a triangle, with its sloping forehead and occiput. In craniostenosis the superior suture lines form a hard, palpable ridge, and the fontanels are closed (Chapters 1 and 13). Other disease conditions also result in enlarged head size, specifically acromegaly and Paget's disease. In acromegaly the head is elongated, and the jaw is enlarged, along with the ears and nose. Additionally, the teeth are separated, increased folds are apparent around the eyes, the skin is coarse, the hands are disproportionately large, and the fingers appear spadelike and blunt on the ends. In Paget's disease the head is enlarged, rounded, and appears reddened and warm, with dilated vessels.

After observing the general appearance, *palpate* the cranium for bony abnormalities. Lesions may be apparent on the cranium from a variety of problems, which are generally categorized as outcomes of congenital, traumatic, postoperative, or erosive processes. When present, these lesions are generally concave and pulsating, except in instances where there is increased intracranial pressure, wherein the lesion feels tense and convex. Bony elevations may also be apparent and may indicate a developmental event of no consequence or a meningioma.

If you are examining an infant, an increase in head size of more than ½ inch per month or an abnormally sized fontanel is cause for further attention. In general the anterior fontanel is closed by 18 months of age. A fontanel that is abnormally large or full and tense indicates increased intracranial pressure. When the anterior fontanel is obliterated prematurely and the head shape is abnormal, the infant may have craniostenosis. Chapter 13 offers further detail on these conditions.

At this point *percuss* the skull with a firm rap of the index and second fingers. In children where sutures are separated or where hydrocephalus has occurred, the sound resulting from percussion is like that of a "cracked pot."

*Auscultation* is an important part of assessment and is performed when one places the stethoscope over the frontal area and occipital regions bilaterally and over each closed eyelid and listens. The object of listening is to detect bruits, which are often faintly heard systolic sounds. If the client cooperates by holding the breath during auscultation, bruits are more readily detected.

Bruits are apparent for a variety of reasons. In young children they are so frequently detected that they are of little value in pointing to a specific diagnostic problem. Bruits are often audible in Paget's disease in individuals with arteriovenous malformations. Individuals with carotid or aortic stenosis may also have a bruit. Bruits are audible when the external vessels dilate to supply the needs of a vascular meningioma. When space-occupying intracranial processes distort blood vessels, a bruit may be detected even though the vascular disturbance is not of the primary type. Bruits are not usually heard in individuals who have a berry aneurysm.

Transillumination is a technique in which an infant is taken into a dark room and a flashlight with a rubber extender is held to the scalp. The circumference of the circle of illumination of the frontal scalp should not extend from the light more than 1 or 2 cm. The parietal and temporal regions should reveal an even more limited extension of light outward. The occipital area reflects the light out into the adjacent scalp less than the other parts of the cranium. When the results of this test do not fall within these guidelines, further assessment is warranted because the infant may have such problems as hydrocephalus, a space-occupying lesion (including a porencephalic cyst), or increased intracranial pressure.

### Meningeal irritability

Next assess the client for meningeal irritation. *Brudzinski's sign* consists in causing the individual in supine position to bend the knees to avoid pain as the neck is flexed. *Kernig's sign* is noted if the client is placed in a supine position with the hip flexed and is unable to extend the knee without pain. Neck rigidity is a response to meningeal irritation that may result from a variety of disorders: inflammatory or destructive processes, cervical spine disease or fusion, and parkinsonism. When meningeal irritation occurs in combination with extreme increased intracranial pressure, it should signal the possibility of herniation of the cerebellar tonsils.

### Spine

Have the client do straight-leg raises if you suspect a prolapsed lumbar disc is present. If this is the case, the client will show a limited capacity for raising the extended leg on the ipsilateral side (*Lasègue's sign*) and often will experience root pain on the involved side when the contralateral leg is raised. If the lesion is in the upper lumbar region, pain is augmented when the hip is hyper-extended. Lasègue's sign differs from Kernig's and Brudzinski's signs by the lack of nuchal rigidity.

Test the jugular compression by occluding the jugular veins digitally or with a sphygmomanometer cuff at 40 mm and noting if pain is produced along the distribution of the sciatic nerve.

These tests are helpful in establishing the diagnosis of a ruptured intervertebral disc.

Note the curves of the vertebral column, particularly normal cervical and lumbar *lordosis,* as well as any deformities, such as *kyphosis* and *scoliosis*. Palpate and percuss the spine for tenderness. Examine the range of motion by having the client bend forward, backward, and to each side.

### Peripheral nerves

Peripheral nerves should be grossly assessed for unusual characteristics. By palpating the ulnar nerve at the elbow and the lateral popliteal nerve at the point where it rounds the fibula, you may assess their vulnerability to trauma by noting the degree to which these structures are superficial. Hypertrophic polyneuritis and leprosy result in thickening of nerves. The superficial lesions of neurofibromatosis are often palpable along a nerve pathway. If the client describes an injury wherein neuronal tissue has regenerated, tapping the point where regrowth has occurred causes the client to experience paresthesia along the newer branches *(Tinel's sign)*. If the ulnar or median nerve is compressed by a deep ganglion, tactile pressure at the wrist frequently results in similar symptoms.

### Auditory capacities and assessment

The examination continues with an evaluation of the ears with an otoscope. Otitis media should be ruled out as a problem, since its presence with neurological symptoms may account for the genesis of facial paralysis, intracranial infection, meningitis, rapidly advancing focal seizures, or an increased cell count in the cerebrospinal fluid.

Hearing capacities should also be assessed grossly by rubbing the fingers on one of the client's ears while the client's eyes are closed. Then ask the client to identify the side where the rubbed fingers are heard. You may also stand behind the client and whisper directions, advising him or her to demonstrate comprehension. Identification of the sound of a ticking watch may also be used. Normally most instances of deafness do not result from disorders of the eighth cranial nerve.

To test hearing, use a tuning fork of 1024 Hertz (cycles per second), since it tests the range of human speech (300 to 3000 Hertz) and does not cause difficulty in distinguishing vibration from sound. Two additional tests are commonly employed at this point: Weber's test for lateral hearing discrimination and Rinne's test to compare air and bone conduction. To perform the *Weber test,* tap the tuning fork on your knuckles to cause light vibrations and then place it soundly on the center portion of the upper head or forehead (Fig. 11-10). Ask the client to describe where he or she hears the sound. The sound is most often heard equally in both ears or is perceived in the midline. If the client does not perceive the sound, press the fork more firmly toward the head.

To perform the *Rinne test,* set the tuning fork into light vibration and place the base on the client's mastoid process (Fig. 11-11), where it remains until the client says the sound is no longer audible. Then set the vibrating fork into motion again and place the U-like aspect near the client's ear canal so that the client reports hearing the sound (Fig. 11-12). Compare the results of these two tests, since normal individuals here the sound through air for a longer period than through bone.

### Skin

A number of characteristic skin lesions and markings accompany neurological diseases. One of the first observations an astute practitioner makes is vasomotor changes and adequacy of the peripheral vascular system. Note brown, discolored areas on the skin, known as café-au-lait spots because they may be present along with subcutaneous nodules in von Recklinghausen's disease.

Angiomatous lesions accompany a number of neurological conditions. A port-wine stain on the face is associated with Sturge-Weber syndrome. Nevi covering a spinal segment are seen in association with the static developmental lesions from faulty neural tube formation, syringomyelia, and spinal astrocytoma (Chapters 1 and 13).

Telangiectases may occur either on the skin or

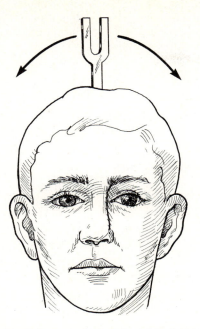

**FIG. 11-10.** Weber test. Evaluation of lateral hearing discrimination.

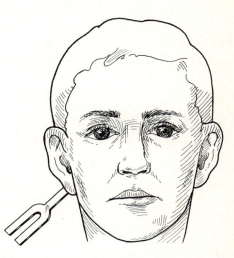

**FIG. 11-11.** Evaluation of bone conduction in audition.

on spinal coverings in association with familial hemorrhagic telangiectasia. At times pregnant women and individuals with hepatic cirrhosis have spider nevi.

Herpes simplex should be assessed carefully, especially if the eruption is in a pregnant woman, to avoid transmission of herpes—possibly in the form of meningoencephalitis—to the fetus. If lesions are in the birth canal, delivery is by cesarean section to prevent the possibility of neonatal incursion of this devastating neurological disease.

Rashes and allergies should be described, since they may be related either to a particular condition or to the reactions an individual has when taking certain medications.

Pellagra-like skin disorders may be caused by deficiencies.

Malignancies of the skin, such as melanoma, are known to metastasize into the nervous system.

Decubiti may be evident in clients who endure prolonged pressure over anesthetic areas of the

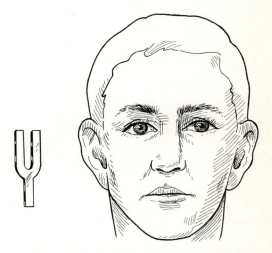

**FIG. 11-12.** Evaluation of air conduction in audition.

skin. Similarly, evidence of burns, scars, and tropic changes in the periphery might lead the practitioner to suspect a disturbance in sensory capacities.

Abnormal pigmentation or tufts of hair along the spinal axis or at the posterior fossa may indicate an underlying neural tube deformity (Chapters 1 and 13).

### Autonomic system

Examine the skin for its general appearance and texture, with emphasis on color (erythema, cyanosis, and pallor), temperature, and sweating. Note the characteristics of the nails and hair. Signs of urinary or fecal incontinence may be evident. Examination of the abdomen may demonstrate bladder or bowel distention.

### Cardiac status

The general examination proceeds to an assessment of cardiac status. It is significant to note changes in rate and rhythm, including extrasystoles. Heart sounds that are irregular or with murmurs should be evaluated more extensively. Pulses should be assessed for quality, variations, and intensity in all extremities, as well as apically. Chapter 24 offers a discussion of cerebrovascular disorders. Pulse rates may also indicate a response to general systemic disturbances, neurological disorders, or interruption in vascular supply, which may impair usual conscious functions.

Carefully measure blood pressure in both arms with the client in the supine and standing positions. The determination of hypertension is important in the identification of disease states and necessary measures of prevention. Blood pressure determinations are necessary as a part of gathering base-line data and also as a vital means for assessment of client response to invasive studies used in diagnosing neurological problems. Additional blood pressure readings may be indicated by the client's condition.

### Pulmonary status

Assessment of the lungs includes the consideration of any infectious process or obstructive condition that might interrupt breathing. Such interruptions affect gaseous perfusion, energy level, cerebral functions, and integrity. Tuberculosis should be ruled out as part of this assessment. The lungs provide one site for the origin of tumors, and malignant processes of the lungs should always be considered when the client has a chronic inflammation of the pulmonary system with signs of decreased appetite, cachexia, and other vague complaints that may accompany cancer.

### Abdomen

Palpate the abdomen. Enlargement of the liver and spleen is a frequent finding in several types of malignancy and in chronic alcoholism.

### Reproductive system

Assess the reproductive system for malignancies, since these lesions often metastasize to the spine. Moreover, review the history of sexual maturity, menses, and childbearing, since a number of chromosomal and single-gene disorders produce abnormalities.

### Other considerations

Carefully palpate the breasts for growths, since secondary metastases to the cerebrum and spine often originate in the breast.

Assess thyroid functions for size and appropriateness of hormonal production.

Palpate the neck, groin area, and axillae to detect any increase in the size of the lymph nodes.

Examine the mouth carefully for infectious processes, localized as abscesses, since these may provide sources of infection for the brain. Assess the bite to ascertain the presence of defective closure and defective teeth, since these may cause undue pressure at the temporomandibular joint.

### Cranial nerves

The assessment continues with the evaluation of the 12 cranial nerves, outlined here.

*Cranial nerve I.* The first cranial nerve, the olfactory nerve, regulates the sense of smell.

ASSESSMENT. Before testing, you must inspect the nasal passages to eliminate the possibility of an obstruction interfering with test results. After patency of the nasal passages has been established, ask the client to identify common scents with the eyes closed. You may use oil of peppermint, coffee, tobacco, cloves, alcohol, or other substances with familiar odors.

## SUMMARY OF CRANIAL NERVES

| Nerve | Tests |
|---|---|
| Olfactory (I) | Smell |
| Optic (II) | Visual acuity, visual fields, and examination of fundi |
| Oculomotor (III), trochlear (IV), and abducens (VI) | Pupillary response, external ocular movements, and nystagmus |
| Trigeminal (V) | Motor functions, sensory functions, and corneal reflex |
| Facial (VII) | Motor function of upper and lower face, taste |
| Acoustic (VIII) | Whispered voice, Rinne, and Weber |
| Glossopharyngeal (IX) and vagus (X) | Motor functions, including vocal cord assessment |
| Accessory (XI) | Strength of trapezius and sternocleidomastoid muscles |
| Hypoglossal (XII) | Strength and ability to extend tongue in midline |

**DISORDERS.** The sense of smell may be interrupted by interferences in the neurons of the olfactory bulb and tract or in the primary olfactory receptors found in the nasal mucosa. Hallucinatory olfactory experiences may result when the disturbance is in the uncus.

*Cranial nerve II.* The second cranial nerve is the optic nerve, which has the primary function of vision.

**ASSESSMENT.** Several tests are done to assess the integrity of the optic nerve's function. Testing begins when the client's ability to read the Snellen charts and ordinary print from a newspaper or magazine is assessed. When the client wears corrective lenses, the nature of the correction is noted, and the client is requested to perform visual testing with and without glasses.

Visual fields are assessed as the client masks one eye and fixates the other eye on your nose. Wiggle a finger starting in the periphery of each visual quadrant and moving inward to the nose. Ask the client to indicate when he or she first sees the moving finger in the periphery. Then repeat the test with the client's other eye. When the client seems to have limited ability to detect the moving finger in a portion of the visual field, refer him or her for more explicit testing through standard perimetric tests.

Assess the point of visual extinction in the periphery by simultaneously moving the fingers in opposite sides of the visual fields and noting the client's response.

The eye assessment continues with an ophthalmoscopic examination, wherein you examine the optic discs, vessels, and periphery of the retina. When the pupils are too small for adequate visualization, they may be dilated pharmacologically by a qualified professional.

**DISORDERS.** The client may have a problem with visual acuity, which requires corrective lenses for remediation.

Disturbances in the visual fields may result from an interruption at several points along the optic pathway, including the occipital lobe, the geniculocalcarine tract, the lateral geniculate body, fibers of the optic nerve and tract, or the neurons or sensory structures of the retina. When a lesion is apparent on the retina, it may result in a blind spot in the ipsilateral eye. If the lesion affects the optic nerve, partial or complete blindness may result in that eye. Blindness in the opposite half of both visual fields occurs when a complete lesion affects either one optic tract or one of the lateral geniculate bodies. Blindness in the upper quadrants of both visual fields contralateral to the side where the lesion is located results from a disturbance in temporal lobe functions. A disturbance of parietal lobe functions results in contralateral blindness in corresponding lower quadrants of the eyes. Central vision remains functional when the lesion interrupts operations at the level of the occipital lobe, but this lesion may result in contralateral blindness in the corresponding half of each visual field (Fig. 11-13).

*Cranial nerves III, IV, and VI.* Cranial nerves III (oculomotor), IV (trochlear), and VI (abducens) are tested simultaneously, since they all cooperate to affect eye movement. Specifically, the oculomotor nerve affects pupillary constriction, elevation of the upper eyelid, and majority of extraocular eye movements. The trochlear nerve is

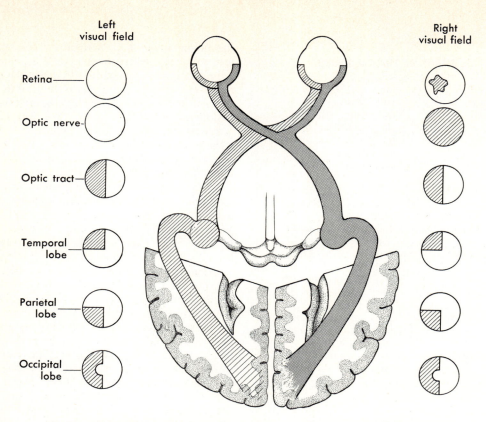

**FIG. 11-13.** Visual field defects in relation to lesions of specific portions of visual pathway.

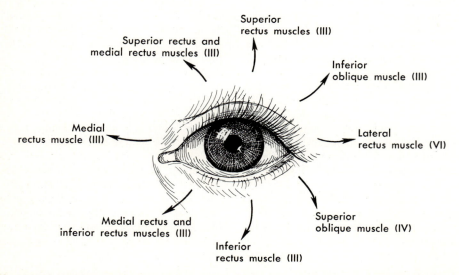

**FIG. 11-14.** Innervation of extraocular muscles. (From Conway, B.L.: Pediatric neurologic nursing, St. Louis, 1977, The C.V. Mosby Co.)

responsible for downward, inward eye movements. The abducens nerve controls lateral deviation of the eye (Fig. 11-14).

ASSESSMENT. The adequacy of ocular movements in all planes is assessed when the client is directed to stabilize the head while moving the gaze to follow your finger through the full range of ocular movement.

The room is darkened for the assessment of pupillary response, which begins with a comparison of size, shape, and equality of pupils. Ask the client to shift the gaze from distant to close objects, so that you may observe the pupillary constriction that normally occurs in the pupillary accommodation reflex. In assessing differences in pupillary size you need to inquire about congenital abnormalities or traumatic events that affected the pupil. Also question the client about any medications, including eye drops, he or she might have received. In general, younger persons have larger, more responsive pupils than elderly ones do.

Direct and consensual pupillary reflexes are assessed when a bright light is shined into each eye after an approach from the side.

DISORDERS. When functional integrity of the oculomotor nerve is disrupted, the client loses the ability to look medially, up, and down in the involved eye. Disturbed functions in the trochlear nerve interrupt the individual's ability to look down and in a lateral direction. A disorder in the abducens nerve results in the inability to look in a lateral direction with the affected eye. In any of these disorders the client reports double vision. In considering the underlying problem, attempt to decide whether the problem is in the nerve proper or in the nuclei of the pons and midbrain.

As eye movements are evaluated, the astute practitioner observes the client for unusual ocular movements. It might be helpful to rapidly move the patterned strip of border fabric across the client's visual field in an even, horizontal fashion. As the client looks straight forward but shifts the eye to follow the pattern, nystagmus may be detected. When nystagmus is present, describe it thoroughly as to direction of eye movements, pattern of unusual movements, and tendency for deviation to be more pronounced in a given direction. If the client is aware of the unusual ocular movements, it is helpful to know when they were first noticed.

*Cranial nerve V.* The fifth cranial nerve, the trigeminal nerve, has a motor and a sensory division. The motor division supplies the temporalis, pterygoid, and masseter muscles, which allow mastication. Assess the motor functions by asking the client to clamp the jaws together and then applying resistance to try to move them apart. As the client clamps and unclamps the jaws, note any distortion in movement or asymmetry.

ASSESSMENT. The jaw jerk *(maxillary reflex)* is assessed when a firm tap is applied with a reflex hammer to the midchin area with the client's mouth slightly open. The normal response is a sudden closing motion of the jaw.

The sensory division of the trigeminal nerve comprises three parts, including the ophthalmic, mandibular, and maxillary branches, which supply superficial sensations to the cornea, the mucosa of the nose and mouth, and the skin of the face and forehead. The pain nucleus is located in the medulla and upper spinal cord, whereas the touch and motor nuclei are situated at the midpons level.

To evaluate sensibility in the trigeminal nerve, employ a variety of sensory tests, bilaterally, to note the presence and symmetry of response. Apply the sensory tests to three areas: jaws, cheeks, and forehead. Sensory tests include touching these areas with wisps of cotton, using pinpricks, and eliciting responses to hot and cold objects. Perform these sensory tests with the client's eyes closed. Finally test the corneal reflex by noting the presence of a blink when a wisp of cotton is lightly moved on the patient's cornea. It is not sufficient for the sclera to be the only part of the eye touched in eliciting the corneal reflex.

DISORDERS. One of the most common disorders of the trigeminal nerve is tic douloureux (trigeminal neuralgia), which is detailed in Chapter 19. Problems in sensibility and motor functions are also reportable. The use of contact lenses may diminish or obliterate the corneal reflex.

*Cranial nerve VII.* Cranial nerve VII, the facial nerve, has a motor and a sensory division. The sensory component supplies a sense of taste to the anterior two thirds of the tongue, maintains some sensation in the external ear canal, and innervates the lacrimal, submaxillary, and sublingual glands. Most of the facial muscles are innervated by the motor division.

ASSESSMENT. To assess the motor portion, ask the

client to elevate the eyebrows, wrinkle the forehead, frown, smile, show the teeth, balloon the cheeks out with air, and close the eyes so that you cannot open them. Note the client's face during relaxation and conversation to see if there are any asymmetrical features, especially in the nasolabial folds.

The sensory component of the nerve is assessed when the client is asked to extend the tongue so that sugar and then salt can be placed on the anterior portion on each side of the tongue. The tongue should remain extended until the client has had adequate time to identify the taste. Swallowing or retraction of the tongue before taste identification results in incorrect test results, since both sides of the tongue become involved in the discrimination of taste. Between applications of sugar and salt, encourage the client to drink water to remove the previous taste. Quinine and vinegar may also be utilized.

**DISORDERS.** When there is a disturbance in the supranuclear fibers that supply the facial nerve, paresis is limited to the lower portion of the face. If the whole face is paralyzed, the interruption in neuronal functions involves the motor nucleus or the peripheral aspect of the facial nerve. The motor nucleus of the facial nerve is located in the posterior aspect of the pons. (Fig. 11-15 shows the clinical features of Bell's palsy.) In contrast to an interrupted neuronal supply at the lower motor neuron, be aware of disturbances in the functions of facial muscles that occur when the neuronal interference is at the upper motor neuron. For example, the client with a unilateral cortical lesion has little or no functional disturbance of the upper face, since muscles of the forehead and eyes are innervated from both sides of the brain. Clinically the individual with a unilateral cortical lesion does the following: (1) When the eyes are closed, the nasolabial fold is flat; also the eyes close weakly. (2) When the eyebrows are raised, the lower portion of the face is paralyzed, but the forehead wrinkles and the eyebrows elevate bilaterally without difficulty.

If there is a disturbance in taste, the problem may be an interference in the sensory nucleus, a portion of the tractus solitarius of the medulla, or the sensory fibers of the facial nerve.

*Cranial nerve VIII.* The eighth cranial nerve,
the acoustic nerve, has two major divisions: the cochlear nerve and the vestibular nerve. The vestibular nerve is not tested in the usual neurological examination but requires assessment through caloric tests when the client has a history of dizziness, disturbed balance, or tinnitus.

**ASSESSMENT.** Test the cochlear nerve by performing a hearing test on the client. Utilize a tuning fork to determine lateral hearing discrimination and air and bone conduction, as previously discussed in the section on auditory assessment and as shown in Figs. 11-10 to 11-12.

**DISORDERS.** Disturbances of the cochlear nerve may occur within the nerve itself or in its nucleus at the pontomedullary junction. Symptoms of disturbed functions may include deafness, diminished hearing, or tinnitis.

*Cranial nerves IX and X.* The ninth cranial nerve, the glossopharyngeal nerve, and the tenth cranial nerve, the vagus nerve, are assessed together.

**ASSESSMENT.** Assess the pharyngeal gag reflex by touching the side of the pharynx with an application stick or a tongue depressor. The palatal reflex is evaluated as the mucous membrane, lateral to the vagus, is stroked, bilaterally, resulting in the stimulated side rising if normal.

The vagal nerve innervates the motor portions of the pharynx, larynx, and soft palate. The vagal nerve is intimately involved in autonomic functions, which are assessed in the general autonomic operation evaluation. The integrity of vagal nerve functions may be evaluated separately from that of glossopharyngeal nerve functions. Vagal functions are intact when the client is able to swallow, speak clearly without a hoarse vocal quality, move the vocal cords symmetrically during speech, and move the soft palate symmetrically when vocalizing the sound "ah."

Autonomic and motor nuclei of the vagus nerve are located in the medulla. Sensory fibers of the glossopharyngeal nerve that innervate the mucosa of the tonsils, soft palate, pharynx, and neighboring areas arise from a nucleus found in the medulla.

**DISORDERS.** In pathological conditions the palate and uvula deviate to the contralateral side when a lesion of the vagal nerve results in paralysis. Vocal cord paralysis caused by an interference with vagal

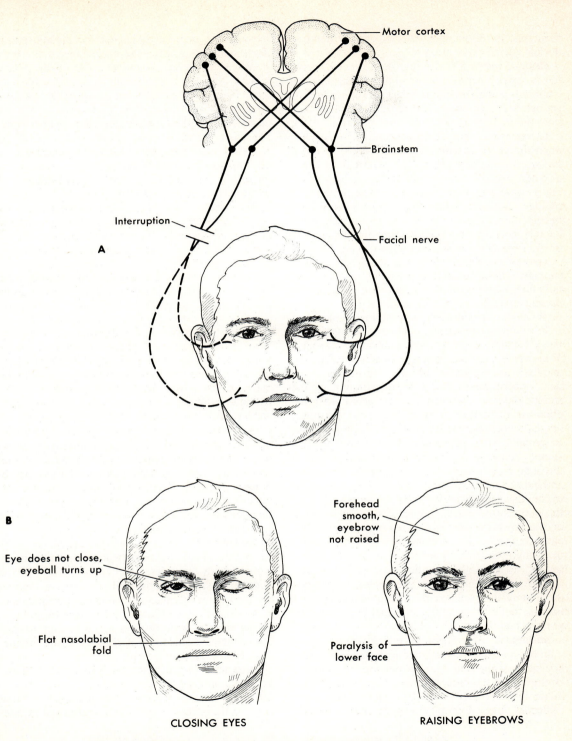

**FIG. 11-15.** Clinical features of Bell's palsy, an outcome of lower motor neuron paralysis.

functions is frequently detected by hoarseness during speech production.

*Cranial nerve XI.* The eleventh cranial nerve, the accessory nerve, has its nuclei in the nucleus ambiguus of the medulla and in the upper five or six cervical cord segments. Its function is to provide motor operation to the upper portion of the trapezius and sternocleidomastoid muscles, wherein posture and movements of the head and shoulder girdles are made possible. This nerve is assessed to determine if there are problems, such as wasting or weakness in the muscles supplied. When a problem is detected, the next step is to further delineate the nature of the lesion (unilateral or bilateral) and its location in the nucleus, nerve trunk, branches, or local muscle.

ASSESSMENT. Severe defects in the involved muscles are quickly detected when the client's head falls forward in extreme weakness of the trapezius muscle and the head falls backward in extreme weakness of the sternocleidomastoid muscle.

In routine assessments, evaluate the integrity of the accessory nerve by performing two tests: (1) The strength of the trapezius muscle is observed and the area palpated as the client shrugs the shoulders against resistance. (2) The strength of the sternocleidomastoid muscle is evaluated when the client turns the face to the right against resistance applied to the right side of the face by your hand. In response the left sternocleidomastoid muscle should stand out prominently. Repeat this test on the opposite side, and evaluate equality of strength and bulk bilaterally. To evaluate both sternocleidomastoid muscles simultaneously, place a hand on the client's forehead and apply resistance while he or she bows the forehead. This maneuver should cause both muscles to stand out, so that equality in strength and bulk may be more accurately assessed. Additionally, ask the client to arise from a supine position. If the sternocleidomastoid muscles are normal, this movement should be done without difficulty, the head being the first part to rise.

DISORDERS. If the client has a birdlike, thin neck with obvious thyroid cartilage and gland, the sternocleidomastoid muscles may be absent or wasted. If the sternocleidomastoid muscles are affected bilaterally, the client raises the lagging head with difficulty after elevating the body from a supine position. A grimace may even accompany the effort, since lifting the head requires such exertion.

When the defect is unilateral, the client is unable to turn the head against resistance to the opposite side. In a unilateral problem the sternocleidomastoid muscle fails to stand out when the client moves the head to the side against resistance.

When the trapezius muscle is affected, the shoulder drops unilaterally and the scapula is displaced in a lateral, downward direction. The client with weakness in the trapezius muscle may still be able to weakly shrug the shoulders, since this function is also controlled to some extent by cervical nerve innervation to the trapezius muscle.

If coarse twitching is evident in the trapezius muscle, it is most commonly caused by a compressive or irritative lesion near the origin of the nerve trunk. Fasciculations in the trapezius muscle indicate a lesion in the nucleus.

Bilateral sternocleidomastoid lesions indicate muscular dystrophy and poliomyelitis. Poliomyelitis or polyneuritis might result in paralysis of the trapezius muscle bilaterally. Unilateral impairment might be caused by such problems as trauma to the neck or base of the skull, space-occupying lesions at the level of the jugular foramen, or body irregularities at the base of the skull.

*Cranial nerve XII.* The twelfth cranial nerve, the hypoglossal nerve, regulates all tongue movement and some movement of the larynx and hyoid bone during and after swallowing. In assessing the integrity of this nerve, inspect the tongue for any abnormalities, including weakness, wasting, and involuntary movement and ascertain the degree of voluntary muscle control.

ASSESSMENT. Test the twelfth cranial nerve by asking the client to extend the tongue. Immediately note atrophy, tremors, or lateral deviation of the tongue. Assess the strength of voluntary movement by having the client move the tongue from side to side against the resistance of a tongue blade.

DISORDERS. A number of nonneurological diseases reveal themselves in changes in the tongue. For example, clients with cretinism or Down's syndrome have characteristic enlargement of the tongue.

A number of conditions may affect the normal movement of the tongue, including trauma, space-occupying lesions, progressive bulbar palsy, extreme hemiplegia from vascular accidents, and amyotrophic lateral sclerosis.

## Cerebellar functions

The cerebellum was introduced in Chapter 1 in relation to embryology, discussed in Chapter 2 concerning anatomy, and detailed in Chapter 3 in relation to integration. A number of tests are employed to evaluate coordination and balance, the main functions of the cerebellum.

To conduct the first test, instruct the client to touch the index finger to the nose with alternating hands. Then have him or her perform the same task with the eyes closed.

Next ask the client to touch the nose and then touch your finger in rapid succession. During this test move your finger to different locations and have him or her perform the task with increasing speed. Repeat the same task with the client's other hand.

Request the client to touch the index finger to the thumb on the same hand in a tapping motion of rapid movements. Repeat the same test with the client's other hand.

Ask the client to sit down. With the hand open, have the client pat his or her thigh in a rapid succession of pronation and supination of the hand. Repeat the test with the client's other hand.

Ask the client to move the heel along the opposite shin and to draw a figure eight in the air with each foot.

Ask the client to rise to a standing position with feet together, first with the eyes open and then with them closed. Ask the client to walk about 20 steps. Note the gait, arm swing, and presence of any associated movements. Cerebellar disorders do not reflect differences in coordination with eyes open or shut. Ask the client to walk in a heel-to-toe (tandem) pattern along a straight line. Observe any undue difficulty with tandem walking. If the client seems unusually unsteady on the feet, stand ready to lend support during tandem walking.

For all tests of locomotion, evaluate smoothness and accuracy of the task and look for any abnormal movements: tics, tremors, ataxia, or exaggerated arm swing. Posture should be maintained in an erect position without difficulty, and the client should be able to judge the distance between two points, as in the finger-to-nose test.

When there is a disturbance of cerebellar function, it is most often manifested in tremors, ataxia, or difficulty with alternating movements. Other signs of impaired cerebellar functions include nystagmus (abnormal rhythmical eye movements) and disturbances in speech and muscle tone.

## Motor integrity

Chapter 3 contains a discussion of motor output. Here, as part of the neurological assessment, both palpate and inspect the muscles for size and tone.

*Muscle size.* Begin the test of muscle size using a tape measure to evaluate the size of corresponding parts in the calves, thighs, and upper arms. Observe the client for posture and adequacy of muscle contours. Observation of missing muscles, estimations of muscle bulk, and nutritional status are also made at this time. In one setting a simple method for determining malnutrition was utilized that could be performed by auxiliary workers. The method is based on a color-coded tape measurement of the middle of the upper arm, which has a relatively stable circumference between 1 and 5 years of age, when malnutrition and growth interferences are most prevalent in children. Children who were malnourished had arm circumferences of 12.5 cm or less. More than 75% of the children who had less severe degrees of malnutrition had arm circumferences of 12.5 to 13.5 cm. Most normal children had arm circumferences between 13.5 and 17.5 cm.

Carefully inspect the hands to detect fine tremors of individual muscle fibers or fasciculations and to evaluate the muscles for wasting. When muscle atrophy is present as an outcome of lower motor neuron disease, fasciculations are commonly present.

Use a percussion hammer to tap the various muscle groups over the body. Note signs of irritability or weakness in response to this stimulus.

More detail on muscle-wasting disorders is available in Chapter 17 and in the sections on muscular dystrophy, syringomyelia, poliomyelitis, peroneal muscular atrophy, polyneuritis, and peripheral nerve disorders. Muscle wasting may also be caused by congential muscle disorders or interruption in growth during muscle development in childhood.

***Muscle tone.*** Muscle tone, the *degree of tension present in a muscle at rest* is difficult to assess, since circumstances inherent in the assessment situation may vary. During this portion of the assessment, make every attempt to create a comfortable holistic climate, wherein relaxation can occur. After the client is relaxed, palpate the muscles in all extremities at rest. Then move the limbs passively and note any resistance to these movements.

Muscle tone is abnormal if it is decreased or increased. When muscle tone is diminished, muscles respond to movement in a lax manner; for example, arms hang in a pendulous fashion when relaxed at the side. Also, resistance to passive movement is decreased, and the possible range of motion at a joint is increased. When a limb is placed in a given position, the client finds it difficult to maintain the position. Thus displacement of the limbs from that position occurs with ease. In instances of tone loss the deep tendon reflexes are absent or diminished.

*Hypotonia,* diminished muscle tone, occurs in a variety of problems. The problem may result from a lesion in the sensory aspect of the reflex arc (tabes dorsalis) or in the motor aspect of the reflex arc (peripheral nerve injuries, poliomyelitis, polyneuritis). At times the hypotonia is caused by a lesion that affects both sensory and motor integrity (extreme cord destruction, cord compression, syringomyelia). Hypotonia may result from a disturbance in the muscle itself (myopathias, muscular dystrophy, myasthenia gravis). In the early stages of neurological shock after severe cord destruction, hypotonia in muscles is apparent. In Sydenham's chorea, involuntary movements occur concurrently with diminished muscle tone, which allows hyperextensibility, particularly at the fingers and wrists.

Tone in muscles may also be increased abnormally. *Three major forms of increased tone* are most common. In the first type, tone and resistance are more pronounced in one group of muscles than in the antagonist group of muscles. In this type of increased tone, resistance to passive movement is initially apparent, but it suddenly gives way. This response is termed *clasp-knife spasticity* and is most obvious at the knee and elbow. At rest, affected muscles are firm on palpation and tend to form contractures. The clasp-knife response is an outcome of upper motor neuron disease and is most pronounced in the extensor muscles of the lower extremities and in the flexor muscles of the upper extremities.

The second form of hypertonicity, *lead-pipe rigidity,* occurs when muscles and their antagonists have an equal amount of resistance. In moving an extremity through passive range of motion the amount of hypertonicity remains constant. In clients with an extreme degree of hypertonicity, muscles remain rigid, and the extremity remains in strict immobility. This type of hypertonicity is apparent in clients with lesions of the extrapyramidal system and with severe upper motor neuron impairments, as evident in extreme spasticity.

The third form of hypertonicity, *cogwheel rigidity,* occurs as muscles and their antagonists contract in a rapid, alternating manner throughout the passive range of motion. This type of hypertonicity appears intermittently and most prominently at the wrist. Its presence indicates an extrapyramidal disorder.

The first type of increased tone is apparent in injury, space-occupying lesions, or degenerative processes affecting the cerebrum. Lead-pipe rigidity is common in the postencephalitic type of Parkinson's disease. Cogwheel rigidity is commonly seen in arteriosclerotic degeneration of the extrapyramidal system, some forms of Parkinson's disease, carbon monoxide poisoning, and ingestion of high dosages of chlorpromazine or reserpine.

Clonus occurs as the stretch on a hypertonic muscle causes reflex contractions that continue until the stretch stimulus is released. The presence of clonus with other abnormal signs, such as Babinski's sign, indicates a pyramidal tract disorder. Clonus may be seen in normal individuals who are very tense, those who have strained muscles in defecating, or those who have been frightened by almost having an accident while driving a car.

Myotonia, a condition wherein the muscle contraction continues into the period of relaxation, may be seen as the client is asked to squint the eyes and let go. On letting go the period of relaxation is delayed. In these clients percussion of the thenar eminence causes the thumb to slowly adduct and the muscle to dimple. Myotonia is most common in individuals with dystrophia myotonica and myotonia congenita. To diagnose true myotonia, the client may be injected with adrenocorticotropic hormone, causing the problem to be less prominent for a few hours.

## Involuntary movements

During the assessment process observe the client to detect the presence of any involuntary movements. When such activity is observed, accurate and precise recordings are important. These observations should include the following:

1. Effect of internal and external environment
2. Precipitating events
3. Nature of movement (constant, intermittent)
4. Time of occurrence (at rest, during movement, in sleep)
5. Alteration in movement with eyes open or closed
6. Alteration related to initiation of voluntary activity or position of trunk or limbs
7. Client's awareness of activity and factors influencing onset

Involuntary movements are detected throughout the assessment process but especially during the cerebellar evaluation and when the client is asked to extend the arms in front palms upward with the eyes open and then closed.

Involuntary movements are evident in many forms. Epileptic episodes are one type of involuntary movement (Chapter 14). Chorea and dystonia are discussed in Chapter 18. Facial tics, or odd facial movements, occurring as a habit spasm do not involve organic disorders. Shrugging movements of the shoulders are another type of tic.

*Tremors* are an additional type of involuntary movement. They are categorized as fine and coarse. A *fine* tremor requires close observation for detection, whereas a *coarse* tremor is observable without particular effort. Anxiety and nervousness may result in a tremor that is often confined to the fingers but may involve all body parts. Other causes of tremors include thyrotoxicosis, alcoholism, amphetamine addiction, primary heredofamilial tremor, Parkinson's disease, intention tremor (a coarse tremor that appears with voluntary movement in conditions where a space-occupying lesion interferes with cerebellar connections), or disseminated sclerosis. Tremors may also be seen in collagen and Wilson's diseases. Searching

movements of the hands resembling athetoid movements may occur in clients who have experienced a severe loss of position sensibility, as in tabes dorsalis, cervical spondylosis, and carcinomatous sensory neuropathy.

*Fasciculations* are irregular contractions of muscle fascicles observable at rest and increased after voluntary activity. This activity, observable as a "jumping muscle," does not cause discomfort. It signals irritation of the anterior root or anterior horn cell degeneration. It is often associated with exaggerated reflexes and wasting of the muscles.

*Fibrillations* are finer movements that may be detected by electromyography.

## Muscle strength

Movement of the major joints, including flexion and extension, is tested as the client moves the body extremity through active range of motion with and without resistance. The strength of corresponding muscles is compared. The following considerations are helpful in evaluating strength: (1) Does the strength vary in corresponding muscles? (2) Is the strength appropriate for the size and age of the client? (3) Does any weakness seem apparent? (4) If so, is it variable, improved by conscious effort or rest, or congruent with capacities detailed by history? (5) Does any deformity, injury, or disease process hamper movement or accurate assessment?

A five-point rating scale is used to assess muscle strength. This scale provides some standardization to the evaluation process and is as follows:

5   Normal strength.
4   The muscle completes its full range of movement but succumbs to resistance.
3   The muscle completes its full range of movement against gravity but not against further resistance.
2   The muscle is unable to complete the portion of movement that goes against gravity.
1   Effort results in attempts at muscle contraction, but the joint or limb fails to move.
0   Complete paralysis.

In a routine assessment of muscle strength the major muscle groups are evaluated. Impairments in muscle strength require referral to a specialist for complete testing of individual muscles.

In appraising young, handicapped, or uncooperative clients, special methods may have to be utilized in estimation of muscle strength. Muscle power in the fingers and hands may be observed as the child is given toys that are manipulated with the hands. Shoulder girdle strength is determined when the child is carefully held by the axillae. When muscle weakness exists, the child tends to slip through the examiner's fingers. Muscles in the pelvic girdle and the proximal lower extremities are evaluated when the child is observed swinging the legs in a rotary fashion to climb steps and the child is observed during the process of rising to a stance from a supine position. When weakness exists, Gowers' sign is present, as detailed in Chapter 17. The distal lower extremities are assessed for muscle power as the child walks on the heels, walks on tiptoe, or demonstrates an usual gait.

Major muscle groups are most frequently assessed in the following order:

| | |
|---|---|
| **Neck** | Extensors and flexors |
| **Shoulder** | Adductors, abductors, and rotators |
| **Elbow, wrist, and fingers** | Extensors and flexors |
| **Hand** | Grip (dynamometer may be used) |
| **Abdominal muscles** | Contraction and relaxation |
| **Spine** | Extensors |
| **Hip and knee** | Flexors and extensors |
| **Toes** | Flexors and extensors, with particular attention to great toe |

## Sensory assessment

Before the tests for sensory integrity are performed, it would be helpful to review the section in Chapter 3 on input and Chapter 15.

In evaluating the integrity of the sensory system it is important to keep several points in mind:
1. Is the client, able to perceive the sensory stimulus?
2. Do distal and proximal portions of the same extremity vary in sensitivity?
3. Are corresponding portions of the body equal in sensitivity?
4. In sensory disturbances a sketch is helpful in circumscribing the affected area.

Several factors affect the accuracy and diagnostic value of sensory evaluation. First, all sensory tests should be performed while the client, has the

eyes closed. Second, total relaxation, understanding, and cooperation are essential in the client, since his or her expectations and accurate perception of sensory stimuli affect the outcome. When sensory problems exist, a diminished capacity in sensibility occurs more commonly than total absence of sensation. When primary sensory modalities are normal, but impairments exist in cortical sensory modalities, the genesis of the problem is in the parietal lobe. Table 11-5 outlines the sensory evaluation plan.

## Evaluation of reflexes

*Assessment.* Assessment of the reflexes should be done when the client is relaxed in order to obtain the most accurate evaluation. Care should also be taken to apply the same degree of stimulation at all points, so that various points are comparable in response. Although a number of tests for reflexes are available, only a few are commonly used to assess reflex status.

Reflexes are divided into two categories, *deep* and *superficial,* as shown here.

| SUMMARY OF REFLEXES | |
|---|---|
| **Deep** | **Superficial** |
| Biceps | Upper abdominal |
| Brachioradialis | Lower abdominal |
| Triceps | Cremasteric |
| Patellar | Plantar |
| Achilles | Gluteal |

*Reflex status.* In addition to cutaneous areas of diminished sensibility or paralysis, reflex changes are also valuable in localizing the level of a spinal cord lesion. Reflex changes are significant, because of the changes that appear when reflex arcs are impinged on or broken. In general, reflexes are diminished or abolished in accordance with the defect in the arc. Table 11-6 lists the common deep and superficial reflexes, points of stimulation, expected results, and involved segments.

Generally the localizing value of superficial reflexes is limited, since they have a superimposed cortical pathway. Thus a change in the superficial reflexes may indicate a lesion at either the cortical or the lower motor neuron level. In contrast, the

**TABLE 11-5.** Sensory evaluation

| Type | Method | Points to evaluate |
|---|---|---|
| **Primary forms of sensation** | | |
| Superficial tactile sensation | Touch hands, forearms, trunk, thigh, lower legs, feet, and perineal and perianal areas with cotton wisp. | Does client perceive stimulus? Do corresponding body parts differ in response? |
| Superficial pain | Apply pin or sharp object to skin. Take care to avoid injury during testing. Test body parts listed in test for superficial tactile sensation. | Do proximal and distal parts of same extremity differ in sensitivity? Do you have adequate cooperation from client? |
| Thermal sensitivity | Touch body parts listed in test for superficial tactile sensation with test tubes of hot and cold water. Take care to avoid injury during testing. | Do sensory changes conform to anatomical pathways? |
| Vibratory sense | Place a vibrating tuning fork on the bony prominences: wrist, elbow, shoulder, hip, knee, shin, and ankle. | Note sensitivity in corresponding body parts. Observe ability to detect cessation of vibration. Compare sensitivity in distal and proximal aspects of same extremity. |
| Deep pressure pain | Squeeze Achilles tendons, calf, and forearm. | Note sensitivity in corresponding body parts. |
| Motion and position | Move fingers and toes passively. To avoid detection of movement through pressure, avoid applying tactile pressure during testing, and grasp each digit on the lateral aspect between your thumb and index finger. | Evaluate client's ability to identify direction of movement and final destination of digit. |
| **Cortical and discriminatory forms of sensation** | | |
| Two-point discrimination | Touch two different body parts simultaneously with sharp objects. Ask clients whether one or two points are being stimulated as testing continues over body surface. | Compare corresponding body parts for sensibility. Remember that areas of body vary in capacity to perceive distances in two-point discrimination. |
| Point localization | Touch client's skin lightly. Ask client to detect point where he or she was touched. | Compare corresponding body parts for sensitivity to like stimuli. |
| Texture discrimination | With eyes remaining closed, place common objects, for example, burlap, silk, or cotton in client's hand. Client is required to identify object. | Can client identify object? |
| Stereognostic capacity | Place familiar objects, for example, dime, comb, or paper clip, in client's hand. Client is required to identify object. | Can client identify object? |
| Graphesthesia | With blunt end of cotton applicator, trace numbers and letters on palms of client's hands or other body parts. Client should be able to identify figures. | Can client identify figures? Compare sensibility in corresponding body parts. Be certain that educational limitations do not interfere with client's ability to complete test. |
| Extinction | Touch two corresponding body parts simultaneously. Client should report being touched simultaneously on both sides. | Does client report being touched simultaneously on both sides? |

**TABLE 11-6.** Deep and superficial reflexes

| Reflexes | | Stimulus | Normal results | Involved segment |
|---|---|---|---|---|
| Deep | Superficial | | | |
| Biceps muscle | — | Tap biceps tendon. | Forearm flexes at elbow. | C5-C6 |
| Forearm pronator muscles | — | Tap palmar side of forearm medial to styloid process of radius. | Forearm pronates. | C6 |
| Triceps muscle | — | Tap triceps tendon. | Forearm extends at elbow. | C6-C7 |
| Brachioradial muscle | — | While holding forearm in semipronated position, tap styloid process. | Forearm flexes at elbow. | C7-C8 |
| Finger (flexion) | — | Tap palm at tip of fingers. | Fingers flex. | C7-T1 |
| Abdominal muscles | — | Tap inferior thorax, abdominal wall, and symphysis pubis. | Abdominal wall contracts; leg adducts when symphysis pubis is tapped. | T8-T12 |
| — | Abdominal muscles | Stroke upper, middle, and lower skin on abdomen. | Abdominal muscles contract with retraction of umbilicus toward stimulated side. | T8-T12 |
| — | Cremasteric muscle | Stroke medial upper leg in adductor region. | Testicles move up. | L1-L2 |
| Adductor muscle | — | Tap medial condyle of tibia. | Leg adducts. | L2-L4 |
| Quadriceps muscle (knee jerk) | — | Tap tendon of quadriceps femoris muscle. | Lower leg extends. | L2-L4 |
| Triceps sural muscle (ankle jerk) | — | Tap Achilles tendon. | Plantar flexion of foot occurs. | L5-S2 |
| — | Plantar area | Stroke lateral side on sole of foot. | Plantar flexion of toes occurs. | S1-S2 |

deep reflexes are elicited by percussion of the muscle tendon or periosteum and are mediated only through the spinal arc. Deep reflexes are therefore more valuable in localizing the level of a spinal cord lesion. When reflexes are asymmetric, diminished, increased, or absent, findings should be compared to the results of the remainder of the neurological assessment, and consultation with a specialist should be utilized as appropriate.

**DEEP TENDON REFLEXES.** Assess the deep reflexes by using a percussion hammer to soundly tap the bony prominence or tendon. The response in the respective muscle is a sudden stretch and contraction.

The *biceps reflex* is elicited when the biceps tendon is percussed after the client has supinated the hand and flexed the elbow. The result is contraction of the biceps muscle. Integrity of the biceps reflex indicates the status of the fifth and sixth cervical segments.

The *brachioradialis reflex* is elicited when the styloid process of the radius is percussed. The normal outcome is pronation of the forearm and flexion at the elbow. This reflex indicates the integrity of the fifth and sixth cervical segments.

The *triceps reflex* is elicited when the triceps tendon is percussed with the elbow flexed above the olecranon groove. The normal response is extension of the elbow. Integrity of this reflex reflects intactiness of C6 through C8.

The *patellar reflex* is elicited when the patellar tendon is percussed while the knee is flexed and dangling free. The typical response is extension of the leg at the knee. The typical response is extension of the leg at the knee. This reflex depends on innervation originating at spinal cord segments L2 through L4.

The *Achilles reflex* is elicited when the Achilles tendon is percussed while the foot is held in neutral position. The normal response is plantar flexion of the foot. S1 and S2 are the spinal cord segments at which the nerves innervating this reflex originate.

SUPERFICIAL REFLEXES. The superficial reflexes are elicited as various points on the skin are stroked with a reasonably sharp object that will not damage the skin. A tongue blade may be an appropriate stimulus. Five reflexes are commonly assessed in an evaluation of the superficial reflexes: upper abdominal, lower abdominal, cremasteric, plantar, and gluteal.

The *upper abdominal reflex* is assessed when a stimulus is moved from the umbilicus outward in a diagonal direction to the northeast and northwest. The typical response is upward movement of the umbilicus toward the area of stimulation. Cord segments including T7 through T9 are involved in this maneuver.

The *lower abdominal reflex* is tested like the upper abdominal reflex, except that the stimulus is moved from the umbilicus in a diagonal direction to the southeast and southwest, with a resulting downward movement of the umbilicus. This reflex depends on the integrity of T11 and T12.

In the *cremasteric reflex,* light scratching on the inner aspect of the upper thigh with the testing object results in elevation of the testicles on the ipsilateral side. This response depends on the integrity of T12 and L1.

The *plantar response* is elicited by firm stroking of the lateral aspect of the dorsum of the foot. Toes should flex after about 18 months of age. This reflex depends on integrity of S1 and S2.

In the *gluteal reflex,* stroking of the skin results in tenseness in the gluteal area. This reflex depends on integrity of the cord segments extending from L4 through S3.

Pathological reflexes are detailed in Chapters 3 and 17.

## Flow sheet

When a chronic process is identified in a client who will be checked at intervals by the practitioner, the use of a chronic disease flow sheet may be helpful in summarizing key points in the disease process and treatment plan over a lengthy period of time. Examples of flow sheets are readily available and are currently recommended as a handy way of maintaining relevant data for research and health care audits, as well as for having quick access to data that may influence decisions in care. In one article by Schmitt, 19 diseases are highlighted with regard to some relevant items for a flow sheet.

## REFERENCES

Alexander, M.M., and Brown, M.S.: Physical examination part 17: neurological examination, Nursing76 **6**:38, June 1976.

Alexander, M.M., and Brown, M.S.: Physical examination part 18: neurological examination, Nursing76 **6**:50, July 1976.

Amiel-Tison, C.: Neurological evaluation of the maturity of newborn infants, Arch. Dis. Child. **43**:89, 1968.

Apgar, V.: The newborn (Apgar) scoring system: reflections and advice. Pediatr. Clin. North Am. **13**:645, 1966.

Babson, S.G., et al: Diagnosis and management of the fetus and neonate at risk: a guide for team care, St. Louis, 1979, The C.V. Mosby Co.

Ballard, J.L., et al.: A simplified score for assessment of fetal maturation of newly born infants, J. Pediatr. **95**:769, Nov. 1979.

Barker, J., et al.: Denver Eye Screening Test manual, Denver, 1972, W.K. Frankenburg.

Barness, L.A.: Manual of pediatric physical diagnosis, New York, 1972, Year Book Medical Publishers, Inc.

Bates, B.: A guide to physical examination, ed. 2, Philadelphia, 1979, J.B. Lippincott Co.

Battaglia, F.C., and Lubchenco, L.O.: A practical classification of newborn infants by weight and gestational age, J. Pediatr. **71**:161, 1967.

Beeson, P.B., and McDermott, W., editors: Cecil-Loeb textbook of medicine, ed. 14, Philadelphia, 1975, W.B. Saunders Co.

Behrman, R.E., editor: Neonatology: diseases of the fetus and infant, ed. 2, St. Louis, 1977, The C.V. Mosby Co.

Bickerstaff, E.R.: Neurological examination in clinical practice, ed. 3, Philadelphia, 1973, J.B. Lippincott Co.

Browder, J.A., and Merchon, P.M.: Speech and language development: the physician's role, Postgrad. Med. **56**:151, 1974.

Capute, A.J., and Biehl, R.F.: Functional developmental evaluation, Pediatr. Clin. North Am. **20**:3, 1973.

Chard, T.: The fetus at risk, Lancet **2**:880, 1974.

Chusid, J.G.: Correlative neuroanatomy and functional neurology, ed. 17, Los Altos, Calif., 1979, Lange Medical Publications.

Conway, B.L.: Neurological assessment during the first year of life in current practice in pediatric nursing, St. Louis, 1980, The C.V. Mosby Co.

Conway-Rutkowski, B., editor: Patient compliance, a symposium, Nurs. Clin. North Am., Sept. 1982.

Desmond, M.M.: Clinical behavior of the newly born, J. Pediatr. **62:**1307, 1963.

Dickson, S.: Communication disorders: remedial principles and procedures, Glenville 1974, Scott, Foresman & Co.

Dobbing, J.: The later growth of the brain and its vulnerability, Pediatrics **53:**2, 1974.

Drage, J.S., and Berendes, H.: Apgar scores and outcome of the newborn, Pediatr. Clin. North Am. **13:**635, 1966.

Drumwright, A.F.: The Denver Articulation Screening Exam, Denver, 1971, University of Colorado Medical Center.

Farr, V., et al.: The definition of some external characteristics used in the assessment of gestational age in the newborn infant, Dev. Med. Child Neurol. **8:**507, 1966.

Forster, F.M.: Clinical neurology, ed. 4, St. Louis, 1978, The C.V. Mosby Co.

Frankenburg, W.K., et al.: The revised Denver Developmental Screening Test: its accuracy as a screening instrument, J. Pediatr. **79:**988, 1971.

Frankenburg, W.K., et al.: Validity on the Denver Developmental Screening Test, Child Dev. **42:**475, 1971.

Haymaker, W.: Bing's local diagnosis in neurological diseases, St. Louis, 1969, The C.V. Mosby Co.

Hiles, D.A.: Strabismus, Am. J. Nurs. **74:**1082, 1974.

Kahn, H.: Visual dysfunctions, Nursing74 **4:**26, 1974.

Koenigsberger, R.M.: Judgment of fetal age. I. Neurologic evaluation, Pediatr. Clin. North Am. **13:**823, 1966.

Korones, S.B.: High-risk newborn infants—the basis for intensive nursing care, ed. 2, St. Louis, 1976, The C.V. Mosby Co.

Kugel, R., editor: Vision screening of preschool children, report of the Committee on Children with Handicaps, American Academy of Pediatrics, Pediatrics **50:**966, 1972.

Mead, M., and Newton, N.: Conception, pregnancy, labor, and the puerperium in cultural perspective, Rev. Med. Psychol. **4:**22, 1962.

Mechner, F.: Patient assessment: neurological examination. Part III, programmed instruction, Am. J. Nurs. **76:**609, April 1976.

Mingeot, R.A., and Herbaut, M.: The functional status of the newborn infant, Am. J. Obstet. Gynecol. **115:**1138, 1973.

Paine, R.S., et al.: Evolution of postural reflexes in normal infants and in the presence of chronic brain syndrome, Neurology **14:**1036, 1964.

Preston, M.S.: Psycholinguistics and the evaluation of language function, Pediatr. Clin. North Am. **20:**79, 1973.

Prior, J.A., and Silberstein, J.S.: Physical diagnosis: the history and examination of the patient, ed. 5, St. Louis, 1977, The C.V. Mosby Co.

Scanlon, J.W.: How is the baby? The Apgar score revisited, Clin. Pediatr. **12:**61, 1973.

Schmitt, B.D.: The chronic disease flow sheet in ambulatory pediatrics, Pediatrics **51:**722, 1973.

Schuring, A.G., and Gunter, J.P.: Paralysis of the facial nerve in children, Clin. Pediatr. **9:**105, 1970.

Seeds, A.E.: Adverse effects on the fetus of acute events in labor, Pediatr. Clin. North Am. **17:**811, 1970.

Shakir, A., and Morley, D.: Measuring malnutrition (letter), Lancet **1:**758, 1974.

Synder, M., and Baum, R.: Assessing station and gait, Am. J. Nurs. **74:**1256, July 1974.

Smithells, R.W., and Speidel, B.D.: Prenatal influences and prenatal diagnosis, Br. Med. J. **4:**105, 1971.

Thuline, H.C.: Color blindness in children: the importance and feasibility of early recognition, Clin. Pediatr. **11:**295, 1972.

Towell, M.E.: The influence of labor on the fetus and the newborn, Pediatr. Clin. North Am. **13:**575, 1966.

Travis, L.E.: Handbook of speech pathology and audiology, New York, 1971, Prentice-Hall, Inc.

Tucker, S.M.: Fetal monitoring and fetal assessment in high-risk pregnancy, St. Louis, 1978, The C.V. Mosby Co.

Usher, R., et al.: Judgment of fetal age and an objective method for its assessment, Pediatr. Clin. North Am. **13:**835, 1966.

Vaughan, V., III, et al., editors: Textbook of pediatrics, ed. 11, Philadelphia, 1979, W.B. Saunders Co.

Warwick, R., and Williams, P.L., editors: Gray's anatomy, ed. 35, Philadelphia, 1973, W.B. Saunders Co.

WIC Currents: News of women, infants, and children programs, Ross Timesaver, vol. 1, No. 2, March-April 1975.

Willis, W.D., and Grossman, R.G.: Medical neurobiology: neuroanatomical and neurophysiological principles basic to clinical neuroscience, ed. 2, St. Louis, 1977, The C.V. Mosby Co.

Zaner, A.R.: Differential diagnosis of hearing impairment in children: developmental approaches to clinical assessment, J. Commun. Disord. **7:**17, 1974.

# 12
# NEUROLOGICAL DIAGNOSTIC TESTS

To institute effective medical and nursing care, an accurate diagnosis must be made. This is accomplished by learning about the illness through questioning of the client, the family, or friends; making observations; and evaluation of the client with physical and neurological examinations. History taking should elicit information as to the nature, onset, extent, and duration of subjective complaints or manifestations of illness that caused the client to seek medical care. Previous illnesses and personal and family health should also be discussed. While this is being done, the physician and nurse establish the type of contact with the client that inspires trust and confidence, which are extremely important in obtaining the client's full cooperation and acceptance of whatever tests and treatments may be necessary.

A positive relationship will be developed and enhanced if the practitioner regards the client as an individual who is greatly concerned about his or her own illness and is generally anxious and apprehensive about the outcome and the future. The client should be actively involved intellectually as well as physically in every procedure done to establish a diagnosis, carry out the treatment prescribed, and assist with the necessary nursing care. Furthermore, the client's emotional reactions should be evaluated in terms of adjustment to the illness, acceptance of the hospital and staff, and separation from his or her family. Every attempt should be made to understand each client in terms of a particular ethnic, cultural, social, and economic background, as well as his or her particular life-style. Effective verbal and nonverbal communication is essential if rapport is to be established, the client's emotional needs are to be satis-

fied, and an accurate diagnosis is to be made. The assessment of the client should lead to the identification and validation of the problems with him or her.

## NEUROLOGICAL EXAMINATION

The neurological examination is performed to determine and localize any disease of the nervous system. It should be preceded by a complete physical examination and history. It begins at the initial encounter and continues during all subsequent contacts. Observations to determine the client's mental status are made during the time the history is being taken (Chapter 11).

## DIAGNOSTIC STUDIES

Numerous diagnostic studies are available to investigate abnormal findings apparent in the history and physical examination. Laboratory studies of blood, urine, and stool are ordered as indicated. Initial radiographic studies frequently include views of the skull and spinal column. In proceeding to further studies physicians tend to order the least invasive procedures first. Thus an electroencephalogram, a brain scan, and even a CAT (computerized axial tomographic) or PET (positron emission tomographic) scan are normally ordered before air studies or cerebral angiography.

Other tests, used frequently by the medical service, are also helpful in the diagnostic study of the client with neurological disease, such as gastric analysis with histamine (should be done to detect and measure hydrochloric acid when subacute combined degeneration of the spinal cord with or without pernicious anemia is suspected); blood chemistry, including glucose, urea nitrogen, calcium, albumin-globulin ratio, and serum protein; serology; basal metabolism; vital capacity; phenol-sulfonphthalein test; urea clearance; urine dilution and concentration tests; intravenous pyelography; electrocardiography; pressor tests; oscillometry; and thermocouple readings.

After completion of the physical and neurological examinations and taking of the history, all data are reviewed, and a tentative diagnosis is made. If further diagnostic evaluation is needed, specific tests may be ordered. This chapter will describe the most commonly used neurological diagnostic procedures.

## Electroencephalography

### Expected outcome
The client should have an understanding of the procedure and be informed of the results.

*Definition.* The electroencephalogram (EEG) consists of a graphic record of the electrical activity of the brain.

*Indications.* (1) To detect electrical abnormalities that may indicate an intracranial pathological or pathophysiological condition. (2) To determine the existence and type of epilepsy.

Usually the EEG is made in a room specially constructed (shielded) to eliminate interference from outside electrical activity (such as elevators and machines). Lighting, external distractions, noise, and interruptions should be minimal. If possible, it should be done in a controlled environment under standardized conditions. If a client is too ill to be moved, the EEG machine may be taken to the bedside. However, allowances should then be made for artifacts.

*Preparation of client.* The test is explained to the client. The explanation is modified according to the understanding and needs of the individual client.

Ideally, especially for hospitalized clients, anticonvulsant medications are discontinued for at least 48 hours before the test. Since there is always the risk of precipitating a bout of seizures, in actual practice medication is rarely omitted. Unless a sleep record is desired or the client is less than 18 months of age, sedatives also are withheld. Young infants may require sedation (usually a sodium pentobarbital [Nembutal] suppository) to eliminate crying and excessive activity.

Unless specifically ordered, the client does not fast before the test, since fasting may affect the brain-wave pattern.

*Procedure.* The client, depending on condition, may walk or be transported by wheelchair or stretcher to the room where the EEG is to be made. The chart is taken along, and the client is introduced to the technician who performs the test. The client is transferred from the stretcher or wheelchair to the bed located in the EEG suite (Fig. 12-1).

Usually 16 electrodes are applied with electrode compound paste to the scalp over corresponding areas (prefrontal, frontal, temporal, parietal, occipital) of both sides of the head, and one may be placed on each earlobe for grounding. After the electrodes have been applied, the jacks of the lead wires are inserted into the appropriate numbered holes (according to the area used) in the jack box. The cable of this box goes to the EEG machine.

After the electrodes have been applied, the client is instructed to keep the eyes closed, relax, and not move any part of the body (muscular activity causes artifacts that may complicate the interpretation of the record).

Generally the technician remains seated at the machine while it is being run. This enables him or her to observe the client through a window and record any movements that may influence the graph.

Approximately every 5 minutes the record is interrupted to permit the client to move if desired. If this is not done periodically, the client may become fatigued, tense, or restless, resulting in artifacts.

As part of the test, the client is asked to hyperventilate to accentuate the abnormalities of the record. The client is asked to breathe rapidly (30 to 40 times per minute) and as deeply as possible for 3 minutes. He or she may become light headed, dizzy, or restless during this period. At times the client may become emotionally disturbed and uncooperative. These are transient symptoms that disappear spontaneously.

*Nursing intervention.* When the test is completed, the paste is washed off with water, and the electrodes are removed.

The client is returned to his or her room and follows the previous regimen. Anticonvulsant medication is resumed. Apart from the fatigue caused

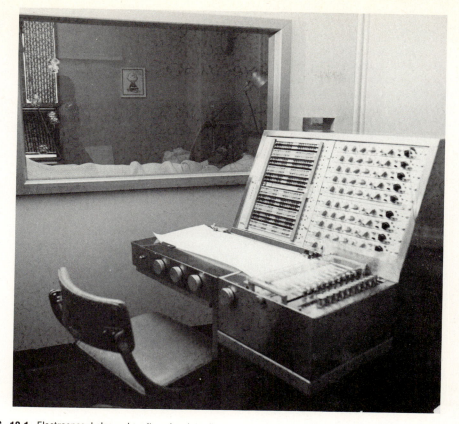

**FIG. 12-1.** Electroencephalograph suite, showing client isolated from equipment; electroencephalograph room is specially constructed to shield out noise and other artifacts.

by maintaining a particular position for an extended period (1 to 2 hours), the client should not suffer any ill effects.

The record (Fig. 12-2) is reviewed and interpreted according to the frequency, amplitude, and characteristics of the brain waves. The client receives the results of the test or is informed that further testing is indicated.

*Documenting death.* The EEG is useful in the documenting of cerebral death through demonstration of electrographic silence. Strict criteria are used to determine the silence, with the equipment being calibrated to maximum amplitude so that artifacts are identified with noncephalic and precordial electrodes, which demonstrate electrocardiographic activity that may be transmitted to

cephalic electrodes and be misinterpreted. The client should receive no medication or ventilation before the test. The criteria for brain death vary from state to state, but clients who demonstrate flat EEG patterns after extensive testing for 24- to 48-hour periods clearly fall into the category of brain death and the need for continued life support should be examined. (Refer to discussion in Chapter 9.)

### Echoencephalography

#### Expected outcome
The client should have an understanding of the test and be informed of the results.

A diagnostic technique that utilizes sound as a basis is especially helpful in the identification of subdural hematomas. Such a technique is echoen-

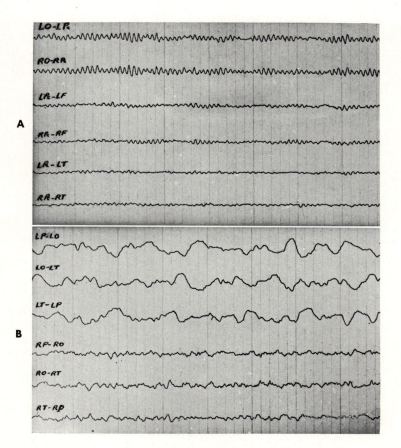

**FIG. 12-2.** Electroencephalographic records. Placements are indicated by *L,* left; *R,* right; *F,* frontal; *T,* temporal; *O,* occipital; *P,* parietal; *Pc,* precentral; calibration for time and amplitude is same for all and can be noted in **E** (see opposite page). **A,** Normal record with regular, 10-per-second alpha waves dominant throughout. **B,** Irregular high-amplitude delta waves (1 to 2 per second) prominent over the left side. This client had intracranial tumor.

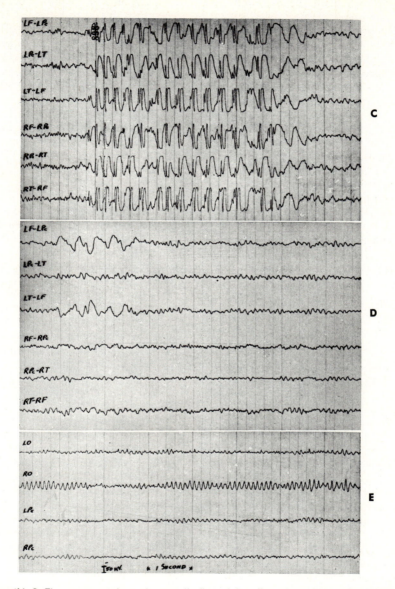

**FIG. 12-2, cont'd. C,** Three-per-second, synchronous "spike and dome" waves present in all areas, as seen in minor epilepsy. **D,** Irregular, high-amplitude, 2- to 3-per-second waves out of phase in left frontal area. Client had jacksonian epilepsy. **E,** Greatly diminished amplitude in occipital area. Client had head injury with fracture of left occipital bone.

cephalography, a method of recording sonic pulses from certain structures in the head by reflection of ultrasonic impulses that have been directed through the client's skull back toward the source, where they are recorded and projected on an oscilloscope screen. The time taken for the impulse to return to the receiver is graphically interpreted as the distance of the reflecting surface from the source-receiver. Since the bones of the skull are reflectors, the distance between these can be projected, and since certain normally midline structures are also reflectors, any shift of these structures from their normal position can be visualized. The advantages of this procedure lie in its simplicity, rapidity, and safety. At the present time, however, in practice it gives no more information than shift of midline structures as determined by a plain radiographic study. Preparation of the client is minimal. The procedure causes little discomfort and may be performed at the bedside if necessary. The client should be informed of the results or that additional tests are necessary.

### Electromyography

**Expected outcome**
The client should understand the test and cooperate to obtain an accurate aid to diagnosis.

Electromyography of the skeletal muscles consists in evaluation of the electrical activity of the motor unit (action potential) detected by needle electrodes inserted into the muscle with the activity displayed on an oscilloscope or oscillograph and heard over a loudspeaker for simultaneous visual and auditory analysis. One measures each motor unit to identify one of the eight or more characteristic patterns to rule out an altered EMG (electromyogram). Electrical activity is measured upon needle insertion, immediately afterward, with muscle at rest, and with minimal and maximal muscle contraction. Abnormalities in the amplitude, duration, wave formation and sound, and motor unit action potential frequency are observed. Photographs or magnetic tape serve as the client's permanent record of the test results.

The EMG serves as a useful means of determining neuromuscular diseases or disorders. Pathological states, medication effectiveness, time and manner of reinnervation of muscles, and aberrent conduction velocities can be estimated through appropriate electrical stimulation of the motor unit.

*Nursing intervention.* The client should receive an explanation of the procedure and its technique. The client should be informed that the test can be seen and heard as it is being performed. Cooperation should be emphasized to accomplish the test by flexion and relaxation of the muscle or lying still. The test is moderately uncomfortable and pain may occur on needle electrode insertion. The client should experience some muscle soreness in the muscles studied after the test. Premedication or sedation is avoided to ensure client cooperation and accurate results. Length and extent of the test vary depending on the history. The test can be performed on an outpatient.

### Muscle biopsy

Whenever the integrity of the motor unit is disturbed at any level (motor neuron, peripheral nerves, myoneural junction, or muscle fibers), a muscle biopsy is indicated to allow identification of the causative problem. At times the motor unit becomes involved secondary to general systemic disease and is evaluated to ascertain the particular outcomes of the disease process on muscle.

Before performing a muscle biopsy, one customarily obtains supporting data from serum enzyme level determinations and electromyography. No particular contraindications exist for muscle biopsies, except the existence of clotting disturbances, wherein severe bleeding might accompany the procedure.

After the practitioner receives the client's permission, the client is cognitively and psychologically prepared for the procedure, which is performed under local anesthesia and may be locally painful afterward.

The muscle for biopsy is carefully selected so that it represents moderate involvement by the disease process. If the muscle is minimally or severely affected, it does not provide adequate data. Consideration should also be given to the fact that muscle traumatized by multiple intramuscular injections or particularly probing with needles during electromyographic studies is not suitable for biopsy.

After site selection is complete, the area is prepared. The site is locally anesthetized without direct injection into the muscle under study. The extremity is positioned so that the selected muscle is at rest.

Care must be taken to preserve the biopsied muscle tissue in a manner that does not interfere with testing procedures. In many institutions the muscle tissue is merely placed in moistened saline gauze and taken to the laboratory for histological and histochemical studies within a 30-minute period. Tissue may also be subjected to ultrastructural and biochemical studies. Less frequently the biopsied muscle is placed in a fixative or clamps. In this instance paraffin sections are also done.

Findings from muscle biopsies are definitive. For example, they allow the practitioner to differentiate myasthenia gravis, muscular dystrophy, and inflammatory myositis. Moreover, these studies on biopsied muscle reveal characteristic findings in congenital disorders resulting in infantile hypotonia, Duchenne type of muscular dystrophy, nemaline myopathy, and infantile spinal muscular atrophy. Through special histochemical staining techniques, inborn errors, such as certain storage diseases and muscle enzyme abnormalities, may be detected. In a muscle undergoing denervation atrophy the extent and chronicity of the problem may be evaluated.

*Nursing intervention.* Complications occurring after the muscle biopsy are related to bleeding dyscrasias or inadequate surgical techniques and may include local infection or hematoma formation. If these develop, surgical intervention may be required. However, for most individuals aftercare merely involves symptomatic relief for pain at the operative site and care to keep the wound area dry and intact. The client should be able to move the muscle immediately after the procedure, and the sutures can be removed in 7 to 10 days. The client should report any signs of infection or bleeding to the physician. Reassure the client that results will be forthcoming, or let him or her understand the need for more testing.

## Brain biopsy

### Expected outcome

The client should be able to describe the procedure and the results within the limits of his or her cognitive and educational capacities.

In certain instances a brain biopsy is obtained to provide data essential to genetic counseling and to determining a prognosis for the client. Although this procedure is rarely performed as a primary diagnostic measure, it is commonly done during intracranial surgery, especially when the problem is a neoplastic space-occupying lesion. Because a brain biopsy is diagnostic rather than therapeutic, the performance of this procedure as a primary diagnostic technique is reserved for rather well-defined situations and circumstances. Brain biopsies should only be performed after informed consent is obtained from the client or responsible family member in a setting where laboratory facilities are adequate to perform the necessary tests. Generally it is done only after several specialists have conferred and agreed to the necessity of the procedure, which might be expected in instances where other means have failed to reveal the diagnosis, where the disease process is chronic and progressive, and where vital data are essential to the identification and possible treatment of a diffuse disease process.

Teaching of the client is done within the limits of the client's capacity, which is often hampered by the nature of the disease process. For later comparison a complete record of vital signs and neurological status is obtained.

*Procedure.* The site of choice for primary neurodiagnostic brain biopsies is the nondominant hemisphere in either the parieto-occipital or the frontal cortex. Alternative sites are selected, since the site of choice may not be appropriate. The specimen is obtained after the neurosurgeon turns back a flap or makes a large bur hole. The specimen commonly measures at least 1 ml and contains white matter, cortex, and meninges. The specimen is then apportioned into samples for a number of studies, including electronmicroscopy and tissue culture, microbiological procedures, chemical analysis, and frozen section and tissue smear tests.

A number of conditions may be diagnosed when data gleaned from the brain biopsy are utilized. A number of inherited disorders, broadly grouped in categories such as the leukodystrophies and storage diseases, are among the identifiable disorders. Common examples contained within these categories include metachromatic leukodystrophy, Tay-Sachs disease, Niemann-Pick disease, and Gaucher's disease. Studies on biopsied brain tissue also identify diseases grouped under the organic dementias, such as Jakob-Creutzfeldt and Alzheimer's disease. Other progressive conditions, such as inflammatory processes, subacute sclerosing panencephalitis, and necrotizing herpes encephalitis, may be diagnosed through these studies.

*Nursing intervention.* Although most experts agree that no complications result from a brain biopsy, it is actually hard to make a clear-cut determination about complications. It should be recalled that clients subjected to this procedure already have such advanced disease states that problems such as seizures, hemiparesis, or hemorrhage may result from the primary disease process itself. Since a surgical wound is involved, observe the client for hematoma formation and attempt to keep the wound dry, intact, and free from infection. Generally, a dressing is placed over the operative site and is changed as necessary in relation to drainage and the need to inspect the wound. Vital signs and neurological status are evaluated serially and compared to preoperative values. The client is placed in bed, made comfortable, and supported symptomatically.

### Nerve conduction studies

Studies designed to provide information primarily about nerve conduction of myelinated fibers are most commonly utilized when a peripheral neuropathy (motor, sensory, or sensorimotor) is suspected because of damage of the myelin-producing Schwann cells or when neuromuscular junction disorders are diagnosed.

**Expected outcome**
The client should have an understanding of the test and that additional tests may be required.

Two tests may be utilized to determine nerve conduction. In the fastest-conducting myelinated fibers, demyelinating peripheral neuropathies usually display slow conduction velocities. Specific diagnosis can be made after the conduction velocity has been calculated through division of the distance between the proximal and distal points by the time required for an electrical stimulus to travel between the two points. A repetitive nerve stimulation test is utilized when a disorder of the neuromuscular junction is suspected. Fatigability of nerve conduction may be attributable to faulty neurotransmitter release or aberrant postsynaptic action.

For both studies, the client is usually placed in a recumbent position with the limb to be tested po-

sitioned to prevent movement artifact. The client should be informed that a tingling or short electrical sensation will be felt when the nerve is stimulated. The limb tested may feel tired or weighty after the test. The test may prove uncomfortable to clients with sensory loss. The client's cooperation to lie still when the nerve is stimulated is necessary for an accurate test. Sedation is usually not given before the test because of the possibility that the client may need to exercise the extremity being tested so that high-frequency stimulation of the neuromuscular junction can be avoided and a less painful test made.

### Nerve biopsy

To establish an accurate diagnosis of peripheral neuropathy, a nerve biopsy may be necessary. This procedure can determine the extent of damage to both myelinated and unmyelinated nerve fibers, axon or myelin damage, or selective injury to nerve fibers of a specific diameter.

**Expected outcome**
Preparation is similar to that of a muscle biopsy and may be incorporated into the muscle biopsy to prevent the need for two test sites. The most common site for a nerve biopsy is the sural nerve. The client usually experiences some degree of sensory loss after the biopsy, but few long-term effects or complications have been reported. This test is usually performed after appropriate nerve conduction studies have shown impaired nerve conduction velocities. Nursing management of the client is similar to that of the muscle biopsy.

### Lumbar puncture
**Expected outcome**
The client should be able to explain the procedure, the cooperation required, and the possible posttest effects.

*Definition.* Lumbar puncture is the introduction of a hollow needle with a stylet into the lumbar subarachnoid space of the spinal canal, with strict aseptic technique being used.

*Indications.* The reasons for doing a lumbar puncture may be diagnostic or therapeutic.

*Diagnostic needs.* (1) To measure the cerebrospinal fluid (CSF) pressure. (2) To obtain CSF for visualization and laboratory examination. (3) To perform spinal dynamics for signs of block caused by a tumor or other pathological conditions of the spinal cord. (4) To inject air, oxygen, or radiopaque substances for radiographic visualization of the nervous system.

*Therapy*. (1) To remove blood or pus from the subarachnoid space. (2) To inject drugs and sera. (3) To reduce intracranial pressure. (4) To produce spinal anesthesia.

*Contraindications*. (1) When a lumbar puncture will not contribute to the diagnosis or treatment of the illness. (2) When an intracranial tumor is suspected and there is clinical evidence of greatly increased intracranial pressure (papilledema). (3) When an infection is present at the site of puncture. (4) When encephalography or myelography is contemplated in the near future, to eliminate subjection of the client to a second puncture.

*Equipment*. When a lumbar puncture is ordered by the physician, a sterile disposable tray is requisitioned from the central supply department and placed conveniently on a sterile field on a movable table.

*Preparation of client*. The client is prepared both psychologically and physically by having the procedure and aftercare explained to alleviate anxiety and ensure cooperation. If the client is prepared adequately, there is less likelihood of having a reaction such as a headache.

In some hospitals, a signed permit must be obtained before the procedure. If the client is mentally incompetent or under 21 years of age (18 years in some states), the closest relative should sign the permission. In any emergency or if a relative is not available, the attending physician responsible for the patient signs the permit.

Before the procedure, the nurse should instruct the client in the process of the procedure thoroughly and honestly. The client should be informed that the body position is or can be uncomfortable. Instruct the client to lie in the lateral recumbent position with the back as near to the edge of the bed as possible. If the mattress sags, the bed may be firmed with bedboards placed under the mattress. The legs are flexed at the thighs, the thighs on the abdomen, and the shoulders and head bent toward the knees so that maximum bowing of the spine is obtained, affording the greatest space between the vertebrae. The position may be maintained when the client clasps the hands below the knees. Inform the client that if the position cannot be maintained someone will help hold the position by putting one arm around the shoulders and the other about the knees. The client may have a small pillow under

the head and a large one between the knees. Some physicians prefer doing the lumbar puncture in the sitting position, if an accurate cerebrospinal fluid pressure is not essential. Instruct the client that the position of immobilization is important and that cooperation will ensure a more accurate test and less trauma, emotionally and to the lumbar area. The client should breathe normally. At some point just before the procedure, the bladder and bowel should be emptied. If the client is very apprehensive, a sedative may be ordered 20 to 30 minutes before the test. Answer all questions that the client may have as honestly as possible. Great fear of paralysis, headache, or severe pain may have been instilled into the emotional repertoire of the client from a previous traumatic lumbar puncture or a person who had had such an experience. The nurse must positively identify these fears or other protective mechanisms and not alienate the client by dismissing the anxiety or fear underlying the client's questions or responses to client teaching.

*Procedure*. The curtain should be drawn around the client's bed. Remove the client's bed linens and cover the client with a bath blanket, and fanfold the bed linens at the foot of the bed. Place the client in the lateral recumbent position with the back as near the edge of the bed as possible. The legs should then be flexed as previously described at the knees with the thighs being flexed on the abdomen and the head bent toward the knees for optimum bowing of the spine. The client should clasp the hands on the knees to maintain the position. Place a small pillow under the head and a large one between the knees. The client should be draped with a bath blanket in such a manner that the lumbar spine and crest of the ilium are exposed. Slip the protective sheet under the client's lower back and allow to hang over the edge of the bed. Arrange the table with the assembled equipment to suit the handedness of the physician. If the client's lumbar area is hairy, a dry shave may be done.

The physician will wash the hands thoroughly and then palpate the client's spinous processes and the interspaces of the lower lumbar vertebrae. An imaginary line drawn at the level of the iliac crests will be at the interspace between the third and fourth lumbar vertebrae, the site at which the needle is generally inserted. The spinal cord ends at the lower border of the first lumbar vertebra or upper border of the second lumbar vertebra; consequently there is minimal danger of injuring the spinal cord. The site selected for infants and young children is usually lower because the spinal cord extends almost to the sacral region. Sterile gloves are applied. The physician will cleanse an area of skin approximately 8 inches square with thimerosal (Merthiolate or Betadine) and discard the applicators into the paper bag or emesis basin. The procaine hydrochloride (Novocain) solution is prepared.

The client is draped with a fenestrated sheet and Novocain drawn into the syringe. Tell the client what is about to be done. A wheal is made under the skin with injection of the solution, usually 2 ml. The physician will insert the lumbar puncture needle into the site chosen. After the subarachnoid space has been entered, the stylet is removed and the fluid begins to drip.

The stopcock with the manometer is connected to the needle, and the initial pressure is recorded. The 6-inch rubber tube is attached to the outlet of the stopcock, and the fluid is collected in a calibrated glass or test tube. By using a stopcock, the manometer is left attached, and the pressure can be checked, if desired, during the removal of the fluid.

An adequate amount of fluid, usually 8 to 10 ml, is removed for laboratory tests (cell count, total protein, colloidal gold, and serology). If the fluid is cloudy or if signs of meningitis exist, a sterile specimen is obtained for culture. The fluid is measured carefully, placed in properly labeled tubes, and sent immediately to the laboratory. If the cerebrospinal fluid is bloody, label one specimen with the client's name, date it, and tape it to the head of the bed. (Laboratory examinations of the bloody fluid are usually invalid and therefore are deferred until the fluid is clear.)

The physician will take the final pressure reading and remove the stopcock, manometer, and needle. Cleanse the disinfected area with alcohol, remove the fenestrated sheet and protective sheet (a Band-Aid will be applied), and cover the client.

*Nursing intervention.* Many believe it is unnecessary to keep the client in bed, flat or otherwise; however, some advocate the facedown position for 4 to 6 hours after lumbar puncture to re-

duce the likelihood of cerebrospinal fluid leakage into the epidural space.

Instruct the client as to the length of time he or she must remain in bed; this may vary, depending on the individual client and the philosophy of treatment. Give a drinking tube to the client if he or she is to remain flat any length of time. Remove the screening.

Clients with intracranial pathological conditions are observed for changes in the level of consciousness and in the vital signs. Hypotension, tachycardia, tachypnea, and an elevated temperature may occur and should be observed with the physician being notified for appropriate intervention as necessary. Headache, nuchal rigidity, and bleeding from the site may require extensive intervention and observation.

The client may need assistance to turn every 2 to 4 hours. Vital and neurological signs must be taken frequently at least for the first 2 hours and then as ordered. Pain medication may be required. Fluids should be encouraged for the first 6 to 12 hours as appropriate. Diet may be as tolerated. Observation of the site for redness, swelling, or drainage is necessary with any symptoms being reported to the physician. The client may ambulate as ordered and resume normal activities of daily living as tolerated.

## CHARTING

**Nurse's notes**

Procedure, practitioner, date, and time
Amount and character of fluid removed
Cooperation of client
Specimens to laboratory and the test or tests ordered
Significant reactions (color, pulse, respiratory changes, headache, nausea, vomiting, dysuria, retention)

*Sequelae.* After lumbar punctures one or more sequelae may occur in approximately 25% of the clients, regardless of the conditions under which they are performed.

Headache generally is believed to be caused by seepage of cerebrospinal fluid through the dural puncture wound. Its incidence can be reduced when a small-bore needle is used. It usually is relieved if the client remains flat in bed and one reestablishes the level of cerebrospinal fluid by forcing fluids.

Other sequelae may be nuchal rigidity caused by

meningeal irritation; a rise in temperature with or without a preceding chill; local pain, trauma, hematoma, or edema, usually the result of faulty technique; pain in the back radiating to the thigh because of irritation of a nerve root; and transient difficulty in voiding caused by psychic trauma, enforced bed rest, or the aggravation of a low-grade bladder disturbance.

If displacement of the brain causes sudden loss of consciousness, emergency treatment consists in maintaining a patent airway and employing artificial respiration as necessary. The removal of cerebrospinal fluid from the lateral ventricles may also be indicated. If the listed contraindications are considered and observed, this emergency situation may be avoided.

The other sequelae may be kept to a minimum with adequate preliminary psychological and physical preparations of the client and the use of good technique on the part of the practitioner.

*CSF analysis.* When the lumbar puncture begins with a determination of the cerebrospinal fluid (CSF) pressure, it is important to take the necessary precautions to ensure an accurate reading. The initial pressure reading is ascertained before CSF is deliberately removed. While the manometer is connected to the needle via a three-way stopcock, check the client to be certain that no excessive intrathoracic or intra-abdominal pressure is being exerted, since these factors falsely elevate CSF pressure. To eliminate these problems assist the client in straightening the legs and neck and in taking slow, deep breaths. Before recording this reading, assess the patency of the system by manually compressing the client's abdomen, asking the client to cough, or requesting the client to do a Valsalva maneuver. Any of these measures should result in a temporary increase in CSF pressure if the system is patent. CSF also rises and falls in the manometer in concert with respiration. The recorded reading should be the lowest pressure measurement. Normally the opening CSF pressure is between 60 and 180 mm $H_2O$. Although closing pressures are also frequently obtained, their value is far less valuable clinically. When the CSF pressure is elevated, consider causative problems, such as an infection, a space-occupying intracranial lesion, or a hemorrhage. In contrast, the CSF pressure may be abnormally low, as in instances of

spinal subarachnoid obstruction above the puncture site. When a spinal subarachnoid obstruction is suspected, assess the CSF dynamics carefully before fluid is removed for study.

After CSF is extracted, a number of tests are employed to analyze the fluid. Abnormal findings are compared to those gleaned from the history, physical examination, and diagnostic tests to gain a more complete picture of the client's problem. Some of the most common tests are reviewed here.

**VISUAL INSPECTION.** CSF is normally clear, odorless, and colorless and looks most like ordinary tap water. The waterlike appearance of the fluid persists even when up to 500 cells/mm$^3$ are contained in the fluid.

At times CSF has a discolored appearance on inspection, known as *xanthochromia.* The pink-red discoloration of CSF occurs when red blood cells have gained access to the CSF within a 3-hour period preceding the test. If frankly bloody fluid is obtained, you need to identify the genesis of the problem. If the bloody fluid is the result of entry into a vertebral or thecal vessel during the puncture, the following characteristics are apparent: (1) the color clears as successive samples are obtained, (2) the bloody fluid frequently clots, (3) red blood cells are normal when examined, and (4) the supernatant fluid is clear. In contrast, if the source of bloody CSF is from hemorrhage in the central nervous system, the following characteristics are observed: (1) the bloodlike appearance of the fluid remains consistent in all samples, (2) if left to stand the bloody fluid infrequently clots, (3) on examination the red blood cells are crenated, and (4) the supernatant fluid appears xanthochromic.

If the CSF is colored brown, orange, or yellow, the abnormal color is the result of the presence of blood that has been in the CSF for 3 to 28 days. The color is caused by red blood cell breakdown. Another possible cause of discolored CSF is bilirubinemia.

At times CSF has a turbid appearance. When CSF appears cloudy, the problem may be increased numbers of white blood cells, elevated protein levels, or the existence of numerous microorganisms.

**COMPONENT PARTS.** Normally CSF is clear, colorless, and free of red blood cells and composed of 0 to 5 white blood cells of the agranulocytic variety per cubic millimeter. The protein count is 15 to 45 mg/dl in samples taken from the lumbar region and 5 to 15 mg/dl in ventricular CSF samples. The glucose level of CSF is roughly 60% to 80% of the blood level. Although a typical CSF glucose level is 40 to 80 mg/dl, the findings have more validity when compared to a blood glucose level obtained just before the lumbar puncture is performed. The presence of microorganisms is not a normal finding.

In summary, the findings in normal CSF are as follows:

| | |
|---|---|
| Appearance | Clear, colorless |
| Red blood cells | None |
| White blood cells | 0 to 5 cells/mm³ (agranulocytes) |
| Protein | 15 to 45 mg/dl (lumbar sample) |
| | 5 to 15 mg/dl (ventricular sample) |
| Glucose | 40 to 8 mg/dl (60% to 80% of current blood glucose level) |
| Microorganisms | None |

RED BLOOD CELLS. Common conditions that introduce blood into CSF include intracranial or subarachnoid hemorrhage and cerebral trauma. In these instances blood enters either the ventricular system or the subarachnoid space to join the CSF. If bleeding is minimal, so that the accumulation is less than 300 to 500 cells/mm³, the color of the CSF will appear normal on visual inspection. As previously mentioned, fresh red blood cells in sufficient quantity will tinge the CSF a pink-red color, whereas red blood cells undergoing breakdown result in CSF discoloration ranging from yellow to brown.

WHITE BLOOD CELLS. ''Leukocytosis'' and ''pleocytosis'' are terms used to describe an increase in the population of white blood cells. White blood cell numbers increase in response to any inflammatory process that interrupts the integrity of the meninges or ventricular lining. Such inflammatory responses may result from an infection (meningitis) induced by fungi, viruses, or bacterial agents or from an irritative focus in or near the pathway of CSF flow, as with space-occupying lesions, brain abscesses, multiple sclerosis, mastoiditis, and other conditions. Chapter 20 presents more detail on abnormal CSF findings. Without detailing the percentages of various cells seen in different conditions, it is sufficient to say that the practitioner is alerted to suspicious activity in the CSF pathway when the white blood cell count is 5 to 10 cells/mm³ and aware that a disease process is active when the count is greater than 10 cells/mm³.

PROTEIN. In normal CSF the protein level is only 1% of the serum protein content. Slight increases of protein occur in connection with a number of conditions. Such increases are regarded lightly, unless they become elevated to 60 mg/dl. Elevated protein levels frequently accompany increases in the number of cells in the CSF, since cells, whether normal or disintegrated, add protein to the total protein count. Some conditions wherein increased cell counts are seen with increased CSF protein levels include leukocytosis, subarachnoid hemorrhage, and meningitis. At other times elevations in the protein level are not accompanied by increased white blood cell counts, as in degenerative processes of the central nervous system (neurosyphilis, multiple sclerosis, superficial brain tumors, and blockage within the subarachnoid space).

Decreased amounts of CSF may also be noted. Although a decreased protein level is of little known significance in clinical diagnostics, it is correlated with the rapid production of CSF.

GLUCOSE. As previously mentioned, fluctuations in the CSF glucose level may be related to systemic blood glucose levels. When hyperglycemia occurs in the circulatory system, there is a concurrent elevation of CSF glucose level. Elevations in CSF glucose levels infrequently indicate pathological conditions in the central nervous system.

Decreases in CSF glucose levels may be related to hypoglycemia or to pathological conditions of the central nervous system. In meningeal infections caused by yeast, protozoa, fungi, or tubercle bacilli the decrease of glucose is not extremely great, if glucose depression is caused at all. However, in bacterial meningitis the drop in CSF glucose levels is striking, and the level of CSF glucose may even drop to 0. In raging meningeal infections a large number of white blood cells are marshaled to fight infection. The metabolic needs of these white blood cells further deplete glucose levels in the CSF. (See comparisons of CSF in various diseases in Tables 20-1 and 20-2.)

COLLOIDAL GOLD. CSF protein content may be altered quantitatively or qualitatively by some diseases. When these changes result in an altered albumin-globulin ratio, the colloidal gold test is utilized to identify these changes. In this test CSF, diluted with successively more saline diluent, is added to 10 test tubes placed in a darkened room at room temperature for 24 hours. In normal CSF the gamma globulins are unable to precipitate the colloidal gold because of the presence of albumin and alpha and beta globulins. If the gamma globulin ratio increases, the solution changes color as evaluated on a five-point scale. Color changes are divided into three zones, which include equal divisions of the three tubes.

Zone I, changes in color in the first three tubes, is often found in individuals with general paresis from syphilis. Thus zone I is frequently referred to as the *paretic curve*. Zone I alterations may also be apparent in multiple sclerosis.

Zone II changes, altered color in the middle four tubes, are associated with tubercular meningitis, polymyositis, encephalitis lethargica, and, most commonly, tabes dorsalis. Because of zone II's association with tabes, it is often termed the *tabetic curve*.

Zone III changes, color alterations in the last three tubes, are most commonly associated with purulent meningitis; this zone is therefore often termed the *meningitic curve*.

MICROORGANISMS. Special studies are available to isolate causative organisms in central nervous system invasion. A discussion of organisms and testing techniques is available in Chapter 20.

SPECIAL STUDIES. Investigators are only beginning to realize the potentials for such sophisticated CSF analyses as are involved in performing amino acid determinations, electrophoresis, and immunoelectrophoresis. Currently some of these studies may be valuable when encephalitis, malignancy, multiple sclerosis, or Guillain-Barré syndrome are diagnosed.

## Spinal dynamics

The spinal dynamics test may also be referred to as the manometric test, Queckenstedt test, or CSF pressure readings.

*Definition.* The determination of variations of CSF pressures read from a calibrated manometer (attached to a needle in the spinal subarachnoid space) in response to timed compression of the jugular veins.

*Purpose.* To determine the presence or absence of a block, partial or complete, in the circulation of the CSF in the spinal (subarachnoid) space.

*Indications.* (1) In the presence of spinal cord disease when a diagnosis of spinal tumor is being considered. (2) After fracture or dislocation of the vertebrae to determine if the spinal cord is being compressed.

*Contraindication.* Any intracranial disease; especially when clinical signs of increased intracranial pressure or hemorrhage are present.

### EQUIPMENT

Same as for lumbar puncture, with the addition of the following:

Sterile No. 18 spinal needle (desirable for free flow of CSF)
Calibrated water manometer and three-way stopcock
Sphygmomanometer
Stopwatch
Pencil
Sheet of paper prepared as shown below

*Procedure.* The steps outlined for lumbar puncture are followed through the connection of the stopcock and manometer to the needle. The air in the manometer is expelled when it is tilted horizontally. Before removing any fluid record the first stabilized reading. This is called the *initial pressure,* and normally, with the client relaxed in the lateral recumbent position, it varies from 60 to 180 mm of CSF. The fluid should oscillate in the manometer and should respond quickly to changes in the client's breathing and with coughing or straining. Before continuing with the manometric readings, the client's position should be checked for comfort, the legs straightened so that the abdomen is not compressed, and the head supported in good alignment with the back so that the neck is straight. The client should be reassured as necessary and instructed as to his or her part in the successful completion of the test. Instructions should be simple but complete so that the client understands them clearly and can cooperate. Without this the test can be equivocal or even worthless. Ideally, three individuals are needed: one to read the fluid pressures, one to time and record, and one to compress the jugular veins.

After the initial pressure has been obtained, the client is told to take a deep breath, hold it, and strain down as though at stool for a period of 10 seconds (referred to as abdominal straining, Table 12-1). A reading is taken at 10 seconds (the cli-

**TABLE 12-1.** Chart for abdominal strain and jugular compression

| Abdominal strain | | Jugular compression (cuff technique) | |
|---|---|---|---|
| Initial pressure | _____ | Initial pressure with cuff on neck | _____ |
| After 10 seconds of straining | _____ | Cuff inflated to 40 mm Hg | _____ |
| 5 seconds after relaxing | _____ | After 10 seconds of compression | _____ |
| 10 seconds | _____ | 5 seconds after releasing cuff | _____ |
| 15 seconds | _____ | 10 seconds | _____ |
| 20 seconds | _____ | 15 seconds | _____ |
| 25 seconds | _____ | 20 seconds | _____ |
| 30 seconds | _____ | 25 seconds | _____ |
| | | 30 seconds | _____ |

ent relaxes), and readings continue at 5-second intervals until the pressure returns approximately to the initial level. This is done to determine the patency of the needle and, depending on the client's ability to cooperate, will always show a sharp rise and rapid fall. Without this assurance that the needle is free and open in the canal, a subsequent subnormal response to jugular compression is meaningless. Abdominal straining should be repeated until the physician is satisfied with the response. When the pressure is again stabilized, a new reading is taken before continuing. Then the client is told what to expect, reassured that nothing untoward will happen, and advised neither to cough nor to hold the breath. Careful digital pressure is applied for 10 seconds to both jugular veins. Readings are taken at 5-second intervals from the time the jugular veins are compressed until the CSF pressure drops and is stabilized. Normally after 10 seconds of jugular compression there should be a rise of at least 100 mm from the initial pressure, with a fall to the previous level within approximately 30 seconds. A sluggish, poor rise with a slow, delayed fall would suggest some interference with the circulation of CSF and is interpreted as a *partial block*. No rise after 10 seconds of correct compression of the jugular veins is interpreted as a *complete block* and suggests obstruction within the spinal canal (Fig. 12-3). If there is any question about an abnormal response, it should be checked with a competent witness. After this, fluid is removed, and the final pressure is read. The remainder of the procedure and the aftercare of the patient are the same as for any lumbar puncture.

For greater facility and validity, the blood pressure cuff is used for jugular compression. The following routine is recommended: After abdominal straining has been completed, explain to the client what you are going to do, prepare him or her for possible reactions (facial warmth, local constriction, fullness in the head), and assure him or her of their transient nature. Wrap the cuff, preferably of medium size, around the neck and secure it in the usual manner. Check the CSF pressure in the manometer and record it (the application of the cuff or the client's emotional reaction may cause a spontaneous rise). Press the bulb and quickly elevate the mercury column to 40 mm, take the CSF reading, maintain the mercury at this level for 10 seconds, take a pressure reading and then quickly release the bulb, and finally read the pressure every 5 seconds until the fluid level is stabilized.

This technique was used in conjunction with digital jugular compression on 30 clients preliminary to iophendylate (Pantopaque) myelography. In this series one experienced nurse did the digital compression on all the clients. The cuff technique was tried in an effort to standardize the results obtained from spinal dynamics when the tests were made by various staff members with various degrees of experience. Maintaining the mercury column at 40 mm for 10 seconds produced CSF pressure elevations comparable to 10 seconds of bilateral digital jugular compression, and in each instance the test interpretations were confirmed by myelography. No adverse reactions occurred when the cuff was used as just described, and little subjective or objective discomfort was noted. Many clients in this series remarked that the digital com-

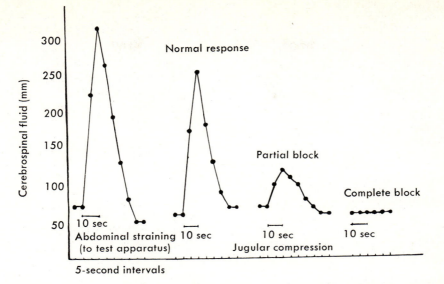

**FIG. 12-3.** Spinal dynamics. Graphic record of measurements of lumbar CSF pressures demonstrating test for patency of apparatus by abdominal straining, normal response on jugular compression, limited rise with partial block, and absence of any change in pressure with complete block. All stimuli are for 10-second intervals, and pressure readings are recorded every 5 seconds.

pression was more bothersome than the cuff pressure. This technique has the added advantage of consistency when done by different members of the team and is less subject to question when abnormal results are reported.

## Lateral cervical puncture

### Expected outcome
The client should have an understanding that the procedure is an alternative to lumbar puncture, but that the procedure and principles are the same with the area being different.

*Definition.* The insertion of a needle into the C1-C2 interspace through to the subarachnoid space to obtain CSF when lumbar puncture is contraindicated.

*Indications.* (1) Superficial infection or acute traumatic damage to the lumbar area. (2) Gross obesity. (3) Arachnoiditis. (4) Spinal column bony deformities. (5) Inability to flex neck for cisternal puncture. (6) Inability to safely perform cisternal puncture without major complications of the procedure. See Contraindications (p. 318).

*Preparation of client.* The procedure is ex-

plained to the client similarly to that for lumbar puncture. Inform the client that he will be lying flat in bed without a pillow and with the neck as straight as possible. The client may feel a few "pops" and an uncomfortable sensation but should feel little pain. The client should lie as still as possible so as not to distort the landmarks for the physician to guide the needle. The client should not cough or breathe abnormally. The client should not move unless the physician directs him to do so. A signed consent should be obtained.

*Procedure.* The client is placed in supine position without a pillow under the head. The neck should be as straight as possible with sandbags used about the head for stability and prevention of movement. A sedative may be ordered for the very apprehensive client. The skin is prepared with an antiseptic solution and local anesthetic injected as in the lumbar puncture. A standard (20-gauge) lumbar puncture needle is passed through the landmark in the cervical spine, 1 cm caudal and 1 cm posterior (Fig. 12-4). As the tissue planes are entered, several "pops" will be felt, necessitating

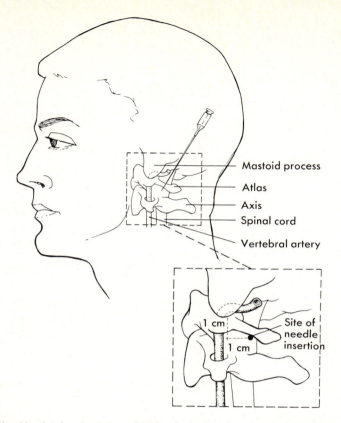

**FIG. 12-4.** Relationship of major structures and landmarks for lateral cervical puncture. Needle is inserted perpendicular to neck with client in supine position.

full cooperation of the client. The subarachnoid space may be already entered, and manual palpation is not an aid in this procedure as it is in the lumbar puncture. The stylet will be removed frequently from this point on to ascertain needle position and flow of CSF. Once the subarachnoid space has been successfully positioned, the needle must be carefully supported because of the lack of surrounding tissue. Subsequent CSF pressure measurement, fluid collection, and spinal dynamics can be performed as in the lumbar puncture.

After the completed procedures, the needle is removed rapidly. The site should be cleansed with alcohol and a Band-Aid may be applied, if the client desires one.

*Nursing intervention.* The nurse should instruct the client to lie flat for 4 to 6 hours. The client should force fluids unless contraindicated. Pain medication may be obtained as necessary. The client may have a small pillow under the head. When the client turns to the side every 2 to 4 hours, the neck may be supported with a small rolled towel, if desired. Vital and neurological signs should be checked frequently for the first two hours and as ordered thereafter. The client should be observed as in the lumbar puncture with notification of the physician as necessary. Ambulation and diet should resume as ordered when the client can tolerate activity.

*Contraindications.* The contraindications are the same as for the lumbar puncture with the addition of puncture of the vertebral artery and spinal cord.

*Results.* At this time, current research indicates

that the values for lateral cervical puncture (LCP) are similar to and within the normal range of the lumbar puncture.

**CHARTING**

Same as for lumbar puncture.

## Cisternal puncture

**Expected outcome**
The client should be able to describe the procedure and co-operate as much as possible for an accurate test.

*Definition.* Introduction of a short-beveled hollow needle with a stylet in the median line below the occipital bone into the cisterna magna. Cisternal puncture is used frequently on ambulatory clients in some outpatient departments in preference to lumbar puncture because, when done by a skilled physician, the risk is negligible and the ill effects minimal.

*Indications.* (1) To remove CSF for laboratory analysis when impossible to obtain it at the lumbar level. (2) To demonstrate subarachnoid block by doing a cisternal puncture simultaneously with a lumbar puncture. (3) To introduce isophendylate (Pantopaque) or air for myelography. (4) To perform encephalography. (5) For drainage of CSF if a lumbar puncture is contraindicated or a subarachnoid block is present.

*Preparation for client.* The procedure is explained to the client and permission is obtained. The nape of the neck is shaved to the occipital protuberance.

*Position.* The client is placed on the side of the edge of the bed or treatment table with the head bent slightly forward and held firmly.

*Procedure.* The preparation of the skin is like that for lumbar puncture. The use of local anesthesia is optional. The needle is inserted to a depth of about 5 cm (adult) in the midline below the occipital bone. The steps of the procedure are as outlined for the lumbar puncture.

*Nursing intervention.* The client should be watched for cyanosis, dyspnea, and apnea. If no adverse reaction occurs, the outpatient is usually permitted to go home; an inpatient is allowed out of bed to resume previous routine. Distressing headache does not occur as a reaction to cisternal puncture, increasing its value as a diagnostic aid.

**CHARTING**

Same as for lumbar puncture.

## Ventricular puncture

**Expected outcome**
The client should understand the test and its complications.

*Definition.* The insertion of a needle into the lateral ventricle. In infants a short-beveled No. 22 needle with a stylet is introduced through the scalp and anterior fontanel. In adults a ventricular needle is directed through an opening in the skull made with a bur or trephine.

*Indications.* (1) If lumbar, lateral cervical, or cisternal punctures are unsuccessful or contraindicated. (2) For the injection of dye into the ventricles of an infant to determine the type of hydrocephalus present. (3) To remove fluid quickly after ventriculography or craniotomy if the client shows evidence of increased intracranial pressure and cerebral decompensation. (4) To inject air or oxygen directly into the ventricles for the localization of a tumor when encephalography is contraindicated. (5) Preliminary to ventricular drainage.

**EQUIPMENT**

**Sterile**
2 No. 22 needles with stylets
Medicine glass
Manometers
Three-way stopcock
6-inch tubing with adapters
6 sponges (3 by 3 inches) or 6 cotton balls
2 ml syringe with 2 needles, No. 25 and No. 22
2 fenestrated sheets
3 pairs of gloves

**Other**
Straight razor
4 gauze squares
Liquid soap
Emesis basin
Thimerosal (Merthiolate) or povidone-iodine (Betadine)
Alcohol, 70%
Collodion
3 test tubes
Adequate lighting
Ampule of dye (neutral phenosulfonphthalein)
Sheet restraint
Stool

## Infants

**PREPARATION OF INFANT.** The physician obtains permission from the responsible adult.

It is generally necessary to give an infant a sedative before a ventricular puncture. Sodium pentobarbital (Nembutal) in solution given orally 30 minutes or, if rectally, about 1 hour before the procedure has proved most satisfactory.

The anterior third of the head is cleansed with soap and water and then shaved. A straight razor is more efficacious than a safety razor.

A wise precaution is to immobilize the infant, even though it is well sedated, by wrapping in a draw sheet. (If dye is to be injected into the ventricle, it normally takes about 3 minutes for it to reach the subarachnoid space of the spinal canal and so there is adequate time to remove the sheet and place the infant in position for lumbar puncture.) This procedure is usually done on the treatment table.

**PROCEDURE.** The infant is placed on the back, and the nurse holds the head to prevent movement. The physician cleanses the area with thimerosal or Betadine, puts on sterile gloves, drapes the infant with a fenestrated sheet, and proceeds to insert the needle with strict aseptic technique. (If the infant does not have hydrocephalus, difficulty may be encountered in obtaining fluid, since normally there are only a few milliliters in the lateral ventricles. The amount is greatly increased in hydrocephalus.) After the initial pressure is noted and fluid has been removed for tests, the dye, diluted with CSF, is injected by means of a 2 ml syringe, and the exact time is noted. The stylet is replaced in the needle, which is then withdrawn. The area is cleansed quickly, carefully dried, and a piece of sterile cotton with collodion is placed over the puncture site. The infant is unwrapped, turned on the side, and kept in position by the nurse, who places one hand across the shoulders, the other under the knees. The physician then proceeds to do a lumbar puncture. Fluid is allowed to drip intermittently from the lumbar needle, and a note is made of the time lapse between the injection of dry into the ventricle and the appearance of the dye in the lumbar spinal fluid. The circulation of the dye is accelerated when the infant's head is raised. If the dye does not appear after a certain interval, approximately 5 minutes, an obstructive type of hydrocephalus is diagnosed. The stylet is replaced, the needle withdrawn, the area cleansed and dried, and the wound protected with sterile cotton and collodion.

The infant is carried to the crib and observed for any untoward reaction to the sedative or to the procedure. Skin color, vital signs, and any leakage of CSF from the wounds are noted. Feedings and routine are resumed when the infant has recovered completely. Specimens are labeled and sent to the laboratory for routine tests.

The dye may also be recovered in urine by insertion of a retention catheter before the procedure is started. The catheter is released every 2 minutes until the dye appears. Urine is collected for a 2-hour period, and the dye excreted is analyzed quantitatively.

## CHARTING

**Nurse's notes**
Procedure, physician, date, and time
Amount and character of fluid removed
Specimens to laboratory
Significant reactions

**COMPLICATIONS.** (1) Fever. (2) Hemorrhage. (3) Wound infection. (4) Oozing of CSF from wounds. (5) Meningitis.

*Adults.* A ventricular puncture on an adult usually follows a craniotomy or craniectomy. The head dressing is removed, and then the steps are followed as outlined for lumbar puncture, with substitution of the ventricular area for the lumbar area.

## EQUIPMENT

Dressing tray, sterile
Lumbar puncture tray plus 2 special brain needles with rounded ends, a 20 ml syringe, and 2 sterile towels

**PREPARATION OF CLIENT.** A permit is obtained from the client or closest relative, or both. If the client is conscious, reassure as necessary. Place the client on the side opposite the ventricle to be tapped. After the head dressing has been removed, support the head firmly in the correct position to prevent sudden movement.

**PROCEDURE.** The physician puts on gloves,

cleanses the area with thimerosal or Betadine, drapes the client with a fenestrated sheet, and places one towel under the head and one over the face. The needle is inserted, the stylet is withdrawn, the stopcock and manometer are attached, and the fluid pressure is measured. Fluid is removed slowly, with frequent check of pressure, until the desired reduction has been achieved. The stopcock and manometer are detached, the stylet is replaced, and the needle is withdrawn. The area is cleansed, and the head is redressed with sterile gauze. A labeled, dated specimen of fluid may be placed in a rack in the treatment room or taped to the head of the bed for comparison with subsequent specimens.

NURSING INTERVENTION. The client is watched closely and checked for signs of shock or increased intracranial pressure. The level of consciousness and vital signs are checked according to the condition and need of the individual client. Usually the client is positioned on the side with the head above the level of the heart.

## CHARTING

**Nurse's notes**
Procedure, physician, date, and time
Amount and character of fluid removed
Observations and significant reactions

## Neuroradiology

Radiographs of the skull are taken routinely in the following projections: lateral, posteroanterior, axial (submentovertical), and half axial (Towne). When indicated, specialized views are made of the optic foramina, petrous bones, and sella turcica. For more detailed information tomograms (selected vertical or horizontal layered exposures at measured depths) are sometimes made. The films are examined for signs of fracture, erosion of the bone (including the size of the sella turcica), position of the pineal body if calcified, unusual calcification, and abnormal vascularity. Additional information, if necessary, can be obtained by contrast studies (encephalography, ventriculography, and angiography, details of which follow in this chapter).

Radiographs are taken of the various regions of the spine, depending on the part involved. These are made routinely in the anteroposterior and lateral projections and, if indicated, in the oblique projection. If the special radiography unit is available, tomograms are made as necessary for more exact information of a particular area. The lateral views give information about the condition of the vertebral bodies and the presence of normal curves. Abnormal lateral curvature (scoliosis) is demonstrated in the anteroposterior view as well as erosion or fracture of the pedicles or laminae. Contrast studies are performed with positive (isophendylate) or negative (air) medium to demonstrate encroachment on the subarachnoid space. This is called *myelography* and is discussed later in this chapter.

In addition to the previously mentioned routine radiographic studies of the skull and spine, special projections, tomography, and contrast techniques have been developed for more accurate diagnosis and have made neuroradiology a special field. These contrast studies are cerebral angiography, pneumoencephalography, ventriculography, myelography, and CAT scans when ordered. Brain scanning, a technique utilized in nuclear medicine, also relies on contrast to specify pathological conditions. Contrast is used for the diagnosis of spinal lesions that compress and distort the spinal subarachnoid space, into which the contrast medium is injected, and leads to the diagnosis of spinal tumors and ruptured discs. The other methods are used for diagnosis of intracranial pathological conditions.

Although ventriculography was for many years the method of choice in the diagnosis of intracranial tumors, cerebral angiography has become increasingly important and is frequently used instead of ventriculography. Pneumoencephalography is used more frequently than ventriculography.

## Cerebral angiography

**Expected outcome**
The client should be able to explain the procedure and possible complications.

*Definition.* The injection of a radiopaque substance into the cerebral circulation in conjunction with special roentgenological studies of the intracranial and extracranial vessels. The injection is made into the carotid system to outline the anterior, middle, and posterior cerebral arteries and returning venous circulation; the injection is made into the vertebral artery to outline the vertebral-basilar system in the posterior fossa.

*Indications.* (1) The visualization of the cerebral arteries and veins to determine the site, size, and nature of pathological processes. (2) The localization of tumors, abscesses, aneurysms, hematomas, or other lesions large enough to distort grossly the normal cerebrovascular pattern.

*Contraindications.* (1) Severe liver, kidney, or thyroid disease. (2) Sensitivity to the contrast material. (3) Age. (4) Anticoagulant therapy. (5) Recent thrombotic or embolic episodes.

*Solutions used.* Although Thorotrast is considered superior to other contrast media from the radiographic standpoint, it is relatively dangerous because of its radioactivity and possible delayed deleterious effect. It is rarely used.

Diatrizoate sodium (Hypaque), 45%, or meglumine diatrizoate (Renografin), 60%, is now most commonly used. Renografin is available in 25 ml vials or ampules, and a 1 ml ampule is available for the sensitivity test. This solution should be warmed to body temperature before being used and should not be left in a syringe exposed to strong light for any prolonged period of time. Although the predictive value of a sensitivity test is questionable, it is recommended that it be done the day before the angiogram is scheduled. Renografin, 0.5 to 1 ml, is injected slowly into a peripheral vein to determine if the client is sensitive to the drug. Special care should be taken if the client has a personal history of bronchial asthma, allergy to seafood or drugs, or a family history of allergy. If either applies, several successive, small, increasing injections of Renografin may be given over a period of several minutes. The client should be observed closely. Sneezing, itching, urticaria, faintness, vomiting, and respiratory difficulty are manifestations of sensitivity. No response to the pretest does not guarantee that the client will not have an anaphylactoid reaction. Renografin should be used with caution in clients who are elderly, severely debilitated, or hypertensive, or in those who have advanced arteriosclerosis, cardiac decompensation, or a recent cerebral embolism or thrombosis. One fatal reaction may occur in approximately every 100,000 examinations in which Renografin is used.

The usual single dose for an adult is 10 ml; a smaller amount, determined in relation to body weight, is given to children.

*Preparation of client.* The procedure is explained to the client by the physician, and a written permission is obtained from him or her or, depending on severity of the condition, the closest relative. The sensitivity test is performed.

If indicated, a sedative is given the night before the angiogram is scheduled. If a general anesthetic is to be given, no food or fluid should be taken for at least 6 hours before the procedure.

Temperature, all pulses, respiration, and blood pressure are measured. The client is encouraged to void. Artificial dentures are removed and placed in a suitable receptacle. If carotid or vertebral puncture is anticipated, the circumference of the neck should be measured.

If the client is a man, his face and the anterior portion of his neck are shaved, and he is dressed in a hospital shirt and pajama pants. If the client is a woman, bobby pins, hairpins, and hairnet are removed. If a femoral approach is to be used, the groin will have to be shaved.

Depending on the client's condition and the type of anesthesia to be used, premedication, such as a small dose of atropine, codeine, meperidine hydrochloride (Demerol), or scopolamine, is given 30 to 45 minutes before the procedure is begun. Empty bowel and bladder.

It is very important that the nurse thoroughly prepare the client before the procedure by instructing him or her in all aspects before, during, and after the test regarding what the client is expected to do and what is going to be done to assess his or her status before and after the test. The client should understand that intensive monitoring will occur after the test and will include at least vital and neurological signs and observation of the puncture site. The nurse should answer as honestly as possible any questions that the client may have. The frequent monitoring of the client status may indicate to the client that he or she is not progressing well. If the client is progressing well, he or she should be told so to allay any possible anxiety about the frequent monitoring.

*Procedure (closed method).* The client is transferred to a stretcher and transported to the radiology department with the chart and prepared movable table. He or she is placed on the back on the table and, depending on the room temperature, is covered with a sheet or blanket.

The client's position is adjusted so that the head is hyperextended, and the arms are removed from the shirt sleeves and placed at the sides. The shirt is draped across the chest and tucked in snugly at the armpits.

The two physicians put on sterile gloves. The nurse uncovers the sterile field and opens two 25 ml ampules of 60% Renografin. Their contents are aspirated into the two marked syringes by a physician. Next the two unmarked syringes are filled with saline solution.

If both carotid arteries are to be injected, the anterior aspect of the neck from the chin line to the clavicles and to an inch behind the ears is painted with thimerosal or with Betadine. If only one side is to be injected, the neck area is prepared to the midline anteriorly and approximately 1 inch behind the ear posteriorly. The prepared area is draped with sterile towels.

The carotid artery is palpated, and, if general anesthesia is not indicated, procaine is injected in the usual manner. (Unless the client is unable to cooperate, local anesthesia is preferred.)

The physician selects a needle (the size varies) and connects it to the Venotube, which is attached to a syringe filled with saline solution. Some of the saline solution is expelled so that no air bubbles remain in the syringe or Venotube; the tube is occluded with a Kelly clamp.

While one physician introduces the needle into the artery, the other holds the attached syringe and the Kelly clamp, which is released after the needle is introduced under the skin. When the artery is entered, blood should flow back into the tubing under considerable pressure. The assistant immediately clamps the Venotube, and the needle is threaded into the artery; the clamp is released, and saline solution is injected to clear the tubing of blood. (Saline solution is used to keep the tubing open, to prevent clotting of the blood, and to ensure the correct placement of the needle in the artery before the contrast material is injected.)

The radiography technician is alerted; the syringe filled with saline solution is replaced with one containing Renografin (10 ml). If an automatic camera is used, timed, repeated radiographs may be taken during the injection of the contrast material. This makes possible the visualization of both arterial and venous circulations; however, if the camera is not available, a single radiographic exposure is made during each injection. The ipsilateral cerebral arteries are thus visualized; the film is changed quickly, and approximately 3 seconds after the injection a second film is exposed to record the venous circulation. As soon as the injection is completed, the syringe is detached and replaced with one containing saline solution.

The needle is left in place; its patency is maintained by the slow injection of saline solution until the wet films have been reviewed. If these are not satisfactory, Renografin is injected again, and more films are taken. The needle is removed; a sterile sponge is applied to the puncture site, and local pressure is maintained for about 5 minutes to prevent bleeding and the formation of a hematoma.

If the other carotid artery is to be injected, this procedure is repeated. The client is then transferred to the stretcher and returned to his or her room.

If is necessary to use the femoral artery for visualization of the vertebral-basilar artery circulation, the same principles apply as in direct carotid puncture, with the exception of the passage of a long catheter. In this manner the femoral artery is the favored site for injection. The common internal and external carotids are better visualized by this method.

A recent coupling of Doppler scanning with angiography has proved to be valuable for those clients who will ultimately require surgery and cannot tolerate two invasive procedures, or both techniques combined also improve the positive diagnosis of the disorder.

*Complications.* If any untoward reactions occur, these generally take place during the procedure or immediately thereafter. They may be local or central in origin and are caused by a local hemorrhage or vasospasm. A hematoma may occur at the puncture site and may be small or of such a size as to compress the trachea and esophagus, thus causing difficulty in breathing and swallowing, necessitating an immediate tracheostomy. Hemiparesis, hemiplegia, aphasia, or changes in the level of consciousness may occur with an adverse intracranial reaction.

If an anaphylactoid reaction occurs, the procedure should be interrupted and treatment started immediately. External cardiac massage and mouth-to-mouth breathing should be adminstered for cardiac arrest. The following drugs may be given intravenously: secobarbital (Seconal), 10 to 100 mg, for severe apprehension; diphenhydramine (Benadryl), 20 mg, for allergic symptoms and methoxamine hydrochloride (Vasoxyl), 5 mg, for shock or air hunger. If methoxamine is not available, phenylephrine (Neo-Synephrine), 0.2 to 0.5 mg, may be substituted. Depending on the severity of the reaction, the administration of oxygen and intravenous fluids may be indicated.

Ephedrine should never be used, since it may induce ventricular fibrillation. Respiratory stimulants should not be used because they may cause convulsions.

*Nursing intervention.* The client is placed in a comfortable position in bed. If a general anesthetic has been given, he or she is kept on the side until fully conscious. Routine observations are carried out as for any client after anesthesia. In addition, as indicated by the client's condition, vital signs are taken; the neck is checked for evidence of swelling and difficulty in swallowing or breathing, and for hematoma or hemorrhage from the puncture site, if it occurs. Notify the physician immediately. The motion and strength of the extremities are tested, and facial mobility is noted. An ice collar may be applied to the neck to relieve superficial swelling and local discomfort. An untoward reaction occurs rarely. Generally this procedure is tolerated well, and the client resumes normal routine a few hours after returning to the room.

If the femoral puncture was used, a sandbag should be kept in place for at least 4 hours and the site observed for hematoma or hemorrhage. Any swelling may indicate arterial occlusion if the pulses distal to the site cannot be detected. Color and temperature of the extremities should also be observed.

*Alternate procedure (open method).* At times, because of technical difficulties or the client's inability to cooperate, it may be considered advisable to expose the internal carotid artery before the contrast material is injected. The procedure would then be performed in the operating room under strict aseptic technique. In addition to the equipment listed under the procedure for the closed method, sterile instruments and silk ligatures are required. After the local skin preparation is completed, the area is draped. An oblique incision, approximately 3 cm long, is made over the external carotid artery, which is then retracted to expose the internal carotid artery. The procedure is continued as previously outlined. After the removal of the needle, gentle pressure is exerted on the wound to accelerate hemostasis. The wound is closed and dressed. The aftercare of the client follows the principles noted under the closed method. Sutures are removed on the third day, and a small protective dressing is applied.

*Additional techniques.* Two other types of angiography are currently available to provide data on blood flow patterns, in addition to the more traditional method, which offers biplane rapid serial angiography. These techniques include cineagiography and subtraction angiography.

*Cineangiography* is a technique wherein 16 mm film records the selected site at a speed of 48 frames per second. Instant replay is possible, since the pictures are videotaped. For more precise detail the sequence of pictures is replayed at a rate of 24 frames per second. Cineangiography is utilized to assist in evaluation of the subclavian steal syndrome, the effect of head positions on vertebral and carotid blood circulation, and the severity of arterial stenosis.

*Subtraction angiography* is useful when the presence of a bone blocks visualization of blood vessels under study. Special film allows one to obtain one film wherein the total radiographic image and subtraction mask are contained.

## CHARTING

**Nurse's notes**
Procedure, physician, date, and time
Vital signs and observations
Significant reactions

## Pneumoencephalography

### Expected outcome
The client should be able to explain the procedure and complications and cooperate as much as possible.

*Definition.* The introduction of filtered room air, nitrogen, oxygen, or other gases into the sub-

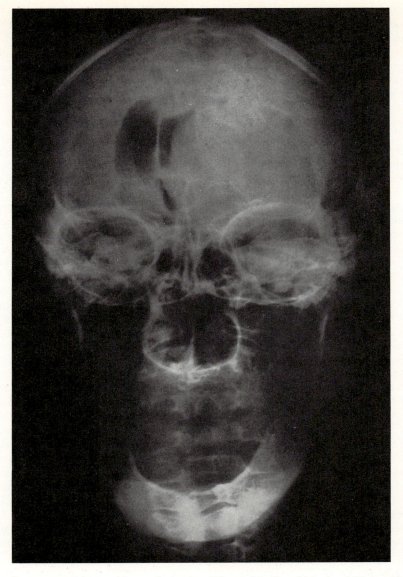

**FIG. 12-5.** Pneumoencephalogram (abnormal) showing shift and distortion of lateral and third ventricles. This was caused by intracranial tumor.

arachnoid space by lumbar or cisternal puncture to outline the ventricular system, and intraspinal intracranial subarachnoid spaces (Fig. 12-5).

*Purposes.* The purposes may be either a diagnostic or a therapeutic radiographic study of fluid spaces within and surrounding the brain.

DIAGNOSTIC. (1) To demonstrate the intracranial subarachnoid space and the ventricular system. (2) To demonstrate cerebral atrophy or porencephaly. (3) To localize an intracranial lesion.

**THERAPEUTIC.** To break up posttraumatic subarachnoid adhesions for relief of headache.

*Contraindications.* Same as discussed under lumbar puncture. Pneumoencephalography may be performed in suspected infratentorial or supratentorial lesions, provided that equipment is available for making bur holes in the skull in the event of an emergency. Recent lumbar puncture (usually less than 10 days) is reason for delaying this procedure.

*Preparation of client.* The physician explains the procedure to the client and relatives. The family should be acquainted with any possible complications. If the client has reached the age of majority (18 years in many states) and is considered legally competent, he or she may sign the necessary permit. If not, the nearest responsible relative should do so. Preferably both should sign.

Necessary orders for the preparation of the client are written by the physician on the day preceding the test. Sample orders with explanatory notes follow:

Sedative should be given at bedtime to ensure a good sleep. Nothing is given by mouth after midnight.

If the test is to be made in the afternoon, the client may have coffee and toast not later than 8 AM and then begin fasting.

If the lumbar area is hairy, it should be dry shaved.

Sedative or ataractic drug may be given 1 hour before the time scheduled, as indicated by individual client's needs.

Atropine sulfate with or without codeine phosphate may be administered 30 minutes before the test.

If the client is ambulatory, he or she should have a tub bath in the morning; otherwise a bed bath is given. A shirt, open in the back, and pajama trousers should be worn to expedite the procedure and prevent unnecessary exposure. Oral hygiene should be administered, and artificial dentures should be removed and placed in a suitable receptacle in a safe place. The hair should be combed and, if long, should be braided neatly and secured with a bandage end. All hairpins, bobby pins, and hairnets must be removed because they may obscure the radiographic findings. Temperature, pulse, respiration, and blood pressure should be measured and recorded on the chart and special pneumoencephalography record as controls. A note is also made of the size and reaction of the pupils, facial symmetry, and the motion and strength of the extremities. The client should be re-

assured as necessary, and medications should be given as ordered.

Some physicians give a general anesthetic such as thiopental sodium (Pentothal) or tribromoethanol (Avertin); others believe that using a local anesthetic with adequate preliminary medication is better. Through personal experience with both methods on adults it has been determined that a client recovers more quickly, has fewer physical ill effects, and requires less special nursing care if a local anesthetic is used. However, since this may be an acutely uncomfortable procedure, there are some adults who are unable to cooperate under local anesthesia. This group of clients and all young children do better under general anesthesia unless it is contraindicated. Regardless of how this procedure is carried out, the client may have a headache or vomit. The danger of aspirating vomitus is negligible under local anesthesia.

If possible, two nurses should be available to observe and emotionally support the client and to assist the physician. The following observations should be made and recorded during the procedure: pulse, respiration, color, diaphoresis, nausea, vomiting, headache, and level of consciousness. Blood pressure readings are taken as indicated by the client's condition; if the client tolerates the procedure well, this may be deferred until after the test is completed. The nurse also records on the special sheet the amounts of CSF removed and air injected.

*Procedure.* The client, dressed in a hospital shirt and pajama pants, is taken to the radiology department with the chart and slippers. The prepared equipment is also taken to the radiology department on a movable table. (The radiology room selected for this procedure should be of sufficient size to permit caring for the client if he or she should have a seizure during the procedure.)

The client is assisted to a sitting position on the side of the stretcher, slippers are put on, and he or she is helped from the stretcher to a foot stool and then to the floor. The client is seated in a specially designed chair with an opening in the lumbar region to facilitate lumbar puncture. The chair is motorized and rotates the client anteriorly or posteriorly through a complete somersault. This rotation will permit the movement of gas without requiring the removal of all CSF.

The physician then performs the lumbar puncture and measures the initial pressure. (In the sitting position the CSF pressure may normally range from 300 to 450 mm $H_2O$.) Before any CSF is removed, 5 cc of air is injected slowly. The stopcock is then turned to prevent escape of fluid, and a sterile sponge is placed over it. The equipment is covered with a sterile towel. The client is cautioned to hold the head still, and a lateral radiograph is taken. The technician then turns the x-ray tube and takes the posteroanterior film. These two films are immediately processed, and the physician interprets them before continuing the procedure. The injection of air without the preliminary removal of CSF generally permits visualization of the third ventricle, the aqueduct, and the fourth ventricle. During this 5- and 10-minute interval the nurse remains with the client and checks vital signs and general condition. The physician removes the protective sponge and puts on sterile gloves. The nurse removes the towel, exposes the equipment, and places it next to the physician. The procedure continues with the gradual introduction of measured amounts of room air to a total of 25 to 30 cc, or 5% less gas injected than CSF withdrawn to allow expansion of gas at body temperature. The rate of exchange of gas for CSF should not exceed 5 ml per minute. The test is terminated as previously outlined. The needle is then removed, and the client is assisted onto the table, where a series of radiographs of the skull is taken.

The identification of a space-occupying mass demands immediate surgery. The pressure alterations within the brain after the introduction of air will increase cerebral edema and the possibility of displacement of the brain, herniation, and compression of the bulb, thus causing acute respiratory failure and death.

***Nursing intervention.*** The client is taken back to the room on a stretcher and returned to bed. The head is laid flat without a pillow, and the client made as comfortable as possible. If the client has a history of seizures, side rails are placed on the bed. The client is instructed so that untoward reactions may be minimized. The position is changed from side to side at least every 2 hours. The bed is kept flat for approximately 12 hours, and, unless contraindicated, fluids are forced to 3000 ml after nausea subsides. These things are done to hasten absorption of the air. The nurse notes possible untoward reactions such as severe prolonged headache, chills, fever, shock, nuchal rigidity, convulsions, continued vomiting, and signs of increased intracranial pressure. Many clients will be febrile as long as 36 to 48 hours with consistent temperature of 101° F.

Reactions are reported to the physician immediately and treated symptomatically. (If the client has been taking anticonvulsant medication, this should be resumed to prevent seizures.)

The routine postencephalography orders are as follows (these orders may be modified for the individual client as necessary):

Keep client flat in bed for 12 hours and then increase the head Gatch bed as tolerated.
Force fluids to 3000 ml.
Measure output (2 days).
Plan diet as tolerated after nausea subsides (the regular diet is usually resumed on the second day).
Check temperature, pulse, respiration, and blood pressure on return to bed, then pulse, respiration, and blood pressure every 30 minutes for 2 hours, and then every hour for 4 hours.
Take temperature (rectally) every 4 hours.

These clients may be acutely uncomfortable with headache and nausea for the first 12 to 36 hours. During this period analgesics, codeine, or meperidine (Demerol) may be administered. Thereafter symptoms gradually subside. Nursing care is directed toward making the client as comfortable as possible. During the first 12 hours the client is fed assisted in changing position and supervised closely. After this interval he or she should be encouraged to become more active and independent. The head of the bed is progressively elevated; the average client is usually sufficiently recovered by the second day to resume previous routine. Air is absorbed from the subarachnoid spaces in 24 hours, from the cisterns in 48 hours, and from the ventricles within 72 hours, and CSF is reformed.

## CHARTING

### Nurse's notes
Procedure, physician, date, and time
Amount of air injected
Cooperation of client
Observations and vital signs
Significant reactions
Treatment (if any)
Instructions given the client

## Ventriculography

### Expected outcome

The client should be able to explain the procedure, complications, and necessity for craniotomy if indicated.

*Definition.* The introduction of gas or positive contrast medium directly into the lateral ventricles by ventricular puncture through the coronal sutures in infants, or through bur or twist drill holes in the older child or adult, or into the frontal posterior parietal, or occipital regions for special radiographic study of the brain (Fig. 12-6).

*Indications.* (1) To localize a brain tumor. (2) To detect cerebral anomalies such as porencephaly and atrophy. (3) To note patency of the ventricular system.

*Purpose.* When pneumoencephalography is contraindicated in the presence of a pronounced increase in intracranial pressure or when a posterior fossa lesion is suspected.

*Contraindications.* (1) When a lesser procedure will suffice. (2) When roentgenological visualization of the intracranial subarachnoid spaces is desired.

*Disadvantages.* (1) Necessitates a surgical procedure (if the client is over 18 months of age and the bones of the skull have fused). (2) Some trauma to the brain may result.

*Preparation of client.* Preparation of the client must be both psychological and physical.

PSYCHOLOGICAL. If the client's condition permits, the procedure should be discussed with him

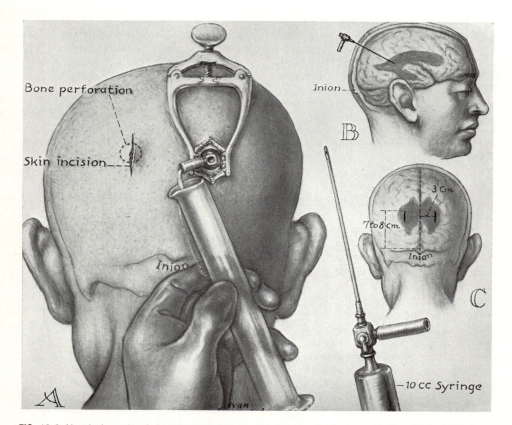

**FIG. 12-6.** Ventriculography. **A,** Location of incisions and burr holes. **B,** shows needle in ventricle. **C** shows further details. (From Sachs, E.: Diagnosis and treatment of brain tumors and care of the neurosurgical client, ed. 2, St. Louis, 1949, The C.V. Mosby Co.)

or her by the physician. In any event the physician should discuss the test and the risk involved with the nearest of kin and have the permit signed. The nurse is prepared to give reassurance as necessary. Pretest teaching should include information regarding the test, and posttest surgery if necessary.

**PHYSICAL (AS ORDERED DAY BEFORE BY PHYSICIAN).** If the client is restless and wakeful, a mild sedative is given. If the test is to be done in the morning, nothing is given by mouth after midnight. If the test is to be done in the afternoon, a light breakfast (coffee and toast) may be given before 8 AM and then nothing by mouth.

On the night before, the appropriate part of the head is clipped and then shampooed. If a craniotomy is to follow or if the client is a man, the entire head is usually clipped. If the client is a woman, her head should be covered with a cap or a wig, if available. It is appropriate for skin preparation and hair removal to be performed in the radiology department or operating room the day of the procedure.

The following instructions are usually included in the preoperative orders:

Have the client sign a permit for ventriculogram and notify family of hour scheduled. Give 0.0004 gm of atropine sulfate (adult dose) 30 minutes before operation. On call to the operating room at _____.

In addition to carrying out the physician's orders, the nurse should give the client a bath and administer oral hygiene. If any hair is left on the head, it should be combed, braided if possible, and secured with a rubber band or bandage. All hairpins and bobby pins must be removed. The client is dressed in a hospital shirt and pajama trousers, and a towel is secured around the head. The client voids before going to the operating room.

The temperature (rectal), pulse, respiration, and blood pressure are measured. Level of consciousness, equality of the pupils, facial symmetry, and strength of the extremities are noted (if a craniotomy is to follow, the detailed preoperative observations listed in Chapters 22 and 26 should be made).

The chart should be completed.

*Procedure.* The client with the completed chart is transported on a stretcher to the operating room.

He or she is then transferred to the operating table and placed in a sitting position with the head tilted slightly forward and supported on the headrest. Body restraints are applied, and a footboard is used to prevent the client from slipping down on the table. The physician scrubs, puts on gloves and, using a sponge stick, cleanses the scalp with pHisoHex or Betadine. The areas to be trephined are anesthetized by injection of lidocaine. Sterile towels are placed over the scalp and secured, with the operative areas being left exposed. Two sterile sheets are draped over the client's body. The physician changes gloves. Saline gauze strips are placed on each side of the line of incision, compression and traction are applied, and simultaneously the incision is made down to the periosteum. This is elevated, and a self-retaining mastoid retractor is inserted. Clients who bleed are given coagulants as necessary. A hole is made in the skull by using a perforator and a bur. The dura is incised, and the underlying pia-arachnoid is coagulated. A ventricular needle is inserted into the lateral ventricle, the stylet is removed, and CSF appears. The procedure is repeated on the opposite side if indicated. The fluid is gradually removed and replaced with filtered air or oxygen. The total amount of fluid removed may vary from 20 to 50 ml, and a smaller amount of air is injected. Sometimes after a ventricle has been tapped, a catheter is inserted in place of the needle. This is left in place until radiographs have been taken and read. It permits the insertion of more air if necessary. Otherwise, the needle is removed after the insertion of air. The galea and skin are sutured with interrupted black silk; sterile dressings are applied. The client is transferred to a stretcher and taken to the radiology department by the physician and nurse. If a general anesthetic has been given, the anesthetist should also accompany the client and remain while the films are taken. The client may then be returned to the operating room for craniotomy if indicated.

*Nursing intervention.* After the radiological studies have been completed, the client is returned to his or her bed, clothing is changed as necessary, and he or she is made as comfortable as possible. Temperature, pulse, respiration, and blood pressure are measured immediately and then at 30-minute or hourly intervals for 4 to 12 hours, depending on condition and the radiographic findings. The head is usually elevated 10 to 15 degrees and the position changed every 2 hours. If the client is unconscious, the routine for posturing clients outlined in Chapter 9 is followed. Diet and fluids are given as tolerated. These clients usually have less reaction than those who have encephalography, but they may have the same type of reactions outlined in the section on encephalography. An ice bag may relieve headache. Analgesics and selected controlled drugs may be given for severe discomfort. The pretest observations are continued, and changes are reported immediately. On the day after ventriculography the head is elevated as tolerated. Depending on the individual client, he or she may be permitted out of bed on the second or third day. Side rails are used as indicated. The most severe complications that may occur are increasing intracranial pressure, hemorrhage, or respiratory collapse. The treatment is symptomatic.

### CHARTING

**Nurse's notes—preoperative**
Complete preoperative checklist
Chart early medications
Chart base-line neurological and vital signs

**Nurse's notes—postoperative**
Procedure by physician, date, and time
Time client returned to room
Amount and character of fluid removed (if catheter in place)
Specimens to laboratory as ordered
Significant reactions

## Myelography

**Expected outcome**
Same as for lumbar puncture.

*Definition.* The introduction of a positive (Pantopaque) or negative (air) contrast medium into the subarachnoid space by lumbar or cisternal puncture for special radiographic study of the spinal canal.

*Indications.* (1) Visualization of the spinal subarachnoid space. (2) Determination of the level of a suspected spinal lesion by the resulting distortion of the outline of the subarachnoid space.

*Purpose.* When rupture of an intervertebral disc or compression of the spinal cord is suspected.

### EQUIPMENT

The same as that listed for lumbar puncture and spinal dynamics, with the addition of the following:

Sterile 20 ml syringe
Sterile towels
Package of sponges (4 × 4 inches)
2 pairs of sterile gloves
3 ampules of isophendylate (3 ml each) or metrizamide (Amipaque)
Procaine (Novocain) and syringe with No. 27 needle
Adhesive tape
Special form for spinal studies

*Preparation of client.* The procedure is explained, and the permit is obtained, as in lumbar puncture.

Food and fluid are omitted for approximately 4 hours before the test. If it is scheduled after lunch, a light breakfast may be given to the client. If the physician is especially interested in the lumbar region, a cleansing enema or colon lavage may be ordered to obviate the possibility of gas shadows on the films.

If necessary, the lumbar area is dry shaved. After voiding, the client is dressed in a hospital shirt (open in the back) and pajama pants, assisted onto a stretcher, taken to the radiology department, transferred to the fluoroscopic table, positioned on the side, and draped as for lumbar puncture.

*Procedure.* This is performed completely in the radiology department to eliminate the need for a second lumbar puncture.

The procedure is the same as for lumbar puncture until the subarachnoid space of the spinal canal is entered. Spinal dynamics are then determined, and approximately 10 ml of CSF, unless previously examined, are removed for chemical and cytological study. After this the stylet is replaced in the needle.

The nurse prepares and opens the ampules of isophendylate or metrizamide (two for lumbar, three to four for cervical visualization), the physician draws the contrast material into the syringe and, after removing the stylet, slowly injects 1 ml into the lumbar puncture needle. After the physician fluoroscopes the client on the tilting table to see if the contrast material is in the subarachnoid space, the remaining 5 ml of contrast material is introduced. The stylet is replaced, and the needle is left in the subarachnoid space. The client is turned onto the abdomen and positioned so that the feet are flat against the upright foot support. (This is to keep the client from sliding off the table when it is tilted to the upright position. A shoulder brace or harness at the opposite end helps maintain the client in the correct position when tilted downward.) The physician drapes the needle with two sterile sponges and the surrounding area by folding up the fenestrated sheet. The sheet is secured to the skin with adhesive tape to avoid its displacement and contamination of the puncture site.

The physician puts on a protective lead apron; extinguishes the lights and, tilting the table to various degrees, fluoroscopes the spinal subarachnoid space and visualizes the surrounding structures. Spot films are made as indicated. When the radiographs are completed, the lights are turned on; the drapes are removed; and, after putting on sterile gloves, the physician removes the stylet, attaches the syringe, and aspirates the contrast material. The stylet is replaced, and the needle is removed. The skin is cleansed with alcohol, and a small cotton collodion dressing may be applied. The patient is returned by stretcher to bed.

*Nursing intervention.* After the isophendylate has been removed, the client may remain flat in bed for a few hours and then resume previous routine. If the material has not been removed, the client's head is kept elevated above the level of the spine to prevent possible gravitation of the isophendylate to the brain. This may cause an irritative cerebral meningitis. The client should be watched for signs and symptoms of meningeal irritation; otherwise no special observations are made. Metrizamide need not be aspirated because it will be absorbed within 48 hours. The client should be observed for headache, nausea, or vomiting.

## CHARTING

### Nurse's notes
Procedure, physician, date, and time
Significant reactions
Specimens to laboratory
Comments

For *air myelography* (negative contrast medium) the client is placed in the lateral recumbent posi-

tion, and the head of the table is tilted down 20 degrees. A needle is introduced into the cisterna magna, and CSF is removed and completely replaced with air. Tomograms passing through the midsagittal plane are then made. In this way the spinal cord is outlined.

The client, with the head lower than the trunk to prevent the trapped air from entering the intracranial subarachnoid space, is then returned to the ward and maintained in this position for 48 hours. Most of the air should be absorbed by this time, and the head may be elevated.

### Brain scanning

Most pathological lesions in the brain accumulate substances, such as vital dyes (trypan blue) or various radioactive isotopes, from the bloodstream. The exchange of these substances between plasma and abnormal tissue is much faster and freer than that between plasma and normal brain tissue. Therefore since the concentration of the tracer substances is greater in the pathological region than in the surrounding brain tissue, an abnormal brain–normal brain concentration ratio exists. It can now be measured for diagnostic purposes. This principle is the basis for radioactive brain scanning.

Brain tumor localization was ushered in with the fluorescence localization work by Moore. This was closely followed by his efforts and others in the study of radioisotopes as a means of lesion identification. In 1946 radioisotopes became available for medical research. Rapid technical developments occurred, producing the rectolinear scanning device; a small crystal moved slowly back and forth across the organ being studied with data recorded on film or paper by dots. This test frequently required several hours, and uncooperative clients were a serious problem. In the 1960s there was developed a large single crystal that permitted almost instant visualization of an organ or region. The development of special isotopes closely followed the imporved instrumentation. Technetium 99m, with a half-life of 5 to 6 hours and good energy output, is now the isotope most commonly used for brain scanning. Because of the associated ability to store information on tape for repeated replays and the ability electronically to select small areas within an organ, blood flow studies are now available. Such information can be plotted on contour maps in such a way as to identify areas of vascular insufficiency in the brain. A bolus of technetium 99m injected intravenously can be followed during its first flow through the brain. A short time later the static scan is obtained for identification of pathological tissue. To enhance the isotope uptake, one administers 0.25 to 0.56 ml of potassium perchlorate to the client to block uptake by the thyroid, choroid plexus, and salivary glands to prevent artifacts on the scan. Similar solutions are used to enhance uptake of the other radioisotopes available and to block irradiation to other organs.

Scanning is preferable to all other techniques because of its minimal morbidity. Accuracy of tumor detection varies but is in the range of 90% to 98% when one is dealing with metastatic tumors, malignant gliomas, or meningiomas. When a tumor remains slow growing and relatively avascular, the level of accuracy decreases. Astrocytomas have been identified with an accuracy of about 80%. Tumors located in the posterior fossa are more difficult to identify because of the muscle mass that obscures tumor uptake.

The combination of brain scan, angiography, air study, and CAT scan offers almost 100% accuracy in localizing tumors. Scanning is useful in search of blood clots, infection, or other abnormalities that either break the blood-brain barrier or displace normal brain tissue.

*Procedure.* A radioactive substance, generally technetium 99m, is given intravenously at a specified time before the test. The client is then sent to the radioisotope laboratory and placed in contact with the sensing device with optical display on a television screen. The brain scanning is completed within a few minutes, and the client is returned to the ward. The client may resume previous activity. Since no adverse reactions are expected, no special observations or aftercare is necessary.

*Nursing intervention.* The client should be assured that there is no pain with the procedure. There are no special preparations other than the potassium perchlorate. The client can ensure an accurate test by only moving when instructed to do so. The radioactive substance will cause no harm to the client or others nearby. There are no aftereffects.

## COMPUTERIZED AXIAL TOMOGRAPHY

One of the greatest breakthroughs in neurodiagnostics occurred in the early 1970s, when computerized axial tomography (CAT) was introduced. Although the equipment required is very expensive, most large centers are now equipped to perform this specialized testing (Fig. 12-7).

CAT scans may be invasive or noninvasive. When they were first introduced, all CAT scans were noninvasive. Currently CAT scans may be done with or without the injection of contrast medium. When contrast medium is used, the same problems and precautions for allergic reactions are taken as they would be in any situation employing dye injection.

One type of CAT scan is the EMI scan, wherein the client lies flat on a hydraulic table with the head resting in a latex cap. The latex cap is located in a methyl methacrylate (Lucite) cube filled with water so that the cap fits snugly about the head. To be held steady, the client is provided with a seat and foot support. Once oriented to the procedure and made comfortable the client is instructed not to move during the 5-minute intervals required for each scan. Talking and breathing do not interfere with testing so long as the client can do this without moving the head.

After EMI scanners were developed a refinement in equipment known as the ACTA (automated computerized transverse axial) scanner was made. In this scanner an x-ray beam enters a computer, which assimilates data onto a black-and-white picture. A second computer analyzes the picture and produces a color picture that reflects the density of tissue in relation to the entry of the x-ray beam rather than actual color. The ACTA scanner has an advantage over the EMI scanner, since it may be used for head or total body scans. The outcome of testing includes data in black-and-white and color pictures, cassette tapes, Polaroid pictures of oscilloscope images, and a numerical printout of the findings.

When the noninvasive approach is utilized, the procedure is painless and involves so little radiation (approximately that necessary for skull roentgenography) that the procedure may be done several times to monitor progress of a disease process. The CAT scan may be performed in less time than either the pneumoencephalogram or the cerebral

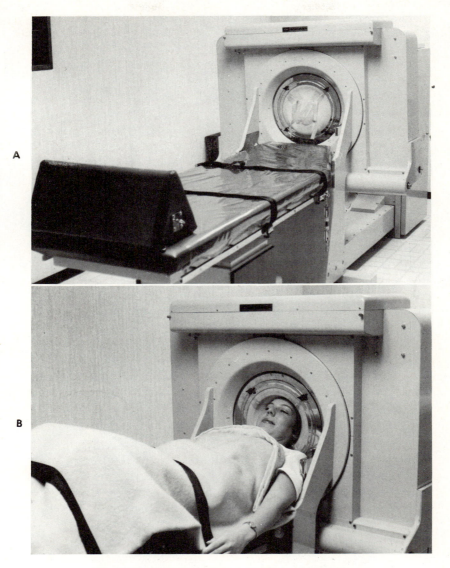

**FIG. 12-7. A,** Scanning equipment. **B,** Client receiving CAT scan.

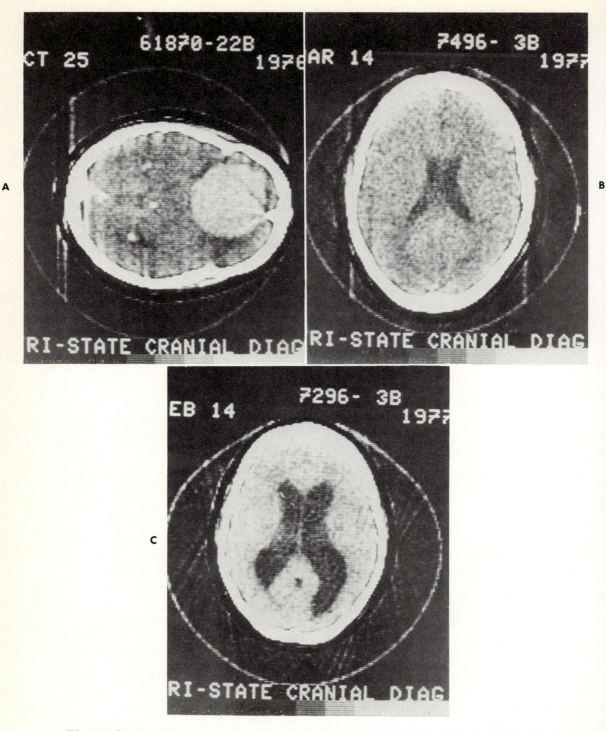

**FIG. 12-8.** Results of CAT scans. **A,** Hematoma behind eye orbit. **B,** Normal. **C,** Ventricular dilatation (hydrocephalus).

angiogram. CAT scans performed by the EMI scanner allow the practitioner to get a 360-degree view of the brain in 1-degree angles. This added dimension provides more definitive data on both the integrity of intracranial structures and the precise location of any abnormalities. Polaroid films of the significant findings are reproduced within minutes of the test, so that the physician receives instant results along with pictures of the problem. Neither pneumoencephalography nor cerebral angiography can provide the same degree of data available from the CAT scan. To date only autopsies and biopsies have been able to provide this amount of data. Some experts believe that even more data will be available from these scans in the future as techniques become refined and as further experience is gained in interpreting test results.

The disadvantages of CAT scanning include the cost of equipment acquisition; the cost of the test to the client; the need for remaining perfectly still during the scanning procedure, which may require 30 minutes (in the young child or uncooperative client heavy sedation may be required to keep him or her motionless, and necessary precautions and adequate monitoring are then required for the sedated client); limited visualization of the posterior fossa; and lack of vessel visualization.

The indications for the use of the CAT scan are increasing daily. Popular uses currently include determination of the presence of a space-occupying lesion, since this process outlines the problem more adequately than either the brain scan or cerebral angiography. In suspected hydrocephalus the CAT clearly outlines the ventricles at least as well as might be expected from a pneumoencephalogram. Porencephalic cysts and abnormal brain development are also problems the CAT scan identifies rather accurately even before visual inspection during surgery is possible. Other indications for the use of the CAT scan include head trauma and cerebrovascular disturbances.

*Client preparation.* If the procedure is noninvasive, there are virtually no contraindications, unless they would pertain to problems with exposure to small amounts of radiation. When the procedure involves contrast media, one takes a history of allergic responses, pretests the client's response to dye, and observes the client for a reaction after the dye is injected. Most CAT scans are done in an outpatient basis with no aftercare, unless sedation is required or contrast is used. The most important part of preparation is to explain the testing procedures, the need to be immobile, the appearance of the equipment, and what the client may expect.

*Findings.* Lesions are evident as alterations of normal tissue absorption (density) relative to water as a standard and are interpreted in groups of disorders that fall into the category of density present (Fig. 12-8).

## POSITRON EMISSION TOMOGRAPHY

The 1980s have been the time when the most recent improvements have been made upon the CAT scan. The PET scan (positron emission tomography) is experimentally being used to spot abnormal regions of brain metabolism in serious mental illnesses and neurological disorders in an effort to study and correlate the pattern and action of pharmaceutical agents with the appropriate effect on neuropathological states. A bolus of deoxyglucose containing radioactive fluorine is injected as in the contrast media in the CAT scan. The procedure is similar to the CAT scan. In the PET scan positrons are emitted and collide with electrons producing photons that are detected and processed by computer. The chemical activity produced during the collision of the positrons and the electrons constructs a composite color picture on a display screen. The various shades of color indicate levels of glucose metabolism. The color pattern levels and colors may be the key in the future to confirm a diagnosis of serious mental illness and neurological disorders. The PET scan has already been used in the diagnosis of epilepsy and may help surgeons to locate and destroy epileptogenic cells. Detection of the postsurgical status of cerebrovascular bypass in clients for localization and adequacy of blood flow is another current use of the PET scan.

Extreme expense and the need for trained manpower and specialized equipment are still problems in widespread utilization. Forty major research centers worldwide have been designated as places for investigational use in technique and treatment utilization.

In some sources PET is termed PETT, which

includes an additional word in the phrase *"positron emission transaxial tomography."* However, PET and PETT refer to the same type of computed tomography. Watch future experiments with *xenon enhancement tomography* (XET), wherein xenon, an expensive substance, requries intubation and anesthesia to enhance the brain image for studies. Perhaps, more practical uses for XET will occur with further study. Practitioners should also be aware of the research which is occurring to develop the NMR, *nuclear magnetic resonance,* of the body. Since NMR is sensitive to edema and ischemia, some believe that it might be a valuable tool for evaluation of various types of disease conditions.

## OTHER STUDIES
### Cystometry

*Bladder functions.* Bladder function is normally regulated through the nervous systems, which are voluntary (conscious control of the external sphincter) and autonomic (automatic control of the internal sphincter and detrusor muscles through the pelvic nerve of the parasympathetic division by way of the sacral segments of the spinal cord). The physiological stimulus for contraction of the bladder is tension on its walls by the fluid within. The spinal cord is responsible for the reflex emptying of the bladder, the contraction of the detrusor muscle, and the relaxation of the internal and the external sphincters. Urination would take place frequently with as little as 50 ml filling if not controlled and conditioned by the higher centers (brain). Voluntary inhibition of bladder function begins with the training of the infant. It is promoted by cultural patterns that dictate appropriate places, situations, and even positions in which micturition may occur.

In adults with normal bladders the intravesical pressure of the empty bladder is approximately 1 cm $H_2O$, and its capacity is about 500 ml. Generally awareness of filling begins with 200 to 250 ml of fluid; desire to void occurs at 250 to 300 ml. With additional filling, this desire becomes increasingly urgent to the point of acute discomfort and obvious distention when capacity is reached.

Neurological disease may produce three types of bladder disturbances—the atonic, the hypotonic, and the hypertonic—with varying degrees of in-

volvement (Fig. 12-9). The *atonic bladder* (associated with the early stage of spinal cord injury) is characterized by the absence of muscle tone and contractility, a greatly enlarged capacity, no feeling of discomfort with distention, overflow with a large residual, and an inability voluntarily or reflexly to empty the bladder completely. The *hypotonic bladder* varies only in degree from the atonic bladder. There may be slight contraction of the detrusor muscle and a rise in intravesical pressure with filling; however, these are not sufficient to empty the bladder spontaneously so that distention results. The *hypertonic bladder* (seen in the late stage of spinal cord injury or in slowly developing spinal cord disease) is characterized by increased muscle tone, diminished capacity, and higher intravesical pressure. Its emptying is on a reflex level and occurs spontaneously with little voluntary control (associated with frequency, urgency, voiding in small amounts, and sometimes incontinence).

In acute, severe vascular and traumatic diseases of the brain no physiological disturbance of the bladder as such occurs; however, the unconscious or stuporous client is unable to control micturition, and incontinence occurs at frequent intervals. Since the bladder empties spontaneously with 50 to 100 ml filling, it contracts progressively and finally simulates the hypertonic bladder just discussed. If a retention catheter is inserted and connected to a tube for free (straight) drainage, the normal bladder may contract and also become hypertonic.

**Expected outcome**
The client should be able to explain the procedure and cooperate for an accurate test.

*Definition.* Cystometry consists of a record of intravesical pressures with various degrees of filling of the bladder. These readings are determined by introduction of measured amounts (usually 50 ml at a time) of a sterile solution through a retention catheter into the bladder until spontaneous emptying takes place or a total filling of 500 to 750 ml is reached.

*Indications.* (1) To determine the muscle tone of the bladder. (2) To determine the capacity of the bladder.

*Nursing intervention.* Explain the procedure to

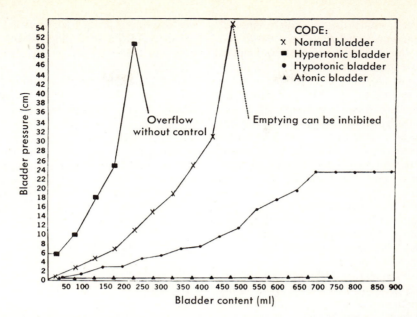

**FIG. 12-9.** Cystometric graph illustrating representative curves for normal, hypertonic, hypotonic, and atonic bladders.

the client. Emphasize the need for cooperation for the successful completion of the test. Instruct him or her to remain very quiet without any movement of the body or extremities and to report the first feeling of bladder fullness, discomfort, or desire to void.

Draw the curtains around the unit. Place the client flat on the back and cover him or her with a bath blanket; fanfold the top bedclothes to the foot of the bed. (Adequate covering should be used to prevent chilling during the procedure, which may last 30 to 60 minutes.)

*Procedure.* Place the infusion standard beside the bed. Note the level of the symphysis pubis, and mark it on the standard with a piece of adhesive tape. Place the cystometric tape on the standard so that the clamp (for a tripe outlet) is parallel with the adhesive tape marker. Remove the protective cap from the bottle. Attach the sterile plastic thiopental-dispensing cap with vent and outlet. Open the sterile bundles. Attach the plastic genitourinary tubing to the outlet of the plastic cap of the bottle. Invert and hang it on the standard according to the manufacturer's instructions.

Adjust the triple outlet into spring clamps on a level with the bladder. Place the 70 cm hollow rod adjacent to the centimeter scale and attach with adhesive tape.

Adjust the client's position and the standing light. Drape the client as for catheterization. Uncover the catheterization tray, put on sterile gloves, and test the balloon of the Foley catheter.

Proceed with the catheterization in the usual manner, substituting the Foley catheter for the nonretention type. Empty the client's bladder; holding the catheter in the left hand, inflate the balloon with 5 ml of sterile water. Pinch the branch firmly, bend it on itself, and fasten securely with a rubber band (not necessary if catheter branch has a terminal plug or valve).

Place a Kelly clamp on the plastic tubing next to the connector.

Holding the connecting tip over the emesis basin, open the clamp and flush the solution through to expel air. (For accurate results it is essential that air be expelled before starting the test.) Close the screw clamp. Attach the connection to the catheter. The physician will release the Kelly clamp and record the pressure within the previously emptied bladder with the nurse unclamping the bottle and manometer at the physician's direction. Place a strip of adhesive tape at the level of the solution in the irrigating bottle.

Open the screw clamp, let 50 ml of fluid enter the bladder, and then close the clamp.

Remove the Kelly clamp on the manometer and record the intravesical pressure. Continue introducing successive amounts of 50 ml of fluid and measuring the pressure until spontaneous emptying takes place or a total filling of 500 to 750 ml (hypotonic bladder) is reached.

At the end of the procedure close the clamps, separate the catheter from the connection tip, and empty the bladder. Measure the return as a check on the procedure. Remove the rubber band from the Foley branch. Deflate the Foley balloon and remove the catheter (unless some form of catheter drainage is indicated). If the catheter is left in the bladder, protect the open end by wrapping it in a sterile 2 by 2 inch sponge or sterile stopper and securing it with a rubber band. Make the client comfortable, rearrange the bedclothes, remove the bath blanket, and draw back the curtains. Collect all equipment and take it to the utility room. Discard soiled sponges and soiled linen. Dispose of equipment in proper receptacle.

### CHARTING

**Nurse's notes**
Procedure, physician, date, and time
Significant reactions

## Caloric tests for vestibular function

### Expected outcome
The client should be able to explain the procedure and cooperate for an accurate test.

*Definition.* Examination of the vestibular portion of the eighth cranial nerve is by injection of cold or hot water into the external auditory canal. Normally stimulation of the canal with cold water produces rotary nystagmus away from the side of the ear being irrigated; with hot water there is rotary nystagmus toward the side of the irrigated ear. If the labyrinth is diseased, no nystagmus is elicited.

*Indications.* (1) To test the function of the ves-

tibular portion of the eighth cranial nerve. (2) To aid in the differential diagnosis of lesions in the region of the brainstem and cerebellum.

*Contraindications.* (1) A perforated eardrum (cold air may be used as a substitute). (2) Acute disease of the labyrinth, as in Ménière's syndrome (before testing, wait until the attack subsides).

### EQUIPMENT

Irrigating can with tubing
Glass medicine dropper with a small rubber tip
Kelly clamp
Gallon pitcher of cold or hot water (depending on the temperature ordered by the physician)
Bath thermometer
Ear bulb syringe
Small bowl of warm water
Stomach tube with V-cut funnel or an emesis basis
Pail
Stopwatch
Pad and pencil
Rubber apron and towel
Cotton
Otoscope
Standard
2 chairs

*Preparation of client.* The procedure is explained to the client. The physician examines the eardrums for perforation and tests the client for nystagmus, Romberg's sign, and past-pointing for later comparison with test results.

The client should wear pajamas.

Food and fluids should be omitted for about 6 hours before the test is done.

*Preparation of equipment.* If the vertical canals are to be tested, all necessary articles should be assembled in the treatment room, whereas if the horizontal canals are to be tested, at the bedside. The solution should be 86° F (30° C) if cold, and 112° F (44.5° C) if hot.

The nurse prepares the caloric sheet shown in Table 12-2 and completes the pretest data.

*Procedure.* The client is taken to the treatment room and seated in a chair with the head tilted slightly forward to test the vertical canals. The rubber apron is adjusted. (If the horizontal canals are to be examined, the client is positioned in bed with the head tilted backward at an angle of 60 degrees.)

**TABLE 12-2.** Record of caloric test

| Observations | Dizziness | Nystagmus | Nausea | Vomiting | Past-pointing | Romberg's sign |
|---|---|---|---|---|---|---|
| Pretest | None | None at rest | None | None | None | Positive; sways to left |
| Left ear Duration of irrigation 3 minutes | None | Unchanged | None | None | None | Positive; sways to left |
| Right ear Duration of irrigation 20 seconds | Present 10 seconds after irrigation ended | To left at 20 seconds | None | 15 seconds after irrigation ended | To right at 20 seconds | Positive; sways to right |

INTERPRETATION: The absence of any response on stimulation of the left side indicates an interruption of the vestibular mechanism probably caused by a destructive lesion, for example, an acoustic nerve tumor, as was found in this client. Stimulation on the right side produced a normal response characterized by spontaneous nystagmus to the left, past-pointing to the right, dizziness, vomiting, and postural deviation to the right.

The physician sits in a chair facing the client and instructs him or her to keep the eyes open, to look straight ahead, and to follow directions as quickly and as accurately as possible. The physician shows the client what he or she will be expected to do (past-pointing, Romberg) and asks him or her to report any unusual feeling or discomfort that may occur after the irrigation is begun.

A second person holds the stopwatch and keeps a written record of the time intervals, the client's complaints, and the physician's observations. The nurse expels air from the tubing by letting some water escape. The funnel tube or emesis basin is placed beneath the ear for the outflow. The ear on the affected side should be irrigated first, since the client's reaction may be negligible. The solution is directed into the external auditory canal and should flow steadily under moderate pressure (the can is approximately 1 foot above the client's head) until the client complains of nausea and dizziness or until nystagmus is present. Normally this takes 20 to 30 seconds.

The irrigation is stopped when the initial symptom appears, and the time is noted or, if there is no reaction, the irrigation is stopped after 3 minutes of stimulation. The physician tests the client for past-pointing and nystagmus and records the time of onset and direction. When all objective findings cease, the ear is irrigated with a small amount of warm water and then dried.

After 5 minutes, or as soon as the client recovers, the procedure is repeated in the other ear. The apron is removed, and the client is helped into a wheelchair and taken back to bed.

*Nursing intervention.* The client should remain in bed with a moderate head elevation until all subjective symptoms disappear. This normally takes 30 to 60 minutes; he or she may then resume previous diet and routine.

*Aftercare of equipment.* The irrigating set should be separated, washed with warm soapy water, rinsed, and dried. The tip should be sterilized. All other equipment should be cleansed as necessary and the tray reset and returned to the cupboard. The treatment room is straightened and left in order.

### CHARTING

**Nurse's notes**
Procedure, physician, date, and time
Significant reactions

### Caloric test (Hallpike)

The Hallpike test is a caloric test with the client lying on a couch with the head raised 30 degrees. (The external canal at this level is most sensitive to thermal stimuli.) This position facilitates the cooperation of the client, the immobilization of the head, and the testing for nystagmus. The client is asked to stare straight ahead at an object while the physician tests for nystagmus at a distance of 12 inches.

The apparatus described on p. 338 may be used. The irrigating can is placed on a standard about 6 feet above the client's head so that the solution will flow freely. Cold or hot tap water approximately 7 Celsius degrees below (30° C or 86° F) or above body temperature (44.5° C or 112° F) may be used.

The solution, 250 to 500 ml, is directed into the canal for 40 seconds. The time interval is recorded from the beginning of the flow to the end of any visible nystagmus with the client looking straight ahead. (This takes about 2 minutes with cold water and about 1 minute 40 seconds with hot water.)

*Nursing intervention.* The care of the client is similar to that for the caloric test.

## Caloric test (Nelson)

Nelson has developed a simple procedure for testing vestibular function that may be performed in the client's home or in the physician's office.

### EQUIPMENT

Tuberculin syringe (plastic)
Paper cup
Frenzel lenses (+20 convex)
Stopwatch or wristwatch with second hand
Cold water and ice cubes
Paper towels
Paper and pencil

*Preparation of client.* After the procedure is explained and the necessary instructions ar given, the client assumes the supine position with the head tilted 30 degrees forward or the sitting position with the head tilted 60 degrees backward. The head is turned to the side during the injection of ice water to facilitate its flow into the ear canal.

*Preparation of equipment.* A paper cup is half filed with cold water, and three ice cubes are added. (The temperature of the water is thus maintained at 1° to 3° C during the testing period.) The tuberculin syringe is placed in the water, filled, and kept immersed for about 30 seconds before the first irrigation.

*Procedure.* The position of the client is adjusted as necessary. The client puts on the special glasses. A paper towel is placed under the ear to be tested (to catch the little water spillage). The filled syringe is removed from the ice water and 0.2 ml (about 4 drops) is injected into the aural canal. If nystagmus does not occur, the procedure is re-

peated with increasing amounts of fluid at 5-minute intervals.

| | |
|---|---|
| Initial injection | 0.2 ml |
| After 5 minutes | 0.4 ml |
| After 10 minutes | 0.8 ml |
| After 15 minutes | 1.6 ml |
| After 20 minutes | 2.0 ml |

If nystagmus still does not occur, the labyrinth tested is rated as not reacting to the thermal stimulus, and a disturbance of vestibular function is present. If indicated, the procedure is repeated in the other ear. After the completion of the procedure, the client's ears are dried and the towels removed. Generally no aftercare is indicated, and the patient may resume normal activity.

This method of testing vestibular function was performed on more than 100 clients. Nelson reported that no uncomfortable level of nausea, no severe vertigo, and no vomiting occurred, although patients reported transient mild ear pain during the injection. Nelson stated that in 75% of the 28 normal subjects tested, nystagmus was present after the initial injection of 0.2 ml of ice water and only a few of this group required the second injection of 0.4 ml.

He recommended the wearing of the Frenzel lenses to decrease the visual fixation effects on vestibular nystagmus and, because the fine eye movements are magnified, to detect the small beats of nystagmus.

## Glucose tolerance test

The glucose tolerance test frequently is made to rule out hypoglycemia if the client has a convulsive disorder. It is also used in the diagnostic study of clients with pituitary disease. After the oral administration of glucose the blood glucose of a healthy adult (70 to 120 mg/dl) will rise to about 200 mg/dl within an hour and should return to the normal level in 2½ hours. In a client with hypoglycemia the fasting blood glucose is lower than normal (40 to 70 mg/dl); after the oral administration of glucose no appreciable rise in its concentration is found, and a fall below the fasting level within the next 5 hours may occur.

*Oral technique.* Fasting blood glucose, 2 ml, is obtained in a fluoride or oxalate tube and shaken well.

An adult is given 100 gm of glucose by mouth, and a child is given 25 gm. It is most palatable if the adult dose is dissolved in two glasses of cold water with the juice of one lemon and kept refrigerated until the scheduled time; the child's dose is dissolved in one-half glass of cold water with the juice of one fourth of a lemon and refrigerated.

After the glucose is taken by the client, blood is obtained at the following intervals: 30 minutes and 1, 2, 3, 4, and 5 hours. A No. 22 needle should be used to minimize the client's discomfort. Each time the blood is taken, a urine specimen also should be obtained.

The client must continue to fast during the 5-hour period. If the glucose is not retained, the test should be interrupted and repeated the following day. The client may have food as desired on completion of the test.

During the test period the client is kept in bed to ensure cooperation and to permit closer supervision.

*Intravenous technique.* If the client is unable to retain glucose taken by mouth, it may be administered intravenously.

The fasting blood glucose is taken; then 0.2 gm of glucose/kg of body weight is given in a 50% solution intravenously.

After the injection of the glucose, blood specimens are taken from the arm opposite the one used for the injection at the following intervals: 3, 4, 5, 10, 15, 60, and 90 minutes.

The blood glucose level of a healthy adult after the intravenous administration of glucose will rise to 300 or 400 mg/dl within 3 to 4 minutes and should return to normal, that is, the fasting level, within 60 to 90 minutes.

## Sweat test (iodine-starch method of Minor)*

### Expected outcome
The client should be able to explain the test and cooperate for an accurate test.

---

*Chinizarin test of Guttmann. Chinizarin is a powder that may be substituted for iodine and starch. It is said to be simpler to use, since the test consists in dusting the fine, absolutely dry powder mixture (sodium salt of chinizarin—2, 6-disulfonic acid, 35 gm; sodium carbonate, powdered, 30 gm; rice starch, 60 gm) over the skin area to be examined. Otherwise the test proceeds as outlined.

*Definition.* The application of iodine and starch to specific areas of the body to demonstrate the distribution and degree of perspiration.

*Purposes.* (1) To determine the location and extent of lesions in the sympathetic nervous system. (2) To evaluate the results of sympathectomy by analysis of the areas of anhidrosis.

*Contraindications.* None.

*Preparation of client.* An explanation of the test is given. Clothing is removed as determined by the area to be examined. The nurse begins to force fluids a few hours before the test. The client voids.

*Procedure (carried out at room temperature).* Bedclothes are folded to the foot of the bed. Protective rubber sheeting is placed on the bed and covered with a bath blanket. Curtains are drawn around the bed, or portable screens are adjusted.

### EQUIPMENT

Large bed cradle
Loin cloth (if area is not included in test)
Large pitcher of fluids at bedside
Iodine mixture: iodine, 1.5 gm; castor oil, 10 ml; absolute alcohol, to 100 ml
Powdered starch
Cotton
6 feet of protective rubber sheeting
2 warm blankets
Sterile 2 ml syringe with No. 25 needle
Pilocarpine, 0.006 to 0.012 gm (adult dose)

---

The client lies on the stomach or back, with the areas to be examined exposed. No skin surfaces should be in contact with each other. The cradle is placed over the client and covered with a blanket.

The iodine mixture is applied to the area to be examined. After the painted area has dried, it is dusted with powdered starch.

Fluid intake is continued. Pilocarpine is given subcutaneously as ordered.

The physician remains with the client to check sweating, its amount and distribution. Normally it takes about 20 to 30 minutes for pilocarpine to stimulate sweating. As the client perspires, the starch dissolves and then reacts with the iodine to produce a dark purple color. When there is little or no sweating, the starch remains white, since no re-

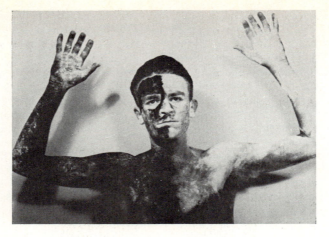

**FIG. 12-10.** Starch-iodine sweat test, demonstrating good sweating in black areas over client's face, chest, and upper extremity on right side and absence of sweat in corresponding areas on left side after sympathectomy at T2-T3 , left.

action takes place with the iodine, and thus clearly demonstrates areas of impaired sweating (Fig. 12-10).

Sweating can also be produced when aspirin and hot tea are used and the nude body is exposed to a controlled room temperature of 120° F. (The use of pilocarpine at room temperature is a simpler and less uncomfortable procedure, but since its action is at the peripheral nerve endings, its use is not satisfactory for a determination of sympathetic denervation. Under such circumstances the use of external heat and aspirin is recommended.)

***Nursing intervention.*** The cradle, blankets, and rubber sheet are removed. A cleansing bath is followed by local application of alcohol to remove all traces of iodine mixture from the skin.

The client is assisted into clean, dry pajamas. The bedding and unit are straightened, and curtains or screens are removed.

***Aftercare of equipment.*** All items used are collected; blankets are discarded into the laundry bag; the rubber sheet is returned to the rack; and the cradle is returned to the closet. The iodine mixture and starch are returned to cabinet. The syringe and needle are discarded in the appropriate manner.

## CHARTING

**Nurse's notes**
Procedure, physician, date, and time
Area prepared
Medication given
Significant reactions

## REFERENCES

Ayer, J.B.: Puncture of the cisterna magna, Arch. Neurol. Psychiatry **4:**529-541, 1920.

Ayer, J.B.: Spinal subarachnoid block, Arch. Neurol. Psychiatry **10:**420-426, 1923.

Basmajian, et al.: Computers in electromyography, London, 1975, Butterworth & Co. (Publishers), Ltd.

Baum, S., et al.: Brain scanning in the diagnosis of acoustic neuromas, J. Neurosurg. **36:**141-147, Feb. 1972.

Blegvad, B.: Caloric vestibular reaction in unconscious patients, Arch. Otolaryngol. **75:**506-514, 1962.

Bligh, A.S., et al.: Computer assisted tomography of the brain, Lancet **2:**1260, 1974.

Bloch, S., et al.: Reliability of Doppler scanning of the Carotid-bifurcation: angiographic correlation, Radiology **132:**687-691, 1979.

Blount, M., et al.: Obtaining and analyzing cerebrospinal fluid, Nurs. Clin. North Am. **9:**593-609, 1974.

Boulay, R.D.: Atlas of normal vertebral angiograms, London, 1976, Butterworth & Co. (Publishers), Ltd.

Brazier, M.: The analysis of brain waves, Sci. Am. **206:**142-153, 1962.

Brown, R.E.: Ultrasonography: basic principles and clinical applications, St. Louis, 1975, Warren H. Green, Inc.

Buchthal, F.: The electromyogram, World Neurol. **3:**16-34, Jan. 1962.

Chesney, D.N., and Chesney, M.O.: Care of the patient in diagnostic radiography, ed. 5, Philadelphia, 1978, J.B. Lippincott Co.

Chusid, J.G., and McDonald, J.J.: Correlative neuroanatomy and functional neurology, ed. 17, Los Altos, Calif., 1979, Lange Medical Publications.

Clarke, T.A.: Observations on caloric tests of vestibular function, J. Laryngol. Otol. **58:**380-386, 1943.

Conway, B.L.: Pediatric neurologic nursing, St. Louis, 1977, The C.V. Mosby Co.

Dandy, W.E.: Ventriculography following the injection of air into the cerebral ventricles, Ann. Surg. **68:**5-11, 1918.

Daube, J.: The description of motor unit potentials in electromyography, Neurology **28:**623-625, 1978.

Di Chiro, G.: Atlas of detailed normal pneumoencephalographic anatomy, ed. 2, Springfield, Ill., 1971, Charles C Thomas, Publisher.

Dix, M.R., and Hallpike, C.S.: Discussion on acoustic neuroma, Proc. R. Soc. Med. **51:**889-899, 1958.

Donohoe, K., et al.: Cerebral circulation and cerebral angiography, Nurs. Clin. North Am. **9:**623-634, 1974.

Feild, J.R., Robertson, J.T., and DeSaussure, R.L., Jr.: Complications of cerebral angiography in 2,000 consecutive cases, J. Neurosurg. **19:**775-781, 1962.

Franckson, J.R.M., et al.: Physiologic significance of the intravenous glucose tolerance test, Metabolism **11:**482-500, 1962.

Gibbs, F.A., and Gibbs, E.L.: Atlas of electroencephalography, ed. 2, vol. 1, 1950, vol. 2, 1952, vol. 3, 1974, Cambridge, Mass., Addison-Wesley Publishing Co., Inc.

Gilbert, G.J.: Pneumoencephalography in normal-pressure hydrocephalus, N. Engl. J. Med. **285:**177-178, July 15, 1971.

Goldensohn, E.S., and Koehle, R.: EEG interpretation: problems of over-reading and under-reading, Mount Kisco, N.Y., 1975, Futura Publishing Co., Inc.

Goodgold, J., and Eberstein, A.: Electrodiagnosis and neuromuscular diseases, ed. 2, Baltimore, 1978, The Williams & Wilkins Co.

Guttmann, L.: Topographic studies of disturbance of sweat secretion after complete lesions of peripheral nerves, J. Neurol. Psychiatry **3:**197-210, July 1940.

Hallpike, C.S.: The caloric tests, J. Laryngol. Otol. **70:**15-28, 1956.

Handa, J.: Dynamic aspects of brain scanning, Baltimore, 1972, University Park Press.

Harmon, V.: Taking the pain out of back procedures, Nursing74 **4:**91, Sept. 1974.

Hecht, A.: Factors influencing oral glucose tolerance: experience with chronically ill patients, Metabolism **10:**712-723, 1961.

Hill, K.R., et al.: The EMI scanner, Radiography **40:**147, July, 1974.

Hyndman, O.R., and Wolkin, J.: The pilocarpine sweating test, Arch. Neurol. Psychiatry **45:**992-1006, 1941.

Kiloh, L.G.: Clinical electroencephalography, London, 1972, Butterworth & Co. (Publishers), Ltd.

King, D.L.: Diagnostic ultrasound, St. Louis, 1974, The C.V. Mosby Co.

Kinney, A.B., et al.: Cerebrospinal fluid circulation and encephalography, Nurs. Clin. North Am. **9:**611-621, 1974.

Langworthy, O., Kolb, L.C., and Lewis, L.G.: Physiology of micturition: experimental and clinical studies with suggestions as to diagnosis and treatment, Baltimore, 1940, The Williams & Wilkins Co.

Lenman, J.A., and Ritchie, A.E.: Clinical electromyography, ed. 2, Philadelphia, 1976, J.B. Lippincott Co.

Lin, J.P.: Angiographic investigation of cerebral aneurysms. Technical aspects, Radiology **105:**69-76, Oct. 1972.

List, C.F., Burge, C.H., and Hodges, F.J.: Intracranial angiography, Radiology **45:**1-14, 1945.

Livanov, M.N.: Spatial organization of cerebral processes, New York, 1975, Halsted Press.

Livingston, K.E.: Technic of lumbar puncture, N. Engl. J. Med. **287:**724, 1972.

Mandrillo, M.: Brain scanning, Nurs. Clin. North Am. **9:**633-639, 1974.

Maravilla, K., et al.: Application of metrizamide in the radiographic evaluation of the neurologically diseased patient, J. Neurosurg. **5:**389-406, 1979.

Mathews, W.B., and Glaser, G.N.: Recent advances in clinical neurology, no. 2, Edinburgh, 1978, Churchill Livingstone (or Longman, Inc., New York).

McDicken, W.N.: The principles and use of diagnostic ultrasonic instruments, New York, 1976, John Wiley & Sons, Inc.

Medical Skills Library: Lumbar puncture, 1972, ROCOM.

Moore, G.: Use of radioactive diiodo-fluorescein in the diagnosis and localization of brain tumors, Science **107:**569-571, 1948.

Munro, D.: Activity of urinary bladder as measured by new and inexpensive cystometry, N. Engl. J. Med. **214:**617-624, 1936.

Naidich, T.P., et al.: Advances in diagnosis: cranial and spinal computed tomography, Med. Clin. North Am. **63:**849-896, July 1979.

Nelson, J.R.: The minimal ice water caloric test, Neurology **19:**577-585, 1969.

New, P.F.J.: Computed tomography: a major diagnostic advance, Hosp. Pract. **10:**55, 1975.

Nomura, T.: Atlas of cerebral angiography, New York, 1970, Springer-Verlag New York, Inc.

Peterson, H.O., and Kieffer, S.A.: Introduction to neuroradiology, New York, 1972, Harper & Row, Publishers.

Ramsey, G.H., French, J.D., and Strain, W.H.: Iodinated organic compounds as contrast media for radiographic diagnosis. IV. Pantopaque myelography, Radiology **43:**236-240, 1944.

Roche Report: Hans Berger, psychiatrist-pioneer of the electroencephalogram of man (special issue), Frontiers of Psychiatry **2:**1-11, May 15, 1972.

Ross, A., et al.: Neuromuscular diagnostic procedures, Nurs. Clin. North Am. **14:**107-121, 1979.

Samaha, F.J.: Electrodiagnostic studies in neuromuscular disease, N. Engl. J. Med. **285:**1244-1247, 1971.

Shapiro, D., and Clark, M.: Scanning the human mind, Newsweek, p. 63, Sept. 29, 1980.

Slaughter, J.: Preoperative neurosurgical diagnostic studies, Point of View **12:**6-8, 1975.

Sodee, D.B., and Early, P.J.: Technology and interpretation of nuclear medicine procedures, ed. 2, St. Louis, 1975, The C.V. Mosby Co.

Spetzler, R., et al.: Computerized tomographic diagnosis: pitfalls for neurosurgeons, J. Neurosurg. **5:**231-236, 1979.

Stone, B.: Computerized transaxial brain scan, Am. J. Nurs. **77:**1601-1604, 1977.

Stookey, B., and Klenke, D.: A study of spinal fluid pressure in the differential diagnosis of diseases of the spinal cord, Arch. Neurol. Psychiatry **20:**84-109, July 1928.

Stookey, B., Merwarth, H.R., and Frantz, A.M.: A manometric study of the cerebrospinal fluid in suspected spinal cord tumors, Surg. Gynecol. Obstet. **41:**429-442, 1925.

Swets, J.: Assessment of diagnostic technologies, Science **205:**753-759, 1979.

Takahashi, M.: Atlas of vertebral angiography, Baltimore, 1975, University Park Press.

Ter-Pogossian, M.M., et al.: Positron-emission tomography, Sci. Am. **243:**171-181, Oct. 1980.

Turner, O., and Byrne, V.C.: The Queckenstedt test—a consideration of the method of application and the nursing problems related to it, Yale J. Biol. Med. **12:**737-741, 1940.

Waddington, M.M.: Atlas of cerebral angiography with anatomic correlation, Boston, 1974, Little, Brown & Co.

Wende, S., et al.: Cerebral magnification angiography: physical basis and clinical results, New York, 1974, Springer-Verlag New York, Inc.

Young, D.A., and Burney, R.E.: Complication of myelography—transection and withdrawal of a nerve filament by the needle, N. Engl. J. Med. **285:**156-158, July 15, 1971.

Zivin, J.: Lateral cervical puncture: an alternative to lumbar puncture, Neurology **28:**616-618, 1978.

# PART FOUR

# DISORDERS AFFECTING FUNCTIONAL CAPACITIES

# 13

# STATIC AND DEVELOPMENTAL LESIONS

Embryonic development is a crucial growth period subject to many potential interferences that may result in long-range consequences. In Chapter 1 the complex interrelationships in the growth process and the precision that earmarks the developmental timetable are discussed. Chapter 5 continues with the multiplicity of factors influencing individual capacities at various developmental stages, and Chapter 11 suggests considerations that may clarify the genesis and outcomes of growth or health interferences during ongoing assessment and client management.

This chapter is divided into three parts: (1) some major anomalies that are direct outcomes of defective development or destruction at certain points in the antenatal period, (2) static factors in the perinatal period that may result in far-reaching health problems, and (3) static problems in infancy and early childhood resulting in long-range health disturbances.

## SPECIFIC ANOMALIES OF DEVELOPMENT OR DESTRUCTION IN UTERO

Since many factors have been identified that may potentially cause growth disturbances in the developing fetus, it is prudent to examine the pregnant woman serially, take a comprehensive history, stress the importance of sound health measures, and monitor psychosocial and physical aspects of living, since they profoundly influence maternal and fetal well-being.

When the pregnant woman is in the high-risk category, where her potential for encountering personal difficulty or producing a growth-retarded or defective fetus is increased, referral to a specialist or a perinatal center may be indicated to ensure the best outcome for the mother and fetus.

In consideration of fetal outcomes associated with developmental errors and destructive antenatal events, defining distinct categories is a difficult task because of the following three facts: (1) Defective growth or destruction of existing tissues may have a profound effect on that tissue, surrounding tissue, and subsequent development that is dependent on previously formed structures. (2) The postnatal consequences may be physically present at birth but not clinically apparent until later, because of differential development and lack of functional influence of some neurological structures at birth. (3) When the interference has been minimal clinically but neuronal damage has resulted, the infant may have poor capacities for coping with a variety of biological stressors, including injuries, toxins, or infections, even though these responses are difficult to document.

Generally, defective fetal development is categorized according to cause, including the following: (1) inheritance, (2) invasive disorders, (3) fetal disturbances caused by transient or chronic interferences, and (4) chromosomal abnormalities. Other specific anomalies are without definable cause, being related to certain developmental errors. These separate discussions are presented in relation to particular impairments of antenatal origin.

## INHERITANCE

Inheritance apparently affects fetal development at the molecular level without known disturbances of the chromosomes, which probably occur during oogenesis. Further discussion on inherited disorders is in Chapter 16.

## INVASIVE DISORDERS

Invasive disorders include lesions that result in displacement of neural tissue and, when located in the head, enlargement in head circumference. During the newborn period, however, abnormal increases in head size are more frequently caused by hydrocephalus than by invasive processes such as brain tumors. The invasive disorders also encompass infectious processes.

### Infectious processes

Epidemiologists have coined the term TORCH to denote the major infections that the mother may transmit to the fetus or newborn and that may result in serious health problems. TORCH represents the first letter of each of the following infections:

Toxoplasmosis
Other virus infections
Rubella
Cytomegalic inclusion disease (CID)
Herpes simplex (HSV)

These infections, which are known to result in acute and long-range health interferences, along with other significant infectious problems, may be divided according to the kinds of agents causing them, namely, viruses, protozoa, and bacteria, as follows:

Viral infections
    Rubella
    Cytomegalic inclusion disease
    Varicella
    Herpes simplex
    Hepatitis B
Protozoal infections
    Toxoplasmosis
Bacterial invasions
    *Escherichia coli* infection
    Congenital syphilis

***Viral infections.*** The major infections composing this category include rubella, cytomegalic inclusion disease, varicella (chickenpox), herpes simplex (HSV), and hepatitis B.

RUBELLA. A woman of childbearing age who lacks immunity for rubella may produce a defective fetus if she contracts rubella infection, commonly called German measles, particularly in the first trimester of pregnancy.

Clinical findings in the fetus may include such anomalies as microcephaly, deafness, cardiac defects, mental retardation, cataracts and other eye problems, autistic behavior, and meningoencephalitis. Cardiac and visual disturbances are more commonly seen when the infection has occurred during the first 8 weeks of pregnancy, whereas hearing is affected most often from infections during the first half of the pregnancy. Low birth weights and immunoglobulin deficiencies are common. Temporary disturbances in the newborn may include pneumonia and hematological problems, such as thrombocytopenic purpura and hepatitis. Far-reaching effects include the lack of immunity by age 4 or 5 years, even though the affected infant has shed the rubella virus during the first year of life. Other undesirable outcomes are the possible development of diabetes, hypothyroidism or hyperthyroidism, and precocious puberty.

When the diagnosis of rubella is suspected in the pregnant woman, serological tests confirm or refute the presence of the virus in the mother. To determine the presence of a fetal infection, amniocentesis may be indicated, since the rubella virus can be isolated from the amniotic fluid. Two major reasons may cause the pregnant woman to elect amniocentesis, including the following: (1) detection of the rubella problem several months after the suspected onset of the virus, since serological techniques do not indicate whether or not the infection was a primary one, and (2) conversion to a positive reaction on serological testing during pregnancy, wherein the mother wants to confirm fetal involvement before deciding on therapeutic abortion.

The disadvantages of amniocentesis are that it takes about 21 days to determine the presence of rubella in amniotic fluid; that positive results indicate fetal involvement, whereas negative results do not guarantee lack of fetal involvement; and that there is currently an inability to distinguish between those infections that have minimal sequelae and those that result in severe defects. However, the gravity of potential anomalies justifies amniocentesis when there is a clinical indication.

Intervention modalities are primarily geared toward prevention through the testing of women who have not had rubella or the immunization, so that counseling or immunization may be offered, depending on the individual situation. Massive rubella immunization has been available since 1969 and is particularly encouraged for every female before adolescence. When neither the immunization has been given nor the virus has been contracted before the childbearing years, an immunization may be given if the woman is protected from becoming pregnant for a minimum of 3 months. Giving the immunization during the first trimester of pregnancy may have undesirable outcomes for the fetus. Another aspect of prevention includes the protection of pregnant women who may become accidentally exposed to an infant shedding the virus. Thus when the practitioner examines infants, it is important to be cognizant of symptoms indicating the possibility of rubella, so that further follow-up and referral of potentially infected infants may result.

When infants and children have congenital defects caused by rubella, they need a carefully planned, individualized program of comprehensive treatment that incorporates all physical and psychosocial needs within the context of the family complex. Educational remediation for mental retardation, apparent in many of these children, is particularly valuable in assisting them toward attaining their maximum functional capacities, especially when special educational techniques are applied from an early age. Mental retardation in early years may even be significantly overcome by the age of 9 years in those who have received special education.

**CYTOMEGALIC INCLUSION DISEASE.** Cytomegalic inclusion disease is currently believed to be the most prevalent congenital infection in modern times. As many as 1% of all newborns secrete cytomegalovirus (CMV) via nose, mouth, or urine, and about 5000 to 8000 neonates are affected with severe defects caused by the virus each year.

Investigators have recovered the virus from as many as one third of the adults tested over 25 years of age and as many as one fifth of those over 35 years of age. The infection is about twice as common as rubella in women. In healthy women the virus is often subclinical and not detected.

Clinically the virus produces symptoms that simulate infectious mononucleosis in some adults. Apparently cytomegalovirus belongs to the group of herpesviruses and remains dormant in the system after the primary infection has occurred, unless it is reactivated by immunosuppression, such as is produced by the hormonal changes associated with pregnancy. The fetus is at greatest risk during primary infection. Effects of a primary infection on the fetus have not been fully determined in the first trimester. However, transmission of the virus to the fetus during the second trimester is associated with brain damage, mental retardation, liver disease, optic atrophy, cerebral palsy, auditory impairment, chorioretinitis, microcephaly, cranial calcification, and thrombocytopenia and erythroblastosis where the direct and indirect bilirubin levels are elevated in the presence of a negative Coombs test and no indication of incompatibility. Cytomegalic inclusion cells may be found in the urine for several months after birth. In adults the virus may be isolated from saliva, breast milk, blood, semen, urine, and the endocervix.

When the infection is transmitted to the fetus during the third trimester, no symptoms may be evident at birth. However, damage in future years may appear in the form of defective hearing, weakened immunity, behavioral disturbances, learning disorders, and intellectual deficiencies. If the infection is transmitted postnatally, no apparent undesirable effects result.

Intervention is limited to early identification of the disease and institution of measures of adequate sanitation, since the infection seems to occur more commonly in conditions of poor sanitation and overcrowding. A vaccine is currently being developed. However, there are many questions to answer before wide-scale immunizations are given, for example, whether a single vaccine would provide protection against all strains of the virus, whether vaccinations given to the pregnant woman would also offer immunity to the fetus, or whether the vaccine would increase the potential for neoplastic diseases.

Evidence of the infection in the neonate requires referral to a specialist for further diagnosis and treatment of acute problems. The nurse practitioner should continue to be involved in the plans for long-range management of this child, especially with regard to interpretation and coordination of the total efforts of the health team, educational specialists, and other community resources for the child within the family context. Emotional support and family guidance are also indicated, particularly during the many crises that may occur in the family with a defective child.

**VARICELLA.** Varicella (chickenpox) poses an infrequent threat to the neonate, because most North American women have had chickenpox well before the time that pregnancy occurs. Thus they transmit antibodies to the neonate and these provide protection for the first 4 to 6 months of life.

When the mother contracts the infection during the first 15 weeks of pregnancy, the fetus is affected. Fetal involvement may include such problems as hypoplastic extremities, scarring of the skin, eye defects, and retardation in growth and motor capacities.

If the virus is contracted during the last half of pregnancy, the infant may manifest the rash some time after the immediate perinatal period. However, when the infection occurs within a few days of delivery, the fetus is unprotected by maternal antibodies and often suffers an extreme case of the disease. Passive immunity induced by zoster-immune globulin provided by the Centers for Disease Control in Atlanta should be given to the neonate shortly after delivery to avoid the development of severe or fatal forms of the disease.

The neonate whose mother has recently had the virus should be isolated from other newborns, though most newborns in a nursery setting would be unaffected by exposure, since they possess antibodies against the virus. If the mother has never had varicella, the neonate is unprotected and should be kept away from siblings or other children who have the virus.

When the immune mechanism is altered through the use of steroids and antimetabolic medications, the individual may have a severe case of varicella that could result in death.

**HERPES SIMPLEX.** Herpes simplex (HSV) is a widespread dermatotropic and neurotropic viral infection that is probably transmitted by direct contact with lesions. Asymptomatic types of the virus infection are rare. In neonates the infection may be present in combination with another infection and remain unidentified. Premature infants have a high incidence of infection, which is probably caused by the fact that they were delivered early because of a maternal infection.

Clinically, recovery from generalized eruptions is usual, though problems resulting from secondary infections need to be controlled. However, when the neonate has systemic involvement or infection in the central nervous system, the prognosis is poor and death may occur rapidly. Diagnosis only at autopsy is not unusual.

When infection occurs during the first trimester, damage to the eyes and central nervous system may occur. However, such damage, secondary to a maternal viremia, is much more common with infection in the second trimester. During the third trimester, infection is transmitted most frequently at the time of delivery. If the mother has lesions, a cesarean section may be done before the membranes have ruptured to avoid fetal contamination. Other sources of infection in the perinatal period include contact with a contaminated internal fetal monitor or contact with infected nursery personnel. Contraction of the infection in the perinatal period may result in severe neonatal infections with potential central nervous system involvement.

Far-reaching effects of the infection include the development of chorioretinitis, the persistence of neurological disturbances, and the eruption of local herpes lesions. At this time no vaccine is available.

**HEPATITIS B.** Hepatitis B, or serum hepatitis, generally spread through contaminated blood or needles and mosquito bites, may also be contracted through intimate contact. The virus has been recovered from breast milk, blood, saliva, and amniotic fluid from individuals in both the acute states of infection and the asymptomatic carrier state.

When the mother is a carrier or contracts the infection during the first trimester of pregnancy, the antigen is not transmitted to the fetus. However, when maternal infection occurs during the second or third trimesters, the fetus is at risk for becoming infected. Infected fetuses may manifest the infection between 14 and 180 days after birth, or they may become asymptomatic carriers of the virus. Symptoms of active infection include jaundice, hepatosplenomegaly, and sometimes coma and death.

When no infection is present, the administration of hepatitis B immunoglobulin or a leukocyte extract results in active immunity. Research and experimentation continue on the use of a killed vaccine, which seems to offer complete immunity in preliminary investigations.

*Protozoal infections.* The chief protozoal infection of concern is toxoplasmosis.

TOXOPLASMOSIS. *Toxoplasma gondii,* a protozoon, was isolated in rodents in 1908. By 1939 Wolf, Cowen, and Paige found the organism in affected neonates, and Sabin, Pinkerton, and others demonstrated the presence of toxoplasma organisms in persons who had acquired the disease. However, the focus remained on the congenital form of the disease, because of the severity of the symptoms and the lack of understanding of neonatal problems at that time.

Most of the research on the disease has been done using Parisian women, since a large group in that locality eat improperly cooked meat. Another source of infection is contaminated cat feces.

In some individuals the only sign of the infection may be lymphadenopathy in the posterior cervical chains. Nodes appear swollen, painful, and nonsuppurative bilaterally within 2 to 4 weeks after the onset of the infection. In other persons, symptoms include fever and swollen lymph nodes resembling those of infectious mononucleosis. However, toxoplasmosis generally has a more prolonged course, which may last from 2 to 6 months with intermittent exacerbations. Another form of the disease includes a febrile course, wherein no organ involvement is evident, and a transient morbiliform rash may occur. This type is neither recurrent nor does it extend for a prolonged period of time.

Whenever acute chorioretinitis is noted as the only symptom in children, possibly in recurrent or prolonged form, toxoplasmosis should be considered as a probable cause. In toxoplasmic chorioretinitis there are large white areas bordered with dark pigmentation. These focal lesions are both severe and extensive and often include both the maculae and the periphery of the retina. There is also evidence of extensive connective tissue growth. Optic atrophy and microphthalmia are fre-

quently associated. The presence of toxoplasmosis may be confirmed by serological studies.

Fetal involvement may be severe when the mother contracts the primary infection sometime during the first two trimesters of pregnancy. When the mother has antibodies before pregnancy, the fetus in the current pregnancy is not affected. Neonates frequently do not have symptoms of toxoplasmosis when their mothers contract the disease during the last trimester.

Fetal involvement may range from intrauterine growth retardation and prematurity to mild disease or major sequelae. In one study wherein 180 women acquired toxoplasmosis during pregnancy, only 20 offspring (11%) of the total number affected acquired severe forms of the disease. Of this number there were 11 abortions, and of the 59 unaborted pregnancies, two died, and seven had a severe form of the disease. Others in the study had mild symptoms of the infection or no involvement at all.

Pathophysiologically the nervous system shows evidence of diffuse inflammation, which is most concentrated in the cerebral cortex, basal ganglia, and periventricular tissues. Necrotic areas are obvious and may eventually become cavities. In the late stages, extreme gliosis occurs and deposits of calcium appear. Miliary tubercles appear in the meninges and ependyma, and ependymitis frequently occludes the aqueduct of Sylvius, causing hydrocephalus. Large retinal lesions, spinal cord involvement, and the formation of large cystic masses by these organisms are not uncommon.

Clinically the congenital type is often chronic, whereas the acute form of toxoplasmic encephalitis, which occurs in persons between 5 and 10 years of age, has a limited course. The adult form also has an acute course. In the chronic form, when infants have survived the initial fever and disease process, the infection becomes inactive, and survival may continue for an indefinite period. However, these children may have the following deficits: mental and speech retardation, hydrocephalus, spasticity in the extremities, microcephaly, chorioretinitis and optic atrophy, convulsions, intracranial calcifications, cerebrospinal fluid abnormalities, impaired immunity, diminished visual and auditory capacities, and hepatosplenomegaly.

The diagnostic triad includes *hydrocephalus, chorioretinopathy,* and *intracranial calcium deposits.* When the calcium deposits are not evident with the other symptoms, another diagnosis should be considered.

Intervention to avoid the disease is limited to encouraging the pregnant woman not to handle cat litter and advising her to eat meat that has been throughly cooked. Spiramycin, an erythromycin type of antibiotic, is available in the United States. Pyrimethamine (Daraprim) is an antiprotozoal medication that is also currently administered.

*Bacterial invasions.* Infection with *Escherichia coli,* a gram-negative organism, and congenital syphilis are two major bacterial threats to the neurological integrity of the neonate.

ESCHERICHIA COLI INFECTION. Most gram-negative infections are diagnosed within the first 2 weeks of life and may occur before an infant obtains sufficient antibodies from the mother's breast milk. Mortality from sepsis, with or without complications, is high. Neonatal meningitis is detailed in Chapter 20.

CONGENITAL SYPHILIS. Congenital syphilis is preventable. Testing for this venereal disease should take place both early and late in the prenatal care, and the disease should be promptly treated when found. When infection occurs either after 16 to 18 weeks of gestation or by contact with lesions during the birth process, the fetus may become actively infected or remain asymptomatic. Practitioners should be aware of the increasing incidence of syphilis among adults and consider the possibility of a congenital infection in infants with symptoms wherein the mother has had inadequate prenatal care and testing for venereal disease. Further information on congenital syphilis is available in other sources.

## FETAL DISTURBANCES

Fetal disturbances with the potential for development of undesirable outcomes may result from (1) maternal ingestion of foreign substances, (2) maternal insufficiencies in blood gas exchanges, nutritional supplies, or waste removal, (3) defective implantation or infarction of the placenta, (4) trauma to the pregnant uterus, (5) exposure to irradiation, (6) blood or blood factor problems, and (7) concurrent maternal illnesses or conditions.

Many times neurological defects may be present in the absence of a family history of such problems. Careful interviewing may reveal a fetal interference, such as those listed, that correlates with a crucial point in embryonic development. However, at times evidence of an interference may be present when a neurological problem is not obvious, or a neurological defect may be apparent in the absence of an identifiable cause. Investigations in cause-effect relationships of factors and outcomes in fetal development remain limited, but new findings continue as techniques in prenatal diagnostics are refined.

## Research

For many years embryologists have caused developmental errors to occur by deliberate interference at crucial points in the fetal growth of laboratory animals. Through these investigations, much information that also seems applicable to human embryonic development has become available.

To confirm these findings in humans, scientists require fetal products. Such products have become more readily available because of more liberal interpretations of present laws and because of the greater accessibility to abortions. However, such research raises many thorny issues pertaining to ethical and moral questions. Strict standards for research on viable fetuses have been devised by the National Institutes of Health.

## Prevention and key nursing interventions

The nurse's role in preventing interferences with fetal growth and development is a large one. Obviously, acceptable prenatal care and preparation of the family group for the new member is a major portion of the role. However, since so much neurological development occurs before many women recognize their pregnancy or have it confirmed, the potential for continuing unacceptable health practices, such as poor nutrition, exposure to harmful agents, or ingestion of foreign materials, is greater during this period than when women receive health information and prenatal care. Another important aspect of prevention hinges on the practitioner's transmission of information to clients about specific positive activites that avoid or minimize developmental defects. Thus the practitioner needs to make an impact on usual health practices and health maintenance in individuals from early childhood, so that the best possible physiologic and psychosocial circumstances exist during the childbearing years. This positive effect on health may be delivered in a variety of situations, including: (1) school and civic group meetings; (2) university- or community college–supported programs; (3) health awareness and specific target group efforts, such as the Childbirth and Parent Education Association; and (4) voluntary agency programs. Other settings wherein primary intervention may occur include home visits, daycare facilities, private offices, and clinics. Information may also be disseminated through the use of media such as lay publications and television.

## DEFECTS FROM IMPAIRED MIDLINE CLOSURE

Defects in the closure of midline structures occur on a continuum from severe to less extensive involvement, with these two primary groups being exemplified by cerebral dysplasias with cranium bifidum and myelodysplasia with spina bifida, respectively. Certain other developmental errors may also occur.

### Cerebral dysplasias with cranium bifidum

Five defects compose this category, as follows: (1) complete cranioschisis, (2) meningoencephalocele, (3) meningocele, (4) cranium bifidum occultum, and (5) porencephaly. These are defined as follows, in order of severity:

*complete cranioschisis* —absence of skull. Three main types of defective development may exist, including anencephaly, hemicephaly, and exencephaly.
*meningoencephalocele* —protrusion of brain tissue, cerebrospinal fluid, and meninges through defective skull. Portion of ventricular system may be included in sac.
*meningocele* —protrusion of saclike structure containing cerebrospinal fluid and meninges through defect in skull. No neural tissue is involved.
*cranium bifidum occultum* —defect in bony structure without herniation of tissue or meninges.
*porencephaly* —bilateral, symmetric, convoluted abnormality supplied by communication with ventricular system.

*Complete cranioschisis* exists when the skull is lacking and the brain is defective. Three major forms may occur, including anencephaly, hemicephaly, and exencephaly. In anencephaly the forebrain and midbrain are absent, and spongy, poorly differentiated tissue occupies the space that normally contains these structures. However, the hindbrain may be present in complete form. In hemicephaly the midbrain may be completely or partially present, but the forebrain is not developed. Exencephaly indicates the presence of the diencephalon and of portions of the hemispheres.

*Meningoencephalocele* is the next defect in order of severity and corresponds to meningomyelocele. The impairment consists of a defective skull, wherein a portion of the brain and meninges has herniated, so that it protrudes from the exterior portion of the head. The saclike protrusion may or may not contain portions of the ventricular system. Defects in the brain are commonly associated with this abnormality.

*Meningocele* refers to an external saclike outpouching that contains the meninges, but no brain tissue, and corresponds to meningocele in the spinal region. Defects in brain tissue may accompany this abnormality.

In *cranium bifidum occultum* the bony structure is defective, but no herniated area of tissue or meninges is involved. However, the skin that covers the defective area may be altered in some way with a marking such as a portwine stain.

*Porencephaly* refers to defects of the cerebrum associated with cranium bifidum, wherein a cleft opens onto the surface of the cerebral cortex, which is convoluted, lined with gray matter, and connected to the ventricular system. This abnormality is bilateral, symmetric, and probably the result of an impairment in the closure of the neural tube.

**Pathophysiology.** This group of defects associated with faulty closure of the skull in the midline is collectively referred to as encephaloceles. The incidence is about 1 encephalocele per 6500 births, and the exact cause is unknown, though recessive factors in inheritance and environmental influences may be implicated in some instances.

Anencephaly is interesting from a developmental viewpoint but is incompatible with life, as are some of the other more severe forms of cranioschisis. However, clients with meningoceles, meningoencephaloceles, and cranium bifidum occultum may have far-reaching health problems that require ongoing provisions for health care related to routine health maintenance, acute problems, and chronic impairments.

In children with cerebral dysplasia and cranium bifidum the skull is generally small and characterized by a diminished cavity and a receding forehead. The bony defect is frequently in the sagittal plane and most often in either the frontal or occipital locations, though it may occur in the parietal, nasal, or orbital areas. The bony defect often appears to be rounded in form with thickened margins. Meningoencephaloceles frequently arise from part of the brainstem. Three types are seen most often, which include (1) growth from the roof of the fourth ventricle, where the meningoencephalocele grows beneath and behind the cerebellum with accompanying cervical spina bifida; (2) saclike growth dividing the cerebellar hemispheres, which are often small with a missing vermis; and (3) growth beginning in the roof of the third ventricle and extending behind the cerebellum. All these types are commonly accompanied by hydrocephalus. If the growth contains choroid plexus and a portion of the ventricle is blocked by constriction at the bony opening, the sac expands rapidly and frequently breaks. In meningoceles the bony opening is usually small, and the sac is covered with meninges and skin.

Three specific defects are frequently associated with cranium bifidum, including microgyria, impaired development of the corpus callosum, and porencephaly. Additionally, sequestration dermoids and epidermoids are often found in the affected cranial area.

Meningoencephaloceles may be formed in areas other than the midline from skull destruction secondary to elevated intracranial pressure associated with severe congenital hydrocephalus. This origin should be differentiated from the type caused by defective development.

*Clinical findings.* Encephaloceles vary in size and shape, but generally continue to grow steadily. The covering may be either a thin membrane or normal skin. When pressure is applied to the growth, it may result in bulging fontanels, disturbed respirations, and impaired consciousness. The growth pulsates simultaneously with the other pulses in the body when the bony opening is of a moderate size. Palpation of the bony defect is usu-

ally possible after the sac has been reduced. Some children have a characteristic facial appearance, which includes protrusion of the eyes as a result of shallow eye orbits and a receding forehead, prominent nose, and wide cheek bones. Generally, most encephaloceles are readily observable.

A variety of problems are frequently associated with cranium bifidum, including varying impairments in mental capacities, cerebral palsy, hydrocephalus, spina bifida, talipes equinovarus (clubfoot), and cleft lip and palate.

*Diagnostic considerations.* One of the most promising findings in open types of cranium bifidum (and spina bifida) is the relationship of elevated alpha fetoprotein (AFP) levels in amniotic fluid to neural tube anomalies, as first described by Brock and Sutcliffe in 1972. Other investigators have confirmed this relationship and have ntoed that the presence of an elevated AFP concentration from the fourteenth week of gestation on indicates anencephaly or open spina bifida cystica.

In closed lesions the AFP concentration determined from fetal cerebrospinal fluid and capillary blood does not have access to the amniotic fluid. Thus a lower AFP level—possibly even a reading in the high normal range—may be present, even when the developmental defect exists. However, amniotic fluid assays are still valuable for mothers in the high-risk group, since the most disabling defects usually accompany the open types of lesions. Elevated levels of AFP in maternal serum are less expensive and more practically available as a screening tool than amniotic fluid determinations but have to be read in the context of other findings.

Both the serum and amniotic AFP determinations yield a false-positive result when multiple pregnancies exist or when the gestational age has been incorrectly computed. Ultrasound may then be employed to determine multiple pregnancies, gestational age, or the existence of anencephalus. Counseling and explanations of fetal outcomes and the course of action, if any, is appropriate in light of the findings.

After birth, transillumination is sometimes valuable in distinguishing meningocele from meningoencephalocele, since meningoceles are usually more opaque. However, at times the involved brain tissue may be thin and appear to be translucent, and so this test should be considered in the context of other findings. Skull films show the size of the cranial opening. Ventricular air studies may also be ordered by the neurologist to assess the extent of brain and ventricular tissue included in the defect.

At times intracranial tumors, cephalhematomas, or abscesses are mistaken for encephaloceles. Cephalhematomas differ from encephaloceles by location, which is usually in the parietal area rather than the midline; by the lack of pulsations; by their decreasing growth; and by the new bone growth that forms in their periphery after several weeks. Abscesses are characterized by the pus that may be removed during needle aspiration. Congenital tumors such as gliomas or hemangiomas may cause local bone destruction that resembles that produced by encephalocele. In these cases, further diagnostic evaluation by a neurologist or neurosurgeon is appropriate.

*Anticipated outcomes.* In severe cases of encephaloceles, death before the age of 1 year is not uncommon. When the saclike growths expand rapidly, the danger of the sac breaking is great. Death is generally associated with complications of hydrocephalus, infection, or rupturing of the encephalocele. For the survivors, problems related to the physical and mental impairments discussed previously may severely limit functional capacities.

*Intervention modalities.* Intervention is divided into the efforts of *early detection and care, acute management,* and *chronic care and health maintenance.*

ACUTE MANAGEMENT. After the presence of the encephalocele has been determined, the practitioner provides care related to protecting the encephalocele from injury, infection, and pressure. Meticulous skin care, provisions for adequate body temperature maintenance, and a reduction to minimum levels of fluid consumption within safe limits is desirable until the neonate is received at an acute care facility for further evaluation, stabilization, and possible surgery.

Acute management may or may not include surgery, depending on the severity of the brain defect, the degree of neural tissue involved in the sac, and the philosophy of the neurosurgeon. Principles related to stabilization of the body processes for surgery should be employed. Postoperatively, vital signs, serial head circumference measure-

ments, wound characteristics, signs of increasing intracranial pressure, and responses to the environmen and usual infant care routines are important indices of functional level and postoperative recovery. Abnormalities in any of these areas should be promptly evaluated and reported to the neurosurgeon, as indicated.

CHRONIC CARE. The provision of chronic care and health maintenance is probably the area of greatest involvement for the practitioner. Certainly the family needs detailed instruction and support in learning to provide the physical care for the infant as they integrate the newborn into the family group. The multiple acute and chronic problems that the family experiences emotionally, socially, financially, and physically provide the practitioner with many opportunities for integrating comprehensive health care delivery into a feasible plan for the infant and family. Counseling and guidance are important to this infant and family, since the multitude of problems they face may cause many acute and chronic periods of crisis. Referral to specialists in rehabilitation, education, surgery, neurology, and psychological and social services may be indicated for the involved mental and physical problems. However, care should be taken to be aware of the master plan of care, so that conflicting methods of management as a result of lack of communication may be avoided.

HEALTH MAINTENANCE. In addition to providing routine health care, programs of stimulation and help to encourage the infant in functioning at the highest level, and assistance of the family as needed, the practitioner should conduct assessments of the infant for changes in neurological status and increasing intracranial pressure and instruct parents as to the significance of these signs. Any changes should be reported to the neurosurgeon or neurologist managing the case.

When the family has had a child with an encephalocele, counseling and evaluation with a geneticist are appropriate. If another pregnancy occurs, the family should be advised about the methods of antenatal diagnosis suitable in their situation. Close follow-up and support are particularly indicated during the prenatal period whether the pregnancy is completed or ends in spontaneous or therapeutic abortion.

In summary, the family retains the ultimate decision-making power about the long-range plan of care and education for the child. (Refer to Chapter 7 for further detail on coping with mental retardation.) Many alternatives are available in working out the problems of living with a child who has limited capacities, and the practitioner can be of great assistance to the family in finding the solution that fits their individual situation best.

## Myelodysplasia with spina bifida

Myelodysplasia with spina bifida is characterized by incomplete fusion of one or more vertebral laminae, which is frequently accompanied by defective development of the spinal cord. While the cause of this condition is not known, the causative factors are generally believed to affect spinal cord development before the end of the third week of gestation by interfering with the closure of the neural tube. Impairment with the growth of the vertebral column probably occurs before the end of the eleventh week, since bony formation from the first cervical to the fourth sacral vertebra is completed by that time.

Whereas about 5% of the population probably has the bony deformity known as spina bifida occulta, only about 1 in 1000 infants has the accompanying protrusion of the meninges and neural tissue. Of the saclike protrusions. meningomyelocele is the most common type. The defect most frequently occurs in the lumbar or lumbosacral area. Location of the defect at the sacral or upper cervical vertebra is less common, whereas involvement of the lower cervical and thoracic regions is rare. After one child has been born with myelodysplasia, the incidence of producing another child with the deformity rises to 10 times the frequency for the general population.

*Pathophysiology.* Myelodysplasias with spina bifida may be divided into five major categories, including the following: (1) complete rachischisis, (2) meningomyelocele, (3) meningocele, (4) spina bifida occulta, and (5) congenital dermal sinuses. These may be defined as follows, in order of severity:

*complete rachischisis* —exposed, red, flattened spinal cord consisting of poorly differentiated neural tissue between bifurcated vertebral laminae.
*meningomyelocele* —soft, saclike protrusion containing meninges, cerebrospinal fluid, and a portion of spinal cord or its roots.

*meningocele* —saclike protrusion that does not contain neural tissue.
*spina bifida occulta* —defect in vetebral laminae without external protrusion. Faulty cord development and defects in overlying skin may be associated.
*congenital dermal sinus* —epithelium-lined tract that may communicate with neural tissue, most commonly in the sacral area of the spine or the posterior fossa of the head.

The most severe deformity in this category is *complete rachischisis,* wherein the spinal cord is exposed, red, and flattened within the groove formed by the bifurcated vertebral laminae. The lesion is composed of poorly differentiated neural tissue that may be at varying stages of development in individual infants. Frequently there is no sac, but the lesion may appear to protrude because of the tendency for it to rest on the cerebrospinal fluid that accumulates beneath it. The lesion is often confused with meningocele, since the external appearance may include the overgrowth of skin and meninges. However, in this highly vascular lesion, paralysis of the legs and other severe neurological symptoms almost always occur. Infections in these lesions are common. Depending on the extent of involvement, which may include the entire spine and cranium, the prognosis may result in either severe neurological defects or it may be incompatible with life.

The next defect in the order of severity is *meningomyelocele,* a soft, rounded protrusion containing a portion of the spinal cord or its roots (Fig. 13-1). Even though the neural groove has closed in this defect, cord damage is often present from adhesions or traction with resulting paralysis below the level of the lesion in accordance with the amount of neural involvement. This sac is characterized by the attachment of portions of the spinal cord to the sac wall as a result of the connection that has been maintained with surface ectoderm, by the thin covering of meninges and skin, and by the cerebrospinal fluid it contains, which is supplied by communication with the subarachnoid space.

In *meningocele* an external protrusion is obvious but does not contain neural tissue. The cord and spinal nerve roots may be normal or defective at the level of the lesion. The external appearance may include a normal skin covering or a thin, atrophied parchmentlike covering. Internally the

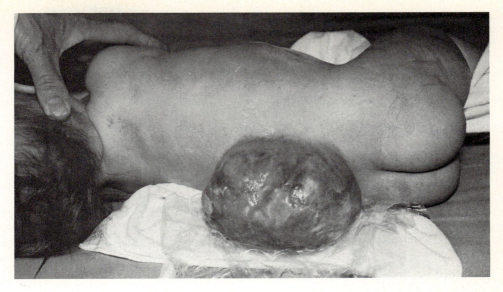

**FIG. 13-1.** Photograph of 6-month-old infant with L2-L4 myelomeningocele. Sac contains spinal elements and cerebrospinal fluid. Infant had bilateral flaccid paralysis of lower extremities.

meninges may fuse to form a single layer, or they may be clearly separated into the dura mater and arachnoid, forming a double sac.

In *spina bifida occulta* there is no external protrusion, but the skin overlying the defective vertebral lamina may display such markings as unusual hair growth, dimpling, or the presence of extra fat deposits or telangiectases. In this defect the neural tube has closed, and no neurological impairments exist in most of the cases. However, faulty cord development may accompany the defect. In these cases the cord may be attached securely to the spinal column by a fibrous mass, preventing normal cord ascension during development. Thus the conus of the cord may be located beneath its usual position. Consideration should be given to this possibility when a lumbar puncture is indicated.

Although *congenital dermal sinuses* might be regarded in the continuum of problems associated with the faulty closure of the neural tube, most of the sinuses are confined to the skin or communication with dermoid or epidermoid cysts and therefore do not penetrate into the nervous system. During the period of embryonic growth the neuro-

ectoderm separates from the epithelial ectoderm along the dorsal aspect of the embryo between the third and fifth gestational weeks. When this separation is not complete, the epithelium-lined tracts or sinuses result. These sinuses are characterized by skin markings, such as port-wine stains, dimpling, or the presence of hair. Although they may occur at any level of the spinal column or on the head, the most common sites are the sacral area of the spine and the posterior fossa of the head. Coccygeal sinuses usually extend only into the fascia and are termed "pilonidal sinuses." These pilonidal sinuses are prone to periodic infections but usually have no neurological significance. Underlying bony defects may also be revealed by roentgenograms.

*Clinical findings.* Several conditions are commonly associated with myelodysplastic problems. A large percentage of clients with meningomyeloceles develop hydrocephalus, which is frequently accompanied by the Arnold-Chiari deformity. Neurological impairment in the majority of children with meningoceles is either absent or minimal. Sometimes cranium bifidum is found in the client with spina bifida, which indicates interference with the same developmental process at two different levels. Progressive gliosis, which results in cavity formation in the gray matter and a clinical picture similar to syringomyelia, is sometimes seen in cases of spina bifida occulta.

Myelodysplastic problems result in neurological impairment in the myotomes innervated by affected spinal cord segments. Such involvement may vary from complete paralysis to little or no deficit, depending on the location and extent of the meningomyelocele. In lesions of the *lumbosacral* area the muscles of the leg are most severely affected, whereas the hip extensors and knee flexors are less involved. Affected muscles are flaccid. In severe cases, paralysis of the lower extremities may be complete. Flexion contractures of the hip and extension contractures of the knee are common. The great toe is usually dorsiflexed. Ankle reflexes are often absent, knee reflexes are frequently brisk, and hamstring jerks may or may not be evident. Electrical responses of muscles vary according to the degree and distribution of paralysis in the muscles. Clubfoot (talipes cavus, equinus, varus, and calcaneus) and hip subluxation are often associated with myelodysplastic lesions in the lumbosacral area. In *thoracic* lesions, pyramidal tract involvement is often observed either as spasticity of one or both lower extremities or as hyperactive reflexes. When the lesion is located in the *upper cervical* area, impaired development of the posterior columns of the spinal medulla and the cerebellum may be evident by such symptoms as cerebellar ataxia and weakness and spasticity of the extremities. If *cervical enlargement* is present, symptoms may be progressive, similar to those associated with syringomyelia. Some investigators attribute the weakness and atrophy in the arms, which is more pronounced in the distal portion; the trophic changes in the digits with potential ulcerative areas and loss of terminal portions; and the spastic paralysis of the lower extremities, which may progress to tetraplegia, to a progressive process of gliosis related to defective congenital development.

Whereas severe defects are obvious in the neonate, the milder impairments may not be evident until later childhood. Early developmental milestones may be normal, but as the sac with the attached spinal cord is stressed by spinal flexion associated with normal activity, the lower extremities develop poorly. Thus the child appears to have disproportionately large shoulders in relation to the small pelvis and thin legs in later life. When sudden, extreme spinal flexion occurs in children with these defects, paralysis may result.

In *lumbosacral* lesions, sensory disturbances are usually bilateral, symmetric, and localized according to affected dermatomes. Assessment of these disturbances is more difficult than determination of muscle involvement because of the limited cooperation from infants and young children. Observation of infants to ascertain the extent of analgesia and thermanesthesia is necessary, so that measures of safety from damaging stimuli might be enacted both in the nursery and by the parents at home. Sensory involvement often includes the feet, ankles, posterior aspects of the legs, thighs, buttocks, and perineal area. In general, pain sensations are affected most, whereas tactile capacities are involved least. Proprioceptive mechanisms are usually abnormal only when neurologic involvement from the myelodysplastic lesion is severe. Distal portions of the lower extremities are frequently mottled or cyanotic and cold. Impaired innervation also predisposes the involved area to skin ulcerations, especially over the bony prominences. In all cases except the mildest ones, defective sphincter control is present. However, the type of involvement varies according to the level of the lesion (see discussion of urination and defecation in Chapter 25). Observation for a relaxed anus and a protruding rectum is important to indicate sphincter involvement. Early detection and management of urinary tract infections are a constant concern.

In lesions of the cervical segments, responses to pain and temperature in the areas innervated by the cervical dermatomes are generally more impaired than tactile sensibility.

Clinical manifestations in *congenital dermal sinus* include the external appearance already described and such acute symptoms as inflammation with or without purulent drainage, drainage of spinal fluid, or recurrent meningitis, especially those types that may be attributed to skin bacteria. When the tract terminates within the cranium or spinal cord, symptoms coincide with those found in tumors. When there is intraspinal cystic expansion of the sinus tract, symptoms include disturbances in reflexes and sensibility, abnormalities in sphincter control, and weakness in the lower extremities. Cystic expansion within an occipital sinus tract leading into the posterior fossa results in symptoms associated with tumors in the cerebellum or fourth ventricle or obstructive hydrocephalus.

*Diagnostic considerations.* The external appearance of a midline sac makes the diagnosis of a myelodysplastic problem generally obvious. These sacs are usually translucent on transillumination, fluctuate with palpation, and cause the fontanels to bulge when pressure is applied to the sac because of their communication with the spinal subarachnoid spaces. Although surgical and pathological data are needed to confirm the presence or absence of neurological involvement in the sac, many of the lesions may be differentiated by usual clinical characteristics, such as the pedunculated, translucent sac, the lack of paralysis, and the small vertebral defect associated with meningocele, as compared to the greater opacity, larger vertebral defect, and paralysis related to meningomyelocele. Congenital lipomas, which may involve the cauda and be associated with spina bifida, are difficult to distinguish from myelodysplastic problems.

Spina bifida occulta is difficult to distinguish from other interferences that may result in congenital paralysis of the lower extremities. Palpation of defective vertebral arches, abnormal skin markings in the affected region, and roentgenography confirm the presence of myelodysplasia. However, radiological studies require the interpretation of a specialist, since a few individuals have spina bifida without symptoms and since ossification of the vertebrae in the lumbosacral area is incomplete until 8 years of age.

Moreover, consideration of mongolian spots, birth injury, and amyotonia congenita should be part of the differential diagnosis. Mongolian spots are brown or bluish skin markings frequently located in the sacral area of dark-skinned neonates or occasionally white newborns; these spots disappear in a short time. Birth injury may result in damage to the thoracic portion of the spinal cord after a breech delivery. This injury causes paraplegia in flexion or paraplegia in extension without muscle atrophy. Amyotonia congenita is characterized by general weakness, extreme loss of muscle tone, and the absence of sensory or trophic impairment. Occasionally, children who have a consistent problem with sphincter control after the function is well established may be found to have a defect in the vertebral laminae.

The diagnosis of *dermal sinus tract* may be made by inspection of the skin in some instances. However, in dermal sinuses of the occipital area these defects may be concealed by hair. Whenever a tumor is excised from either the posterior fossa or the cauda equina, the area should be carefully inspected with a strong light to ascertain the presence of a sinus. The same careful scrutiny of the area is warranted in cases of recurrent pyogenic meningitis. Roentgenograms of the spine and skull are valuable in revealing the bony abnormalities that frequently accompany dermal sinus.

*Anticipated outcomes.* The prognosis in the cases of myelodysplasia with a saclike protrusion depends on the degree of neural involvement, the presence of other anomalies, the size and location of the sac, and the complications that result. Convulsions and death may result if the sac ruptures suddenly, whereas meningitis may occur when the sac leaks slowly. When neurologic symptoms accompany spina bifida occulta, the potential for increasing deficits should be considered.

In cases of dermal sinus tract the prognosis is generally good when the tract is removed. However, neurological damage may occur as a result of meningitis or surgical removal of a cyst that is firmly attached to the spinal cord or meninges.

*Intervention modalities.* Surgical removal and plastic repairs are recommended for all simple meningoceles. However, surgical intervention in meningomyeloceles may not be appropriate when neurological involvement is extreme, when an infection of the lesion is present, or when associated problems such as hydrocephalus are severe. Decisions are made on an individual basis after such specialists as physical therapists, orthopedists, neurosurgeons, and urologists have conferred. If there is an immediate danger of the sac rupturing, surgery is performed quickly. However, when the covering over the sac is adequate, the time of surgical intervention varies according to the philosophy of the neurosurgeon and the symptoms that the child displays. Although supportive care and surgery are the only treatments, neither can reverse the damage and paralysis that exist. However, one may prevent further paralysis by surgical removal of fat deposits that compress the cord and adhesions that cause injury by traction. Surgical intervention may result in secondary damage and further neurological sequelae or in improvements where there was cord compression. These possibilities should be understood by the family before surgery.

Surgical intervention in cases of spina bifida occulta is appropriate when neurological symptoms progress. At times, inspection during surgery reveals a cyst, lipoma, or congenital defects in conjunction with the bony abnormality.

Prevention is not possible, except in those cases where high-risk maternity clients have undergone amniocentesis and elevated alpha fetoprotein (AFP) levels have indicated an open type of lesion, so that the decision to abort the fetus by therapeutic means is made. Beyond this secondary type of prevention, no means of predicting which pregnancy will produce an infant with dysplasias of the spine or cranium is currently available.

General principles of care may be summarized as acute intervention, transitional aspects, and long-range maintenance. *Acute intervention* implies the initial phase of neonatal assessment, stabilization, and treatment of early problems to maximize potential capacities and minimize conditions that may result in further deformity or untoward outcomes. This aspect of care is usually provided in a hospital. During this phase, emotional support for and involvement of the family in normal care and special procedures are vital in assisting them toward independence in physical care and acceptance of the defective child as an individual within their family context. Before the child's discharge the family needs to have a thorough understanding of the child's problems and potential capacities, so that they may utilize every resource to ensure maximum growth and development. The family also needs to be completely confident in the ability to provide the physical care that the child requires and to identify the conditions that indicate the need for medical attention—urinary tract infections, constrictive casts, wound infections, increasing intracranial pressure, meningitis, or any other unusual change in the child.

Ideally the nurse practitioner is familiar with the case at this time and is able to effect a smooth *transition* to home and long-range care by developing an acceptable working relationship with the infant and family, by assessing the entire range of needs in the infant and family, by conferring with the hospital personnel and specialists involved, and by organizing all of this information into a plan of care that incorporates and integrates acute and chronic situational needs with available resources and services.

The practitioner continues to have a major role in the *long-range maintenance* of myelodysplastic children and their families. One of the primary problems in these families is the splintered care that they receive as a result of the involvement of several separate specialists without intercommunication. The practitioner may be the central figure in integrating total care and in interpreting priorities and information to the family. Also, the practitioner plays an important role in assisting the family in the psychosocial and economic realms by offering counseling, guidance, and referral as they face the multitude of financial, social, and psychologic problems inherent in accepting the child with limited capacities into the family group. Additionally, the practitioner suggests ways to stimulate and offer the growing child as many normal interactions with siblings, peers, family, and others as possible, so that development may be consistent with the child's potential capacities. Furthermore, the practitioner provides routine health maintenance for the child, monitors chronic problems, and initiates appropriate referrals for untreated, acute, or changed problems. The practitioner also assists the family in learning techniques that facilitate physical care and promote the highest functional level within the child throughout the entire course of management. The practitioner maintains ongoing communication with such specialists as educators, urologists, orthopedists, neurologists, neurosurgeons, hospital personnel, physical therapists, and psychosocial professionals in order to have current information on the needs and objectives of the child and family. Contact with religious leaders may be appropriate for some persons as well. Finally, the practitioner assists the family in arriving at a decision to maintain the child in the home setting, in a day-care setting, or in an institution providing full-time care, as appropriate for the individual family and child. See Table 13-1.

**TABLE 13-1.** Long-term management in myelodysplasia

| Concern or problem | Nursing intervention | Expected outcome |
|---|---|---|
| A. Guilt or concerns about coping with child and having other children. | 1. Inform parents about multifactorial genesis of neural tube defect; statistics about recurrence in other offspring and future generations. | 1. Parents will be able to explain the cause of the defect. |
| | 2. Explain prenatal diagnostics available:<br>  a. Ultrasound.<br>  b. Blood serum screening test done from the fourteenth to sixteenth week of pregnancy to pinpoint women with elevated alpha-fetoprotein (AFP) levels (emphasize low cost and ease of doing test)<br>  c. Amniocentesis for high-risk clients done at about 16 weeks of gestation to determine elevated AFP levels. Note: Discuss false-positive results caused by multiple pregnancies or misjudged gestational date. | 2. Parents will utilize the nurse and other members of the health team to determine family planning goals and follow through with implementation. |
| | 3. At appropriate time, discuss all aspects of therapeutic abortion. | 3. Parents will be able to explain essential prenatal care for future pregnancies in themselves or their children. |
| | 4. Provide guidance and counseling as parents emotionally and practically confront problems and responsibilities of bonding to and caring for an affected child. | 4. Parents will identify their feelings of acceptance or rejection of their child, and their current problems and concerns. |
| | | 5. Parents will state that they have adequate guidance to cope with their personal feelings, problems, and fears; work cooperatively with spouse or significant other; assist siblings and other family members in coping; and approach the practical issues of caring for the myelodysplastic child. |
| B. Diminished sensory awareness in areas affected by the lesion. | 1. Feet, lower extremities, perineum, and buttocks will be inspected three times daily (more if incontinence, orthopedic appliances, or immobility cause increased susceptibility to skin breakdown) by caretaker and older child, as appropriate to ensure adequate skin integrity. | 1. The child will remain free of skin breakdown and injury. |
| | 2. Instructions in hygienic care; bowel habits and urinary routines will include the importance of practices that promote good skin integrity. | 2. The child will adequately accomplish self-care. |
| | 3. Warnings will be issued on the importance of avoiding temperature extremes, that is, hot water bottles, heating pads, hot bath water, frigid weather, wherein exposure is prolonged or clothing is inadequate, since the client may be unable to detect skin damage because of impaired sensibility. | 3. Weight will be within normal limits for height, age, and sex. |

*Continued.*

**TABLE 13-1.** Long-term management in myelodysplasia—cont'd

| Concern or problem | Nursing intervention | Expected outcome |
|---|---|---|
| | 4. Provide the parent and client with ongoing assistance in weight control to enhance self-concept and decrease the chance of skin breakdown related to obesity. | |
| C. Potentially lower self-esteem caused by physical problems, response patterns of significant others, and delayed development or limited physical, social, and intellectual capacities. | 1. Provide practical help and referrals for social, educational, and vocational experiences with others in light of developmental age.<br>2. Pinpoint child's capacities through testing. | 1. Child will play with age-appropriate friend twice weekly.<br><br>2. Client education, activities, and responsibilities for self-care and decision-making will be appropriate to client capacities and functional level. |
| | 3. Emphasize child's positive points: (a) talents, (b) physical features by choosing stylish clothes and hair designs and emphasizing good hygiene, (c) encourage the child to verbalize feelings about self and about acceptance by others. | 3. The family relationship will be warm and loving and supportive. |
| | 4. Assist the child and family in forming close ties in a healthy manner, so that as the child grows toward independence the family may relinquish appropriate responsibilities for daily care, decisions, and activities to the client. | 4. Feelings about child's condition will be openly verbalized and accepted. |
| | 5. Provide guidance to the parents to stabilize their marriage, relationships with children, and coping mechanisms in rearing a child with many problems. | 5. Child will be socially acceptable. |
| | 6. Provide parents with adequate information on psychosexual development so that they or the nurse may assist the client with age-appropriate issues. (Refer to Chapters 6 and 15 for information related to paralysis and functional potentials.) | 6. Child will become independent in activities of daily living. |
| | 7. Refer child and family to appropriate specialists when the parental marriage is threatened, when the client must adjust to lack of a partner because of social or intelligence-level problems, or when the client has selected a partner with similar problems. | 7. Client will become self-supporting.<br>8. Sexuality will be freely discussed at each developmental stage by the nurse, selected specialists, the parents, and the client as appropriate. |
| D. Increased numbers of musculoskeletal problems. | 1. Assist parents in identifying musculoskeletal problems—clubfoot, subluxated hip, scoliosis, contractures, other joint deformities.<br>2. Provide adequate client and family teaching and supportive and cooperative care planning at all points of intervention. Refer to specialized orthopedic books for detailed care. | 1. Achieve independent locomotion. |

**TABLE 13-1.** Long-term management in myelodysplasia—cont'd

| Concern or problem | Nursing intervention | Expected outcome |
|---|---|---|
| E. Impaired bowel and urinary functions. | 1. Establish an individually tailored bowel routine in concert with the physiological capacities, developmental age, and needs of the client. (Refer to Chapter 25; Vigliarolo, 1980.) | 1. Client will maintain good renal and bowel tone. |
| | 2. Initiate a bladder-training routine that minimizes the potential for urinary tract infections. | 2. Client will be independent in bowel and bladder functions. |
| | 3. Teach client and family intermittent catheterization technqiues, if applicable. | 3. Client will have socially acceptable bowel and bladder care, that is, in relation to odor, soiling, and so on. |
| | 4. Prepare client and family for the care of a permanent catheter or have urological surgery, as needed. Use other references to formulate detailed plans on urological care. (See Chapter 25 for information.) | |
| F. Development of hydrocephalus. | Refer to section on hydrocephalus. | |
| G. Development of hydrosyringomyelia in children who do not have shunts or who have compensated hydrocephalus. | 1. Observe child for progressive symptoms, that is, increasing spasticity, weakness in extremities, scoliosis, and behavioral changes. | 1. Child and family will be able to explain problem and treatment. |
| | 2. Explain this condition of older children to families with a vulnerable child. | 2. Disability will be avoided by prompt intervention. |
| | 3. When condition occurs, refer child to a neurosurgeon for insertion of shunt. | |
| | 4. Involve child and family in total care planning at all points of the problem. | |

**Presurgical expected outcomes**

1 Neonate's general condition will be stable.
2 The highest level of health and well-being will be promoted in all body systems.
3 Infection will be absent.
4 The sac will be intact.
5 Physiotherapy will be done according to individual prescription to avoid deformity and loss of function.
6 Any change in the client's condition will be noted and promptly reported to the physician.
7 Head circumference and serial evaluations for increased intracranial pressure will be performed.
8 Symptomatic nursing intervention will include consideration to all concerns and problems (physical, intellectual, spiritual, socioeconomic, cultural) in the client and family.

*Acute intervention.* The protective skin of the sac may be paper thin; therefore it should be carefully and frequently inspected for evidence of irritation, abrasion, rupture, leakage of cerebrospinal fluid, and infection.

MOTOR AND SENSORY FUNCTIONS. Accurate observation of motor and sensory functions is required, with testing and charting of the degree of motion, strength, and sensation of the extremities. These are evaluated in terms of spontaneous movement and activity in response to unpleasant stimulation or bodily restriction. These observations should be made three or four times a day, and any change should be reported.

SPHINCTER CONTROL. The amount and frequency of urination is noted as accurately as possible, and the number of wet and soiled diapers are recorded. The infant is examined for distention because of the possibility of urinary retention with overflow. Describe stools carefully as to consistency, frequency, and amount. Note and report symptoms of diarrhea or constipation. Not only can you aid in the prevention of cystitis and impactions, but you can also be of great help to the physician in the evaluation of sphincter control and in the decision regarding surgical treatment.

**ORTHOPEDIC APPLIANCES.** Splints and casts are frequently required during infancy when the commonly associated problems of subluxation of the hip or clubfoot occur.

**HEAD.** Measure the head and chest in centimeters every morning. Since hydrocephalus may be a secondary complication (developing in 80% of children with myelomeningocele defects, generally within the first month of life), the fontanels are examined at least three times a day, and signs of tension or bulging are reported.

**BEHAVIOR.** The nurse can help the psychologist evaluate the mental status of the infant by observing and recording activity in response to feeding, bathing, and other environmental stimuli. Nurses caring for these infants or children with other developmental diseases should know what behavior to expect from a normal child at different age levels. This knowledge will make their observations more pertinent and meaningful.

**MENINGITIS.** The nurse should be alert for early symptoms of meningeal irritation such as hyperirritability, increased sensitivity to noise and light, fever, restlessness, increased crying and fretfulness (probably caused by headache), nuchal rigidity, and vomiting. Meningitis may be a secondary complication after rupture or infection of the sac.

**VITAL SIGNS.** Rectal temperatures are taken every 4 hours. Pulse, respiration, and blood pressure are measured as ordered, depending on the age of the child.

**POSITION.** Before operation the infant with a meningocele is postured in the following manner to prevent irritation, contamination, or rupture of the sac: Place the infant on the abdomen with the head turned to the side and the hips and pelvis elevated to prevent contamination of the sac by urine or feces. Place sandbags at the sides to maintain position and prevent rolling. Support the lower extremities so that the feet are free from pressure and at right angles to the legs for prevention of foot drop. Posture the upper extremities for comfort and prevention of wristdrop. Depending on the age and size of the infant, a small support may be required under the chest to maintain good alignment. Keep a cradle over the involved area to support the weight of the bedclothes. The use of cotton doughnuts is not recommended. A padded strainer or a sufficiently thick foam rubber pad with a center opening large enough to permit protrusion of the sac may be used to protect it when the infant is being transported. This pad should be at least 3 inches wide so that it may be held in place by soft cotton straps that are wrapped around the infant.

**CLOTHING.** Do not put diapers and shirts on these infants until the surgical repair has been done. They add to the dangers of local irritation. Adjust the environment to the infant's needs, regulate the temperature as indicated, and, if necessary, use an Isolette to provide warmth. This may be tilted so that the infant's head is elevated and still not interfere with the position previously outlined. The mattress and pillow should be protected with Pliofilm, or plastic sheeting, rather than rubber sheeting.

**HYGIENE.** Hygiene depends on the age of the infant and the condition of the skin. Cleanliness and changing whenever the infant is wet are essential for the prevention of local and general breakdown of the skin. Oil is used as necessary. If the sac is intact, it is left dry and exposed; if the sac is abraded or oozing, gentle cleansing with hydrogen peroxide helps prevent crusts. Some physicians believe the sac should be protected by a dry dressing; others recommend petrolatum gauze. Complications are less likely to arise if no dressing is applied. There may be sensory involvement with local anesthesia; therefore great care must be exercised to prevent burns.

**NUTRITION.** The formula and supplementary feedings are generally regulated by the pediatrician or neonatologist after consultation with the nursing staff. The nurse is responsible for reporting feeding problems, regurgitation, vomiting, and anorexia. The infant is weighed as ordered, depending on age and progress. Measure fluid intake accurately, and report early signs of dehydration.

**ELIMINATION.** Note bladder and bowel function as detailed in the discussion of observations. If there is retention, manual expression of the bladder contents by local pressure (Credé's method) at 2-hour intervals may reduce the amount of residual urine and the danger of urinary tract infection. If the anal sphincter is relaxed, care should be used to prevent local irritation. Zinc oxide ointment applied locally may be used as a preventive and curative measure. Diet may be adjusted to combat the extremes of diarrhea or constipation. Mild laxatives are used to prevent constipation or impactions. Low enemas or suppositories may be necessary for regular evacuation of the bowel. Prevent contamination of the lesion by the infant's excretions.

MEDICAL TREATMENT. Medical treatment is supportive during the preoperative interval; maintenance of good nutrition is emphasized. Some physicians advocate limitation of fluid intake. The child should have plenty of fresh air. Development should be checked periodically. Every attempt should be made to foster normal maturation within the regimen necessitated by the infant's disability.

If the sac is leaking cerebrospinal fluid or if a superficial infection is present, powdered boric acid, sulfadiazine, or alcohol dressings may be applied three to four times a day. Aspiration of the sac may help reduce local tension, prevent enlargement, decrease the amount of leakage, and arrest an early hydrocephalus. If the infant becomes dehydrated as a result of the aspirations, subcutaneous injections of physiological sodium chloride solution may be given as necessary.

The discussion of surgery with the parents informs them of the probable outcome and the possibility of residual disabilties. The permit for operation is obtained and arrangements made for transfusions according to the needs of the individual patient.

PREPARATION FOR SURGERY. Omit feedings 6 to 12 hours before the scheduled time. Evacuate the lower bowel with an enema the evening before operation. Check the permit and the reports of blood typing, cross matching, Rh factor, and urine. Depending on the type of anesthesia to be used, mild sedative medication may be given with atropine sulfate.

Local preparation is usually done in the operating room. The infant is transported to the operating room in the prone position in the crib. This eliminates unnecessary handling and reduces the hazards of local trauma.

After the infant is transferred to the operating table, the nurse rearranges the Isolette, changing linen as necessary and checking supplementary equipment. It is left in the recovery room to receive the infant directly from the table at the end of the operation.

*Postoperative nursing intervention.* The necessary observations are as outlined previously, with special emphasis on the early recognition of complications such as shock, acute hydrocephalus, wound rupture, infection, meningitis, hyperthermia, loss of sphincter control, pressure sores, dehydration, and respiratory infections. The dressings are checked frequently for evidence of drainage, which may or may not be cerebrospinal fluid.

POSITION. Some surgeons advocate keeping the head lower than the spine to maintain the pressure of cerebrospinal fluid within the brain and to lessen the possibility of loss of cerebrospinal fluid through the wound. If the infant has hydrocephalus, the head is elevated to increase drainage from the brain. The prone position is advocated until the wound is well healed; if primary healing takes place without complication, this generally is accomplished within 5 to 7 days. Change the position every 2 hours, with special attention to weakened or paralyzed extremities. The principles outlined in Chapter 9 for posturing clients are followed and modified according to the needs and size of the infant. The combinations of wristdrop, footdrop, muscle stretching, decubitus ulcers, or other deformities may be prevented when these principles are applied. After the wound is well healed, the head is elevated at all times for the subsequent 9 to 12 months. For this reason the mother should be taught the importance of holding and carrying the infant in the upright position.

NUTRITION. Feedings are resumed and supplemented as needed. If the fontanels become tense, the infant is placed on a restricted fluid intake to obtain the optimum degree of dehydration. This should be accomplished under the guidance of a pediatrician and is contraindicated if hyperthermia develops.

HYGIENE. The care of the skin is continued as previously outlined. A diaper and shirt may be used.

ELIMINATION. Sphincter control is evaluated and secondary complications watched for and treated immediately. The principles of care outlined under preoperative care are applied.

WOUND DRESSING. The dressing is protected from

external contamination by the use of Pliofilm or other nonpermeable material. This should be secured to the skin with a hypoallergenic adhesive to eliminate the danger of skin irritation such as may be caused by adhesive tape. Examine dressings meticulously at frequent intervals for any sign of cerebrospinal fluid leakage. Report a wet dressing immediately so that the physician can examine the wound for possible rupture and institute the necessary treatment. Sutures are removed between the fifth and seventh days, depending on the condition of the wound. A protective dressing is kept on the wound for at least 2 weeks.

**TREATMENT OF COMPLICATIONS.** The early detection of complications will facilitate their successful treatment.

SHOCK. Symptomatic and systemic treatment is instituted, depending on the age of the child and the degree of shock. Loss of cerebrospinal fluid may precipitate shock; to prevent this the head is maintained in a position lower than the spine.

ACUTE HYDROCEPHALUS. Fluid intake is limited unless contraindicated, and the head is elevated. Ventricular or lumbar punctures may be done to remove excess cerebrospinal fluid. A shunt may be needed.

WOUND RUPTURE WITH LEAKAGE OF CEREBROSPINAL FLUID. The head is kept lower than the spine, and prophylactic chemotherapy is instituted to prevent infection. The wound is resutured unless contraindicated.

WOUND INFECTION OR MENINGITIS. Symptomatic treatment is administered with suitable chemotherapy and the use of local antiseptics as indicated. (Many of the deaths that occur during the first year of life may be caused by meningitis.)

RESPIRATORY INFECTIONS. Respiratory treatment is directed by the pediatrician.

HYPERTHERMIA. Tepid or cool sponge baths are given when the temperature reaches a certain point, often arbitrarily set at 103° F. Fluid intake is maintained. Bedclothes are reduced to a minimum. Low, cool colon lavages and antipyretic medication such as aspirin or acetaminophen (Tylenol) may be given by rectum. If a hypothermic unit is available, it may be employed effectively to reduce high temperatures.

PARALYSIS. Supportive posturing of the extremities is indicated to prevent deformities and footdrop or wristdrop. Basswood or cockup splints may be used to support the upper extremity and molded posterior casts to support the lower extremities. Passive exercise directed toward maintaining the normal range of motion of the joints of the affected extremities also reduces complications.

BLADDER AND BOWEL DISTURBANCES. The treatment for bladder and bowel disturbances is the same as that suggested for preoperative care and must be modified according to the age of the child.

Unless complications develop, the infant is ready for discharge by the middle or end of the third postoperative week. The nurse should ascertain if the mother fully understands the needs of the child and instruct her regarding any special care required. Both practitioners enlighten parents as to any secondary ill effects that may occur and arrange for a follow-up appointment. If the child shows evidence of mental or physical retardation, arrangements should be made for periodic psychological tests to evaluate progress.

If an adult has surgical repair of a spina bifida occulta, the nurse applies the principles of nursing care as outlined in Chapter 22.

In January 1973, a new national group, the Spina Bifida Association of America, was organized to develop better educational and occupational opportunities for persons with spina bifida and to improve medical techniques and facilities.

*Other conditions associated with spina bifida.* *Status dysgraphicus* is a term that includes all of the defects involved in the category of myelodysplasia with spina bifida that may be attributed to impaired closure of the neural tube. The most common conditions have been discussed in the previous section, but defects are possible in all portions of each segment. The most frequently involved areas are the cervical and lumbosacral regions. Mental deficiencies and cerebral defects are often associated with these cases. Clinical findings include concurrent errors in development, such as trophic and sensory changes in the extremities, anomalies in skeletal formation, malformed ears, asymmetric features, atrophied muscles, unusual hair growth, and faulty genital organ development.

*Myelodysplasia with Klippel-Feil syndrome* is a rare congenital anomaly wherein the cervical vertebrae may be reduced in number and fused together and wherein the posterior wall of the spinal canal is usually defective, resulting in spina bifida occulta. One makes the diagnosis by noting the triad of common symptoms: shortening of the neck, lowering of the hairline, and limitations in head movement. Mental impairments, congenital deafness, squints, and retractions of the eyeball may be associated. Neurological deficits may or may not be noted. However, syringomyelia may result in progressive paralysis as an associated consequence of the development defect. Mirror movements of the hands—movements in one hand being imitated exactly by movements in the opposite hand—are reported in a number of cases.

Myelodysplasia may also be present when the sacrum and coccyx are absent. The cause of this problem is unknown. Clinically the iliac crests are in a more medial, vertical placement, resulting in loss of the normal curvature of the buttocks and absence of the intergluteal fold. Dislocated hips, impaired bowel and bladder functioning, and paralysis and anesthesia in areas innervated by affected segments are common findings. The lack of bone may be determined by palpation and demonstrated by roentgenography.

**DIPLOMYELIA.** Diplomyelia refers to the duplication of the spinal cord. Generally this double cord is located beneath the midthoracic area. Normal functioning of the double cord is possible. Neurological symptoms occur when there are associated malformations of the cord or congenital tumors. Spina bifida, most commonly of the occult type, occurs in about half of the cases. Meningoceles and the various forms of clubfoot are also connected with this condition in some clients.

**DIASTEMATOMYELIA.** Diastematomyelia is a congenital defect caused prenatally when abnormal mesodermal cells protrude into the tissue of the neural tube rather than assuming their usual arrangement around the periphery. These cells gradually form a bony or cartilaginous spur that extends only one or two segments, generally, to divide the spinal cord into two separate portions. Each portion of the spinal cord has its own complete dual sac. Various other defects in the vertebral bodies and arches, including spina bifida, are commonly associated with this condition. Cutaneous lesions in the median part of the back, such as nevi, abnormal hair growth, dimples, lipomas, dermal sinus tract, or telangiectasis, may be observed. Although the symptoms are not always apparent at birth, many children with diastematomye-

lia have symptoms indicating interferences with innervation to the sphincters and lower extremities. These symptoms may include an abnormal gait and problems in attaining bowel and bladder control. Physical examination may reveal atrophy of one or both extremities, weakness or spasticity in one or both extremities, changes in deep tendon reflexes, and various foot deformities, including trophic ulceration in the feet. Roentgenograms and myelography reveal the extent and location of the defect. Treatment consists of surgical excision of the bony or fibrous septum and closure of the posterior dura in order to place the two sections of cord in a single canal. Although surgery does not correct prior damage, it does avoid further progression of symptoms by eliminating the source of fixation, stretching, and compression of involved portions of the spinal medulla. Nursing care is directed to preoperative and postoperative measures commonly used for spinal surgery and long-range intervention in the multiplicity of problems created by impaired bowel and bladder operations and defective functional capacities in the lower extremities.

## Other developmental errors

When the corpus callosum is absent, other errors of growth are often present, including absence of the gyrus fornicatus and falx and fusion of the frontal hemispheres.

Heterotopias, displacements of tissue or organ growth, are caused in development when abnormal migration of the neurons occurs. This migration results in the formation of nuclear masses in the white matter with peripheral borders of glial cells. Other errors in the formative period are commonly associated.

The cortical ageneses may encompass several developmental problems, including poorly developed, simplified cortical patterns (macrogyria), overly complicated cortical patterns (microgyria), incomplete formation of associational or projectional tracts, and cellular abnormalities in the cortex or motor tracts. Problems related to degenerative rather than developmental problems are detailed in Chapters 16 and 17.

Defects in the basal ganglia, which occur in the development of the forebrain, encompass several syndromes that are characterized by impaired muscle tone and frequently by involuntary movements.

Some of these conditions are included in the section on specific problems in the perinatal period.

Cranial nerve nuclei may be underdeveloped or absent. The resulting problems are related to the nerves involved. Defective development in either one or both sides of the cerebellum is often accompanied by faulty growth in the pons and olives.

The special senses — vision, olfaction, and audition — may not be intact because of faulty development of the brain.

# DEFECTIVE HEAD GROWTH

Four major problems account for the continuum involved in abnormal head growth. At one end there is the head that is smaller than normal and at the other end the head that is larger than normal. The problem of cranial underdevelopment may be caused by faulty brain development or impaired growth patterns in the skull and may be divided into microcephaly and craniostenosis. Two problems are typically identified as causes of enlarged head growth: macrocephaly and hydrocephalus.

## MICROCEPHALY

Underdevelopment of the brain is termed "microcephaly." Within this category there is the true form of microcephaly and multiple conditions that result in secondary microcephaly.

True microcephaly is a recessive inherited disorder wherein the mature brain attains a weight of less than 1000 gm. When brains of microcephalic individuals are examined during autopsy, they are found to be developed to a level usually seen at 3 to 4 months of gestation. Impairments in brain growth may also occur as outcomes of porencephaly, intrauterine growth disorders resulting in lobar agenesis or abnormal cortical patterns, and cystic degeneration resulting from birth injury.

In examining the true microcephalic infant the practitioner notes that the head circumference is small at birth and destined to reach a maximum of 17 inches by maturity and that the infant has unusually small fontanels. The face is normal and provides a striking contrast to the abnormal skull, so that the infant appears to have a flat occiput, a pointed vertex, a receding forehead, and a narrow head with a definite slant in the lateral aspects. A variety of abnormalities are present as primary problems, including impairments in growth and development, disturbances in locomotion, speech disorders, and variable deficiencies in cognitive and mental capacities. Seizures are typically present. In the neurological examination, deep tendon reflexes are exaggerated in early childhood but seem to become diminished as growth continues to maturity.

The diagnosis is confirmed by the features noted on physical examination when such problems as disease processes or cerebral trauma have been excluded. By the time diagnosis is made the fontanels are usually either small or closed prematurely. Intrauterine diagnosis is not possible, since the interferences with head growth are not usually significant until after birth, when head growth is abnormal as determined by comparison with normative patterns. As the diagnosis of microcephaly is confirmed, the practitioner should construct a pedigree of the family to evaluate the possibility of an inherited disorder.

### Expected outcome

The major objective of the health team in managing the microcephalic individual is to promote the highest level of development, functional capacities, and psychosocial-family adaptation possible. A holistic approach to the child and family is essential as efforts of the total health team are utilized in maintaining normal health, avoiding and treating infections, and promoting an optimal pattern of living for both the child and family. Cooperation and communication between all involved professionals assist the family in adjusting to the mentally retarded child, coping with acute and chronic problems, and moving in a directed manner toward long-range objectives. The practitioner who works with these clients should refer to the discussions and references on mental retardation and specific learning disabilities.

## CRANIOSTENOSIS

Craniostenosis denotes a group of conditions wherein two or more cranial bones unite prematurely so that cranial appearances are distorted. The brain is normal in these cases, and symptoms are related to inadequacy of cranial capacity. The names of the various types of craniostenosis are derived from the sutures involved in the premature closure. Distortion of the head and face depends on which sutures are involved.

Diagnosis is made when clinical observation of the head and face reveals characteristic abnormalities compatible with growth disturbances caused by premature closure of one or more sutures. Palpation and skull radiographs confirm the closure of the suture or sutures. Increased intracranial pressure is often present. Differential diagnostic considerations include the following: (1) hydrocephalus, which also includes increased intracranial pressure; (2) space-occupying lesions, which usually do not result in changes in head shape; and (3) microcephaly, which also may include premature closure of the sutures and a pointed vertex. Microcephaly is excluded because it includes the following physical findings that are not apparent in craniostenosis: smaller cranial capacity, mental retardation, and absence of papilledema and exophthalmos. Spastic paralysis may be an additional finding in microcephaly.

Changes in the face and head may not be apparent in craniostenosis when diagnosis and surgical intervention occur early in infancy. Early detection minimizes secondary changes from bony distortion and increased intracranial pressure and subsequent problems and is promptly followed by surgical separation of fused cranial bone and replacement in the suture region with a polyethylene film. This surgical procedure prevents union of the bones and provides adequate space for brain growth.

The management protocol is individualized, since children are diagnosed at various points and thus have varying problems in relation to delay in diagnosis and surgical intervention. After surgery is completed the practitioner monitors the child for signs of rejection of the polyethylene strip as well as infection and continued approximation of the sutures. At the time of discharge, parents are given verbal and written instructions on signs of increased intracranial pressure so that they may know when to seek medical assistance. Families should also receive assistance on coping with the child's changed image. Because this condition seems to have possible inherited qualities, a detailed family history is important. The practitioner will also want to examine subsequent children early in life to detect any cranial abnormalities. Refer to the article by Humphrey et al. for detailed preoperative and postoperative care.

## Macrocephaly

Macrocephaly is a primary problem related to embryonic growth or progressive disease processes that results in abnormal cellular and structural changes in brain tissue. In contrast, hydrocephalus is a condition wherein brain tissue is normal but an abnormality exists in the flow of cerebrospinal fluid through the ventricular system. Neuronal dysfunction from hydrocephalus is not primary, as is that found in macrocephaly, but instead is secondary to complications and outcomes of increased intracranial pressure (Table 13-2).

In macrocephaly the problem resulting in abnormal brain growth may be the result of a disturbance in the developmental period wherein defects in cellular and structural formation are observed or may be the result of a degenerative process such as the lipoidoses, Schilder's disease, or Green-

**TABLE 13-2.** Head enlargement—comparison of macrocephaly and hydrocephalus*

| Macrocephaly | Hydrocephalus |
|---|---|
| Abnormal head size as a result of tissue defects secondary to developmental error or progressive destructive process | Abnormal head size as a result of ventricular enlargement |
| Large symmetrical head | Head growth lateral and asymmetrical |
| No increased intracranial pressure | Primary increased intracranial pressure |
| Primary mental retardation | Possible secondary mental retardation |
| Primary growth retardation | Possible secondary growth retardation |
| Primary convulsions | Possible secondary convulsions |
| Primary problems in attaining independent mobility | Possibly secondary problems in attaining mobility |
| Primary behavioral, visual, and communication deficiencies | Possible secondary behavioral, visual, and communication deficiencies |
| Delayed closure of fontanels | Full, tense fontanels and widespread sutures |

*From Conway, B.L.: Pediatric neurologic nursing, St. Louis, 1977, The C.V. Mosby Co.

field's disease. In these destructive processes, brain size becomes abnormally large, causing cranial sutures to remain open beyond the usual time and the head circumference to be unusually large. In the secondary type of macrocephaly, clinical findings are related to the causative disease process.

In the primary type of macrocephaly the findings are consistent with the symptoms presented in Table 13-2. To differentiate primary macrocephaly from hydrocephalus and secondary types, a ventriculogram is required.

The type of intervention is related to the individual pattern of disease presentation. Generally, treatment is symptomatic and premised on a multidisciplinary base geared to meeting acute and chronic needs of the child with severe impairments within a family context.

## HYDROCEPHALUS

*Etiology and pathology.* Hydrocephalus may be caused by an excessive production or inadequate absorption of cerebrospinal fluid in the brain or an obstruction that interferes with the circulation of cerebrospinal fluid through the ventricular system; either condition in the infant is followed by enlargement of the head. Obstruction at the narrower pathways (foramina of Monro, aqueduct of Sylvius, foramina of Magendie and Luschka) of the ventricular cerebrospinal fluid circulation causes the so-called *noncommunicating* (internal) *hydrocephalus* (Fig. 13-2). The obstruction occurs most

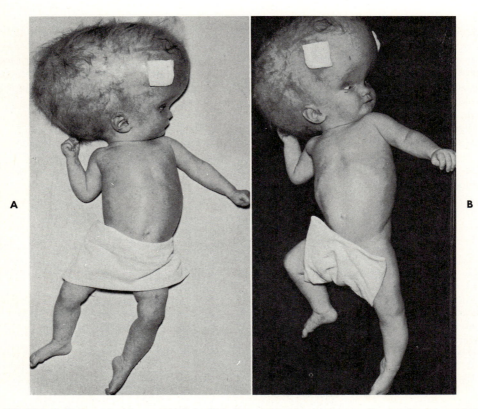

**FIG. 13-2. A,** Photograph of 1-year-old infant with hydrocephalus, showing extreme disproportion between head and body. **B,** Note distention of frontal veins, depression of eyeballs, and projection of forehead.

frequently in the aqueduct of Sylvius between the third and fourth ventricles; it may be the result of a maldevelopment, infection, or tumor. Because the cerebrospinal fluid is unable to circulate from the ventricular system to the subarachnoid circulation, where it is normally absorbed into the blood vessels, the lateral and third ventricle become dilated, and the intracranial pressure increases. Another type called *communicating* (external) *hydrocephalus,* in which the fluid circulation through the ventricular system into the subarachnoid space is not impeded, is probably the result of faulty absorption of the fluid by the venous circulation. This communicating type of hydrocephalus is frequently seen in association with the previously mentioned cerebrospinal malformations.

*Signs and symptoms.* The head may be of normal size with bulging fontanels, though in time it becomes strikingly enlarged and assumes a shape characterized by an increase in the vertical, lateral, and anteroposterior dimensions out of proportion to the size of the face and body of the infant (Fig. 13-2, *A*). The roof of the orbit is depressed, and the eyes are displaced downward and outward with unusual prominence of the whites of the eyes. Distention of the superficial veins is apparent, and the scalp is thin and fragile (Fig. 13-2, *B*). Radiographic examination of the skull shows thinning of the bones with separation of the sutures and widening of the fontanels. A ventriculogram would demonstrate enlargement of the ventricular system. Computerized axial tomography provides a picture of the ventricular system along with tissue densities and the presence of any space-occuping masses. The child is sluggish and lies quietly in bed without normal activity. The process, if of the communicating type, may become arrested spontaneously or may go on to cause optic atrophy, spasticity of the extremities, convulsions, malnutrition, and death. If the child lives, mental and physical retardation may occur.

*Treatment.* The noncommunicating, obstructive type of hydrocephalus is treated by elimination of the obstruction, if this is possible. In some cases this is done by removal of tumors that fill the ventricles or compress them from without.

A temporary treatment termed ''ventriculostomy'' may also be used. Ventriculostomy is an opening into the lateral ventricles for purposes of providing external continuous ventricular drainage (CVD) and is important for (1) temporary drainage of cerebrospinal fluid in certain conditions (nonfunctional shunts, central nervous system infection, postinfectious hydrocephalus, normal pressure hydrocephalus, papillomas of the choroid plexus, hydrocephalus from tumors affecting central nervous circulation), (2) establishing an opening to sample cerebrospinal fluid and instilling medications or inject contrast media for diagnostic studies, and (3) a portal of entry useful in continuous intracranial pressure monitoring.

More permanent methods usually involve shunting. One method of treatment is the insertion of a tube into the occipital horn of the lateral ventricle, the other end of which is fixed into the cisterna magna (Torkildsen) thus obstruction in between is bypassed. The treatment of choice consists of the insertion of a siliconized rubber catheter into a lateral ventricle, the other end of which is passed through the external jugular vein into the right auricle (auricular ventriculostomy). With this system, normal ventricular pressure can be maintained and the excess cerebrospinal fluid channeled through the auricle into the general circulation and excreted (Table 13-3).

**Expected outcomes**

1 Complications will be prevented.
2 Parent-child bonding will be facilitated.
3 Infant will be in optimal physical and emotional condition for surgery.
4 Family will be involved in all aspects of care.
5 Family will be able to explain diagnostic studies, purposes of shunt, hydrocephalus, signs of increased intracranial pressure and infection.
6 Family will be able to identify age and developmentally appropriate activities of multisensorial stimulation.
7 Family will be able to identify child's psychosocial, physical, and intellectual capacities and appropriate utilization plan for community resources.
8 Family relationships will be harmonious and mutually supportive.

*Preoperative nursing intervention*

ENVIRONMENT. The environment is controlled as for any young infant. Room temperature is regulated according to the infant's needs. Exposure to drafts is avoided. The infant's clothes do not require modification from those in routine use in a nursery.

**TABLE 13-3.** Procedures for surgical correction of hydrocephalus*

| Procedure | Problem | Description | Purpose |
|---|---|---|---|
| Choroid plexectomy (Dandy) | Communicating type | Transcortical exposure of lateral ventricles to coagulate or excise choroid plexuses | Reduces cerebrospinal fluid production |
| Lumbar subarachnoid ureterostomy (Heile) | Communicating type | After lumbar laminectomy and left nephrectomy, polyethylene tube passed from lumbar subarachnoid space through paraspinal muscles into free ureter | Excess cerebrospinal fluid drained through ureter to bladder |
| Lumbar subarachnoid peritoneostomy | Communicating type | After lumbar laminectomy, polyethylene tube passed from subarachnoid space around flank and into peritoneum | Less effective method of draining cerebrospinal fluid that spares kidney; may be used when temporary shunt needed |
| Third ventriculostomy (Dandy) | Obstructive type | Opening made on anterior wall of floor of third ventricle into interpeduncular cistern | Cerebrospinal fluid drained into cisterna chiasmatis of subarachnoid space; not commonly done; used when cisterna magna not available for Torkildsen procedure |
| Ventriculocisternostomy (Torkildsen) | Obstructive type | Polyethylene tube extended from lateral ventricle through bur hole in occipital skull area under scalp to posterior fossa, where inserted into cisterna magna or cervical subarachnoid space | Successful method for diverting fluid past obstructed third ventricle or aqueduct of Sylvius |
| Auriculoventriculostomy (Matson) | Both types | Tube passed from lateral ventricle through bur hole in parietal skull area under skin for continuation down jugular vein to discharge cerebrospinal fluid into superior vena cava or right atrium by one-way valves (such as Spitz-Holter, Heyer-Pudenz) to avoid reflux of blood into ventricles and to drain excess cerebrospinal fluid into blood when ventricular pressure increases | Cerebrospinal fluid directed into general circulation |
| Ventriculoureterostomy (Matson) | Obstructive type | Polyethylene tube passed from lateral ventricle down dorsal spine subcutaneously below to twelfth rib, where inserted through paraspinal muscles into free ureter (after nephrectomy) | Rarely used; alternative to auriculoventriculostomy, especially if obstruction includes basilar and cerebral subarachnoid spaces, posterior fossa, and spinal subarachnoid spaces |
| Ventriculoperitoneostomy (Cone) | Obstructive type | Tube passed from lateral ventricle subcutaneously down dorsal spine for reinsertion into peritoneal cavity | Temporary measure of diverting cerebrospinal fluid that spares kidney; commonly used in children |
| Ventriculofallopian or spinofallopian tube shunt | Both types | Tube passed from lateral ventricle or spinal subarachnoid space into ligated fallopian tube and finally into peritoneal cavity for absorption | Diverts cerebrospinal fluid into peritoneal cavity; method of limited effectiveness |
| Ventriculopleural shunt | Both types | Diverts cerebrospinal fluid from lateral ventricle into pleural cavity | Unpopular method for diverting cerebrospinal fluid from engorged ventricles |

*Modified from Conway, B.L.: Pediatric neurologic nursing, St. Louis, 1977, The C.V. Mosby Co.

POSITION. Frequent change of position is stressed to eliminate prolonged pressure on the head. The scalp, usually thin and fragile, is sensitive to pressure and becomes reddened, and bedsores occur very quickly. The weight of the head can be distributed more evenly if a small sponge rubber or water pillow is used. Keep the head elevated 20 or 30 degrees to increase drainage from the brain. The principles of posturing previously outlined may be applied in a modified form. When the child is picked up and held, support the head carefully.

OBSERVATIONS. The child's general behavior and reactions to care are noted. Daily measurement of the head and chest is made to note changes. (Comparison of these is important during the first 2 years of life, since they enlarge at approximately the same rate; for example, at birth the head measures 33 to 35 cm, the chest 31 to 35 cm; at 3 months the head measures 39 to 41 cm, the chest 38 to 43 cm; at 6 months the head measures 41 to 43 cm, the chest 42 to 45 cm.) Frequent checking of the size, fullness, and tension of the anterior fontanel is done to gauge more effectively the degree of pressure. It is important to watch for symptoms of increasing intracranial pressure as manifested by changes in alertness, anorexia, vomiting, convulsions, or changes in the vital signs.

NUTRITION. Diet generally is regulated by the pediatrician and individual infant needs. Hold the infant during a feeding. Fluids may be restricted, unless contraindicated by fever or dehydration. If the infant is vomiting, feedings are administered by nasal tube, or intravenous injections. Weigh the infant at least once weekly and more often if indicated.

HYGIENE. Bathing and special skin care are given according to the routine of the nursery.

ELIMINATION. Elimination is usually not a problem unless there is a coexisting spinal anomaly.

DIAGNOSTIC STUDY. The diagnostic study includes complete physical, psychological, and neurological examinations, radiographic examination of the skull, ventricular dye test (Dandy), lumbar puncture (or ventricular puncture depending on degree and chronicity of increased intracranial pressure), complete blood count, urine examination, blood Kahn testing, blood typing, and Rh-factor determination. Pneumoencephalography, ventriculography, or CAT scans may be done in certain cases, especially when hydrocephalus is secondary in type and believed to be the result of an intracranial lesion. These tests are discussed in detail in Chapter 12.

PREPARATION FOR OPERATION. Check the operative permit. Notify the family of the hour of the operation. Check the typing and cross matching of blood. Make arrangements for blood should transfusion be necessary. Cut the infant's hair and gently shampoo the scalp the night before operation. Omit feedings for the 12-hour period preceding operation. Shave the infant's head in the morning. Measure temperature, pulse, respiration, and blood pressure as ordered.

A sedative may be given on the day of operation as indicated (usually given to the young infant with minimal water in a bottle). Specific medication such as atropine sulfate also may be given.

Change the infant's clothing as necessary; wrap in cotton blankets and take to the operating room with completed chart. It is important to note the infant's current weight on the chart. This frequently serves as a guide to the anesthetist in the administration of the anesthetic.

While the infant is in the operating room, every effort is made to prepare the environment most conducive to an uncomplicated postoperative course. Emergency equipment such as the following should be checked and kept in a place quickly and easily accessible:

Oxygen with funnel or Oxyhood attachment
Hypodermic tray with stimulating drugs
Suction machine with a catheter (No. 10 or 12 French)
Intravenous stand and intravenous regulator

The postoperative bed should be made according to the routine being practiced. The prepared crib should be taken to the operating room to receive the infant directly and to eliminate needless jarring and moving. The infant is returned to a room that facilitates close observation by the nurse.

*Postoperative nursing intervention.* It is recommended that the infant or child have a nurse in constant attendance during the first 24 hours after operation. The aspects of nursing care that follow are stressed.

OBSERVATIONS. If the following observations are

made accurately, the early recognition of complications will be facilitated.

GENERAL. Notes are made regarding the condition, color, and temperature of the body, the quality and rate of respiration and pulse (usually taken at the apex for accuracy), the rectal temperature, and blood pressure.

SPECIAL. Signs and symptoms of increasing intracranial pressure (drowsiness, irritability, apathy, vomiting, or convulsions) are noted, and the dressing is observed for the kind and amount of drainage. If the dressing permits, check the fontanels for fullness and tension at regular intervals. Daily measurement of the head and chest is continued. Note behavior, and chart pertinent data to determine the progress made by the infant. Care for the shunt, that is, pump, according to physician's and manufacturer's directions.

POSITION. Unless contraindicated, keep the head of the bed elevated 20 to 30 degrees. This position increases drainage from the brain, reduces venous congestion, and lowers intracranial pressure. Care is exercised to prevent unnecessary jostling and jarring of the infant's head. Change the position every hour, and support the head during each turning. Principles of posturing may be modified and applied as necessary to the individual infant. Every infant whose spontaneous activity is limited or whose motor function is impaired should be postured to prevent complications. A small sponge rubber pillow is used under the head to aid in the prevention of pressure sores. If there is difficulty in keeping the infant postured on the side, obtain an order for cloth restraints. Apply these loosely around the wrist and the knee of the uppermost extremities and secure them to the side of the crib. The restrained extremities should be checked and exercised frequently to prevent complications.

HYGIENE. Hygienic measures are carried out as in the preoperative period with special attention to all pressure areas, especially the scalp, to prevent breakdown. Cook's mouth ointment may be used on the lips and mucous membranes of the mouth as necessary to counteract the effects of dehydration or fever.

NUTRITION. Oral feedings, regulated by the pediatrician, are resumed as soon as the infant is completely conscious. If vomiting occurs, supplementary feedings may be given by nasogastric catheter.

Depending on the results of the operation, fluids may be restricted. After the third postoperative day the child, with the head well supported on the nurse's arm, should be picked up for feedings.

ELIMINATION. Generally no disturbance of bladder or bowel function is present. Routine observations are made and treatment given as necessary.

EMOTIONAL SECURITY. As the child convalesces, it is important to administer to emotional needs of sensory stimulation, acceptance, security, and parent-infant bonding. Regardless of age, a definite period of the day should be set aside for playing with him or her. Toys appropriate to mental age are provided to develop manipulative and discriminative skills. During the child's playtime the nurse can better observe and evaluate the progress being made. The infant should never be approached abruptly or noisily. Good physical support is maintained at all times to prevent precipitating the fear of falling. The nurse can make a definite contribution to the maintenance of emotional security by a positive physical and psychological approach.

COMPLICATIONS. (1) Shock, (2) meningitis, (3) pneumonia, (4) fever, (5) decubitus ulcers, (6) visual loss, (7) impairment of motor function, (8) spasticity, (9) contractures, (10) progressive mental deterioration.

The nurse plays an important role in the prevention and early recognition of these complications by maintaining a suitable environment, protecting the child from drafts, turning and posturing frequently, observing and reporting early signs, and making certain that nutrition is maintained.

DRESSING. Unless complications arise, the sutures are usually removed on the third postoperative day and the dressing on the seventh postoperative day. If the operation (coagulation of the choroid plexuses of the lateral ventricles) is done in two stages, the second stage follows 7 to 10 days after the first operation. The interval between depends on the individual child's recuperative powers and the absence of complications.

FOLLOW-UP CARE. At the time the child is discharged, the parents are given the necessary instructions regarding the care of the child. Examinations are planned at regular and frequent intervals for proper evaluation of progress. Psychological and developmental tests are administered at intervals of 2 to 6 months, depending on the child's age and rate of development.

## ARNOLD-CHIARI DEFORMITY

The Arnold-Chiari deformity frequently accompanies hydrocephalus and myelodysplasia, particularly in instances where the individual has a meningomyelocele. Other defects commonly associated include bony abnormalities in the base of the skull or at the site of the upper vertebrae and forking or stenosis in the aqueduct of Sylvius.

In the congenital problem known as the Arnold-Chiari deformity there is a tonguelike downward displacement of the cerebellar tonsils and medulla oblongata through the foramen magnum into the cervical area of the spinal canal. Crowding in the lower area is on a continuum and, depending on the situation, may cause the foramina of Luschka and Magendie to remain open or closed. In cases of severe compression the medulla may become twisted on the cord. The cisterna magna may be obliterated by adhesions between the cerebellum and medulla. The pathways of the upper cervical nerve roots are altered to an upward direction as they course to their intervertebral exits.

Many symptoms of the Arnold-Chiari deformity are frequently masked by concurrent symptoms of hydrocephalus and myelodysplasia. However, a few additional symptoms are evident in individuals with this problem, including nuchal rigidity, noisy respirations, weak suck reflex, irritability, vomiting, and preference for hyperextended posturing of the neck.

The diagnosis of this deformity is confirmed through roentgenography and ventriculography. Other entities that are ruled out in the differential evaluation are degenerative cerebellar diseases, space-occupying lesions in the posterior fossa, platybasia, and chronic adhesive arachnoiditis.

Relief of symptoms frequently occurs when compression from above is minimized after associated hydrocephalus is corrected surgically. When shunting does not correct the symptoms associated with the Arnold-Chiari deformity, suboccipital and upper cervical decompression may be indicated. The outcome is related to the severity of the deformity and the response to surgical correction.

Medical and nursing care includes the measures detailed in the discussions of spinal dysplasias and hydrocephalus. Because of the anatomical location of the problem, emphasis is placed on maintaining a patent airway and avoiding choking and aspiration during feedings. Special feeding techniques—thickened feedings, manual chin traction—are helpful in facilitating swallowing. Other techniques include slow feeding, frequent bubbling, and posturing the infant in an upright semi-Fowler's position during feeding.

## DEFECTS IN CEREBROVASCULAR DEVELOPMENT

The nervous system is affected by a number of disorders that alter the blood or the cerebrovascular system. Some of these problems, such as hemorrhage, embolism, or thrombosis, are detailed in Chapter 24. Other conditions that may also affect functions of the nervous system include anemias, problems that alter blood viscosity or its components, and disturbances related to intoxication or infection.

Additionally, there are six types of vascular abnormalities caused by faulty embryonic development, including meningeal angiomatosis, telangiectases, saccular aneurysms, venous angiomas, and arteriovenous fistulas.

*Meningeal angiomatosis* is more commonly termed "Sturge-Weber syndrome" and includes the following features: port-wine stain (facial nevus flammeus), mental retardation, seizures, hemiplegia on the side contralateral to the port-wine stain, calcium deposits in the cerebral cortex (seen on roentgenography), and characteristic eye changes (buphthalmos). Treatment is supportive, directive, and symptomatic.

Extensive occurrence of *telangiectases* (Osler-Weber-Rendu disease) is an autosomal dominant condition wherein small blood vessels contain calcium deposits and frequently dilate so that the walls become thin and vessels burst, with ensuing hemorrhage. Any body organ may contain these abnormal vessels. When they are in the brain, they are most often found in the pons, cerebrum, or cerebellum. Focal findings, cranial nerve disorders, clear or bloody spinal fluid, and late elevations of intracranial pressure are typical findings. Because of multiple points of involvement, sur-

**TABLE 13-4.** Comparison of venous angiomas and arteriovenous fistulas*

| Venous angiomas | Arteriovenous fistulas |
|---|---|
| Capillaries connecting arteries and veins | Communication between veins and arteries larger than capillaries |
| Veins containing venous blood | Arterial and venous blood mixed and brighter red, samples from jugular vein having higher oxygen concentration than normal |
| No pulsations or bruits | Frequently associated with pulsations and bruits |
| Nerve cells or glial fibers often between loops of veins, possibly calcium deposits in lesion | Possibly calcium deposits in walls of affected vessels |
| Rarely increased intracranial pressure | Frequent increased intracranial pressure, papilledema |
| No dilatation of vascular channels in vault and scalp | Often associated with increased vascularity of scalp and vault |
| Focal seizures | Focal seizures |
| Recurrent hemiplegia | Recurrent hemiplegia |

*From Conway, B.L.: Pediatric neurologic nursing, St. Louis, 1977, The C.V. Mosby Co.

gery is not feasible, and management is limited to measures that stop the bleeding. Death often occurs from hemorrhage.

*Saccular aneurysms* most typically affect the carotid arteries and the circle of Willis. Basilar and vertebral arteries of the posterior fossa are affected less often. Several problems may be responsible for saccular aneurysms, including congenital weakness of the vessel wall, processes like degenerative diseases, infectious processes (syphilis), overload from coarctation of the aorta, and emboli from bacterial endocarditis. Aneurysms are more fully discussed in Chapter 24.

A comparison between *venous angiomas* and arteriovenous fistulas is presented in Table 13-4. Generally, venous angiomas are not progressive, and problems are secondary; that is, hydrocephalus occurs if the abnormal vessels interfere with local ventricular functions, and mental retardation may result from the deformity causing prolonged convulsions. Intervention is supportive, aimed toward seizure control and assisting the individual in attaining the highest level of functioning in all areas of living. Surgical intervention and roentgenography are of limited value. When death occurs, it is related to complications arising secondary to the deformity.

*Arteriovenous fistulas* may result from congenital malformations or trauma. Arteriovenous malformations from congenital causes are discussed more fully in Chapter 24. Trauma in skull fractures accounts for the acquired type, since the fractures lacerate the internal carotid artery, allowing communication with the cavernous sinus.

About 90% of the individuals with a congenital arteriovenous malformation experience symptoms after 10 years of age. The type of symptoms depends on the location of the lesion. In many cases as much as 10 years lapse between the onset of symptoms and the development of impairments. For up to 40% of affected individuals the first indication of an arteriovenous malformation is a hemorrhage into the subarachnoid space. These hemorrhages are discussed in Chapter 24.

Familial cerebellar ataxia is an inherited disorder that progresses until death occurs.

## VASCULAR ABNORMALITIES OF THE SPINAL CORD

Telangiectases may be evident in the spinal cord. Sudden hematomyelia without blood in the spinal fluid is a common finding. Acute evidence of symptoms is followed by improvement. Cord compression results if these lesions are located in the vertebrae or epidural coverings. Cutaneous nevi are commonly associated.

Venous angiomas, most often found in men, are located below the fifth thoracic segment. Symptoms include severe root pain and cord damage in rounds of acute episodes with periods of improvement. About two thirds of these individuals have elevated protein levels in the spinal fluid, whereas the other third exhibits normal findings with occasional alterations in the lymphocytes.

Arteriovenous malformations are most commonly found between the upper lumbar segments and the seventh cervical segment in the distal cord or in the cervical enlargement of the proximal cord. Symptoms may be abrupt or insidious and may be related to compression, hemorrhage, or thrombosis of a blood vessel. Episodes begin before 15 years of age and wax and wane through the years in the insidious type. Audible bruits are not found. Findings include bloody spinal fluid and symptoms related to an obstruction in the spinal canal. Chronic damage over several years usually results in paraplegia.

## CEREBRAL PALSY

Cerebral palsy, also called *Little's disease,* or *spastic paralysis,* is primarily a disorder of the pyramidal motor system that may involve one, two, three, or all four extremities. The three major clinical types of cerebral palsy are spastic (about 65%), athetoid (25%), and ataxic (10%). Cerebral palsy is generally believed to be the largest single cause of the crippling of children. Seven out of 10 cases result from prenatal factors or trauma during delivery. A higher incidence occurs in breech and midforceps than in normal deliveries and in premature (almost 50%) than in full-term births. A birth weight of less than 5 pounds may also be an important factor in the incidence of cerebral palsy.

Oxygen deprivation (anoxia) of the brain is believed to be an important causative factor. If the expectant mother is afflicted with rubella virus (German measles), cytomegalovirus (salivary gland virus), or *Toxoplasma gondii* during her pregnancy, serious harm may be done to the developing nervous system of the fetus. Toxemia of pregnancy or maternal diabetes also may affect the fetus adversely and predispose it to cerebral palsy.

Scientists at the Laboratory of Perinatal Physiology in Bethesda have found in their research on rhesus monkeys that hormones released under psychological stress can cause physiochemical reactions in the mother that result in less oxygen to the fetus, thus causing brain damage. The implications of this discovery in primates have not yet been determined for the human.

The practice of doing tests routinely on all pregnant women has resulted in the detection of parental blood incompatibilities and made possible massive exchange blood transfusions in the newborn. Consequently, the previous incidence of cerebral palsy from this cause has been reduced.

It has been established that the age of the mother, sibling rank, race, and economic status are not causative factors. However, developmental disorders occur more frequently in infants whose mothers are in their teens or over 35 years of age. Cerebral palsy is not hereditary and is not contagious. It can afflict anyone at any time before, during, or after birth.

Cerebral palsy commonly occurs in the postneonatal period after encephalitis, meningitis, or cerebral trauma.

The pathological condition consists of localized or widely distributed cerebral atrophy. The lesions, which primarily affect the control of the voluntary motor system, may be found in various areas of the brain (motor cortex, basal ganglia, and cerebellum).

***Signs and symptoms.*** The symptoms of cerebral palsy may range from a mild muscular incoordination to severe spasticity or violent convulsions. No two clients present the same picture. Depending on the extent and location of the cerebral atrophy, a tremendous range and variety exist in the symptoms and in the combination and number of symptoms. The most common symptom is an awkward ataxic gait. Lack of muscular control and lack of balance may be present. From 25% to 50% of the persons with cerebral palsy have seizures; more than 60% are mentally retarded; about 50% have speech problems (dysarthria, aphasia, agnosia, apraxia); more than 33% have visual disorders; and 20% have hearing difficulties. Perceptual disabilities and dental anomalies may be present. Choking and difficulty in swallowing may also occur. Because of the motor, sensory, and intellectual manifestations, the individual with cerebral palsy may develop serious emotional and social problems.

In severely afflicted infants the condition is obvious at birth. Cyanosis, feeble crying, and the inability to nurse are seen early. The head may be retracted, the body arched, and the extremities spastic. Depending on the areas involved, the following also may be present: tumors, athetoid movements, incoordination, and ataxia. The outlook is poor, and the child may die within a year. In less severe cases the abnormality is not noticeable for several months and then only because the child cannot hold the head up properly, is usable to sit or stand, or exhibits a prolonged and exaggerated asymmetric tonic neck response. Because of spasticity, the legs may criss cross (the scissors position). As he or she becomes older, the child stands on the toes when trying to walk. Mild cases have been noted in which the spasticity is minimal, and the gait is only slightly disturbed.

The child's muscular control and coordination may be abnormally slow in developing. Although these tend to improve with age, the lag in motor performance increases.

About 20% of the persons who have cerebral palsy are ambulatory and fairly independent; 50% are moderately handicapped; and 30% are severely handicapped.

More than 60% of those afflicted with cerebral palsy show some degree of mental retardation, and less than 40% show no impairment of intellectual function. The intellectual level should be established by a battery of psychological tests. Often a child seems duller than he or she actually is because of an associated speech disorder. Mental age as well as physical disabilities should be considered before recommendations are made for treatment and care.

Generally this disease is not progressive, though the abnormal motor and sensory functions are more obvious as the child grows; the rate of development of motor, speech, intellectual, and social abilities is delayed. Cerebral palsy is the end result of some process that interferes with the normal development of the brain.

### Expected outcomes

Use outcomes 1, 4, 6, 7, and 8 under the discussion of hydrocephalus. Use the following outcomes from Table 13-1 (A, 1, 2, and 5; B, 1 to 3; C, 1 to 5; D, 1 and 2). Refer to client outcomes listed under mental retardation. The family will be able to explain causes of cerebral palsy, subsequent individual outcomes, current treatment, and specific ways that they may improve functions in their child. The family will have comprehensive assistance and awareness of applicable resources in the community for all their needs.

***Treatment and management.*** No cure for cerebral palsy and no effective treatment have been found. However, recent developments offer some hope for the future treatment of cerebral palsy victims. Levodopa has been used to treat nine clients with athetoid cerebral palsy at the Hospital for Special Surgery in New York. The investigators reported that eight of these clients showed varying degrees of improvement; symptoms were decreased, and their ability fo function improved. Dantrolene sodium is effective in decreasing muscle tone and spasticity but causes severe short-term effects. Diazepam (Valium) is also helpful in improving function in some clients.

Stereotactic thalamotomy has been performed to relieve spasticity with some success. A few researchers have reported that a peripheral nerve block with phenol has alleviated spasticity in selected clients.

Striking improvement in motor capacities has occurred from the insertion of cerebellar stimulators and appropriate physiotherapy. This surgery, though relatively new in human beings, offers great promise for the young child who has exhausted other modes of treatment. Although the long-term implications of these implants are as yet unknown, the resulting improvement in functional capacities in surgical candidates is both welcome and encouraging to the child and family who previously held little hope for improvement to this level of functioning.

Therapeutic intervention is directed toward fostering the normal development of the child and toward preventing secondary complications. Early diagnosis and individual management are imperative if the child's potentialities are to be developed and if physical complications and emotional and social maladjustment are to be prevented.

Each person with cerebral palsy presents a unique problem of treatment. One cannot make a plan for the victims of cerebral palsy as a group because their motor, sensory, intellectual, emotional, and social handicaps are varied in number, in nature, and in degree. They share in common with each other and with persons who do not have cerebral palsy the needs for affection, love, friendship, support, self-identity, respect, a feeling of worth and accomplishment, education, recreation, and satisfying and productive work. They react in the same way if their needs are not fulfilled, are subject to the same frustrations and anxiety, and, because of their disabilities, are especially vulnerable in their relationships with others. Ultimately social deprivation and isolation may be greater handicaps than the physical disability.

*Nursing interventions.* In common with parents of children with other chronic, handicapping disorders the parents of children with cerebral palsy have guilt feelings and are ambivalent toward the afflicted child. Unfortunately each parent tends to blame the other for the defective child, and their relationship may be in jeopardy because of feelings of anger, resentment, guilt, and inadequacy. If these feelings are not shared and resolved, the child will be aware of the conflict and lack of harmony. He or she may capitalize on the situation and manipulate one parent against the other or feel rejected and withdraw from interpersonal contacts.

Because the sharing of problems are resources was seen as helpful, many states and communities have organized parent groups. They provide not only support to parents but also information and a variety of services for those who have cerebral palsy.

To be effective the treatment program must include guidance and support of the parents and siblings of the afflicted child. The parents are the core of the program and must be helped to create the type of family setting in which love, reasonable discipline and freedom, and appropriate stimulation and outlets for self-assertive and self-directive behavior are provided so that the handicapped child and brothers and sisters may develop into well-adjusted adults. Parents need emotional as well as intellectual understanding of their child and themselves if they are to work through their negative feelings, frustrations, and anxiety and accept him or her and the limitations imposed by the disease. The parents' attitude toward the child influences personality growth and development and, to a large extent, adjustment to the disability, to the family, to society, and to life. Parents who capitulate to the child's whims and demands overlook their own needs and rights. This attitude of oversubmission generally results from a feeling of guilt. The growing child who has all requests satisfied tends to make increasingly unreasonable demands and, if they are not fulfilled, reacts with temper tantrums. Furthermore, since the child has not learned to respect the rights of others, he or she is inconsiderate of them and preoccupied with the immediate satisfaction of personal needs. Overin-

dulgence, manifested by showering toys and services on the handicapped child indiscriminately, tends to perpetuate dependence on others and to prevent the development of independent thinking and mature behavior. Both these parental attitudes inhibit the child's normal emotional development, and, because of the associated learned behavior, he or she is alienated from other children.

If the handicapped child is rejected by parents and siblings, he or she becomes hostile and anxious, tending to isolate himself or herself from contacts with others in order not to be hurt by their rejection.

Depending on their level of maturity and the nature and degree of disability, parents tend to react differently toward the child. The parents of a mildly handicapped child have considerable difficulty in accepting the reality of the child's disabilities and have a strong need to prove there is nothing wrong and he or she is normal. As a result, they expect competition with normal children and set standards for performance beyond achievement. The child faced with repeated failure becomes anxious and insecure and is unable to accept the disability. If parents set realistic goals and help the child to develop at his or her own rate and level, through successful experiences the child can become self-confident, independent, and well adjusted.

The mother especially must be helped to foster progressive independence within the capability of the child. Setting limits for a disabled child poses a real problem for most parents. They may be overprotective or too permissive and afraid that discipline will hurt the child. As do normal children, the disabled child needs consistent and reasonable discipline in order to feel secure and develop normally.

The parents of the severely handicapped child have low expectations and foster his or her dependency on them. This child is secure in their love and has little anxiety but is immature and will not develop whatever potentialities he or she may have.

An integrated program of physical therapy, speech therapy, occupational therapy, psychotherapy, play, and education is directed toward helping the child to develop, within the limitations imposed by disease, the skills needed to deal with the activities of everyday living and to adjust to the environment. Goals are related to the meeting of needs and must be achievable in a short time in order to provide motivation. Each child should participate in his or her own care, do as much as possible alone, and receive only the amount of help and direction absolutely necessary to supplement his or her own efforts. Depending on the extent of intellectual and physical disability, opportunities for educational and social activities are provided and utilized within as normal a setting as possible. It is desirable for the child, whenever possible, to attend school with brothers, sisters, and playmates. He or she must learn how to get along with others, how to communicate, how to get about, how to use leisure, how to live safely, how to stay healthy, how to take care of physical needs, and how to become as self-controlling, self-directing, and self-supporting as possible.

Training in walking, acquiring balance, and the coordinated use of muscles and exercises is directed toward reducing disability and increasing motor performance. Braces, the surgical lengthening or shortening of a tendon, or the fusing of a joint also may improve the individual's level of function and decrease the disability. The production of lesions in the thalamic nuclei employing stereotactic surgical techniques has offered significant benefits by the reduction of the involuntary activity associated with severe athetoid movements or hemiballismus.

The child may have difficulty in swallowing because the wave motion of the tongue, which normally pushes the food back and down the throat, is reversed, and the food is pushed forward and out. This creates a feeding problem in the infant and young child; artificial methods (such as tube and intravenous feedings) of maintaining an optimal level of nutrition may be necessary. When the child grows older, he or she is taught to place food on the back of the tongue and to tip the head backward, thus inhibiting the reversed action of the tongue. At least 1 hour is needed for each meal. If choking is a problem, puree the food, and supervise the child closely during meals.

If the child has athetoid movements and is constantly in motion, he or she will need a high caloric diet to prevent weight loss. If he or she is spastic and moves about with difficulty, less food is needed, and caloric intake should be regulated so that excess weight will not further increase the disability.

Occupational therapy may be prescribed to train the child to use the hands in creative and practical activities, help develop good work habits, improve span of attention and concentration, determine capacity for work, evaluate assets and liabilities, and provide opportunities to work and socialize with other persons. The ultimate aim of any program is to develop abilities so that the individual can be employed and be economically independent. Depending on particular capacities, with vocational training he or she should be able to function in almost any type of occupation. In appropriate jobs the individual with cerebral palsy is as efficient as others without any handicap.

## Cerebral palsy associations and research

The United Cerebral Palsy Associations, Inc.,* a national, voluntary, nonprofit organization, was founded in 1949 to alleviate, control, and prevent cerebral palsy. It has the following specific objectives:

To direct and unify the overall, long-range attack on the entire problem of cerbral palsy
To help provide the needed treatment, care, and education
To train the disabled for employment and help them find jobs
To foster and finance research in causes and treatment
To help solve the critical shortage of therapists, vocational counselors, teachers, and other specialists
To give guidance to the parents of children with cerebral palsy
To encourage legislation to help those who have cerebral palsy
To furnish information
To promote public understanding of the problems and special needs of those who have cerebral palsy
To help local affiliated associations provide direct services to persons with cerebral palsy: treatment, guidance, education, recreation, and transportation
To raise funds to carry on its activities and achieve its aims

In 1955 the United Cerebral Palsy Research and Educational Foundation was established as an in-

---

*The United Cerebral Palsy Associations, Inc., 321 W. 44th St., New York, N.Y., 10036.

dependent subsidiary of the United Cerebral Palsy Association, Inc. It sponsors research in normal and abnormal brain functions and professional training in various scientific, medical, and paramedical disciplines.

The National Institute of Neurological Diseases and Stroke is closely associated with the United Cerebral Palsy Research Foundation, the National Association for Retarded Children and Adults, and the Association for the Aid of Crippled Children in seeking to overcome these disorders.

Since 1960 the NINDS has sponsored a nationwide study, *Collaborative Project on Cerebral Palsy, Mental Retardation, and Other Neurological and Sensory Disorders of Infancy and Childhood* (also called *Collaborative Perinatal Project*). Fourteen major obstetrical centers conducted detailed studies on more than 58,000 women and their infants who were followed up until they were 8 years old. In addition to prenatal and delivery data, periodic special examinations were done to detect any neurological defect that may have resulted from unfavorable events of pregnancy. The mothers participating in this study have been studied extensively, completing records of drugs taken and of any accidents, infections, or illnesses occurring during pregnancy.

The data collection on the follow-up study of the children was completed in 1974, and an exhaustive analysis of all the data was then accomplished. It is hoped that the identification of cause-and-effect relationships will make it possible to take steps toward preventing disease and injury in the prenatal period, thus averting permanent brain damage.

Researchers at the NINDS Laboratory of Perinatal Physiology in Bethesda are continuing their studies on rhesus monkeys relating to birth defects, reproduction, and social behavior. They are attempting to create nervous system disorders in these monkeys comparable to those in humans to develop better understanding of the brain and behavior.

Investigators in the Surgical Neurology Branch, Section on Children, are collecting histological, histochemical, and biochemical data from autopsies on children who had neurological disorders. These data are being correlated with clinical data in an effort to develop knowledge that will lead to effective preventive and therapeutic measures.

# HEMORRHAGES

Birth trauma may result in bleeding most commonly into the sternocleidomastoid muscle and cranium. Bleeding into the sternocleidomastoid muscle results in torticollis, or "wryneck," a condition wherein the child holds the head tilted to one side. Exercises and encouragement to shift the head by rotation of the crib are conservative modes of treatment. Persistent cases may require surgery.

When blood accumulates under the skull, it forms a soft, fluctuating mass that is unaltered by pressure changes from crying and does not pulsate. No treatment is required, since the accumulation reabsorbs in several weeks to a few months.

Although the most common intracranial bleeding disorders involve hemorrhage into the subarachnoid and subdural spaces, bleeding may also occur in other portions of the brain. Common clinical signs include restlessness, irritability, lethargy, opisthotonus, disturbed respiratory and cardiac functions, high-pitched cry, poor feeding patterns, muscle twitching, meningeal irritation, and seizures. Retinal hemorrhages and inadequate pupil response are other common findings. Paralysis may be seen if compression occurs from accumulating fluids. The Moro reflex may be absent or abnormal. Treatment regimens vary but often include lumbar punctures to reduce increased intracranial pressure and remove blood in the subarachnoid space. Subdural hematomas are treated by subdural punctures and occasionally, in persistent cases, by surgery.

Chronic subdural hematomas in an infant signal the practitioner to evaluate the infant in light of the possibility of child abuse wherein repeated insults to the cranium have occurred. In older individuals, chronic subdural hematomas are more commonly related to such problems as alcoholism, wherein the inebriated individual strikes the head repeatedly without awareness of injury as he or she stumbles about.

Nursing care emphasizes physical and psychological support of the infant, along with emotional support and explanation for the family. In addition to maintenance of body processes, the practitioner is concerned about the infant's warmth and rest. Elevation of the head and minimal handling are important. Antibiotics are administered prophylactically along with vitamin K. Sedation may be needed for the restless infant. Serial neurological observations are imperative to detect any accumulation of blood and problem of local compression at an early point. If this buildup affects the hindbrain, respiratory problems may result.

In extreme cases of intracranial hemorrhage the prognosis is grave, and death is a common outcome. In less severe cases problems such as cerebral palsy, seizures, mental retardation, or communicating hydrocephalus may result.

## REFERENCES

Asher, M., et al.: The myelomeningocele patient: a multidisciplinary approach to care, J. Kans. Med. Soc. **80:**403-408, 413, July 1979.

Avey, M.: Primary care for handicapped children, Am. J. Nurs. **73:**658-661, 1973.

Babson, S.G.: Diagnosis and management of the fetus and neonate at risk: a guide for team care, ed. 4, St. Louis, 1979, The C.V. Mosby Co.

Bensman, A., et al.: Myelomeningocele birth defect: habilitation of the child, Minn. Med. **54:**599-604, 1971.

Bierbauer, E.: Tips for parents of a neurologically handicapped child, Am. J. Nurs. **72:**1872-1874, 1972.

Blatz, R.: Advice to volunteers working with cerebral palsy patients, Hosp. Community Psychiatry **22:**7-8, Oct. 1971.

Bonine, G.N.: The myelodysplastic child, Am. J. Nurs. **69:**541, March 1969.

Boone, D.: Cerebral palsy, Studies in Communicative Disorders Series, Indianapolis, 1972, The Bobbs-Merrill Co., Inc.

Bracke, M., et al.: External drainage of cerebrospinal fluid, Am. J. Nurs. **78:**1355-1358, Aug. 1978.

Braney, M.L.: The child with hydrocephalus, Am. J. Nurs. **73:**828-831, 1973.

Chaube, S., et al.: The present status of prenatal detection of neural tube defects, Am. J. Obstet. Gynecol. **121:**429, Feb. 1975.

Clausen, J., et al.: Maternity nursing today, New York, 1976, McGraw-Hill Book Co.

Cooper, I.S., editor: Cerebellar stimulation in man, New York, 1978, Raven Press, Publishers.

Cruickshank, W.M., editor: Cerebral palsy: a developmental disability, ed. 3 (rev.), Syracuse, N.Y., 1976, Syracuse University Press.

Culp, D., Bekhrad, A., and Flocks, R.: Urological management of the meningomyelocele patient, J.A.M.A. **213:**753-758, 1970.

Dandy, W.: Diagnosis and treatment of hydrocephalus due to occlusion of the foramina of Magendie and Luschka, Surg. Gynecol. Obstet. **32:**112-124, Feb. 1921.

Dandy, W.: The brain. Section V. Hydrocephalus. Section VI. Encephalocele and meningocele. In Lewis' practice of surgery, vol. 12, Hagerstown, Md., 1944, W.F. Prior Co., Inc.

Davies, P.A., et al.: Very low birthweight and subsequent neurological defect, Dev. Med. Child Neurol. **17:**3, Feb. 1975.

Day, H.: Setting small goals: an effective way of providing nursing care for children, Hosp. Community Psychiatry **23:**126-128, April 1972.

Fisch, C.B.: Intellectual development of children with cerebral palsy. Presented at the annual meeting of the American Academy for Cerebral Palsy and Developmental Medicine, 1978.

Ford, F.R.: Diseases of the nervous system in infancy, childhood and adolescence, ed. 6, Springfield, Ill., 1973, Charles C Thomas, Publisher.

Grabow, J.D., et al.: Cerebellar stimulation for the control of seizures, Mayo Clin. Proc. **49:**759, Oct. 1974.

Hall, P., et al.: Scolosis and hydrocephalus in myelocele patients, J. Neurosurg. **50:**174-178, Feb. 1979.

Humphrey, P., et al.: Craniofacial malformations, Am. J. Nurs. **79:**1230-1234, July 1979.

Hardgrove, C., and Dawson, R.: Parents and children in the hospital, Boston, 1972, Little, Brown & Co.

Haynes, U.: Overview of the National Collaborative Infant Project, New York, 1974, United Cerebral Palsy Associations, Inc.

Hughes, J.G.: Synopsis of pediatrics, ed. 5, St. Louis, 1979, The C.V. Mosby Co.

Jabbour, J.T., et al.: Pediatric neurology handbook, New York, 1976, Medical Examination Publishing Co., Inc.

Kalisch, B.: Nursing actions in behalf of the battered child, Nurs. Forum **12:**365, 1973.

Keats, S.: Cerebral palsy, Springfield, Ill., 1977, Charles C Thomas, Publisher.

Landrieu, P., et al.: Hydrocephalus: a secondary phenomenon, Dev. Med. Child Neurol. **21:**637-642, Oct. 1979.

Lindenberg, R.E.: The need for crisis intervention in hospitals, Hospitals **46:**52-55, 110, Jan. 1, 1972.

Loetterle, B.C.: Cerebellar stimulation: pacing the brain, Am. J. Nurs. **75:**958, June 1975.

Marks, N.C.: Cerebral palsied and learning disabled children: a handbook guide to treatment, rehabilitation and education, Springfield, Ill., 1974, Charles C Thomas, Publisher.

Matson, D.D.: Surgical treatment of myelomeningocele, Pediatrics **42:**225-227, Aug. 1968.

McAndrew, I.: Adolescents and young people with spina bifida, Dev. Med. Child Neurol. **21:**619-629, 1979.

Miezio, P.: Care of the child with myelomeningocele: an overview, Nurs. Digest **1:**45, Nov. 1973.

Minde, K.K.: Coping styles of 34 adolescents with cerebral palsy, Am. J. Psychiatry **135:**1344, Nov. 1978.

New, P.F.J.: Computed tomography: a major diagnostic advance, Hosp. Pract. **10:**55, Feb. 1975.

NINDS Research Profiles: 1972: Summary of research at the National Institute of Neurological Diseases and Stroke, Cerebral palsy, 44-45, DHEW Publication No. (NIH) 72-323, USDHEW, Public Health Service, Washington, D.C., 1972, U.S. Government Printing Office.

Nogen, A.G.: Medical treatment for spasticity in children with cerebral palsy, Child's Brain **2:**304-308, 1976.

Passo, S.D.: Positioning infants with myelomeningocele, Am. J. Nurs. **74:**1658, Sept. 1974.

Passo, S.D.: Malformations of the neural tube, Nurs. Clin. North Am. **15:**5-21, March 1980.

Perkins, W.H.: Speech pathology: an applied behavioral science, ed. 2, St. Louis, 1977, The C.V. Mosby Co.

Petrillo, M.: Preventing hospital trauma in pediatric patients, Am. J. Nurs. **68:**1469-1478, 1968.

Petrillo, M., and Sanger, S.: Emotional care of hospitalized children, Philadelphia, 1972, J.B. Lippincott Co.

Pohutsky, L.C., and Pohutsky, K.R.: Computer axial tomography of the brain: a new diagnostic tool, Am. J. Nurs. **75:** 1341, Aug. 1975.

Salmon, J.H., Gonen, J.Y., and Brown, L.: Ventriculoatrial shunt for hydrocephalus ex-vacuo: psychological and clinical evaluation, Dis. Nerv. Syst. **32:**299-307, May 1971.

Samaha, F.J.: Electrodiagnostic studies in neuromuscular disease, N. Engl. J. Med. **285:**1244-1247, 1971.

Sanner, G.: Pathogenic and preventive aspects of nonprogressive ataxic syndromes, Dev. Med. Child Neurol. **21:**663-671, Oct. 1979.

Shalit, M.N., et al.: The management of obstructive hydrocephalus by the use of external continuous ventricular drainage, Acta Neurochir. **47:**161-172, 1979.

Shydro, J.: Child abuse, Nursing72 **2:**37, Dec. 1972.

Smolock, M.A.: The nurse's role in rehabilitation of the handicapped child, Nurs. Clin. North Am. **5:**411-420, Sept. 1970.

Swaiman, K.F., and Wright, F.S.: Pediatric neuromuscular diseases, St. Louis, 1979, The C.V. Mosby Co.

Teter, A.R., and Sawitzke, S.: Arteriovenous malformations of the brain, Cardiovasc. Nurs. **16**(3):13-17, May-June 1980.

Vaughan, V.C., III, and McKay, R.J., editors: Nelson textbook of pediatrics, ed. 11, Philadelphia, 1979, W.B. Saunders Co.

Vigliarolo, D.: Managing bowel incontinence in children with meningomyelocele, Am. J. Nurs. **80:**105-107, Jan. 1980.

Willson, N., editor: Infections of the nervous system, Philadelphia, 1979, F.A. Davis Co.

# 14

# PAROXYSMAL DISORDERS

In this chapter intense, periodic episodes involving the brain are discussed. Basically this category of problems encompasses the epilepsies and related disorders, headaches, and psychogenic problems that overlap these organic disorders. Psychogenic problems are covered in the discussions of the specific problems to which they relate.

## EPILEPSY

Epilepsy is a term first used by Hippocrates to denote a condition that *seizes* the client. Considered at one time to be of divine origin, it was called the *sacred disease*. In early English writings this condition was referred to as the *falling sickness*. Not until the latter part of the nineteenth century was a distinction made among the variations of this manifestation, which may be a symptom of some other disorder or a disease entity. At least 50 conditions are known that may cause seizures. The most common of these are cerebral trauma, cerebral vascular disease, cerebral atrophy, congenital defects, intracranial tumor, meningitis, encephalitis, diabetic acidosis, poisoning, and acute alcoholism. If meticulous medical and neurological evaluation fails to reveal the cause of the seizure, the diagnosis of *idiopathic epilepsy* is made. Some authorities do not classify individuals who have symptomatic seizures related to a known cause as epileptics and apply this term only to those who have idiopathic seizures.

The most suitable term for this condition is *seizure,* the English translation of the Hippocratic *epilepsy*. Other synonyms are *fit* and *convulsion*.

Hughlings Jackson's definition, a physiological one, is very much to the point: "Occasional, sudden, excessive, rapid, and local discharges of grey matter."* This applies whether the seizure is caused by a focal lesion such as a tumor or is without known pathological cause. It is now believed that any type of brief disturbance in consciousness or in autonomic, motor, or sensory function may be a convulsive manifestation. Generally, convulsive episodes of all types are accompanied by cerebral dysrhythmia.

## CATEGORIZATION

Since a seizure is to its cause as a sneeze is to a cold, seizures are categorized differently by various authors. The major ways of classifying seizure disorders are by clinical patterns, EEG tracings, and etiology. The most prevalent method is the international classification of seizures. (See boxed outline.) With regard to clinical patterns, a seizure represents a neuronal disturbance that results in abnormal electrical discharges. Involved neurons may recover with subsequent cessation of excessive electrical activity, or they may die, leaving an impairment in functional capacities behind. However, the seizure pattern that is clinically apparent is only the manifestation of an underlying problem. When the causative process is demonstrable, the disorder is termed *organic* or *secondary epilepsy*. If the cause remains undetermined, the seizure is termed *cryptogenic* or *idiopathic epilepsy*.

Although each of these paroxysmal disorders affects the cerebrum in characteristic patterns,

---

*From Selected writings of John Hughlings Jackson, vol. 1, On epilepsy and epileptiform convulsions, London, 1931, Hodder & Stoughton, Ltd.

---

**INTERNATIONAL CLASSIFICATION OF SEIZURES**

I. Focal or partial seizures
  A. Simple
    1. Motor
    2. Sensory
  B. Complex
    1. Psychomotor
  C. Extension of simple or complex partial to generalized convulsive activity
II. Generalized seizures
  A. Tonic-clonic (grand mal)
  B. Absence (petit mal)
  C. Infantile spasms
  D. Myoclonic
  E. Akinetic
III. Miscellaneous
  A. Unclassified
  B. More than one type occurring in the same client

---

evoking unusual motor, sensory, visceral, or psychological outcomes, a discussion of seizures solely by clinical classification is not sufficient for the description of seizure disorders in children. However, when these categories are applied to children after one considers anatomic origin, EEG tracing, and causative factors, along with characteristic clinical findings, a relevant description of seizure disorders in these children is possible.

Other conditions that need to be distinguished from classical seizures include reflex seizures, narcolepsy, abdominal epilepsy, breath-holding spells, hysterical fits, tonic fits, and various syncopal problems.

## INCIDENCE

Some 4 million individuals in the United States are afflicted with some type of seizure disorder. Whereas about 6% of all children experience a febrile convulsion once, only about 50% of these individuals have a subsequent seizure, which may or may not be accompanied by an elevated temperature. Although seizure disorders tend to occur in some families more frequently than in others, the exact mode of inheritance remains elusive. However, some experts theorize that persons with tendencies toward seizure disorders probably have a lower neuronal threshold, which results in vulnerability to abnormal neuronal discharges.

## PATHOGENESIS OF SEIZURE DISORDERS

Five basic problems are identified as causative factors underlying convulsive disorders. First, pathological processes, including (1) *errors in formation,* for example, arteriovenous malformations, porencephaly; (2) *infectious problems,* for example, meningitis, encephalitis; (3) *space-occupying lesions,* for example, tumors, hematomas, abscesses, cystic masses; (4) *hemorrhages into the cranial cavity;* (5) *head trauma;* (6) *neuronal damage from deficient supplies,* for example, anoxia or hypoglycemia; (7) *acute cerebral edema,* for example, that secondary to acute glomerulonephritis; (8) *degenerative disorders,* for example, the leukodystrophies; or (9) *cerebrovascular accidents,* for example, emboli or thrombosis, may result in seizures. Second, *toxic endogenous* (uremia) or *exogenous* (the ingestion of such substances as pentylenetetrazol [Metrazol], alcohol intoxication, or abrupt withdrawal, especially when disulfiram (Antabuse) is taken, or lead ingestion, resulting in encephalopathy) substances may result in seizures. *Disturbances in metabolic capacities* that result in interferences with such essential supplies as calcium, oxygen, and glucose may precipitate seizures. Included in this metabolic category are the inborn errors of metabolism. *Fever* is another factor that may precipitate a convulsion in some individuals with decreased neuronal thresholds. Finally, many seizures are termed *idiopathic.*

## FACTORS INVOLVED IN SEIZURE DISORDERS

In making the differential diagnosis with regard to the causative factors and type of seizure patterns in a child, several factors should be considered during the history-taking process and the performance of the physical evaluation, namely, age, type of seizures, history, physical assessment, laboratory data, and direct precipitating events.

### Age

Convulsive disorders are caused by very different problems at various ages. For example, in the neonatal age group, oxygen deficiencies to the brain and traumatic hemorrhages are the two major causes of convulsions. However, such abnormalities as hypoglycemia, hyperbilirubinemia, or decreases in ionized calcium are other important causes of seizures in the perinatal period. Congenital abnormalities resulting in seizures in young children may be easily mistaken for sequelae of trauma occuring during the labor and delivery process. Other common causes of seizure disorders in this age group include narcotic withdrawal in infants born to addicted mothers, neonatal tetanus, pyridoxine dependency, or meningitis.

A second arbitrary age group comprises children from the ages of 1 month to 3 years. During this period, idiopathic seizures are often seen for the first time. Diseases that result in major functional impairments in brain activities, that is, Sturge-Weber syndrome, phenylketonuria, or tuberous sclerosis, are associated with convulsive episodes that begin at this time. When prior neuronal damage has occurred, initial evidence of the resulting convulsive disorder may be observed at this time. This age group is also one wherein acute illnesses, such as gastrointestinal disorders with subsequent electrolyte imbalances, meningitis, or the ingestion of toxic foreign substances, may result in a convulsion. Hypoglycemic episodes and subdural hematomas are other important causative factors in this age group.

In children more than 3 years of age, residual neuronal damage from former injuries may be evident in convulsions. However, idiopathic problems or identifiable disease states are far more significant contributors to a convulsion. Disease states that may produce a convulsion include a renal disorder (such as uremia or hypertension), hypoglycemia, metabolic disorders, degenerative disease processes, space-occupying lesions, or inflammatory disorders such as meningitis.

Seizures may occur any time from infancy to old age, but most commonly the idiopathic disorder begins at puberty or in the 5 years before or after it. About 70% of all convulsive disorders begin before the age of 20 years. The onset of convulsions after 30 years of age in the absence of a head injury calls for most careful diagnostic scrutiny to determine if a discrete organic lesion is present. Cerebrovascular or neoplastic diseases are the most frequent cause of convulsions after 50

years of age. The frequency of seizures varies greatly; they may occur at intervals of minutes or hours to months or years. Female epileptics have a predilection to convulsions just before the menstrual period; sometimes during pregnancy they have been free from attacks that before and after had been numerous. Although convulsions may occur at any time of the day, they are more common at night or in the early morning. An objective change of personality or behavior or a subjective feeling of distress may be noted a day or more before the seizure is experienced.

## Type of seizure

Grand mal (tonic-clonic) and focal motor convulsions are not age specific but may be seen at all ages. Other types of seizures are confined primarily to certain ages.

In the neonatal period, seizure activity may be characterized by a period of sucking, apnea, unresponsiveness, or rigidity. However, at times these behaviors occur normally. To detect which of these behaviors constitutes a seizure disorder, it is necessary to have an EEG tracing recording brain-wave activities during the suspicious activity.

In the second age group, comprising children from 1 month to 3 years of age, so-called minor motor seizures—myoclonic seizures, akinetic spells, or head dropping— may occur in conjunction with a hypsarrhythmic wave configuration on the EEG tracing. This type of seizure disorder may be related to an unknown cause or to known metabolic factors or cerebral trauma. Febrile convulsions are also prevalent in this age group. Breath-holding spells are often observed in this age group and, although they are not seizures, are still given due consideration in the differential diagnosis.

In children more than 3 years of age, three other distinct types of seizure disorders may be observed, including petit mal (absence), temporal lobe (psychomotor or complex partial), and focal sensory seizures. Although focal sensory seizures may actually occur before this age, evaluation of these phenomena are difficult because the young child is unable to describe the sensory experience. The incidence of convulsions occurring after head trauma depends on the type of injury and the severity of brain damage and ranges from 1% to 50%. If epilepsy is a complication, the first seizure occurs within 6 months in more than 50% of those who sustain severe head injuries.

The symptoms and signs may be considered according to whether the seizure is a tonic-clonic or an absence spell. A person with convulsions may be subject to both major and minor seizures or to one type only. Men appear more susceptible to the psychomotor type and women to petit mal (absence).

### History

A thorough history is the cornerstone of a precise diagnosis. (Chapter 11 offers details on the neurological history.) Since so many processes may result in seizure disorders, one should carefully elicit any specifics on the prenatal and perinatal periods, capacities related to patterns of growth and development, and any problems requiring medical or surgical intervention that potentially predispose to seizures. Patterns of family inheritance should also be considered, since many inherited problems are related to seizure disorders.

### Physical assessment

When the client is evaluated during wellness, great pains may be taken in conducting a thorough assessment. However, if the client is convulsing, the physical assessment is necessarily limited to essential components related directly to treatment. After a major motor seizure, confusion, lethargy, agitation, or other postictal changes may be observed. However, neurological abnormalities that persist beyond this period indicate a preexisting cause other than the immediate convulsive episode. Dermal changes—rashes, signs of infectious processes, or other markings (port-wine stain, petechiae, and so on)—may provide clues to the underlying disease process. Refer to Chapters 13 and 20.

### Laboratory data

A complete blood count and urinalysis are valuable in indicating the presence of a systemic problem. Special studies, such as amino acid screening, may be indicated in some children. An evaluation of the individual's ability to metabolize glucose is valuable in determining the possible existence of hypoglycemia. A serum calcium and blood urea nitrogen analysis may reveal the cause of seizures in the neonate as well as in the older child, who may have a disturbance of the parathyroid glands or the renal system. Many agencies run a chemistry profile rather than the individual studies. Thus additional data on the client's condition is also available.

The lumbar puncture may yield valuable data on abnormal processes involving the central nervous system, as detailed in Chapters 12 and 20. Radiographic studies of the skull are utilized to detect such problems as separation of the sutures, bony erosion, and unusual areas of calcification. Electroencephalography represents brain-wave patterns for processes affecting the cerebral cortex. Invasive techniques—ventriculography, pneumoencephalography, and cerebral angiography—are usually reserved until computerized axial tomography, brain scan, or other diagnostic studies indicate the need for further evaluation. It should be mentioned that computerized axial tomography may or may not include dye injection.

### Direct precipitating events

In considering factors that might precipitate a seizure, one should give due consideration to trauma and inflammatory processes affecting the central nervous system, the prenatal and perinatal history, previous seizures, age of onset, presence of auras, and the relationship of these episodes to meals, time, illness, emotion, external stimuli, or menstrual periods.

In idiopathic seizures the actual precipitant remains unidentified. However, investigators believe that a specific gene may be responsible for determining seizure thresholds. Febrile convulsions and breath-holding spells seem to have a recessive pattern of inheritance.

Factors that predispose neurons to damage and subsequent seizure disorders include a wide variety of problems—infections, deficiencies in oxygen, trauma, or hemorrhage—that may occur in association with the many acute and chronic disorders detailed throughout this book.

When key problems related to seizure disorders are considered in a logical age progression, several distinct entities earmark each age. In the formative period, errors of development resulting in such defects as cortical atrophy, agenesis of the corpus callosum, porencephalia, or hydrocephalus may account for the seizure focus. Problems related to the pregnancy itself—abruptio placentae, placenta previa, maternal bleeding, or concurrent maternal health disorders—may interfere with fetal oxygen supplies and neuronal integrity. The next stage of emphasis is the birth process, when injury may occur from prolonged or difficult labor and delivery, abnormal fetal presentations, prolapsed cord, or excessive, poorly timed, or inadequately controlled administration of analgesics, oxytocin (Pitocin), or sedatives.

Major problems that are commonly linked to seizure disorders in the neonate include hypoglycemia, hyponatremia, hypernatremia, hypocalcemia, hyperbilirubinemia, respiratory distress syndrome, sepsis, and infectious problems in the central nervous system. Vitamin $B_6$ deficiencies, hypertensive encephalopathies, diphtheria-pertussis-tetanus immunization reactions, sickle-cell disease, excessive salicylate ingestion, aminoacidopathies, and lead encephalopathy are less frequent causes of seizures during this age.

In children, seizures occur frequently during sleep or as the child is either drifting off to sleep or waking up. Unusual activity, noise, or enuresis after training is complete are indicators of possible nocturnal seizures. Complaints of excessive fatigue or undue sleepiness on awakening should also arouse suspicion as to possible nocturnal seizures.

Photic stimuli, noises of various types, music, and reading have all been implicated as stimuli that may induce seizures in some individuals. In this reflexive type of seizure, every attempt is made to identify the precipitating stimulus so that measures may be taken to either avoid the stimulus or desensitize the child to it. Of these stimuli, photic input and music are regarded as the more common precipitants of seizures. When intermittent sources of light or photic stimuli, such as those provided by a flickering television, rays of sunlight, fluorescent lighting, or psychedelic lights at varying frequencies, are received by the eyes, impulses apparently travel down a thalamocortical pathway associated with the occipital region and spread from these subcortical areas in a diffuse, synchronous manner to involve the cerebral cor-

tex and brainstem. Seizure disorders caused by photic stimuli are comparable to centrencephalic discharges apparent in infantile spasms, absence, or generalized epilepsy. Musicogenic epilepsy is the term utilized to describe any child stimulated to convulsions in response to music. In the instances of photic stimulation, sunglasses with light-polarizing lenses may alleviate the problem, whereas in musicogenic types, programs of avoidance or desensitization are utilized.

At any age the threshold for seizures in susceptible persons may be decreased by such factors as electrolytic, water, or glucose imbalances; fever; inflammatory processes; fatigue; or emotional extremes, such as stress or excitement. Hyperventilation should be avoided in susceptible persons, since the resulting alkalosis may precipitate a seizure. Such medications as the phenothiazines, chlorpropamide (Diabinese), and isoniazid (INH) are also known to reduce the convulsive threshold.

Humoral and metabolic changes associated with puberty and adolescence may also reduce the threshold for seizures. Menstruation may lower the threshold, as serum levels of sodium, potassium, and water are altered by excessive fluid retention.

## GENERAL EVALUATION

Meticulous attention in recording details surrounding seizure activity is designed to exclude problems other than seizures that may alter the conscious state. The goal in the general evaluation is to detect any underlying pathological condition and correct it while symptomatic treatment is provided to relieve the seizures. Refer to Chapters 5, 8, and 11 for techniques in evaluation; refer to the sections on learning disabilities, mental retardation or specific diseases, as applicable.

## MULTIFACTORIAL CLASSIFICATION

Four major groups of seizure disorders are recognized, comprising those representing simple or complex focal (partial, or cortical) disorders, those representing generalized or centrencephalic disturbances, and mixed types of seizures (Table 14-1).

Focal, partial, or cortical, seizures include the focal motor (jacksonian "march," adversive, and tonic postural) and focal sensory types, which account for about 15% of the childhood seizures.

Psychomotor (complex partial) seizures account for another 35% of the convulsive problems, whereas convulsive equivalents such as abdominal epilepsy compose some 10% of the convulsive disorders in children. (See Table 14-1, numbers 1-6.)

Centrencephalic convulsive disorders include the mixed type of problem wherein focal motor or psychomotor seizures may exist with either generalized or myoclonic convulsions in about 5% of the seizure disorders. Generalized, grand mal, or major motor types account for another 20%, whereas the petit mal lapses make up 5%. The remaining 10% comprises myoclonic convulsions, including salaam type, and akinetic varieties. (See Table 14-1, numbers 7-11.)

## Focal (partial or cortical) seizures

*Focal motor types.* Scars in neuronal tissue of the cerebrum result in localized increases in electrical activity. The specific area of cerebrum stimulated determines the nature of the seizure experience, that is, motor, visceral, sensory, or psychological. The clinical assessment, history, and EEG tracing are all helpful in determining the location of the cerebral scar. Although these focal motor convulsions are not age specific, they do tend to occur more frequently in males than in females.

The so-called *jacksonian march seizures* result from an epileptogenic area in the motor strip of the cerebral cortex. In this type, seizures begin with tonic-clonic activity in either one extremity or in the facial muscles. Early seizure activity may be apparent as twitching around the mouth or ocular region. As the seizure proceeds, the activity spreads to other body parts of the ipsilateral side. However, movement of the seizure activity to the other side of the body may occur. When both sides of the body become involved, the seizure is generalized. After the seizure has subsided, a transient weakness or postictal paralysis (Todd's paralysis) may be apparent for as long as a few hours. If the convulsion has been limited to one side of the body, the conscious state is not usually impaired. Observation of weakness or diminished tone in an extremity after a generalized seizure is indicative of a focal seizure disorder.

The pharmacological agent of choice in managing march seizures is usually phenytoin (Dilantin), though combinations of phenytoin, primidone (Mysoline), diazepam (Valium), and barbiturates may be indicated when these seizures have a generalized manifestation. Focal excisions or hemispherectomies are sometimes indicated when medical treatment is not effective.

*Adversive seizures* may differ slightly, depending on which portion of frontal area 8 is injured. In these seizures the head and eyes move in a direction away from the side with the cerebral lesion, unless a destructive process is present, which results in movement of the head and eyes toward the side containing the lesion. The head turning precedes the eye movement when the lesion is located in the frontal area, whereas the opposite is true for lesions in the occipital area.

When the neuronal damage is in the paracentral motor cortex, it may result in a *tonic postural seizure*. In this type of seizure the EEG tracing reveals a focus of spikes or slow-wave activity in the frontal lobe. The actual seizure episode consists of turning the head to one side with accompanying tonic extension of the ipsilateral extremities to the same side. In the interview with the parents, the practitioner typically elicits information about motor development impairments such as limping or dragging of one leg during efforts at walking or the noticeably better functioning of one extremity. Changes in hand preference are also commonly associated with this type of seizure disorder. Other concurrent difficulties include problems in behavioral, learning, or verbal capacities.

Pharmacological support in adversive seizures includes the use of phenytoin and mephobarbital (Mebaral), whereas combinations of phenytoin and diazepam tend to be more effective in managing the postural type of seizure disorder.

*Focal sensory types.* Focal sensory seizure disorders are characterized by an EEG tracing of spikes and slow waves over the epileptogenic focus, which may be located in the occipital or parietal regions. When the seizure has an occipital focus, visual experiences such as awareness of flashing kaleidoscopic colored lights are possible in one or both visual fields. More sophisticated images result if the focus is in the distal aspect of the temporal-occipital area. When the abnormal focus is located in the parietal sensory cortex, sensory experiences such as tingling, numbness, prickling, pain, or paresthesias may occur. Tonic-

**TABLE 14-1.** Characteristics of seizure disorders

| Disorder | Areas involved | Changes in consciousness | Preferred medications | EEG findings | Other impaired capacities |
|---|---|---|---|---|---|
| **Partial seizures (simple)** | | | | | |
| 1. Focal motor (jacksonian march seizures) | Motor strip of cerebral cortex focus | If unilateral, no impairment; when bilateral, consciousness lost and postictal state as in major motor seizure | Phenytoin (Dilantin), primidone (Mysoline), diazepam (Valium) | Focal waves, slow waves, or spikes | Disturbances in motor or behavioral capacities |
| 2. Adversive | Frontal area 8 focus | No loss | Phenytoin (Dilantin), mephobarbital (Mebaral) | Focal waves, slow waves, or spikes | Disturbances in motor or behavioral capacities |
| 3. Tonic postural | Paracentral motor cortex focus | No loss | Phenytoin (Dilantin), diazepam (Valium) | Spikes or slow waves, or both, in frontal lobe | Behavioral, verbal, and learning impairments |
| 4. Focal sensory | Focus in occipital or parietal areas | No loss | Phenytoin (Dilantin), primidone (Mysoline) | Spikes and slow waves over epileptogenic focus in occipital or parietal areas | Ability to recall phenomena occurring during the seizure |
| **Partial seizures (complex)** | | | | | |
| 5. Psychomotor (temporal lobe seizures) | Anterior or posterior temporal lobe focus | Various amounts of awareness during episode; postictal drowsiness or desire to sleep | Phenytoin (Dilantin), primidone (Mysoline), barbiturates, ethosuximide (Zarontin), succinimides, carbemazepine (Tegretol)* | Temporal spike or slow waves | May occur in combination with generalized or focal motor seizures; wide variety of symptoms characteristic of these seizures |
| 6. Psychic seizure | — | No loss | — | — | Feeling that an unknown conversation or situation is overwhelmingly familiar |
| **Generalized seizures** | | | | | |
| 7. Generalized (grand mal, tonic-clonic, major motor) | Cortex, spinal cord, centrencephalon | Loss of consciousness during seizure; postictal sleep after seizure | Phenobarbital, primidone (Mysoline), clonazepam (Clonopin), phenytoin (Dilantin), carbemazepine (Tegretol)* | Variety of findings, depending on cause of seizure | Psychosocial or learning disorders |

| Type | Location | Consciousness | Drugs | EEG | Effect |
|---|---|---|---|---|---|
| 8. Petit mal (absence seizures) | Centrencephalon, cerebral cortex | Transient losses of consciousness; no postictal state | Ethosuximide (Zarontin), trimethadione (Tridione), paramethadione (Paradione), methsuximide (Celontin), chlordiazepoxide (Librium), dextroamphetamine (Dexedrine), acetazolamide (Diamox), phensuximide (Milontin), sodium valproate (Depakene), clonazepam (Clonopin) | 3-per-second spikes and waves | May become a generalized seizure; interferes with conscious responses to environment when uncontrolled |
| 9. Infantile spasms† (salaam, headdrop) | Centrencephalon, spinal cord | None; no postictal state | Diazepam (Valium), metharbital (Gemonil), phenytoin (Dilantin), mephobarbital (Mebaral), steroids, ketogenic diet | Multiple spikes and waves; hypsarrhythmia | Severe mental and developmental deficiencies eventually replaced by focal, psychomotor, or generalized seizures |
| 10. Myoclonic seizures† | — | No detectable loss | (See just below.) | — | Impairments in capacities related to intelligence, perception, motor, or mental functions |
| 11. Akinetic spells | Centrencephalon with spread to brainstem and peripheral muscles | None; no postictal state | Methsuximide (Celontin), clonazepam (Clonopin), diazepam (Valium), metharbital (Gemonil), steroids, methylprednisolone (Medrol) | Normal to slow background with polyspike or multiple spike and wave configurations | — |
| **Miscellaneous** | | | | | |
| 12. Mixed | Frontal, temporal, or occipital focus with spread to centrencephalon | Consistent with types of seizures involved | Primidone (Mysoline), phenytoin (Dilantin), diazepam (Valium), barbiturates, methsuximide (Celontin), ketogenic diet | Spike, polyspike, or spike-wave patterns with progression of focus to a generalized pattern | Interferences with behavior, learning, or motor functions |
| 13. Incomplete data | | | | | |

*Effective; use judiciously because of blood dyscrasias.

†Some infants and young children may experience myoclonic seizures (mild to severe), wherein rapid, brief contractions of the flexor muscles in the upper extremities occur. The trunk and lower extremities are sometimes involved. A forceful episode may cause the child to fall or throw an object being held. Infantile spasms are usually symmetric, whereas myoclonic seizures may be either symmetric or asymmetric, synchronous or asynchronous.

clonic movement or odd posturing may also be associated with these sensory seizures. Sensory focal convulsions are not common in children less than 8 years of age. Older individuals who experience these seizures ably describe the phenomena that characterize their individual experiences.

Pharmacological management of focal sensory seizures oftne revolves around the successful combination of phenytoin and primidone.

### Complex partial (psychomotor) seizures

Psychomotor convulsions have also been termed "temporal lobe" or "limbic convulsions." These seizures, commonly seen in children between 3 years of age and adolescence, consist of bizarre behavioral, motor, sensory, or autonomic manifestations lasting from minutes to several hours. Although individual seizure patterns vary greatly in temporal lobe epilepsy, all these seizures are similar because of their lack of interference with consciousness during the seizure; their postictal sleepiness, which may appear as drowsiness or the desire to sleep for several hours; and their amnesia for the events that occur during the seizure. The focus on the EEG tracing is often in either the anterior or posterior aspects of the temporal lobe. Psychomotor seizures may be seen in combination with generalized or focal motor seizures. When a child has more than one type of seizure disorder, the problem is termed "mixed convulsions."

When the episode lasts for a few seconds and consists of an aura of headache, abdominal disturbances, and feelings of nausea followed by a short period of confusion, lethargy, or staring with subsequent alterations in body postures— stiffness, limpness, or peculiar posturing—during an intact conscious state, many individuals mistake the spell for petit mal epilepsy. During these episodes, motor activity may also be observed. Such activity may be limited to swallowing, lip smacking, or chewing motions, or it may include automatisms and quasi-purposive movements of the extremities, such as walking, running, or kicking, that occur concurrently with inappropriate emotions or expressions. These psychomotor seizures may also be characterized by a wide variety of olfactory, visual, or auditory hallucinations, illusions, and intense feelings that provoke fear and anxiety in the child. In other instances, dizziness

may cause the older child to sit on the floor to regain equilibrium and the younger child to cling fiercely to the parent. Nausea, vomiting, and headache are commonly associated in cases where these seizures are accompanied by vertigo. Another manifestation of this seizure disorder includes a rampage where the child becomes enraged and hyperactive and lacks selection in striking out at those in the environment. After the verbal, active episode the child falls into a period of sleep, as is common in many of these varieties of psychomotor seizures.

Pharmacological management of psychomotor convulsions often begins with phenytoin or primidone. However, other medications, such as barbiturates, ethosuximide (Zarontin), or succinimides, in combination with phenytoin and primidone, may be required to control the seizures. Carbemazepine (Tegretol) may be effective. However, the potential for serious blood dyscrasias makes it a last choice. When Tegretol is used, frequent complete blood counts with differential and liver function studies are necessary. Unfortunately, even when seizures are controlled in children with psychomotor epilepsy, impaired behavioral capacities that interfere with social relations and school performance may persist.

Abdominal pain may be reported before a seizure in some children with psychomotor or generalized convulsive disorders. When abdominal pain with a headache does not occur with nausea and vomiting, the underlying problem may be migraine headache.

Interferences with cognitive, behavioral, and psychological capacities may also characterize abdominal epilepsy. Medications such as phenytoin, mephobarbital, and diazepam teamed with methylphenidylacetate (Ritalin), thioridazine (Mellaril), or chlordiazepoxide (Librium) may be required to alleviate the abdominal discomfort and related problems that interfere with normal functioning. This therapy may be slowly tapered off after 2 to 4 years of treatment.

### Centrencephalic seizures (generalized)

*Tonic-clonic disorders.* The most common type of centrencephalic seizure is the generalized convulsion. This seizure, which may occur at any time, is often preceded by a warning (aura), which may include an odd feeling, nausea, dizziness, tingling sensation, or faintness. After this aura the person quickly loses consciousness and frequently falls. Injury may occur if his or her body strikes an object during the uncontrolled fall. The pale color changes to that of cyanosis because of the hypoxia. The eyes roll up, and the pupils dilate. Muscle spasms and rigidity are observed. As the jaws clamp down, the tongue may be caught between the teeth, so that the tongue is lacerated. After these few seconds of tonic phase there is a clonic phase wherein the muscles twitch. During the period when the person lacks control, incontinence of urine and feces and the inability to handle saliva may be observed. After the tonic and clonic phases have ended (usually 5 minutes or less) the person sinks into a period of deep sleep or confusion for several hours. A headache may be apparent when he or she awakens.

Generalized convulsions that begin after 4 years of age are less commonly associated with deficiencies in mental capacities or perceptual-motor-cognitive domains.

The EEG shows a variety of patterns, depending on the cause of the seizure. Generalized or focal spikes, paroxysmal slowing, or diffuse disorganization may be observed. A focal motor or psychomotor disorder may thus spread to become a generalized seizure. Basically when these discharges spread to the cortex, there is an alteration in the conscious state. If they spread to the brainstem or spinal cord, tonus, clonus, or myoclonus may be observed.

Although treatment in major motor seizures is directed toward elimination of the cause, anticonvulsants may be required in the absence of specific therapy to provide relief from seizures. Phenobarbital, phenytoin, primidone, and clonazepam are the most frequently used anticonvulsants.

***Absence (petit mal) epilepsy.*** Absence (petit mal) epilepsy, most commonly seen in children between the ages of 5 and 12 years, is often discovered when the child seems to daydream and appears to be unable to stay tuned into the train of thought in the classroom long enough to perform adequately. On closer inspection the child has staring or blinking spells accompanied by a transient loss of consciousness lasting for a few seconds. Since falling, incontinence, and postictal states do not accompany these disorders, they often go unobserved. Because they may number in the hundreds per day, they interfere greatly with normal functioning. Clinically these seizures may often be induced by hyperventilation. On EEG tracings there is a characteristic pattern of spikes and waves occurring at a rate of three each second. The petit mal disorder may be most noticeable on an EEG taken during either sleep or hyperventilation.

In this type of seizure disorder the abnormal neuronal discharge spreads rapidly from the centrencephalic origin to the cerebral cortex, so that interferences with consciousness are brief. About 50% of these children experience no further seizures after having petit mal epilepsy for 2 years. However, the changes associated with adolescence may cause petit mal episodes to become generalized seizures. When petit mal seizures are recognized and controlled, no further problems with functional capacities seem to occur.

Although trimethadione (Tridione) and paramethadione (Paradione) have been effectively utilized to control these seizures, associated side effects make these medications less desirable than ethosuximide. When ethosuximide or trimethadione are used to treat these seizures, mephobarbital or phenobarbital should be administered concurrently, since there is always the risk that ethosuximide or trimethadione may induce a generalized seizure. Bone-marrow depression may be another problem in the use of ethosuximide or trimethadione. In the event that trimethadione, ethosuximide, or paramethadione has not proved to be effective in controlling the seizure disorder, methsuximide, chlordiazepoxide, dextroamphetamine (Dexedrine), acetazolamide (Diamox), phensuximide (Milontin), sodium valproate (Depakene), or clonazepam (Clonopin), may be utilized. When females are encountering menarche or growth spurts, a combination of acetazolamide, ethosuximide, and mephobarbital may be effective.

***Infantile spasms.*** Infantile myoclonic seizures, also termed "salaam or head drop seizures" or "infantile spasms," are usually apparent in affected infants from 3 to 12 months of age. During this episode the head, trunk, and limbs may either flex or extend symmetrically, or the head and trunk may quickly extend while the limbs remain flexed and extended. These rapid seizure episodes may number in the hundreds per day. No postictal lethargy or sleep and no interference with consciousness is evident during the seizure activity.

At times the cause of these infantile spasms may be traced to a disorder that has resulted in severe damage to the brain tissue. However, the origin of these seizures may also remain unknown, as is the case in so many children.

Even when spasms are decreased or controlled by pharmacological means, severe mental and developmental deficiencies are apparent in the majority of affected infants. The irregular, high-voltage spikes and waves from both sides of the cerebrum (hypsarrhythmia) and the bursts of high-voltage spikes and waves from the cerebrum or centrencephalon typify the EEG pattern. Between the bursts an interval of electrical quiescence may occur.

Clinically these infants may seem colicky, jittery, and manifest spells of smiling and laughing. Normal activity and attention to the environment are constantly interrupted with these rapid spells, which seem to increase when the infant is stimulated or fed. Other findings depend on the underlying problem.

After the infantile spasms no longer occur, they are replaced with focal, psychomotor, or generalized seizures.

Although attempts at pharmacological control are often frustrating or met with varying degrees of success, persistence in combining the available treatment modalities allows one to find a combination that reduces the number of seizures as much as possible without sedating the infant into an unresponsive state. Diazepam, metharbital (Gemonil), phenytoin, and mephobarbital may be combined in a variety of ways. If the seizures are caused by a pyridoxine deficiency, administration of pyridoxine is effective. Prednisone or an ACTH preparation (Acthar Gel) may reduce the number of seizures as well. In some infants, medications are combined with a ketogenic diet or acetazolamide. Although this is often effective in reducing seizures, urine testing should be done, and the condition of the infant should be monitored for evaluation of the degree of ketosis.

*Myoclonic seizures.* See Table 14-1 and discussion under akinetic spells.

*Akinetic spells.* Akinetic spells, most commonly observed in children between the ages of 3 and 12 years, consist of a transient loss of trunk and limb tonus with or without a myoclonic spasm, which forces the child to fall. Parents often describe an affected child as one who is clumsy and constantly falling for no obvious reason. Since no postictal phenomenon or impairment in consciousness occurs, actual seizure episodes may go unnoticed before diagnosis calls attention to the problem. These episodes may also number in the hundreds per day. A variety of impairments in functional capacities, including intelligence and perceptual, motor, and mental modalities, are frequently associated with these seizures, which involve an electrical discharge beginning in the centrencephalon and extending to the brainstem and peripheral muscles. The EEG tracing often reveals a normal to slow background with patterns of polyspike or multiple spike and wave configurations. In the differential diagnosis, hypoglycemia and basilar artery insufficiency should be excluded. Effective medications include methsuximide, diazepam, metharbital, steroids, methylprednisolone, and clonazepam.

### Miscellaneous mixed convulsive problems

Mixed seizure disorders, frequently seen in children from 2 to 10 years of age, consist of either a focal motor or psychomotor seizure in combination with generalized or myoclonic seizures. The pathophysiology underlying this phenomenon explains the occurrence of these combinations in the same child. First, the epileptogenic focus, which may be located in the frontal, temporal, or occipital cerebrum, is activated, causing a focal motor, psychomotor, adversive, or tonic-postural seizure. The impulse from the abnormally activated neuronal tissue then reaches the centrencephalon to cause a petit mal lapse or generalized or myoclonic seizure.

When performing the clinical assessment, spastic paresis or muscle atrophy may be obvious on one side with accompanying hypertonia and hyperreflexia. Parents may also report falling secondary to a major motor episode, a loss of muscle tone, or a myoclonic seizure. Additionally, they may report a variety of problems related to interferences with school adjustment and performance in the perceptual, cognitive, behavioral, and functional domains.

The EEG tracing, which remains relatively unaltered with medications, may consist of spike, polyspike, or spike-wave patterns that begin at a focal point in one half of the cerebrum and often spread to the centrencephalic area to involve the cerebrum equally. The synchronous spread may result in an EEG tracing typical of generalized seizures.

Since mixed seizure disorders involve more than one type of seizure in a child, a combination of anticonvulsants is indicated. Although many children are successfully controlled using primidone, phenytoin, and diazepam, those with focal, petit mal, and tonic-clonic seizures may be more effectively treated with phenytoin, a barbiturate, and methsuximide (Celontin).

When the seizure disorder remains unclassified, the nurse should consider the possibility that data collection is incomplete.

## Abdominal epilepsy

Abdominal epilepsy (autonomic or visceral diencephalic epilepsy) is termed an epileptic equivalent. By definition it includes recurring abdominal pain without convulsive activity and may or may not be accompanied by a headache and sleepiness as postictal phenomena. In this disorder the EEG appears abnormal, but improvement occurs when anticonvulsants are administered. This problem is most often seen in children between 4 and 12 years of age.

## RELATED PROBLEMS

In this section, cursory attention is given to narcolepsy, reflex seizures, night terrors, nocturnal jerks, hysterical fits, and syncope. Status epilepticus, seizure disorders in adolescence, convulsive problems in the neonate, febrile convulsions, and breath-holding spells are highlighted because of the management problems they present.

## Narcolepsy

Narcolepsy, a disorder more commonly seen in late adolescence or adulthood, is a sudden uncontrollable desire for sleep that may occur while the individual is involved in talking, wakeful activity, or driving. The sudden falling off into a shallow, easily arousable state of sleep is followed by normal functioning on awakening. Although narcolepsy is often unrelated to physiological requirements for sleep, it may be part of a toxic-infectious condition, a posttraumatic state, an endocrine disorder, a neoplasm, a psychological disturbance, or an unknown problem.

When this disorder is apparent, one should consider sudden changes in the emotional climate, depression, inadequate sleep, or other disturbances in the family dynamics, since these problems most often constitute the cause for narcolepsy. Minimal dosages of amphetamines have been utilized in some cases with dramatic results. However, management of the underlying problem—organic or psychogenic—is essential.

## Reflex seizures

Reflex seizures, already mentioned in the discussion of focal sensory disorders, may be precipitated by a variety of sensory stimuli—photogenic auditory, and tactile. General body conditions related to increased temperature, infectious processes, certain medications, excessive hydration, alkalosis, and hypoglycemia may also precipitate a reflexive seizure disorder. These disorders, usually manifested as major motor disorders, may require medication and desensitization to the stimuli. Psychological assessment and treatment may be necessary for success in long-range control of these seizures when they represent the attempt of an emotionally troubled child to gain attention.

## Night terrors

Some children have bad dreams or nightmares with accompanying inappropriate behavior during sleep. During such an episode the child may talk, walk, open the eyes, or exhibit a rigid posture or muscle jerking. Since these seizures are not unlike a state occurring with psychomotor seizures, an EEG is often performed. When these episodes are alleviated by anticonvulsants, they are termed nocturnal seizures.

## Nocturnal jerks

Almost everyone can recall the spontaneous jerks that occur when one is either drifting off to sleep or waking up. Some nervous children seem to have an increased number of these bodily jerks, which resemble myoclonic seizures. Although this is an innocuous, common problem, evaluation of myoclonic seizures is still a consideration in the differential diagnosis.

## Hysterical fits

Hysterical, or functional, seizures, most common in girls between 7 and 15 years of age, are often seen in children who have seizures or who have observed seizure disorders in other family members.

Quite often a "motive" may be established for having the seizure, and an audience is at hand. Episodes may appear to be seizures, but on closer inspection are distinguished by the following characteristics: (1) Emotional problems are apparent in the child. (2) Sensory and motor disorders reported between episodes may not conform to neural pathways. (3) Pallor and pupil dilatation seen in a true major motor seizure are not obvious. (4) Sphincter control is maintained. (5) Movement during the episode does not result in bodily injury. (6) Inappropriate crying and verbalization may continue for an extended period after the momentary episode. Although EEG abnormalities may be evident, treatment is related to solving the underlying psychogenic disturbance.

During the clinical assessment these episodes may be induced and stopped by verbal suggestion or by the application of pressure or painful stimuli over the Achilles tendon.

## Syncope

Syncope in childhood is most often a simple fainting spell that represents a reflexive response to painful or frightening events or procedures performed in the upright position. The underlying mechanism is a disturbance in the reflexive regulation of the vascular system, which leads to the spontaneous relaxation of the visceral-venous system with subsequent slowing of the pulse, falling blood pressure, and transient cerebral ischemia. This type of fainting may be avoided by having the child assume a recumbent position during painful procedures and by allowing crying. Crying tends to reduce the incidence of fainting. Older children faint less often when they grasp an object tightly or willfully contract their abdominal musculature. Hypoglycemia from such habits as skipping meals may also result in syncope. Recovery is enhanced by lowering the child's head beneath the level of the heart.

A short seizurelike reaction often accompanies the Stokes-Adams syndrome that occurs with heart block. Syncopal episodes may also be associated with paroxysmal tachycardia and with physical exertion in children affected with some congenital cardiac disorders, such as tetralogy of Fallot.

A hyperactive carotid sinus reflex, though quite rare, may result in a lack of consciousness with or without tonic-clonic seizure activity.

An apneic spell may also be associated with competitive swimming, especially in activities such as the breast stroke, wherein forced hyperventilation before submerging results in dramatic lowering of the carbon dioxide level, so that hypoxia interferes with stimulation of the respiratory center and further breathing. These episodes, more common in adolescent boys, result in unconsciousness and clonic movements. Prompt efforts at resuscitation are indicated. Ventricular fibrillation may be a problem when rapid repsonse to artificial ventilation is not evident.

## Status epilepticus

Status epilepticus refers to a convulsive series wherein a conscious state is not regained between seizures. About 5% to 10% of the pediatric population with epilepsy have had status epilepticus at some time. About 50% of all individuals with this condition are under the age of 2 years, probably because of their immature nervous systems. The mortality may be as high as 50%. Death is often caused by cardiac or respiratory depression or arrest, which may occur as a result of the combination of medications utilized to stop the convulsions. Other complications include hemiparesis and respiratory infection from compromised respiratory capacities and aspiration from incorrect posturing or acute care techniques.

Prompt treatment is emphasized to avoid irreversible brain damage. Management includes supportive symptomatic intervention, cessation of seizure activity, investigation into causative factors, and the initiation or resumption of a daily long-range program of pharmacological therapy. In the acute period an intravenous line is promptly established, so that body needs may be monitored and supplied with regard to anticonvulsive medication, fluids, nutrients, and electrolytes. Provisions for adequate respiratory exchange and cardiovascular support are two other considerations during the acute period. Along with seizure control, attempts are made to determine the underlying problem. Some common causes of status epilepticus include drug withdrawal, inadequate levels of certain body substances (calcium, sodium, glucose, and so on), head injury, infection, elevated temperature, or response to a toxin. The family may also be questioned about any recent change in the child's pattern of taking anticonvulsive medications, including dosage revision, change to a new medication, or omission of a medication.

Two types of convulsion compose the true status epilepticus, a condition that constitutes a medical emergency. They include grand mal and focal seizures. Diazepam by the intravenous route is the medication of choice in stopping this seizure activity. However, it should be given cautiously and slowly, since rapid infusion may cause respiratory depression and hypotension. When diazepam is either contraindicated or ineffective, phenobarbital or parenteral paraldehyde may be utilized. Phenobarbital or phenytoin is also generally initiated as maintenance therapy after initial control is established.

During the preliminary diagnostic evaluation some immediate laboratory work is indicated, including analysis of electrolytes, glucose and calcium levels, blood urea nitrogen (BUN), and cerebrospinal fluid. Other laboratory work may be needed after information is gleaned from the family. An EEG is usually not helpful at this time, unless the condition is caused by petit mal status epilepticus, which is a blurring of consciousness with a rapid flutter of the eyelids and mouth movements. During these episodes the affected individual may seem to be retarded or psychotic. The usual pattern of three spikes each second seen in true petit mal epilepsy is also seen in this type of state. After initial control has been reestablished, the long-range management is the same as that suggested to control the particular seizure disorder in the individual.

### Seizure disorders in adolescence

Seizure disorders are one of the most common chronic disorders in adolescence. In 50% of the individuals affected with petit mal epilepsy, spontaneous improvement and cessation of the seizure activity, with subsequent changes on the EEG, occur at puberty. One seizure problem that may have its onset during the early part of middle childhood is the type that has its focus in the midtemporal area. During these episodes, which usually occur at night, the child has conscious experiences with such problems of the oral cavity as drooling, odd sensations, and the lack of speech. From this point the seizure may become generalized, or it may merely be followed by a postictal period in which dysarthria without amnesia occurs. Even though the incidence is rare, some children with chronic epilepsy may also develop a neoplasm, which suddenly alters their seizure control. For some children with focal seizures or cerebral palsy, the period of early adolescence may include the occurrence of seizures in response to sensory stimuli.

When the initial onset of epilepsy occurs in adolescence, there are a number of considerations. If the episode is a major motor seizure, is it secondary to another type of seizure disorder that is undiagnosed, such as petit mal? Consideration should also be given to a progressive focal disorder in the brain, which may be evident clinically as an aura or focal phenomenon. Idiopathic epilepsy is another type that may be seen for the first time in adolescence.

*True petit mal (absence) seizures,* primarily a disease of childhood, are manifested in an irregular pattern when seen in the adolescent age group. Instead of the multiple daily episodes obvious in childhood, seizure episodes may occur infrequently or as a prolonged confusion or fuzzy mental condition with flickering of the eyelids and rolling of the eyeballs. During these episodes the EEG shows a continuous pattern of bilateral spike-wave discharges interspersed with occasional interruptions of normal background activity.

*Vasovagal syncope* is a common occurrence in adolescence. At times the reason for the fainting spell may be evident when an emotional and family history is taken. Endocrine problems, such as the hypoglycemia associated with diabetes, may also result in syncope. Tonic stiffening of the trunk and extremities during these episodes appears similar to that taking place during a seizure but is actually caused by upper brainstem ischemia.

Seizures precipitated by sensory experiences are also seen either late in childhood or during adolescence.

*Psychomotor seizures* are frequently seen in adolescents and adults. Since these temporal lobe disorders are quite similar clinically to behavioral disorders, careful scrutiny should be given to the problem during the clinical evaluation. Several pertinent questions are relevant in relation to the seizures themselves. Are the seizures controlled? Does the adolescent have problems typical of the age, and if so, does the seizure activity affect usual behavior? Is there any type of postictal phenomenon, and is it identified as such? For example, aggression may be a behavior associated with these seizures that is sometimes mistakenly evaluated by parents and others as an independent, willful state in the child. Behavioral disorders may also be seen in the adolescent with temporal lobe epilepsy when seizures are out of control. When behavior is an ictal event, brain-wave abnormalities show the unusual activity.

Omission of medications is the most frequent cause of recurring seizures in adolescence. The premenstrual period is associated with an increase in seizures as well; these seizures respond well to acetazolamide. Nocturnal epilepsy is often effectively controlled by long-acting barbiturates (Stental Extentabs, Eskabarb). When barbiturates are used for control of epilepsy in the adolescent, their use should be carefully regulated, since they are the most lethal type of anticonvulsants when they are utilized in a nonprescriptive manner.

Phenytoin, a most effective anticonvulsant, has numerous side effects, including gingival hyperplasia, hirsutism, and rash. It is also associated with Stevens-Johnson syndrome on rare occasions and should be discontinued when these symptoms occur. Vitamin D deficiency, osteomalacia, and lymphoma syndrome may also occur. Practitioners should observe the adolescent for signs of phenytoin intoxication, which include lethargy, increasingly inadequate school performance, and sometimes ataxia and nystagmus.

Certain psychosocial implications should be considered when one is evaluating the adolescent who has seizures. Since seizure episodes are both unpredictable and unremembered by the affected individual, the adolescent may have concerns about personal appearance, sexual capacities, emerging identities, and ability to continue a pattern of increasing independence from the family.

During the early adolescent period, key problems may include poor school performance from excessive anticonvulsant medications, subclinical seizure activity, and specific learning disabilities. Later in adolescence the individual may want to become involved in competitive sports. Such activity should be discouraged, unless the individual is persistent in these desires, and the seizure disorder is well controlled using anticonvulsants. Activities such as swimming, climbing, and driving should be avoided, or if done, the buddy system should be utilized. Alcohol and tranquilizers tend to have a cumulative effect when combined with anticonvulsants, and adolescents should be warned of the potential outcomes.

### Neonatal seizures

About 5 to 10 neonates of every 1000 live births experience a seizure during the first month of life, especially within the first week.

During the *first day* of life, seizure disorders are most often caused by sepsis, bacterial or viral meningoencephalitis, central nervous system abnormalities, hypoglycemia, hypoxia related to birth trauma, and drug withdrawal in infants born to addicted mothers. Seizures occurring during the *first week* may be attributed to hypocalcemia, sepsis, aminoacidurias, pyridoxine deficiencies, and bacterial or viral meningoencephalitis.

Neonatal seizures are manifested differently from those occurring later because of the immaturity of the brain structures during this period. Thus little cortical activity is apparent as a result of the primitive state of cerebral synapses. Seizure activity may be mainly confined to brainstem and spinal cord reflexive responses. Seizures of the motor and limbic systems tend to be limited to the motor area or temporal lobe, since these areas become myelinated and mature early. Clinically, neonatal seizures in these areas may be evident as unusual visceral or autonomic responses and swallowing or chewing activities.

The importance of recognizing the underlying problem, which may result in either a focal or a generalized problem, cannot be overemphasized, since a prolonged disorder may result in permanent neuronal damage.

Correct identification of a seizure in a neonate is difficult, since neonates normally have random movements. Rapid tonic-clonic movements intermingled with this random activity may go unnoticed. Other indications of seizure activity include unusual or rigid posturing, facial grimacing, production of grunting noises, chewing and mouthing movements, and pedaling motions in the legs. Along with these motor disturbances, vasomotor changes, including rubor, cyanosis, pallor, and intermittent apnea, may be observed. Myoclonic, focal, or major motor seizures of the tonic-clonic type are also noted in the neonatal age group.

*Causative factors.* Several problems have been identified as major causes of seizures in the neonate. Injury during the gestational or perinatal period that results in cerebral hypoxia may cause functional impairments in the newborn. These abnormal activities are frequently obvious as a lowered Apgar rating. However, the full extent of damage cannot be assessed until brain structures mature sufficiently to perform at full capacity. The pathogenesis of the subsequent seizure disorder is based on the hypoxia, which causes degenerative neuronal changes and capillary endothelium damage, leading to petechial hemorrhages. Cerebral trauma also results in subsequent hemorrhages. The degree of these hemorrhages is related to neurological impairments and future seizures.

METABOLIC DISORDERS. Metabolic disorders represent a large group of problems that are frequently amenable to therapeutic intervention. In the first few days after protein feedings, seizures are most often associated with phenylketonuria and maple syrup urine disease. First indications of these seizures include impaired consciousness, feeding disorders, and myoclonic seizure activity.

Other metabolic problems, which present a particular problem in this age group, include hypocalcemia, hypomagnesemia, and hypoglycemia. Pyridoxine deficiencies are another problem that may underlie seizures.

*Hypocalcemia* results in tetany in the neonate, which is obvious at about 3 days of life as twitching, tremors, irritability, and focal or major motor seizures. This inadequate serum calcium level may be caused by a transient interference with parathyroid functioning. The pathogenesis of the problem may be most commonly related to a feeding of cow's milk containing a high quantity of phosphorus. Because of renal immaturity, phosphate is retained rather than excreted. The resulting elevation in the serum phosphate level causes a reduction in the calcium level. Levels of serum calcium lower than a range of 7 to 7.5 mg/dl may result in tetany.

When the phosphorus level is normal and the administration of calcium does not alleviate the neonate's seizure disorder, decreased levels of magnesium may be the underlying problem. *Decreased magnesium levels* in the neonate are most often seen after an exchange transfusion of citrated blood or in neonates born to diabetic mothers.

When seizures are related to *hypoglycemia,* convulsive episodes may be seen from 2 hours to 7 days of age. Although no definite point is universally related to the production of seizures, glycogen levels lower than a range of 30 to 50 mg/dl after 2 days of life are considered to be the theoretical indication of hypoglycemia in children this age. Neonates with low birth weights for gestational age may experience hypoglycemic seizures from insufficient quantities of glycogen in the liver and muscles or malnutrition during the gestational period.

If seizures are caused by hypoglycemia, intravenous glucose produces a rapid end to the seizures. Thus intravenous glucose administration has both diagnostic and therapeutic value.

The presence of pyridoxine, vitamin $B_6$, an essential coenzyme in gamma-aminobutyric acid (GABA) production, raises the seizure threshold. *Inadequate supplies of vitamin $B_6$* may result in convulsions both in utero and in the neonatal period. These inadequate supplies may be the result of unavailable supplies from the mother during gestation or an inadequate supply within the neonate.

An important diagnostic clue to the underlying cause of seizures in the neonate is the failure to respond to anticonvulsant medications. This lack of response is usually caused by the uncorrected metabolic disorder that has triggered the seizure episode.

ELECTROLYTIC IMBALANCE. Electrolytic imbalances, especially hypernatremia and hyponatremia, may result in seizure disorders in the neonate. *Hypernatremia,* a disproportionate increase in salt with a concurrent decrease in water, may include convulsions and an altered state of consciousness that may progress from lethargy to coma as sodium levels increase to a high level.

*Hyponatremia* appears the same clinically but is usually caused by sodium losses associated with diarrhea or hypotonic fluid administration.

*Exogenous problems,* such as withdrawal from dependency on substances such as phenothiazines, barbiturates, heroin, morphine, or cocaine, may reduce the seizure threshold. A neonate experiencing withdrawal may seem jittery and irritable and may have convulsions. Paregoric, diazepam, naloxone (Narcan), and barbiturates have all been utilized to treat affected infants. Although symptoms of withdrawal are apparent in a newborn after several days of life, a lack of therapeutic intervention may result in a 50% mortality if interim supportive therapy is not administered.

**INFLAMMATORY PROCESSES.** Inflammatory processes also account for some seizure disorders in the newborn. Moreover, a seizure may be the only clinical symptom indicating a bacterial meningitis. Because of the poorly established blood-brain barrier at this age, 25% of those affected with sepsis have meningitis. Viral and bacterial agents that result in meningitis are detailed in Chapter 20. Toxoplasmosis and cytomegalic inclusion disease, discussed in Chapter 13, may produce neonatal seizures as well.

Developmental defects in the cerebrum, that is, cerebral atrophy, porencephaly, and agenesis of the corpus callosum, may also result in neonatal seizures.

Idiopathic seizures in the neonatal age group may account for as much as 30% of all seizures.

*Management.* Although the management of neonatal seizures requires prompt intervention and control, a physician attempts to diagnose the underlying cause of the seizure while halting the abnormal neuronal discharges. A thorough family and neonatal history and a physical examination with particular emphasis on the neurological assessment are often helpful in pinpointing the causative factor. Laboratory determinations of glucose, calcium, phosphorus, BUN, and electrolyte levels may also be helpful. Routine urinalysis and a complete blood count with a differential analysis are also valuable in assessment of the neonatal condition. Analysis of the spinal fluid reveals the presence of any inflammatory process. Urine and blood may be subjected to screening tests for detection of inborn errors of metabolism. Other laboratory studies are performed as indicated.

Radiographic studies may be done to survey the general structure of the skull, spine, or bones, or they may be ordered to reveal a particular problem using a specific process, that is, pneumoencephalogram or chest film. EEG's, usually delayed until seizure control is attained, may be valuable in localizing the seizure focus. Computerized axial tomography (CAT scans), subdural taps, and other procedures are performed as the individual case indicates.

When seizures of unknown cause are occurring, a five-step plan is enacted to stop the seizure activity. If seizures are controlled at any point, completion of the entire sequence is not warranted. Conditions that may be diagnosed and treated in the same step include the following:

1. *Hypoglycemia*
   a. From 2 to 4 ml of 15% glucose in distilled water per kilogram of body weight is administered intravenously.
   b. Child is observed for 5 minutes.
   c. If seizures continue, the practitioner proceeds to step 2.
2. *Hypocalcemia*
   a. From 2 to 6 mg of 10% calcium gluconate is slowly administered intravenously.
   b. Child is observed for bradycardia and for the cessation of seizures.
   c. If seizures continue after 3 to 4 minutes, the practitioner proceeds to step 3.
3. *Pyridoxine deficiency*
   a. From 20 to 50 mg of pyridoxine hydrochloride is administered.
   b. Child is observed for 5 minutes.
   c. If seizures continue, the practitioner proceeds to step 4.
4. *Hypomagnesemia*
   a. From 2 to 6 ml of magnesium sulfate is administered.
   b. Child is observed for 10 minutes.
   c. If seizure activity continues, the practitioner proceeds to step 5.
5. *Stop seizures*
   a. Diazepam infusion of 0.5 mg/kg is given slowly intravenously.
   b. Maintenance dose may consist of 1 mg/kg/24 hours in evenly spaced doses.

Adjunctive medications for seizure management include phenobarbital for major motor seizures and phenytoin for focal convulsions.

***Outcomes.*** Since seizures are merely symptoms of an underlying problem, the prognosis is related to the cause and the promptness of appropriate intervention. Generally, neonatal seizures occurring during the first week of life that extend over less than 1 week without retinal changes, abnormalities in cerebrospinal fluid, or bulbar or facial weakness tend to result in a better outlook for the individual. Seizures caused by vascular problems, trauma, or deficient oxygenation may result in impaired mental and neuromuscular capacities. Convulsions related to irreversible structural abnormalities from defective development carry an even bleaker outlook.

## Febrile convulsions

A commonly encountered pediatric condition is the febrile convulsion, which may be caused by a temperature elevation to about 104° F (40° C) or more. Twice as many males as females experience febrile convulsions. Nearly one third of the affected children have had a prior history of seizures in their families. Although fever is associated with about 50% of all seizures in children less than 6 years of age, some of these fever-related seizures may be associated with an ongoing convulsive disorder that has been triggered by the febrile state.

When the seizure is a true febrile convulsion, the neurological examination and EEG are normal, and the single episode may be clearly correlated with the increased temperature. This episode of a tonic-clonic nature may be followed by a postictal period of somnolence. Seizures that occur more frequently may indicate an underlying convulsive disorder.

Investigators believe that febrile states reduce the seizure threshold, though the exact mechanism underlying this process has not been delineated. The degree of temperature elevation is apparently more related to seizures than is the speed of temperature elevation.

Management is geared toward control of temperature and seizures and treatment of the causative process. As in any major motor seizure, every attempt is made to minimize cerebral hypoxia, aspiration pneumonia, and weakness in one half of the body.

Physicians differ about whether to utilize phenobarbital or phenytoin continuously in the years when febrile seizures occur most frequently or whether to restrict treatment to an antipyretic agent and phenobarbital only when the child has an elevated temperature. Control of most uncomplicated febrile seizures is possible with phenobarbital.

Although 50% of children with febrile seizures have only one seizure, the remaining 50% have more than one. However, only about 10% of the total number of children exhibit defective EEG patterns and underlying convulsive disorders.

## Breath-holding spells

Most breath-holding spells are obvious before 1 year and are infrequently seen after the third year of life. In these episodes an emotional or painful situation is followed by a short period of crying; complete expiration with cyanosis, pallor, or a respiratory arrest; and a restless phase earmarked by twitching, clonus, opisthotonos, cyanosis or pallor, and incontinence. After this point the young child may be quite limp. A deep, quick breath ends the episode. As breathing resumes, the appearance normalizes, and the child either seems fatigued or returns to usual play. Abnormal neurological findings are not apparent in most children. Medications are not usually required. Parental support and counseling about the individual situation seem to be most beneficial.

## MEDICAL MANAGEMENT

A thorough neurological examination should be performed. Special attention should be directed toward the evaluation of receptive and expressive language and the identification of discrete motor impairments and cerebral dominance (eye, hand, foot). Radiographic examination of the skull should be made to determine the presence of calcium deposits or abnormalities of the bone. A complete cerebrospinal fluid examination, unless contraindicated, should be made to determine whether there are changes in the number of white cells or the chemical constituents. The electroencephalogram may show a brain-wave pattern (Fig. 14-2, *C*) that is generally considered characteristic of idiopathic epilepsy (petit mal). A focus of abnormal electrical discharge may localize a specific lesion (Fig. 14-2, *B*). Pneumoencephalography or ventriculography may be necessary to rule out neoplasms, abscesses, or hematomas, as well as to demonstrate congenital abnormalities or atrophy. Hyperventilation, hydration, sugar tolerance, serum calcium determination, basal metabolism, and psychological tests may also contribute valuable information and should be done in the basic study of every client with a convulsive disorder.

The study of the individual with a convulsive disorder is directed toward a careful search for precipitating causes such as neoplasms, abscesses, vascular anomalies, hematomas, depressed fractures, or scarred cortical areas that can be removed. When the diagnosis of idiopathic epilepsy is definitely made, the most effective type and dosage of anticonvulsant drug or combination of drugs are determined for the client who is then maintained indefinitely on a regimen of anticonvulsant medications. Depending on the severity and frequency of seizures and the response to the medication regimen, the client should be seen at set intervals by the physician, and nurse, who adjust the medication as necessary, monitor the physical condition and psychological status, and examine the client for specific toxic reactions to the anticonvulsant drugs (especially blood dyscrasias). Every individual taking anticonvulsant medication should have white blood cell counts and hemoglobin levels checked every 6 months. Even though the individual has no seizures, treatment should be continued at least 3 years after the last attack occurred. The use of the serum scan (gas-liquid chromatography) permits the physician to obtain an accurate reading of the drug level in the client's blood. Gas-liquid chromatography has become a valuable adjunct for determination of the optimal dosage of the anticonvulsant drug. Recently available is a new method, enzyme multiple immunoassay technique (EMIT), that speeds the process of analysis to a few minutes while only 200 $\mu$l of blood are used.

Hypertonic glucose or mannitol in sterile saline solution intravenously or magnesium sulfate (50%) intramuscularly may be given as a dehydrating agent to reduce cerebral edema. The early administration of sodium phenobarbital (Luminal Sodium) subcutaneously or phenytoin (Dilantin) intramuscularly may be successful in terminating attacks; the intravenous administration of Urevert, urea, lidocaine, or sodium phenobarbital may also be effective. Paraldehyde (2%) solution also has been effective when administered by an intravenous drip

method. This drug is particularly valuable because it is rapidly dissipated by way of the pulmonary tree; thus continuous dosage is possible without sustained deleterious effects. Diazepam (Valium) administered intravenously (0.2 mg/kg) has proved effective. It acts more quickly than the other drugs and has the greatest margin of safety between the desired therapeutic effects and the possible dangerous toxic effects, such as respiratory or vasomotor depression, if administered slowly.

If all else fails, it may be necessary to anesthetize the client. Thiopental (Pentothal) and tribromoethanol (Avertin) have been used successfully. Oxygen may also be indicated. If the client in status epilepticus does not receive vigorous treatment and intensive nursing care, he or she is in grave danger of respiratory depression and death.

Some clients have dramatic emotional and behavioral changes during the convulsive period. Approach and therapy must be modified according to the needs of the individual client and the judgment of the physician and nurse. The nurse can do much to help the client and family through these difficult periods by offering understanding support and willingness to listen and spend time with them.

If neurosurgical treatment is indicated, the principles of nursing care outlined in Chapter 26 concerning the postoperative nursing care of patients with disorders of the brain should be followed.

During the past few years more emphasis has been placed on the well-balanced diet than on the ketogenic (high-fat) diet, which was at one time used in the treatment of clients with epilepsy, though the ketogenic diet still enjoys wide use in infantile spasms.

Clients with seizures should be taught to avoid extreme emotional or physical excitement and excessive fatigue, since these may precipitate an attack. Stimulants in the form of alcohol should be avoided for the same reason. (The use of alcohol is a controversial issue. It should be forbidden if one drink precipitates a seizure; otherwise, an occasional social drink may be permitted. Excessive drinking is contraindicated.) The epileptic should take good care of him- or herself and exercise reasonable precautions to prevent injury. Normal activity seems to act as a deterrent to seizures. The epileptic should not be treated as an invalid but should be expected to participate in the normal routines of play, school, work, recreation, and sleep.

Although the condition of about 80% of the 4 million epileptics is well controlled with medication, psychotherapy may be an important adjunct to the treatment of a client with a convulsive disease.

It is good practice to advise clients with convulsive disorders always to carry a typewritten card on their persons. The American Medical Association has designed an identification card with an emergency medical symbol and recommends that everyone with a health problem that may require emergency care carry a card designating pertinent data. On written request the AMA will supply a single copy of this card and a list of the manufacturers who sell it. The information on this card should include the following items:

Name and address
Nearest relative, telephone number, and address
''I am subject to seizures.''
Medication being taken
Physician to be called for information

This card will safeguard the client and ensure the administration of proper treatment in case an attack or accident occurs on the street. The family will be notified immediately and will not be subjected to needless and prolonged anxiety. Some clients, especially after being in an accident, are not able to give reliable information for hours, days, or even weeks. Under these circumstances, valuable time may be lost while trying to identify the client, notify the family, and make a diagnosis.

During the period the epileptic is in the hospital, every effort is made by the medical and nursing staff to impress on him or her the importance of taking the anticonvulsant medication as ordered. Even though free of seizures for a long time, the epileptic must be warned not to omit a dose or stop taking the medication until told to do so by the physician. The consequences of the abrupt withdrawal of anticonvulsant drug should be described. He or she is thus prepared for possible toxic reactions to the particular drug or drugs being taken and instructed to notify the physician if any occur.

He or she is also instructed as to the nature of the disorder and informed realistically of the possible problems for an epileptic and the available community resources and agencies.

On discharge the client is given adequate instruction and an appointment for future treatment. Regular visits to the physician are most important. The development of trust and confidence in the physician and nurse will enable the epileptic to ask questions and obtain the information vital for adaptation to the limitations imposed by seizures, for optimal psychological and social adjustment, and for establishment of realistic, achievable vocational goals.

A definite attempt is made to help the family to adjust to the disability and to adopt a positive attitude toward the client's future way of life. Every facility is utilized and directed toward helping the client become a useful and well-adjusted member of society.

Several films have been produced concerning the manifestations of epilepsy and the social, economic, and emotional problems of the epileptic. Some of these films are directed toward the lay public and others toward the professionals who treat and care for the epileptic. These visual aids can be valuable adjuncts to any educational program for nursing students or community groups.

### Expected outcomes
The client will:

1 Adjust to life with acceptance of a seizure disorder so that all activity and developmentally appropriate behaviors, tasks, and issues will occur within normative limits.
2 Comply with directions on treatment and medications and will not interrupt this regimen without physician consent.
3 Accept the responses of those who witness an attack and work to help them understand the situation and any measures that they may implement during future attacks.
4 Continue a successful academic or vocational career wherein situational limitations are contingent only on specific functional problems in the individual.
5 Enjoy unqualified acceptance and accurate knowledge in family members and significant others.
6 Be observed so that all seizure-related activities may be observed by or reported to the physician and nurse.
7 Be safeguarded from psychological and physical injury during attacks.
8 Be able to explain all diagnostic and therapeutic procedures utilized in his treatment.
9 Participate in identifying special needs and in developing a nursing care plan as appropriate.

10 Develop realistic current and long-term plans in psychosocial, economic, health, recreational and educational-vocational aspects of living.

*Nursing intervention.* Two aspects of nursing management for the care of the child with seizures is apparent, including intervention during the actual convulsion and long-term planning essential to successful functioning in daily living.

ACUTE INTERVENTION. Certainly concurrent management of the disease process, trauma, or other event that has precipitated the seizure is essential in avoiding a recurrence of the convulsive episode. The actual nursing management of the convulsive episode requires prompt, deliberate attention and astute observation. The main goals during the episode are directed toward ensuring client safety, observing the events of the episode, and calming witnesses after the client has received adequate attention.

A client having a convulsion should never be left alone.

First, the nurse protects the head by placing padding beneath it. Restrictive clothing should be loosened, and objects that the client might strike during the period when control is lost should be moved from reach. If the teeth are not clamped down, a firm, soft object—padded tongue depressor, the leather part of a belt, or other object—may be placed between the teeth. Force should not be used to place anything in the client's mouth or to open the jaw once the teeth have become tightly clamped, since this only increases the amount of injury to the tongue and teeth. Restraint of moving extremities is never advised. When more than one nurse is available, the client may be screened from the view of others, or bystanders may be escorted from the scene. Since so many misunderstandings prevail about seizures, all involved persons should have an explanation and an opportunity to ask any questions they might have. If the significant others are present, the experience might be utilized to assist in teaching the measures to take at home if the seizure pattern occurs again.

After the constant attendance required during the tonic-clonic episode, close attention is continued as the client enters the postictal phase. During this period, the client is turned to the side to facilitate the drainage of the secretions that have collected in the oropharynx. Suctioning may also be helpful in the removal of these excessive secretions.

Should the episode occur when the child is sitting in a chair, he or she should be assisted to the floor so that the nurse managing the episode might have better control.

If the seizure episode occurs repeatedly without the client regaining consciousness between episodes (status epilepticus), a nurse should remain in constant attendance to maintain the airway, administer medications, protect the client from injury, observe and record events of an episode, and provide the care needed by the client, who is essentially an unconscious client. Since a lack of control of the secretions is often part of the client's problems, periodic suctioning is often required. The nurse also carefully monitors the general condition of the client and reports any changes. In addition to providing care for the unconscious client (refer to Chapter 9), the nurse emphasizes oral hygiene, administers medications, and supports clients through diagnostic testing and any special treatments.

Some important observations made by the nurse caring for the client with a major motor seizure include the following:

1. Aura, including subjective sensations, odd feelings, change in mood, outcry, and so on, before the seizure occurs
2. Position of extremities, trunk, and head during the episode
3. Kind of movements occurring during the episode
4. Deviations in the eyes
5. Pupil response and equality
6. Any alteration in color, particularly in the face and lips
7. Clamping closure of jaw and, if so, any injury to the mouth, tongue, teeth, or lips
8. Impairments in the control of saliva
9. Twitching or jerking, particularly origin, duration, spread, and progression of these movements, if applicable
10. Interferences with consciousness
11. Respiratory interferences, including labored breathing, apnea, and rate of respiration
12. Responses during seizure
13. Incontinence

14. Postictal state
15. Alterations in motor power after the seizure
16. Impaired speech after the seizure
17. Length of time entire event lasted
18. Subjective complaints of odd feelings, discomfort, or transient paralysis occurring after the seizure
19. Recall of events occurring during the seizure, or description of the aura by the client after the seizure
20. Specific management modalities during the event with a description of the client's response
21. Education and emotional support of the client, family, and observers with appropriate charting
22. Any precautions taken to avoid future seizures or decrease problems during future episodes
23. Time, length of event, period elapsed since last seizure

Sometimes a client enters the acute care setting for evaluation, regulation of medications, or treatment of an unrelated medical or surgical problem. When the nurse discovers that the client may have seizures, a number of steps are appropriate. First, a tongue blade should be kept with the client at all times. Activity should be geared to the capacities of the client. Those with no apparent seizure activity may have full ambulatory privileges. Assessment of the understanding of the condition by the client and family is important so that realistic plans may be made for living with the problem. Attempts should be made to avoid situations of unusual stress, delayed medications, or overhydration, situations that may add to the client's discomfort or result in an actual seizure. If the client has been admitted for a surgical procedure or extensive radiological and laboratory studies, the nurse and physician should plan adequate coverage using anticonvulsants during the preoperative and postoperative procedure period. The client should also be taught to seek immediate assistance when an aura occurs. As a helpful guide to staff members, pertinent points of this client's seizure experiences—time, aura, precipitating events, and other characteristics—should be listed on the individual nursing care plan.

The nurse is responsible for the administration of medications at regular intervals, for the early recognition of their toxic effects, and for teaching the client to assume responsibility gradually for medications and hygiene. Oral hygiene is stressed in preventing the complications of hypertrophy of the gums or gingivitis that may occur after phenytoin therapy.

***Psychosocial and educational interventions for client and family.*** Probably the most important aspect of overall seizure management is the psychosocial adjustment, which is essential to every affected client and family. When the condition is first diagnosed, time spent in assisting the family in acceptance, understanding, and planning saves many hours and problems later.

During the initial assessment, efforts should be made to elicit the emotional meaning of the seizure disorder to the client and family. Some persons will think that a convulsion is not a seizure. Thus semantics should be carefully explored. Others might say that a major motor seizure is a convulsion, whereas other types are spells but not convulsions. Thus when asking the family about seizure episodes, careful attention should be paid to answers, so that all seizure events may be noted. Since many myths have been propagated from earliest times, listening to the family for their views on the scope of seizures and their reaction to the event in the client is very important.

Next, attention should be directed to a discussion of why the client and family believe that the seizure episode occurred. Some may have ideas that it is related to punishment deserved for an undesirable act of some kind, or they may feel a sense of guilt for having caused it or for permitting a certain event that coincided with the seizure. Other fantasies may prevail about causation of the seizure. Exploration of these beliefs is important, since the family may relate to the client in an unhealthy manner when these mistaken ideas go unexpressed and remain harbored within. Overprotection is a particular outcome of these feelings. Another problem may arise when relatives lay blame on specific members of the client's family and arouse feelings of guilt for transmitting the problem.

When parents are unable to express some of the feelings or problems inherent in living with the child who has seizures, the interviewer may continue the session by using a third party technique. For example, ''Many people think that . . .'' or ''Some families have concerns about . . .'' are good ways to lead into the discussion of essential information including brain damage, effect on intelligence, neuronal cause, and restrictions on the usual life-style. These explanations should be individualized to include the problems that the particular child may encounter in view of the unique seizure problem.

The client often has many questions and concerns about what the seizure is doing inside the brain. Sometimes an abnormal physiological event in the brain may be equated with mental illness in the mind of a client, since both events involve nerves and the brain. These conclusions may cause the client to feel great concern about himself and his future. Another possibility is that the client may feel that the seizure is a form of punishment for something that he has done wrong. The client needs an explanation about the scope of the problem, essentials of control, and effects that the seizure disorder might have on his life-style. This discussion should be geared to the client's developmental level and should be casual enough so that the client may express feelings, ask questions, and indicate the level of understanding and acceptance of the discussion. As treatment progresses, subsequent visits may be used to allow the client to continue his acceptance and discussion of the disease process. They may also be utilized to ask the client about his subjective ideas on the effectiveness of seizure control. In cases of psychomotor seizures, wherein sensory events or intense anxiety may precede the seizure, the client may be able to describe a continuation of these events, which may be controlled by adequate medication.

The EEG provides another area that is interpreted in a wide variety of ways by clients and families. Although the EEG is a valuable diagnostic tool, it has to be interpreted by the physician in the context of the client's performance capacities and the findings seen in the clinical assessment. However, some individuals misunderstand the significance of the EEG. They may construe a normal tracing to be a reason to think that the seizure problem is finished or to independently stop the medications. An abnormal tracing may cause anguish about the possibility of brain damage or worsening of the condition. In explaining the EEG the nurse should be certain that they do not think that the EEG shocks the client, has therapeutic value, or removes something from the brain. The explanation should also include a description of the procedure, with emphasis on the fact that the study does not involve pain. Practice in how to cooperate with the technician may assist the client in getting a better tracing over a shorter time period.

In the first discussion of the seizure disorder with the client and family a wide range of emotional responses may be evident, including fear, anger, guilt, or false notions about impending insanity, death, or brain damage. The patterns of subsequent acceptance are similar to those seen in any process of crisis or grief about loss. In the instance of seizures the loss is probably the loss of ''good'' health. When the process of grief and acceptance is blocked and the family denies the existence of the problem, effective communication and seizure management cannot be instituted.

Clues about disease acceptance may be elicited when one asks the family what the client has been told about seizures. Feelings of overprotection, communication capacities, and psychological responses often come through when the client offers this explanation. However, the nurse should realize that the acceptance process takes time and repeated explanations of pertinent facts, so that individuals should not be expected to grasp the whole problem or their response to it after the first few encounters. Reinforcement of the importance of taking the medication according to prescription is essential; that is, the client should not stop taking the medication even when seizures have not occurred for a long time or as a test to see if the seizures are still present.

When there is poor acceptance of the problem, the client may harbor many unfounded feelings that interfere with normal functioning. For example, he may presume that avoiding play will keep him from having a seizure. He may fear the response of others or fear death and insanity from a seizure. The main fear underlying the client's viewpoint is often the fear of loss of control. The nurse should ask the client to explain why he comes to the physician or clinic and what his plans for a future career and involvement in extracurricular activities are. Sometimes the client has selected dangerous sports or a career that involves climbing, driving, and so on. These activities might best be replaced by other safer activities unless the client cannot accept alternatives. In that case such activities should not be performed without another person in attendance. Realistic acceptance of the seizure problem and its limitations are goals toward which the nurse should carefully guide the client.

Whether or not the client consistently takes medication becomes an important consideration in interviewing the client and family. Many authorities believe that acceptance of the seizure disorder is expressed by patterns of taking medications. Taking an anticonvulsant causes the client and family to realize that a problem exists, since they have a daily reminder in the medication. At times the inability to take the medication is evidence of denial of the problem or the overt expression of an underlying problem in the family-client relationship. Some worry about addicting the client to these medications, and an appropriate discussion of these attitudes is warranted.

When seizures are not controlled, the time that the nurse spends in talking with the family frequently reveals the fact that current medications are not being taken rather than the fact that more or different combinations of medications are required.

***Psychosocial and educational interventions beyond the family.*** Since epilepsy is so widespread among all races of mankind, it is an important problem of public health and preventive medicine. The ignorance and misunderstanding of this disease by the public and professional persons are appalling and, in large part, are the cause of the social ostracism of the epileptic. To be sure, some progress has been made since the days when epileptics were believed to be possessed by devils, but in light of our present knowledge, this progress is negligible. The public still retains many misconceptions of this disease; they range from insanity to criminality.

The epileptic child has the same needs for love, understanding, setting of limits, consistent discipline, and recognition as other children. If the seizures are not completely controlled by medication, climbing trees, riding a bicycle, and swimming may have to be restricted.

It is important that nurses, whether in the clinic, hospital, school, or a community agency, help to educate these families so that epileptic children are afforded opportunities to assume responsibility and to participate actively in a therapeutic regimen directed toward controlling their seizures. Only in this way can these children learn to accept their attacks and adjust to them as to any other disabling illness and ultimately become productive, self-respecting members of society.

Most medical authorities maintain that seizures are less likely to occur when the mind and body are active. Recent legislation provides the client whose seizures are reasonably well controlled with medication the opportunity to attend school.

The school nurse should be notified when a child subject to convulsive seizures is enrolled. The teacher also should be informed of the child's condition, the nature and type of seizure, and what to do if one occurs. By maintaining a calm, matter-of-fact attitude, the teacher can exert a positive influence on the epileptic's classmates. Depending on the age of the children, he or she should show them what to do if an attack occurs. If a seizure occurs, the teacher should discuss the episode with the children, answer their questions, and assure them that the child will be all right. Educators are beginning to recognize that epilepsy is not more complicated than any other health problem and frequently is much less disabling. The presence of an epileptic child in the classroom can serve as an educational experience for classmates by helping them to develop understanding and acceptance and to prepare them more realistically for life. However, even though prepared, children may taunt, ridicule, or reject a classmate who has seizures. If this happens, the teacher should intervene and through discussion and role playing help them gain an understanding of their behavior and its harmful impact on the epileptic child.

The presence of epilepsy by itself does not call for modification in teaching methods, curriculum, or classroom placement. Epileptic children without severe brain damage have the same intellectual ability as normal children and should have the same opportunity to learn and develop within the same school setting.

Many references to the so-called epileptic personality are found in the literature. It is rarely well defined. Moreover, study populations selected from such places as state hospitals may result in findings that cannot be attributed to the typical seizure client. Some believe that undesirable behavioral responses in clients may be attributable more to society's attitude and lack of acceptance, rather than to organic problems.

In an earlier publication Frank described the results as the client matures and seeks employment:

The unemployed person with epilepsy is caught in a vicious and somehow cumulative dilemma: (1) his epilepsy severely affects his early social functioning, which, as it deteriorates, promotes further withdrawal and increasing dependence, (2) if he did not, in the meantime, acquire a skill or education, he is, in reality, multihandicapped, and finally (3) chronic unemployment and lack of income worsens an already weakened self-image and quite probably deprives him of adequate medical care as he increasingly became less and less ''employable.'' The subject person therefore becomes a candidate for the stereotyped epileptic—unkempt appearance and frequent seizures. This unfortunate picture is a reflection of the harsh fact that today's existing public and private programs do not adequately meet the needs of this population of handicapped jobseekers.*

Records show that epileptics, when given an opportunity to work, have a good attitude toward work and a better than average attendance rate.

Every state has a vocational rehabilitation service for the disabled. This service is available free of charge to anyone who is handicapped regardless of the nature of the disability and includes a medical evaluation as well as aptitude and occupational inventories. Guidance in selecting the right job and training for it are also provided. The vocational counselor works with the state employment service to find jobs for the disabled person and the person with controlled epilepsy. New legislation puts more pressure on those discriminating against the handicapped.

Other resources for the epileptic and family are available in public health facilities, sheltered workshops, various specialized private organizations, and welfare agencies. If given the opportunity, more than 80% of the epileptics could be employed, could do a good job, and could become self-supporting, respected, contributing members of society.

## CHILDBEARING

Some evidence exists regarding the fact that the effectiveness of oral contraceptives may be reduced when they are taken concurrently with anticonvulsants.

In pregnancy, the epileptic needs to be monitored by monthly plasma level determinations and appropriate dosage adjustments, to avoid loss of seizure control. Failure to increase medications may result in status epilepticus.

The goal of management is to provide a seizure-free pregnancy on the least number of anticonvulsants possible, with avoidance of trimethadione, a drug known to cause fetal malformation.

Neonates should be examined carefully for abnormalities and treated symptomatically for elevated substance levels, that is, barbiturate withdrawal. Clotting abnormalities may be a serious problem for the neonate.

Serum levels of anticonvulsants are gradually returned to the lower nonpregnant state in the mother.

## LAWS AFFECTING EPILEPTICS

The various states differ in their laws concerning epileptics with respect to driving a vehicle and marrying. The nurse should become familiar with the laws of the state, so that effective counseling of children and parents may occur. Unfortunately some employers still practice discriminatory hiring practices with regard to individuals who have seizures, even though these individuals work effectively when given the opportunity.

## MEDICATIONS

The control of seizures in most epileptics is based on the regular administration of anticonvulsants. The goal of treatment is to prevent seizures while avoiding as many side effects as possible.

Principles of anticonvulsant usage include the following:

*From Frank, D.S.: Rehabil. Rec. **9:**36, Jan.-Feb. 1968.

1. The recommended anticonvulsant is the first one given to the client. When control is not achieved, the dosage is increased to a point just below the toxic level. The gradual increase in dosage requires up to 6 weeks before this medication is termed ineffective.
2. If a medication is stopped, gradual withdrawal is the method of choice, even when the discontinued medication is being replaced by another medication or medications, to avoid status epilepticus.
3. Blood level determinations should be performed to measure all anticonvulsants in order to adequately monitor and evaluate drug therapy.
4. Anticonvulsants are selected so that the least toxic, most effective medication is utilized. When this medication is not effective, the second choice is used.
5. The capsule or tablet form provides a more accurate dose for home use. Young children may need medications to be crushed in fruit to accept the anticonvulsant.

## RESOURCES

The epilepsy Foundation of America (EFA) is working to repeal discriminatory laws, improve the psychosocial and economic outlook for epileptics, and change public attitudes.

Printed and audiovisual materials are available from this organization on request. Anticonvulsants at lower costs and life insurance at reasonable rates are also available from the EFA. Persons desiring more information should specify their professional position and the use for requested materials when they contact the local epilepsy agency or write to the following:

Epilepsy Foundation of America
4351 Garden City Drive
Landover, Maryland 20785

## HEADACHE

Headache is discussed as a discrete entity because it is a very common problem. Studies reveal that headache may be the major subjective complaint in as many as 50% of all persons seen in typical office practice. As is true of seizures, headaches do not constitute a disease entity but rather a symptom indicative of a wide range of underlying problems. Headache may also be part of a syndrome such as migraine, wherein it is the most characteristic symptom. Headache represents the disease to the client, but it signifies the need for investigation into underlying causes to the practitioner. Although the cause of headaches may be either functional or organic, most headaches are found to be of a functional origin.

Before proceeding to a discussion of headache types, it is important to understand the anatomical mechanism of head pain.

## ANATOMICAL MECHANISM OF HEAD PAIN

One of the most intriguing facts about head pain is the number of cranial tissues that are insensitive to pain. These include the skull, the parenchyma of the brain, a great portion of the dura and pia mater, the ependymal lining of the ventricles, and the choroid plexus. The following outlines pain-sensitive cranial tissues:

*Intracranial structures*

Afferent veins
Cranial sinuses
Arteries of dura mater
Arteries and major branches at base of brain
Portions of dura mater near large vessels

*Extracranial structures*

Mucosa
Arteries (more sensitive than veins)
Muscles
Fascia
Scalp
Skin

*Nerves*

Second and third cervical nerves
Trigeminal, facial, glossopharyngeal, and vagal cranial nerves

In considering the pathways of headaches one speaks of headaches resulting from structures that are either above or below the tentorium cerebelli. Pain emanating from structures above the tentorium is conveyed through the trigeminal nerves for expression in the parietal, temporal, or frontal aspects of the skull. Pain originating from the structures below the tentorium is conveyed through upper cervical spinal roots and the glossopharyngeal and vagal nerves for expression in the occipital portion of the cranium.

To better understand the cause of various headaches in relation to the probable underlying mechanism, it may be helpful to relate a few examples. The first broad category of causes is intracranial problems such as (1) meningeal processes (hemorrhage, meningitis), (2) decreases in intracranial pressure (as after a diagnostic study such as pneumoencephalography or lumbar puncture), or (3) space-occupying lesions (hematomas, tumors, abscesses, or aneurysms). In instances of intracranial problems the underlying mechanism may probably be attributed to direct stimulation of pain-sensitive structures from processes resulting in dilatation, distention, or traction.

The second category encompasses a wide range of extracranial causes, which include disorders involving the eye, nasal sinuses, teeth, mouth, ears, cervical spine, muscles of the neck and head, and inflammation of cranial arteries. Pain in this category may be attributed to more than one mechanism. Pain may result from direct stimulation to pain-sensitive structures, from reflex muscular contractions or vascular spasm, or from another area as referred pain.

The third category of causes consists of generalized conditions that include headaches. One major condition in this category is arterial hypertension, wherein the headache is the outcome of dilatation of intracranial and extracranial arteries, with the additional factor of cerebral edema in malignant cases. Headaches may also result from dilatation of intracranial arteries as might occur from pyrexia and hypoxia or intoxication by vasodilator substances such as alcohol, nitrates, and histamine.

## CLASSIFICATION

Headaches are classified according to facts gleaned from the history and to descriptive data. For the purposes of this text, headaches are categorized into three major groups: vascular, muscle contraction, and traction-inflammatory (Table 14-2).

Vascular dilatation characterizes all vascular

**TABLE 14-2.** Headaches: types and intervention modalities

| Classification | Possible interventions |
| --- | --- |
| **Vascular** | |
| Migraine: common, classic complicated (hemiplegia, ophthalmoplegia) | Analgesics |
| | Sedatives |
| Toxic vascular | Antihypertensives |
| Hypertensive | Mood elevators, antidepressants |
| Cluster (histamine) | Cyproheptadine |
| Secondary to infectious process, fever | Ergotamine |
| **Muscle contraction (tension)** | |
| Psychogenic problems: depressive responses, conversion reactions | Methods to relax client |
| | Physical therapy |
| | Antidepressants |
| Posttraumatic response | Analgesics |
| Cervical arthritis | Sedation |
| Chronic myositis | Counseling to alter or remove psychic stressors or change coping patterns |
| **Traction-inflammatory** | |
| Intracranial lesions | Investigation into underlying disorders |
| Extracranial lesions | |
| Disease of facial structures, throat, and ears | Correction of disorder |
| Infection | Symptomatic support |
| Occlusive vascular disorder | |
| Phlebitis, arteritis | |

headaches and is the phenomenon that occurs during the painful phase of the migraine attack. When vasoconstriction is evident, it is often the cause of the sensory experiences that occur before the migraine attack. In extreme cases of migraine attacks, ophthalmoplegic and hemiplegic migraine episodes occur.

### Vascular headache

*Migraine (familial sick headache).* Migraine is a recurring paroxysmal headache with familial predisposition usually preceded by an aura, especially visual phenomena (such as stars, zigzag lines, and transitory impaired vision), and associated with nausea and possibly vomiting. An attack may last for hours or days. If at the first sign of an aura the individual takes the prescribed medication and lies down in a dark, quiet room, the attack may be prevented.

The cause is unknown, but an attack is frequently precipitated by emotional disturbances, fatigue, and tension. External stimuli such as noise, bright lights, and crowds also may precipitate an attack in a susceptible person. The onset is usually about the time of puberty, and the episodes generally terminate at the climacteric. Women are afflicted three times more frequently than men.

There is no known pathological condition, but the mechanism is considered to be vascular, since migraine may be treated effectively by the administration of vasoconstricting drugs.

**PHYSIOLOGICAL PHENOMENA.** As a result of contemporary research on migraine headaches, investigators have concluded that during a migraine attack the dilated migrainous artery is hyperpermeable while undergoing a sterile local inflammatory response. Vasoactive substances operate during this inflammatory response as follows:

1. Levels of plasma serotonin, a substance that normally constricts scalp arteries, decrease at the onset of a migraine attack.
2. A vasodilating polypeptide, related to bradykinin, is found in increased quantities beneath the surface tissues in clients experiencing a migraine attack.
3. In individuals who have migraine attacks, a disorder in the capacities of tyramine to conjugate has been observed. Tyramine, a pressor amine, frees norepinephrine from tissues and is capable of triggering migraine in clients predisposed to this problem. This finding causes some investigators to suspect that migraines are possibly a problem of genetic abnormalities.
4. In instances wherein temporal arteries have been removed during the painful aspect of a migraine attack, increased norepinephrine uptake has been observed.
5. When cluster headaches occur in association with migraine attacks, whole blood histamine levels are elevated during the initial stages of the episode.
6. The injection of prostaglandins, histamine, and other vasodilatating substances may result in a headache in individuals with a predisposition to the problem.

Although vasoactive substances do not account for the total sequence of events inherent in a migraine attack, they do participate in that aspect of the attack related to increased vascular permeability. Knowledge of these substances is valuable in understanding the objectives of pharmacological intervention, which include inhibition of vasoactive substances, stabilization of membranes, reduction in vasomotor functions, and blockage of chemical products that augment the inflammatory process. Because several pharmacological objectives may be met simultaneously, management may include a combination of therapies (Table 14-2).

**TREATMENT AND NURSING INTERVENTION.** Medical treatment is based on the elimination of predisposing factors, both physical and psychological. This requires a complete medical diagnostic study, including history; physical examination; allergy tests, if indicated; histamine test to determine sensitivity; psychological tests; and psychiatric evaluation.

The drug that has been most beneficial in the treatment of migraine is ergotamine tartrate (Gynergen) used alone or in combination with caffeine (Cafergot). This must be administered as early as possible after the beginning of an attack for the most effective therapeutic result.

Methysergide (Sansert) has been used for the prevention or reduction of the intensity and frequency of vascular headaches. It is indicated if the individual has one or more severe vascular headaches a week or if the headache is so severe and uncontrollable that preventive therapy is indicated. It is not recommended for the therapeutic management of the client with an acute vascular headache. The client receiving Sansert as a prophylactic and preventive measure must be closely supervised by the physician and monitored for adverse reactions, especially retroperitoneal fibrosis or related conditions. The manufacturer recommends that Sansert be discontinued at 6-month intervals and that a medication-free interval of 3 to 4 weeks should intervene before Sansert is again administered.

Psychotherapy is being used more frequently in an attempt to demonstrate to the client the influence personality and methods of adjustment have on precipitating or aggravating the recurrent attacks of pain. The physical and emotional environment may contribute exciting factors. These

**TABLE 14-3.** Summary of pharmacological therapies for migraine attacks

| Substance | Action |
|---|---|
| Antihistamines | Interfere with vasoactive amines |
| Antiserotonin compounds | Interfere with vasoactive amines |
| Corticosteroids | Stabilize lysosomal membranes, reduce inflammatory response, lower complement titer |
| Phenylbutazone | Anti-inflammatory, interrupts functions of kinin |
| Aspirin | Anti-inflammatory, stabilizes proteins, decreases formation of active prostaglandins, decreases platelet aggregation, exerts indirect effect on release of vasoactive substances |
| Indomethacin | Anti-inflammatory, stabilizes proteins, inhibits active prostaglandin formation |
| Ergot | Vasoconstrictor, alpha adrenergic blocker |
| Cyproheptadine | Stops action of serotonin and histamine |
| Propranolol | Beta adrenergic blocker |
| Methysergide | Serotonin antagonist, indirectly blocks histamine release, promotes vasoconstriction |

should be evaluated and the client guided, as he or she develops insight, so that he or she can better formulate attitudes and goals and regulate activities in achieving them. Relaxing baths (98° F) twice a day for 30 minutes may help relieve the client's general tension and reduce the frequency of attacks. Chapter 10 offers techniques on biofeedback in relation to migraine attacks. This chapter details some biofeedback techniques in relation to migraine headaches.

The nurse is responsible for assisting the physician with the administration of tests and treatments and for making observations of the client's attitudes, behavior, and reaction to drugs. Nursing care is symptomatic during the attacks. The nurse, under the direction and guidance of the psychiatrist or psychologist, may be able to help the client to adjust psychologically as well as physically to this disease.

*Toxic vascular headache.* A variety of conditions result in systemic vasodilatation and cause one to experience a toxic vascular headache. Some conditions that underlie this type of headache include fever, alcohol consumption, and retention of such agents as nitrates or carbon dioxide.

## Muscle-contraction headaches

Most individuals have experienced a headache related to muscle contraction, since it is the most prevalent type of headache. Some refer to this type of headache as a tension headache. This type of headache is often described as a dull, bandlike ache that has a persistent quality. These headaches are known to last for a few days or up to a period of years. On closer questioning, one finds that the pain is ill defined, bilateral, and characterized by a pattern of gradual onset. The client does not seem to gain relief from the headache without medication. However, the headache does not interrupt sleep. When the headache is the result of tension, sleep does not solve the problem. Instead the headache remains as the client awakens. Sedatives and analgesics are effective in relieving the pain. Ergotamine and vasoconstrictors do not affect this type of headache. In reviewing the client's history, one notes that the headaches are not particularly correlated with a family history of the problem. Moreover, there is a strong connection between tension headaches and situational stresses inherent in many life events.

Because of the strong correlation between situational factors and tension headaches, during the assessment the practitioner gives particular weight to moods, behavioral patterns, and thoughts of the client. Depression is a frequent companion of tension headaches and should certainly be considered during the assessment process.

Posttraumatic headache is often included with muscle-contraction headaches. In considering this type of headache, investigate and palpate for points of tenderness and pain in the neck and head. Arthritis of the spine should also be a major consideration when one is evaluating a possible focus of pain.

*Mechanisms and treatment.* The muscle-contraction headache takes place as the gamma efferent system persists in firing beyond the point where relaxation is indicated. This prolonged period of firing, to the point where tightness in the muscle eventually causes a painful contraction, results from a complex set of steps involving cortical influences or local or systemic disease affecting the muscle spindle. The pain sets into motion a cycle wherein pain results in increased spasms and anxiety—hence, more pain.

A number of measures are available to break this

vicious cycle. One group of measures designed to promote relaxation includes a wide variety of techniques: heat applications, massage, exercise, and posture improvement programs during wakefulness and sleep.

Central influences underlying the initiation of muscle spasm may be negated when the mood and emotional status of the client are altered. When the headaches are triggered by adverse emotional states, therapeutic intervention often includes pharmacological agents such as tranquilizers, sedatives, antidepressants, and analgesics. When the headache seems to be related to a persistent psychological problem, the client should be referred to a qualified therapist for more intensive evaluation and management.

Local instillation of corticosteroids in anesthetics is also effectively utilized to alleviate the pain associated with low-grade inflammation of tendons, muscles, or subcutaneous tissue.

### Traction-inflammatory headache

In some texts the traction-inflammatory category is further subdivided by underlying causes. Since you would not be in a position to identify the discrete cause contributing to a traction or inflammatory headache in more than a general way, the broadness of the category should not pose a problem.*

Organic disease processes of the brain or its components may result in traction-inflammatory headaches. These cranial components include the paranasal sinuses, teeth, nose, ears, eyes, blood vessels, meninges, and brain tissue itself. So-called traction headaches refer to nonspecific head pain that accompanies any space-occupying process in the cranium, including cerebral edema. When headache results from the presence of a subarachnoid hemorrhage, the pain is quite severe. Traction headaches may result from processes contributing to increased intracranial pressure, such as hydrocephalus, or from processes that cause a decrease in intracranial pressure, such as lumbar punctures or fractures at the base of the spine. Traction headaches may also result from inflam-

matory processes such as meningitis, encephalitis, arteritis, or phlebitis of intracranial or extracranial origin. Some of the more severe cranial neuralgias, such as tic douloureaux, are also included in this category. Chapter 19 contains a discussion of cranial nerve disorders.

Earlier there was given a list of the pain-sensitive tissues in the scalp and cranium. In the traction-inflammatory type of headache, pain results from either traction or torque on these structures or acute or chronic inflammatory responses. In these instances, medical or surgical intervention requires a two-pronged approach designed at symptomatic relief along with assessment and management of the underlying condition.

### HISTORY

The history is exacted carefully from the client because it is extremely important in the definition of the headache. However, beyond its relevance to the assessment process, the history is also an excellent means of establishing rapport with and gaining the confidence of the client. Because headaches necessarily involve the head, a portion of the anatomy wherein problems take on particular relevance with relation to personality, intelligence, and so on, disorders involving the head may have special significance for the client. If the headache has persisted for any length of time, the client may be anxious or conceal data because of fears of the gravity of the condition or of the potential of its being a malignant tumor. Once the client's concerns have been aired, the early periods of contact are more valuable both in data collection and in defining the possibilities for the therapeutic relationship.

The headache history begins with the subjective description of headache types and duration of the problem. It is not unusual for the same individual to experience more than one type of headache. The discussion then centers on onset, since data on initiation of symptoms and duration of the disorder are important in identifying the type of headache. If the headache has existed for a relatively short period and seems to be of a progressive nature with associated neurological signs, the chances are quite good that the individual has an organic disturbance. Vascular headaches most often have their onset between childhood and the fourth decade of life. Headaches that have their genesis in

---

*For a more definitive system of classification, consult J.A.M.A. **179:**717, March 3, 1962, and the *Classification of Headache* compiled by the Committee on Classification of Headache of the National Institute of Neurological Diseases and Blindness (Dr. A.P. Friedman, Chairperson).

the fifth decade or afterward are most commonly caused by psychogenic problems, but organic disease is also a cause in a smaller number of cases. Depression as the underlying cause of a headache is suspect when the headache originates after a situational or physiological crisis in an individual's life.

The next task is to determine whether the headache has a focus or is generalized. Does the headache recur in the same place or does it switch sides, a typical finding in migraine headaches? In the absence of increased intracranial pressure a generalized headache is usually related to psychogenic disease, wherein a localized type of pain is more often the result of organic disorders of migraine.

The time of occurrence and the intervals between head pains provide valuable clues to the type of headache. Sinus headaches have their onset in the early morning and increase in severity as the day wears on. Migraines are typified by their tendency to occur in an intermittent pattern. Migraine headaches tend to be absent during happy times and vacations, whereas psychogenic headaches tend to be chronic and worse during holiday periods, when depression may be a factor.

The nature of the head pain should be fully described, since each type has individual qualities. Vascular headaches are intermittent but intense when present. Head pain from organic disease tend to be constant and progressive in contrast to the pain of psychogenic headaches, wherein symptoms are dull, aggravating, and constant.

In some headaches the head pain is preceded by visual or olfactory sensations or more rarely dizziness, paresthesias, and interruption of motor functions. The classic migraine is the most common type of head pain with prodromal symptoms. However, such symptoms may also precede headaches related to some tumors or vascular disorders.

Some headaches consistently occur concurrently with other symptoms. Psychogenic headaches commonly appear in conjunction with behavioral disturbances, whereas migraine headaches are often associated with nausea and vomiting. Focal signs, in combination with a headache, would cause the practitioner to consider the possibility of an underlying organic disturbance.

Situational, physiological, or psychological events frequently trigger headaches. Tension headaches are associated with certain types of employment wherein activity level, noise level, and high pressure for production or public contact create an atmosphere of high anxiety. In women, migraines are commonly associated with the initiation of menstruation. Pregnancy, after the third month, and menopause tend to alleviate migraines associated with menses. Migraines may also be precipitated by a variety of other factors, including stress; fatigue; photic stimuli, such as direct sunlight; and foods containing such vasoactive substances as tyramine. Headaches may be precipitated by the ingestion of monosodium glutamate, sodium nitrate in cured meat, and alcoholic beverages; by excessive amounts of sleep; or by extended periods without food. When workers inhale toxic fumes with inadequate ventilation as a part of their employment, headaches may result. In some individuals, headaches are related to psychosocial problems. When a headache is severe enough to warrant medical attention, the practitioner should inquire about the occurrence of similar episodes in other family members. Migraine headaches have an inherited component, whereas depression headaches tend to a pattern of response in some family situations.

When headaches are associated with interruptions in sleep, the problem is most often related to anxiety or depression. The other types of headaches that may arouse the client from sleep include the cluster headache and occasionally a migraine attack.

If headaches have a focal quality, especially with seizures or additional abnormal findings, the practitioner should rule out the possibility of an organic disorder. Individuals with seasonal allergies may experience more intense head pain in a seasonal pattern. If a client has a past history of tuberculosis, surgical removal of a malignancy, or prior intracranial problem, the onset of headaches would cause the practitioner to assess the possibility of a recurring problem. A number of systemic disorders may include headaches as a part of the symptoms, for example, hypothyroidism. If a client has repeatedly sought medical assistance for evaluation of a headache, the problem may be the result of minimal trauma from an obscure incident or a psychogenic disorder.

As a final part of the assessment, the practitioner needs to carefully elicit any relationship of headaches to pharmacological agents, whether these agents caused or alleviated symptoms. Current usage of medication may also shed light on the cause of a headache. In women of childbearing age the onset of migraine headaches or the increased frequency and intensity of attacks may be related to the use of oral contraceptives. When reserpine is taken as the medication controlling hypertension, the incidence of migraine headaches and depressive episodes may be increased. If the client has previously taken antidepressants with subsequent relief of head pain, the cause may be related to depression.

## EXAMINATION

During the physical examination, several points are worthy of observation to confirm the presumptive diagnosis established during the history.

1. Carefully observe the behavior of the client and the body language in relation to the description of head pain. Detailed complaints of extreme head pain accompanied by a relaxed demeanor indicate a psychogenic origin.
2. Organic or vascular disturbances that result in head pain are usually accompanied by obvious discomfort, especially during locomotion, wherein movements tend to be gauged and guarded. Moreover, the photic stimulation of bright lighting tends to aggravate these types of headaches.
3. Observation of gait is significant, since an intracranial space-occupying lesion may result in disturbed motor functions along with head pain.
4. General observation of the skin of individuals with migraine attacks often reveals vasomotor disturbances such as moist palms or blotchy areas.

The general examination continues with vital sign measurement. Vital signs may reveal several things about the client. If the client is anxious, the pulse and respiration may be accelerated. Increases in the diastolic blood pressure may result in an increased incidence of migraine headaches for the individual prone to these attacks. A temperature elevation or a low-grade fever may be indicative of either a systemic or a neurological infection.

The assessment continues with an evaluation of the head. At this point the practitioner notes facial asymmetry characteristic of a facial palsy, deep furrows on the forehead, and the presence of prominent superficial arteries in the temporal region—an indication of temporal arteritis or migraine headaches.

The eyes are assessed for disorders in extraocular eye movement and defects in the visual field. If palpation of the closed eye reveals increased intraocular tension, referral to an ophthalmologist is indicated for testing through tonometry. Examination of the fundi may reveal such disorders as diabetes, hemorrhage, increased intracranial pressure, or hypertension.

Externally the eyes are inspected for injection of the sclera and lacrimation. If ptosis occurs in association with a cluster or migraine headache, it should resolve spontaneously within a couple of days.

The nasal area is inspected for evidence of sinusitis or inflammation, since these conditions may contribute to a headache. The ears are assessed for the presence of infectious processes and hearing losses.

The mouth is assessed for infection, which may result from a neglected caries that has become abscessed. The client is asked to bite normally, and the practitioner observes the bite for the presence of distortion, which might cause chronic discomfort at the temporomandibular joint.

The entire head is then palpated for defects, crepitus, or overly tender points. Auscultation of the head, eye orbits, neck, carotid arteries, and supraclavicular areas reveals any bruits that may be present.

The neck is rotated and palpated. Tension, limited range of motion, or discomfort may be noted, especially in clients with cervical arthritis or muscle-contraction headaches. In individuals prone to tension headaches the tenderness on palpation often extends to include palpation of the trapezius muscle.

Other systems are reviewed through the history and physical assessment to rule out the possibility of a concurrent problem in another system that may be causing the individual to experience headaches.

The assessment is completed as the remaining portions of the neurological assessment are performed. Abnormal findings in any portion of the neurological examination may cause the practitioner to suspect an organic disorder as the underlying disease condition contributing to head pain.

## DIAGNOSTIC STUDIES

Which diagnostic studies are to be performed is dictated by the findings in the history and physical assessment. When an organic disorder is suspected, further studies are indicated to delineate the problem. Testing begins with laboratory studies on the blood and urine. When indicated, a chest radiograph or skull series may be done. If a vascular problem is suspected, especially in relation to an arrhythmia, an electrocardiogram is taken.

Specific neurological studies begin with the least dangerous and invasive procedures and may involve more elaborate testing when neurological disturbances are apparent. The initial battery of neurological studies often includes such procedures as (1) an electroencephalogram, (2) a brain scan, (3) paranasal sinus radiographs, and (4) cervical spine radiographs. A psychiatric evaluation may be necessary if headaches seem to have a psychogenic focus.

When headaches seem to be related to an intracranial process, further testing may include (1) computerized axial tomography, (2) lumbar puncture, (3) carotid arteriography, (4) ventriculography, or (5) pneumoencephalography.

## INTERVENTIONS

The following outline provides the necessary points for intervention:*

1. Thorough diagnostic evaluation
   - Tests to eliminate the possibility of disease processes or space-occupying lesions
   - Allergy tests
   - Histamine test to ascertain sensitivity
   - Psychological assessment
2. Support during diagnostic workup
   - Assist the client or significant others in understanding each procedure and its personal significance
   - Provide physical support and reassurance before, during, and after procedures
   - Monitor client and act cooperatively with the physician in appropriate interventions for significant findings

*From Conway-Rutkowski, B.: Am. J. Nurs. **81:**1848, Oct. 1981.

3. Assistance during an attack
   - Administer appropriate medication
   - Darken room
   - Reduce environmental noise
   - Provide symptomatic supportive and relief measures
4. Comprehensive treatment plan
   - Provide pharmacological support
   - Enlighten client about precipitating factors, events in daily living, and behavioral patterns contributing to the episodes
   - Work with clients to develop concrete goals and attainable schedules to reduce the stress in their lives
   - Practice *shiatsu* (finger pressure), relaxation, and biofeedback techniques with the client
5. Ongoing interventions—provide client with sufficient information for him to explain:
   - Significance of adequate, prompt intervention
   - Relationship of medications and adjunctive treatment techniques to the prevention or relief of pain
   - Problems with concurrent and/or general relief of pain
   - Problems with concurrent and/or prolonged use of nonprescriptive medications
   - Need to seek a cause for the headache
   - Importance of seeing appropriate health care professionals on a continuing basis to plan and jointly coordinate a therapeutic regimen
   - Dosage, action, and adverse and desirable outcome of medications prescribed
   - Treatment modification in certain situations, such as pregnancy

**Expected outcomes**

The client will:

1 Experience, receive appropriate health care intervention for, and be able to thoroughly explain, all diagnostic tests.
2 Participate in planning care for painful episodes and preventive aspects for thwarting future pain, and in instituting appropriate interventions as needed.
3 Describe all prescribed medications according to dosage, effect, frequency, special information, side effects, and physician-reportable problems.
4 Adjust life style to minimize precipitating events to headaches.
5 Identify specific measures and behaviors that he or she implements that cause, prevent, and alleviate headaches.

Refer to the previous key nursing interventions in clients with headaches. Related information may also be found in Chapter 10 (pain), Chapter 11 (assessment), Chapter 12 (diagnostic tests), and Chapter 27 (adjunctive interventions).

## HEADACHES IN CHILDREN

The organic headache is generally characterized by a dull, throbbing, or bursting sensation, whereas the functional type includes a feeling of pressure. Adults generally detail their symptoms more accurately than children do. Whenever the child offers great detail about the headache, it is often not organic in nature.

The headaches associated with increased intracranial pressure are detailed in Chapter 21. Vascular headaches, aggravated by activity, are often associated with the increased cerebral need for oxygen and distention of the blood vessels in children with cyanotic heart disorders.

Assessing the headache may present a problem in the very young child who cannot describe symptoms. However, observation in these instances reveals such behaviors as irritability, a troubled facial expression, ear-pulling, or head banging or rolling.

A careful history and assessment may be valuable in identifying the child with neurotic headaches. In these instances, episodes bear a relationship to environmental events and last for varying periods of time. The episode may be ended abruptly if the child is deliberately led into a diversionary activity or interest.

In cases of migraine headaches there is usually a family history of related problems. These headaches tend to recur and are seen after an aura occurs. Before the diagnosis is made, the parent may not be aware of the quiet behavior that precedes this headache. The characteristic symptoms of these headaches include photophobia, head pain, lethargic behavior, and nausea or vomiting. Vomiting often results in relief, and after sleeping the child wakes up feeling as he usually does.

## REFERENCES

Addy, D.P.: Childhood epilepsy, Br. Med. J. **2**:811-812, Sept. 1978.

Annegers, J.F., et al.: The risk of epilepsy following febrile convulsions, Neurology **29**:297-303, March 1979.

Blount, M., and Kinney, A.B.: What to remember about EEG, Nursing74 **4**:36, 1974.

Branson, H.: The epileptic. How you can help, RN **35**:48-58, June 1972.

Bruni, J., and Willmore, L.J.: Epilepsy and pregnancy, J. Can. Sciences Neurologiques **6**:345-349, Aug. 1979.

Buckingham, D.: Wigs that replace protective helmets, Nurs. Outlook **19**:118-119, Feb. 1971.

Childhood migraine, N. Engl. J. Med. **276**:56, 1967.

Conway-Rutkowski, B.L.: Getting to the cause of tension headache, Am. J. Nurs. **81**:1846, Jan. 1981.

Coulam, C.B., and Annegers, J.F.: Do anticonvulsants reduce the efficacy of oral contraceptives? Epilepsia **20**:519-526, 1979.

Current concepts of headache, Postgrad. Med. **56**:entire issue, Sept. 1974. (Symposium issue.)

Dalessio, D.J.: Mechanisms and biochemistry of headache, Nurs. Digest **3**:30, May-June 1975.

Diamond, S., and Dalessio, D.J.: The practicing physician's approach to headache, ed. 2, Baltimore, 1978, The Williams & Wilkins Co.

Diamond, S., and Medina, J.L.: Abortive therapy for vascular headaches, Consultant **16**:156-165, 1976.

Diamond, S., and Medina, J.L.: Migraine can be treated, The Female Patient **1**:11-13, 1976.

Draper, I.T.: Lecture notes on neurology, ed. 4, Philadelphia, 1974, J.B. Lippincott Co.

Dreifuss, F.E., and Sackellares, J.C.: Treating epilepsy in children: current prescribing, J. Practical Ther. **5**:63-77, 1979.

Dreifuss, F.E.: The nature of epilepsy. In Wright, G.N., editor: Epilepsy rehabilitation, Boston, 1975, Little, Brown & Co.

Forsythe, W.I., et al.: Phenytoin serum levels in children with epilepsy: a microimmuno-assay technique, Dev. Med. Child Neurol. **21**:448-454, 1979.

Frank, D.S.: Group counseling benefits jobseekers with epilepsy, Rehabil. Rec. **9**:36, Jan.-Feb. 1968.

Frank, D.S.: The multi-troubled jobseeker: the case of the jobless worker with a convulsive disorder, Washington, D.C., 1969, The Epilepsy Foundation of America.

Gascon, G.G.: Epilepsy in the adolescent, Postgrad. Med. **55**:111, 1974.

Graef, J.W., and Cone, T.E.: Manual of pediatric therapeutics, ed. 2, Boston, 1980, Little, Brown & Co.

Graham, J.R.: Cluster headache, Headache **11**:175, 1972.

Hawken, M., and Ozuna, J.: Practical aspects of anticonvulsant therapy, Am. J. Nurs. **79**:1062-1068, June 1979.

Henderson, W.R., and Raskin, N.H.: Hot dog headache: individual susceptibility to nitrite, Nurs. Digest **1**:54, June 1973.

Holowach, J., Thurston, D., and O'Leary, J.: Prognosis in childhood epilepsy: follow-up study of 148 cases in which therapy has been suspended after prolonged anticonvulsant control, N. Engl. J. Med. **286:**169-174, Jan. 27, 1972.

Jabbour, J.T., et al.: Pediatric neurology handbook, Flushing, N.Y., 1976, Medical Examination Publishing Co., Inc.

Kiloh, L.G., McComas, A.J., and Osselton, J.W.: Clinical electroencephalography, ed. 3, London, 1972, Butterworth & Co. (Publishers), Ltd.

Lennox-Buchthal, M.A.: Febrile convulsions, New York, 1973, American Elsevier Publishing Co.

Lindsay, J., et al.: Long-term outcome in children with temporal lobe seizures. II. Marriage, parenthood and sexual indifference, Dev. Med. Child. Neurol. **21:**433-440, 1979.

Livingston, S., et al.: No proven relationship of carbamazepine therapy to blood dyscrasias, Neurology **28:**101, Jan. 1978.

Livingston, S.: Comprehensive management of epilepsy in infancy, childhood and adolescence, Springfield, Ill., 1972, Charles C Thomas, Publisher.

Livingston, S.: Living with epileptic seizures, Springfield, Ill., 1963, Charles C Thomas, Publisher.

Livingston, S., and Livingston, H.: Hyperplasia, Am. J. Dis. Child. **117:**265, 1969.

Masland, R.L.: Commission for the control of epilepsy, Neurology **28:**861-862, Sept. 1978.

Modell, W., ed.: Drugs of choice 1974-1975, St. Louis, 1980, The C.V. Mosby Co.

Montouris, G.D., et al.: The pregnant epileptic: a review and recommendations, Arch. Neurol. **36:**601-603, Oct. 1979.

National Migraine Foundation, 2422 West Foster Ave., Chicago, IL 60625.

New, P.F.J.: Computed tomography: a major diagnostic advance, Hosp. Prac. **10:**55, 1975.

Norman, S.: Surgical treatment of epilepsy, Am. J. Nurs. **81:**994, 1981.

Pharmacology and therapy No. 1: Headache, Hanover, N.J., 1967, Sandoz Pharmaceuticals.

Philips, C.: Headache in general practice, Headache **16:**322-329, Jan. 1977.

Pohutsky, L.C., and Pohutsky, K.R.: Computer axial tomography of the brain—a new diagnostic tool, Am. J. Nurs. **75:**1341, 1975.

Rodin, E.A.: Psychomotor epilepsy and aggressive behavior, Arch. Gen. Psychiatry **28:**210, 1973.

Ruuskanen, I., et al.: Side effects of sodium valproate during long-term treatment in epilepsy, Acta Neurol. Scand. **60:**125-128, 1979.

Selected writings of John Hughlings Jackson: On epilepsy and epileptiform convulsions, vol. 1, London, 1931, Hodder & Stoughton, Ltd.

Shamansky, S.L., and Glaser, G.H.: Socioeconomic characteristics of childhood seizure disorders in the New Haven area: an epidemiologic study, Epilepsia **20:**457-474, Oct. 1979.

Shope, J.T.: The clinical specialist in epilepsy: patients, problems, and nursing intervention, Nurs. Clin. North Am. **9:**761, Dec. 1974.

Still, J.M.: Misuse of psychotrophic drugs, J. Practical Therap. **5:**57-59, Aug. 1979.

Swift, N.: Helping patients live with seizures, Nursing78 **8:**35-31, June 1978.

Troupin, A.S., et al.: Clinical pharmacology of mephenytoin and ethotoin, Ann Neurol. **6:**410-414, 1979.

Troupin, A.S., et al.: Evaluation of clorazepate (Tranxene) as an anticonvulsant—a pilot study, Neurology **29:**458-466, April 1979.

Valproic acid and sodium valproate approved for use in epilepsy, FDA Drug Bull. **8:**14-15, March/April 1978.

Walsh, G., and Mersky, Z.: Seizures and nursing care (videocassette with study guide), AVC Corporation, 4 Commercial Boulevard, Novato, California.

Whitehouse, D.: Psychological and neurological correlates of seizure disorders, Johns Hopkins Med. J. **129:**36-42, July 1971.

Wiley, L.: The stigma of epilepsy, Nursing74 **4:**38, 1974.

Williams, A.: Classification and diagnosis of epilepsy, Nurs. Clin. North Am. **9:**747, Dec. 1974.

Williams, D.: Sleep and disease, Am. J. Nurs. **71:**2321-2324, 1971.

Wilkins, A.J., et al.: Television epilepsy—the role of pattern, electroencephalography and clinical neurophysiology **47:**163-171, 1979.

Wilson, D.H., et al.: Division of the corpus callosum for uncontrollable epilepsy, Neurology **28:**649-653, July 1978.

Wolf, S.: Controversies in the treatment of febrile convulsions, Neurology **29:**287-290, March 1979.

# PART FIVE

# DISORDERS AFFECTING INPUT, INTEGRATION, AND OUTPUT

# 15

# ASSESSING SENSORY, MOTOR, AND SENSORIMOTOR DISORDERS

Whenever the flow of neuronal impulses is interrupted at any point along the pathway from reception to motor response, an alteration in motor response occurs. This functional alteration may be expressed as a sensory, motor, or sensorimotor disturbance, depending on the location of the neuronal interruption. In this chapter, various areas of the nervous system are reviewed in relation to problems that alter normal response patterns. Although some neurological disorders are cited to better illustrate a particular point, detailed coverage of these entities is reserved for other sections of this text. Refer to Chapter 11 for further information on assessment.

## INTERRUPTED TRANSMISSION TO SPINAL MEDULLA SEGMENTS
### Motor disturbances

Muscles have both radicular and peripheral nerve innervation. To explain the difference between these two types of innervation, it is necessary to recall embryonic development and anatomical placement of nerves arising from the spinal medulla.

In embryonic development the spinal cord is divided into somites. Within each somite is a neurotome (a unit of nervous tissue), a dermatome (a unit of integument), and a myotome (a unit of muscle tissue). As development continues, centripetal fibers transmit sensory impulses through posterior roots from corresponding cutaneous segments of each body aspect, and motor fibers travel through anterior roots to corresponding segments of muscle

on both aspects of the body. Although the zones supplied by cutaneous radicular nerves remain circular in the trunk, those in the limbs undergo peripheral displacement. This phenomenon is explained as one observes limb growth during embryonic development. Limb buds originating as right-angled buds to the trunk are innervated by radicular zones that become displaced peripherally in proportion to the degree of limb growth. Because of this displacement caused by limb growth, at maturity muscles are not innervated in accordance with a strict segmental pattern. Therefore radicular innervation of a single muscle may require innervation from more than one segment. The following listing illustrates how some muscles may require neuronal input from as many as four myotomes:

| Muscle | Myotomes |
|---|---|
| Anterior tibialis | L4, L5 |
| Biceps femoris | L4 through S2 |
| Gluteus maximus | L4 through S2 |
| Semimembranosus | L4, L5, and S1 |
| Semitendinosus | L4, L5, and S1 |

These same muscles also have peripheral innervation. Therefore the deep peroneal branch of the common peroneal nerve innervates the anterior tibialis, biceps femoris, and semimembranosus, semitendinosus muscles, whereas the inferior gluteal nerve supplies the gluteus maximus muscle.

Both the common peroneal and the inferior gluteal nerves are composed of motor fibers aris-

**421**

ing from spinal roots from levels L4 through S2. Mediation of these peripheral motor nerves is achieved through nerve plexuses. All peripheral motor nerves have a similar organizational pattern. In general as motor nerves branch, they supply smaller muscles and muscles involved in fine activity with the largest number of fibers. Because of the division and anastomosis of the funiculi composing a nerve trunk, funicular patterns may vary greatly even at distances separated by only a few millimeters.

Mixed spinal nerves, composed of a union between anterior and posterior roots within the intervertebral foramina, course into the periphery to be continuous with plexuses and then course into the peripheral nerves. Thus motor fibers from cell bodies in the anterior horn and sensory fibers from cell bodies in the posterior root ganglia are found in both plexuses and peripheral nerves. Because of this pattern of neuronal supply, one anterior horn may innervate portions of several peripheral nerves, whereas a single posterior root ganglion may gather impulses from fibers arising from several peripheral nerves.

If a practitioner detects flaccid paralysis in a muscle, recall of patterns of radicular and peripheral innervation will prompt the realization that the lesion responsible for this interruption in motor function may possibly be located at the spinal cord (whereby the muscle's nuclear center is devastated), at the root, at the plexus, or at the peripheral nerve supply. When the lesion interferes with neuronal transmission from one anterior root, partial loss of power in a muscle occurs, particularly in the limbs, where each muscle is supplied by more than one spinal segment. Total loss of muscle power in a limb from interferences with radicular supply requires damage to more than one anterior root.

Tables 15-1 and 15-2 summarize lesions affecting muscles innervated by anterior horns or roots. Table 15-3 details the spinal nerves, muscles supplied by them, and actions of these muscles. In determining the origin of paralysis—radicular or peripheral—for a muscle or muscles one should review these tables to identify whether involved muscles have a common peripheral or radicular nerve supply.

If a lesion in the spinal medulla extends to in-

clude the adjacent lateral pyramidal tract, muscles at the level of the lesion undergo radicular paralysis, whereas muscles supplied by anterior horn cells beneath the level of the anterior horn lesion are paretic. A handy reference for identifying which cord areas affect various movements (helpful in making a rapid assessment of the cord area involved in paralysis) is available in the following list and in Chapter 23.

| Cord area | Gross movements |
|---|---|
| Upper cervical | Neck and head movement; elevation of shoulders |
| Middle cervical | Movement of upper arms and forearms; diaphragmatic breathing |
| Lower cervical | Movements in fingers and hands |
| Thoracic | Intercostal muscles involved in respiration; muscles involved in abdominal contractions |
| Upper lumbar | Leg flexion at hip; adduction of thigh |
| Lower lumbar | Remaining thigh movements; movements in lower legs |
| Sacral | Foot and toe movements; sphincter and perineal muscle contraction |

When the spinal cord is damaged because of a fracture or dislocation of a vertebra or because of a space-occupying lesion in the spinal cord, paralysis of muscles in the involved segments occurs. Paralytic contracture and spasticity of muscles beneath the level of the lesion also occurs. When muscle contractures occur in muscles serving opposing functions, the most pronounced contracture occurs in the muscle group that is most powerful. An example of this phenomenon is the flexion contracture of the hip when neuronal impulses from the lower thoracic spinal cord are interrupted. This deformity is the product of unopposed activity of the iliopsoas muscle innervated by segments L1 and L2. Further discussion of flexion versus extension contractures is available in the section describing transverse lesions of the spinal cord.

## Sensory disturbances

The sensory nerve supply of the peripheral nervous system travels a course similar to that of the nerves in the motor system in that radicular sensory fibers also communicate with peripheral nerves and plexuses. However, sensory fibers, despite their complex courses, usually arrive at the

*Text continued on p. 428.*

**TABLE 15-1.** Segmental innervation of trunk muscles*

Segmental columns: Cervical segments (1–8), Thoracic segments (1–12), Lumbar segments (1–5), Sacral segments (1–5), Coccyx.

| Muscle | Segmental innervation |
|---|---|
| Short deep neck muscles | Cervical |
| Splenius muscles | Cervical |
| Deep long muscles of back | Cervical–Lumbar (throughout) |
| Serratus posterior superior | T1–T4 |
| Serratus posterior inferior | T9–T12 |
| Trapezius | C2–C4 |
| Latissimus dorsi | C6–C8 |
| Levator scapulae | C3–C5 |
| Rhomboids | C4–C5 |
| Longus capitis | C1–C4 |
| Longus coli | C2–C7 |
| Scalenes | C3–C8 |
| Pectoralis major | C5–T1 |
| Pectoralis minor | C7–T1 |
| Subclavius | C5–C6 |
| Serratus anterior | C5–C7 |
| Diaphragm | C3–C5 |
| Rectus abdominis | T6–T12 |
| External oblique, abdominal | T5–T12 |
| Internal oblique, abdominal | T7–L1 |
| Transverse abdominal | T7–L1 |
| Quadratus lumborum | T12–L4 |
| Intercostal muscles | T1–T12 |
| Levator, sphincter ani, perineal, and coccygeal | S2–Coccyx |

*From Haymaker, W.: Bing's local diagnosis in neurological diseases, ed. 15, St. Louis, 1969, The C.V. Mosby Co.

**TABLE 15-2.** Segmental innervation of muscles of extremities*

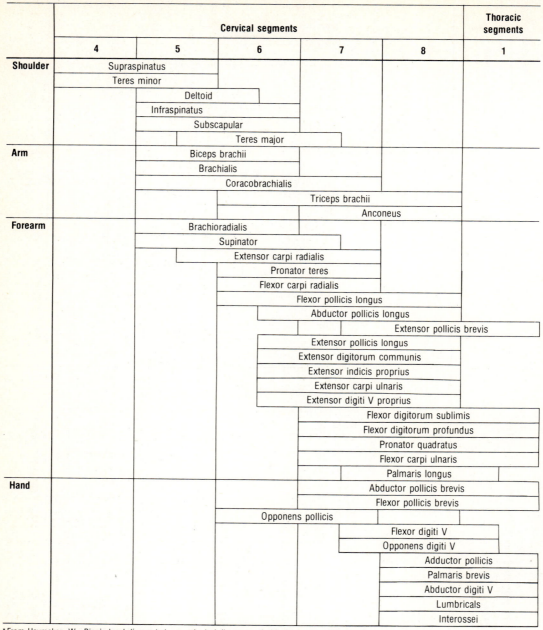

| | Cervical segments | | | | | Thoracic segments |
|---|---|---|---|---|---|---|
| | 4 | 5 | 6 | 7 | 8 | 1 |
| **Shoulder** | Supraspinatus | | | | | |
| | Teres minor | | | | | |
| | | Deltoid | | | | |
| | | Infraspinatus | | | | |
| | | Subscapular | | | | |
| | | | Teres major | | | |
| **Arm** | | Biceps brachii | | | | |
| | | Brachialis | | | | |
| | | Coracobrachialis | | | | |
| | | | Triceps brachii | | | |
| | | | Anconeus | | | |
| **Forearm** | | Brachioradialis | | | | |
| | | Supinator | | | | |
| | | Extensor carpi radialis | | | | |
| | | Pronator teres | | | | |
| | | Flexor carpi radialis | | | | |
| | | Flexor pollicis longus | | | | |
| | | | Abductor pollicis longus | | | |
| | | | | Extensor pollicis brevis | | |
| | | | Extensor pollicis longus | | | |
| | | | Extensor digitorum communis | | | |
| | | | Extensor indicis proprius | | | |
| | | | Extensor carpi ulnaris | | | |
| | | | Extensor digiti V proprius | | | |
| | | | | Flexor digitorum sublimis | | |
| | | | | Flexor digitorum profundus | | |
| | | | | Pronator quadratus | | |
| | | | | Flexor carpi ulnaris | | |
| | | | | Palmaris longus | | |
| **Hand** | | | | Abductor pollicis brevis | | |
| | | | | Flexor pollicis brevis | | |
| | | | Opponens pollicis | | | |
| | | | | Flexor digiti V | | |
| | | | | Opponens digiti V | | |
| | | | | | Adductor pollicis | |
| | | | | | Palmaris brevis | |
| | | | | | Abductor digiti V | |
| | | | | | Lumbricals | |
| | | | | | Interossei | |

*From Haymaker, W.: Bing's local diagnosis in neurological diseases, ed. 15, St. Louis, 1969, The C.V. Mosby Co.

**TABLE 15-2.** Segmental innervation of muscles of extremities—cont'd

| Region | Muscle | Thoracic 12 | Lumbar 1 | Lumbar 2 | Lumbar 3 | Lumbar 4 | Lumbar 5 | Sacral 1 | Sacral 2 | Sacral 3 |
|---|---|---|---|---|---|---|---|---|---|---|
| **Hip** | Iliopsoas | X | X | X | X | | | | | |
| | Tensor fasciae latae | | | | | X | X | X | | |
| | Gluteus medius | | | | | X | X | X | | |
| | Gluteus minimus | | | | | X | X | X | | |
| | Quadratus femoris | | | | | X | X | X | | |
| | Gemellus inferior | | | | | X | X | X | | |
| | Gemellus superior | | | | | X | X | X | X | |
| | Gluteus maximus | | | | | X | X | X | X | |
| | Obturator internus | | | | | | X | X | X | |
| | Piriformis | | | | | | X | X | X | |
| **Thigh** | Sartorius | | | X | X | | | | | |
| | Pectineus | | | X | X | | | | | |
| | Adductor longus | | | X | X | | | | | |
| | Quadriceps femoris | | | X | X | X | | | | |
| | Gracilis | | | X | X | X | | | | |
| | Adductor brevis | | | X | X | X | | | | |
| | Obturator externus | | | | X | X | | | | |
| | Adductor magnus | | | | X | X | | | | |
| | Adductor minimus | | | | X | X | | | | |
| | Articularis genu | | | | X | X | | | | |
| | Semitendinosus | | | | | X | X | X | | |
| | Semimembranosus | | | | | X | X | X | | |
| | Biceps femoris | | | | | X | X | X | X | |
| **Leg** | Tibialis anterior | | | | | X | X | | | |
| | Extensor hallucis longus | | | | | X | X | X | | |
| | Popliteus | | | | | X | X | X | | |
| | Plantaris | | | | | X | X | X | | |
| | Extensor digitorum longus | | | | | X | X | X | | |
| | Soleus | | | | | X | X | X | X | |
| | Gastrocnemius | | | | | X | X | X | X | |
| | Peroneus longus | | | | | | X | X | | |
| | Peroneus brevis | | | | | | X | X | | |
| | Tibialis posterior | | | | | | X | X | | |
| | Flexor digitorum longus | | | | | | X | X | X | X |
| | Flexor hallucis longus | | | | | | X | X | X | X |
| **Foot** | Extensor hallucis brevis | | | | | X | X | X | | |
| | Extensor digiti brevis | | | | | X | X | X | | |
| | Flexor digiti brevis | | | | | | X | X | | |
| | Abductor hallucis | | | | | | X | X | | |
| | Flexor hallucis brevis | | | | | | X | X | X | X |
| | Lumbricals | | | | | | X | X | X | |
| | Adductor hallucis | | | | | | | X | X | X |
| | Abductor digiti V | | | | | | | X | X | X |
| | Flexor digiti V brevis | | | | | | | X | X | X |
| | Opponens digiti V | | | | | | | X | X | X |
| | Quadratus plantae | | | | | | | X | X | X |
| | Interossei | | | | | | | X | X | X |

**TABLE 15-3.** Motor functions of spinal nerves*†

| Nerves | Muscles | Function |
|---|---|---|
| **Cervical plexus (C1-C4)** | Deep cervical | Flexion, extension, and rotation of neck |
| Cervical | Scalene | Elevation of ribs (inspiration) |
| Phrenic | Diaphragm | Inspiration |
| **Brachial plexus (C5-T1)** | | |
| Anterior thoracic | Pectorales major and minor | Adduction and depression of arm downward and medially |
| Long thoracic | Serratus anterior | Fixation of scapula on raising arm |
| Dorsal scapular | Levator scapulae | Elevation of scapula |
| | Rhomboid | Drawing scapula upward and inward |
| Suprascapular | Supraspinatus | Elevation and outward rotation of arm |
| | Infraspinatus | Outward rotation of arm |
| Subscapular | Latissimus dorsi ⎫ | |
| | Teres major ⎭ | Inward rotation and adduction of arm toward back |
| | Subscapularis | Inward rotation of arm |
| Axillary | Deltoid | Rising of arm to horizontal |
| | Teres minor | Outward rotation of arm |
| Musculocutaneous | Biceps brachii | Flexion and supination of forearm |
| | Coracobrachialis | Elevation and adduction of arm |
| | Brachialis | Flexion of forearm |
| Median | Flexor carpi radialis | Flexion and radial deviation of hand |
| | Palmaris longus | Flexion of hand |
| | Flexor digitorum sublimis | Flexion of middle phalanges of second through fifth fingers |
| | Flexor pollicis longus | Flexion of distal phalanx of thumb |
| | Flexor digitorum profundus (radial half) | Flexion of distal phalanges of second and third fingers |
| | Pronator quadrantus | Pronation |
| | Pronator teres | Pronation |
| | Abductor pollicis brevis | Abduction of metacarpus I at right angle to palm |
| | Flexor pollicis brevis | Flexion of proximal phalanx of thumb |
| | Lumbricals I, II, III | Flexion of proximal phalanges and extension of other phalanges of first, second, and third fingers |
| | Opponens pollicis brevis | Opposition of metacarpus I |
| Ulnar | Flexor carpi ulnaris | Flexion and ulnar deviation of hand |
| | Flexor digitorum profundus (ulnar half) | Flexion of distal phalanges of fourth and fifth fingers |
| | Adductor pollicis | Adduction of metacarpus I |
| | Hypothenar | Abduction, opposition, flexion of little finger |
| | Lumbricals III, IV | Flexion of first phalanx and extension of the other phalanges of fourth and fifth fingers |
| | Interossei | Same action as preceding; also spreading apart of fingers and bringing them together |

*From Haymaker, W.: Bing's local diagnosis in neurological diseases, ed. 15, St. Louis, 1969, The C.V. Mosby Co.
†Various muscles may receive still other nerve supplies than those mentioned. The following are the principal accessory nerve supplies: the *brachial muscle* receives fibers from the radial nerve; the *flexor digitorum sublimis,* from the ulnar; the *adductor pollicis,* from the median; the *pectineus,* from the femoral; the *adductor magnus,* from the tibial.

**TABLE 15-3.** Motor functions of the spinal nerves—cont'd

| Nerves | Muscles | Function |
|---|---|---|
| Radial | Triceps brachii | Extension of forearm |
|  | Brachioradialis | Flexion of forearm |
|  | Extensor carpi radialis | Extension and radial flexion of hand |
|  | Extensor digitorum communis | Extension of proximal phalanges of second through fifth fingers |
|  | Extensor digiti quinti proprius | Extension of proximal phalanx of little finger |
|  | Extensor carpi ulnaris | Extension and ulnar deviation of hand |
|  | Supinator | Supination of forearm |
|  | Abductor pollicis longus | Abduction of metacarpus I |
|  | Extensor pollicis brevis | Extension of proximal phalanx of thumb |
|  | Extensor pollicis longus | Abduction of first metacarpus and extension of distal phalanges of thumb |
|  | Extensor indicis proprius | Extension of proximal phalanx of index finger |
| **Thoracic nerves** | | |
| Thoracic | Thoracic and abdominal | Elevation of ribs, expiration, abdominal compression, etc. |
| **Lumbar plexus (T12-L4)** | | |
| Femoral | Iliopsoas | Flexion of leg at hip |
|  | Sartorius | Inward rotation of leg together with flexion of upper and lower leg |
|  | Quadriceps femoris | Extension of lower leg |
| Obturator | Pectineus | |
|  | Adductor longus | |
|  | Adductor brevis | Adduction of leg |
|  | Adductor magnus | |
|  | Gracilis | |
|  | Obturator externus | Adduction and outward rotation of leg |
| **Sacral plexus (L5-S5)** | | |
| Superior gluteal | Gluteus medius | Abduction and inward rotation of leg; also under certain circumstances, outward rotation |
|  | Gluteus minimus | |
|  | Tensor fasciae latae | Flexion of leg at hip |
|  | Piriformis | Outward rotation of leg |
|  | Gluteus maximus | Extension of leg at hip |
| Inferior gluteal | | |
| Sciatic | Obturator internus | |
|  | Gemelli | Outward rotation of leg |
|  | Quadratus femoris | |
|  | Biceps femoris | |
|  | Semitendinosus | Flexion of leg at hip |
|  | Semimembranosus | |
| Peroneal | Tibialis anterior | Dorsiflexion and supination of foot |
| Deep | Extensor digitorum longus | Extension of toes |
|  | Extensor hallucis brevis | Extension of great toe |
| Superficial | Peroneus | Pronation of foot |
| Tibialis | Gastrocnemius | Plantar flexion of foot |
|  | Soleus | |

*Continued*

**TABLE 15-3.** Motor functions of the spinal nerves—cont'd

| Nerves | Muscles | Function |
|---|---|---|
| **Sacral plexus (L5-S5)—cont'd** | | |
| | Tibialis posterior | Adduction of foot |
| | Flexor digitorum longus | Flexion of distal phalanges II through V |
| | Flexor hallucis longus | Flexion of distal phalanx I |
| | Flexor digitorum brevis | Flexion of middle phalanges II through V |
| | Flexor hallucis brevis | Flexion of middle phalanx I |
| | Plantar | Spreading, bringing together, and flexion of proximal phalanges of toes |
| Pudendal | Perineal and sphincters | Closure of sphincters of pelvic organs; also participation in sexual act; contraction of pelvic floor |

same cutaneous area (dermatome) designated by the posterior spinal root from which they arise (see Figs. 3-4 and 3-5). Although this pattern of nerve supply leads one to believe that damage to a posterior root results in a discrete area of sensory disturbance, this phenomenon fails to occur because of the overlap of radicular zones. Thus in most cases an area of skin is supplied by two posterior roots. An exception to this rule is when compression of a single posterior root, secondary to a herniated nucleus pulposus at the level of the limb, results in decreased amounts of sensibility.

Radicular anesthesia occurs if more than one neighboring posterior root is damaged. If cutaneous anesthesia results from disturbances in the peripheral supply, the involved areas include two or more adjacent radicular zones and usually extend to cutaneous areas supplied by the affected peripheral nerve. When one posterior root does not transmit neuronal impulses, hyperesthesia results. Since the phenomenon of radicular overlap often results in practical difficulty in identification of the upper limits of a lesion in relation to the spinal segments involved, the clinical assessment should include careful testing of segments above the level of the lesion to ensure accurate identification of the upper limits of the problem (Chapters 4 and 23).

Two exceptions to the situation just described occur in instances of irritative phenomena involving one root and in referred pain. In considering irritative phenomena one notes that a space-occupying lesion, a spondylitic process, or a herniated intervertebral disk may compress one root and cause anesthesia and pain to specified regions. Thus compression of the root at the level of C2 results in pain in the occiput, whereas compression of the root at the level of L1 results in pain in the inguinal region. When these individual posterior spinal roots are compressed, the resulting pains and dysesthesias from the irritative problem travel to the periphery along the usual peripheral nerve routes. However, the brain confuses the focus of pain origin and projects the pain to the dermatome innervated by the affected spinal root rather than to the region in the root where the problem actually lies. This phenomenon is distinguished from referred pain, since the course of transmission does correspond to the root-nerve system.

Referred pain differs from instances involving irritative phenomenon because the origin of the pain is outside the root-nerve system, namely, viscera or muscles. Although referred pain is also projected to the dermatomes, it may not be limited to a particular region or to only the segments involved through its original point of innervation. Three principles probably explain the mechanism of referred pain, including set-point view, convergence-projection, and convergence-facilitation. Chapter 10 gives additional detail.

To review, the term "*set-point view*" refers to the idea that afferent impulses coming into the spinal cord or supraspinal structures may predetermine the presynaptic filter level so that pain occurs when the total effect of incoming impulses on all fibers exceeds this predetermined level. The term *"convergence-projection"* refers to the idea that because of the Sherrington neural pool concept of pain previously discussed and further discussed in Chapter 10, the brain may interpret pain from certain visceral afferents as if it originated from the skin. The explanation for this phenomenon is that these visceral afferents connect with the same neurons as the cutaneous afferents at some level—spinal, thalamic, or cerebral cortex. In the concept of *convergence-facilitation,* which explains hyperesthesia more than referred pain, impulses from the viscera result in pain in the radicular cutaneous area corresponding to the segment at which they enter the spinal cord.

Since a detailed description of exact sites of referred pain from somatic and visceral afferents is beyond this text, the reader interested in further information is advised to seek additional references. Suffice it to say that visceral structures may be involved in both referred and nonreferred pain when pathological disturbances exist. Additionally, impulses from both sources course to central structures for transmission to spinal and supraspinal structures. Although referred pain may originate from the viscera, the converse is also true. Thus pain from superficial sources may also be referred to and experienced in the deep structures. An example of this might be the instance wherein a client is erroneously believed to have angina until the appearance of herpes zoster vesicles of the upper thoracic segments are found to be the actual origin of the pain.

## Reflexes

Reflex changes are also valuable in localizing the level of a spinal cord lesion. A discussion of reflexes is available in Chapter 11 along with Table 11-6, which summarizes both deep and superficial reflexes as well as methods of eliciting these reflexes and which segments are involved in each one.

### REFERENCES

Chusid, J.G.: Correlative neuroanatomy and functional neurology, ed. 16, Los Altos, Calif., 1976, Lange Medical Publications.

Haymaker, W.: Bring's local diagnosis in neurological diseases, ed. 15, St. Louis, 1969, The C.V. Mosby Co.

Peele, T.L.: The neuroanatomic basis for clinical neurology, New York, 1976, McGraw-Hill Book Co.

Seddon, H.: Surgical disorders of peripheral nerves, ed. 2, New York, 1975, Churchill Livingstone, Division of Longman, Inc.

# 16

# DISORDERS ARISING FROM CHANGES IN SENSIBILITY, NUTRITION, AND METABOLISM

This chapter presents an overview of several situations involving metabolism, growth, nutrition, disease processes, muscle atrophy, and trauma as they relate to interferences with neuronal activity and untoward trophic outcomes.

## INBORN ERRORS OF METABOLISM

The combination of all physical and chemical processes cooperating to effect the growth, maintenance, and transformation of organized substance in living systems is termed *metabolism*. The complex, genetically controlled biochemical processes form a sequential network of reactions, wherein each step in the metabolic pathway requires an enzymatic catalyst to move it to completion. When a given gene malfunctions, the necessary enzyme at a point in the metabolic pathway is either absent or inadequate to effect the required biochemical process. Thus the individual has modified physical characteristics (phenotype). This explanation essentially describes the one gene—one polypeptide principle that underlies the operations of both structural proteins and enzymes.

When a single gene is mutated, it interferes with only the specific protein it controls. However, if this protein, an enzyme, is responsible for a sequence of chemical reactions, the total metabolic pathway may be adversely affected (Fig. 16-1). The phenotypic changes or disease states resulting from this blocked pathway may be attributed to excessive production preceding the block, to in-

adequate enzymatic responses in subsequent reactions, to lack of an essential product, or to accumulations of excessive products in alternate pathways (Fig. 16-2). In such instances, attempts are made to either supplement deficient products or to avoid the ingestion of substances the individual is unable to metabolize.

Although inborn errors of metabolism are rare, there are many of these autosomal recessive disorders that interfere with either the buildup or the breakdown of reactions involved in protein, fat, or carbohydrate metabolism. A detailed discussion of the disease entities involved in the inborn errors of metabolism is beyond the scope of this text. Interested readers should pursue this topic in the references.

## GROWTH

Growth in the context of morphogenesis was discussed in Chapter 1. In this regard, growth and normal cell proliferation are contingent on a number of factors, of which nutrition is one. Interferences from erroneous chemical messages or environmental or nutritional inadequacies have grave outcomes, particularly when they are prevalent during the formative period for body structures. For the nervous system the critical formative period occurs during the first 5 weeks of fetal life, as described in Chapter 1. A discussion of the congenital malformations that may occur from interferences at this point is beyond the scope of this

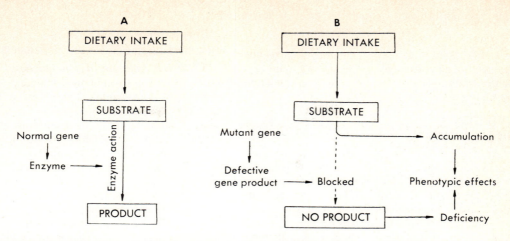

**FIG. 16-1.** Metabolic pathway. **A,** Normal pathway. **B,** Effect of defective gene action. (From Whaley, L.F.: Understanding inherited disorders, St. Louis, 1974, The C.V. Mosby Co.)

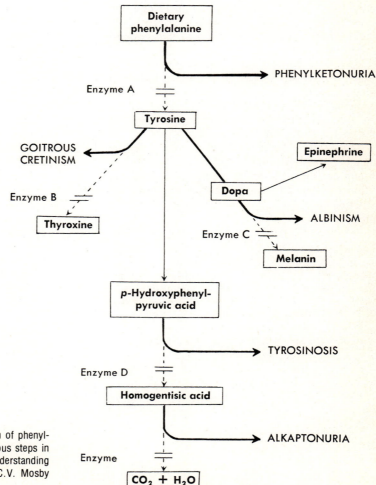

**FIG. 16-2.** Some basic steps in metabolism of phenyl-alanine and consequences of blocks at various steps in metabolic pathway. (From Whaley, L.F.: Understanding inherited disorders, St. Louis, 1974, The C.V. Mosby Co.)

text. Interested readers are encouraged to pursue the mentioned references in Chapter 13, with particular emphasis on the book and slide presentation by Moore.

## NUTRITION
### Dietary patterns

Although a complete discussion of dietary preferences, excesses, and deficiencies is beyond the scope of this text, issues and problems resulting from these patterns daily affect the decisions of practitioners in clinical situations. The concern for a youthful, attractive image leads millions of North Americans into complying with dietary fads. Most of the effort commonly associated with "diet" in the lay sense involves countless methods—pills, books, clinics, organic products, salons, gimmicks, and various dietary plans—designed to eliminate obesity. Because individuals desire to lose weight in a dramatic manner, they may ignore the need for balance in the diet and thus compromise their health.

Another consideration is the current trend toward eating fast foods. One prominent basketball player, Quinn Buckner, was observed by his coach as being "off" on his quickness and reflexive responses. The cause of "Buckner's syndrome" was the excessive consumption of fast foods.

The safety of the diet and the suitability for any dietary program with respect to physiological health or illness should be monitored by the practitioner, especially when the diet requires a restriction in one category or an excess in another product.

Megavitamin therapy and the promotion of various health foods have been prevalent in the last few years. Adele Davis is a proponent of this type of therapy (Davis, 1970). The outcomes of deficiencies or excesses in the various vitamins may be gleaned from sources specific to the topic or from most medical texts describing common medical conditions (Tatkon, 1967; Wade, 1972; Dietary Allowances Committee and Food and Nutrition Board, 1974; Rosenberg and Feldzaman, 1974, 1975; Netter, 1975; Levy and Bach-y-Rita, 1976; Thiele, 1976). Some common neurological disorders related to vitamin deficiencies are briefly presented here.

## Disorders related to vitamin deficiencies

*Thiamine (vitamin $B_1$) deficiency.* The most common reason for thiamine deficiency in normal individuals is inadequate dietary intake. However, there are several conditions that either increase the vitamin requirement or interfere with absorption. Hyperthyroidism, pregnancy, lactation, fever from any source, and mental impairments resulting in increased psychomotor activity may all increase thiamine requirements. Interferences with thiamine absorption may result from chronic diarrhea. Liver disease may account for decreased vitamin utilization. In alcoholism, diminished intake of thiamine combined with impaired absorption and utilization account for the deficient quantity of thiamine. Another cause of thiamine deficiency is frequent or continued dextrose infusions accompanied by low thiamine intake, since dextrose needs thiamine to complete the process of oxidation.

Thiamine is required for the final metabolism of carbohydrates and protein, for functional integrity in nervous tissue, and for other specific enzymatic functions. Cardiac, gastrointestinal, and neurological disorders are manifested when the deficiency of thiamine results in a lack of the coenzyme carboxylase (thiamine pyrophosphate). Severe and prolonged thiamine deficiency results in beriberi, a condition manifested by a predominance of cardiovascular disorders along with polyneuritis and gastrointestinal disturbances. Since this text focuses on the nervous system, the only disturbances detailed are those involving the nervous system.

Because the central nervous system depends almost totally on carbohydrate metabolism for energy supplies, neurological functions are greatly hampered when thiamine deficiencies reduce the glucose utilization in the central nervous system by as much as 60%. At the cellular level, neurons evidence chromatolysis and swelling, which interrupt neuronal transmission at many points in the central nervous system. An additional outcome of thiamine deficiency is the degeneration of myelin sheaths in both the peripheral and central nervous systems. When peripheral nerves become involved, they manifest signs of extreme irritability, and clients have clinical symptoms compatible with polyneuritis, which includes pain radiation along one or more peripheral nerve pathways.

When fiber tracts of the spinal cord become involved, the client may experience muscle atrophy, severe weakness, and even paralysis.

*Nicotinic acid (niacin) deficiency.* When an extreme deficiency of niacin or its amide (niacinamide or nicotinamide) coupled with its precursor tryptophan occurs, pellagra may result. Pellagra is a disorder involving mental, neurological, mucous membrane, cutaneous, and gastrointestinal disturbances. To avoid a deficiency, individuals need to consume tryptophan-containing protein such as that found in milk, wheat, and egg. When high maize diets are eaten, primary deficiencies associated with pellagra are more common. Secondary sources or niacin deficiency include such contributing conditions as chronic diarrhea, alcoholism, cirrhosis of the liver, and extended use of intravenous dextrose infusions without the concomitant administration of vitamins.

Three types of central nervous system problems are noted in connection with a niacin deficiency. First, there may be a rather nonspecific neurasthenic syndrome comparable to that seen in cases of thiamine deficiency. Second, one may note an encephalopathy that includes interferences with consciousness, cogwheel rigidities in the extremities, and automatic grasping and sucking reflexes. This encephalopathy is frequently heralded by delirium, elevated temperature, or prolonged administration of dextrose without temperature, or prolonged administration of dextrose without vitamin therapy. Third, the client may become psychotic.

Although the expression of symptoms varies greatly with individuals, many are noted to have disturbances in memory and orientation and experience confusion and confabulation. When a peripheral neuropathy is apparent or spinal tract involvement seems to be indicated, the cause of these problems is probably a simultaneous deficiency in thiamine. Since no laboratory test is definitive in diagnosis, the practitioner must rely on history and other characteristic symptoms associated with this deficiency to identify the condition.

*Vitamin $B_6$ deficiency.* The vitamin $B_6$ complex is an integral part of skin, blood, and neural metabolism, and consists of three related compounds: pyridoxine, pyridoxal, and pyridoxamine. In the bound form, pyridoxine becomes pyridoxal phosphate, a coenzyme that participates in a number of reactions, including decarboxylation, transamination, synthesis of a minimum of one amino acid (tryptophan), and conversion of several other amino acids into essential substances required by the body. This vitamin is also essential as a coenzyme in the desaturation of fats in the liver. Although many foods contain vitamin $B_6$ and the state of deficiency is rare, individuals with highly processed or restricted diets may be subject to this deficiency. Occasionally an infant on a highly restricted formula deficient in vitamin $B_6$ will have infantile spasms. Although most of these myoclonic episodes are idiopathic, difficult to control, and apt to convert to major motor seizures around 2 years of age, a child who has these convulsions from a lack of vitamin $B_6$ will experience a spontaneous cessation of seizures when pyridoxine hydrochloride is injected. Usually when a clinical picture of myoclonus is seen along with a hypsarrhythmic pattern on electroencephalogram, pyridoxine is injected during the tracing to see if it affects the pattern of the brain waves. When it does, the infant is quite fortunate because further seizures may be controlled by the administration of vitamin $B_6$, even though damage that has already occurred is not reversible.

Vitamin $B_6$ deficiency in adults may be evident as a peripheral neuropathy in clients receiving isoniazid. However, the administration of pyridoxine alleviates the neurological disturbance. In alcoholics the major motor convulsions are believed to be related to a vitamin $B_6$ deficiency. Essentially, these and other symptoms associated with a vitamin $B_6$ deficiency may be diagnosed by observation of characteristic clinical features and confirmation of the response to this vitamin as part of a therapeutic trial to alleviate symptoms.

*Vitamin $B_{12}$ deficiencies.* The vitamin $B_{12}$ complex comprises a number of cobalamin compounds that affect the metabolic cellular organization in an unconfirmed way. However, experiments to date indicate that vitamin $B_{12}$ is active as a coenzyme in the conversion of amino acids and other compounds into essential body substances. Because vitamin $B_{12}$ is believed to play a vital role in reducing ribonucleotides into deoxyribonucleotides, an essential phase in gene development, it is commonly believed to influence growth promotion and red blood cell formation.

When individuals have pernicious anemia, they experience a vitamin $B_{12}$ deficiency that may result in demyelination of the large nerve fibers in the posterior and lateral columns of the spinal cord. Whether the genesis of the problem is dietary consumption or deficiencies related to a total or partial gastrectomy, the symptoms remain the same. Typically the condition continues for a number of years before the myelopathy becomes apparent. At this point the following symptoms are common: reduction in deep sensibility, ataxia, and muscle weakness. Specific symptoms depend on whether the lateral or posterior columns are affected. When the lateral columns are affected, there is pyramidal tract involvement so that the client may experience a spastic-ataxic paraplegia with less obvious signs of interferences with sensibility. If the posterior columns are involved, disorders in deep sensibility, areflexia, ataxia, and motor weakness predominate. Even when the posterior column seems most affected, the practitioner may elicit pathological reflexes that indicate pyramidal tract involvement. When these pyramidal tract signs are evident, the practitioner realizes that the extensive damage of the posterior columns has extended to include the lateral columns.

• • •

Before leaving the topic of vitamins the practitioner should be made aware of the extensive research effort currently taking place to identify the number of points in the metabolic pathways that utilize vitamins and minerals as coenzymes to complete their reactions. In the area of inborn errors of metabolism, information is constantly becoming available that identifies the administration of vitamins—especially the B complex—as a means of completing reactions in metabolic pathways and alleviating symptoms related to disorders at affected points.

### Interferences with cellular nutrition

Another level of consideration is nutrition at the cellular level. When nutritional supplies or sensory input to an identified area is inadequate, the outcome may include major trophic changes in the skin, fingernails, digits, bones, and muscles.

*Decubitus ulcer.* The decubitus ulcer, a preventable but common problem caused by pressure to a cutaneous area, results as ensuing ischemia causes impaired tissue nutrition. As deprivation of the tissues continues, cutaneous tissues lose their integrity and undergo destruction. Progressive destruction of underlying soft tissue continues when the problem remains undetected and/or uncorrected.

Many clients with neurological problems are at increased risk for the development of decubiti because they must be immobilized in some way, whether in recumbency, a wheelchair, or an orthopedic device or cast. Individuals with sensory impairments or alterations in their states of consciousness are particularly vulnerable, since they are often unable to report the discomfort associated with the developing lesion as an aid to early prevention and/or intervention.

Another type of client who might have difficulty in realizing the pain generally associated with the beginning lesion is the client who has a disturbance in sensibility. Incontinent individuals also have special problems, since the constant presence of urine as an irritant on the skin creates an even more difficult challenge in maintaining skin integrity. Nutritional capacities are systemically strained in the emaciated, debilitated, and malnourished individual, so that local pressure as an added stressor may effectively break skin integrity in a relatively short period of time.

The aged client has an even greater predisposition to decubitus formation, since skin in the elderly becomes less elastic, and such an individual loses subcutaneous fat, evidences a decrease in glandular secretions, and displays a general state of atrophy in the skin.

Once the decubitus ulcer forms, it is slow to heal. The overriding objective of nursing care is to promote positive efforts to heal the ulcer. If the ulcer is large, the loss of serum protein is continuous and places a drain on the essential body protein supply. In some clients these problems are further compounded by poor circulation and unusually poor capacities for tissue healing. Individuals with diabetes mellitus are one group of clients in whom the reestablishment of skin integrity is most difficult because of poor healing capacities. Unfortunately, also, sensory losses are present in these clients, so that pain is minor or does not exist in the area of the ulcer. The client often prefers no treatment to this site because of pain or discomfort elswhere.

**PREVENTION.** The treatment of choice, of course, is to prevent decubitus ulcers by stimulation of the circulation, maintenance of a dry skin, and alleviation of pressure, particularly to bony prominences. When a client is immobilized in such a way that movement and position changes are restricted, the practitioner should assess the status of the client, including the skin, and establish a regular regimen for inspection and stimulation of compromised areas. A routine of every 2 hours is usually sufficient, but certain clients may require more frequent attention. Because of the vast differences in skin and local nutritional status, the "2-hour rule" should serve only as a guideline. Careful inspection and assessment of skin condition reveals criteria about the local skin condition, so that the practitioner may decide if the 2-hour schedule is applicable in each case. When an individual tolerates one position for a longer period without difficulty, the practitioner might consider leaving the client in that position at night to allow for a longer period of uninterrupted sleep.

In positioning a client, one should refer to a fundamental text for detailed coverage of appropriate techniques. The overall objective of utilizing these fundamental techniques is to maintain good anatomical alignment and distribute pressure from body weight more evenly. One may protect the bony prominences such as the ankles from undue pressure by propping them on rolled small towels, encircling them in foam rubber encased in a stockinette, and painting them with tincture of benzoin to toughen the skin. Applications of tincture of benzoin may also aid the heels and elbows in remaining intact. Other bony prominences may be protected through the use of a clean, dry sheepskin. Additional methods of total body pressure relief include the use of an air mattress or a water bed. CircOlectric beds and various types of frames have also been used to offer positional relief to selected clients with limited mobility.

Bed linen should be kept free of debris, excess perspiration, and moisture. Bulky padding and wrinkles should also be avoided. Sometimes the roughness of the sheets laundered by commercial means provides a source of irritation to skin. When the client seems to experience skin irritation from rough linens, the practitioner may reduce the friction by thoroughly rubbing a sparing amount of cornstarch into the bottom sheet.

Of particular importance in the facility caring for clients affected by decreased mobility is the provision of a nursing care standard that includes regular inspection of all compromised clients, with special attention to pressure points and bony prominences; a regular program for hygiene and stimulation; and a routine for providing extra care and linen changes to the individual who may require assistance between times when daily care is provided. When possible, the client should be instructed to assist in the skin care program and to detect early signs of local circulatory embarrassment.

Concurrently, the practitioner attempts to provide a diet high in protein and adequate in fluid within the client's limitations. Caloric intake should also be sufficient to prevent the loss of subcutaneous tissue. Adequate nutrition is a helpful adjunct in promoting tissue anabolism.

Brainstorming in team conferences may be helpful in finding better ways of solving individual problems related to disease condition, positional limitations imposed by the problem or treatment modality, and urinary or fecal incontinence. A regular bowel evacuation routine may prevent involuntary defecation. If a condom or catheter is not feasible for the treatment of urinary incontinence, placement of the head of the bed on shock blocks might facilitate the downward flow of the urine. In clients exposed to constant drainage there is an increased need for skin hygiene. The use of a heat lamp may also be an aid in drying a moistened, erythematous area.

Since many neurological impairments result in chronic immobility to varying degrees, the practitioner should educate significant caretakers and the client in methods designed to prevent or minimize opportunities for decubitus ulcer formation. Written instructions for the client and family include recommendations for the treatment of the beginning decubitus ulcer.

Several measures are not generally advocated. These include (1) doughnuts around the area, since they compress the surrounding skin and further compress the skin and further compromise circulation; (2) powder to the skin, since it cakes with moisture and may hasten skin breakdown; and (3) applications of heat and cold to skin areas in clients who have diminished states of consciousness or sensation, since they may not perceive the painful warnings of impending tissue damage. Refer to Chapter 25 for further information.

## NEUROPATHIES RELATED TO DISEASE PROCESSES

Two of the more common disease processes that result in trophic changes are diabetes mellitus and atherosclerosis. Since insulin has become available to diabetics, the incidence of chronic complications related to neural and vascular abnormalities has increased. The segmental demyelination of neurons that results in a neuropathy is believed to be caused by accelerated activity in the polypoid pathway. In cells fully permeable to glucose the following reaction occurs:

$$\text{D-Glucose} + \text{NADPH} + \text{H}^+ \rightarrow \text{Sorbital} + \text{NADP}^+$$
$$\text{Sorbital} + \text{NAD}^+ \rightarrow \text{D-Fructose} + \text{NADH} + \text{H}^+$$

Thus sorbitol and fructose are unable to depart from the cell, and subsequently the osmotic pressure increases. This elevation of osmotic pressure attracts water into the cell and causes swelling. The first indication of this abnormal cellular activity is in diminished nerve conduction velocity. The condition may be improved as hyperglycemia is reduced by dietary or medical therapy. However, in instances of severe neuropathies, a reduction in hyperglycemia does not seem to alleviate the neurological disturbances.

The condition known as diabetic amyotrophy is characterized by weakness and wasting of the proximal muscle groups in rapid succession in diabetics whose conditions are poorly controlled. Muscle involvement may be symmetrical or asymmetrical. The muscles in the pelvic girdle or shoulder are often the first to become involved. The client may also have the additional problems of hypesthesia in distal areas, paresthesias, and lateral pallanesthesia. The practitioner may elicit a positive Babinski sign on clinical examination. When a lumbar puncture is performed, the protein level of the cerebrospinal fluid is elevated. Some individuals believe that this disorder is not a peripheral nerve degeneration in the strictest sense but rather an amyotrophic condition because of the lack of muscle fasciculations and the presence of fibrillation in electromyographic studies.

Atherosclerotic vascular disease has been observed in diabetics at an earlier age than is evident in the remaining population. Epidemiological studies point to hyperglycemia as one of the risk factors contributory to atherosclerosis. However, normalization of blood glucose levels may or may not prevent further vascular abnormalities. In affected persons, symptoms include cold feet, intermittent claudication, paresthesias, slow healing capacities, increased local infections, ulceration, and gangrene caused by the interrupted arterial blood supply to the lower extremities.

Clients with diabetes mellitus may also have a thickening of the basement membrane of the capillaries in tissues. This abnormal thickening results from the accumulation of a glycoprotein in the membrane, which may be the result of glucose entering the glucuronic acid pathway, where it contributes to the eventual synthesis of mucopolysaccharides and glycoproteins. The outcome of thickening in the basement membrane is neuropathy, retinopathy, and renal disease.

Atherosclerosis is discussed in Chapter 24. It is mentioned in this context as a common cause of myelopathy, particularly in senior citizens. In these instances the myelopathy results when the blood vessels feeding various portions of the spinal cord become sclerosed, so that blood supplies are diminished. The myelopathies that result are quite diverse in symptomatology and may include distal amyotrophy, atypical paraparesis, or quadriparesis without sensory disturbances. In disorders of this type, symptoms indicating incomplete transverse cord damage are frequently noted.

### Vascular diseases of limbs

Two vascular diseases of the limbs, Raynaud's disease and Buerger's disease, cause symptoms related to circulatory interferences in the periphery. Both of these conditions are responsive to sympathectomy. Peripheral arteriosclerosis, a third vascular problem, is not responsive to sympathectomy, since this condition affects mostly the large arteries. Large arteries are less responsive to sympathectomy and may be dilated even before the sympathetic nerves are removed. However, as in other conditions that interfere with blood supply, the individual with arteriosclerosis in the periphery may experience pain secondary to ischemia, gangrene, and ulcerated areas in the skin. Chapter 24 contains additional information on peripheral vascular disorders.

*Raynaud's disease.* In Raynaud's disease, exposure to cold causes some clients, especially women who live in northern climates, to experience pronounced local vasoconstriction, particularly in the hands and occasionally in the feet. As the hands become even slightly cool, one may observe severe vascular spasm that interrupts blood flow to the hands. As blood flow and subsequent metabolic activities are interrupted, deep tissues and bones develop pain secondary to ischemia.

After the initial ischemic episode occurs, a second phase of hyperemia takes place, wherein the vessels of the hands dilate, causing them to appear very reddened. During this second phase the client experiences even more intense pain, possibly because of the increase in blood pressure occurring with dilatation of all the arteries or the sudden movement of metabolic products accumulated during the phase of vasoconstriction. Although Raynaud's disease presents only momentary discomfort and alteration of skin color in the early stages of disease, this condition may progressively worsen until vasoconstriction becomes a continuous state. In this instance the blood flow may be impaired to the extent that gangrene becomes a critical danger.

To treat this condition the sympathetic chain at the level of T2 and T3 is removed to interrupt sympathetic impulses to the hand. Although the stellate ganglion contains many of the postganglionic fibers to the hand, it is left intact to avoid excessive sensitization of postganglionic sympathetic fibers to circulating norepinephrine and epinephrine. When the stellate ganglion is removed, the client may experience a recurrence of Raynaud's syndrome each time the adrenal gland is stimulated.

*Buerger's disease.* Buerger's disease (thromboangiitis obliterans) results when an inflammatory response occurs in the triangular sheaths housing the nerve, artery, and vein in some peripheral areas. Nicotine, most commonly used in the form of tobacco, aggravates the problem, which is most often seen in Jewish persons and in the legs rather than the arms. Intermittent claudication is the major symptom that earmarks this disease. Intermittent claudication means that when the client walks, the calf muscles become very painful because of the decreased blood flow that hampers the removal of ischemic products accumulating in muscle. The intensity of the pain has been likened to that of angina pectoris.

To avoid the possibility of loss of the toes or legs from this condition, neurosurgeons offer the client a sympathectomy of the L1 to L3 ganglia of the sympathetic chain. Although the untoward outcomes in this disease are not the result of sympathetic activity, the sympathectomy effectively inhibits normal vasomotor tone, so that vasodilatation in affected portions of the leg may occur.

## Trophic changes related to neurological disease

*Tabes dorsalis.* Neurosyphilis may result in interference with functions of the nervous system at the cerebral (general paresis) or spinal (tabes dorsalis) level. Tabes dorsalis includes a chronic inflammatory reaction in dorsal root ganglia wherein there are degenerative changes in the posterior tract of the cord and the dorsal roots.

The insidious course of tabes dorsalis begins as so-called lightening pains of a momentary, intense shooting type and occurs in both the extremities and the trunk. Paresthesias and numbness of the face and feet may also be prominent at this point. Gastric episodes consisting of abdominal pain, retching, and vomiting are also common complaints of clients affected by this condition. These various manifestations of pain are believed to occur as destruction of pain fibers results in bursts of impulses along those fibers that remain intact.

With time the large myelinated (fast) fibers, mainly in the lower thoracic and lumbar roots, are disturbed, and degenerative changes become apparent in the posterior column. Such interruptions in neuronal function include pallanesthesia, loss of appreciation of the position when the eyes are closed, and Romberg's sign (the inability to stand with the feet close together when the eyes are closed without losing balance). The characteristic slapping gait allows the client to hear when the feet have touched the ground. As ataxia progresses, the client may require two canes or crutches to continue walking. If immobilized in bed for some condition, the client frequently loses the ability to compensate for the lost sense of balance and is unable to learn to walk again.

This degenerative process further interferes with the course of the reflex act as impulses travel from the posterior roots to the anterior horn cells. The result of this interference is the loss of the ankle jerk, knee jerk, and other deep reflexes. Hypotonia, caused by interferences in these same fibers, is most apparent in muscles of the anterior thigh and causes a backward bowing of the legs known as *genu recurvatum*.

Appreciation of deep pain is lost at an early point; pinching of the Achilles tendon (Abadie's sign) or ulnar nerve (Biernacki's sign) or compression of the testes does not induce pain.

As fast fibers undergo destruction, slow fibers remain to carry pain impulses. The result is a disturbance in superficial pain perception. At first the interruption is often most obvious in the side of the nose, the lateral aspect of the arm and leg, and the dorsum and sole of the foot. If pain is perceived after stimulus application in these areas, it is often apparent after a long interval between stimulus and response. Other abnormal changes include the loss of sexual potency and libido and the occurrence of individual disturbances in bladder functions, which include a large residual after voiding and secondary chronic cystitis caused by urinary stasis.

Tabes also results in enlargement of the haversian canals and thinning of the compact layer of bone so that the bones become brittle. Painless, sudden fractures may then occur as a result of normal activity. As the fracture heals, callus formation may be either scant or excessive. Other bone changes include the possible destruction of the head of the humerus or femur. Arthropathies such as effusion and edema result in painless swelling of the joints (Charcot's joints). Clients with tabes commonly have perforating ulcers, particularly on the sole of the foot. More general considerations on tabes are available in Chapter 16.

***Disseminated sclerosis.*** Disseminated sclerosis (multiple sclerosis) is a disease wherein patches of demyelinating lesions of the long conducting pathways of the central nervous system develop as fatty substance around the axons, leaving areas of sclerotic tissue that cause the nerve fibers to degenerate. As neuronal degeneration occurs, functional disturbances and trophic changes appear and persist. Chapter 17 contains a complete description of the disease. Trophic changes that may occur with disease progression include hair loss, unusual brittleness of the fingernails, effusion within the joint capsules, epidermolysis, and, in the last stages of the disease, decubitus ulcers.

***Poliomyelitis.*** Poliomyelitis, an acute infection resulting from a viral invasion, may affect the anterior horns of the spinal cord, the motor cells of the brainstem, and the motor cells in other portions of the brain. The three types of poliomyelitis are termed *bulbar, encephalitic,* and *spinal.* Each of these types is characterized by its invasion of different portions of the nervous system and by special signs related to involvement in that location. Chapter 13 gives additional detail.

In relation to the trophic changes apparent during attacks of poliomyelitis the clinician might note mottling or flushing of affected portions of the body during the acute phase and cool, livid or mottled, smooth and thin, and frequently hairy skin during later stages of the disease. Rarefaction of bone and muscle atrophy are also prevalent in affected limbs. When this condition affects children, bone growth lags, and bones become so much smaller and rarefied that even the jolts of normal activity may result in a fracture.

***Hysterical palsy.*** Hysterical palsy is the term describing the trophic changes, such as those involving the nails, relatively painless ulceration; and digital atrophy seen in some functional conditions. Trophic problems arising in this context respond totally to appropriate psychotherapeutic intervention.

***Syringomyelia.*** A chronic, slowly progressive disease of the spinal cord, syringomyelia may also involve the lower brainstem (syringobulbia). Its cause is unknown, though there is some evidence that it may be a congenital condition affecting the cells of the central canal of the spinal cord. The progressive nature of the disease results from the development of a cyst within the spinal cord or gliosis (scar tissue), with damage to the nerve fibers that cross within the cord (pain and temperature conduction).

The clinical picture is characterized by the loss of the perception of pain and temperature, which makes these clients susceptible to burns and other injuries; ordinary touch sensation is preserved. Also, weakness and atrophy of the hand muscles may be present as well as evidence of autonomic dysfunction (absence of sweating, hyperkeratosis, trophic ulcers, sluggish intestinal activity, and poor bladder tone). Early in the disease the loss of pain and temperature sensibility may be apparent. Weakness and atrophy in the hand muscles may also be apparent, though touch appreciation is preserved. The dorsal aspect of the hand may also appear swollen and glossy and feel cold. Affected body parts usually evidence a cutaneous area that is dry, scaly, and grooved, as the skin of a toad might appear. White layers of epidermis also separate. Other obvious problems include loss of fingernails, formation of Dupuytren's contracture of the palmar surface of the hand, loss of cutaneous hair, and abnormal growth in the soft tissues of the hand. Regardless of the location of the lesion — cervicothoracic or lumbosacral — the progressive type of trophic problems that occur may include incomplete or total loss of the digits on either the upper or lower extremities. Musculoskeletal abnormalities are frequently associated, including scoliosis, clubfoot, and asymmetries of the cranium. Autonomic abnormalities are also evident in the form of absence of sweating and diminished bladder and bowel control. The diagnosis is made on the basis of the abnormal neurological signs and symptoms.

**TREATMENT AND NURSING INTERVENTION.** There is no specific treatment. If the spinal dynamics disclose a block, a laminectomy should be done, and the cyst of the spinal cord opened and drained. Radiation therapy, since it has been helpful in a number of cases, may be given over the area of the spinal cord affected.

The nursing care is directed toward the prevention of complications, especially burns. If the brainstem is involved, the client will have progressive difficulty in eating, swallowing, and talking. Regurgitation of food and fluids may occur, and aspiration may result, making the client more susceptible to respiratory tract infections. The nurse should take every precaution to prevent the aspiration of food or fluid, and, at the first indication of swallowing difficulties, the client should be closely supervised during meals. He or she may have to be fed artificially. The suction machine is always at hand for emergency use. Special mouth care is given to prevent excess dryness of the mucous membranes and formation of crusts and sordes. (If a laminectomy is done, see Chapters 22 and 27 for the nursing care.)

Effective psychological and physical nursing care is given to these clients, just as it should be given to any other client suffering from a chronic, slowly progressive disease.

***Subacute combined degeneration.*** Subacute combined degeneration, a condition affecting the peripheral nerves and the posterior and lateral tracts of the spinal cord, is progressively incapacitating and fatal unless treated. It is frequently, though not invariably, associated with pernicious anemia.

Its cause is the deficiency of vitamin $B_{12}$ because of the failure of the gastric mucosa to produce a substance, the "intrinsic factor" essential for the absorption of vitamin $B_{12}$ from food. The pathological condition is characterized by early degeneration of the sensory fibers of the peripheral nerves. Later the posterior and lateral tracts degenerate. Although only the myelin is lost in the early stages, the nerve fibers themselves are finally involved, and, as a result, there is no hope of recovery of spinal cord function.

The symptoms begin with paresthesias in the hands and feet and around the abdomen, which may be associated with lassitude (a result of pernicious anemia). As the disease progresses, difficulty in walking that may progress to paraplegia will occur.

The diagnosis is made on the basis of the neurological examination, which reveals impairment of the perception of touch, position, passive motion, and vibration (signs of posterior tract involvement) and impaired muscular power and spasticity (signs of interruption of the pyramidal tract). The laboratory is especially helpful, since blood studies reveal the pernicious anemia (diminished number of red blood cells with large abnormal forms containing more hemoglobin than usual), and examination of the gastric juice shows an absence of free hydrochloric acid even after administration of histamine.

**TREATMENT AND NURSING INTERVENTION.** The treatment is specific, consisting of the intramuscular administration of vitamin $B_{12}$. One determines the dosage by finding the amount necessary to reach and maintain a normal blood picture and doubling it. It is usually 30 to 60 $\mu$g of vitamin $B_{12}$ intramuscularly daily for 3 days and then 30 $\mu$g once a week for 6 months, followed by a maintenance dose of 30 $\mu$g once a month for life. The therapeutic effect is most favorable; and the client can continue a normal existence while he or she takes vitamin $B_{12}$. Massage and warm baths may be given to relieve spasticity.

The nursing care is based on the symptoms of disturbed function and is directed toward the prevention of complications and the alleviation of emotional distress.

## THEORETICAL BASIS OF TROPHIC CHANGES

Trophic changes have been ascribed to the disturbed operations of sensory fibers, motor neurons, and sympathetic fibers that regulate circulatory functions. However, no one actually knows how each of these factors specifically relates to the trophic outcomes commonly associated with a variety of disease conditions.

Most information about trophic changes in humans is the result of experimental investigations in animals. Although trophic changes are believed to be quite similar in humans and animals, definitive evidence is hampered by the inability to replicate experimental conditions in humans.

In investigations of the muscles of dogs after cord sections, alterations in metabolic processes are observed in muscles located distal to the level of transection. For example, instead of giving up creatinine as muscle usually does, affected muscle exudes creatine for a period of up to 3 weeks. An interference with vascular permeability is probably also evident along with the metabolic disruptions.

When individuals are confined to bed rest status for an extended period, bone resorption occurs as a direct result of mechanical inactivity and subsequent circulatory disturbances. Experimentally the relationship of trophic changes to interruptions in circulation was demonstrated as Geiser and Trueta

(1958) severed the Achilles tendon of a rabbit and observed changes by monitoring the microopaque material injected into the vascular system. In summary, they observed rapid bony deterioration and reduction in bone mass within a 6-week period. Concurrently, blood vessels in the locality became extremely enlarged. Urist (1967) has done similar studies that show that oxygen tension is significant in cellular processes in bones. In studies on bone cultures, osteoprogenitor cells were found to differentiate into osteoclasts rather than osteoblasts when the oxygen concentration in the experiment was elevated from 35% to 95%.

The relationship of sympathetic nerve interferences in relation to abnormal circulation and subsequent trophic changes has been studied by various investigators. There remains a large gap in understanding about the significance of interrupted sympathetic nerve functions and trophic changes. In early studies by Atlas (1938) an attempt was made to explain late tissue and vascular abnormalities in relation to increased epinephrine sensitivity. Preganglionic sympathectomy does not seem to interfere with this phenomenon. Moreover, the resulting sensitization causing vasoconstriction may explain the nutritional and vasomotor alterations observed in denervated tissue. Tower (1935, 1937) noted that trophic changes in muscle and other tissue did not result from interferences in impulses after interruption of posterior roots.

Contemporary investigators thus believe that trophic changes related to such disease processes as multiple sclerosis, poliomyelitis, tabes dorsalis, syringomyelia, and peripheral nerve injury are explained by their combination of motoneural, sensory, and circulatory interferences. The exact interrelationship of these factors probably varies with the location of the lesion in the axis of the nervous system. However, with regard to neuronal influences on trophic changes in tissue, the opinion expressed by Sherrington in 1900 still has great relevance. He stated that by the very nature of neuronal functions being totally responsible for precise and specific tissue capacities, nerves have the ability to effect trophic responses in tissues.

Trauma has been cited as a precipitating factor in causing further damage. When animals with a denervated limb are given unrestricted space to ambulate, bone and joint disturbances occur that are not evident in animals confined in activity through placement in a small cage.

## Peripheral nerve damage

Severe trophic changes may be evident when lesions of the peripheral nervous system interrupt normal neuronal functions. When a peripheral nerve such as the ulnar or sciatic nerve is interrupted through trauma, a so-called warm phase of dry, flushed, warm skin is apparent for about 3 weeks. During this time the skin is not responsive to mechanical means of cooling. After the warm phase a cool phase ensues, wherein trophic changes become more evident, particularly in the digits. When damage to the median and sciatic nerves is partial and causalgia is a concurrent phenomenon, the persistence of the warm phase and sweating may be noted. In instances of causalgia, skin and bone changes are frequently more pronounced than those occurring in painless nerve injuries of like proportion.

Chapters 2 and 3 discuss the anatomy and physiology of afferent and efferent peripheral nerves. It is important to restate the fact that afferent and efferent nerves of the peripheral nervous system have a cellular sheath (sheath of Schwann) that encircles them and permits successful regrowth after destruction of a neuronal fiber. Neuronal fibers within the central axis lack this sheath of insulating myelin and do not regenerate after damage.

As an axon emerges from a peripheral nerve cell, it is sheathed by myelin and encased in neurilemma. As the axon continues outward, there are narrowed areas, known as nodes of Ranvier. At these nodes the continuity of myelin is broken, but the neurilemmal covering remains continuous. The neurilemmal encasement at each node consists of a single flattened cell that is essential to the restoration of functions in damaged neuronal fiber. Myelin, an insulating substance, is present in greater quantities around nerves engaged in rapid conductions and discrete functions. For example, fibers involved in touch have more substantial quantities of myelin.

When a nerve with mixed functions—motor and sensory—is severed by accident, the client reports anesthesia in the regions supplied by sensory portions of the nerve and interference with motor functions in areas served by motor components of the nerve. An accident involving the radial nerve would result in such sensory and motor deficits in the hand. When electric current is applied to affected parts, a response to faradic current is apparent, but galvanic current elicits no response. This electrical activity confirms the presence of a degenerative response, wherein muscles do not respond to incoming stimuli of the radial nerve because of denervation.

To comprehend the process of neuronal regeneration it is easiest to limit the explanation to a single axon of the radial nerve as an example. After the axon has been severed, the distal portion of the axon becomes swollen, the myelin disintegrates, and the products of destruction are removed by phagocytosis. However, the neurilemma remains viable. This process is termed *wallerian degeneration* (Fig. 16-3).

On the proximal aspect of the severed nerve, altered functions also become apparent. The cell body evidences shock as the Nissl substance experiences chromatolysis and the nucleus of the cell moves from its central position. In the proximal end of the axon near the point of damage the degenerative pattern is similar to that occurring in the distal fragment, except that the axonal swelling and disintegration of myelin extend only to the adjacent node of Ranvier.

After several days the nerve cell demonstrates normal functions again, and small fibrils emerge from the node proximal to the point of injury. Of the many fibrils formed, only a small number connect with the neurilemma of the distal stump for the redirection and myelination necessary to revitalize the muscles they supply.

Those fibrils that fail to contact neurilemma disappear. Regenerating fibrils that must course more than a few millimeters between proximal and distal fragments continue to grow and, after missing connection with the distal stump, form a matted lesion (neuroma) that may result in pain. (Chapter 10 offers more detail on pain.) However, because they are unable to reestablish contact, the affected part (in this instance the hand) remains denervated and thus without function.

If initial response to injury does not include (1) first aid that further damages tissue, such as a tight tourniquet that impedes nutritional supplies to tis-

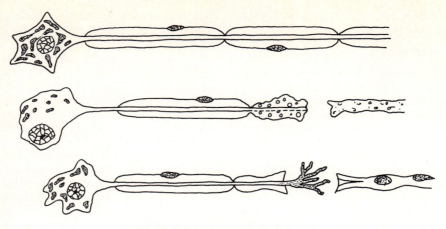

**FIG. 16-3.** Diagram of nerve regeneration.

sues; (2) inadequate surgical intervention in the wound; (3) infection; (4) secondary thermal or mechanical injury during healing; or (5) overall poor health status, the neuronal regeneration proceeds. Evidence of regained neuronal integrity includes prickly sensations, tingling, and pain in the hand and gradual reestablishment of function.

Another factor affecting reestablishment of functional integrity in a nerve fiber is neuronal specialization. In general the more highly specialized peripheral nerves are the least likely to reestablish functional integrity successfully. As described, the establishment of function in other neurons proceeds only when inhibitory factors such as those just detailed do not interfere.

### Polyneuritis

The distal portion of an axon may also be interrupted by a disease process so that symmetrical polyneuritis occurs. In this instance, as in trauma, the distal portion of the axon is the most affected because protein synthesis occurs in the cell body. Thus protein and other vital substances necessary to the integrity of the axon and myelin sheath are passed distally by a process termed *axoplasmic flow*. When this vital flow is interrupted anatomically by trauma or a disease process, unsupplied areas of the axon and myelin sheath degenerate uniformly first in segmental demyelination, which is early and reversible. If neuronal distress con-

tinues, wallerian degeneration of distal portions occurs, as detailed in the previous section.

### Carpal tunnel syndrome

The carpal tunnel syndrome (CTS), a disorder resulting from compression of the median nerve at the wrist, results in early symptoms such as numbness and tingling augmented by repetitive motor activity, stiff edematous fingers upon awakening that become more functional with use, and burning sensations during slumber that cause the client to awaken. If CTS is recognized and treated at this point, all adverse symptoms may be abated.

Burning sensations of pain that radiate to the elbow, forearm or shoulder may cause the practitioner to be concerned about such differential considerations as cervical arthritis, thoracic (first-rib) syndrome, or other conditions related to sensory and functional disorders of the upper extremity.

The diagnostic assessment includes recognition of the symptoms described, diminished sensory response to pinpricks in the fingers and palmar aspect of the hand, weak and atrophic thenar (thumb) muscles in chronic cases, and a positive response in Phalen's and Tinel's signs.

Phalen's sign is positive when the client, who has the forearms vertically positioned in an upward direction with hands lowered into complete flexion, feels burning pain and numbness soon after assuming this position. Individuals with a normal response should be able to maintain this posture for a while before experiencing numbness and pain.

Tinel's sign is elicited when the practitioner barely taps the median nerve at the wrist. An abnormal response is one wherein a tingle moves quickly throughout the hand.

If atrophy is present, it is obvious in the thumb muscles and in the thenar eminence between the thumb and wrist on the backside of the hand. It is helpful to compare both hands to make this determination.

Diagnostic studies that confirm the clinical impression include hand and wrist roentgenograms, electromyography (EMG), and nerve conduction time tests. EMG testing is painful and requires the emotional support of the nurse during and after testing.

In a study done by Gainer and Nugent on 326 clients with CTS, the age of onset varied from 14 to 84 years and 119 (37%) experienced CTS during the sixth decade. Half of the clients had endured CTS for up to 1 year. Forty percent of those affected were housewives and cooks. It is significant to note that 78% of those involved worked at a job requiring extensive hand usage. More than two thirds of the clients had CTS in the dominant hand. Eighty-two percent benefited from surgery, whereas 51% of those reported abatement of CTS symptoms.

Conservative treatment consists of avoiding repetitive activities such as typing or crocheting. It may also include a hand-and-wrist splint that maintains the wrist in neutral position, while one avoids flexion. An injection of water-soluble cortisone into the carpal canal may provide short-term relief. Treatment of systematic disorders like gout, hormonal imbalances, and rheumatoid arthritis may decrease CTS symptoms. If these measures fail, surgical intervention is indicated. While the surgeon is decompressing the median nerve, correction of growths, tendon ruptures, or other abnormalities may be corrected.

Nursing intervention includes informing the client about the condition and activities that diminish or augment symptoms. Nursing care during surgery is the same as any orthopedic surgery of the hand. Include care to ensure functional and sensory integrity of the hand, adequate circulation, and precautions in infection control to diminish the possibility of a postoperative infection. Refer to Larson and Gould's *Orthopedic Nursing* for further detail on general care of musculoskeletal problems.

## INTERVENTION MODALITIES

### Expected outcomes

The client will:

1 Specify preventative or health promotion available, and comment on ways that he or she integrates them into daily living.
2 Describe the components of an adequate diet and the pros and cons of fad diets, fast foods, and vitamin supplements.
3 Identify problems, concerns, and outcomes related to individual physiological disturbances.
4 Discuss strengths, limitations, and specific needs in relation to identified problems.
5 Describe care and medications within a realistic framework for implementation.
6 Utilize genetic counseling or other directive and supportive services as needed.

In each problem affecting disturbances in function or sensibility and related trophic changes the genesis of the problem; the course of the disease process or problem; and the outcome in terms of acute, chronic, or increasing disability varies. Thus nursing care in relation to psychosocial, vocational, and economic factors is premised on a thorough understanding of problems and outcomes related to physiological disturbances in the context of the affected individual. Physical limitations may be assessed through thorough comprehension of the disease process coupled with an adequate history and physical examination and appropriate diagnostic studies. The complete plan of care should utilize services of all helping professionals in combination with client and family capacities and objectives in a realistic program that emphasizes (1) reestablishment of function, (2) maintenance of function, and (3) instruction in new patterns, as applicable.

## REFERENCES

Atkins, R.C.: Dr. Atkin's diet revolution: the high calorie way to stay thin forever, New York, 1977, Bantam Books, Inc.

Atlas, L.N.: Etiology of vasomotor and nutritional changes following peripheral nerve section, Surgery **4:**718, 1938.

Atlas, L.N.: Further observations on etiology of vasomotor disturbances following peripheral nerve section, Surgery **10:** 318, 1941.

Berger, M.R., and Froimson, A.I.: Hands that hurt: carpal tunnel syndrome, Am. J. Nurs. **80:**264-66, Feb. 1980.

Corbin, K.B., and Hinsey, J.C.: Influence of the nervous system on bone and joints, Anat. Rec. **75:**307, 1939.

Davis, A.: Eat right and keep fit, New York, 1970, The New American Library, Inc.

Dietary Allowances Committee and Food and Nutrition Board: Recommended dietary allowances, ed. 8, Washington, D.C., 1974, National Academy of Sciences.

Dyck, P.J., et al.: Peripheral neuropathy, Philadelphia, 1975, W.B. Saunders Co.

Feingold, B.F.: Why your child is hyperactive, New York, 1974, Random House, Inc.

Fuerst, E.V., et al.: Fundamentals of nursing: the humanities and sciences in nursing, Philadelphia, 1974, J.B. Lippincott Co.

Gainer, J.V., Jr., and Nugent, G.R.: Carpal tunnel syndrome: report of 430 operations, South. Med. J. **70:**325-28, 1977.

Geiser, M., and Trueta, J.: Muscle action, bone rarefaction and bone formation, J. Bone Joint Surg. **40B:**282, 1958.

Guthrie, R., and Guthrie, D.: Nursing management of diabetes mellitus, ed. 2, St. Louis, 1982, The C.V. Mosby Co.

Guyton, A.C.: Textbook of medical physiology, ed. 5, Philadelphia, 1976, W.B. Saunders Co.

Guth, L., and Windle, W.R., editors: The enigma of central nervous regeneration, Exp. Neurol. (suppl.) **5:**1043, 1970.

Holling, E.H.: Peripheral vascular diseases: diagnosis and management, Philadelphia, 1972, J.B. Lippincott Co.

Kremer, W., and Kremer, L.: Doctor's metabolic diet, New York, 1974, Crown Publishers, Inc.

Landon, D.H., editor: Peripheral nerves, New York, 1976, Halsted Press.

Larson, C.B., and Gould, M.: Orthopedic nursing, ed. 9, St. Louis, 1978, The C.V. Mosby Co.

Levy, J.V., and Bach-y-Rita, P.: Vitamins: their use and abuse, New York, 1976, Liveright.

Netter, F.: Fad diets can be deadly: the safe and sure way to weight loss and good nutrition, Hicksville, N.Y., 1975, Exposition Press, Inc.

Passwater, R.: Supernutrition: megavitamin revolution, New York, 1975, The Dial Press.

Rosenberg, H., and Feldzaman, A.N.: Doctor's book of vitamin therapy, New York, 1974, G.P. Putnam's Sons.

Rosenberg, H., and Feldzaman, A.N.: The book of vitamin therapy, New York, 1975, Berkley Publishing Corp.

Sherrington, C.S.: Trophic changes of the spinal cord. In Schafer, E.A., editor: Textbook of physiology, Edinburgh, 1900, Pentland.

Stillman, I.M., and Baker, S.: Doctor's quick inches off diet, New York, 1975, Dell Publishing Co., Inc.

Sunderland, S.: Nerves and nerve injuries, ed. 2, New York, 1979, Churchill Livingstone, Division of Longman, Inc.

Tatkon, D.: Great vitamin hoax, New York, 1967, Macmillan Publishing Co., Inc.

Thiele, V.F.: Clinical nutrition, St. Louis, 1976, The C.V. Mosby Co.

Tower, S.S.: Atrophy and degeneration in skeletal muscle, Am. J. Anat. **56:**1, 1935.

Tower, S.S.: Function and structure in chronically isolated lumbosacral spinal cord of dog, J. Comp. Neurol. **67:**109, 1937.

Tower, S.S.: Trophic control of non-nervous tissues by the nervous system: a study of muscle and bone innervated from an isolated and quiescent region of the spinal cord, J. Comp. Neurol. **67:**241, 1937.

Urist, M.R.: Bone-body fluid continuum as influenced by prolonged inactivity. In Calloway, P.H., editor: Human ecology in space flight—second conference proceedings, vol. 2, New York, 1967, Gordon & Breach Science Publishers, Inc.

Wade, C.: Fact-book on vitamins and other food supplements, New Canaan, Conn., 1972, Keats Publishing, Inc.

Whaley, L.F., and Wong, D.: Nursing care of infants and children, St. Louis, 1979, The C.V. Mosby Co.

Willis, W.D., and Grossman, R.: Medical neurobiology: neuroanatomical and neurophysiological principles basic to clinical neuroscience, ed. 2, St. Louis, 1977, The C.V. Mosby Co.

# 17

# DISORDERS AFFECTING MOTOR OUTCOMES

This section begins with a discussion of motor neuron disturbances, specifically upper and lower motor neuron disorders and peripheral nerve disorders. Disturbances at the neuromuscular junction are discussed. Finally problems of the muscle are detailed.

## MOTOR NEURON DISTURBANCES

Motor neuron disease includes a number of disturbances that may involve changes in muscle function, tone, and reflexes, as well as the appearance of involuntary movements, muscle atrophy, or electrical reactions. The resulting damage depends on whether the lesion affects the upper motor neuron, the lower motor neuron, or both areas. The upper motor neuron refers to the descending motor pathway (pyramidal tract). Damage to the pyramidal tract may occur at various points between its origin in the cerebral cortex and its termination at various points in the spinal cord. The level of the lesion interfering with pyramidal tract functions may often be identified by the problems that occur concurrently. Within the cord, corticospinal fibers are disturbed when a lesion impinges on the lateral column. Lower motor neuron lesions affect spinomuscular fibers. Damage to anterior horns or anterior roots makes up the category of lower motor lesions. At times lesions affect both the upper and lower motor neurons. Before defining the diagnostic problem, the practitioner is faced with the problem of identifying which category that explains the source of the motor system lesion.

## Upper motor neuron disorders

Paralysis in the upper motor neuron is characterized by a number of changes below the level of the lesion, including an incomplete loss of power, a more bilateral and diffuse involvement of muscles in a limb in comparison to the situation with lower motor neuron lesions, little atrophy, an increase in muscle tone, an increase in deep reflexes, a decrease or absence of the abdominal reflex, a positive test for the pathological reflexes detailed in Chapter 11, a lack of electrical changes, no fasciculations, mild vasomotor phenomena, and the presence of Strümpell's sign.

Although only a neurologist should make the final definition of where the disturbance lies, particularly in relation to interferences with the pyramidal tract, which courses the long route from the cerebral cortex to the spinal medulla, interested readers may refer to lengthy discussions of the various portions of the central nervous system in *Bing's Local Diagnosis in Neurological Disease* (Haymaker, 1969) for differences in symptomatology related to various locations for possible lesions and to appropriate sections in this textbook.

Since the spinal cord is the modality for connecting all portions of the nervous system, profound changes occur when an individual experiences acute cord transection. Outside the military service, most injuries involving the spinal cord occur from indirect violence that results in either flexion or extension of the spinal cord. One way this type of injury commonly occurs is in automobile accidents, where a whiplash of the head and neck occurs (see Chapter 10). However, other examples might include trauma related to diving into a pool with insufficient water or free-falling from an airplane when the parachute does not open in time to slow the rate of fall. Refer to Chapter 23 for clients' problems and immediate aspects of assessment and intervention of spinal shock.

Whatever the cause, the individual suffering acute cord transection experiences a variable degree of spinal shock from the interrupted transmission of descending supraspinal impulses, from inhibition of spinal segments below the level of the lesion, and from axonal degeneration in interneurons. During this state of spinal shock, severe functional impairment below the level of the lesion is obvious, including paralysis and flaccidity in muscles; absence of sensation; loss of bladder and rectal control; transient drop in blood pressure; and poor venous circulation, which results in cold cyanotic limbs, absence of sweat, and potential skin breakdown. Priapism in male subjects and an absence of perspiration and reflexes are also evident during the early hours after injury. Extreme pain may additionally be experienced by the client at the level of the lesion. (Refer to Chapter 10).

When the lesion is located at the cervical level, these symptoms may include all four extremities as well as the trunk. In these instances, accessory muscles in the nose, mouth, and neck may be attempting to carry on the process of respiration. Thus efforts to breathe are inadequate, and respiratory failure becomes imminent when ventilatory assistance is not utilized.

When injury involves the thoracic spine, muscles of the upper extremities and those involved in respiration are spared. After the early stage of spinal shock has passed, the flaccid muscles becomes spastic. The atonic bladder becomes hypertonic but may be made to function automatically with appropriate intervention.

If the injury involves the lumbar spine, the cauda equina and conus medullaris are affected. This trauma to the lumbar spine results in continuing flaccidity of the lower extremities, bladder, and rectum. Bladder control is not possible in this type of injury.

*Spinal shock.* Spinal shock results in paralytic ileus, which occurs at different times because of the course of the splanchnic nerves to the viscera. For the thoracic injury, the elapsed time is at least 24 hours; for the cervical injury, it is 48 hours; and for the lumbar injury, paralytic ileus occurs quickly after the injury. At the first sign of nausea, vomiting, or distention, a nasogastric tube is inserted. Because of the time lapse and depending on other individual factors, the nasogastric tube may be inserted in the client with cervical injury after traction has been applied.

Because of adrenal and pituitary functions during spinal shock, urinary retention occurs. A Foley catheter should be inserted for 2 to 4 days after injury, at which time the endocrine levels stabilize and diuresis occurs. Urinary control should then be maintained with an intermittent catheter routine, as suggested in Chapter 25. Bowel management, problems in mobility, and skin care are further defined therein. Chapters 9 and 27 provide additional care interventions for clients with limited mobility. Chapters 11 and 12 provide the practitioner with essential information on assessment and diagnostic tests that may be performed. Sexuality, as discussed in Chapter 6, answers specific questions that a client may have. Chapters 6 and 7 detail responses to illness and hospitalization that may occur in the client.

Spinal shock also results in disturbed thermal control (poikilothermy) because the sympathetic nervous system is damaged. This damage causes an interruption in the mechanism controlling sweating and radiation through capillary dilatation. The hypothalamus cannot keep body heat through vasoconstriction and increased metabolism. Thus the client assumes the temperature of the air. Temperature needs to be normalized. However, one should be very cautious with heating devices to avoid burns.

The practitioner should also be aware of the prevalence of stress ulcers, particularly after 7 to 10 days have elapsed from the injury or after surgery. This ulcer, caused by the embarrassed circulation existing in the stomach area after blood has been shunted to the traumatic area of need, is manifested by abdominal and shoulder discomfort before other signs appear.

Begin prescribed exercises assisted by a physical therapist under the neurologist's or neurosurgeon's direction. Resistive exercise is needed to maintain muscle strength.

If possible, contemporary practitioners either stabilize the client and transport him or her to a spinal cord center, or continue treatment if a qualified staff and facility is available. Surgery is usually delayed until the client has achieved stability in electrolytes, blood gases, renal function, gastrointestinal persitalsis, and cardiovascular and respiratory status. In partial lesions, where normal functional return is possible, surgery is avoided. Surgery is designed to remove any projectile that obstructs spinal functions and to use various types of internal fixation devices to stabilize the vertebral column. The type of device is dictated by the type of damage and the level of the lesion.

One current practice that has greatly improved the treatment and outcome for clients is the trend toward using devices, such as the halo ring, that becomes part of the plaster-cast jacket. This jacket, which is removable for skin care, provides needed support during bone healing. The halo brace also improves care for the elderly and frail by decreasing respiratory problems. Rehabilitation may begin as early as 2 to 3 weeks after injury.

Mentally, the early responses to paralysis, which include shock and panic, give way to realization about the injury and finally to defensive retreat. Defensive retreat is a particularly hard phase to cope with in that it includes combinations of denial, avoidance of reality, anger, and continual repetition of factual information that the client must assimilate. The last two phases of psychological response are acknowledgment of the condition and adaptation to it. These last steps may extend over a period of years after injury, and, for many, ideal adjustment and response never exist. (Refer to Chapter 25 for further detail.)

A plan of comprehensive health care intervention for the client and significant other should be mutually developed at the time of injury and extend for as long as there is a need. In this plan special individual and group sessions should be arranged to assist spouses, families, and significant others in coping with the physical, emotional, financial, and psychosocial aspects of the problem.

Although spinal shock usually continues for 2 to 3 weeks, it may persist for as short a time as a few days or as long as 3 months. As the stage of spinal shock wanes, reflex activities reappear first, often within 1 to 3 weeks of the injury. The reappearance of the reflexes occurs in the following manner: flexor responses precede extensor ones, superficial reflexes go before deep ones, and distal responses are evident before proximal ones. When the client is tested clinically, painful plantar stimuli are found to cause slight movements of the feet and toes, and anal and erection reflexes may be noted at this time, if not earlier. Crossed reflexes may not be elicited before about 3 months have passed. If the client demonstrates a return in muscle functions originating in the proximal limbs, a partial transection of the cord has probably occurred.

***Types of paralysis.*** Both partial and complete transections may result in either paraplegia in flexion or extension. When a transection occurs in the cervical area, paraplegia in extension often results, whereas a transection in the thoracic area may result in either paraplegia in flexion or extension. Paraplegia in flexion generally occurs when the transection is in the midthoracic region.

The mass reflex may be elicited after the client recovers from spinal shock. The mass reflex refers to the synergistic movement of muscles beneath the level of the lesion when appropriate stimuli are provided. In the mass reflex, or withdrawal response, the reflexogenic zone increases so that there is withdrawal of the lower extremities in response to plantar stimulation. This response is particularly evident in complete transections. When the transection is in the lower cervical area, the withdrawal response includes the stimulated lower limb, the trunk muscle, and often the fingers and thumb extensors of either side.

In both extensor and flexor types of paraplegia Babinski's reflex may be elicited, even though a flexor response in the great toe is present, for 2 to 3 weeks after injury before the pathological reflex is detected.

As new axonal growth occurs, the client, who may have initially been flaccid, may experience spasticity. When flaccidity is a persistent state, one observes areflexia, adynamia, extreme muscular atrophy, and an absence of synergistic reflex activity.

To complete this section, it seems important to

compare the characteristics of partial and complete transections.

In a partial transection the paralysis is asymmetrical. The client may experience some sensation and possibly have a return of some voluntary activity within a week. On assessment the practitioner notes that the paralyzed region is larger than the anesthetic area. In evaluating the mass reflex one notes that the reflexogenic zone that participates in the flexor response is smaller than that seen in complete transections. Reflexes are asymmetrical, and few flexor spasms occur. Vasomotor and sphincter disturbances are less obvious than in complete transections. When the mass reflex is elicited, the flexor response is followed by extension. When plantar pressure is applied to a flexed limb, bilateral movements of the legs result.

In complete transection there is asymmetrical paralysis. No sensation or voluntary movement is present. The reflexogenic zone is larger than that seen in partial transections, and the paralyzed and anesthetic areas cover the same region. Flexor spasms are frequently evident, and vasomotor and sphincter disturbances are pronounced. Responses to stimulation and reflex testing are symmetrical. When the mass movement is elicited, the result is limited to a flexor response. No marching movements of the legs occur when plantar pressure is applied. Flaccidity, areflexia, and complete sensory loss persist for more than 5 days after injury.

*Stroke.* Although stroke is detailed in Chapter 24, it is mentioned here since it is a common example of a problem that affects the upper motor neuron.

### Lower motor neuron disorders

Interruption in motor function may also occur as the result of a disturbance in the final common pathway. In this situation the disturbance may involve the peripheral motor nerves or the anterior horn. Some conditions that result in abnormal motor responses may even include involvement of the entire reflex arc. When the anterior motor neuron, or lower motor neuron, is affected, the following abnormalities result: complete absence of power; local, unilateral involvement of muscles; local atrophy; decreased tone and flaccidity; abdominal reflex changes when the lesion involves that level; absence of pathological reflexes; degenerative changes as detected by electromyography;

presence of muscle fasciculations; and absence of Strümpell's sign.

*Anterior horn disorders.* Denervation at the level of the anterior horn results in characteristic problems, including paralysis, atrophy, loss of reflexes, and fasciculations. If the disorder also involves the peripheral nerve, pain and sensory disturbances may additionally be evident.

Muscle fasciculations characterize anterior horn cell disease. When they are attributed to peripheral nerve disease, further study has revealed involvement of the entire reflex arc or involvement of the anterior horn through retrograde degeneration. These fasciculations seen in denervated muscle are the result of isolated contraction of one or more motor units. Such activity is readily observable by visualization and may be documented by electromyography. Fasciculation is evident when several motor units contract, with resultant muscle twitching observable under the surface of the skin.

Fibrillation occurs when individual muscle fibers contract. Such activity is present after the fifth day of denervation and is demonstrable only through electromyography.

Investigators still are unable to determine the origin of the fasciculations by site in striated muscle wherein anterior horn cell disease has occurred, as in amyotrophic lateral sclerosis. It is presumed that fasciculations begin at the myoneural junction. Several agents affect the production of fasciculations: (1) curare and denervation of muscle eliminate them; (2) neostigmine, acetylcholine, and methacholine (Mecholyl) increase them; and (3) spinal anesthesia and direct injections of procaine into the muscle produce no effect on them. Prolonged fibrillation occurs with acetylcholine; thus it is believed that fibrillation is augmented by the acetylcholine usually present in tissue fluids, which represents the degree of muscle fiber excitability seen after denervation. After denervation, sustained fibrillation potentials are not usually evident until after the third week.

Little information is available on the atrophy that develops after muscle denervation. The time of onset of muscular atrophy varies with the causative lesion. Vascular lesions may result in atrophy in a few days to a few weeks, whereas progressive problems such as tumors may result in a delayed onset of atrophy.

Atrophy in denervation is attributed to fibrillary

activity wherein glycogen is decreased or depleted along with other muscle substances. Some investigators dispute this theory by citing cases of atrophy that is apparent within 10 days in denervated muscle and in inactive muscle wherein the nerve supply is normal. When disuse atrophy has been investigated, researchers have found that activity and maintenance of muscle tension are the most crucial factors in avoiding muscle atrophy.

The development of atrophy occurs at differing rates in the various disorders of the anterior horn and peripheral nerves. Although the rate of trophic changes cannot be estimated, there is general agreement about the direct relation of the degree of atrophy to the number of motor units destroyed.

A number of chemical changes accompany the process of muscle atrophy. Potassium levels decrease, whereas calcium and chloride levels increase. A rapid decrease occurs in phosphorus levels, particularly in adenosine triphosphate and phosphocreatine. As fibrillation begins, glycogen and phosphocreatine levels decrease sharply, whereas creatine levels begin to drop after the fifteenth day. The degree of muscle loss determines the decrease in potassium, creatine, and phosphate compounds.

Examples of clinical forms of motor neuron disease are progressive muscular atrophy, amyotrophic lateral sclerosis, and bulbar palsy. Progressive muscular atrophy and amyotrophic lateral sclerosis are primarily lower motor neuron diseases, whereas bulbar palsy may involve both the upper and lower motor neurons. Multiple sclerosis is also a condition that is characterized by scattered neurological lesions.

**INFANTILE SPINAL MUSCULAR ATROPHY (WERDNIG-HOFFMANN DISEASE).** Werdnig-Hoffmann disease is an autosomal recessive disorder that results in obvious muscle weakness and other abnormalities such as generalized floppiness as early as 3 months of age. Subsequent life is characterized by symptomatic supportive management for the progressive downhill course. Numerous upper respiratory infections occur before death at about 3 years of age.

**AMYOTROPHIC LATERAL SCLEROSIS.** Amyotrophic lateral sclerosis (ALS) is a severe form of anterior horn disease, wherein the cause and cure remain elusive. The onset of ALS is between 40 and 70 years of age. About 2 or 3 males are affected to each female with ALS. ALS has an incidence of 2 to 7 cases per 100,000 in the general population. Although affected individuals may survive for a number of years, death frequently occurs about 3 years after diagnosis. When atrophic changes occur in the brainstem, death often follows within 12 to 18 months. Aspiration pneumonia or respiratory failure may be the immediate cause of death.

The disease now identified as amyotrophic lateral sclerosis was first reported by James Bell in 1830. Almost 40 years later Charcot described it in his writings. It was dramatically brought to the attention of the public when Lou Gehrig, Hall of Fame baseball star and a victim of amyotrophic lateral sclerosis, died in 1941.

Although comparatively rare in the United States (an estimated 5000 to 10,000 cases), this disease is prevalent on the island of Guam and some of the nearby Mariana Islands. In these places a form of amyotrophic lateral sclerosis is a hundred times more common than that in the continental United States.

Because of studies performed on those affected with amyotrophic lateral sclerosis in Guam, a genetic basis or external agent is possible as a causative agent. No definitive evidence is available to support either possibility. Other proposed causes include inappropriate nutrition; ingestion of uncooked meat; metabolic disturbances such as metal imbalances; and responses to systemic stimuli such as spinal anesthesia, infection, trauma, or electric shock. Recent attention has also been focused on chronic viral infections or abnormal immune response to a virus.

CLINICAL COURSE. The symptoms vary from individual to individual, depending on which motor nerve cells in the brain and spinal cord are involved. The first symptom may be irregular twitchings (fasciculations) of the muscles, which may be accompanied by muscular weakness. Frequently the muscles of the lower arms and hands are involved, and atrophy of the muscles is evident on both sides of the thumbs and in the palms. Leg muscles may become spastic and progressively weaker until flaccidity and atrophy occur. If the brainstem is affected, speech, chewing, swallowing, and even breathing are difficult. Excessive drooling may occur.

Once the motor nerve cells are damaged, the symptoms increase progressively in severity, and paralysis of the involved muscles results. Although because of damage to higher nuclear centers in the brain the client may be subject to involuntary outbursts of laughing and crying without external stimuli, the mental faculties are not affected. Even in the terminal stages of the illness he or she can hear and understand and is acutely aware of the condition. However, the person may not be able to communicate in any way except by movement of the eyes and eyelids.

The helplessness, powerlessness, and absolute dependency of the client with amyotrophic lateral sclerosis during the last weeks and months of life are even more tragic because he or she remains mentally alert and aware of what is happening.

MANAGEMENT. Although laboratory tests may be performed to rule out other diseases, the diagnosis is made on the history and examination of the client.

There is no known medical treatment that will arrest, modify, or cure amyotrophic lateral sclerosis. The physician treats the client symptomatically, maintains an optimal level of health and well-being, monitors nutrition, treats any infection promptly, and gives the client and family emotional support as necessary.

Nursing intervention is directed toward the (1) prevention and early recognition of complications; (2) adaptation of hospital routines as necessary to meet the special needs of the client and family; (3) administration of skilled physical and psychological nursing care according to the severity and extent of the symptoms and the progress of the disease; (4) fulfillment of emotional needs by making every effort to understand the client's reactions to the illness, perceiving and accepting changes in mood, showing interest and concern, encouraging verbal and nonverbal expression of anxiety and fear, and, above all, spending time with him or her; and (5) preparation of the family, significant others, and client to manage at home where the bulk of life occurs for the client with amyotrophic lateral sclerosis. After diagnosis, hospitalization is typically limited to those wherein surgery occurs for dysphagia or acute care intervention is needed for a problem such as an upper respiratory infection.

HOME MANAGEMENT

*Psychosocial adjustment.* ALS is probably one of the worst neurological diseases. In advanced disease not only is the sensory status intact making interminable hours in bed miserable and demands for frequent reposturing and skin checks a mandate (see Chapter 9), but also the daily knowledge of decreasing function and impending death create added, continual difficulty to emotional acceptance and adjustment for both the client and significant others. The expected outcomes suggested for multiple sclerosis are applicable for ALS. When the brainstem is involved, involuntary laughing or crying may occur, as it does in multiple sclerosis.

*Communication.* Ours is a very verbal society. Social rejection commonly occurs as an additional insult to the ALS client who looses speech along with other functional abilities. Beginning as hoarseness, speech continually worsens, as muscles weaken, until it is gone. The electrolarynx is of no use in facilitating vocalization. Alternate methods—commercial or homemade—need to be explored. When communication is restricted to movements of the eyes and eyelids, a code may be devised.

*Dysphagia.* In ALS progressive difficulty in swallowing occurs. At first impaired swallowing may be managed by informed significant others who learn that thickened liquids and pureed foods placed on the posterior aspect of the tongue reduce feeding problems. After the gag reflex is gone, normal eating patterns must be modified. The nasogastric tube is usually unacceptable for long-term use because of physical irritation and lack of social acceptance. Postsurgical problems that may be encountered with the placement of a gastrostomy tube result in abandonment of this procedure in favor of cervical esophagostomy. Like other alternative feeding methods, special instructions and return demonstrations are required for those who will care for the client with cervical esophagostomy.

Dysphagia caused by spasm of the cricopharyngeal muscle may be relieved by cricopharyngeal myotomy.

*Other problems.* Secretion control is a major problem as the disease advances. Medications such as atropine are a mixed blessing. Although atropine dries secretions, the thickened secretions may complicate the client's respiratory status. Oral suctioning may be helpful, when significant others learn correct usage methods. If further intervention is required, a surgical procedure, transtympanic neurectomy, is indicated to control the neurological supply to the parotid glands.

Respiratory embarrassment is another serious concern. Weakened muscles also affect normal respiration. Failure in respiratory muscles frequently results in death. Although opinions vary on the use of heroic measures, such as ventilatory assistive devices, for a terminal client, consideration should be given to the need for excellence in nursing care and supportive assistance, devices, and measures that facilitate client comfort.

*Multidisciplinary cooperation.* The physician and nurse need to introduce the client to any resources and personnel that may provide physical aids, assistance in environmental rearrangement to facilitate safety and independence at home, psychosocial support, and economic assistance. Agencies such as community health and visiting nurses should cooperate with the physician and nurses in the office and the acute care facility to monitor client progress and alter management as required in the individual case.

Clients and significant others may benefit by writing (1) ALS Society of America, 15300 Ventura Boulevard, Suite 315, Sherman Oaks, CA 91403, and (2) National ALS Foundation, Inc, 185 Madison Ave., New York, NY 10010.

## Mixed disorders

*Bulbar paralysis.* Bulbar paralysis is characterized by weakness and spasticity of the muscle groups innervated by the affected nuclei of the lower brainstem (the bulb). The symptoms most frequently found are difficulty in articulation and swallowing. These may progress to the point that articulate speech and swallowing are impossible. Drooling of saliva is inevitable. There may be episodes of explosive crying and laughing as seen in pseudobulbar paralysis (vascular origin). As a result the client presents serious problems in nursing care. The client must be observed carefully during mealtime to guard against aspiration and choking. A suction machine should be kept at the bedside continually. Secondary to aspirating food

or fluid, acute respiratory complications may ensue.

Nursing care is directed toward the prevention of complications, maintenance of morale, comfort, and therapeutic effect. The principles of care outlined for clients with disseminated sclerosis also may be used in the care of these clients.

*Disseminated (multiple) sclerosis.* Disseminated sclerosis, or multiple sclerosis (MS), may be an acute disease, with periods of remissions and exacerbations, but it is most frequently seen as a chronic disease of unknown cause affecting the white matter of the brain and spinal cord. It was first described by Charcot in 1868. It is characterized by the scattering of demyelinating lesions of the long conducting pathways of the central nervous system. This destruction of the fatty substance around the axons leaves patches of sclerotic tissue; the nerve fibers degenerate, and disabilities increase and persist. Spontaneous remission of symptoms may occur at any time and may last from a few weeks to many months or even years. Although apparently complete recovery may take place from particular episodes, the general nature of the disease is progressive. The course and prognosis of multiple sclerosis cannot be predicted: the manifestations vary from person to person in number, severity, and duration. About 50% of those affected become incapacitated within 10 years after the onset of the disease. The scattering of lesions and variable periods of freedom from, and adjustment to, symptoms as well as their multiplicity give the disease its name.

The intermittent episodes may be trivial or severe, depending on the size, number, and location of the lesions, which may appear at any time from childhood to old age. Although it is difficult because of the nature of the disease to determine accurately how many persons in the United States have multiple sclerosis, the number is estimated at about 500,000.

The onset in about 75% of the cases occurs between 20 and 40 years of age.

Multiple sclerosis is believed to be a major cause of chronic disability among young adults and is known as a crippler and not a killer. The average duration of the illness is about 27 years; there are cases on record of persons with multiple sclerosis who have lived as long as 60 years after the diagnosis was made. The survival rate is about 85% of that for the general population. Multiple sclerosis is not contagious.

Extensive multidisciplinary efforts have been expended to specify the precise cause and pathogenesis of multiple sclerosis. Two main points represent the major thrusts of researchers. First, there is evidence that humans experience changed immunological capacities, as found by extension of the allergic encephalomyelitis research conducted on animals. However, although some believe that experimental allergic encephalomyelitis and multiple sclerosis may begin by a similiar mechanism, the disease courses differ. One finding that presents difficulty in utilizing these animal studies as a definitive model is the recent data from brain scans and CAT scans with contrast media indicating that the blood-brain barrier evidences altered capacities at different points in the course of multiple sclerosis. Second, there is a quest for one causative "slow" agent with an extended latency period. Large numbers of studies provide conflicting findings on viral agents and their immunological significance and response patterns in humans. Measles in relation to multiple sclerosis has been studied extensively. The consensus is that inadequate cellular responses in clients with multiple sclerosis may be linked more to the outcome of the disease process (multiple sclerosis), rather than to the cause. Whatever the connection, viruses are probably related to multiple sclerosis in some way. Many believe that more than one virus may be involved. Until multiple sclerosis can be reproduced in an animal, researchers will be hampered in these experiments.

Extensive attempts to correlate immunogenetic, infectious processes, histocompatibility antigens with elevated viral antibody titers, and geographic locale with multiple sclerosis have occurred. The answer? A large scale effort needs to be organized wherein adequate research techniques, study populations, and complete evaluations are made of all factors over a long period of time. Then statements about specific populations, relationships of climate, house pets, and other factors may be accurately discussed. Moreover, the role of factors such as chemical, metabolic, and enzymatic disturbances; allergic reactions; viral infection; autoimmune responses; inadequate blood circulation;

nutritional deficiency; and constitutional vulnerability need to be assessed.

The National Institute of Neurological Diseases and Stroke (NINDS) reported that an epidemiological survey of 600,000 government workers and their families in Mexico City revealed an incidence rate of multiple sclerosis of only 1.5 per 100,000, a rate among the lowest reported anywhere in the world. Japan also has a low incidence rate. Since the level of environmental sanitation in Mexico and Japan is below that of the United States and many other countries where the incidence rate of multiple sclerosis is higher, it has been suggested that "environmental sanitation is inversely related to the frequency of multiple sclerosis."*

Multiple sclerosis is also more common in the northern countries of Europe than in the hot Mediterranean basin; Italy is part of the low-incidence area, whereas Ireland is in the high-incidence area. The occurrence of the disease on the Shetland and Orkney Islands is reported to be at least 200 per 100,000, a rate three times higher than in any other known population.

Emotional stress, overwork, fatigue, lowered vitality, and acute respiratory tract infections have precipitated exacerbations of the disease.

**SYMPTOMS.** The signs and symptoms may vary in character, number, and duration. They may be transient, lasting only a few hours or many weeks. The most common initial symptom is sensory impairment, which is manifest by numbness and tingling sensations (paresthesias). Transient muscular weakness may occur, and, with repeated exacerbations, it may culminate in the paralysis of one, two, three or all four extremities. Nystagmus, diplopia, and blurring or loss of vision occur frequently. Poor coordination, impaired position sense, loss of balance, spasticity, ataxia, and difficulty in walking may be present. Articulatory speech defects (scanning) are common. Urinary and fecal incontinence, pronounced fatigability, and inappropriate affect may be present.

Investigators maintain that there is no characteristic multiple sclerotic personality. Symptoms of mental illness are not common; psychosis is ex-

---

*From U.S. Department of Health, Education, and Welfare: NINDS research profiles, Washington, D.C., 1971, U.S. Government Printing Office.

tremely rare. Mood swings, euphoria or depression, and irritability are at times evident and are believed to be psychological reactions to the nature of the disease, its uncertain course, and its chronicity.

As the disease progresses, secondary complications may ensue: urinary tract infections, metabolic or nutritional disturbances, joint contractures, deformities, and emotional problems. As remissions become fewer and shorter, the client becomes increasingly disabled and physically incapacitated.

**DIAGNOSIS.** In its early stages, multiple sclerosis is rarely recognized and diagnosed. An average interval of about 6 years exists between the onset of the initial symptoms and the diagnosis of multiple sclerosis. Diagnosis depends on a careful history and the multiplicity of scattered neurological signs that cannot be explained on the basis of a single lesion or a systemic disease. No laboratory tests are specifically indicated, but many may be done to rule out infectious or neoplastic disease of the nervous system. Studies of cerebrospinal fluid may furnish valuable confirmatory information. Frequently in multiple sclerosis an increase in the number of white blood cells in the cerebrospinal fluid has been found. Some investigators have observed a significant increase in gamma globulin in 85% of their clients with multiple sclerosis. An abnormal colloidal gold curve in the absence of neurosyphilis may also confirm the diagnosis. Willmon maintains that an absolute diagnosis can only be made at autopsy; otherwise, diagnosis of multiple sclerosis is actually an educated opinion.

Evoked response measurements are a major breakthrough in objective assessment of neuronal disorders, such as multiple sclerosis where lesions may not be apparent clinically. Results of stimulus-controlled, evoked-response measurements are compared to responses from normal individuals. Thus the practitioner gains valuable data on new and existing lesions to validate the symptoms subjectively reported.

If lesions are 1.5 cm in diameter or larger, a brain scan may be useful as an objective way to document new lesions.

Contrast-enhanced CAT scans provide an important way of locating new lesions. Questions on the association of multiple sclerosis lesions to subjective signs, the relationship of CAT-scan images and the integrity of the blood-brain barrier, especially in relation to multiple sclerosis and ACTH, still remain open to investigation.

Another diagnostic tool is a bath for the client wherein the water is at 40° C. Hot water or prolonged exposure to the hot sun may cause a recurrence of symptoms or the presentation of new symptoms that can be noted objectively by the practitioner.

Rate all new symptoms and changes in functional abilities by using a graph and scale, such as that suggested by Poser (1979). Record data about the client at specified intervals to remain objective about progress or changes.

**TREATMENT AND NURSING INTERVENTION.** Since the beginning of the twentieth century about 200 different treatments have been tried on clients with multiple sclerosis. These treatments were related to the different theories of the cause of multiple sclerosis. Because of the nature of this disease, its characteristic remissions, and its unpredictable course, it has been difficult to evaluate the effect of medications and other treatments. The administration of one of the adrenocortical steroids (usually prednisone) by mouth or ACTH by intramuscular injection may be effective in lessening the intensity or shortening the duration of an acute exacerbation of symptoms. Corticosteroid use remains controversial. To date, no effective specific treatment has been identified. However, improved care and the use of chemotherapeutic and antibiotic agents in the treatment of secondary complications have prolonged the lives of many victims of multiple sclerosis. Considerable research is being focused on attempts to find an effective preventive or curative treatment for those afflicted with this disease.

The program of treatment should be planned according to the particular needs of each client, the extent of the disability, and the symptoms. The client's emotional, intellectual, social, and spiritual resources and level of motivation also must be considered. The aims of treatment are to help the client achieve maximum physical capacity and optimum psychosocial adjustment by maintaining general health, increasing resistance to infection, and mobilizing community resources as necessary.

Treatment should include an integrated program of physical, educational, occupational, and recreational therapies. Individual or group psychotherapy also may be indicated for the client or family or both. The client with multiple sclerosis should be encouraged to live and work up to capacity. Every effort should be directed toward establishing and maintaining good health and preventing complications.

Physical therapy in the form of massage; active, resistive, and stretching exercises; and relaxing baths may be used to increase the client's physical comfort, maintain muscle tone and the range of motion of the joints, reduce spasticity, improve coordination, and build up morale. Swimming and walking barefoot also have been of help in improving muscle tone, coordination, and walking. Mephenesin (Tolserol), chlorpromazine (Thorazine), or other muscle-relaxing drugs may be given for the relief of spasticity.

Dantrolene sodium (Dantrium) and baclofen (Lioresal) are also helpful in relieving such components of spasticity as resistance to passive movement, flexor spasm, and clonus. The disadvantage of these drugs is that they may limit mobility, since spasticity essential to locking the knee and hip joints in ambulation is not present. An adverse outcome of these drugs is gastrointestinal problems. Refer to the explanation of spasticity in Chapter 25.

Vitamins B and $B_{12}$ are generally used for their systemic effect. For persistent spasticity of the lower extremities, it may be necessary to section lumbosacral nerve roots (rhizotomy) for the relief of pain. Since this results in paralysis, it should be done only as a last resort.

Every effort is made to assist the client in adjusting to the vagaries of this illness. Excessive physical fatigue, rundown physical condition, emotional stress, and extremes of environmental temperature should be avoided because they may precipitate in exacerbation. The client should remain an independent, functioning member of the family and community as long as possible. The tendency to be overdependent is characteristic of persons with this chronic disease. Independence may be fostered by encouragement of the client to participate actively in family life and to take care of him- or herself to the greatest extent possible. Realistic self-care goals are set so that they can be achieved and the motivation of the client strength-

ened in the process. The public health nurse is a valuable resource for the client and family and can help them understand the nature of multiple sclerosis and the client's emotional reactions and changing needs. The public health nurse can help the family to establish a schedule of daily activities, to arrange or modify the home setting as necessary to facilitate the client's ambulation and increase independence, and to encourage him or her in the development of new interests and hobbies to replace those no longer possible. Prepare the family for the changes that may occur in their treatment of the client. The education of the family is directed toward helping them understand the client's needs to realize potentialities for independent living and to continue as an active, respected member of the family; they also must adjust to any changes that must be made in the home and in family life.

Supportive and symptomatic clinical treatment may not only minimize the client's disability but also may be of definite psychological value in helping to mobilize remaining capabilities, to develop new skills, and to achieve an optimum level of adjustment.

Many communities have multiple sclerosis groups that meet regularly and afford clients opportunities to discuss and solve their common problems.

NURSING CARE. The nursing care of clients with advanced degenerative diseases is based on the symptoms of disturbed function and the prevention of complications, with recognition of the emotional problems that may be present in any chronic or recurrent illness.

ENVIRONMENT. It is believed by some physicians that a cold damp climate may act as a precipitating factor in this disease. Since it is economically impossible to send all these clients to warm dry areas such as Arizona, the client should be protected as much as possible from the vicissitudes of the climate to which he or she is exposed. The client should be instructed to wear adequate clothing whether inside or outdoors, not to go out during inclement weather, and to avoid exposure to drafts or other situations that may cause a chill.

OBSERVATIONS. The nurse is responsible for noting the client's emotional and physical behavior, reactions to medication and physical therapy, and alterations of old, and appearance of new, symptoms.

ACTIVITY. During the early stages of the illness the client is generally able to be up and about with supervision and slight assistance.

Since one side is usually more involved, the client may improve balance during walking by leaning to the less involved side. Additionally, the slapping gait may be minimized if the client places the heel on the floor first and then rolls the weight forward on the lateral aspect of the foot. Refer to Chapter 25 for other techniques on assisting the client in movement.

Activity is encouraged within the limitations imposed on the individual client by the disease. Physical exertion is avoided, and planned periods of rest are enforced to prevent fatigue. As the disease progresses and disability increases, the regimen is modified. The client, when in bed, is postured to increase comfort and prevent complications. However, even the most helpless client, who may not be able to get out of bed without considerable assistance, is lifted into a large comfortable armchair or wheelchair at least twice a day. This is important not only because of the physical and environmental changes that ensue but also because of the psychological effect on morale. Active and passive exercises of the extremities and joints should be continued to prevent complications. Dorsiflexion of the ankles several times every hour may prevent stasis of the large veins of the calves. The client is encouraged to be as independent as possible. If there are tremors of the upper extremities, manual dexterity may be so impaired that the client depends on others for the performance of all activities related to dressing, changing of position, bathing, reading, writing, and eating. These tremors are usually aggravated by purposive acts but may be lessened by rest. The client should not be presented with situations, obstacles, or challenges with which he or she cannot cope, since failure may increase discouragement and depression. The nurse's approach in aiding the client to follow a certain regimen is directed toward the achievement of certain goals without precipitating any untoward emotional reactions. When the client is no longer able to do certain things alone, his or her needs should be anticipated and satisfied in an inconspicuous and matter-of-fact manner.

To decrease the mental fatigue secondary to facing the problems of everyday living when one is physically handicapped, it is recommended that all clients with chronic, disabling diseases be placed on a regulated daily schedule. This should make provisions for a routine time for getting up in the morning; bathing and dressing; meals and interval feedings; and occupational therapy in the form of light work in or about the home when possible, supplemented by selected reading (using special devices to eliminate the fatigue of holding the book and turning pages), hobbies, especially those related to collecting things, doing jigsaw puzzles, listening to radio programs, watching television, exercising, and taking walks outdoors if possible (otherwise, even a few steps at frequent intervals indoors will have a definite psychological and physical value). If the client is confined to a wheelchair, a regular time is set aside for going outdoors or, if the weather is inclement, moving into another room for a change of scenery. A regular time is also set for serial assessment of skin and joint integrity, so that treatment and activity may be appropriately planned.

Diplopia may hamper participation in activities. Utilize an eye patch to improve vision.

NUTRITION. A well-balanced diet that is easily assimilated is provided for the client. If there is difficulty in swallowing or chewing, the diet should consist of soft semisolid foods. If this presents difficulties, the soft food may be liquefied in an electric blender and taken by mouth or administered through a Levin tube. Vitamin B is frequently used to supplement the diet. It is imperative that bodily nutrition be maintained to ensure physical well-being and maximum resistance to infection. If a tendency for stones to be formed in the bladder is discovered, a high-protein, low-ash diet may be used as a preventive measure.

Obesity must be avoided so that the client may maintain optimal mobility, appearance, and self-concept assessments.

Avoid very hot foods because they may precipitate a sudden emotional outburst of crying or laughing. If such an outburst occurs, the client becomes embarrassed. Shorten this episode by reminding the client of something sad to stop laughter and by asking the client to hold his mouth open to stop crying.

**HYGIENE.** Whenever possible and unless contraindicated, bathing is done in a bathtub. Some clients have impairment of the perception of temperature; therefore one should regulate the bath water by testing it with a bath thermometer. Warm, but not hot, water is generally used for cleansing purposes because of its additional relaxing effect on spastic muscles. If the client can bathe him- or herself at all, he or she should be encouraged to do so with supervision and assistance as necessary. If there is weakness of the lower extremities, the water is drained from the tub before the nurse or orderly assists the client out of it. Every attempt is made by the nurses and auxiliary workers to maintain the client's interest in his or her personal appearance. This is especially important in caring for women affected with this disease. Anything that results in improving personal appearance, such as the arrangement of the hair or the use of cosmetics, may do much to build morale.

**ELIMINATION.** During the course of the disease the client may have urinary tract difficulties characterized by urgency, frequency, and periods of incontinence. These may be partially controlled by a regulated intake of fluid, anticholinergic medication, generally atropine, and the development of habitual emptying of the bladder at regular intervals. (It is important that the client not dwell on the possibility of being incontinent and curtail social activities because of the fear of being embarrassed. He or she should be helped to depersonalize such an experience so that self-esteem is not damaged.) If incontinence continues or progresses, the use of catheter or condom drainage is recommended to prevent emotional trauma, breakdown of the skin, and retention. Rarely do these clients have involuntary defecations. If they do, enemas or colon lavages (Chapter 27) should be used as necessary to prevent the occurrence of accidents. Some clients may be trained to empty their bowels at a certain time each day. This is done whenever possible in the bathroom or on a commode. If the client is constipated, an anticonstipation diet, cathartics, and colon lavages may be used to prevent fecal impactions. If the client is incontinent, a program of bowel training is initiated.

**REHABILITATION.** Occupational therapy should be used in the treatment of every client with a chronic illness and should be adjusted to abilities, interests, and needs. It can be employed as a means of rehabilitation by increasing the scope of activity, stimulating the muscle tone of weakened muscles, and training the client to utilize remaining functions to the maximum degree. A definite program of diversional activity is planned whether the client is treated in the hospital or at home. He or she should not be permitted to feel sorry for him- or herself, to be unnecessarily dependent, or to be continually preoccupied with self and illness. The family, understanding the illness and accepting the client as he or she is, can do much to maintain morale and interest in life by their firm positive approach and by stimulating and directing interests toward outside matters. Excessive sympathy and oversolicitude will increase emotional problems and hinder the acceptance of and adjustment to the disease.

**COMPLICATIONS.** (1) Incontinence with incomplete emptying of the bladder, often resulting in cystitis and the formation of calculi, (2) injuries from falls caused by gait disturbances, (3) pain, (4) decubitus ulcers, (5) contractures, (6) footdrop and wristdrop, (7) fecal impactions, (8) dysphagia, (9) regurgitation, (10) aspiration, (11) respiratory tract infections, (12) depression or other emotional disturbances, (13) nutritional or metabolic disturbances.

**Expected outcomes**
The client with multiple sclerosis will:
1 Identify specific ways of maintaining the highest level of well-being.
  a Make a realistic schedule that takes the need for rest, recreation, prescribed exercises and activities, and work, or avocational goal-related activities, into consideration.
  b Discuss ways of reducing pressure, stress, and anxiety in relationships and activities of daily living.
  c Specify techniques that promote relaxation, energy conservation, and an even distribution of energy expenditures.
  d Identify specific ways to set an unhurried pace.
  e Describe a balanced diet that is individually suitable.
  f Identify activities that may be integrated into the activities of daily living to improve mental health.
2 State specific safety measures that require compliance:
  a Environmental safety in relation to sensory deficits, gait, and mobility and necessary special equipment.
  b Prescribed physiological exercises to improve functional ability.
  c Activities appropriate or inappropriate to health status.
  d Modification plan related to individual dysfunction.
3 Identify issues related to emotional status such as the following:

a Need to or methods for maintaining maximum independence.

b Acceptance of multiple sclerosis.

c Avoidance of obesity.

d Problems related to stimuli such as hot foods.

e Situations and issues involving significant and distant others and their attitudes toward client disability.

f Need to utilize health professionals to include family and significant others in physical care and coping mechanisms for the present and for the increasing problems in the future.

4 Explain the importance of infection control and avoidance of general complications in relation to specific measures in the following:

a Skin integrity.

b Joint contractures and orthopedic deformities.

c Urinary tract care.

d Avoidance of infectious illness.

e Eating wherein swallowing is impaired.

f Fatigue.

g Regular bowel movements.

h Appropriate psychotherapy.

5 Comply with total treatment protocol in regard to the following:

a Prescriptions from physical and occupational therapists, nurses, dieticians, physicians, and so on.

b Utilization of appropriate medications and dosages at the correct time.

c Remodeling of the home environment to improve safety and independence.

d Utilization of needed special equipment.

e Identification and use of health care agencies, special equipment, rehabilitative programs, and financial resources as appropriate.

f Exploration and use of local and National Multiple Sclerosis Society resources.

g Continual contact with the physician and nurse practitioner to report progress, needs, concerns, adverse outcomes to treatment and inappropriate responses to treatment.

**NATIONAL MULTIPLE SCLEROSIS SOCIETY.** The National Multiple Sclerosis Society (NMSS), a voluntary, nonprofit organization, was founded in 1947. It helps support clinics, centers, and special programs for the evaluation and treatment of clients with multiple sclerosis. The national society helps clients and their families secure appropriate medical supervision. It sponsors grants for research throughout the country and fellowship grants and has 6 regional offices. Other services such as counseling, recreational programs, special equipment, and aids for activities of daily living also are provided. Considerable effort is expended to educate the public about the problem of multiple sclerosis

and to obtain funds to carry on its many activities.

The national society cooperates with the NINDS in continuous and coordinated nationwide research programs directed toward finding the cause and effective treatment of multiple sclerosis; it also cooperates with the International Congress of Neurology and the International Panel on Multiple Sclerosis, which it founded.

*MS Keynotes,* a quarterly publication, provides the newest information on multiple sclerosis research, therapy, and rehabilitation techniques. It also serves as a vehicle to build the morale of clients with multiple sclerosis and their families.

In 1967 16 foreign countries joined with the NMSS of the United States to form the International Federation of Multiple Sclerosis Societies. This organization has eight objectives: (1) stimulating greater worldwide interest in research on multiple sclerosis by the medical and scientific community and the general public; (2) helping to establish standards for forms of treatment and treatment facilities; (3) acting as a medium for the exchange of information on research, client services, professional and public education, and organizational and fund-raising methods; (4) helping to strengthen existing national societies; (5) stimulating and aiding in the development of new national societies; (6) gaining recognition of the importance of the multiple sclerosis problem by international groups, such as the World Health Organization (WHO), so that they may help in combating this disease; (7) developing new methods of informing the public about the problem, and (8) recruiting new and influential leadership on behalf of the national societies.

Descriptive pamphlets, manuals on home care, reprints of articles on multiple sclerosis, and slides and films may be obtained from the national society.

## PERIPHERAL NERVE DYSFUNCTION

In peripheral nerve dysfunction, one nerve may be involved *(mononeuritis),* or two or more nerves in separate areas may be involved *(mononeuritis multiplex),* or the problem may include a syndrome of structures affecting sensory, motor, reflex, or vasomotor functions *(polyneuritis).*

Four types of agents may be responsible for these neuropathies, namely, mechanical, vascular, infectious, and metabolic factors.

*Mechanical agents* include trauma, tumors, cast, crutch, or traction pressure; local compression from other sources; violent muscular activity; and cramping postures, inherent in some occupations and tasks. The outcome of mechanical agents is a mononeuritis, wherein symptoms include pain, weakness, and paresthesias.

*Vascular agents* may include such factors as arteriosclerosis, hemorrhage, refrigeration, or radium. The outcome in these situations is a neuritis in those nerves with a common blood supply. An example of this problem is Volkmann's ischemic paralysis.

*Infectious agents* usually result in local involvement of a nerve. One example might be a disturbance of the facial nerve secondary to mastoiditis. Polyneuritis has been attributed to a variety of causative agents, including systemic infection, diphtheria, scarlet fever, typhoid fever, flu, vaccines, upper respiratory infections, measles, and infectious mononucleosis. In polyneuritis it is probably the hypersensitivity to the agent that produces the toxic effect.

*Metabolic agents* are also frequently responsible for polyneuritis. Some examples of these agents include nutritional deficiency secondary to alcoholism, vitamin $B_{12}$ deficiency, gastrointestinal interruptions, chronic disease, toxemia associated with pregnancy, diabetes mellitus, and pernicious anemia.

Mononeuritis may be single or multiple. When it is multiple, the findings on physical assessment are asymmetrical. In polyneuritis, symptoms are bilateral and symmetrical. Polyneuritis begins in the fingers and toes and progresses upward. First sensations include numbness and tingling, which give way to anesthesia. If pain is associated, it is of a burning nature. Muscle weakness is peripheral and results in muscle tenderness, decreased deep tendon reflexes, edema, discolored skin, and diaphoresis.

EVALUATION. When a peripheral neuropathy is suspected, the history, physical assessment, and laboratory data are geared toward identification of the cause and problem and elimination of similar diagnostic possibilities. By analyzing the data gleaned from the history and physical assessment, one can usually identify the causative agent. The assessment continues with the analysis of laboratory data. A blood count may reveal anemia; stippling of red blood cells, as seen in lead poisoning; or eosinophilia, as might be found in polyarteritis. Urinalysis may reveal the presence of porphyrins if the client has experienced heavy metal poisoning or certain infections. An elevated glucose level in the urine may indicate the presence of diabetes mellitus. Radiographic studies of the bones may reveal trauma, malignancy, or hypertrophic arthritis.

The cerebrospinal fluid remains normal in mononeuritis but reveals an elevated protein level in Guillain-Barré syndrome, diphtheria, and diabetes mellitus. A VDRL test rules out the possibility of syphilis.

Differential diagnoses that must be ruled out when one is evaluating polyneuritis include poliomyelitis, tabes dorsalis, multiple sclerosis, progressive muscular atrophies, and muscular dystrophy.

### Neuritis

Infections of the nerves and nerve roots (radiculitis) are not common, though the term *neuritis* is applied loosely to many pains caused by muscle and joint diseases. (In association with inflammation of muscles, nerves are frequently involved secondary to the disease of the muscle, but that situation and the neuritides caused by avitaminosis are not included here.)

*Alcoholic polyneuritis,* caused by a nutritional deficiency secondary to prolonged and excessive alcoholic intake, is a slowly progressive, chronic disease primarily involving the extremities. Pain, paresthesia, and muscle tenderness with subsequent loss of sensation and motor power characterize this peripheral neuritis.

*Infectious polyneuritis* (Guillain-Barré syndrome) is a fairly acute involvement of the motor components of the spinal and cranial nerve roots that is presumed to be caused by a virus. This disease may occur at any age, but it is more common in the age group from 30 to 50 years. Both sexes may be infected. The pathological manifestations are inflammatory and degenerative changes in the roots and nerves.

The onset is acute, with fever, severe pain in the muscles, and weakness or paralysis of individual muscle groups, including those about the head and face. No loss of sensation is incurred, and the client usually recovers with little, if any, residual disabilities. If the seventh, ninth, and tenth cranial nerves are involved, disturbances of varying degrees in swallowing, speaking, and breathing caused by paralysis of the vital centers in the medulla oblongata may be present and may culminate in death. The rate of recovery is related to the extent and degree of involvement. Motor function may begin to return 2 days to 2 weeks after the onset of the symptoms. In some instances full recovery may take up to 18 months.

The diagnosis is clarified by a study of the cerebrospinal fluid that shows a characteristic dissociation between the white blood cells and protein. The cell count may increase slightly (10 to 50), and the total protein may be elevated to as much as 750 mg/dl.

*Treatment and nursing intervention.* Treatment for alcoholic polyneuritis consists of controlling the alcoholic intake and overcoming the nutritional deficiency with an adequate, balanced diet and supplementary vitamins. Bed rest is usually imperative during the acute stage. Control of pain is effected by administration of drugs and correct posturing of the client. Nursing care is directed toward maintenance of the client's comfort and prevention of complications (foot drop and wrist-drop).

The treatment for infectious polyneuritis is palliative and symptomatic. The principles of nursing care are the same as those applied to clients with serious spinal cord injuries, especially those involving the cervical area (Chapters 23, 25, and 27) and, if cranial nerves are involved, as described in Chapter 19.

## NEUROMUSCULAR JUNCTION DISORDERS

Four possibilities account for problems in transmission at the myoneural junction. First, acetylcholine production at the motor nerve terminals may be insufficient. Second, acetylcholine production may be adequate, but it may be destroyed before reaching the motor end plate where it is normally reactive. Third, acetylcholine may be in competition with another substance at the reactor site. Fourth, acetylcholine production and reaction processes may be normal, but acetylcholine may persist for an abnormal period of time before enzymatic destruction.

Abnormal production of acetylcholine is most commonly observed in botulism. No known exam-

ples are available to illustrate the destruction of acetylcholine before it reaches the end plate. The competitive situation at the receptor site is best seen in response to the administration of curare. An example of excessive persistence of acetylcholine is seen when the anticholinesterases such as neostigmine, edrophonium (Tensilon), eserine, and diisopropyl fluorophosphate (DFP) are administered, since these agents combine with cholinesterase to prevent the destruction of acetylcholine.

When diagnosticians are investigating the nature of myoneural dysfunctions, edrophonium is frequently administered. If the problem is caused by a competitive block, this anticholinesterase permits acetylcholine to achieve a sufficient level to overcome the competitive inhibition. If the problem is caused by a depolarization block, edrophonium administration further aggravates the condition.

Myasthenia gravis is an example of a myoneural problem.

### Myasthenia gravis

Myasthenia gravis, though not a degenerative disease, is included in this chapter because of its chronic nature. Although the degree of weakness present may level off, it is slowly progressive, and remissions rarely occur. Thomas Willis, a British physician, first described this disease in 1672; during the next 250 years only 300 cases were identified. It is a disease characterized by a chemical (acetylcholine) deficiency at the point where the motor nerve joins a skeletal muscle (myoneural junction) as a result of which the muscle does not receive the motor impulse properly and does not contract well, if at all. The cause or explanation of this deficiency is not fully known. Three possible explanations of the pathological condition have been offered: (1) it is caused by a deficiency of acetylcholine production (presynaptic), (2) it is caused by a disturbance of the end plate (postsynaptic), and (3) it is caused by an abnormality in the muscle fiber itself. Since there is increasing evidence that the thymus (which may be implicated in myasthenia) plays an important role in immunological processes, it also has been suggested that myasthenia gravis is produced by an autoimmune mechanism that destroys or inactivates the sensitive receptor substance in muscle. Although weakness of skeletal muscle is a primary manifestation of this condition, there is no evidence of disease of the central or peripheral nervous system. There is no muscular atrophy, no loss of sensation, or any manifestation other than extreme fatigability of muscles, which often is so severe that it merges into transitory paralysis.

Since myasthenia gravis is not always recognized and diagnosed, it is not possible to determine its incidence accurately. It is estimated that about 50,000 persons in the United States have myasthenia gravis. It is not hereditary. It is three times more common in young women than in older ones and three times more common in men over 40 years of age than in those under 40 years of age. It generally occurs in young persons, mainly between the ages of 15 and 50 years, and in women slightly more often than in men.

The symptoms are caused by progressive weakness of the muscles as they are being used. The degree of weakness varies in each client and may be mild, moderate, or severe. Muscles affected vary from client to client but most frequently are the extraocular muscles and those used for chewing, swallowing, speaking, and breathing. There may be ptosis of the eyelids, double vision, impaired swallowing, and weakness of the voice. If the neck muscles are involved, the head bobs and cannot be maintained in one position without support. When other muscle groups are involved, fatigue may be general, and physical activity may be limited. The muscles are strongest in the morning but become exhausted with effort and finally do not function. At the height of an attack the client presents a characteristic picture: a blank, ironed-out facial mien, ptosis of the eyelids, the head tilted back to facilitate seeing, inability to chew or swallow, frequent nasal regurgitation of fluids, and a pronounced nasal tone to the voice, if it is audible at all. If the accessory muscles of respiration are involved, respiratory difficulties will ensue. Symptoms may increase during menses and under emotional stress. There may be exacerbations when the client suddenly becomes more disabled. These may be associated with respiratory or other infections, may follow major surgical procedures, or may occur without any overt precipitating cause. The mortality is 15 times that of the general population.

The diagnosis is made on the basis of the history and physical findings and confirmed by the client's response to a test dose of neostigmine (Pro-

stigmin) or edrophonium (Tensilon), which revives the function of the exhausted muscle dramatically within a few minutes. Tensilon is a valuable diagnostic aid because of its rapid and brief action. The intravenous dose for the adult client is 2 mg; if there is no response within 30 seconds, an additional 8 mg may be given during the ensuing 60 seconds. It is especially effective in the evaluation of the degree of weakness of the oropharyngeal or ocular muscles. The improvement lasts about 5 minutes. Neostigmine (Prostigmin), 1.5 to 2 mg, given intramuscularly produces the maximum therapeutic effect from 30 to 60 minutes after it is injected. Since its effect persists for several hours, it is most valuable in evaluating the motor function of the extremities.

Frequently as an associated finding there may be an enlargement or tumor of the thymus. In these instances, especially if the client is a woman and less than 35 years old, surgical treatment may be beneficial. A survey of 1355 female myasthenic clients after surgical removal of the thymus gland revealed that 89% of them were improved or completely recovered.

In a 5-year follow-up study of 111 myasthenic clients who had thymectomies, Papatestas and his associates reported that 75% were in remission or improved at the end of the period, half of those in remission had to wait until 2 years after surgery for this to occur, and only seven clients had remissions within a month after surgery.

The effects of pregnancy on myasthenic women are not predictable; generally, if the myasthenic symptoms are aggravated, they may be controlled by regulation of the dosage of the specific medication on which the client is being maintained. The delivery process should not present any particular problems. The newborn infant may have a weak cry, suck poorly, move the legs feebly, and have respiratory difficulty. These manifestations usually subside within 7 to 14 days. In the interim the infant can be maintained with small doses of neostigmine to ensure adequate ventilation of the lungs and adequate nutrition.

***Treatment and nursing intervention.*** There is no known cure. However, with drug treatment the mortality has been reduced from 90% to 10%. It is palliative and must be continuous. Although physiological rest with avoidance of physical and emotional strain are important, the use of anticholinesterase drugs such as neostigmine (Prostigmin), pyridostigmine (Mestinon), or ambenonium (Mytelase) is imperative to counteract the symptoms of fatigue and weakness. The optimal maintenance dose of the drug must be established and regulated for each client (with the continued use of a cholinergic drug, the majority of myasthenic clients can be restored to 80% of the normal level of function). Neostigmine has been generally the most effective; many clients prefer pyridostigmine because they tend to have less diarrhea and abdominal cramping. Mestinon, available in a slow-release tablet for sustained action, if taken at bedtime will prevent the morning weakness that some clients complain of on awakening. Ephedrine sulfate and potassium chloride may be used to supplement the anticholinesterase medication. The potassium helps prevent hypokalemia, which, if it occurs, increases muscle weakness. Diplopia is rarely abolished with medical treatment. Covering one eye with an eye patch or, if the client wears glasses, frosting one lens is preferable to increasing the amount of the drug. Certain drugs (magnesium sulfate, morphine or its derivatives, curare, procainamide, quinine, quinidine, and chlorpromazine) have been known to increase the muscular weakness of myasthenic clients and generally should not be administered. Smoking, drinking, prolonged exposure to the sun, and cold weather may also increase symptoms.

For several years different investigators have reported unfavorable results after the treatment of myasthenic clients with corticosteroids. Warmolts and Engel of the Medical Neurology Branch, National Institutes of Health, have successfully treated a small group of adult myasthenic clients with high single-dose, alternate-day oral prednisone. These clients also received potassium supplements, antacids, and a diet low in sodium and carbohydrates. Research on the use of oral prednisone therapy in myasthenia gravis is being continued on inpatients to determine its effects over a prolonged period and to identify the precautions that must be followed. The effect of prednisone is antipathogenic rather than antisymptomatic. It may lead to remission or improvement even after the drug is discontinued because of immunosuppression.

Plasma exchange, a method that removes autoantibodies from the plasma, is an important treatment in myasthenia gravis. Although it is not a cure, it results in clinical improvement in some clients. Immunosuppressive therapy is an important adjunct to plasma exchange. Refer to the article by Blount et al. for specific detail on nursing management during the procedure.

The nurse is responsible for administering all drugs on time, usually 20 to 30 minutes before meals; noting their therapeutic effect; and observing the client for toxic manifestations (increased peristalsis, abdominal cramps, diarrhea, sweating, nausea, vomiting, or fibrillary twitchings of the muscles). Atropine sulfate has been used as an antidote for the toxic symptoms; on occasion it may be necessary to reduce or discontinue the cholinergic drug temporarily. With continued use of one of these drugs, these clients, previously chronic invalids and frequently bedridden, can become ambulatory and often lead an economically useful life.

If hyperthyroidism is present (estimated incidence, 5%), the client may be treated with radioiodine therapy or antithyroid medication while receiving an anticholinesterase drug.

If an acute exacerbation is accompanied by respiratory insufficiency, it should be considered a "crisis," and vigorous emergency treatment should be administered. Respiration must be maintained with a positive-pressure machine. A tracheostomy may be indicated for the prevention of an obstruction and to facilitate the removal of pulmonary secretions by suction. While the respirator is being used, the cholinergic medication should be drastically reduced so that pulmonary secretions and any gastrointestinal side effects will be diminished. During this period the client should receive professional nursing care of the highest level. With treatment the client should improve within a few days, and the medication should be resumed.

While the client is in the hospital, the nurse has an excellent opportunity to help him or her adjust to the restrictions imposed by this disease. Strenuous activity is contraindicated, and periods of rest should be planned. Every effort should be made to build up general resistance, and exposure to persons with upper respiratory tract infections should be avoided. Because of the involvement of the respiratory muscles, these clients have an increased susceptibility to pulmonary infections.

The diet should be adjusted to the individual

needs; if the muscles of swallowing or chewing are affected, the food should be soft, semisolid, or fluid until neostigmine is given. A regular diet may be tolerated with the use of this medication. If the dysphagia persists even after intramuscular medication is given, a Levin tube may be inserted. The tablet medication may be ground up, and regular food may be mixed in an electric blender and given by tube three times a day or more frequently if necessary.

The activity of the client depends on the degree of muscular involvement and the response to therapy. The nurse assists with hygiene and should administer any special care as necessary. Unless toxic symptoms develop after the prolonged use of medication, excretory functions present no specific problems.

Light occupational therapy and other forms of diversion such as books, puzzles, television, and radio are provided as indicated by the client's needs and interests. Although morale is generally good, every effort is made to aid the client to function as normally as possible.

While the client is in the hospital, he or she and the family should be instructed about the nature of myasthenia gravis; the importance of following the medication regimen; the significant adverse reactions to the specific drug or drugs; the necessity to plan activities according to the maximum therapeutic effect of the drug and to set reasonable, reachable goals; the community resources; activities and medications that may increase fatigue; the danger of complications (aspiration, choking, respiratory tract infection, respiratory difficulties); and what to do in an emergency.

This disease may last for years. The prognosis for relief of symptoms is good with medical therapy. These clients are observed and examined at regular intervals, and adjustments are made in their medications and activities as indicated. With moderate care they should be able to enjoy a happy, useful life.

The Myasthenia Gravis Foundation, Incorporated (MGF)* was founded in 1952. It has three primary objectives: (1) education, (2) the aid and treatment of persons with myasthenia gravis, and (3) research. It gives grants to clinics and research

---

*MGF, Inc., 230 Park Avenue, New York, NY 10007.

centers. Research studies are focused on a search for more effective treatment methods, testing new drugs, and finding the cause. The MGF publishes a newsletter and a handbook for clients that are available on request. Medications also may be purchased at reduced cost. MGF chapters may be found in most states.

## MUSCLE DISORDERS

Particularly in children, distinguishing muscle disease (myopathy), spinal cord disorders (myelopathy), and peripheral nerve disturbances (neuropathy) may be rather difficult during the initial assessment, since these entities all may include symptoms of weakness and hypotonia. Clinical and laboratory tests are utilized when one makes the differential diagnosis. Table 17-1 shows some diagnostic manifestations and Table 17-2 some common findings.

In electromyographic studies, intrinsic muscle disease (myopathy) results in a picture different from that of denervation. In myopathy, no fibrillations or fasciculations are detected. The basic change in electromyographic studies seems to be in the action potentials themselves.

Most defects in muscle seem to be related to inheritance, whether the problem is a deformity or an intrinsic disease of the muscles. Examples of muscle diseases include pseudotrophic muscular dystrophy (Erb's dystrophy), limb-girdle muscular dystrophy (Leyden-Moebius dystrophy), facioscapulohumeral muscular dystrophy, myotonia congenita, myotonic dystrophy, ocular myopathy, dermatomyositis, and polymyositis.

### Muscular dystrophy

Muscular dystrophy is a chronic disease with bilateral symmetrical wasting of the skeletal (voluntary) muscles. The affected muscles are frequently hypertrophic or pseudohypertrophic (enlarged because of connective tissue and fatty deposits that replace the striated muscle). The nervous system is not affected, and no sensory or neural disturbances exist. No fibrillation and no qualitative electrical abnormalities are found in clients with muscular dystrophy. Muscle fibers worn out or injured in normal use cannot be reconstructed. Controlled research studies have proved that no deficiency of vitamin E exists. However, some evidence has

**TABLE 17-1.** Diagnostic manifestations of motor system lesions

| | EMG | Peripheral nerve conduction time | Muscle biopsy | Cerebrospinal fluid protein level | Serum enzyme levels |
|---|---|---|---|---|---|
| Myelopathy | Neurogenic findings | Normal early, decreased in later stages | Nerve disorder | Sometimes elevated | Generally normal |
| Polyneuropathy | Neurogenic findings | Decreased | Nerve disorder | Sometimes elevated | Generally normal |
| Myopathy | Neurogenic findings | Normal | Muscle disorder | Normal | Often elevated |

been found to support the theory of faulty metabolism, and current investigations are attempting to discover whether the utlization of vitamin E in the conversion of foods into tissues and energy is a factor in this disease. Research on the use of certain drugs that influence protein metabolism is also in progress.

There are four major types of muscular dystrophy.

*Pseudohypertrophic* (Duchenne) muscular dystrophy affects more boys than girls (3:1); the onset is usually between the ages of 3 and 10 years. This type runs a more rapid course and accounts for about 50% of all cases. Involvement of all the voluntary muscles is progressive, and death usually occurs within 10 to 15 years of the onset of symptoms. The involved muscles are weak but contain fat that enlarges them and gives an impression of strength. This is especially evident in the calf muscles. Weakness of the pelvic muscles results in difficulty when one is rising from the floor and climbing stairs. Lordosis and a waddling gait are pathognomonic of this type.

*Juvenile* (Erb, limb-girdle) muscular dystrophy affects both sexes equally and is transmitted (autosomal recessive) to children only when both parents carry the defective gene. Up to 50% of the offspring may be carriers, 25% may be disabled, and 25% may be completely free of the hereditary defect. Onset generally occurs during the teens or twenties. This type takes a slower course and first involves muscles of the upper arms and pelvis. It may cause only slight disability, which may persist for many years.

*Facioscapulohumeral* (Landouzy-Déjerine) muscular dystrophy affects either sex and may be

**TABLE 17-2.** Clinical findings in myelopathy, polyneuropathy, and myopathy

| Disorder | Clinical findings |
|---|---|
| Myelopathy | Possible sensory change |
| | Possible weakness |
| | Possible deep tendon reflexes |
| | Possible pathological reflexes |
| | Possible spasticity |
| | Negative abdominal reflexes |
| | Possible fasciculations |
| | Sphincter involvement |
| Polyneuropathy | Sensory changes |
| | Distal, symmetrical weakness |
| | No deep tendon reflexes |
| | No pathological reflexes |
| | Positive abdominal reflexes |
| | Rare fasciculations |
| | Rare sphincter involvement |
| Myopathy | No sensory change |
| | Proximal, symmetrical weakness |
| | Increased deep tendon reflexes |
| | No pathological reflexes |
| | Positive abdominal reflexes |
| | No sphincter involvement |

transmitted (autosomal dominant) by either parent; 50% of the offspring may inherit it. Onset occurs during adolescence or early adulthood. This type is slowly progressive from initial involvement of face, shoulders, and upper arms, spreading to all the voluntary muscles. Despite this, few persons who have this type of muscular dystrophy are incapacitated before they reach an advanced age.

The *mixed type* of muscular dystrophy occurs after 30 and before 50 years of age in both sexes. It is not hereditary and runs a rapid downhill course; death may occur within 5 years of onset.

The cause of muscular dystrophy is not known. It occurs in all races throughout the world. About 200,000 persons are afflicted with this disease in the United States; about 50,000, or 25%, are completely disabled; approximately 66% are between the ages of 3 and 13 years.

About 66% of the muscular dystrophies (Duchenne) are inherited through a sex-linked recessive gene carried by the unaffected mother. About 50% of the sisters of boys with muscular dystrophy will be carriers, and about half their male offspring will inherit muscular dystrophy. Several persons in the same family may be afflicted. Diagnostic tests that permit the identification of carriers of muscular dystrophy have been developed. It has been established that 65% of the suspected genetic carriers of the pseudohypertrophic type may be identified; thus genetic counseling can be used.

The disease may last for 30 years or longer without any remission. Some afflicted persons may become helpless and completely disabled in a few months, whereas others, depending on the disease type, may lead useful and reasonably long lives. In general the prognosis is worse if muscular dystrophy occurs in infancy rather than during adolescence.

There is no associated mental defect. The level of intelligence follows that of the general population. About 50% of those who have muscular dystrophy have "normal" personalities.

The nature of the disease, its progression, chronicity, and associated motor disabilities, tend to foster dependency, emotional immaturity, and other unhealthy personality traits. These traits can be prevented to a large extent by providing the family with the necessary diagnostic and treatment services for the client and sufficient knowledge to help them understand and accept the disease and by encouraging normal family life and activities.

**Symptoms.** The symptoms of muscular dystrophy are related to the voluntary muscles involved. Depending on the type, some symptoms are primary and appear earlier than others. Some individuals may have limited pathological muscular involvement with little progression, whereas others may become severely disabled with all the skeletal muscles in a dystrophic state.

The symptoms and signs most frequently found are difficulty in raising the arms above the head, sitting up from a reclining position, standing up, climbing stairs, or running, as well as lordosis, scoliosis, waddling gait, poor balance with a tendency to fall, winged scapulas, blank facies, flat smile, and inability to whistle. The muscles of the hands, feet, tongue, palate, mastication, and chest are rarely involved.

**Diagnostic evaluation.** The diagnosis of muscular dystrophy is made primarily through observation of the child's voluntary movements and gait. The medical and family histories are important. A muscle biopsy may reveal the presence of fat, thus confirming the diagnosis. The electromyogram of the affected muscles demonstrates shorter, weaker bursts of electrical activity than those seen in healthy muscles. Chemical changes in the blood and urine may also aid in making the diagnosis.

**Management.** No cure is known for muscular dystrophy, and no treatment will arrest the course of the disease. Every effort should be directed toward developing the dystrophic child's optimal physical and emotional health, helping him or her adjust to the disability, and creating the home and social environment in which he or she can use the muscles as much as possible and as long as possible

Since bed rest and periods of inactivity accelerate the progress of the disease, they are avoided. The physician may prescribe physical therapy, especially resistive and stretching exercises, to preserve the range of motion of the joints, prevent or minimize contractures (ankles, knees, hips, elbows), prevent atrophy of disuse, and stimulate muscular action. The goals of treatment are to help the child with muscular dystrophy develop maximum physical capacity, become as independent as possible, and achieve healthy psychosocial adjustment.

Although the young child with muscular dystrophy may be awkward and may take a long time to do anything, he or she should be taught how to take care of him- or herself and be given enough time to succeed in so doing.

The child's mother is especially important in influencing development and should participate actively in any treatment plan. Her attitude toward the child will help him or her become, despite the disability, an independent and mature adult or will make him or her dependent and perpetuate immaturity. Both parents must be informed of the nature and course of muscular dystrophy and helped to accept the prognosis and to cope with the problems that arise within the family because one of its members has this disease. Furthermore, they should be told that considerable research is being directed toward finding its cause and cure but that at present no treatment is effective. Helping the parents accept this reality is essential. Otherwise they may expend all their resources, time, and money in a fruitless search for a cure by taking the child to a succession of clinics and hospitals. Not only is the life of the family disrupted, but also the afflicted child is emotionally drained and deprived of the opportunity to make the most of remaining physical, intellectual, and spiritual resources.

The parents should be helped to establish realistic goals for the child and encouraged to set limits as for their other children. He or she has the same basic needs as they do and requires the same love and consistent discipline in order to become well-adjusted and self-directing.

Parents tend to overprotect a handicapped child and thus deprive him or her of normal play activities and social contacts. Most of these parents need help if they are to understand and work through their feelings of guilt, resentment, and pity. Only after they do this will they be able to provide a healthy family life for the dystrophic child and brothers and sisters.

The physician should tell the parents about the services provided by the state agency for crippled children and by the local or state muscular dystrophy association. He or she should encourage them to enroll in the local muscular dystrophy association and join a group of parents of dystrophic children so that their mutual problems can be shared and solved. As the disease progresses, they may be referred to the public health nursing agency.

The child with muscular dystrophy should attend public school as long as possible. This individual needs the stimulus provided by competing with classmates in the school environment. The opportunities for play and social activities as well as for learning are essential for the development of personality.

Every effort is directed toward the development of interests, creative hobbies, and reading and writing skills. These will sustain the individual with muscular dystrophy when the disability increases and physical activity is curtailed.

As the disease progresses, braces may be prescribed to prevent slumping and spinal curvatures and to facilitate standing. In the home, various innovations such as grab bars, overhead slings on the bed, and raised toilet seats help lessen the dystrophic person's dependency on others. The use of a footboard and bed cradle may add to comfort in bed and prevent footdrop. Ultimately, it may be necessary to resort to a wheelchair for locomotion. If, from the onset of the disease, the individual is impressed with the importance of using the muscles as much as possible, muscular strength will be retained. Once strength is lost through inactivity, there is no hope of regaining it.

If the adult with muscular dystrophy must change jobs, the state vocational rehabilitation agency will help this individual prepare for and find a job within his or her capacity.

Generally the person with muscular dystrophy does not need a special diet. In some circumstances, depending on the level of activity and the utilization of food for energy, it may be necessary to limit caloric intake. Since any excess weight tends to increase the problem of ambulation, it should be controlled.

*Nursing intervention.* The basic principles of nursing care for the individual with muscular dystrophy have been implied in the discussion on treatment and management. The nurse must foster independence on the part of the client, must stimulate activity, and must ensure maximum participation in self-care activities. Since bed rest and prolonged sitting or watching television can work irreparable damage on the dystrophied muscles, these activities are supervised and limited. The nurse's attitude and approach toward the client and family can further their acceptance of the disease and can help them adjust to it. The nurse's awareness that a normal family life helps the mental health of all its members is a guide in helping the client develop personal resources and skills so that he or she, too, can be a contributing and respected member of the family.

*Muscular Dystrophy Association.* In 1950 in New York a small group of parents of children with muscular dystrophy formed what is now the Muscular Dystrophy Associations of America, Incorporated. Its aims are to foster and support research in an attempt to discover the cause and cure of the disease.

In 1959 this association established the Institute for Muscle Disease in New York City, the first research center in the world devoted exclusively to the study of muscles. It conducts and supports basic and applied research studies in nerve, muscle, and metabolism and has developed an immense reference library on the subject of muscles in health and disease.

Affiliated muscular dystrophy chapters are located throughout the United States, along with residential summer camps and clinics. Educational* and recreational programs, diagnostic services, special equipment, physical therapy, transportation, and orthopedic appliances are provided or arranged for on request without cost.

## RESEARCH PROGRAMS RELATING TO NEUROMUSCULAR DISORDERS

The NINDS research program relating to neuromuscular disorders includes the support of individual investigators and the training of clinical researchers in basic neurophysiology and neurochemistry techniques. Two clinical research centers, at the University of Pennsylvania and at Columbia University, have been established with NINDS support to study these diseases. A third center, at Harvard, is concerned with the chemical aspects of neuromuscular transmission.

Under Public Law 480 the institute has also developed a collaborative project at the Academy of Medicine in Warsaw, Poland. A clinic in Warsaw has been designated as a study center for clients with neuromuscular diseases from the entire country.

Research is progressing in an effort to reduce the number of unidentified carriers of muscular dystrophy to zero and simplify the methods used to detect carriers. In addition to serum creatine kinase studies, histochemical analyses of muscle biopsies

---

*Audiovisual aids, slides, posters, exhibits, pamphlets, recordings, and films may be obtained from the Muscular Dystrophy Associations, Inc., 1790 Broadway, New York, NY 10019.
*Progressive Muscular Dystrophy* (16 mm, color, silent, 24 minutes) shows the course and progression of muscular dystrophy in 10 young boys ranging in age from 6 to 13 years and may be obtained on loan.

of carriers and electromyograms of clients are being evaluated. Thus far the search for effective drug therapy has been unsuccessful.

## INHERITED DISORDERS

In the past few years, great emphasis has been placed on understanding the relationship of many neurological entities to preventive problems and inheritance. Journals and textbooks in the past few years have abounded with information on prenatal diagnostics and perinatal care. All this is geared toward anticipating potential problems and minimizing undesirable outcomes in both the mother and child. Newborn care has become so specialized that a new area of perinatology, or neonatology, has become a discrete specialty. For detail in intensive care of the neonate refer to *High-Risk Newborn Infants —the Basis for Intensive Nursing Care* (Korones, 1976).

Apart from the untoward outcomes of the prenatal and perinatal periods that may occur from mechanical agents, environmental factors, and effects of toxic substances (Chapters 1 and 13), there is a whole area of inherited disorders. Many of these entities have either primary or secondary neurological problems.

Although it is beyond the scope of this book to do more than touch on this area, it is important to realize that a good understanding of inherited problems is fundamental to organizing many of the neurological entities within logical categories.

Inherited problems are organized under two headings: chromosomal disorders and single-gene disorders. When the problem is a *chromosomal aberration,* it may affect either the autosomes or the sex chromosomes. Alterations in the chromosomes are problems of either structural or numerical changes.

By far the largest group of inherited disorders are *single-gene problems*. These problems account for the vast number of metabolic diseases representing problems in areas such as protein, lipid, or glycogen chains.

Whatever the mode of inheritance, the informed practitioner needs a thorough understanding of what this problem may mean to the affected individual and to individuals within the family who are considering marriage and having children. Although many of these inherited disorders are apparent in the pediatric age group, some of them do not become evident for many years. Consider the autosomal dominant condition known as Huntington's chorea. The average age of onset is 35 years, though it may occur between 25 and 55 years of age. By the time the client is aware of the disease, the family has already been produced. The outcome will be that half of the offspring of that heterozygous individual will be affected.

Most single-gene disorders are autosomal recessive, so that there is not a vertical progression of the problem through the family generations, as is the case in dominant inheritance. As a matter of fact, when an individual is believed to have a disease of this type, the family is often surprised and cannot find the trait within previous generations.

Once the problem is known, the practitioner may be asked to assist in genetic counseling. With the public focus and the number of lay articles available on this subject, questions are being directed from all age groups: young persons considering marriage, pregnant women who suspect an inherited disorder, and older individuals who are concerned about other family members. Moreover, a group of inheritance factors may assist the client in planning future pregnancies in relation to the disease process. Diagnostic testing, such as amniocentesis, may provide the pregnant woman with data about how the disease process has affected a given fetus.

## REFERENCES

Adornato, B.T., et al.: Abnormal immunoglobulin bands in cerebrospinal fluid in myasthenia gravis, Lancet **2:**367-368, Aug. 12, 1978.

Aita, J.F.: Cranial CT and multiple sclerosis (Letter), Neurology **28:**202, Feb. 1978.

Alexander, M.A., et al.: Mechanical ventilation of patients with late stage Duchenne muscular dystrophy: management in the home, Arch. Phys. Med. Rehabil. **60:**289-292, 1978.

Alter, M., and Kurtzke, J.: The epidemiology of multiple sclerosis, Springfield, Ill., 1968, Charles C Thomas, Publisher.

Alter, M., et al.: Migration and risk of multiple sclerosis, Neurology **28:**1089-1093, Nov. 1978.

Archibald, K., and Vignos, P.J., Jr.: A study of contractures in muscular dystrophy, Arch. Phys. Med. **40:**150-157, 1959.

Baer, A.S.: The genetic perspective, Philadelphia, 1977, W.B. Saunders Co.

Bamford, C.R., et al.: Aids in the diagnosis of multiple sclerosis, Ariz. Med. **36:**365-370, May 1979.

Bardossi, F.: Multiple sclerosis: grounds for hope, Public Affairs Pamphlet No. 335A, New York, 1971, Public Affairs Committee, Inc.

Bauer, H.J.: Problems of symptomatic therapy in multiple sclerosis, Neurology **28:**8-20, Sept. 1978.

Beebe, G.W., et al.: Studies on the natural history of multiple sclerosis: epidemiologic analysis of the army experience in World War II, Neurology **17:**1-17, 1967.

Bennett, M.V., editor: Synaptic transmission and neuronal interaction, New York, 1974, Raven Press.

Blount, M., et al.: Management of the patient with amyotrophic lateral sclerosis, Nurs. Clin. North Am. **14:**157-172, March 1979.

Blount, M., et al.: Plasma exchange in the management of myasthenia gravis, Nurs. Clin. North Am. **14:**173-190, March 1979.

Booker, H., Chun, R., and Sanguino, M.: Myasthenia gravis syndrome associated with trimethadione, J.A.M.A. **212:**2262-2263, 1970.

Brain, W.R.: Diseases of the nervous system, ed. 8, New York, 1977, Oxford University Press, Inc.

Brain, Lord: Brain's clinical neurology, ed. 4, New York, 1973, Oxford University Press, Inc.

Bromley, I.: Tetrapegia and paraplegia: a guide for physiotherapists, New York, 1976, Longman, Inc.

Buetner, E.H., et al.: Studies on autoantibodies in myasthenia gravis, J.A.M.A. **182:**46-58, 1962.

Carlson, C.E., coordinator: Behavioral concepts and nursing intervention, Philadelphia, 1970, J.B. Lippincott Co.

Carroll, B.: Fingers to toes, Am. J. Nurs. **71:**550-551, 1971.

Christopherson, V.A.: Role modifications of the disabled male, Am. J. Nurs. **68:**290-293, 1968.

Comebecker, R.B.: Thoughts of an A.L.S. patient, RN **35:**44-45, 83, June 1972.

Compston, A.: HLA and neurologic disease (Guest editorial), Neurology **28:**413-414, May 1978.

Crate, M.: Nursing functions in adaptation to chronic illness, Am. J. Nurs. **65:**72-76, Oct. 1965.

Davidites, R.M.: A social systems approach to deviant behavior, Am. J. Nurs. **71:**1588-1589, 1971.

Davidoff, R.A.: Pharmacology of spasticity, Neurology **28:**46-51, Sept. 1978.

Desmedt, J.E.: New developments in electromyography and clinical neurophysiology, vol. 1-3, White Plains, N.Y., 1973, Phiebig.

Dore-Duffy, P., et al.: Lymphocyte adherence in multiple sclerosis, Neurology **29:**232-235, Feb. 1979.

Dubowitz, V., and Brooke, M.H.: Muscle biopsy—a modern approach, Philadelphia, 1973, W.B. Saunders Co.

Dworkin, J.P., and Hartman, D.E.: Progressive speech deterioration and dysphagia in amyotrophic lateral sclerosis: case report, Arch. Phys. Med. Rehabil. **60:**423-425, 1979.

Dyck, P.J., et al.: Peripheral neuropathy, Philadelphia, 1975, W.B. Saunders Co.

Eldridge, R., et al.: Amyotrophic lateral sclerosis and parkinsonism dementia in a migrant population from Guam, Neurology **19:**1029-1037, 1969.

Enstrom, J.E., and Operskalski, E.A.: Multiple sclerosis among Spanish-surnamed Californians, Neurology **28:**434-438, May 1978.

Feldman, R.G., et al.: Baclofen for spasticity in multiple sclerosis: dougle-blind crossover and three-year study, Neurology **28:**1094-1098, Nov. 1978.

Ferguson, F.R.: A critical review of the clinical features of myasthenia gravis, Proc. R. Soc. Med. **55:**49-52, Jan. 1962.

Flacke, W.: Drug therapy: treatment of myasthenia gravis, N. Engl. J. Med. **288:**27-31, Jan. 1973.

Fredericks, E.J., and Russman, B.S.: Bedside evaluation of large motor units in childhood spinal muscular dystrophy, Neurology **29:**398-400, March 1979.

Gaspard, N.: The family of the patient with long-term illness, Nurs. Clin. North Am. **5:**77-84, March 1970.

Glaser, G.H.: Crisis, precrisis and drug resistance in myasthenia gravis, Ann. N.Y. Acad. Sci. **135:**335-345, 1966.

Goodgold, J., and Eberstein, A.: Electrodiagnosis of neuromuscular diseases, Baltimore, 1972, The Williams & Wilkins Co.

Goss, C.M., editor: Gray's anatomy of the human body, ed. 29, Philadelphia, 1973, Lea & Febiger.

Goust, J.M., et al.: Abnormal T cell subpopulations and circulating immune complexes in the Guillain-Barré syndrome and multiple sclerosis, Neurology **28:**421-425, May 1978.

Grabow, J.D., et al.: Cerebellar stimulation for the control of seizures, Mayo Clin. Proc. **49:**759, 1974.

Hall, P.V., et al.: Glycine and experimental spinal spasticity, Neurology **29:**262-267, Feb. 1979.

Hardgrove, C., and Dawson, R.: Parents and children in the hospital, Boston, 1972, Little, Brown & Co.

Hardy, A.G., and Rossier, A.B.: Spinal cord injuries: orthopedic and neurological aspects, 1975, Publishing Sciences Group, Inc.

Harmetz, A.: Must they sacrifice today because of threatened tomorrows? Today's Health, Nov. 1971.

Harrower, M.: Mental health and MS, New York, 1971, National Mutiple Sclerosis Society.

Hauser, S.L., et al.: Lymphocyte capping in muscular dystrophy, Neurology **29:**1419-1429, 1979.

Haymaker, W.: Bing's local diagnosis in neurological diseases, ed. 15, St. Louis, 1969, The C.V. Mosby Co.

Herz, E., and Glaser, G.H.: Spasmodic torticollis (clinical evaluation), Arch. Neurol. Psychiatry **61:**227-239, 1949.

Hirschberg, G., Lewis, L., and Thomas, D.: Rehabilitation. A manual for the care of the disabled and elderly, Philadelphia, 1964, J.B. Lippincott Co.

Hubbard, J.L.: Peripheral nervous system, New York, 1974, Plenum Publishing Corporation.

Johnson, W., Schwartz, G., and Barbeau, A.: Studies on dystonia musculorum deformans, Arch. Neurol. **7:**301-313, 1962.

Kahana, E., Leibowitz, U., and Alter, M.: Cerebral multiple sclerosis, Neurology **21:**1179-1185, 1971.

Keane, J., and Hoyt, W.: Myasthenic (vertical) nystagmus: verification by edrophonium tonography, J.A.M.A. **212:**1209-1219, 1970.

Kempton, J.W.: Living with myasthenia gravis; a bright new tomorrow, Springfield, Ill., 1972, Charles C Thomas, Publisher.

Kirschner, P.A., Osserman, K., and Kark, A.: Studies in myasthenia gravis transcervical total thymectomy, J.A.M.A. **209:**906-910, 1969.

Kisonak, R.: He's had his last Christmas with his family, The Hartford Courant **6B:**April 30, 1972.

Knott, H.S.: Crisis in myasthenia, Med. Clin. North Am. **53:**285-291, 1969.

Kondo, K.: Does gastrectomy predispose to amyotrophic lateral sclerosis?, Arch. Neurol. **36:**586-587, Sept. 1979.

Korones, S.B.: High risk newborn infants: the basis for intensive nursing care, ed. 2, St. Louis, 1976, The C.V. Mosby Co.

Landon, D.H., editor: Peripheral nerve, New York, 1976, Halsted Press.

Leinonen, H., et al.: Capillary circulation and morphology in Duchenne muscular dystrophy, Eur. Neurol. **18:**249-255, 1979.

Lindenberg, R.E.: The need for crisis intervention in hospitals, Hospitals **46:**52-55, 110, Jan. 1, 1972.

Lindh, K., and Rickerson, G.: Spinal cord injury: you can make a difference, Nursing74 **4:**41, Feb. 1974.

Loree, K., et al.: The challenge of multiple sclerosis by and for its patients, New York, 1972, National Multiple Sclerosis Society.

Marchant, M., et al.: Interdisciplinary learning on a neurological service, Am. J. Nurs. **72:**1638-1639, 1972.

Masaoka, A., et al.: Spontaneous remission of myasthenia gravis in patients with thymoma (Brief communications), Neurology **28:**495-496, May 1978.

McFarland, H.F., and McFarlin, D.E.: Cellular immune response to measles, mumps, and vaccinia viruses in multiple sclerosis, Ann. Neurol. **6:**101-106, Aug. 1979.

McQuillen, M.P.: Hazard from antibiotics in myasthenia gravis, Ann. Intern. Med. **73:**487-488, 1970.

Muscular Dystrophy Associations of America, Inc.: Patient and community services program, New York, 1971, The Associations.

Myasthenia Gravis Foundation, National Medical Advisory Board: Myasthenia gravis: manual for the physician, New York, 1970, The Foundation.

National Multiple Sclerosis Society: Amyotrophic lateral sclerosis: a concern of the National Multiple Sclerosis Society, New York, 1972, The Society.

National Multiple Sclerosis Society: Annual report, 1971, New York, 1972, The Society.

Newsom-Davis, J., et al.: Function of circulating antibody to acetylcholine receptor in myasthenia gravis: investigation by plasma exchange, Neurology **28:**266-272, March 1978.

Ogg, E.: Milestones in muscle disease research, New York, 1971, Muscular Dystrophy Associations of America, Inc.

Osserman, K.E., and Genkins, G.: Studies in myasthenia gravis: review of a twenty-year experience in over 1,200 patients, Mt. Sinai J. Med. N.Y. **38:**497-537, 1971.

Papatestas, A.E., et al.: Studies in myasthenia gravis: effects of thymectomy, Am. J. Med. **50:**465-474, 1971.

Paty, D.W., et al.: Chronic progressive myelopathy: investigation with CSF electrophoresis, evoked potentials, and CT scan, Ann. Neurol. **6:**419-424, 1979.

Perlo, V., et al.: The role of thymectomy in myasthenia gravis, Ann. N.Y. Acad. Sci. **183:**308-315, 1971.

Petrillo, M., and Sanger, S.: Emotional care of hospitalized children, Philadelphia, 1972, J.B. Lippincott Co.

Phillips, D.F.: The hospital and the dying patient, Hospitals **46:**68, 72-75, Feb. 16, 1972.

Poser, C.M.: A numerical scoring system for the classification of multiple sclerosis, Acta Neurol. Scand. **60:**100-111, 1979.

Poser, C.M.: Clinical diagnostic criteria in epidemiological studies of multiple sclerosis, Ann. N.Y. Acad. Sci. **122:** 506-519, 1965.

Price, J.: Patient care classification system, Nurs. Outlook **20:**445-448, 1972.

Putnam, T.J., Herz, E., and Glaser, G.H.: Spasmodic torticollis; surgical treatment, Arch. Neurol. Psychiatry **61:**240-247, 1949.

Reid, D.E., et al.: Principles and management of human reproduction, Philadelphia, 1972, W.B. Saunders Co.

Rowland, L.P.: Drugs in the management of myasthenia gravis. In Modell, W., editor: Drugs of choice 1972-1973, St. Louis, 1972, The C.V. Mosby Co., pp. 275-280.

Russell, A.S., and Lindstrom, J.M.: Penicillamine-induced myasthenia gravis associated with antibodies to acetylcholine receptor, Neurology **28:**847-849, Aug. 1978.

Sawa, G.M., and Paty, D.W.: The use of baclofen in treatment of spasticity in multiple sclerosis, J. Can. Sciences Neurologiques **6:**351-354, Aug. 1979.

Scadding, G.K., et al.: Humoral immunity before and after thymectomy in myasthenia gravis (Brief communications), Neurology **29:**502-506, April 1979.

Schumacher, G.A.: Multiple sclerosis. In Conn's current therapy, Philadelphia, 1970, W.B. Saunders Co.

Sears, T.A., et al.: The pathophysiology of demyelination and its implications for the symptomatic treatment of multiple sclerosis, Neurology **18:**21-26, Sept. 1978.

Seay, A.R., et al.: Serum creatine phosphokinase and pyruvate kinase in neuromuscular disorders and Duchenne dystrophy carriers (Brief communications), Neurology **28:**1047-1050, Oct. 1978.

Shaternick, J.: Living with myasthenia gravis, Am. J. Nurs. **63:**73-75, Feb. 1963.

Shibasaki, H., et al.: Multiple sclerosis among Orientals and Caucasians in Hawaii: a reappraisal, Neurology **28:**113-118, Feb. 1978.

Stackhouse, J.: Myasthenia gravis, Am. J. Nurs. **73:**1544, Sept. 1973.

Symington, G.R., and Mackay, I.R.: Cell-mediated immunity to measles virus in multiple sclerosis: correlation with disability, Neurology **28:**109-112, Feb. 1978.

Tagliavini, J., et al.: Carrier detection in Duchenne muscular dystrophy, Neurology **29:**1423-1425, 1979.

Terry, F.J., et al.: Principles and technics of rehabilitation nursing, ed. 2, St. Louis, 1961, The C.V. Mosby Co.

Test yourself: myasthenia gravis, Am. J. Nurs. **79:**659, April 1979.

Thompson, C.E.: Reproduction in Duchenne dystrophy (Brief communications), Neurology **28:**1045-1047, Oct. 1978.

Tindall, R.S.A., et al.: Serum antibodies to cytomegalovirus in myasthenia gravis: effects of thymectomy and steroids, Neurology **28:**273-277, March 1978.

Toglia, J.U.: Electronystagmography in neurological diagnosis, Appl. Neurophysiol. **42:**257-266, 1979.

U.S. Department of Health, Education, and Welfare: Multiple sclerosis: hope through research, DHEW Publication No. (NIH) 72-75, Washington, D.C., 1971, U.S. Government Printing Office.

U.S. Department of Health, Education, and Welfare: NINDS Research Profiles: 1971, DHEW Publication No. (NIH) 72-53, Multiple sclerosis, Washington, D.C., 1971, U.S. Government Printing Office, pp. 48-53.

Viets, H.R., editor: Myasthenia gravis: the second international symposium proceedings, Springfield, Ill., 1961, Charles C Thomas, Publisher.

Viets, H.R., and Schwab, R.S.: Thymectomy for myasthenia gravis, Springfield, Ill., 1960, Charles C Thomas, Publisher.

Walton, J.: Muscular dystrophy and its relation to the other myopathies: neuromuscular disorders, Res. Publ. Assoc. Res. Nerv. Ment. Dis. **38:**378-421, 1961.

Warmolts, J., and Engel, W.K.: Benefit from alternate-day prednisone in myasthenia gravis, N. Engl. J. Med. **286:**17-20, Jan. 6, 1972.

Weiner, H.L., et al.: Decreased lymphocyte transformation to vaccinia virus in multiple sclerosis, Neurology **28:**415-420, May 1978.

Willard, H.: Occupational therapy, ed. 4, Philadelphia, 1971, J.B. Lippincott Co.

Willis, W.D., and Grossman, R.G.: Medical neurobiology: neuroanatomical and neurophysiological principles basic to clinical neuroscience, ed. 2, St. Louis, 1977, The C.V. Mosby Co.

Wishik, S.M.: How to help your handicapped child, Public Affairs Pamphlet No. 219, New York, 1970, Public Affairs Committee, Inc.

Young, R.F., and Goodman, S.J.: Dorsal spinal cord stimulation in the treatment of multiple sclerosis, Neurosurgery **5:**225-230, Aug. 1979.

# 18

# DISORDERS OF REFINED MOVEMENTS

The last three chapters have been organized to separate disorders of sensorimotor systems so that the reader might identify a logical division for various disorders. This chapter continues to expand on dysfunctions interfering with normative precision in motor movements.

Basically, the basal ganglia and the cerebellum operate together to regulate movement and control involuntary activity. The basal ganglia seems to control total movement, whereas the cerebellum regulates and constantly modifies refined motor activity.

The cerebellar dysfunctions are obvious in nystagmus and in instances of normal proprioception wherein opening or closing the eyes fails to correct ataxia. Extrapyramidal disease consists of a number of involuntary movements, which may include chorea, parkinsonism, athetosis, dystonia, tremor, ballism, and tics.

### Expected outcomes
The client or significant others will:

1 Explain the pathophysiology, clinical outcomes, current understanding of disease by professionals, and available treatments.
2 Describe his or her individual symptoms, problems, and concerns and state specific measures to alleviate them.
3 Discuss ways that maximum independence in socioeconomic functions and activities of daily living may be attained and maintained.
4 Specify the positive and negative outcomes from each type of treatment and medication, and the limitations of each method.
5 Explain the dosage, desired effects, adverse outcomes, special instructions or precautions, and storage directions for each medication as well as reasons to notify the physician.

6 Demonstrate specific therapy protocols for exercise, speech, or activities of daily living.
7 Identify specific schedules that have been written to show how therapy protocols will be integrated into life outside of the health care agency.
8 Discuss specific community agencies that offer services commensurate with client needs.
9 Explain the importance of and specific daily ways of maintaining the highest possible level of physical and psychological functioning.
10 Identify the specific hazards of impaired mobility that are individually applicable and state specific ways to prevent physical complications.
11 State specific measures needed to promote safety in mobility and in eating, if impaired functions exist.
12 Demonstrate at least three ways that stress from continual motor performance may be alleviated. Utilize relaxation therapy techniques, control of the daily calendar, and adequate rest periods to diminish stress.
13 Work to develop positive, open, and accepting relationships with significant others in regard to self, the disease state, and any limitations that this condition might impose.
14 Identify detail as to exact ways that helping professionals will be utilized.
15 Establish an open, trusting, therapeutic relationship with the nurse and the physician in charge, wherein dialog occurs freely when assistance is needed or when questions occur.
16 Continue to be involved in some type of regular social interchange with appropriate individuals.
17 Discuss the impact of the disease state and associated concerns with issues of total sexuality and control of one's life space.

## CEREBELLAR DISORDERS

The cerebellum is an extraordinarily interesting structure to study because of its intricacy and complexity of function. Chapters 1 through 3 give details on embryology, anatomy, and physiology, and Chapter 11 offers guidelines in assessment. Because the cerebellum is the structure that refines motor activity, it is used to adaptation. Thus when a lesion interrupts its functional integrity, the cerebellum may make adjustments that mask symptoms until the lesion has expanded to a large size.

Much of what has been learned about cerebellar disorders is the outcome of animal studies. Monkeys have been utilized to study the outcome of removal of the nodulus, flocculus, and uvula, which results in a discrete syndrome of the flocculonodular lobe. Resulting symptoms include impaired posture and equilibrium without the loss of motor power. The outcome is impaired capacities in standing and walking, with a concurrent inability to run.

In the early stages of midline tumors in childhood, especially medulloblastomas, which arise in the nodulus of the inferior vermis, a discrete set of symptoms is seen, including truncal incoordination without limb involvement. Such lack of coordination is not evident when the child reclines but becomes particularly obvious during standing and walking. Tumor expansion in later stages does not make the detection of these symptoms as discrete.

When a disturbance occurs in the cerebellar hemispheres, it is termed the syndrome of the neocerebellum. Symptoms in this syndrome consist of hypotonia, dyssynergia, and tremor. *Hypotonia* is usually less prominent than the other symptoms.

Investigators do not understand how the functional breakdown of movement known as *dyssynergia* occurs. Some believe it results from a loss of postural tone in muscles, wherein hypotonia contributes to the weakness, and involuntary movements are the attempt of the cerebellum to compensate for the lack of tone by voluntary efforts. Others believe dyssynergia is related to the inability of the cerebellum to balance the inhibitory and facilitatory impulses necessary to the execution of smooth, coordinated motor activity.

When *tremor* occurs in association with a disturbance in the neocerebellum, intention tremor is apparent with voluntary movement but not at rest. The movements often follow voluntary movement and may consist of any degree of movement up to and including rather extreme tremor. A number of conditions result in this type of tremor, even when distinct disturbances of the cerebellum are not necessarily detected. Some examples of causative disease entities include senile tremor, hereditary tremor, idiopathic tremor, multiple sclerosis, cerebellar tumor, and parenchymatous cerebellar degeneration.

When disorders of the cerebellar type result in a tremor, the tremor is more intense if there is involvement of the nuclei, particularly the dentate nucleus. Severe tremors occur in Benedikt's syndrome, a disturbance of the superior cerebellar peduncle, and in occlusion of the superior cerebellar artery, where there is also a disturbance in the superior cerebellar peduncle. When cerebellar nuclei are involved, recovery from symptoms is never complete.

Little is known about the origin of cerebellar tremors. Investigators have discovered that areas 4 and 6a of the cerebral cortex are involved in tremor production by noting that the tremor abates when these areas are surgically extirpated after contralateral section of the cerebellar peduncles. When intention tremors occur as a part of a cerebellar disturbance, the genesis of the problem is believed to be related to inadequate compensatory mechanisms within the cerebral cortex. Little explanation is offered in instances of senile tremor, since pathological changes have been primarily found in the corpus striatum, not the cerebellum.

In studying infratentorial tremors one may find reference to cerebellar fits. In actuality the cerebellum is not the genesis of this activity. Instead the fit probably results from a precipitous neuronal discharge in the area of the upper pons or lower region of the midbrain. Symptoms include the spontaneous onset of body rigidity, wherein there is extension of the arms and legs. During the episode the body is postured in a position of decerebrate rigidity. These episodes often result in a loss of consciousness and may last for a period of minutes or hours.

***Differential considerations.*** Disturbances in tone, balance, and coordinated movements may result from a lesion either at the cerebellar level or in the periphery. When the lesion is in the cerebellum, acute or chronic problems may occur in relation to balance and integrated movements (ataxia). Assessment reveals such symptoms as broadbased, staggering gait and intention tremor unaffected by conscious control. Chapter 11 details the complete assessment of cerebellar functions. To summarize probable findings, one would note a disturbance in the exercise wherein the client touches the finger to the nose in rapid succession, in regulating extraneous movements, in correctly gauging the distance of an object so that reaching out does not result in overshooting the object, and in walking, particularly in a heel-to-toe pattern along a straight line. When the client is a child or seems uncooperative in testing, some of these capacities may be assessed as the practitioner observes the individual while utilizing eating utensils. Other symptoms commonly associated include nystagmus, dysarthria, pendular knee reflexes, and hypotonia.

Similar symptoms result when the interruption in function occurs at the level of the spinal cord or within the reflex arc. At times the level of the lesion may be determined as the history points to a particular diagnosis, which may be verified by laboratory and diagnostic testing. However, in the initial attempt to differentiate a peripheral lesion from a central lesion the examiner may utilize the Romberg test. When the lesion is in the spinal cord or arc, the individual is unable to maintain balance without utilizing vision. In addition, changes in vibration sense and joint position are noted on testing.

Common causes of cerebellar ataxia include birth trauma, congenital disorders (Dandy-Walker syndrome or hydrocephalus), infections (cerebellar abscesses, parasitic disease, and poliomyelitis), metabolic problems (Hartnup's disease), degenerative disorders (ataxia-telangiectasia, Friedreich's ataxia, metachromatic leukodystrophy), neoplasms of the posterior fossa, and toxic substances or medications in high dosages (phenytoin [Dilantin], acetazolamide [Diamox], piperazine, thallium, chlorophenothane [DDT], and lead). Head injuries may also result in ataxia.

*Scientific advances.* Individuals with intractable seizures and severe spasticity from cerebral palsy have received profound relief from the functional incapacity secondary to abnormal muscle tone and involuntary muscle activity as a result of the surgical insertion of a cerebellar implant (pacer, stimulator). Work on the concept of cerebellar stimulators dates back to AD 15, when shocks from electric fish were used to remedy gout and headaches.

In 1897 Charles S. Sherrington won the Nobel Prize for implanting animals with a stimulator in the anterior lobe to diminish exterior hypertonus found in decerebrate rigidity. Cooper and Davis are the two physicians who have successfully implanted cerebellar pacers in individuals of all ages to treat seizures, spasticity associated with stroke or cerebral palsy, and generalized myoclonus, which evades control under usual treatment regimens.

After the cerebellar stimulator is inserted, electrical current adjustments are made on an external pack, and intensive physical therapy is utilized to assist the individual in gaining functional capacities. Many associated changes have also been noted in individuals who have implants, including alterations in posture, electroencephalographic tracings, seizure discharges, evoked responses, pain threshold, and behavior. Although the cerebellar stimulator has offered promising results in many individuals to date, a number of questions still remain unanswered about the long-term effects of cerebellar implantation.

## EXTRAPYRAMIDAL DISORDERS

Authorities vary as to what is included in the extrapyramidal system. Although some use the term to include the basal ganglia and the extrapyramidal structures in the cerebral cortex, others interpret the extrapyramidal system to include structures and neurons of the motor system excluding the pyramidal tract. As mentioned in Chapter 1, the basal ganglia consist of the corpus striatum, globus pallidus, and substantia nigra. Others may include the red nucleus, corpus subthalamicum, and cerebellum as parts of the extrapyramidal system. Although areas of the cortex that contribute to the extrapyramidal system are not well delineated, an important linkage is believed to exist between the corpus striatum and the premotor cortex.

When the functions of the extrapyramidal system are disrupted, problems with associated movements occur. The disorders that may result include a paucity of movement (*paralysis agitans*) or involuntary movements (*chorea, athetosis* and *dystonia,* and *tremor*).

### Paralysis agitans

A paucity of movement may occur in paralysis agitans, wherein muscle tone is abnormal. In this instance the client is rigid, demonstrates plastic resistance to passive movement, and shows the cogwheel phenomenon. However, the clasp-knife response associated with spasticity from interrupted pyramidal tract functions is not evident. The rigidity in this disorder is of myotatic genesis, whereas the posterior roots and proprioceptive nerve ending of muscle remain intact. When voluntary activity is attempted, several points may be noted, including synchronization of impulses, augmented myotatic reflexes, and augmented activity in protagonists and antagonists.

Other disorders that result in similar rigidity are dystonia musculorum deformans and hepatolenticular degeneration.

## Chorea

Evidence is unclear as to whether chorea is caused by lesions in more than one area. In arguing this point proponents direct attention to lesions in the corpus striatum in clients with Huntington's chorea. Others argue that vascular softenings are known to occur in the corpus striatum without subsequent chorea. Moreover, choreiform movements have been documented in lesions of the thalamus. Experimental studies on lesions in the basal ganglia continue. The role of gamma-aminobutyric acid, a neurotransmitter, will continue to be the subject of future research.

Chorea is most commonly associated with either Huntington's disease or Sydenham's chorea. Huntington's disease is discussed extensively in the next section. Sydenham's chorea, occurring after rheumatic fever, is usually of a mild, transient type that requires no pharmacological control. The ingestion of certain pharmacological agents may also incude chorea. These include methylphenidate, amphetamines, oral contraceptives, phenytoin, anticholinergics, levodopa, and certain anticonvulsants. Treatment in drug-induced chorea is to stop ingestion of the implicated medication. Treatment of the causative disorder is indicated when chorea is the result of a systemic disease process, such as systemic lupus erythematosus, thyrotoxicosis, or hepatolenticular degeneration. Methods outlined under the care of the client with Huntington's disease are utilized when chorea is associated with senility or the benign inherited form.

***Huntington's chorea.*** Huntington's chorea, also called *Huntington's disease,* is a rare, familial, progressively degenerative disease of adults characterized by violent choreiform movements, akinesia, and mental deterioration.

This disease was first described more than a hundred years ago (1872) by a 22-year physician, George Huntington, who practiced in Long Island, New York. He called it *hereditary chorea* and at that time identified three of its major characteristics: (1) its hereditary nature, (2) its onset in adult life, and (3) its frequent progression to insanity and suicide. In recognition of his contribution to medicine the disease was named after him.

Before 1968 the public knew very little about Huntington's disease. Families generally tried to conceal the afflicted members and rarely admitted that they had a history of the disease. There was little understanding of the disease; in its early stages it was often misdiagnosed.

In 1967 Woodrow (Woody) Guthrie, composer and singer of folk songs, died at the age of 55 from Huntington's disease. (His mother also died of the disease in a mental institution.) Woody, when only 34 years old, began to experience periods of depression and temper outbursts. At times his gait was peculiar, his speech was slurred, and he had involuntary jerky movements of his arms. He was admitted to a hospital for 3 weeks and diagnosed an alcoholic. The physical and psychological manifestations persisted, and he and his family suffered for 7 years without knowing what he had. After being told that he had Huntington's disease and after talking it over with his wife, he decided that the only way their three children could have a relatively normal life was for him to spend the rest of his life in a hospital. During the subsequent years his condition progressively deteriorated until he was completely helpless and speechless. His wife Marjorie visited him every day, sometimes with the children. Woody's intellectual abilities were not impaired. He lived long enough to know that his son Arlo also had become a successful folk singer and had given a concert at Carnegie Hall.

After his death, Marjorie Guthrie started a vigorous campaign to stimulate scientists to do research on Huntington's disease and help families face the same crisis she had faced and continues to face knowing that her children have a 50% chance of inheriting the affected gene.

Mrs. Guthrie founded the Committee to Combat

Huntington's Disease (CCHD)* in 1967 and became its executive secretary. It now has chapters in large cities throughout the United States and affiliated chapters in Austria, England, and Scotland. The purpose of CCHD is to educate the public, help clients and their families, and encourage and support research programs and scientific conferences. She and CCHD are dedicated to the detection and care of sufferers from Huntington's disease† and its eradication through research.

*Huntington's Disease,*‡ a film produced by Eaton Laboratories in 1971 and narrated by George Paulson of the Ohio State University College of Medicine, is available without charge.

The onset of symptoms most frequently occurs between the ages of 25 and 55 years; the average age of onset is 35 years; about 5% of the identified victims of Huntington's disease were 60 years old before manifestations appeared; and 2% were afflicted during childhood. Huntington's disease may last 10 to 20 years. Death usually results from exhaustion, heart failure, pneumonia, or suicide.

The condition is hereditary through a dominant autosomal gene. It may be transmitted by either a male or female parent; each offspring, regardless of sex, has a 50% chance of inheriting this disease. It does not skip a generation; therefore those who do not inherit the disease cannot transmit it, and their heirs, unless another carrier of the gene marries into the family, also will be free of the affected gene.

Based on a review of published articles, it is estimated that about 14,000 Americans have Huntington's disease. The CCHD believes the number to be more than 50,000. The pathological condition is a degenerative process that involves the cells and nerve fibers of the cerebrum, brainstem, and cerebellum. Diffuse cerebrocortical atrophy results from the progressive destruction of the neurons.

This disease develops gradually in adult life

---

*The national headquarters is at 200 W. 57th St., New York, NY 10019.
†An official registry of affected families is maintained at the Creedmoor Institute, Station 60, Jamaica, NY 11427.
‡One may borrow this film (16 mm, 14 minutes, sound, and color) by contacting the local Eaton sales representative or writing to the Eaton Medical Film Library, Eaton Laboratories Division, The Norwich Pharmacal Co., Norwich, NY 13815.

with choreiform movements in the face and upper extremities. These are purposeless, at first slow, but later become violent in nature and involve the entire body. The person may be hurled out of bed by the force of the uncontrollable activity. The gait is bizarre. Facial grimacing and smacking of the tongue are frequent; speech is dysarthric and unintelligible; personality may change radically, with intermittent periods of apathy, irritability, depression, elation, hostility, and aggression; the individual may become irresponsible and use poor judgment, often necessitating social and legal supervision; he or she may become untidy and careless in personal appearance and personal habits; and intellectual functions may deteriorate progressively. The physical and psychological symptoms may be equally severe, or either the involuntary abnormal movements or the personality changes may be more prominent. At first spontaneous movements may be inhibited with considerable effort, and the person may be able to perform certain tasks independently (such as eating and dressing); ultimately all movements are aggravated by attention, effort, and emotional upsets, and the individual becomes completely helpless and is unable to do anything alone. The movements may diminish appreciably or even disappear during sleep.

Diagnosis depends on recognition of the clinical picture and the family history.

**NURSING INTERVENTION.** The treatment is protective, preventive, symptomatic, and supportive. There is no known cure. The nursing care of clients afflicted with this illness embodies the use of all the skills, attitudes, and principles previously described for the care of clients with other chronic, progressively disabling diseases. As the bizarre, jerking movements increase in degree, the nurse controls the physical environment so that the client will not sustain injury. If he or she is confined to bed, well-padded side rails should be in place at all times to prevent his or her being thrown out of bed by the spasms. Restraints are never used because of their tendency to increase movements and the possibility of causing an injury. There may be personality changes, increasing irritability, forgetfulness, apathy, and depression. The client requires close supervision, and precautions should be taken to prevent suicidal attempts. The nurse is responsible for the maintenance of good hygiene, good nutrition, and adequate elimination; the observation of behavior; and the prevention of complications. Since many clients have difficulty in speaking and communicating, the nurse must develop sensitivity in perceiving and meeting their emotional, intellectual, physical, and social needs. Not only the client but also the family require considerable emotional support.

Since there is generally progressive mental deterioration, these clients ultimately reach the point at which they cannot be cared for at home or in a general hospital and must be committed to a facility equipped to handle complex physical and emotional disturbances.

Current research indicates that the disease process is directly related to an increased amount of dopamine in comparison with normative acetylcholine and GABA supplies. Various attempts have been employed to increase and maintain GABA supplies. However, none have been successful yet. Some of the substances that have been part of these recent experiments include sodium valproate, muscimol, L-glutamate, and pyridoxine administration. Loeb et al. utilized low doses of bromocriptine to achieve dopamine antagonism while enjoying phenothiazine-like outcomes, and reported some success for a small group of clients.

Thus pharmacological support is currently a constant balancing process geared toward decreasing chorea while one takes care in not worsening depression or in promoting tardive dyskinesia. Medications either antagonize dopamine by depletion (that is, tetrabenazine) or by receptor blockade (that is, phenothiazines, such as perphenazine [Trilafon], or the butyrophenones, such as haloperidol [Haldol]). Tetrabenzine may exaggerate depression, whereas the phenothiazines and the butyrophenones may cause tardive dyskinesia.

## Parkinson's disease (paralysis agitans or "shaking palsy")

Persons have been known to be afflicted with the "shaking palsy" since at least the second century. At that time it was described by Galen, a Greek physician, who was practicing medicine in Rome. In 1817 James Parkinson, an English physician, wrote such an accurate description of the "shaking palsy" as a separate disease entity that in recognition of his contribution it was given his name. He was the first writer to identify three of the most frequent signs of this disease: the involuntary tremulous motion, the muscular weakness, and the bending forward of the trunk, with uncontrollable acceleration of gait.

In 1862 Charcot, a French neurologist, added muscular rigidity and deformity of the extremities to the symptoms described earlier by Parkinson. Nine years later Minart, a German neurologist, reported shrinkage of the corpus striatum and the lenticular nucleus on the side opposite the tremor. This was the first recognition that the parkinsonian tremor might be linked to a disorder of the basal ganglia. Previously it was generally believed that the site of the pathological lesion was in the cerebral cortex or spinal cord. In 1919 Brissaud and Tretiakoff of France reported cell loss in the substantia nigra in the brains of clients who had parkinsonian symptoms before they died.

Akinesia and rigidity are most likely associated with the function of the system composed of the substantia nigra, corpus striatum, globus pallidus, and thalamus; the origin of the other symptoms, especially tremors, has not been established.

In 1959 Carlsson noted that about 80% of the dopamine in the brain is concentrated in the caudate nucleus and putamen. In Parkinson's disease the level of dopamine in the corpus striatum is reduced by more than 50%. Hornykiewicz, stimulated by the work of Carlsson and his own observations of clients with hypertension who developed parkinsonism after treatment with reserpine, concluded that reserpine depletes brain dopamine levels. In 1959 he examined the brains of clients who had died of Parkinson's disease or an associated complication to confirm his theory of the relationship between dopamine and extrapyramidal function. He quickly discovered that the extrapyramidal centers of the autopsied brains, especially the substantia nigra, showed a loss in pigmentation that was characteristic of a serious deficiency of the amino acid dopamine.

Animal research demonstrated that dopamine did not cross the blood-brain barrier and that the administration of an enzyme called *monoamine oxidase* to healthy animals caused an increase in the amount of dopamine in the brain. However, when monoamine oxidase was given to clients with Parkinson's disease, it was ineffective. Although it diminished the further breakdown of dopamine, the deficiency was already so great that no therapeutic effect resulted.

It is now well established that the deficiency of dopamine in the nigrostriatal complex in clients with Parkinson's disease is both characteristic of and specific for this syndrome. No other extrapyramidal disorder has been found to exhibit such a severe loss of dopamine.

*Types.* Although the cause of parkinsonism has never been determined, many specialists subdivide it into three categories, which include the primary (idiopathic) type, the secondary (symptomatic) type, and the paraparkinsonism syndromes. The primary type comprises the majority of all cases. Of these primary cases a few reveal a family history wherein inheritance is attributable to autosomal dominance with incomplete penetrance. The secondary type, often associated with afterinfection, especially after von Economo encephalitis, is more commonly linked to a drug reaction from reserpine, tetrabenazine, the phenothiazines, or the butyrophenones. The third category, paraparkinsonism, is reserved for those cases wherein parkinsonism is merely part of the symptomatology of other disease entities. Wilson's disease, normal pressure hydrocephalus, and toxic reponses to manganese, carbon monoxide, and carbon disulfide are only a few of the disorders resulting in parkinsonian-like symptoms.

It has been demonstrated that regardless of whether the client is afflicted with postencephalitic or arteriosclerotic parkinsonism or that associated with chronic manganese poisoning, each one has a dopamine deficiency. This theory is also reinforced by the fact that all artificially produced parkinsonism in man or in animals seems to act directly through striatal dopamine mechanisms. Phenothiazines, such as chlorpromazine and haloperidol, that block the dopamine-sensitive cellular sites of the *corpus striatum* produce a functional deficiency of dopamine and symptoms of parkinsonism.

Testing out this theory in 1961, Barbeau in Canada and Birkmayer and Hornykiewicz in Austria administered L-dopa, a metabolic precursor of dopamine that crosses the blood-brain barrier and is converted into dopamine, to clients with Parkinson's disease. They observed a significant decrease in rigidity in some of the clients. Subsequent studies on the clinical use of L-dopa in parkinsonism showed that, when administered intravenously or orally, it produced a transient decrease in parkinsonian symptoms—rigidity or akinesia, or both.

In 1966 it was clearly recognized that if the amount of dopamine in the brain could be increased and maintained for a prolonged period, significant relief of parkinsonian symptoms would result.

*Current research.* Current research reveals that although great strides have been made in symptomatic relief, primary parkinsonism remains as a progressive disorder. Levodopa and dopamine agonist substances are still the most effective pharmacological agents, but practitioners now believe that their use should be more limited because of the long-term problems resulting in behavioral alterations and fluctuating symptomatic relief. Moreover, surgical intervention is appropriate for only a few clients. Future studies should offer increased promise as researchers pursue the hypothesis that there is more than one type of dopamine receptor.

*Clinical symptoms.* This chronic disease state may remain stationary for many years. However, it is one of the most crippling diseases of the nervous system and may lead to a fatal outcome. Estimates of its incidence in the United States vary from 900,000 to more than 1 million cases, with from 40,000 to 50,000 newly diagnosed cases each year. This number will increase as the life-span increases.

The peak onset of Parkinson's disease is in persons over 50 years of age. Estimates of the prevalence of Parkinson's disease range from 1 case per 1000 to 1 case per 200 population. Furthermore, epidemiologists maintain that a higher incidence of Parkinson's disease occurs among relatives of the clients who develop tremor and related symptoms after ataractic drug therapy. (About 15% of those who take certain tranquilizers develop tremors and signs of parkinsonism; fortunately these disappear with the discontinuance of the medication.) The abnormal signs and symptoms resulting from impaired control and regulation of movement may occur as early as 1 year or as late as 25 years after an attack of encephalitis.

The symptoms are slow to develop and may be

tremor (usually most noticeable in the fingers, which perform involuntary pill-rolling movements) or rigidity. The tremor is exaggerated when the client is under emotional stress, fatigued, or cold and may disappear during purposeful activity and sleep. Coordinated voluntary muscular activities which previously were accomplished together without conscious awareness, are no longer possible. These must be broken down into steps and performed deliberately. For example, the client cannot rise automatically from a chair and simultaneously take a handkerchief from a pocket and blow the nose. The mere act of rising from the chair must be done slowly and deliberately and completed before the client can attempt any other act. He or she must learn to perform slowly a single motor act. The rigidity will affect posture and gait to such an extent that the individual bends forward increasingly as he or she walks at a progressively more rapid rate that is uncontrollable (propulsion), or the stride is so shortened that locomotion is accomplished with short steps (*marche à petit pas*). Progressive loss of automatic movements is observed; the normal swinging of the arms while walking is absent. Voluntary and automatic movements are reduced in frequency and take longer to perform. Generally as the disease progresses, writing, speaking, eating, chewing, and swallowing are considerably impaired. There is loss of reflex blinking, and facial mobility is impaired. Consequently, the client presents a mask-like facies with a staring, fixed gaze; the face does not express any emotion. Salivation, believed to be caused by infrequent swallowing, may be a problem. It can be reduced somewhat if the client is instructed to swallow at frequent intervals. If it is not controlled, drooling results. This may cause local skin irritation and be a source of embarrassment to the client, thus increasing the physical and emotional discomfort.

When this disease occurs in an arteriosclerotic client, some impairment of memory and thinking and some mental confusion may occur. Otherwise intellectual functions are not affected. Some clients demonstrate a characteristic muffled and monotonous speech with a nasal quality. As in other chronic neurological diseases, some of these clients may manifest changes in mood and behavior. In addition, the client with postencephalitic par-

kinsonism may experience oculogyric crises (painful upward rotation of the eyes into a fixed position).

*Diagnosis.* The diagnosis depends on the clinical history of an insidious onset of progressive stiffening of the muscles; difficulty in initiating movements (akinesia); postural abnormalities; gait disturbances; loss of normal, spontaneous, coordinated movements; and tremors of the fingers, which is verified on examination. Laboratory tests are not helpful.

*Treatment and nursing intervention.* No cure is known for Parkinson's disease. Treatment of this disease consists of physical therapy to help neutralize the muscular rigidity and prevent musculoskeletal complications; drugs, especially L-dopa (levodopa or Sinemet) to replace and maintain dopamine in the basal ganglia and substantia nigra, thus relieving rigidity and akinesia; and selective thalamic surgery for destruction of a tiny area in the brain by heat, freezing, or other methods, thus eliminating the tremors, and rigidity of contralateral limbs. Nonlateral problems with gait, speech, and posture are minimally alleviated by surgery. When bilateral surgery is performed, complications are more severe and more prevalent. Supportive psychotherapy for both client and family may be an important adjunct to the therapeutic regimen.

A program of physical therapy including preventive and corrective exercises is essential for every client with Parkinson's disease regardless of whether it is caused by arteriosclerotic changes or a viral infection, whether the client is in his or her thirties or sixties. It is important that physical therapy be maintained to preclude the development of ankylosing fibrotic changes about the joints as a result of the existing immobility of muscles. If a physical therapist is not available, a member of the client's family should be taught how to massage and stretch the affected muscles. The client should perform every physical act that presents difficulty from 12 to 20 times a day. Goals of treatment are to keep muscles alive, improve efficiency; prevent contractures and deformities, and reduce dependency on others. Speech may be improved if one instructs the client to read aloud and to use the lips in an exaggerated manner.

Both the client and the family should be informed about the diagnosis and about the nature of the illness so that they will be better prepared to participate in the prescribed treatment program. Helping them to understand and face the diagnosis of Parkinson's disease also serves to allay any unexpressed fears of insanity, brain tumor, or imminent death.

More than 90% of all persons with Parkinson's disease are cared for at home. Whether this poses a serious economic, physical, social, or psychological burden on the family depends on the home situation, the presence and age of children, their appreciation of the nature of the illness, their willingness to participate cooperatively in the treatment program, and the recognition that the client can be best helped when encouraged and permitted to do things independently. It may take the client three or four times longer to do things, but it is imperative that he or she does them or face the prospect of becoming a helpless invalid. A time schedule for the activities of everyday living should be arranged so that there is no hurry or pressure.

It is especially important that the client eat a well-balanced diet. If he or she has trouble cutting food, it should be cut beforehand. An electric warming tray may be used to keep food warm. Some clients may prefer and are less fatigued eating six smaller meals than three large ones. If the client has difficulty in chewing, the food may be prepared in a blender. Because of diminished physical activity and the use of certain drugs, constipation may be a problem. The inclusion of adequate fluid and fruit in the diet and the establishment of regular habits of elimination are important preventive measures. Stool softeners, mild cathartics, and rectal suppositories are usually preferable to reliance on enemas. Some clients tend to be preoccupied with their bowels and need to be reeducated about the notion that health depends on a daily bowel movement.

Prolonged sitting in a chair may cause edema of the feet and should be avoided. (Some physicians advocate the use of a rocking chair as a circulatory stimulant and a psychological relaxant.) A knotted sheet tied to the bottom of the bedpost can be used by the client to attain a sitting position before he or she gets out of bed. The client will have less difficulty in getting out of a straight chair if 2-inch blocks are placed under the back legs and the chair is tipped slightly forward.

Falls may be prevented when scatter rugs and doorsills are removed and railings on the stairs are added. Self-care can be facilitated by instillation of a raised toilet seat and wall handles and by use of special clothing with zippers instead of buttons and moccasin type of shoes without shoelaces.

The client should not be isolated from social activity but should be involved in the daily life of the family and participate to the extent of his or her capacity. Emphasize abilities, not disabilities. The tremor and other symptoms should be accepted and discussed without embarrassment. Relationships with members of the family will determine the level of adjustment; if the individual is content, happy, and secure in their love, he or she will be better able to cope with the problems posed by the illness and will function more effectively.

Psychotherapy, with control of the environment and personal relationships to avoid emotional upsets, has proved helpful. These clients are encouraged to be physically and economically independent as long as possible. As the clients become increasingly incapacitated because of postural defects and gait disturbances, all ambulatory activity should be supervised to prevent falls. An electric rocker may be used to stimulate circulation. These clients seem unduly sensitive to weather changes and are usually more comfortable in a warm, temperate climate.

As the disease progresses, clients generally develop a personality characterized by increased irritability, querulousness, hypersensitivity, and stubbornness. They frequently make excessive demands on their nurses, families, and friends and become increasingly dependent. Insomnia is a prominent symptom; sedatives are given with questionable effect. Ultimately, the medical and nursing care of these clients is directed toward making them less miserable and as comfortable as possible.

***Pharmacological therapy.*** Each individual needs a thorough base-line evaluation and subsequent periodic evaluations for assessment of disease progress and psychosocial, economic, and functional capacities. If the life-style of the individual is such that functions of daily living may continue with minimal disruption, the use of levodopa should be postponed.

Because of the basic neurotransmitter discrepancy, wherein too much acetylcholine and too little dopamine exist, agents affecting the cholinergic system, as well as those acting on the dopaminergic system, may be employed.

AGENTS AFFECTING CHOLINERGIC ACTIVITY. Three types of agents are effective in relieving parkinsonism—anticholinergic agents, tricyclic antidepressants, and antihistamines.

Anticholinergic agents such as trihexyphenidyl and benztropine work by blocking muscarinic receptors. (Refer to Chapter 4 for further detail on the cholinergic system.) Adverse outcomes may include dry mouth, blurred vision, urinary problems, constipation, and behavioral changes such as forgetfulness, confusion, drowsiness, delusions, or hallucinations.

Amantadine, a drug that works by an unknown mechanism attributable to its anticholinergic properties, is effective in clients affected by mild to moderate symptoms. Along with its tendency to be less effective after a few months of treatment, toxic effects may include blurred vision, dry mouth, delusions, confusions, livedo reticularis, and edema.

Tricyclic antidepressants serve the dual purpose of affecting desired motor outcomes while elevating the mood. Sedation and hypotension may occur as undesirable side effects.

The mild anticholinergic effect of antihistamines result in their effectiveness in parkinsonism, but their main drawback is sedation.

AGENTS AFFECTING DOPAMINERGIC ACTIVITY. When treatment is necessary to provide adequate client functioning, levodopa may be utilized. To improve the effectiveness of levodopa while decreasing adverse outcomes such as glaucoma, vomiting, cardiac arrhythmias, and hypotension, decarboxylase inhibitors such as benserazide in Madopar and carbidopa in Sinemet are administered. Even though this results in one-fourth the dosage requirement to produce the same effects as levodopa, problems such as psychosis and dyskinesia persist.

Researchers continue to seek ways to improve outcomes from levodopa. Experiments are being conducted in methods to promote enzymatic inhibition and to effect selective dopamine receptors. Bromocriptine, a dopamine agonist, has been used with some success, whereas lergotrile results in serious adverse outcomes. Experts hope that experimental studies will prove the effectiveness of tiapride and oxiperomide. Until some treatment is found, practitioners will continue to be plagued by problems of trading off parkinsonism symptoms with grave behavioral disorders in clients who require maximal treatment to function in activities of daily living.

LEVODOPA. The potency of levodopa (Larodopa, Levopa, and Dopar) and the high incidence of adverse reactions make it almost mandatory that the client be admitted to the hospital so that reactions to this drug can be closely monitored and the optimal, safe maintenance dosage determined. The drug manufacturers recommended that hematopoietic, hepatic, cardiovascular, and renal functions evaluations be done before levodopa therapy is initiated and periodically thereafter as long as the client is maintained on the drug. Most adverse reactions are reversed by reduction of the dosage. However, levodopa is not a cure for Parkinson's disease; if it is discontinued, the symptoms recur.

Individual reactions to and tolerance of this drug vary considerably. Improvement and control of some of the symptoms range in degree from slight to complete. Levodopa has not been effective when the client is suffering from drug-induced parkinsonism.

Levodopa, though not a panacea, has revolutionized the treatment of clients with Parkinson's disease and enabled many persons to resume their activities of daily living, to work, to socialize, and to love and be loved. Carbidopa-levodopa (Sinemet) offers further improvements over levodopa.

The physician and nurse play important roles in helping the client receiving levodopa and the family become familiar with the drug and its therapeutic and adverse effects, understand changing needs as the condition improves, and adjust to the gradual transition from being a dependent person to an independent one capable of again assuming responsibility. (On occasion the resumption of responsibility associated with the role and position in the family has been resisted by the person who has acquired them; the equilibrium of the family has been so threatened that the client and spouse have requested a discontinuance of levodopa so that the client can return to dependent status.)

When the client with advanced Parkinson's disease is admitted to the hospital for evaluation and treatment, he or she may manifest severe physical and psychological problems. The individual may be unable to take care of his or her own needs and may be uncommunicative, depressed, and withdrawn. There may be an inability to walk without assistance and even to change position. He or she may have a history of constipation, incontinence, and skin breakdown. This person presents an unattractive appearance: the face is expressionless; there is drooling, stooping, and tremulousness. He or she appears disinterested and neglected. Generally this person has been rejected and has become isolated from social contacts. He or she has lost dignity, self-esteem, and hope.

The nursing staff must be helped to accept this client as a person who deserves and needs the highest degree of understanding and nursing skill. Their attitudes toward the client with Parkinson's disease can facilitate or hinder adjustment to the hospital. He or she has been sensitized to the feelings of others and will quickly perceive negative, rejecting attitudes. The nursing staff communicate their feelings nonverbally by the way they act in the presence of the client; by expression, mannerisms, avoiding eye-to-eye contact, being in a hurry, and reactions to the person's negative behavior, dependence, and depression.

When possible, the nursing staff should be assigned to the client on a consistent basis. They should have a good knowledge of Parkinson's disease, its manifestations and associated complications; the aging process; the psychological impact of a chronic, progressively disabling disease; defense reactions and dependency needs; and the therapeutic and adverse effects of levodopa is this therapy is to be instituted.

Although the physician is responsible for evaluating the mental, physical, and neurological status of the client on admission and periodically during levodopa therapy, the nurse plays a significant and important role in assessing the client's abilities, closely observing and monitoring reactions to the drug, reporting changes in condition, helping with the activities of daily living, providing emotional support, and preparing the client adequately for all tests and procedures. The physical therapist is also an important member of the team. Because of the possibility of osteoporosis, contractures, and postural abnormalities, the physical therapist must evaluate the client and prescribe a regimen of corrective and remedial exercises and activity to be

implemented gradually as the client's rigidity and akinesia are reversed by levodopa. Staff and client must be cautioned against the too rapid resumption of physical activity so that spontaneous fractures and phlebothrombosis may be prevented.

Not all clients with Parkinson's disease manifest the classic symptoms to the same extent and degree. Rarely do these clients have intellectual impairments. If they exist, they may be attributed to cerebral cellular changes that are associated with old age. Some clients may be confused and have mood swings. The nurse must be aware of the client's need for intellectual stimulation and diversion and must provide opportunities for these needs to be satisfied.

After the nurse has admitted the client, oriented him or her to the physical setting, and informed him or her of rights and privileges and the hospital regulations, as assessment of physical limitations and existing complications such as constipation, incontinence, malnutrition, insomnia, contractures, and depression is made. The nurse identifies existing problems, validates these with the client, and initiates a written nursing care plan. Priorities and realistic short-term goals are established. As the client responds to levodopa, these are changed to reflect decreasing dependence. Retraining programs to reestablish bladder and bowel control and self-care activities are utilized as necessary. The principles of physical and psychological nursing care associated with the care of any disabled, chronically ill client should be applied.

The nurse is indispensable when the client is receiving levodopa therapy. The nurse's approach to the client and the administration of nursing care are influenced by the possible adverse as well as therapeutic reactions to the drug. Objective assessment of these reactions and changes in the client's physical and emotional status, as well as the meticulous administration of the drug as ordered, are important nursing responsibilities.

The most frequent adverse reactions to levodopa may be classified under four major headings: gastrointestinal, cardiovascular, neurological, and psychiatric.

*Gastrointestinal reactions*. Nausea, vomiting, anorexia, and loss of weight may occur early in the course of treatment. Constipation may be increasingly a problem. The nausea and vomiting may be lessened by administration of the medication with or immediately after a meal. If a dose is given at bedtime, milk and crackers or other nourishment should also be given. All meals should be closely supervised to ensure an adequate nutritional and fluid intake. If necessary, the client should be spoon-fed. The client should be encouraged to drink 6 glasses of water each day, and selected fruits and vegetables, low in vitamin $B_6$ content, should be included in the diet to combat constipation.

*Cardiovascular reactions.* Orthostatic hypotension, dizziness, arrhythmias, tachycardia, palpitations, and syncope may occur. Generally a reduction in the dosage will control these adverse effects. The nurse is responsible for measuring pulse, respiration, and blood pressure four times a day and reporting changes promptly. The client who has bouts of hypotension should be closely supervised and instructed not to rise abruptly from a recumbent or sitting position to an erect position. Support and panty hose or elastic bandages may help to avert a drop in blood pressure with position change. Abdominal binders also may be useful.

*Neurological reactions.* Some aged clients with organic brain disease tend to become more confused and disoriented. Insomnia may become a real problem. Usually eliminating the bedtime dose and reducing the total daily dosage are effective in controlling this symptom. Involuntary abnormal movements may occur as the total dosage of levodopa is increased. These may become more severe the longer the client receives the drug. These movements may include exaggerated swinging of the arms, grinding of the teeth, smacking of the lips, grimacing, intermittent turning of the head, and torticollis and choreiform twitchings of the fingers. These abnormal movements are exaggerated under emotional stress, may be accompanied by muscle spasms, and are most severe at the end of the day. Phenothiazines, barbiturates, and other drugs have been used without success. The gradual reduction of the dosage of levodopa to the level at which the abnormal movements cease is an effective treatment. However, if the amount of levodopa then administered has no therapeutic effect, the physician, client, and family must decide whether the dosage should be increased and whether the increased mobility and lessening of the parkinsonian symptoms are important enough to tolerate the abnormal movements.

*Psychiatric reactions.* Changes in mood and behavior may occur. These include agitation, aggression, hypersexuality, hallucinations, paranoid or grandiose delusions, nightmares, depression, and catatonic stupor. These manifestations may be alleviated by reduction of the dosage of levodopa. These clients must be closely supervised at all times so that they are protected from hurting themselves and others. The nurse who is familiar with the possible effect of the drug will be better prepared to cope with the erotic client without overreacting.

*Other considerations.* The nurse, client and family should be prepared for color changes in body fluids caused by the metabolic by-products of levodopa. The urine may appear rusty brown and become black on standing; saliva may be black, and underclothing may be blackened by sweat.

Certain medications that counteract the therapeutic effects of levodopa are contraindicated. Monoamine oxidase inhibitors, alpha-methyldopa, and reserpine are especially contraindicated. When other drugs are administered to the client taking levodopa, the individual should be closely monitored for untoward effects. Alcohol should be avoided in large quantities, since it is an antagonist to levodopa.

It has been established that pyridoxine hydrochloride (vitamin $B_6$) reverses the effect of levodopa; therefore certain multivitamins, iron supplements, and foods containing pyridoxine in large amounts should be eliminated. Foods that contain *large* amounts of pyridoxine are malted milk, dry skim milk, cowpeas, lentils, lima beans, navy beans, split peas, soybeans, kidney beans, sweet potatoes, yams, avocados, bran products, wheat germ, oatmeal, baker's yeast, brewer's dry yeast, soy flour, pork, beef liver, beef kidney, bacon, fresh salmon, tuna, molasses, and walnuts. Certain foods containing less pyridoxine may be used moderately: dry milk, yellow corn, canned tomatoes, bananas, prunes, dried apricots, dried dates, whole wheat and rye breads, lamb, veal, ham, cod, canned salmon, crab, peanuts, and peanut butter. The foods just listed are those most available and not all inclusive. The ingredients of packaged foods should be checked before being added to the diet of the client taking levodopa. The client should be informed that the ingestion of large amounts of chocolate, old cheese, and Chianti may also neutralize some of the effects of levodopa. Eaton Laboratories has published informational pamphlets available without charge to clients taking levodopa and their families. In addition, clients should realize that ingesting a high protein meal at once can block the effects of levodopa, whereas a great reduction in protein consumption may have the opposite effect, even when levodopa is given with a decarboxylase inhibitor. If Sinemet is used, dietary restrictions are not necessary.

SINEMET. Sinemet is a registered trademark for a combination of carbidopa and levodopa in a proportion of 1 to 10. Before Sinemet is administered, clients should have discontinued levodopa therapy for at least 8 hours.

Sinemet is available in tablet form in two strengths: (1) 10 mg of carbidopa and 100 mg of levodopa and (2) 25 mg of carbidopa and 250 mg of levodopa.

The main indication for Sinemet is in the treatment of Parkinson's disease, wherein dopamine is depleted in the corpus striatum. When dopamine is administered, it is ineffective in restoring brain levels, since it does not cross the blood-brain barrier. Thus levodopa, the precursor of dopamine, is administered, since it crosses the blood-brain barrier to be converted to dopamine in the basal ganglia, thereby probably relieving symptoms of Parkinson's disease.

One of the disadvantages of using levodopa is the large doses required to achieve the desired effect. Thus nausea and other adverse symptoms frequently accompany its administration. When levodopa is taken orally, it rapidly converts to dopamine in extracerebral tissues so that only a fraction of the dosage is available in unchanged form for use in the central nervous system. Some of the undesirable symptoms are caused by this conversion to dopamine in the extracerebral tissues.

Carbidopa does not cross the blood-brain barrier to influence levodopa metabolism in the central nervous system but does inhibit decarboxylation of peripheral levodopa.

When carbidopa and levodopa are administered simultaneously, the action of carbidopa results in greater availability of levodopa to the brain tissue. Carbidopa may possibly have the advantage of preventing dopamine-induced cardiac arrhythmias. Carbidopa is known to reduce the quantity of levodopa required to achieve a therapeutic effect by 75%. Carbidopa also inhibits the action of pyridoxine (vitamin $B_6$), so that its simultaneous administration does not reverse the effects of levodopa.

When carbidopa and levodopa are administered simultaneously, symptoms such as nausea and vomiting are decreased, but there are no conclusive data to support any increase in overall effectiveness in relation to the disease process. However, since carbidopa only affects peripheral levodopa, it does not reduce adverse symptoms that may occur within the central nervous system, such as dyskinesias that may become evident earlier with Sinemet than with singular administration of levodopa. Although some clients improve with the substitution of Sinemet for levodopa, others do not.

Sinemet is contraindicated in clients with melanoma or unevaluated skin lesions, since levodopa may stimulate activity in malignant melanoma. Specific hypersensitivity to Sinemet and narrow-angle glaucoma are other contraindications. When a client is going to receive Sinemet, monoamine oxidase inhibitors should be discontinued 2 weeks before Sinemet is administered.

Sinemet may be associated with the occurrence of involuntary movements and mental disturbances. Thus clients should be closely observed for signs of depression and potential suicidal thoughts, particularly when a history of psychiatric disturbance exists. Care is taken when Sinemet is administered to known cardiac clients, such as those with a history of myocardial infarction with subsequent atrial, nodal, or ventricular arrhythmias. As early therapy commences, intensive cardiac care facilities should be readily available. Other clients who require close observation during Sinemet administration include those with bronchial asthma, extreme pulmonary or cardiovascular disturbances, and renal, hepatic, or endocrine disorders. Clients with a history of peptic ulcer should be carefully monitored, since Sinemet therapy may result in gastrointestinal hemorrhage.

At this time the effect and safety of Sinemet on children under 18 years of age and in pregnant or lactating women is not established. However, there is some experimental use of Sinemet in comatose children who do not respond to other forms of therapy. In these cases, investigators hope to replenish dopamine stores, if they are depleted, and activate the reticular activating system to encourage arousal. Responses of these comatose children seem to include restlessness, a catlike cry, increased muscular tension, and sometimes arousal (in the limited number of cases observed by this author).

During Sinemet administration the client should have serial assessments of hepatic, renal, cardiovascular, and hematopoietic functions. If the client has chronic wide-angle glaucoma, the intraocular pressure needs to be controlled and monitored. If the client receives concurrent medications for hypertension, these drugs may need to be regulated again after the initiation of Sinemet. In hypertensive clients the tendency of Sinemet to cause orthostatic hypotension may present a problem. If the client receives phenothiazines and butyrophenones, the effect of Sinemet on parkinsonian symptoms may be negated.

Some of the adverse reactions have been previously mentioned, but a number of others have also been reported, including dry mouth, sialorrhea, dysphagia, abdominal disturbances, ataxia, increased hand tremor, weakness, headache, numbness, bruxism, nightmares and insomnia, confusion, hallucinatory and delusional experiences, increased irritability and anxiety, malaise, fatigue, euphoria, blepharospasm, muscle twitching, trismus, odd sensations of the tongue, including burning and bitter taste, gastrointestinal symptoms such as constipation, diarrhea, and flatulence, skin rash, flushing, diaphoresis, urinary incontinence or retention, unusual breathing rhythms, blurred vision, diplopia, dilated pupils, hot flashes, changes in body weight, darkened color of perspiration and urine, oculogyric crisis, hiccups, hair loss, hoarseness, edema, priapism, and stimulation of latent Horner's syndrome. A number of laboratory studies may also reveal abnormalities.

For clients previously taking levodopa the Sinemet dosage will be 25% of the levodopa dosage. A typical adult dosage is three to six tablets of Sinemet 25/250 daily in equal doses. At this time, eight tablets daily is the maximum dose advised. Usually, Sinemet therapy is started gradually (Sinemet 10/100 twice daily) and increased every day or every other day until the desired dosage is achieved. Blepharospasm is an early indication of an excessive dosage for that client.

When a client receiving Sinemet requires general anesthesia, Sinemet therapy is interrupted until the client can resume oral intake.

If overdosage results, intervention is supportive and symptomatic and includes cardiac monitoring, maintenance of adequate respiratory capacities, gastric lavage, and careful use of intravenous fluids.

Other indications for the use of Sinemet include postencephalitic and symptomatic parkinsonism, such as that associated with central nervous system trauma, carbon monoxide intoxication, or manganese intoxication.

***Surgery.*** As long as the client is maintained on levodopa, clinical and laboratory evaluations must be continued. The long-term safety of the drug has not been established.

Various neurosurgical procedures have been developed in an attempt to alleviate the disabling manifestations of this disease. These have included ligation of the anterior choroidal artery and stereotaxic measures of varying refinement. The latter have utilized electrical coagulation, fixation of the tissues with alcohol, freezing, radioactivity, and ultrasound to achieve a therapeutic effect through the destruction of the ventrolateral nucleus of the thalamus. The use of electroprobes to identify and correlate electrical impulses with the tremulous arm or hand movements has increased the accuracy of the surgical procedures. In this regard the freezing of the area localized is the preferred treatment.

Only about 12% of the clients with Parkinson's disease are considered suitable candidates for surgical treatment. It is generally limited to the younger, healthy person with unilateral tremor or rigidity. It is contraindicated when bilateral manifestations are severe and when the lower cranial nerves (vagus and glossopharyngeal) are involved. The mortality in selected cases ranges from 0.5% to 2%; the risk of serious complications ranges from 1% to 2%.

When clients have been properly selected, about 75% of them have been benefited by pallidal and thalamic surgery. It is believed that surgery reduces the abnormal inhibitory effect the disease exerts on the nerve circuits and restores functional and balanced nerve activity, thus reducing rigidity and muscular weakness. Clients perform better, gain weight, and are no longer depressed.

*Continuing research.* The Parkinson Disease Foundation, a voluntary association, was established in 1957. Its purpose is to promote and support research in the cause, prevention, and cure of Parkinson's disease. It has developed a "brain bank" at Columbia University Medical School to study the nerve tissues and biochemistry of the brain. To further this scientific research, persons with Parkinson's disease are asked to make provision in their wills for their brains to be donated to the brain bank.

In 1964 the NINDS established the Parkinson's Disease Information and Research Center at Columbia University in New York. This center, supported by NINDS, has two primary functions: (1) to develop a comprehensive automated library service of the scientific literature on Parkinson's disease and to publish bibliographies, indices, and critical reviews and (2) to conduct a comprehensive research program in an attempt to determine the cause of Parkinson's disease and more effective evaluative and treatment methods.

This center also conducts large research conferences focusing on research on Parkinson's disease for scientists from the United States and other countries. Conference proceedings have been published.

The NINDS now supports four clinical research centers at Columbia University, the University of Colorado, Brookhaven National Laboratory, and the Albert Einstein College of Medicine in New York City.

The film, *Management of Parkinson's Disease and Syndrome with Levodopa,** describes the pharmacological research that led to the discovery of the therapeutic impact of levodopa on parkinsonian symptoms. Dr. Melvin Yahr and Dr. Roger Duvoisin of the Department of Neurology, Columbia University, discuss their experiences in treating clients with this drug and show five clients before and after levodopa administration. They discuss the dosage, side effects, and contraindications, as well as therapeutic responses.

In 1971 Eaton Laboratories produced a film, *Treatment of Parkinsonism with Levodopa,** which is narrated by Dr. George Paulson of the Ohio State University College of Medicine. He describes the history and treatment of this disease during the last 150 years. The three classic symptoms of tremor, rigidity, and akinesia are demonstrated. The historic work of Hornykiewicz that identified the role of dopamine in Parkinson's disease and the use of levodopa are discussed.

## Athetosis and dystonia

The physiological theory underlying athetosis and dystonia remains unclear. Lesions in athetosis have been located in the corpus striatum, thalamus, and globus pallidus. Because of the increase in medullated fibers, the corpus striatum takes on a marbled appearance in congenital double athetosis.

During sleep neither chorea nor athetosis is apparent. Moreover in cases where the individual becomes hemiplegic, chorea and athetosis are no longer apparent in the involved extremities.

One theory of explanation for athetoid movements is the proposal of a pathway wherein nerve impulses course from the pyramidal tract through parapyramidal fibers in areas 4 and 6, from which they continue on to subcortical centers and then to the anterior columns of the spinal cord.

*Athetosis and its variants: dystonia and torticollis.* *Bilateral athetosis* is seen principally as a variant of infantile cerebral palsy. Symptoms usually appear during childhood or early adolescence. It is characterized by slow, writhing, purposeless movements of the limbs with bizarre posturing. Voluntary activity and emotional stimuli aggravate the movements, which then become exaggerated in range and force. Since coordinated movements are impossible, a serious degree of disability follows. Movements of the face, tongue, and thorax interfere with speech, eating, and smooth respira-

---

*This film (16 mm, 34 minutes, sound, and color) is available on loan, without charge, from the Roche Film Library, % Association-Sterling Films, Inc., 600 Grand Ave., Ridgefield, NJ 07657, or may be obtained through the local Roche sales representative.

---

*This film (16 mm, 20 minutes, sound, and color) may be obtained without charge if one contacts the local Eaton representative or writes to the Eaton Medical Film Library, Eaton Laboratories Division, The Norwich Pharmacal Co., Norwich, NY 13815.

tion. The involuntary muscular action is of longer duration than the short jerks of chorea, and during the manifestations all muscles of the part involved are in strong tonic contraction (chorea has associated hypotonia), which results in characteristic posturing of the fingers. As the disease progresses, various postural abnormalties affecting the neck, trunk, and extremities may develop.

The cause is prenatal, and the pathological condition includes lesions in the basal ganglia as well as in the cerebral cortex. The diagnosis is made by observation of the characteristic movements. (Refer to Chapter 13.)

*Torticollis* (wryneck) consists of repeated tonic or clonic movements of the head to one side. It may involve the sternocleidomastoid muscle alone or the entire distribution of the eleventh cranial nerve and the upper cervical nerves. It may occur as a single disease entity or a manifestation of bilateral athetosis.

**TREATMENT AND NURSING INTERVENTION.** Since all clients with athetosis have some grotesque or bizarre manifestation of muscular activity or posture, the nurse should develop an objective attitude toward them. They are generally very sensitive about their appearance and are easily hurt and embarrassed by the demonstration of a thoughtless, tactless attitude by the persons around them. Being observed by others generally increases the abnormal movements with which they are afflicted. The nurse can, by a calm, matter-of-fact, kind approach, do much to alleviate their psychological distress and develop a feeling of rapport.

Medical treatment with drugs and muscle reeducation has been of little, if any, help. However, the administration of high dosages of anticholinergic drugs to children have had a positive outcome (Fahn). With torticollis there may be local pain because of spasm of the muscles involved; this may be dystonic in nature or a symptom of an emotional disturbance. If the latter, psychiatric evaluation and treatment are indicated. Emotional upsets tend to aggravate the spasm and movements; rest and isolation tend to lessen their severity and frequency. Psychotherapy is an important adjunct to treatment.

Surgical treatment consists of the interruption of the extrapyramidal tracts in the brain or spinal cord or partial section of the spinal accessory and upper cervical nerves on the affected side (torticol-

lis). The degree of postoperative improvement is minimal. Nursing care after this type of operation is similar to that after any craniotomy (Chapter 26) or laminectomy (Chapter 22).

Cooper reports that dystonia has been successfully treated by cryothalamotomy (surgical destruction of selected areas of basal ganglia and thalamus with liquid nitrogen).

*Tremor.* Tremor, apparently the result of a lesion in the globus pallidus or substantia nigra, or both, is a problem that greatly interferes with functional capacities. When hemiplegia affects an individual with a tremor associated with paralysis agitans, the tremor ceases. Rhythmical bursts of motor-unit discharges are evident in electromyographical studies of muscles with tremors.

Experimental efforts to produce tremors have been largely unsuccessful except in the case of intention tremor, wherein the disturbance has been created by the production of a lesion in the cerebellum or its pathways.

Surgical procedures have been attempted in the effort to relieve individuals of tremors. Removal of the precentral cortex results in cessation of tremors, whereas injections of procaine and alcohol into the opposite globus pallidus abate symptoms temporarily in some individuals and permanently in others. Surgical ablation of tremors has also been seen with destruction of the contralateral ansa lenticularis and the opposite thalamus, including the ventrolateral nucleus. The explanation behind the success of these surgical procedures may be accounted for by the interruption of afferent systems, such as the cerebellothalamic, pallidothalamic, and rubrothalamic tracts, to the thalamus. When tremors are halted by ansotomy, the rationale for success lies in the effective interruption of pallidofugal facilitating impulses that course to lower centers.

*Ballism.* In this disorder the client typically flings one arm outward in abrupt rotation. Although hemiballism is more common and is caused by a vascular lesion of the dorsomedial nucleus of the thalamus, symptoms abate—sometimes forever—when therapy is comprised of one course of perphenazine or haloperidol administration for a few months.

*Tic.* Tics may be misdiagnosed as a psychological disorder when they include involuntary words or noises. Such treatment can be very upsetting and frustrating to the client and family.

Tics are defined as rapid, erratic, purposeless movements. Sweet has categorized tics into four major types: (1) transient tic of childhood, (2) chronic simple tic, (3) persistent simple and multiple tic of childhood and adolescence, and (4) chronic multiple tic (Gilles de la Tourette's syndrome). Because of spatial limitations only Gilles de la Tourette's syndrome is briefly discussed.

Gilles de la Tourette's syndrome is a disorder of movement wherein the client often utters strange sounds or words involuntarily. It is often misdiagnosed, so that clients and families endure a long period of unsuccessful treatment. Although the cause of this disorder is unknown, it is believed to be related to a chemical or physiological abnormality. Adverse psychological circumstances can aggravate symptoms however. Haloperidol is the medication most commonly used to treat this condition. However, the client should be fairly disabled by the condition before haloperidol is tried, since there are such adverse outcomes associated as akathisia, dyskinesia, akinesia, and constipation. When haloperidol is ineffective, clonidine has been of value in some clients.

One may obtain further information on this syndrome by writing The Tourette Syndrome Association, Bell Plaza Building, 42-40 Bell Boulevard, Bayside, NY 11361. A major goal of this organization is the education of the public and health care professionals to the existence of this disorder. They also publish a quarterly newsletter.

## REFERENCES

Barr, A.N., et al.: Long term treatment of Huntington disease with L-glutamate and pyridoxine (Brief communications), Neurology **28**:1280-1282, Dec. 1978.

Chouza, C., et al.: Tratamiento del parkinsonisma con bromocriptina, Acta Neurol. Lat. Am. **24**:193-204, 1978.

Cohen, D.J., et al.: Clonidine in Tourette's syndrome, Lancet **2**:551-553, 1979.

Cole, W.: Marjorie Guthrie fights against her husband's killer, Good Housekeeping, pp. 64-74, March 1973.

Cooper, I.S., editor: Cerebellar stimulation in man, New York, 1978, Raven Press, Publishers.

Cooper, I.S.: Dystonia reversal by operation on basal ganglia, Arch. Neurol. **7**:132-145, 1962.

Eaton Laboratories: Caring for the parkinsonian patient on Dopar (levodopa, Eaton) capsules: a nurse's guide to therapy, Norwich, N.Y., 1970, Eaton Laboratories.

Elizan, T.S., et al.: Viral antibodies in serum and CSF of parkinsonian P and S and controls, Arch Neurol. **36**:529-534, Sept. 1979.

Erb, E.: Improving speech in Parkinson's disease, Am. J. Nurs. **73**:1910, Nov. 1973.

Fahn, S.: Treatment of dystonia with high dosages of anticholinergic medication, Neurology **29**:605, 1979.

Fischbach, F.T.: Easing adjustment to Parkinson's disease, Am. J. Nurs. **78**:66-69, Jan. 1978.

Fos, G.: Postural drainage, Am. J. Nurs. **73**:666-669, 1973.

Garron, D., Klawans, H., and Narin, F.: Intellectual functioning of persons with idiopathic parkinsonism, J. Nerv. Ment. Dis. **154**:445-452, 1972.

Halgin, R., et al.: Levodopa, parkinsonism, and recent memory, J. Nerv. Ment. Dis. **164**:268-272, 1977.

Huntington, G.: On chorea, Med. Surg. Reporter **26**:317-321, April 13, 1872.

Klawans, H.L., editor: Clinical neuropharmacology, New York, 1976, Raven Press, Publishers. (The work of Sweet et al. on tics is on pp. 81-105.)

Klawans, H.L., et al.: Lergotrile in the treatment of parkinsonism, Neurology **28**:699-702, July 1978.

Klawans, H.L., et al.: Treatment and prognosis of hemiballism, N. Engl. J. Med. **295**:1348-1350, 1976.

Klawans, H., et al.: Use of L-dopa in the detection of presymptomatic Huntington's chorea, N. Engl. J. Med. **286**:1332-1334, 1972.

Klawans, H.L., Jr.: The pharmacology of extrapyramidal movement disorders, White Plains, N.Y., 1973, Phiebig.

Korenyi, C., Whittier, J., and Conchado, D.: Stress in Huntington's disease (chorea) (review of the literature and personal observations), Dis. Nerv. Syst. **33**:339-344, 1972.

Lieberman, A.N.: Bromocriptine in Parkinson's disease: current prescribing, Practical Therap. **5**:37, 40-41, 45, 1979.

Lieberman, A.N., et al.: Bromocriptine in Parkinson disease: further studies, Neurology **29**:363-369, March 1979.

Lieberman, A.N., et al.: Lergotrile in Parkinson disease: further studies, Neurology **29**:267-272, Feb. 1979.

Llinás, R.R.: The cortex of the cerebellum, Sci. Am. **232**:56, Jan. 1975.

Loeb, C., et al.: Bromocriptine and dopaminergic function in Huntington disease, Neurology **29**:730-734, May 1979.

Loelterle, B., et al.: Cerebellar stimulation: pacing the brain, Am. J. Nurs. **75**:958, June 1975.

Lynch, H., Harlan, W., and Dyhrberg, J.: Subjective perspective of a family with Huntington's chorea. Implications for genetic counseling, Arch. Gen. Psychiatry **27**:67-72, July 1972.

Mandell, A.J., editor: New concepts in neurotransmitter regulation, New York, 1973, Plenum Publishing Corporation.

Mena, I., and Cotzias, G.C.: Protein intake and treatment of Parkinson's disease with levodopa, N. Engl. J. Med. **292**:181, Jan. 23, 1975.

Nausieda, P.A., et al.: Bromocriptine-induced behavioral hypersensitivity: implications for the therapy of parkinsonism, Neurology **28**:1183-1188, Nov. 1978.

Nutt, J., et al.: Treatment of Parkinson's disease with sodium valproate: clinical, pharmaceutical and biochemical observations, J. Can. Sciences Neurologiques **6**:337-343, Aug. 1979.

Perry, T.L., et al.: Isoniazid therapy of Huntington disease, Neurology **29:**370-375, March 1979.

Poirer, L.J.: Extrapyramidal system and its disorders, New York, 1979, Raven Press, Publishers.

Roaf, R., and Hodkinson, L.J.: The paralyzed patient, Philadelphia, 1977, J.B. Lippincott Co.

Robinson, M.B.: Levodopa and parkinsonism, Am. J. Nurs. **74:**656, April 1974.

Salter, R.B.: Textbook of disorders of the musculoskeletal system, Baltimore, 1970, The Williams & Wilkins Co.

Schmorl, G., and Junghanns, H.: Human spine in health and disease (translated by E. Besemann), ed. 2, New York, 1971, Grune & Stratton, Inc.

Shapiro, A.K.: Gilles de la Tourette syndrome, New York, 1978, Raven Press, Publishers.

Stipe, J., et al.: Huntington's disease, Am. J. Nurs. **79:**1428-1433, Aug. 1979.

Stevenson, A.C., et al.: Genetic counselling, ed. 2, Philadelphia, 1977, J.B. Lippincott Co.

Strohfus, S.: L-Dopa therapy and intensive individual care help Parkinson patients gain function and control, Mod. Nurs. Home **24:**37-40, July 1970.

Weiner, W.J., et al.: The effect of levodopa, lergotrile, and bromocriptine on brain iron, manganese, and copper (Brief communications), Neurology **28:**734-737, July 1978.

Wells, R.W.: Huntington's chorea: seeing beyond the disease, Am. J. Nurs. **72:**954-956, 1972.

Yahr, M.D., editor: Current concepts in the treatment of parkinsonism, New York, 1974, Raven Press, Publishers.

Yahr, M., and Duvoisin, R.: Drug therapy of parkinsonism, N. Engl. J. Med. **287:**20-24, July 6, 1972.

Young, P.: Woody Guthrie's widow: she mobilizes a battle on a brain disease, National Observer, June 3, 1972.

# 19

# DISORDERS ARISING FROM CRANIAL NERVES

The cranial nerves may be involved in association with or as a part of other disease conditions, but some have disorders peculiar to themselves, and only these are considered here. (Refer to Chapter 11 for discussion of assessment of cranial nerves.)

## TRIGEMINAL NEURALGIA (TIC DOULOUREUX)

Trigeminal neuralgia is a severely distressing affliction of middle life and old age consisting of disabling and recurring bouts of pain in one side of the face along the sensory distribution of the fifth cranial (trigeminal) nerve. The trigeminal nerve comprises three branches that convey impulses related to heat, cold, pain, and touch from the scalp, face, and mucous membranes of the head. Of these three roots, one is of unknown significance, one is a motor branch, and one is a sensory branch. The motor and sensory roots combine with the mandibular branch to innervate the muscles of mastication. (If trigeminal neuralgia occurs in a person younger than 40 years of age, it may be symptomatic of a mass lesion within the brain. Facial pain has been associated with acoustic tumors; meningiomas of the middle fossa, tentorium, and cerebellopontine angle; and vascular lesions of the posterior fossa. Therefore special diagnostic studies should be performed whenever the client is younger than 40 years of age to determine whether the trigeminal pain is primary and idiopathic or secondary to an intracranial lesion.)

Nothing is known of the etiology or pathology of this condition (it is not the pain associated with disease of the teeth, tongue, jaws, eyes, sinuses, or ears).

It is estimated that 15,000 persons in the United States are afflicted with trigeminal neuralgia each year. As the number of individuals 65 years of age and older increases, the incidence of this disease also may be expected to rise. Women are afflicted more frequently than are men.

The symptoms begin without apparent relationship to any circumstance or incident, though subsequent attacks may be precipitated by a cold breeze, taking food or fluid of extreme temperature, or touching a particular part of the face (trigger point) from which the paroxysm starts. The bouts may occur at irregular intervals of days, weeks, or months. Each episode consists of a series of paroxysms of extremely severe shooting pain that starts in a particular point with a nagging, pecking, repetitive "tic," increasing in severity to the point where the pain shoots violently with explosive force through the face on the affected side; the pain may last for days or weeks. Each paroxysm may last only for seconds or minutes, but the client continues to have discomfort in the region involved. This is magnified by apprehension about future attacks. The paroxysms occur in the distribution of the three divisions of the trigeminal nerve, almost always on one side of the face. The third (mandibular) division is most frequently affected; the second (maxillary) is next in order; and least frequently involved is the first (ophthalmic) division. Not uncommonly the disorder extends into a division adjacent to the one in which it began and occasionally into all three. The trigger point, stimulation of which may precipitate pain, is most frequently that part of the skin or mucous membrane close to the point of appearance of the branch of the nerve concerned, such as the supraorbital notch (first division), the infraorbital foramen near the junction of the nose and cheek (second division), and the mental foramen or the side of the tongue (third division).

The diagnosis can be made on the history and is confirmed when one witnesses a typical attack. Between paroxysms the client manifests apprehension by the care with which he or she protects the face from any stimulation (a draft of air, movement of the face during eating, speaking, brushing the teeth, washing the face, or shaving). Examination discloses no impairment of motor or sensory function. Careful study should always be made to eliminate dental and sinus infections as aggravating factors; therefore radiographic examination of the skull, teeth, and sinuses should be included.

## Treatment

The treatment is palliative during the acute episodes. The inhalation of trichloroethylene (10 to 15 drops on cotton) has been tried with variable success in relieving the pain. Carbamazepine (Tegretol) has been used for the treatment of severe trigeminal pain with good results. It is metabolized in the liver, and, because of the serious adverse reactions (aplastic anemia, agranulocytosis, thrombocytopenia, and leukopenia) that may occur, the client's cardiac, hepatic, and renal functions should be evaluated before this drug is started, and closely monitored while he or she is receiving it. Cobra venom, nicotinic acid, thiamine chloride, potassium iodide, analgesics, and narcotics have been administered for relief of the paroxysms with little, if any, impact. Sedatives may be given to ensure adequate sleep. Phenytoin (Dilantin) has also been widely used in the treatment of trigeminal neuralgia. Although the action of phenytoin is poorly understood, it has been effective in achieving some pain relief for selected clients. However, relief is not usually sustained. The numerous side effects inherent in the use of phenytoin often cause clients to discontinue use of this medication.

Propranolol hydrochloride (Inderal) is also being used to treat trigeminal neuralgia, though dosages are usually lower than those for hypertensive clients. Because of the prevalence of this condition in older individuals, some may already be on Inderal for hypertension and get relief from both problems. Hypoglycemia is a particularly troublesome side effect because it may cause symptoms that only compound a client's discomforts, at a time when eating may be avoided because of pain. With all treatments, be sure to help the client break the cycle of symptom chasing. Substitute planned interventions that affect client needs holistically.

Interruption of the peripheral trigeminal branches of the affected part is accomplished by injection of the particular division with absolute alcohol. This gives relief that may last from a few weeks to several months, at which time the treatment may be repeated. By specific radiographic procedures, absolute alcohol in very small amounts can be injected into the gasserian ganglion. In one study, this procedure was accompanied by thorough sensory assessment. In 309 clients not responsive to pharmacological therapy, treatment continued for up to 20 years without serious complications or fatality. Of these clients, 12 developed keratitis. This method of injection provides more long-lasting relief than do injections outside the ganglion. One problem described in other reports of alcohol injection is the flow of alcohol into the subarachnoid space and damage to other cranial nerves.

Two techniques may be employed for temporary relief. In one, peripheral branches of the nerve are avulsed, but branches regenerate, causing a return of pain. The rootlets may also be decompressed and manipulated in such a way that sensory functions remain intact. However, this second approach often results in recurring pain. Ultimately, an operation must be done and consists in dividing the sensory root of the trigeminal nerve intracranially. Usually if all three divisions of the trigeminal nerve are not involved, a partial section is carried out to spare the division or divisions not affected. Because of the permanent anesthesia that results and the associated peculiar sensations of numbness, heaviness, and stiffness of the involved areas, some clients are disappointed in the operative result and complain bitterly of these residuals. To obviate the occurrence of this emotional reaction, it is recommended that an alcohol injection precede any surgical therapy to acclimate the client to these sequelae. When the pain recurs, the sensory root can be divided, but the client should be informed of the permanent aftereffects.

During the past few years a surgical technique developed by two neurosurgeons, Rand of the University of California at Los Angeles and Jannetta of the University of Pittsburgh, utilizing an operating microscope, which provides magnification of the area and up to 2000 footcandles of light, has been successful in the treatment of clients with trigeminal neuralgia. Microsurgery permits greater precision in the selective cutting of fibers within the trigeminal nerve; sensations of pain and temperature are eliminated; the sensation of touch and the corneal reflex are preserved. Microsurgical techniques are being perfected and utilized in other neurosurgical procedures.

One of the most promising breakthroughs in surgical management of trigeminal neuralgia was re-

ported in work done on 310 clients at West Virginia University Hospital. The surgery, known as *radio frequency retrogasserian rhizotomy*, requires only local anesthetic or analgesics and an overnight hospital stay. Since it does not involve the problems of major surgery, previously poor surgical risks may be good candidates for the procedure. Of the 310 clients treated, only 22 required a second surgical procedure.

In this technique the neurosurgeon relies on radiographic techniques to insert an electrode through the cheek into the foramen ovale and onto the gasserian ganglion and the rootlets posterior to it (Fig. 19-1). Electrode placement is determined when the nerve is stimulated. When placement is exact, a surgical lesion is made by radiofrequency current. The regulation of current allows the neurosurgeon to make as many lesions as desired to achieve the appropriate degree of anesthesia. Clients must adjust to the permanent numbness that results. When the ophthalmic division is involved,

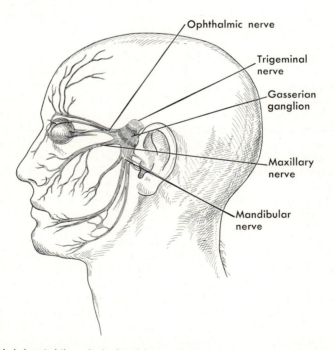

**Fig. 19-1.** Electrode is inserted through cheek and foramen ovale to gasserian ganglion, so that lesion is created electrically for control of pain.

the surgical lesion may frequently be made so that the corneal reflex remains intact. Odd sensations such as burning, scratching, or itching (anesthesia dolorosa) in the numb areas may be eliminated by regulation of the extent of the surgical lesion.

## Preoperative nursing intervention

### Expected outcomes

1 Nursing care routines will be done when pain is absent.
2 Normal physiological routines and activities of daily living will be continued or scheduled so that they do not interfere with the postsurgical status or augment pain.
3 Stimulation that augments pain will be absent or as minimal as possible.
4 Inadequate hygienic and nutritional status will be corrected and maintained.
5 Nutritional and hygienic needs will be satisfied in a manner that minimizes client pain.

*Observations.* Before operation the nurse notes the characteristics of the attack (description of the pain, area involved, precipitating factors, frequency, and duration), the emotional attitude of the client, difficulty in eating or in performing oral hygiene, and the condition of the affected eye (especially early signs of inflammation or corneal irritation).

*Position and activity.* Unless otherwise incapacitated, these clients, who are usually in the fifth, sixth, or seventh decade of life, are encouraged to be up and about and as active as possible. Their ambulation is emphasized because of their advanced years and because of the psychological benefits derived from following as normal a routine as possible. The paroxysmal nature of the pain may permit some of them to continue to be economically independent for some time. Outdoor activity during cold, windy, or rainy weather may precipitate an attack and should be avoided.

*Nutrition.* In most of these clients the act of chewing precipitates an attack, and for this reason, many of them refrain from eating an adequate amount because of fear that pain may ensue. The client's diet is planned according to individual needs based on general physical condition, activity, and occupation. It consists of food easily and quickly masticated. A semisolid, fluid diet is usually ordered for the preoperative client. Chewing may cause less discomfort if limited to the unaffected side. The temperature of the food and fluid is extremely important. Since hot and cold nourishments may precipitate an attack of pain, these should be avoided. Nourishment given to the client at room temperature is recommended. Ice is avoided in water or other fluids for the same reason. Frequent, small feedings may be better tolerated than three large meals. If because of the inability to control the pain the client is unable to take adequate nourishment by mouth or shows signs of malnutrition or dehydration, nutritional needs are maintained by administration of the feeding through a retention nasal tube. This tube is inserted in the nostril on the unaffected side of the face. This may be particularly indicated for the period preceding surgical treatment to improve the client's general condition.

*Hygiene.* Unless contraindicated, a cleansing tub bath is recommended daily. Since the mere act of touching the affected area may precipitate pain, many of these clients refrain from washing their faces, brushing their teeth, or shaving. Emphasize the importance of good oral hygiene in preventing complications, and encourage the client to perform these measures despite discomfort. Mouthwash is used after each meal. Extremes of temperature of the water used for cleansing are avoided. The use of a soft material for a washcloth may help to avoid precipitating an attack. If there is corneal anesthesia, special eye care is given to prevent excessive dryness of the cornea. Special cleansing and lubrication of the nostril on the affected side may be indicated to combat excessive dryness of the mucous membrane and crust formation, which may cause local discomfort or difficulty in breathing. All hygiene is accomplished when the client is free from pain, interrupted if pain occurs, and resumed after it passes.

*Elimination.* Elimination is not usually a problem. The client's normal habits of elimination are maintained insofar as possible. If diarrhea or constipation develops, it may be the result of an inadequate or poorly balanced diet. A change of diet should suffice to correct it.

*Psychological and physical preparation.* The psychological and physical preparation of a client for surgery follows the principles outlined in earlier chapters. To avoid unnecessary reiteration, this discussion will be limited to the preparation of the operative area. Determination of when the operative site is prepared and who does the preparation is according to institutional policy. Generally, shaving of the hair is carried out by the neurosurgeon after the client is anesthetized to decrease the trauma. The following procedures are usually acceptable.

FOR TEMPORAL OPERATIVE PROCEDURE. A minimal amount of hair should be removed. This is particularly important if the client is a woman, since subsequent concealment of the area will be facilitated. A rectangular area 2 by 5½ inches is prepared in the temporoparietal region. Its posterior boundary divides the ear, and the upper boundary is 2½ inches from the midline. The area is outlined after the hair is parted at its outer limits. If the client is a woman, the hair outside this area is fastened away from the field. The hair within the area is removed with a clipper (if long it should be braided and cut off with scissors before being clipped). The scalp is then scrubbed. For a female client the remainder of the hair should be combed, braided if long, and secured away from the operative area.

FOR SUBOCCIPITAL APPROACH. Again for cosmetic reasons, minimal hair is removed. The upper boundary of the area to be prepared extends from just about the external occipital protuberance to the top of the ear. Using the midline as a boundary, all hair is removed below this level on the affected side. Parting the hair, clipping, scrubbing, and shaving are done in the manner described for the temporal approach.

## Postoperative nursing intervention
### Expected outcomes
1 Complications will be absent.
2 When present, complications will be observed early, monitored, reported, and treated to minimize undesirable outcomes.

The postoperative nursing care depends on the operative site. If suboccipital, refer to Chapter 26 for the nursing care after infratentorial surgery. If the temporal operation is done, the principles of nursing care described here are followed.

*Observations.* The vital signs, including the blood pressure, are checked every 30 minutes until the client has fully recovered and then every hour for 6 hours or longer, depending on the condition. Symptoms of increasing intracranial pressure are watched for because they may develop after a middle meningeal hemorrhage (a rare complication). Signs of facial weakness are noted when the client smiles, raises the eyebrows, or closes the eyes. The eye on the affected side should be examined frequently for the early recognition of a complication. Note and report facial edema, herpes, sordes, parotid swelling, and subjective complaints.

*Position.* The client usually remains in bed for 24 to 48 hours. During this period the head is elevated to a 30-degree angle, and frequent change of position and deep breathing are encouraged to obviate the danger of respiratory complications. Thereafter, activity is progressively increased. Unless complications occur, the client usually is discharged 7 to 10 days after the operation is performed and should then be able to resume normal routine.

*Nutrition.* As soon as the client is convinced that eating will not bring back pain, the maintenance of adequate nutrition will cease to be a problem, and a diet is planned to suit individual needs. By the third postoperative day, regular food should be well tolerated. Because of the anesthesia of the inner cheek and mucous membrane of the mouth on the affected side, instruct the client to chew food on the opposite side to avoid biting the cheek and to avoid hot liquids or food because of the danger of burning the desensitized tissues.

*Hygiene.* Routine care is administered. Provide special oral hygiene five times daily (on awakening, after eating, and on retiring). Because of the persistent anesthesia of the mouth, residuals of food may accumulate and cause complications. The mouth should be kept clean and well lubricated at all times. Special eye care is given as indicated. It is vitally important if the ophthalmic division has been sectioned and the cornea is insensitive.

*Dressing.* Sutures usually are removed on the third day, and the dressing is removed on the fifth day.

For all clients and especially those who will have minimal hospital stays because of their candidacy for radio frequency retrogasserian rhizotomy, the practitioner may be most therapeutic by empathizing with the client and listening to reports of extreme pain, subsequent therapies, and coping mechanisms that have resulted in alterations in life-style. Chapter 10 gives further detail on the dynamics of pain. The practitioner may then assist the client in adjusting to postsurgical impairments and in reordering daily patterns to improve the quality of life.

*Additional considerations.* Other aspects of nursing care are based on the individual client's needs and are similar to the principles recommended for the care of a convalescent elderly client within the hospital. During the hospital stay the client should be well indoctrinated with the necessary information to prevent complications after discharge. Instructions regarding special eye care are outlined in Chapter 27.

*Complications.* Complications that may occur postoperatively have already been mentioned in passing. However, for emphasis they are repeated here: (1) postoperative hemorrhage from the middle meningeal artery; (2) facial paresis or paralysis caused by edema of the seventh cranial nerve; (3) herpes caused by injury of the gasserian ganglion or dehydration and hyperthermia (can be eased by the application of Tanac or phenol and camphor [Campho-Phenique]); (4) Irritation or ulceration of the cornea because of loss of sensation and dryness (can be prevented by vigilance and special eye care); (5) local trauma such as burning of the external cheek or the inner mucous membrane because of loss of temperature perception or biting of the inner cheek, which may result in ulcer formation (this trauma may result in part from inadequate instruction of the client); (6) respiratory infections (increased susceptibility because of the age group).

Treatment of these complications is symptomatic; their prevention and early recognition are emphasized. This responsibility to a large extent rests on the nurse.

## GLOSSOPHARYNGEAL NEURALGIA

Glossopharyngeal neuralgia, a paroxysmal pain that occurs in the throat and ear and may be precipitated by swallowing, coughing, sneezing, talking, turning the head toward the affected side, or clearing the throat, is comparable to trigeminal neuralgia but involves the sensory distribution of the glossopharyngeal (ninth cranial) nerve. In addition to pain, there may be loss of the gag reflex and loss of taste on the posterior one third of the

tongue. Glossopharyngeal neuralgia is caused by compression, inflammation, or injury of the ninth cranial nerve. In some cases, carbamazepine (Tegretol) has been used to relieve the pain. (This drug, which is discussed in Chapter 28, is used with considerable caution.) This condition is treated surgically by division of the cranial nerve intracranially after a hemisuboccipital craniectomy. Occasionally the vagal nerve is also involved. If it is, the upper two rootlets of the vagus are also sectioned.

The principles of nursing care after intracranial surgery are described in Chapter 26.

## FACIAL PARALYSIS (BELL'S PALSY)

Bell's palsy is a suddenly developing loss of the ability to move the muscles of one side of the face. As a result of this, the client presents a grotesque picture characterized by the loss of expression of one half of the face, the displacement of the mouth toward the unaffected side, and the inability to close the affected eyelids.

In the absence of involvement of the facial (seventh cranial) nerve secondary to an intracranial hemorrhage or tumor, meningitis, or focal trauma, the cause and disease process are unknown, though in some cases herpetic vesicles are seen in the external auditory meatus. This has led to the theory that a viral infection of the geniculate ganglion is responsible for the condition. DeWeese has claimed that Bell's palsy is caused by local ischemia and edema. Based on his own studies on clients with facial paralysis and a review of the literature, Goldberg suggests that emotional trauma and the resulting vasoconstriction may be a mechanism that causes facial paralysis.

The symptoms begin with discomfort behind the ear, which may or may not be accompanied by herpetic vesicles in the external ear. Within a period of hours there is a complete paralysis of the same side of the face. All the muscles of the involved side are powerless and flaccid. No movement is elicited when attempts are made to raise the eyebrow, close the eyelids, smile, show the teeth, or blow out the cheek. Saliva may drool from the angle of the mouth and tears trickle from the eye on the affected side. The client cannot whistle or manage fluid or food without difficulty, since liquids may dribble from the lips on the affected side and food may collect in the paralyzed cheek.

Taste is lost over the anterior two thirds of the tongue on the affected side.

Ordinarily the condition appears to be static for about 2 weeks, at which time the muscles begin to regain tone. Voluntary movement may appear within 3 to 4 weeks, and complete recovery may occur within 3 to 4 months. However, some clients manifest no recovery for almost 6 months, and maximum recovery, which may not be complete, may occur in about a year. It is in this group of clients that the reaction of degeneration is present during the third week. If at this time the muscles respond to faradic stimulation, the outlook is good. More than 80% of the clients with primary Bell's palsy recover without residuals.

Other conditions that may interfere with the functional integrity of facial muscles include space-occupying lesions, demyelinating disease, trauma, cerebrovascular accidents, and infectious processes.

### Treatment and nursing intervention

**Expected outcomes in nursing intervention**
1 Complications will be absent.
2 The client will adjust to temporary or permanent facial disfigurement.
3 Nutritional intake will be adequate.

The treatment is palliative and stresses the prevention of complications. Massage and electrotherapy have been used to maintain and stimulate muscle tone and to impede atrophy. Some physicians advocate the administration of vasodilating drugs to stimulate circulation and to restore the blood supply to the affected area. Steroids and streptokinase-streptodornase (Varidase) also have been used to reduce edema of the nerve. A facial sling may be used to prevent stretching of the muscles and, by improving lip alignment, to facilitate eating. Warm, moist heat applications may reduce associated pain. Supportive psychotherapy generally is of value to the client.

Nursing intervention is directed toward alleviation of the client's disability and the prevention of complications. If the involvement of the facial nerve is secondary to a systemic or neurological disease, nursing care is given accordingly.

*Complications.* The following complications may occur: (1) emotional reactions, (2) stretching of weakened muscles and loss of tone, (3) eating and drinking difficulties, (4) trauma to the mucous membrane, (5) anorexia and weight loss, (6) keratitis, (7) facial spasm or contracture.

The client may react emotionally to the change in appearance. Strong positive reassurance based on probable recovery must be given. If removal of the cause is impossible or if the paralysis does not recede because of irreversible trauma to the facial nerve, the client should be told of the possibility of having reparative (an anastomosis of the facial nerve with the eleventh or twelfth cranial nerve) or plastic surgery performed. Matter-of-fact acceptance of the client's disfigurement by family and friends may help minimize the emotional reaction.

Stretching of weakened muscles and loss of tone can be prevented by the use of a facial sling.

Eating and drinking difficulties can be minimized when a facial sling is used to improve lip alignment and the client is taught to take food on the unaffected side. A soft diet may be more easily consumed. Privacy at meals minimizes embarrassment from drooling. Special mouth care is always indicated.

Trauma to the mucous membrane can be prevented when the client is instructed to chew food on the unaffected side to eliminate biting of the inner cheek and to avoid hot foods and fluids that may cause burns in the insensitive areas.

Anorexia and weight loss can be prevented when one supervises the meals, seeing that they are attractively served and easily assimilated and adding supplementary feedings as indicated. The client should be weighed at definite intervals.

See Chapter 27 for prevention of keratitis and special eye care.

### MÉNIÈRE'S SYNDROME

Ménière's syndrome is a disturbance of the peripheral elements of the eighth cranial (acoustic) nerve within the internal ear. The cause is unknown. There are several unproved theories of the cause of Ménière's syndrome: an allergy, toxicity, localized ischemia, hemorrhage or hypoxia, viral infection, or edema as the result of a disturbance of salt and water metabolism. The pathological condition is characterized by a dilatation of the endolymphatic channels in the cochlea, with resulting atrophy of the hearing mechanism. The damming up of fluid is caused by obstruction of its drainage by the vascular tissues around the endolymphatic duct. This obstruction is caused by scarring of the vascular mechanism, probably as a result of infection.

The majority of persons who have Ménière's syndrome are between 30 and 60 years of age. No sex or race is immune. Generally the involvement is limited to one side; only about 10% of those afflicted have a bilateral disorder.

The signs and symptoms are of sudden onset, with severe vertigo that recurs in bouts lasting from minutes to days. They are precipitated by sudden movements of the head and usually associated with severe nausea and some vomiting. Considerable noise in the head (tinnitus) is experienced, and hearing is impaired in the affected ear. Nystagmus usually occurs during the attack. The frequency, severity, and duration of the attacks vary with each client.

These bouts of spontaneous vertigo, nausea, and vomiting (with tinnitus and impaired hearing) occur in attacks that may come at intervals of weeks or months and ultimately may disappear. The attacks cease when complete deafness occurs. The diagnosis is made on the basis of the history and the minimal physical signs as mentioned. Ménière's syndrome must be distinguished from tumors of the posterior fossa in the cerebellopontine angle, which simultaneously involve adjacent cranial nerves and the cerebellum. Caloric and audiometric tests should be performed to assist in making the diagnosis. Electronystagmography (ENG) is also commonly used.

## Treatment and nursing intervention

The client outcomes for treatment are the identification of specific circumstances that precipitate an attack, listing of measures implemented during an attack, detailing of symptoms requiring medical intervention, and specification of actions and principles related to safety during vertigo. Clients should also be able to inform you on the use, dosage, side effects, and therapeutic outcomes related to their prescriptive medications.

The treatment is directed toward reduction of the endolymphatic pressure by opening up the impaired drainage system. This is accomplished by the use of vasodilator drugs, of which nicotinic

acid is often administered. Other commonly used antivertiginous medications include dimenhydrinate (Dramamine), diphenhydramine hydrochloride (Benadryl), nicotinyl alcohol–trimethobenzamide hydrochloride (Tigacol), and meclizine–nicotinic acid (Antivert). In more severe attacks, Dramamine or Benadryl may be given parenterally. Intramuscular injections of atropine sulfate abate symptoms in about 20 minutes by controlling causative impulses from the autonomic nervous system.

Diuretics and the restriction of fluid intake are also advocated, but their therapeutic effect is questionable. Simultaneously, sedation is given as necessary as a palliative measure, and fluids are administered parenterally if vomiting has persisted for some time. Since the excessive use of tobacco and alcohol may be a contributing factor, they should be used with moderation.

The severe cases may have to be treated surgically by the intracranial division of the vestibular portion of the acoustic nerve. This is performed through a small opening in the occipital bone of the side affected. The dura is incised, and the cerebellum is retracted medially to expose the lower cranial nerves. The acoustic nerve is identified, and its vestibular portion is divided between the internal auditory meatus and the pons. The wound is closed with interrupted silk sutures in the various layers, and a dressing is applied. Dietary measures based on low salt intake with supplementary ammonium or potassium chloride have been tried.

During the past few years, another surgical treatment has been developed with some success. With the client under local anesthesia the mastoid bone is opened, and sufficient bone is removed to permit the introduction of a treatment rod and an ultrasonic beam into the lateral semicircular canal. (This technique is described by James and his associates.) The ultrasonic beam causes selective destruction of the vestibular apparatus without injuring the cochlear division. Labyrinthine circulation is improved, the attacks cease, and hearing is progressively restored. Extreme care must be exercised during the procedure to prevent trauma to the facial nerve. After this treatment, fluids are limited to 1 liter each 24 hours. Salt, tea, and coffee are prohibited. (It is believed that these measures are necessary to prevent an increase in the secretion of endolymph.) Vitamin B complex is given for 3 months.

Another type of surgical treatment has been developed, but its use is limited to clients with unilateral symptoms and signs. The function of the inner ear is destroyed by transtympanic labyrinthotomy; the bouts of paroxysmal vertigo cease, and hearing is lost. This result also can be achieved by daily intratympanic injections of streptomycin for 1 week. Bilateral Ménière's syndrome may be treated by the parenteral administration of streptomycin sulfate. The labyrinth is destroyed selectively without destroying hearing.

Cryosurgical labyrinthectomy is another procedure accomplished through the ear canal without mastoidectomy. The procedure simulates that of ultrasonic surgery.

Nursing care is symptomatic and emphasizes the prevention of injury secondary to falling. When free of symptoms, the client is usually permitted to be ambulatory under supervision. If an attack occurs, encourage bed rest until all symptoms have disappeared. Some clients will need the added protection of side rails during this period. The duration of the paroxysmal vertigo and the associated symptoms may vary from minutes to hours to days. The individual client may receive some subjective relief by assuming certain positions and curtailing activity. If an operation has been performed, the nursing care is the same as that outlined in Chapter 26.

## BULBAR PARALYSIS (NINTH AND TENTH CRANIAL NERVES)

Involvement of the lower cranial nerves, principally the ninth and tenth, occurs in association with neoplastic, infectious, vascular, or degenerative diseases. The specific nursing care must be elaborated on according to the needs of the individual client and the presenting symptoms. Any or all of the manifestations discussed here may be present to a slight or pronounced degree.

The symptoms of *glossopharyngeal paralysis* are absent pharyngeal (gag) reflex; anesthesia of the base of the tongue, tonsils, and posterior part of the palate; loss of taste on the posterior part of the tongue; difficulty in swallowing; and increased salivation.

Symptoms of *vagal paralysis* are as follows:

speech difficulty (hoarse, nasal quality or loss of voice) caused by involvement of the muscles of the larynx, pharynx, or soft palate; difficulty in breathing; and vomiting or regurgitation of fluids and food.

### Treatment and nursing care

Medical and surgical treatment are directed toward removal of the cause if possible. The nursing care is symptomatic. The expected outcome is the prevention of complications.

*Complications.* (1) Aspiration of food or fluid after regurgitation, (2) respiratory difficulties, (3) swallowing difficulties, and (4) depression and fear.

Remain with the client whenever oral feedings are consumed to prevent aspiration of food or fluids after regurgitation. A suction machine should be available at the bedside at all times and used whenever necessary. The client is fed while lying on the side with only a 10-degree head elevation. Tube feedings may be necessary; insert the nasal tube with great care because of the laryngeal paralysis. Special oral hygiene is administered at least every 2 hours and after each oral feeding.

Respiratory difficulties may be further aggravated by the aspiration of fluid or food. Tracheostomy may have to be resorted to as a preventive or therapeutic measure. Increased susceptibility to infection is present. Respiratory failure may occur, but the respirator is of little, if any, avail. It is important for the nurse to note and report any change in respiratory function.

To prevent swallowing difficulties, make food puréed, moist, and easily assimilated. Observe the client for choking. Keep an accurate record of intake. Diet should be regulated according to the client's needs.

The client may be apprehensive and fearful of dying. Refer to the section on death for therapeutic considerations. If death is imminent, an opportunity should be afforded the client to see his or her spiritual advisor.

### REFERENCES

Abbott, M., and Killeffer, F.A.: Symptomatic trigeminal neuralgia, Bull. Los Angeles Neurol. Soc. **35:**1-10, Jan. 1970.

Ariagno, R.: Four years of ultrasound in Ménière's disease, Arch. Otolaryngol. **76:**18-22, 1962.

Barnett, S.B., and Kossoff, G.: Round window ultrasonic treatment of Ménière disease, Arch. Otolaryngol. **103**:124, March 1977.

Barraquer, B.: The physiopathogenesis of idiopathic trigeminal neuralgia and its bearing on the effect of carbamazepine in this indication. In Birkmayer, W., editor: Epileptic seizures—behaviour, pain, Baltimore, 1976, University Park Press.

Bonduelle, M.: Current approaches to the treatment of trigeminal neuralgia. In Birkmayer, W., editor: Epileptic seizures—behaviour, pain, Baltimore, 1976, University Park Press.

Cambier, J., et al.: Trigeminal neuralgia in comparison with other forms of lightning pain. In Birkmayer, W., editor: Epileptic seizures—behaviour, pain, Baltimore, 1976, University Park Press.

Carney, L.R.: Considerations on the cause and treatment of trigeminal neuralgia, Neurology **17**:1143-1151, 1967.

Chawla, J.C., and Falconer, M.A.: Glossopharyngeal and vagal neuralgia, Br. Med. J. **3**:529-531, 1967.

Coleman, C.C., and Walker, J.C.: Technic of anastomosis of the branches of the facial nerve with the spinal accessory for facial paralysis, Ann. Surg. **131**:960-968, 1950.

Cracovaner, A.J.: Nonsurgical management of Ménière's disease, N.Y. State Med. **62**:1435-1439, 1962.

Crary, W.G.: Ménière disease and cerebral impairment, Arch. Otolaryngol. **102**:368, June 1976.

DeWeese, D.D., and Saunders, W.H.: Textbook of otolaryngology, ed. 4, St. Louis, 1973, The C.V. Mosby Co.

Dix, M.R., and Hallpike, C.S.: Discussion of acoustic neuroma, Proc. R. Soc. Med. **51**:889-899, 1958.

Dohlmann, G.F.: On the mechanism of Ménière attack, Arch. Otorhinolaryngol. **212**:301, Sept. 16, 1976.

Dooley, D., and Browder, J.: A modification of the Tiffany operation for tic douloureux, J. Neurosurg. **19**:414-418, 1962.

Ecker, A., and Perl, T.: Alcohol injection for trigeminal neuralgia, J.A.M.A. **231**:811, Feb. 24, 1975.

Freese, A.S.: Microsurgery: new insight in medicine, Today's Health **46**:43, 80-82, Oct. 1968.

Frew, J.C.: Betahistine chloride in Ménière's disease, Postgrad. Med. J. **52**:501, Aug. 1976.

Garcia-Bengochea, F.: Surgical avenues leading to relief of trigeminal neuralgia, Geriatrics **30**:99, Aug. 1975.

Geldard, F.A.: Sensory saltation: metastability in the perceptual world, New York, 1976, Halsted Press.

Goldberg, M.J.: Emotional factors contributing to facial paralysis, J. Am. Geriatr. Soc. **20**:324-329, July 1962.

Goldstein, N.P., Gibilisco, J.A., and Rushton, J.G.: Trigeminal neuropathy and neuritis, J.A.M.A. **184**:458-462, 1963.

Hallpike, C.S.: The caloric tests, J. Laryngol. Otol. **70**:15-28, 1956.

Hanes, W.: Tic douloureux: a new theory of etiology and treatment: report of 40 cases, J. Oral Surg. **20**:222-232, 1962.

Haye, R., and Quist-Hanssen, S.: The natural course of Ménière's disease, Acta Otolaryngol. **82**:289, 1976.

Herman, L., et al.: Static compliance of the eardrum in Ménière's disease, Arch. Otolaryngol. **103**:84, Feb. 1977.

Klockhoff, I.: Diagnosis of Ménière's disease, Arch. Otorhinolaryngol. **212**:309, Sept. 16, 1976.

Leibowitz, U.: Bell's palsy—two disease entities? Neurology **16**:1105-1109, 1966.

McKenzie, K.G., and Alexander, E.: Restoration of facial function by nerve anastomosis, Ann. Surg. **132**:411-415, 1950.

Nelson, J.R.: The minimal ice water caloric test, Neurology **19**:577-585, 1969.

Ostrow, L.S.: New hope for patients with trigeminal neuralgia, Am. J. Nurs. **76**:1301, Aug. 1976.

Rothman, K.J., and Manson, R.R.: Epidemiology of trigeminal neuralgia, J. Chronic Dis. **26**:3-12, 1973.

Sheldon, M., et al.: Treatment of Bell palsy with prednisone: a prospective, randomized study, Neurology **28**:158-161, Feb. 1978.

Stahle, J.: Ménière's disease: allergy, immunology, psychosomatic, hypo- and hypertonus, Arch. Otorhinolaryngol. **212**:287, Sept. 16, 1976.

Taarnhøj, P.: Decompression of the trigeminal root, J. Neurosurg. **11**:299-305, 1954.

Tytus, J.S.: Trigeminal neuralgia. In Youmans, J.: Neurological surgery, vol. 3, Philadelphia, 1973, W.B. Saunders Co.

Wepsic, J.G.: Tic douloureux: etiology, refined treatment, N. Engl. J. Med. **288**:680-681, 1973.

Wersäll, J.: Ménière's disease—concluding remarks, Arch. Otorhinolaryngol. **212**:393, Sept. 16, 1976.

Whiteman, M.: Bell's palsy, Am. J. Nurs. **71**:2139-2140, 1971.

Wilbrand, J.: Ménière's disease, Arch. Otorhinolaryngol. **212**:331, Sept. 16, 1976.

# PART SIX

# INVASIVE DISORDERS

# 20
# INFECTIOUS PROCESSES

Infectious agents that invade the body may cause various abnormal neurological responses. When the meninges of the spinal cord or brain are involved, the outcome is meningitis, encephalitis, or a combination of the two, unless the infectious process is localized into an abscess. Primary or secondary involvement of the nervous system may occur when acute myelitis exists. Undesirable neurological responses are also evident with the cutaneous eruptions of herpes zoster. Normal pressure hydrocephalus is included here because it is a possible outcome of bacterial meningitis. Rheumatic fever may be associated with extreme discomfort and involuntary movements of Sydenham's chorea. Preventable infectious processes include poliomyelitis, botulism, rabies, and tetanus.

## INFLAMMATORY DISORDERS

### MENINGITIS

Meningitis is an acute inflammation of the pia-arachnoid membrane in the spinal cord or brain. A variety of agents may be responsible for meningeal infection, including bacteria, protozoa, yeasts, viruses, and fungi. These agents most commonly affect the meninges as a secondary site, with the primary force remaining elsewhere in the body. Meningitis is a possible outcome of a variety of clinical conditions. Some of these are infections involving the head and face: otitis media, mastoiditis, ruptured brain abscess, sinus infections, orbital infections, and tonsillitis. Individuals who have a generalized sepsis may also experience involvement of the meninges. Infections in the bones, skin, lungs, or heart valves may be conveyed to the meninges by the vascular system. Meningitis

caused by skin flora may result when a dermal tract or sinus connects the skin to the spinal coverings. Contamination of the meninges may also be an outcome of a skull fracture in a few instances. Meningitis may result from direct implantation of the infectious agent through such mechanisms as trauma or surgery. Military personnel in combat situations may develop meningitis because penetrating head wounds provide a portal of entry for infectious agents. One of the most virulent, rapidly progressing forms of bacterial meningitis is meningococcal meningitis. It is encountered in "pockets" of the population in a sporadic form. At times other bacterial meningitides, such as *Haemophilus influenzae,* may have a rampant course resembling that of meningococcal meningitis, but the rapid picture of deterioration is not so common. Various forms of viral meningitis are prevalent, especially during the warm summer months.

### Characteristic findings

When an individual has meningitis, symptoms are contained in four main categories, including (1) infection, (2) meningeal inflammation, (3) alterations in behavioral capacities and the level of consciousness, and (4) abnormal neurological findins.

*Infection* is evident by a gradual onset of fever of either high or low grade, though temperature changes are just as commonly absent in infants. The practitioner may also be aware of a possible infection as a seemingly minor ailment results in progressively severe symptoms. As the temperature rises, the metabolic rate increases, with resulting presence of such symptoms as rash, malaise, lethargy, tachycardia, and chills.

*Meningeal inflammation* is evident clinically in

the form of fever, headache, stiffness in the back and neck, and pain on forced movement of the neck. Two classic signs—Kernig's and Brudzinski's—are utilized to ascertain the presence of meningeal inflammation. *Kernig's sign* is elicited as the client lies in a supine position while the practitioner flexes one leg at the hip and knee and then straightens the knee. Pain caused by or resistance to this maneuver indicates the presence of disc disease or meningeal inflammation.

To elicit *Brudzinski's sign,* the client is placed in a dorsal recumbent position. The practitioner puts the hands behind the client's head and flexes the neck forward, noting any pain or resistance, since these signs indicate the presence of meningeal irritation, neck injury, or arthritis. Moreover, the practitioner should note whether the maneuver results in flexion at the client's hips and knees, since such reactive flexion indicates the presence of meningeal inflammation.

*Alterations in the level of consciousness or in behavioral capacities* are frequently observed in cases of meningitis. Because of limited capacities for verbalization and immaturity, such changes are more difficult to evaluate in infants and young children. However, age-appropriate tests and activities and reports from parents assist the practitioner in assessing such abnormalities.

*Abnormal neurological findings* may include a broad spectrum of symptoms that vary from case to case. Interruption in cranial nerve, sensory, or motor functions; alterations in deep and superficial reflexes; and the presence of specific foci resulting in seizures are some of the main types of problems that occur. Although convulsions may accompany meningitis at any age, the occurrence of generalized convulsions is a frequent event in infants who have meningitis.

Increased intracranial pressure often accompanies meningitis. (Chapter 21 offers a complete discussion of increased intracranial pressure.) If infants have increased intracranial pressure, they may not have the total number of symptoms spelled out in textbooks. Thus it is easy to disregard the presence of increased intracranial pressure in the early stages. When present, infants often have symptoms that include full, tense fontanels, irritability, crying on position change, headache, vomiting, diplopia, and other ophthalmic problems, as discussed in Chapter 13.

In older children and adults with increased intracranial pressure the sutures in the cranial vault are securely knit. Thus signs of increased intracranial pressure proceed more rapidly and often include behavioral changes, papilledema, cracked-pot sound when the skull is percussed, slowed pulse, and changes in the breathing pattern.

*In summary,* infants with meningitis may have few concrete signs of meningeal irritation and frequently have a temperature that is either normal or minimally altered. Early signs often include decreased desire and quantity of feeding, irritability, grimacing, lethargy, high-pitched cry, and crying when the position is changed. Fontanels may be full and tense, but vomiting may or may not be present. In older individuals, neurological abnormalities and meningeal irritation are obvious at an early point. Early signs often include headache, low-grade fever, and a stiff neck that becomes painful with movement. However, practitioners should be alert to the fact that shock may be the first recognizable symptom in meningitis, especially in infants with fulminating cases.

### Cerebrospinal fluid analysis

Once meningitis is suspected, the client should receive priority attention in having spinal fluid drawn and analyzed, since promptness is imperative in some types of meningitis to minimize neurological sequelae and severity of the disease process.

In Chapter 2 the cerebrospinal fluid was discussed in relation to normal components. In this section it is discussed in relation to invasive and inflammatory processes.

Before the spinal fluid is obtained, the practitioner should examine the eyes for papilledema. When papilledema is present, the puncture site of choice may be the cistern or ventricles instead of the lumbar area. Wherever the site, the cerebrospinal fluid is obtained *before* antibiotics are administered and *analyzed immediately* for cell types and quantity, gross appearance, quantity of glucose and protein, and presence of microscopic organisms. An immediate determination of the presence and type of bacterial organisms is made as a stained smear of centrifuged sediment is viewed microscopically.

Manometric pressure determinations are made, especially at the beginning of the procedure, since differences in pressure add data assistive in distinguishing space-occupying lesions from meningitis.

Simultaneously, cerebrospinal fluid is placed in aerobic and anaerobic cultures, so that ideal growth conditions prevail to provide proliferation for identification of the causative agent. Because these tests require time, results are not available when the initial treatment begins. Thus initial therapy is formulated when the data immediately available are considered: gross appearance of fluid, type and number of white blood cells, glucose and protein count, and prevalence of certain meningitides in a given age group.

Tables 20-1 and 20-2 are valuable in determining cerebrospinal fluid characteristics in health and disease. However, there are some general facts that assist in identifying the causative problem in a presumptive manner before the availability of cultures.

If the cerebrospinal fluid appears grossly normal on visual inspection but the manometric pressure reading is elevated, bacterial meningitis, except for the tubercular form, is excluded. To distinguish the tubercular form from another nonbacterial inflammatory agent, one need only look at the glucose content in cerebrospinal fluid. When the glucose content is normal, attention is focused on such differential considerations as mumps meningoencephalitis, subdural hematoma, syphilis, lead poisoning, neoplasm, meningism, and brain abscess, wherein no meningeal inflammation is evident.

Three conditions produce cerebrospinal fluid that has a milky, iridescent quality: tuberculous meningitis, meningococcal meningitis, and poliomyelitis. In *tuberculous meningitis* the abnormal appearance of cerebrospinal fluid is accompanied by a disturbed sensorium, a diminished glucose content, and a dominance of lymphocytes, even though polymorphonuclear cells may be more abundant in the early stages of disease. When tuberculous meningitis is suspected, one carefully evaluates the history, chest radiograph, and tuberculin test for positive findings. Even when none of these factors points to tuberculosis, one cannot disregard tuberculous meningitis as a diagnostic possibility. Although the cerebrospinal fluid in *meningococcal meningitis* is visibly like that found in tuberculous meningitis, the similarity only lasts for the first few hours. By that time the cerebro-

spinal fluid analysis in meningococcal meningitis is strikingly different. Although the appearance of cerebrospinal fluid is similar in tuberculous meningitis and *poliomyelitis,* such features as normal sensorium and normal to elevated cerebrospinal fluid glucose content quickly distinguish these two problems. At a preliminary glance, tuberculous meningitis may also resemble lymphocytic choriomeningitis, except that the second condition is characterized by rapid onset of symptoms and a normal cerebrospinal fluid glucose content.

It is also helpful to know what the various forms of bacteria look like when stained and studied under the microscope. *Meningococcal organisms* are the only gram-negative cocci; other common meningitis-producing organisms such as streptococci, staphylococci, and pneumococci are gram positive. Meningococci are also characterized by a location within a pus cell. At times *Haemophilus influenzae* has been mistaken for meningococci because of its pleomorphic shape. However, *H. influenzae* is easily distinguished from meningococci because of its location outside pus cells and because it stains gram negatively. A further bit of evidence may be had if a drop of *H. influenzae* is mixed with *H. influenzae* type B antiserum, since this mixture results in a swollen capsule around the organism.

Although pneumococcal, streptococcal, and staphylococcal organisms are all gram-positive cocci, they are readily distinguished when stained and studied under a microscope. *Pneumococci* are lancet-shaped gram-positive cocci that appear most commonly in pairs. *Streptococci* are gram-positive cocci that appear in chains, and *staphylococci* are gram-positive cocci found in clumps.

If *tubercle bacilli* are suspected, the routine culture procedure does not reveal these organisms. Thus cerebrospinal fluid should be allowed to stand for 12 to 24 hours to form a web (pellicle), and staining for acid-fast bacteria should be done.

## Major types of meningitis

*Meningococcal meningitis.* Meningococcal meningitis, a virulent, rampant disease originating in the nasopharynx, is also termed cerebrospinal fever, epidemic meningitis, and spotted fever. Most of the material reaching the public refers to this type of meningitis when this subject is addressed, and this fact is not surprising in view of

*Text continued on p. 508.*

**TABLE 20-1.** General profiles of common neurological problems*†

| Condition | Pressure (mm H₂O) | Appearance | Cells | Protein levels (mg/dl) | Glucose levels (mg/dl) | Culture | Chloride levels | Comments |
|---|---|---|---|---|---|---|---|---|
| Normal | 40-200 | Clear | 0-5/mm³ lymphocytes | 15-40 | 40-80 | Negative | 110-128 mEq/L, 650-750 mg/dl | CSF glucose level varies with blood glucose level |
| Normal for perinatal period | 40-200 | Clear or blood-tinged | Varies; 0-25/mm³ polymorphonuclear neutrophils; 0-700/mm³ red blood cells | 40-120 | 40-80 | Negative | Normal | CSF glucose level varies with blood glucose level |
| Normal for neonate | 40-200 | Clear | 0-15/mm³; mainly polymorphonuclear neutrophils | 20-70 | 40-80 | Negative | Normal | CSF glucose level varies with blood glucose level |
| Meningism | Increased | Clear | Normal, lymphocytes | Normal | Normal | Negative | Normal | No pathogenic organisms |
| "Bloody tap" | Normal | Red, clears in later tubes | Red and white blood cells same as peripheral circulation | Normal or slightly increased | Normal | Negative | Normal | Negative benzidine reaction on supernatant |
| Bacterial | Usually increased | Turbid | 500/mm³, mainly polymorphonuclear neutrophils | High | Low or absent | May be aerobic or anaerobic growth | 103-116 mEq/L, 600-680 mg/dl | Stained smears and cultures positive (Table 20-2) |
| Viral | Normal or moderately increased | Clear | Usually less than 500/mm³; early more polymorphonuclear neutrophils, later more lymphocytes | Slightly increased | Normal | Negative | Normal | Special techniques needed to isolate virus |
| Mycotic | Moderately increased | Clear or cloudy | Normal or increased, lymphocytes alone or mixed with polymorphonuclear neutrophils | Elevated | Low | | | Need Sabouraud's agar to culture fungi: India ink preparation for cryptococci |
| Spirochete (syphilis) | Normal or slightly increased | Clear or turbid | 25-2000/mm³; mostly lymphocytes | Normal to elevated | Normal | Negative, occasional spirochete | Normal | CSF and serum Wassermann tests often positive |
| Acid-fast bacteria (tuberculosis) | Increased | Clear or opalescent | 30-500/mm³; early mostly polymorphonuclear neutrophils; later all lymphocytes | Increased | 10-20 | Dubos medium results in growth | Early normal; later 94-110 mEq/L, 550-650 mg/dl | Undisturbed CSF often forms pellicle |
| Poliomyelitis | Normal to increased | Clear or opalescent | 15-400/mm³; early polymorphonuclear neutrophils, later mainly lymphocytes | 30-60; later 100-600 | Normal | | Normal | Special studies needed on stool and serum from clients in acute and convalescing stages |

*From Conway, B.L.: Pediatric neurologic nursing. St. Louis, 1977, The C.V. Mosby Co.
†Research continues on the practicality and reliability of counterimmunoelectrophoresis (CIE) of urine, gastric aspirate, blood, serum, and

**TABLE 20-2.** General findings in meningitis*

| Problem | Infectious agent | Classification | CSF findings | Comments |
|---|---|---|---|---|
| Meningococcal meningitis (spotted fever; epidemic meningitis; cerebrospinal fever) | *Neisseria meningitidis (intracellularis)* | Bacteria | Gram-negative cocci found, in pus cells<br>Pressure increased<br>Appearance purulent<br>Cells 500-20,000/mm³; predominately polymorphonuclear neutrophils<br>Protein levels increased<br>Glucose level diminished or absent | Transmission by droplet spray; meningitis preceded by meningococcemia<br>Associated problems: conjunctivitis, joint effusion, Waterhouse-Friderichsen syndrome, toxic myocarditis, or other complications of meningitis; purpuric lesions containing microorganism associated<br>Course rapid and often fulminating; immediate treatment with penicillin G or sulfonamides required |
| Pneumococcal meningitis | Pneumococcus *(Diplococcus pneumoniae)* | Bacteria | Lancet-shaped gram-positive cocci often in pairs<br>Pressure increased<br>Appearance purulent<br>Cells 500⁺/mm³; mainly polymorphonuclear neutrophils<br>Protein levels increased<br>Glucose levels diminished or absent | Characteristic cocci apparent on stained smear; growth of cocci on cultures<br>Frequently follows pneumococcal infection of lungs, upper respiratory tract sinuses, or middle ear or skull fracture<br>Associated problems: abscess, empyema, or general complications of meningitis, mastoidectomy possibly needed<br>Treatment with penicillin therapy required<br>Onset less pronounced than meningococcal type |
| Streptococcal meningitis | Streptococcus | Bacteria | Gram-positive cocci appearing in chains<br>Pressure increased<br>Appearance purulent<br>Cells 500⁺/mm³; mainly polymorphonuclear neutrophils<br>Protein levels increased<br>Glucose levels diminished or absent | Characteristic cocci apparent on stained smear and in growth on cultures<br>Secondary to primary infection of upper respiratory tract, sinuses, or mastoid process; may be transmitted to neonate through infected cord or break in integrity of mother's genital or breast skin |
| Staphylococcal meningitis | Staphylococcus | Bacteria | Gram-positive cocci in clumps<br>Pressure increased<br>Appearance purulent<br>Cells 500⁺/mm³; mainly polymorphonuclear neutrophils<br>Protein levels increased<br>Glucose levels diminished or absent | Cocci on stained smears and culture; *Staphylococcus aureus* coagulase-positive meningitis rare, severe, and requires rapid, vigorous treatment with penicillin or sulfadiazine |

*From Conway, B.L.: Pediatric neurologic nursing, St. Louis, 1977, The C.V. Mosby Co.          *Continued.*

**TABLE 20-2.** General findings in meningitis—cont'd

| Problem | Infectious agent | Classification | CSF findings | Comments |
|---|---|---|---|---|
| Staphylococcal meningitis— cont'd | | | | Staphylococcal meningitis of coagulase-negative type associated with breaks in skin integrity (dermal fistula, open myelodysplastic problem); insertion of foreign object through neurosurgery, that is, shunt; *Staphylococcus aureus* coagulase-positive infection after furuncles, bacteremias, and so on<br>Associated problems: abscesses, empyemas, and general complications of meningitis<br>Course depends on disease severity and success of treatment<br>Treatment with penicillin therapy of choice |
| Tuberculous meningitis | *Mycobacterium tuberculosis* | Acid-fast bacteria | Culture of tubercle bacillus on Dubos medium grows more rapidly; CSF sitting undisturbed for 12-24 hours forms web (pellicle)<br>Pressure increased<br>Appearance clear or opalescent<br>Cells 30-500/mm³; early up to 30% polymorphonuclear neutrophils, later all lymphocytes<br>Protein levels increased<br>Glucose levels diminished | Stain for acid-fast bacteria and culture positive<br>History of exposure to infected adult; positive chest radiograph or tuberculin test<br>Prolonged treatment with isoniazid (INH), *p*-aminosalicylic acid (PAS), streptomycin sulfate, or rifampin<br>Course usually involves recovery with adequate treatment; recurrence possible |
| *Haemophilus influenzae* meningitis | *Haemophilus influenzae* type B | Bacteria | Pleomorphic, gram-negative rods resembling cocci but found outside pus cells<br>Pressure increased<br>Appearance purulent<br>Cells 500⁺/mm³; mainly polymorphonuclear neutrophils<br>Protein levels increased<br>Glucose levels diminished or absent | Stained smear and culture positive; swollen capsule when mixed with type B antiserum; cultures of nose, throat, and blood often positive<br>Especially common from ages 3 months to 6 years<br>Accompanies upper respiratory infection of agent<br>Course insidious or fulminating<br>Associated problems: general complications of meningitis<br>Disease severity proportional to degree CSF glucose levels lowered<br>Treatment of choice usually ampicillin, unless strain is resistant |
| *Escherichia coli* meningitis | *Escherichia coli* | Bacteria | Gram-negative rods<br>Pressure increased<br>Appearance purulent<br>Cells 500⁺/mm³; mainly polymorphonuclear neutrophils<br>Protein levels increased | Smear of CSF showing many microorganisms; growth on culture media rapid<br>Often associated with history of urinary tract infection, infected cord, open myelodysplastic problem, or diaper rash pyoderma |

**TABLE 20-2.** General findings in meningitis—cont'd

| Problem | Infectious agent | Classification | CSF findings | Comments |
|---|---|---|---|---|
| *Escherichia coli* meningitis—cont'd | | | Glucose levels diminished or absent | Complications are those generally associated with meningitis<br>Course depends on disease severity<br>Antimicrobial therapy determined by sensitivity testing |
| *Klebsiella pneumoniae* (Friedlander's bacillus) meningitis | *Klebsiella pneumoniae* | Bacteria | Gram-negative rods<br>Pressure increased<br>Appearance purulent<br>Cells 500$^+$/mm³; mainly polymorphonuclear neutrophils<br>Protein levels increased<br>Glucose levels decreased or absent | Clinically similar to *E. coli*<br>Culture and sensitivity testing required to identify microorganism and appropriate antimicrobial therapy |
| *Listeria monocytogenes* meningitis | *Listeria monocytogenes* | Bacteria | Nonsporeforming gram-positive rods<br>Pressure increased<br>Appearance purulent<br>Cells 500$^+$/mm³; mainly polymorphonuclear neutrophils<br>Protein levels increased<br>Glucose levels decreased or absent | Rod found on stained smear and in culture<br>Course similar to other purulent meningitides<br>Treatment possibly including penicillin and erythromycin or tetracyclines |
| Acute syphilitic meningitis | *Treponema pallidum* | Spirochete | Occasional spirochete found; Wassermann CSF test often positive<br>Pressure normal to increased<br>Appearance clear or opalescent<br>Cells normal to 200/mm³; mostly lymphocytes<br>Protein levels normal to increased<br>Glucose levels normal | Wasserman blood test often positive<br>Acute or subacute onset<br>Three main types: (1) acute basilar meningitis, involving meninges at base of brain and causing cranial nerve impairment; (2) acute vertical meningitis, involving meninges over vertex and causing headache, nausea, vomiting, and convulsions; and (3) acute syphilitic hydrocephalus, involving meninges of posterior fossa and resulting in headache, nausea, vomiting, and choked discs<br>Incidence of this type of menigitis decreased by adequate treatment of primary syphilis; vigorous treatment with penicillin results in rapid recovery; residual damage possibly remaining |
| Benign lymphocytic choriomeningitis | Virus | Virus | Culture negative<br>Pressure increased<br>Appearance clear or cloudy<br>Cells 100-1500/mm³; mostly lymphocytes | Transmission by infected mice or blood-sucking insects that bite infected dogs, then humans; rare west of Mississippi river<br>Acute course lasting about 1 week |

*Continued.*

**TABLE 20-2.** General findings in meningitis—cont'd

| Problem | Infectious agent | Classification | CSF findings | Comments |
|---|---|---|---|---|
| Benign lymphocytic choriomeningitis—cont'd | | | Protein levels elevated<br>Glucose levels normal<br>Chloride levels normal | Treatment symptomatic; recovery usually complete |
| Aseptic meningitis syndrome | Enteric cytopatho-genic human orphan (ECHO) virus | Virus | Pressure normal or increased<br>Appearance clear<br>Cells less than 1000/mm³; early mainly polymorpho-nuclear neutrophils, later 85⁺% lymphocytes<br>Protein levels normal or slightly high<br>Glucose levels normal | Special studies on stool or antibody studies on serum from clients in acute and convalescing stage required to isolate organism<br>Transmission by enteric-oral pathway<br>Possible morbilliform rash that does not itch; mainly on face and trunk<br>Rapid onset<br>Acute course lasting about a week<br>Treatment symptomatic only |
| Aseptic meningitis syndrome | Coxsackie group A or B virus | Virus | Pressure normal or increased<br>Appearance clear<br>Cells 500 or less/mm³; mainly lymphocytes<br>Protein levels normal or increased<br>Glucose levels normal | Special studies on stool or antibody studies on serum from clients in acute or convalescing stage required to isolate organism<br>Transmission by enteric-oral pathway<br>Chest or abdominal pain possibly evident early; rapid onset of disease<br>Process lasting about 1 week<br>Transient paresis occurring rarely<br>Treatment symptomatic |

the rampant course and extreme effect that this organism has on the client. Weather conditions in winter and spring and crowded living conditions are factors that enhance the incidence of the four types of meningitis, resulting from *Neisseria meningitidis (intracellularis)*. This organism spreads by droplet spray from the mouth and nose of either healthy carriers or individuals with a mild upper respiratory infection caused by this organism. Before symptoms of meningitis are evident, mild to severe meningococcemia occurs. During this time a lumbar puncture may yield normal findings in cerebrospinal fluid even though this changes within a few hours when the meninges are invaded. When meningococcemia is present, the condition may be so severe that Waterhouse-Friderichsen syndrome (hemorrhages in the adrenal cortex with possible fatality) may occur even before the meninges are invaded. When the meninges do become involved, large amounts of purulent inflammation are evident. There are several undesirable

outcomes that frequently accompany this disease, including the flattened, engorged gyri related to increased intracranial pressure evident on autopsy, communicating hydrocephalus from destruction of the subarachnoid space, abnormalities in the cranial nerves, deafness, arthritis, toxic myocarditis, and conjunctivitis.

Within hours of onset the client experiences a rapid downhill course that often includes severe headache, projectile vomiting, high fever, and rapid alterations in the level of consciousness up to and including coma. Rigidity of the neck and back is often noticeable, and convulsions are common. The characteristic purpuric skin lesions may occur either during the fulminating stage of meningococcemia or during the meningeal invasion. Whenever they occur, the lesions should be aspirated for culture and microscopic study, since the organism resides within them.

Because of limited communication capacities, any infant or young child with a fever, an increased white blood cell count, and changes in behavior and level of consciousness who has a concurrent upper respiratory tract infection should have a lumbar puncture performed to discount the possibility of a meningococcal invasion.

In treating this virulent disease the antibiotics of choice are penicillin G and the sulfonamides. Sterile, painful joint effusions occur in about 5% of the clients affected with meningococci. Symptomatic relief may be provided by paracentesis, but spontaneous reabsorption of fluid occurs even without intervention. If the client develops conjunctivitis, the treatment includes cool compresses, the instillation of prescribed pharmacological agents, eye rest, and dark glasses. No known treatment is available for toxic myocarditis. If the client is affected by the Waterhouse-Friderichsen syndrome, the outcome is poor. In these cases, adrenal steroids and epinephrine have been utilized as part of the intervention modality. For individuals who have had intimate contact with the client affected by meningococci, see Table 20-4.

Nursing management is outlined in a general section at the end of the specific meningitides. Naturally, holistic nursing approaches and total support, both physically and psychologically, are essential during the acute infectious process. Emotional support and education about the disease process are appropriate for the client, family, and community. This condition is reportable to public health authorities and should be reported promptly, so that contacts might receive immediate follow-up care.

*Gram-positive coccal meningitis.* The gram-positive cocci, including *pneumococci, streptococci, staphylococci,* result in a similar clinical picture and are frequently discussed together.

Usually the onset and course of the disease caused by these three agents are less severe than meningococcal meningitis, and a petechial rash is rare. The immediate history frequently includes infections in the ears, sinuses, upper respiratory tract, or other areas of the body. These agents are also common invaders in skull fractures and open types of myelodysplasia. Symptoms of meningitis are detailed earlier in this chapter.

A few characteristic features assist the practitioner in distinguishing these three agents. Pneumococcal meningitis most frequently occurs in children with sickle-cell disease, mastoiditis, or previous skull fractures and in those who have had two or more cases of purulent meningitis. A petechial rash and acute endocarditis are common findings in the child with streptococcal or staphylococcal meningitis. *Staphylococcal meningitis* of the coagulase-negative variety is often found wherein the subarachnoid space has a portal at the skin, as in instances of dermal fistulas (Chapter 13). When this problem is evident, wherein a foreign body has not been introduced through prior neurosurgery, the practitioner should carefully examine the client to eliminate the portal of contamination and subsequent infections. *Staphylococcus aureus* meningitis is a rare, rampant, infectious process that begins in the upper respiratory tract and results in bacteremia and abscesses in the central nervous system.

The characteristics that are assistive in diagnosis have been previously discussed. Treatment usually involves large doses of penicillin but is symptomatic for concurrent problems. For example, incision and drainage are indicated in empyema or abscess formation, mastoidectomies are performed if meningitis is caused by pneumococci or streptococci. Complications include perceptual, motor, intellectual, and neurological dysfunctions to a different degree in each situation.

*Tuberculous meningitis.* Mycobacterium tuberculosis is the causative organism for tuberculous meningitis, a condition that is a distinct possibility in any child exposed to the adult form of pulmonary tuberculosis or who demonstrates a positive tuberculin skin test with disturbances in central nervous system functions.

The onset is gradual, and symptoms include irritability, drowsiness, and personality changes. As the disease course progresses, drowsiness proceeds to stupor, the temperature becomes elevated, and the associated increased intracranial pressure results in convulsions.

Ordinarily the symptoms normally associated with meningitis occur, with the addition of a tuberculous lesion and characteristic dermatographia, termed *tache cérébrale*. Diagnostic confirmation occurs when the tubercle bacillus is isolated from a pellicle of cerebrospinal fluid and when the culture or guinea pig inoculation with cerebrospinal fluid yields positive results.

The treatment regimen is prolonged and includes the necessity for long-term follow-up to detect recurrences. Several medications are effective against the tubercle bacillus, including isoniazid (INH), *p*-aminosalicylic acid (PAS), streptomycin sulfate, rifampin, and, in extreme cases, the addition of cortisone. Since the disease process is prolonged, positive steps, such as adequate diet, should be planned to maintain and promote health. Plans should also allow for diversion and reentry either into school or the vocational setting. Follow-up of possible contacts is imperative. Recovery is expected if intervention occurs in the early stages of disease. Death is certain in untreated clients.

*Haemophilus influenzae meningitis.* The type B strain of *Haemophilus influenzae* meningitis, a common problem in children from 3 months to 6 years of age, is suspected when irritability, unexplained temperature elevations, and high white blood cell counts accompany an upper respiratory tract infection. Other signs of meningitis may or may not be present. In certain clients, *H. influenzae* has a virulent course wherein there is high temperature, seizures, and delirium. As previously discussed, the working diagnosis is initially established as stained microorganisms appear as gram-negative pleomorphic rods under microscopic study. Although *H. influenzae* is sensitive to several antibiotics, ampicillin is usually the agent of choice, either alone or in combination with other antibiotics. The decision to use one or more antibiotics depends on the severity of the disease process and on the age of the child. In this disease, cultures of the nose, throat, and blood frequently reveal proliferation of the *H. influenzae* organism. Even in the elevation of the initial glucose count, one can gauge the severity of this disease process, since it is directly proportional to the decrease in cerebrospinal fluid glucose levels.

Complications occur in this type of meningitis, as in others. One particular problem frequently seen in this type of meningitis is subdural effusions, especially in those cases where treatment has been delayed or not vigorous enough. Another common problem is the development of otitis media, which may be treated with a myringotomy. Educators are noting a significant number of minor perceptual-motor and learning problems in the primary years of school, even in those children who seem to have weathered the infection without sequelae. However, in addition to these problems, one must carefully consider the care required by the client with an acute infection of the central nervous system as a priority.

*Gram-negative meningitis.* Several gram-negative organisms are common causative agents in meningitis, including *Escherichia coli, Pseudomonas aeruginosa, Klebsiella pneumoniae,* and *Proteus morgani.* Individuals with an inadequate immune mechanism are particularly susceptible to both enteric flora and pathogens prevalent in the hospital setting. These infections are most commonly associated with urinary tract infections in older children and with open myelodysplastic lesions, diaper-area pyoderma, and cord infection in infants.

In the majority of cases of sepsis or meningitis caused by a gram-negative organism the causative agent is *E. coli.* Gram-negative organisms present a particular threat to the neonate; thus a national neonatal meningitis study group has been formed to evaluate pharmacological intervention. The mortality in neonates has been sharply reduced by treatment combining ampicillin and gentamicin with or without intrathecal injections.

The source of contamination is usually revealed in the history. Symptoms are congruent with those seen in any type of meningitis. The treatment modality is contingent on the sensitivity of the bacteria to the antibiotic, client age, and disease severity. The outcome is directly related to disease severity and adequacy of management. Chronic problems and complications are related to the severity of the disease process. Nursing management is geared toward usual care of the client in the acute phase of meningitis, toward treatment of individual complications, and toward the developmental age of the child.

*Other bacterial meningitides.* *K. pneumoniae* (Friedländer's bacillus) may be a causative organism that produces a meningitis clinically similar to those types resulting from gram-negative rods. Only laboratory analysis distinguishes this type from that caused by gram-negative rods. Sensitivity tests should be performed to see if the medications prescribed at the time of the presumptive diagnosis are effective.

*Listeria monocytogenes* meningitis is a purulent bacterial type caused by gram-positive, rod-shaped, nonsporeforming bacteria. Pharmacological agents of choice include the tetracyclines or a combination of penicillin and erythromycin.

In rare instances, *acute syphilitic meningitis* develops within 1 to 2 years after the occurrence of a primary infection. This meningitis may be an outcome of either congenital syphilis or primary infection in an adult. This type of management may be prevented by adequate treatment of early syphilis.

***Benign lymphocytic and viral meningitides.*** Some types of meningitis require only symptomatic support during the acute stage of illness. These include benign lymphocytic choriomeningitis and meningitis related to the coxsackievirus and ECHO virus.

In benign lymphocytic choriomeningitis, viral transmission occurs through contact with infected mice or through dogs who have been bitten by blood-sucking insects and convey the virus to humans. Symptoms of meningitis and infection occur, such as fever, malaise, general aching, headache, fatigue, vomiting, nuchal rigidity, Kernig's sign, and alterations in the deep tendon reflexes that remain for 3 to 4 weeks. As is typical in viral meningitides, the cerebrospinal fluid is under increased pressure, and analysis reveals a normal glucose level and a slight increase in protein content. The cell count may vary from 100 to 1500 cells/mm$^3$, but lymphocytes outnumber other types. Acute symptoms are present for about 1 week. Clients typically recover completely.

The enteric cytopathogenic human orphan (ECHO) viruses are transmitted by the enteric-oral route. ECHO viruses are most prevalent during the summer months. When an ECHO virus is responsible for aseptic meningitis, the symptoms include high fever, headache, stiff neck, and the possible presence of a morbilliform rash on the face and trunk. Although the onset of symptoms is rapid, the acute phase is complete within 1 week. Intervention is symptomatic, and total recovery is usually anticipated. The cerebrospinal fluid reveals a normal to elevated pressure, a normal glucose level, and a normal to slightly elevated protein level. The cell count generally numbers less than 1000/mm$^3$, with a majority of polymorphonuclear cells early and a predominance of lymphocytes

later in the disease course. Although ordinary techniques for cultures do not reveal the organism, the virus can be isolated in feces or antibody studies of blood from clients during the acute stage or the period of recovery.

Like ECHO viruses the *coxsackieviruses* typically are present during the summer months and are transmitted by the enteric-oral pathway. Coxsackieviruses are either of the group A or B variety and may be responsible for a number of illnesses, including meningitis. In this type of meningitis the onset of symptoms is rapid and may include fever, nausea, vomiting, and headache. Chest or abdominal pain is commonly seen in the early stages of illness, with a subsequent stiffening of the back or neck within 1 day. In examining the cerebrospinal fluid one finds that except for pleocytosis, up to about 500/mm$^3$ with lymphocytes predominating, the cerebrospinal fluid is essentially normal. Preventive management includes maintenance of health through adequate nutrition and rest and avoidance of large crowds when the virus is prevalent. Intervention is symptomatic and may include such measures as the administration of analgesics or the application of warmth to the uncomfortable areas of the back or chest. Recovery is usually complete in this self-limiting illness, though transient weakness may result from the condition. Table 20-3 shows the distinguishing factors among the enteric viruses.

***Other types.*** In *partially treated meningitis,* enough pharmacological agents have been administered to confuse the picture without relieving the problem. The cerebrospinal fluid picture in these cases usually shows a relatively normal glucose level and a predominance of mononuclear cells. When further treatment is not administered, a re-

**TABLE 20-3.** Differentiating enteric viruses

| Virus | Characteristic |
|---|---|
| Poliomyelitis | Paresis or paralysis occurring more commonly than with coxsackieviruses |
| ECHO | Nonpruritic, red, discrete maculopapular rash often evident in first 5 days |
| Coxsackie | Often associated with herpangina or pericarditis-pleurodynia |

lapse occurs wherein the cerebrospinal fluid glucose level dips, and granulocytes predominate in the cerebrospinal fluid count.

*Fungal meningitis* occurs less often than bacterial and viral meningitis. However, when it is evident, it should be treated vigorously.

### Probability of age

Certain meningitides are most prevalent in given age ranges. When the initial studies of the cerebrospinal fluid do not indicate a specific pathogen, the practitioner orders an antibiotic or combination of medications that will combat the statistically most probable organism. In the age group from birth to 3 months, penicillin G and kanamycin or gentamicin are used. In the age group ranging from 3 months to 6 years, ampicillin is recommended. In the group from 6 to 21 years, penicillin G is utilized. However, practitioners should have current information to the effectiveness patterns of antibiotics, since resistant strains of organisms are being seen increasingly and since new medications are constantly becoming available.

### Pathology

Meningitis is an infection of the pia-arachnoid membrane caused by specific organisms, the most frequent of which are the meningococcus, staphylococcus, streptococcus, and pneumococcus. The pathology consists of an inflammatory reaction in the pia-arachnoid. The subarachnoid space contains cerebrospinal fluid, which is cloudy to milky white in appearance because of the abnormal increase of white blood cells. These may vary in number from a few hundred to 50,000/mm$^3$. Congestion of the adjacent brain tissue and degeneration of some nerve cells are present. The meningeal infection may be subsequent to a systemic infection disseminated through the bloodstream or by direct extension, as from infected paranasal sinuses.

### Treatment and nursing intervention

*Specific treatment* depends on the organism responsible for the infection, but general supportive measures such as bed rest, blood transfusions, necessary fluids, and nourishment should be administered. Specific antibiotic therapy is employed according to the causative organism. Anticonvul-

sant medication may be given to control seizures. Other manifestations or sequelae of meningitis are treated symptomatically. The client is placed in isolation of a respiratory type during the acute stage and as long as the cultures of the nasal secretions are positive (Table 20-4).

Since meningitis usually occurs after a primary infection, its *prevention is emphasized,* and the following practices are recommended: effective use of chemotherapy in the treatment of clients with sinus and ear infections; maintenance of strict aseptic technique during all intracranial, intraspinal, mastoid, and sinus operations; use of prophylactic antibiotics in the treatment of clients with head injuries accompanied by bleeding from any orifice; avoidance of overcrowding in schools, camps, and public gatherings, especially during the winter months; and protection of young children who live in a temperate zone by maintaining an adequate diet, wearing adequate clothing, and using supplementary vitamins as necessary to build up resistance to infection.

*Successful treatment depends on the early recognition and diagnosis of the disease.* The nurse, through observation of the client with an acute upper respiratory tract, sinus, or ear infection after severe head injury or after certain neurosurgical operations have been performed, can detect the onset of meningitis early and greatly expedite the administration of effective therapy by reporting significant symptoms to the physician immediately.

The *sequelae* that may persist are visual impairment, optic neuritis, hearing loss, personality changes, headache, convulsions, motor loss, and endocarditis. Their treatment is symptomatic and essentially supportive.

*Observations.* Variability of symptoms (such as nuchal rigidity, photophobia, irritability, headache, malaise, and changes in level of consciousness) is noted. The nurse watches for chills, body-temperature changes, and convulsions and describes them accurately; notes the amount of vomiting; checks the client for signs of dehydration; and records reactions to the medications administered orally, intramuscularly, or intravenously.

*Position.* The principles of posturing and turning should be applied and supportive devices used as described in Chapter 22 to ensure the client's

**TABLE 20-4.** Summary of nursing interventions and outcomes in meningitis

| Intervention | Expected outcome |
|---|---|
| 1. Data will be rapidly collected on:<br>  a. General physical condition, history, vital signs, neurological signs.<br>  b. Presence of meningitis alone or as outcome of another disease.<br>  c. Client age.<br>  d. Infectious agent.<br>  e. Time of disease existence.<br>  f. Responses to prior treatment.<br>  g. Severity and symptoms.<br>  h. Changes in behavioral patterns and levels of responsiveness, signs of bacterial shock, focal abnormalities, seizures, vomiting, increased intracranial pressure, other complications. | 1. Complications and disease severity are minimized. |
| 2. Appropriate treatment is instituted rapidly; monitoring continues as appropriate. | 2. Complications and disease severity are minimized; client will have total base-line and continuing assessments. |
| 3. Client is informed about meningitis and specific treatments; individual needs are met.<br>  a. Touch is used to reassure client.<br>  b. Age-appropriate techniques (games, conversation) are used to coach the client through novel and painful situations.<br>  c. Client and family are encouraged to verbalize and participate in needs assessment, diagnosis, care planning, implementation, and evaluation. | 3. Anxiety and fear of the unknown are decreased.<br>Client and family can describe disease process, individual response, treatment, and expected outcomes within the limits of illness and age levels. |
| 4. Physical needs are met.<br>  a. Room darkened for client with photophobia.<br>  b. Noise level decreased and cool head cloth provided for client with headache.<br>  c. Adequate body alignment, back rubs, and reposturing done to promote comfort.<br>  d. Bedding and clothing dry and free of wrinkles.<br>  e. Ambulation progresses from bed rest according to individual needs and capacities.<br>  f. Diet returns to predisease status in relation to disease and client response.<br>  g. Hydration status is adequate as determined by urinary quantity and concentration, skin turgor, condition of mouth and mucous membranes, and body weight.<br>  h. Overhydration is avoided.<br>  i. Bowel habits are regulated individually.<br>  j. Laboratory data is closely monitored and considered in treatment plans.<br>  k. Complications and worsening condition are detected and treated promptly.<br>  l. Temperature is normalized.<br>  m. Mouth and lip care are provided as a part of normal hygiene.<br>  n. Intake and output are monitored during the acute phase and throughout the illness for certain clients and children.<br>  o. Unit routines and isolation policies are explained and modified as possible to meet individual needs.<br>  p. Supportive treatment measures are based on symptoms and on client needs. | 4. Avoidable problems and discomforts are prevented.<br>Client cooperates with treatment plan.<br><br><br><br><br><br>The possibility of cerebral edema is decreased.<br>Client will have the benefit of any appropriate, available treatment. |
| 5. Safety.<br>  a. Respiratory isolation and contact isolation for lesions is maintained according to agency policy.<br>  b. Contacts are identified and treated with rifampin, therapeutic dosages of penicillin, or merely observed, according to physician or agency policies, when meningococcus is the infectious agent. | 5. The client will not harm self or others. |

*Continued.*

**TABLE 20-4.** Summary of nursing interventions and outcomes in meningitis—cont'd

| Intervention | Expected outcome |
|---|---|
| 5. Safety—cont'd | |
|    c. Cases of meningococcal and tuberculous meningitis are reported to the health department. | |
|    d. Seizure precautions are implemented when appropriate. | |
|    e. Measures appropriate to age, awareness, and orientation are taken to make the environment safe for the client and others. | |
| 6. Follow-up. | 6. The client will be free of infection. The effects of meningitis will be assessed. |
|    a. The client with recurring meningitis will be evaluated to find the reservoir of infection. | |
|    b. Testing and treatment will continue as appropriate while the client is infected. | |
|    c. Functional and intellectual testing will be done after the client is free of infection to ascertain any deficits in operational capacities. | |
| 7. Significant others. | 7. Fear of the unknown will be decreased. Individual will have access to all needed supportive services. |
|    a. Will be oriented to the unit and its routines. | |
|    b. Will be provided with assistance from helping resources, that is, social services, chaplain as required. | Negative feelings, misinformation, and blame-setting will be decreased. |
|    c. Receive thorough explanations of disease, treatment, and outcomes and will have opportunity for appropriate health care participation. | Continuity in interpersonal relations between significant others and health care personnel will be maintained. |
|    d. Will be able to express feelings of guilt, shock, disbelief, worry, and so on and receive factual information and therapeutic intervention as needed. | |
|    e. Be approached personally and systematically as they are involved in various aspects of the nursing process. | |
|    f. Have constant dialog with nurse and physician on disease process, client status, response to treatment, and individual needs. | |
|    g. Will receive written and verbal discharge plans and some type of planned follow-up after hospital discharge, as possible. | |

comfort and to prevent the development of complications.

*Nutrition.* A well-balanced diet, regulated to the needs of the client in the febrile and afebrile stages, is important in maintaining nutrition and in increasing resistance to the infection. Parenteral fluids may be necessary to supplement oral intake. If the client is receiving sulfonamide therapy or has an elevated temperature, the fluid intake is maintained at a level of 2500 to 3000 ml in each 24 hours. (Kidney complications are less likely to occur if adequate fluid is administered.) Small supplementary feedings are given between meals. If vomiting is a problem or if the client is unable to take oral feedings, a retention nasal tube is used, and a well-balanced tube feeding mixture is given. Supplementary vitamins may also be given to improve the metabolism of the nervous system.

*Hygiene.* Hygiene is administered as for any acutely ill febrile client. Special oral hygiene should be given every 2 to 3 hours. The regimen for the prevention of decubitus ulcers should be followed as indicated by the needs of the individual.

*Elimination.* Urinary output is measured carefully and, if the client is receiving sulfonamide therapy, a specimen is examined daily for hematuria. Fluid intake is regulated to ensure an output of approximately 1000 ml each 24 hours. Mild cathartics and enemas are used as necessary to establish adequate bowel evacuation. If there are clinical signs of increased intracranial pressure, enemas may be contraindicated.

*Diversion.* During the acute stage the client

should be kept quiet, in a darkened room, and at complete physical rest to conserve strength. As the person convalesces, occupational therapy may be used as a diversion. During this period he or she may enjoy reading, visiting with friends, and watching television. Periods of rest should be scheduled to avoid fatigue.

*Education.* The *public conception of meningitis* is one of both fear and misconception. Education in the disease process and emotional support are very important. Disease outcomes should not be firmly promised, since this may be false reassurance. Reassurance may be provided as the practitioner points out the improvement the client has made during the disease process. After hospital discharge, the client should be advised in measures to build immunity and avoid infection.

*Evaluation.* After treatment has begun, it is exceedingly important to monitor the effectiveness of the intervention modality. In older children and individuals a second lumbar puncture performed 24 hours after the initiation of therapy should result in a negative culture, a Gram stain free of organisms and an increase in white blood cells, glucose, and protein in comparison to the initial lumbar puncture. Infants undergo the same changes, which, however, may not be evident for a few days. When this picture is apparent, antimicrobial therapy is considered effective.

Certain criteria assist the practitioner in determining when antimicrobial therapy may be safely stopped. In infants, antimicrobial therapy continues for 3 weeks because of the high incidence of recurrence in young infants. In individuals beyond the infant age range, treatment is stopped if the cerebrospinal fluid cell count is less than $30/mm^3$, glucose and protein levels are normal, microorganisms are absent, and the client has been afebrile for 5 days.

After therapy has ceased the client is observed for 2 days so that symptoms of illness do not return.

At times the client does not improve with antimicrobial therapy, as evidenced by continued temperature elevations and worsening of symptoms. The problem may be the outcome of a concurrent infection in another part of the body or ineffective therapy. Drug fever may also be the cause of continuing fever, wherein the client who is unaffected has temperature elevations until the drug is discontinued.

*Follow-up.* The necessity to rebuild one's health and resistance to infection has been previously discussed. In addition, long-range serial assessments should be done in cognitive, motor, perceptual, sensory, and developmental domains to detect early problems. Vision and hearing tests should be performed after the acute process has ended. Referrals are made according to situational findings.

*Meningism.* Before this topic is ended, it will be helpful to consider meningism, since it is quite similar clinically to meningitis. In meningism, meningitis-like symptoms occur in association with a febrile illness in the individual. At times, convulsions and coma may be seen in this condition. The cerebrospinal fluid is under increased pressure, is normal in appearance, and reveals a normal cell count and glucose level but a slightly increased protein level. The diagnostic lumbar puncture frequently relieves the symptoms. Remaining symptoms and discomforts are managed symptomatically.

## ENCEPHALITIS

Encephalitis is an infection of the brain caused by a virus. A few specific types have been identified in particular epidemics. One type found in horses, pheasants, and occasionally other birds in many states along the Atlantic seaboard is called *eastern equine encephalitis*. This viral disease, primarily of birds, is passed to horses and humans only by mosquitoes. The incubation period ranges from 5 to 15 days. Human cases of eastern equine encephalitis have been confirmed in Massachusetts and New Jersey. The disease in humans is often severe and frequently fatal. The disease may also occur in a nonepidemic form as a complication of a systemic viral infection such as measles, chickenpox, or mumps.

The pathological condition is characterized by diffuse damage to the nerve cells of the brain, with perivascular cellular infiltration, proliferation of glia, and increasing cerebral edema.

### Acute type

The onset may be insidious or sudden, with headache, high fever, convulsions, and lethargy or restlessness progressing, if untreated, to stupor and coma. After the acute phase is over, the client may remain comatose for days, weeks, or longer (the condition popularly called *sleeping sickness*). Death may occur, though recovery is generally the rule. Personality changes, behavior disturbances, parkinsonism, mental deterioration, psychotic manifestations, paralyses, or convulsions may persist in 60% of the cases. The nonepidemic type is not so serious or so likely to be followed by sequelae as the epidemic type. Table 20-5 gives common findings in encephalopathies.

The diagnosis depends on the clinical signs, but the specific virus may be identified only by specific immunological reactions or by isolation of the causative agent from the blood or spinal fluid.

The type of encephalitis resulting from the bite of a mosquito that previously had bitten an infected bird can be prevented. Young children, the most frequent victims, should be kept indoors during early morning and evening hours when mosquitos are most active. During the day they should play in sunny areas away from bushes, trees, and swampy areas. Stagnant pools should be sprayed; windows and doors should be screened.

*Treatment and nursing intervention.* Treatment is supportive and symptomatic. Isolation of the client during the acute infectious stage is regulated by the type of encephalitis. The administration of hypertonic solutions, steroids, or both intravenously may combat cerebral edema effectively. If respirations are impaired, a tracheotomy and artificial mechanical respiration may be indicated. Vaccines may be helpful, and sedatives may be indicated for the control of restlessness and sleeplessness. Anticonvulsants are given to control seizures. Aspirin and cool alcohol sponges may be given to reduce the fever. If they are not effective, hypothermia may be initiated. Physical therapy and graduated exercises should be continued until optimal spontaneous activity is resumed.

OBSERVATIONS. The client's general condition is noted. Watch for signs of meningeal irritation and symptoms of increasing intracranial pressure (headache, vomiting, convulsions, and changes in the level of consciousness). Take the rectal temperature at the intervals ordered, and report changes in the vital signs, including blood pressure rates. Signs of cranial nerve involvement (ptosis, strabismus, nystagmus, diplopia, dysphagia,

and aphonia), abnormal patterns of sleep, and manifestations of behavioral disturbances should be noted.

POSITION. The client is kept in bed in a quiet, dimly lighted room. Posturing and turning of the client every 2 hours during the period of enforced bed rest is recommended strongly to increase comfort and to prevent complications. The interval in bed depends on the client's progress after becoming afebrile.

NUTRITION. Nutrition is maintained in the same way as outlined for the care of the client with meningitis.

HYGIENE. Hygiene is the same as described for the care of the client with meningitis.

ELIMINATION. If the client is unconscious, some form of catheter drainage may be used to maintain normal bladder function and to keep the client dry. If he or she is conscious, urinary output is measured and retention watched for. Unless contraindicated by greatly increased intracranial pressure, colon lavages, enemas, or mild cathartics may be used to maintain adequate bowel evacuation.

SLEEP. Many clients with encephalitis have a reversal of the sleep pattern and tend to sleep during the day and to remain wakeful and restless at night. As the client convalesces, an activity schedule should be planned to occupy him or her during the day hours; this may help to keep the client awake and facilitate sleeping at night.

DIVERSION. Occupational therapy is indicated during the convalescent and chronic stages. If residual disabilities are present, it should be directed to ameliorating them or to developing compensatory skills. If indicated, it may be used as a reeducational and vocational aid in the rehabilitation of the client. Diversional activities, insofar as possible, should follow the trend of the client's normal interests and pursuits. During the hospital stay the librarian and the physical therapist, as well as the occupational therapist and the nurse, may make valuable contributions toward improving morale and accelerating convalescence.

PSYCHOLOGY. The psychological care of the seriously ill client with an infection is also important. When the client is conscious, emotional needs should be assessed and met. He or she should have opportunities to talk about the illness and the problems associated with it and be helped to solve

**TABLE 20-5.** Common findings in encephalopathies*

| Problem | Causative mechanism | Course | CSF findings | Comments |
|---|---|---|---|---|
| Infectious encephalitis | Arthropod-borne viruses; includes western equine, eastern equine, St. Louis infections | Acute after direct invasion of brain tissue | Pressure increased<br>Appearance often clear<br>Cells normal early but 20-500/mm³, mainly lymphocytes, seen later<br>Protein levels normal or increased<br>Glucose levels normal | Special viral tests required to demonstrate organism<br>Long-term sequelae frequent<br>No specific treatment known; early treatment similar to that for bacterial meningitis until diagnosis established by viral studies; treatment for convulsions or increased intracranial pressure possibly required<br>Abnormal EEG<br>Acute course lasting about 10 days to 2 weeks |
| Infectious encephalitis | Enteric-oral transmission; includes ECHO, coxsackie, poliomyelitis infections | Acute after direct invasion of brain tissue | Pressure increased<br>Appearance often clear<br>Cells in coxsackie infection less than 400/mm³; in ECHO infection between 200 and 1000/mm³; and in poliomyelitis less than 200/mm³<br>Protein levels normal or increased<br>Glucose levels normal | Differences in three virus as follows: *ECHO* often associated with red, discrete maculopapular rash that does not itch in first 5 days; *coxsackie* often associated with herpangina, pleurodynia, and pericarditis; *poliomyelitis* most common cause of sporadic asymmetric flaccid paralysis with elevated temperature and meningeal irritation |
| Infectious encephalitis | Miscellaneous viruses; includes herpes simplex and rabies | Acute after direct invasion of brain tissue | Essentially normal; in herpes simplex count less than 200/mm³; in rabies less than 100/mm³ | Special viral studies required<br>In herpes simplex external lesions often associated; diagnosis made by noting EEG changes in temporal lobe, doing brain biopsy, using fluorescent staining techniques on initial cerebrospinal exam; treatment with 5-iodo-2'- deoxyuridine (IUDR)<br>High mortality and morbidity<br>Rabies transmitted by bite from rabid animal with 4- to 8-week incubation period; death occurring within 5 days from beginning symptoms; prophylactic treatment available |
| Infectious encephalitis | Myxovirus; including mumps and measles | Acute course long after virus introduced; mumps | SSPE† showing sharp increase of gamma globulin and rise in measles antibody titer | Both disease processes caused by "slow viruses" |

*Continued.*

*From Conway, B.L.: Pediatric neurologic nursing, St. Louis, 1977, The C.V. Mosby Co.

†SSPE, Subacute sclerosing panencephalitis.

**TABLE 20-5.** Common findings in encephalopathies—cont'd

| Problem | Causative mechanism | Course | CSF findings | Comments |
|---|---|---|---|---|
| | | having short course as other meningitides and resulting in recovery; measles possibly resulting in SSPE and eventual deterioration and death | In mumps: Pressure normal or increased Appearance clear or slightly cloudy Cells 0-2000/mm³, mainly lymphocytes Protein levels often increased Glucose levels normal | |
| Infectious encephalitis | Consuming infected brain tissue cause of kuru | Acute course long after virus ingested; characterized by deterioration and death | | Slow viral disease |
| Parainfectious encephalitis | Antigen-antibody reaction; includes rubeola, rubella, herpes zoster(?), infectious mononucleosis | Reaction associated with systemic infection | Pressure normal, but frequently increased Appearance clear or opalescent Cells 15-1000/mm³, early mainly polymorphonuclear neutrophils, later mainly lymphocytes Protein levels 60-150 mg/dl Glucose levels normal, sometimes diminished Chloride levels normal | Special methods required in serological testing techniques Symptoms of causative systemic infection apparent and may be confirmed by history and complete blood count Long-term sequelae frequent No specific treatment known, except Vidarabine (Vira-A) for herpes simplex causing encephalitis; early treatment similar to that for bacterial meningitis until diagnosis established by viral studies; treatment for convulsions or increased intracranial pressure required Abnormal EEG Acute course lasting about 10 days to 2 weeks |
| Parainfectious encephalitis | Postvaccinal reaction; includes vaccinia inoculation, rabies vaccine, yellow fever vaccine, pertussis vaccine reactions | Reaction follows administration of vaccine | Pressure normal but frequently increased Appearance clear or opalescent Cells 15-1000/mm³, early mainly polymorphonuclear neutrophils, later mainly lymphocytes | Special methods required in serological testing techniques Symptoms of causative systemic infection apparent and may be confirmed by history and complete blood count Long-term sequelae frequent |

| | | | | |
|---|---|---|---|---|
| | | Protein levels 60–150 mg/dl; Glucose levels normal, sometimes diminished; Chloride levels normal | | No specific treatment known; early treatment similar to that for bacterial meningitis until diagnosis established by viral studies; treatment for convulsions or increased intracranial pressure required; Abnormal EEG; Acute course lasting about 10 days to 2 weeks |
| Parainfectious encephalitis | Toxic response to by-product of systemic infection; includes scarlet fever, shigellosis, salmonellosis, influenza | Glucose levels normal; Cells less than 50/mm³ | Toxic response associated with clinical evidence of disease process | Positive cultures |
| Uremia | Toxic condition secondary to renal insufficiency and retention of nitrogenous waste products in blood | Pressure increased; Appearance clear; Cells normal; Protein levels normal to slightly elevated; Glucose levels normal; Chloride levels normal to slightly elevated | Central nervous system signs dependent on severity of uremia | Treatment of underlying disease process as possible; Fluid and electrolyte balances to be restored; Dietary management possibly needed; Central nervous system signs (seizures, emotional changes, restlessness) and elevated blood pressure to be monitored and managed |
| Diabetes mellitus | Metabolic disease | Pressure normal; Appearance clear; Cells normal; Protein levels normal; Glucose levels vary with blood glucose levels; Chloride levels normal | Central nervous system signs related to hypoglycemia, hyperglycemia, and complications of disease process | Appropriate studies necessary to identify metabolic disease process (diabetes mellitus); Treatment to normalize energy-insulin use desirable in children |
| Lead encephalitis | Ingestion of lead over period of time; includes lead acquired from toys or furniture painted with lead-based paint, crayons colored with lead-based substances, fruit-tree sprays | Pressure normal to high; Appearance clear; Cells to 100/mm³, mainly lymphocytes; Protein levels elevated; Glucose levels normal; Chloride levels normal | Insidious; encephalopathy usually precedes peripheral nerve disturbances; course often precipitated by acute condition, that is, acidosis or infection | Increased coproporphyrin and lead levels in urine; Changes on radiographic examination; Lead line on gums; Urine containing increased amounts of amino acid, glucose, protein, and blood; Increased lead concentration on blood; Later anemia; More common in children under 5 years of age because of tendency to mouth objects; Pica often described in history |

Continued.

them. The family should be supported during the acute phase of illness and, as the client convalesces, progressively involved in the care and the planning for discharge. If the client has residual paralysis or other disabilities requiring special appliances, services, or home care, the Visiting Nurses Association and other community agencies should be contacted and also be involved in predischarge conferences.

### Chronic type

Some of the so-called slow viruses have afforded scientists valuable data that may lead to a better understanding of some of the progressive degenerative diseases of the nervous system. The commonly known chronic types of encephalitis include subacute sclerosing panencephalitis (SSPE), kuru, and mumps meningoencephalitis. *SSPE* is a deteriorating condition resulting in death that follows even years after a case of the measles. Care is symptomatic and supportive. *Kuru* was a disease of a tribe of New Guinea highlanders who consumed brain tissue of their deceased and thereby ingested the slow virus, which resulted in neurological deterioration. Since the cause of this isolated disease has been identified, the practice has stopped, and the disease process has been eradicated. *Mumps meningoencephalitis* may be virtually prevented by the administration of vaccine and has a favorable prognosis when it occurs. The mumps virus, however, like the others, often remains dormant and invades the central nervous system even years after the clinical case of mumps has occurred.

### ABSCESS

An abscess is a collection of exudate (pus) and may occur in any part of the body as a result of local or systemic infection. Abscesses are found in and around the nervous system (extradural or subdural) or within the nervous tissue itself. They may be intracranial or intraspinal.

The cause may be any of the organisms that cause meningitis, as described earlier. The pathological condition may be a pocketed mass of exudate outside the dura resulting from infection of the overlying bone, a localized collection trapped in the subdural space as a complication of meningitis, an intracerebral abscess (intraspinal abscess is rare) secondary to a sinus or middle ear infection,

or an embolus from a pulmonary infection. The cerebral abscess may be a diffuse early softening of the infected brain, or it may localize itself in time into a restricted area and develop a capsule within which the exudate is contained.

The signs and symptoms vary with the location of the abscess. If intracranial, in addition to the signs and symptoms of meningitis, there may be hemiplegia, hemianopia, speech disturbances, unconsciousness, and papilledema. The spinal abscesses cause pain in the back and flaccid paralysis of the extremities with bladder and bowel disabilities.

The diagnosis depends on the history of preceding infection, evidence of osteomyelitis (bone erosion) by radiographic examination, and localizing signs found on neurological examination. Electroencephalography, ventriculography, brain scanning and computerized axial tomography may be helpful in localizing the cerebral lesion.

### Treatment and nursing intervention

The treatment consists of all the measures indicated for the care of clients with meningitis with the addition of specific antibiotic medication and the elimination of any focus that may be propagating the infection, such as osteomyelitis of the skull or spine or infections of the sinuses, ears, and lungs. The most important aspect of treatment is the drainage and elimination of the abscess by neurological surgery.

For the preoperative and postoperative care of a client with an intracranial abscess see Chapters 21 and 26; for care of a client with a spinal abscess see Chapter 22.

### MYELITIS

Myelitis is an acute inflammation of the spinal cord that may occur in association with an acute infectious disease (such as measles, influenza, erysipelas, pneumonia, gonorrhea, or neurosyphilis) or as a primary infectious process. The resulting necrosis may result from the inflammatory agent itself or a secondary embolic or thrombotic complication.

The onset is rapid, and the signs reach their maximum within 1 or 2 days. The infection may involve the spinal cord completely or partially at any level. There is relatively little back pain. Flaccid paralysis of the extremities is the dominant part of the picture and depends on the location and extent of the pathological process. This is most frequently in the midthoracic region. Sensory disturbances and loss of sphincter control are invariably present.

The diagnosis is made on the history of sudden paraplegia corroborated by the neurological examination and other signs of acute infection. There is no block with spinal dynamics, and the cerebrospinal fluid, on laboratory examination, may be within normal limits.

The prognosis depends on the severity and extent of the lesion and the prevention and control of complications. Rarely does the client recover completely without residual disabilities.

### Treatment and nursing intervention

Treatment is supportive and symptomatic; it consists of bed rest and prevention of complications. Rehabilitation should be planned for the individual client in light of needs and residual disabilities.

Refer to the discussion of disturbances in motor integration in Chapter 15, the discussion of sexuality in Chapter 6, and the principles of preoperative nursing care outlined in Chapters 22 and 26.

### HERPES ZOSTER (SHINGLES)

Herpes zoster is a cutaneous eruption of vesicles in the area of distribution of a particular spinal or cranial nerve root that is presumed to be a viral infection of the posterior root ganglion. Pathological studies demonstrate swelling, hyperemia, and changes in the cells of the ganglion with associated inflammatory reaction. The onset may be fever and malaise followed by pain with intense itching in the skin area where the vesicles will later appear (about the fourth day). The vesicles last about 5 days and then dry and disappear, but they may leave scars. The pain generally disappears after about 2 weeks; however, in about 50% of the clients, over 60 years of age it may persist for 1 to 2 years as a disturbing postherpetic neuralgia. The diagnosis is made on the basis of the clinical findings.

### Treatment and nursing intervention

Treatment consists of local care of the vesicles, instructing the client not to scratch the lesions, bed rest during the acute period (first week), and such analgesics as may be necessary. The administration of oral corticosteroids in otherwise healthy clients is believed to shorten the duration of postherpetic neuralgia. Generally, narcotics or other drugs that may produce dependency with prolonged use are avoided. If the vesicles are unbroken, they may be painted with collodion or tincture of benzoin; otherwise wet dressings may be applied. Corticosteroid lotions and sprays also have used to relieve local discomfort and to hasten the resolution of the herpetic lesions. The postherpetic neuralgia must sometimes be relieved by neurosurgical measures (division of the posterior root or roots involved). Nursing intervention is symptomatic and directed toward increasing the client's comfort and preventing secondary infection. If the client receives corticosteroid therapy, he or she is closely monitored for adverse reactions.

#### Expected outcomes
1 Secondary infection will be absent.
2 Client will describe rationale for each health care intervention.

## SECONDARY PROBLEMS

### NORMAL PRESSURE HYDROCEPHALUS

Normal pressure hydrocephalus (NPH) refers to a condition in adults wherein the ventricles enlarge, with subsequent compression of adjacent cerebral tissue, whereas the cerebrospinal fluid pressure remains within normal limits. This entity is controversial in that the exact causative mechanism remains unknown. Other names for this condition include occult hydrocephalus, low pressure hydrocephalus, adult hydrocephalus, hydrocephalic dementia, and hydrocephalus ex vacuo.

The cause of NPH is unknown, but often several causative factors are evident involving obstruction and impaired cerebrospinal fluid absorption in the cerebral subarachnoid spaces. Some conditions resulting in these factors include trauma, subarachnoid hemorrhage, thrombosis of the superior sagittal sinus, and complications that stem from bacterial meningitis.

In NPH the onset of symptoms is gradual, and the symptoms often include what is termed the classic triad: (1) mental changes, (2) gait disturbances, and (3) urinary incontinence. Other common symptoms may include nystagmus, speech impairments, paroxysmal episodes, pronounced bilateral pyramidal and extrapyramidal disturbances, and abnormal reflexes. In NPH there is always an absence of papilledema and headache.

## Diagnosis

NPH is not a discrete entity, but several studies may be done to support the diagnosis, which is suspected when the onset of symptoms is gradual. These studies include a lumbar puncture, pneumoencephalogram, arteriogram, radioiodinated human serum albumin (RISA-131) scan, electroencephalogram, and skull radiographs.

Although the cause and diagnosis of NPH are poorly defined, the treatment of NPH is specific and well accepted. Treatment is highly successful and involves the surgical insertion of a shunt, the ventriculovenous shunt being the most common. Chapter 13 gives further detail on hydrocephalus and shunting procedures.

## SYDENHAM'S CHOREA (ST. VITUS'S DANCE)

Sydenham's chorea is seen in children 5 to 15 years of age, frequently in association with rheumatic fever (which may or may not be obvious at the time) as a manifestation of cerebral involvement by the same organism. Girls are affected more often than boys. Some investigators maintain that a severe emotional shock may cause chorea in a susceptible child. Some evidence has been presented that sibling rank may be a precipitating factor; the first or second child with younger siblings is apparently more predisposed to chorea.

The disorder is characterized by involuntary, purposeless, rapid expressions of normal motion such as flexion and extension of the fingers, raising and lowering the shoulders, grimacing, and exaggerated purposeful movements. The involuntary movements may occur during sleep (the only ones to do so except those of convulsions).

The pathogenic agent is a viridans streptococcus, the same as for rheumatic fever. The pathological condition is diffuse perivascular and vascular involvement of the brain.

The symptoms are restlessness, fretfulness, irritability, and emotional instability, followed by generalized weakness, increasing severity of the choreiform activity, and awkwardness in handling objects. Associated symptoms of rheumatic fever including cardiac involvement are frequently seen.

The choreic manifestations may develop progressively over a 2-week period, achieve a plateau of severity, and recede gradually until recovery occurs about 10 weeks from the onset. Recurrence of symptoms may take place weeks or months after recovery from the initial attack.

## Treatment and nursing intervention

The treatment is directed to the complete illness, including cardiac and joint involvement. The neurological aspects of the illness should be managed by good nursing care, bed rest, and moderate sedation as necessary.

*Environment.* The client with chorea should be in a single room that is kept quiet, and external stimuli should be reduced to a minimum. Whenever possible, the same nurses and physicians are present, and the number of personnel is reduced to the fewest necessary to accomplish care. During the acute stage, visits from the client's family are limited, and at times it may be necessary to prohibit them. Friends are not permitted to visit during the client's stay in the hospital, and other clients should not socialize with him or her. Maximum mental, emotional, and physical rest is emphasized. Supportive psychotherapy is important during the acute phase of treatment. The client may react emotionally to the restrictions of the therapeutic regimen and separation from family; therefore the staff must, insofar as possible, furnish the interest, warmth, and affection normally supplied by parents. The nurse should be sensitive to this client's needs at all times and should afford opportunities to talk about things that interest or trouble him or her relevant to the level of growth and development.

*Observations.* Note the nature and extent of the involuntary movements, the amount of muscular weakness, any speech defect, subjective complaints (especially those referred to the joints, heart, or throat), the client's reaction to drugs and other treatment, appetite, and any behavior or personality problems.

*Position and activity.* During the acute stage the client is on complete bed rest with exceptional curtailment of activity. For the first week or so he or she should be spoon-fed and bathed. Activity aggravates the motions, further fatigues the client, and thus increases the danger of complications. A bed cradle supports the weight of the bed-clothes, increases comfort, and lessens the danger of skin irritation as a result of the restless, uncontrollable movements of the extremities. Principles for posturing the client outlined in Chapter 22 are applied and modified as indicated. As the client convalesces, activity is progressively but slowly increased. Bed rest is continued until the client is free of symptoms.

*Nutrition.* A high-calorie, high-vitamin diet is ordered. The nurse is responsible not only for feeding the client during the acute stage of this illness but also for supervising every meal during the convalescent period to ensure adequate nourishment. Encourage fluid intake to maintain body needs. It is important for the client to maintain weight and resistance to infection. Vomiting, anorexia, anemia, and loss of weight are treated symptomatically and vigorously.

*Hygiene.* A cleansing bath is given daily, with alcohol rubs as necessary. Oral hygiene is administered three times a day. If the client's skin is dry or if he or she is losing weight, massages with a lubricating solution or baby lotion may be given to improve the nutrition of the skin.

*Elimination.* Urinary output is measured. Since these clients are frequently constipated, mild cathartics may be necessary for effective evacuation of the bowels.

*Medications.* A mild sedative such as phenobarbital is given two or three times a day to ensure adequate rest. Fowler's solution, sodium salicylate, and calcium lactate also have been used as symptomatic treatment with questionable therapeutic effect. Administration of aspirin is especially indicated if signs or symptoms of rheumatic fever are present.

*Diversion.* During the convalescent period, light age-appropriate occupational therapy may be used to keep the client busy and diverted. Selected reading is permitted for definite periods each day. All new therapy is instituted gradually, and the client is observed closely for evidence of fatigue or the recurrence of symptoms.

*Rehabilitation.* After the client's discharge from the hospital, physical activity should be curtailed for at least a month. The family is instructed as to their responsibility for protecting the client from undue emotional strain and strenuous physi-cal activity and for recognizing early evidence of recurrence. The client needs definite follow-up appointments for the ensuing year wherein special attention is paid to the heart and any residual complications.

**Expected outcomes**

1 Environmental stimuli is minimized.
2 Objective and subjective complaints and symptoms are rapidly reported and treated.
3 Activity, nutrition, and hygiene are planned to conserve energy, avoid complications, and aid the client in coping successfully with all phases of illness and recuperation
4 Client will describe the use of prescribed medications.
5 The client will have knowledge of an individualized, specific plan for follow-up care after the acute phase of illness has passed.

## PREVENTABLE NEUROLOGICAL DISORDERS

### POLIOMYELITIS (INFANTILE PARALYSIS)

Poliomyelitis is an acute infection caused by a virus that attacks principally the cells of the anterior horns of the spinal cord, though the motor cells of the brainstem and brain may also be involved. This selective involvement of different parts of the central nervous system led to the identification of three different strains of the virus that causes poliomyelitis. The three types of poliomyelitis are called *bulbar, encephalitic,* and *spinal;* each type is characterized by special signs and symptoms, depending on which cells are affected. Although children and young adults are most susceptible, no age group is naturally immune to the poliomyelitis virus. More than one third of all cases occur after the age of 15 years.

For the 5-year period immediately preceding the introduction of the Salk vaccine in 1955, yearly average of almost 39,000 poliomyelitis cases was reported in the United States. The highest number, almost 58,000, occurred in 1952. In 1962, years after the advent of the Salk vaccine and 4 years after the introduction of the oral Sabin vaccine, only 910 cases, or 0.5 per 100,000 population, were reported. There were 47 deaths, or 0.3 per million persons. Most cases that now occur in the United States are among young persons who have not been adequately immunized. This disease has become less virulent and is now a relatively rare cause of death in our country.

With the increasing public recognition of the importance of effective immunization for children and young adults and with the development of an oral vaccine that in one dose gives prolonged protection against the three types of poliomyelitis, it is hoped that this immunization will become so routine and widespread that new cases of poliomyelitis will not occur.

Although this disease occurs less frequently in adults, it is recommended that everyone up to 50 years of age be immunized. National, state, and local medical associations have endorsed the use of the oral Sabin vaccine. After extensive testing of this live polio virus in accordance with federal regulations, Dr. Luther Terry, then Surgeon General of the U.S. Public Health Service, announced in July 1963 that a license had been granted for the production and sale of this trivalent vaccine gainst poliomyelitis. The American Academy of Pediatrics recommends that the oral Sabin vaccine be initially administered at 2 months of age.

Poliomyelitis is most communicable in its early stages. The incubation period is 5 to 12 days. It may be transmitted through direct contact with the pharyngeal secretions or feces of infected persons.

Some public health officers recommend isolation during the acute, febrile phase of this illness; others insist on isolation for a 2-week period. Mask and gown technique should be used, and if a single room is not available, there should be an 8-foot area around the bed. Body excreta should be disinfected before disposal. Bed linen and all articles used within the room should be considered possible sources of infection and treated accordingly.

Healthy children should be protected further by the following precautions: (1) Public bathing should be prohibited if a case of poliomyelitis has been reported in the area; (2) any child or adult suspected of having poliomyelitis should be placed on strict isolation; (3) any person who has been in direct contact with a client with suspected or diagnosed poliomyelitis should take precautions to prevent further spread of the disease during the incubation period.

The manifestations of poliomyelitis are related to the particular strain of the causative virus. If the spinal cord is involved, pain and weakness of the muscles of the trunk and extremities are dominant; if the higher centers of the brain are involved, delirium, drowsiness, and, at times, unconsciousness are primary; if the brainstem is involved, respiratory and swallowing difficulties occur.

Some medical experts maintain that only 1 of every 10 cases of poliomyelitis progresses to the stage at which the disease is recognized. Some children may have mild symptoms of headache, nausea, a low-grade fever, and sore throat; may improve after 24 hours in bed; and then may manifest more severe symptoms, including stiff neck and muscular pains. Other children recover completely after the onset of the early symptoms without any further discomfort. Adults tend to be more uncomfortable, are irritable, and complain initially of headache, fatigue, and malaise. After several days, paralysis may occur. Muscle spasms and hypersensitivity to touch may be associated with the muscular weakness.

Pathological examination reveals necrosis of the cells of the anterior horns of the spinal cord with associated congestion and cellular infiltration.

Since the early clinical picture may be similar to meningitis, the diagnosis may be difficult to establish. A lumbar puncture should be performed. The cerebrospinal fluid reveals an increase of white blood cells and protein and will help determine the diagnosis.

### Treatment and nursing intervention

The following discussion of treatment and nursing care is focused on the management of a client with a virulent form of poliomyelitis. Today most clients would not require this level of treatment and nursing.

Treatment is symptomatic and palliative and directed toward the prevention of complications such as deformities, contractures, stretching of weakened muscles, footdrop and wristdrop, and respiratory failure. Pain is relieved by the application of heat by means of a cradle with electric lights.

Posturing the client in a neutral position, massage, active and passive exercises, muscle reeducation, and electrical stimulation are directed toward promoting the return of muscular function without complications. Postural drainage and the cautious use of suction are indicated if mucus accumulates in the throat or if bulbar involvement is evident. The respirator is indicated if the diaphragm and intercostal muscles are affected. Signs of respiratory distress are manifested by increasing restlessness, a peculiar grunting type of breathing with increasing difficulty, and slight cyanosis. If the respiratory nucleus in the medulla oblongata is destroyed, the respirator will be of no avail. Complete bed rest is vital during the acute phase. Adequate nutrition is maintained by a special diet as indicated for the individual client. The convalescent period may last for months or years; physical therapy and remedial exercises are continued until maximum function has returned to the affected muscles.

*Observations.* The nurse observes the vital signs (temperature generally is taken every 4 hours), the quality and rate of respirations, and signs of involvement of the diaphragm and intercostal muscles. The nurse notes the muscles involved and the presence of spasm or pain, weakness or paralysis, the mental attitude (especially anxiety, emotional tension, or irritability), malaise, headache, vomiting, signs of meningeal irritation, cranial nerve involvement, and sphincter disturbances.

*Position.* After fracture boards have been placed under the mattress, the client is put to bed at complete rest. A firm mattress prevents sagging and ensures effective support of the entire body. A footboard (36 by 18 inches) is placed at the foot of the bed and arranged to afford a 4-inch space between the end of the mattress and the board. This facilitates effective posturing of the client in the prone and supine positions. During the acute phase the client is placed in the side-lying position only when necessary for administration of nursing care or treatments. He or she is always maintained in a neutral position, with the muscles of the extremities supported to prevent stretching and contracture. The correct alignment of the body is emphasized and maintained within the restrictions imposed by painful muscular spasms. A turning sheet is used at all times to minimize handling of affected muscles. These muscles are usually very tender and sensitive to touch; if the position of an extremity is changed, the nurse effects this change by supporting the extremity at the joints, never using the muscle belly for this purpose. During the acute phase the Stryker frame may be used to

great advantage. It minimizes handling of the client and facilitates the frequent change of position. (See Chapter 27 for discussion of the Stryker frame.) The upper and lower extremities are postured as outlined in Chapter 22. The space between the board and mattress leaves the heels free from pressure when the feet are placed in dorsiflexion against the board; when the client is lying on the face, the board serves as a floor and the feet are placed at right angles to it, with the intervening space utilized to prevent pressure on the toes. The head of the bed is not raised during the acute phase.

If bulbar signs are present, the foot of the bed is raised and the client's head turned to the side to facilitate drainage of mucus from the throat and mouth, thereby preventing choking and aspiration.

An air-fluidized bed may be used to increase the comfort of the client during the acute stage of poliomyelitis. The position must be changed much less frequently, and there is less possibility of skin breakdown.

Special physical therapy (massage, active and passive movements) is usually started early in the treatment and may be continued for months or years until maximum function has returned to the affected muscles. After the acute phase, which may last from a few to several weeks, underwater exercises such as those done in the Hubbard bath or in a warm pool (85° to 92° F) further facilitate the reeducation and rehabilitation of the client in a psychological as well as in a physical sense.

*Nutrition.* The diet should be high in vitamin and caloric content with adequate protein; as the client convalesces, it is increased or modified according to individual needs. Its consistency may be modified; a client with bulbar involvement may have to be fed by a nasal tube, intravenously, or by other artificial means. Vitamins $B_1$ and $B_{12}$, because of their direct effect on the central nervous system, may also be given. Fluids are encouraged unless there are signs of edema of the cerebrum or spinal cord; under these circumstances they may be restricted and dehydration measures instituted. Measure and record the fluid intake carefully.

*Hygiene.* Bathing the client during the acute stage generally is restricted because of the sensitivity and tenderness of the affected muscles. Use alcohol with minimal pressure and without any friction. Special oral hygiene, supplemented by the use of suction as necessary, is important if there are signs of bulbar involvement. As the pain recedes, scrupulous skin care is given to prevent the development of pressure sores. Frequent change of position is essential during this period to prevent redness and induration of vulnerable areas; it can be effected with minimal fatigue and discomfort by using the Stryker frame. Adequate caloric intake is maintained to retard wasting of the subcutaneous fat over prominent bones as an added measure to prevent breakdown of the skin. Warming the hands before giving any nursing care may decrease the client's uncomfortable reaction. Nightgowns, shirts, and pajamas should be omitted during this period to eliminate unnecessary moving of the client. The client who tends to perspire should lie between cotton blankets rather than sheets because these absorb excess moisture and prevent chilling. If the individual complains about the blankets, they should be removed. The use of Pliofilm to protect the bed in place of heavier rubber sheets will contribute to the client's comfort and may decrease the amount of sweating.

*Elimination.* Measure the urinary output accurately, and observe the bladder for distention. If retention occurs, catheter drainage of the bladder may be instituted after the initial catheterization, which should always be done with a retention catheter. Check the client for abdominal distention; treatment is started immediately. Usually a rectal tube and fomentations to the abdomen will be effective. The diets for these clients are regulated to eliminate gas-forming foods and fluids. If the client is constipated, mild cathartics may be given. A prolonged interval on the bedpan is avoided. Improper use of the bedpan may produce lumbar spasm and pain; this can be avoided by use of the Stryker frame, which is so constructed that direct contact with the bedpan is unnecessary. Colon lavage is recommended in preference to an enema because it is less fatiguing, and it is then not necessary to place the client on a bedpan.

*Rest.* During the acute phase, while pain and muscle spasm persist, all nursing care is directed toward reducing the discomfort of the client, achieving a good therapeutic effect, and preventing complications. No care, unless absolutely essential, is administered when the client is tired; every attempt is made to plan nursing care so that minimal fatigue and discomfort will result. During this phase of the illness merely touching a client may cause a painful reaction.

If the client is an infant or small child, separation from the mother at the onset of the illness may increase fear and counteract the desired therapeutic effects of medical and nursing care. Therefore arrangements should be made so that the mother can spend long periods of time with him or her and assist with the required care. During this period the mother can instruct the nurse about feeding and play routines and special needs. Meanwhile the nurse has an opportunity to develop a trusting relationship with the child. If there are other children at home, the assistance of relatives, homemakers, or friends may be obtained, so that the mother can devote time to the sick youngster without needless anxiety about the rest of the family.

*Diversion.* During the early weeks of illness, depending on the type and degree of involvement of the nervous system, the client can rarely participate in any activity, diversional or otherwise. The room should be kept quiet and external stimulation reduced to a minimum to avoid fatigue and excitement. The responsibility for maintaining the client's morale, for giving reassurance as necessary, and for allaying any anxiety or fear rests on the nurse to a considerable degree. By attitude and approach the nurse can do much to instill hope and confidence within the client. When attending him or her, every word uttered and every motion executed should be planned ahead with this purpose in mind.

As he or she convalesces and function returns, activity is progressively increased. Occupational therapy may be initiated and increased progressively. Visitors may be permitted for short periods. Watching television and light reading may be added to the schedule. Each new activity should be supervised to evaluate the client's reaction and to avoid fatigue. Physical therapy and reeducation play important roles in the ultimate recovery of the patient, and cooperation and interest must be retained to promote the maximum return of function to the involved muscles. Most clients enjoy exercises performed in a warm pool and find them less tiring than other forms of physical therapy.

## Expected outcome in prevention

Since mass immunization programs will progressively reduce the incidence and virulence of poliomyelitis, all health workers, educators, and religious leaders should direct their efforts toward facilitating and perpetuating the routine administration of trivalent vaccine against poliomyelitis to 2-month-old infants and immunizing pregnant women and every man, woman, and child not already protected against this disease. If this is accomplished, this disease will be eradicated.

### Expected outcomes in disease
1 Complications will be absent.
2 Client will be free of pain.
3 Subjective and objective disease-related problems and discomforts will be minimized.
4 Client will be able to explain the disease process accurately and will be involved in planning, implementing, and evaluating his or her own care.

## NEUROSYPHILIS

Neurosyphilis is an affliction of any part of the nervous system resulting from infection by *Treponema pallidum*. It develops after inadequate treatment of early syphilis.

The pathological condition is extensive and may include the meninges, blood vessels, brain, spinal cord, and peripheral nerves. The meninges are congested, and the pia-arachnoid is infiltrated with lymphocytes that gather around the blood vessels. The vessels show proliferation of the intima, splitting of the elastica, and cellular infiltration of the tunicae media and adventitia, resulting in a severe panarteritis. The nervous tissue itself offers poor resistance to the organism, and as a result the cytoplasm of the cells and the myelin of the nerve sheaths degenerate. The added effect of impaired blood supply caused by the arterial disease results in areas of softening that lead to atrophy. This is most striking in the frontal lobes. The spinal cord shows degeneration of the posterior tracts, and the peripheral nerves show loss of the large-calibered sensory fibers.

The signs and symptoms are of great variety. In the early stages there may be only a mild meningeal reaction with minimal discomfort, though with a severe meningitis the clinical picture described previously will be evident. Should large arteries become occluded to the point of thrombo-sis, hemiplegia, or other disturbances commensurate with the location and size of the vessel affected may result.

This disease has two large subdivisions, depending on whether the disorder is principally cerebral (*general paresis*) or spinal (*tabes dorsalis*). The pathological condition of general paresis consists of a diffuse, chronic meningitis; the pia-arachnoid is thick, milky, and adherent to the brain. The frontal convolutions are atrophied, and the temporal and parietal convolutions may also be affected. The vascularity of the cortex is increased, with perivascular infiltration by round cells, disorganization of the cortical layers, and increase of the glia with resultant scarring.

The symptoms and signs of paresis are many and varied, as may be anticipated from the disease condition. The principal characteristic is progressive mental deterioration with physical debilitation leading to death within 3 to 5 years after onset unless treated. Emotional changes may occur, as well as impairment of judgment, concentration, and memory. The client's standards of moral and social behavior deteriorate; he or she becomes boastful and euphoric or may be unsociable and silent. At the same time the lips, tongue, and hands become tremulous and speech slurred. Vision may fail because of optic atrophy, and double vision may be present because of extraocular nerve involvement. The pupils are irregular, small, and unequal and do not react to light though they do on convergence (Argyll Robertson pupil). The client may develop convulsions and paralysis with incontinence of urine and may ultimately become bedridden. Early and adequate treatment can obviate the progress of symptoms.

*Tabes dorsalis* is a spinal cord disorder, and the pathological condition consists of a chronic inflammatory reaction in the dorsal root ganglia with degeneration of the dorsal roots and the posterior tract of the spinal cord. An associated mild degree of meningitis may be present.

The symptoms of tabes develop slowly, with fleeting, sharp, shooting pains (called lightning pains) in the extremities and around the trunk, and paresthesias and numbness of the feet and face. Painful visceral episodes may occur, especially gastric crises characterized by retching, vomiting, and abdominal pain. The gait becomes uncertain (ataxic), especially in the dark, and the inability to stand with the feet together and the eyes closed (Romberg's sign) is demonstrable. There is loss of libido and sexual potency; variable bladder dysfunction with a large residual volume is manifest as well as chronic cystitis. The knee jerk reflexes are lost. Loss of sensation can be shown with regard to deep pain, position, passive motion, and vibration. Hypotonia may appear as well as arthropathies (Charcot's joints), painless swelling of joints caused by effusion and edema.

The diagnosis of neurosyphilis depends on the history and the findings just enumerated, but it is confirmed by the complement fixation (Wassermann or Kahn) reactions of the blood and cerebrospinal fluid. The cerebrospinal fluid also contains an increased number of white cells and increased protein levels, and the colloidal gold curve is positive.

The colloidal gold curve test consists of adding cerebrospinal fluid, increasingly diluted with normal saline solution from 1:10 to 1:5120, to 10 tubes containing a measured amount of colloidal gold solution. An additional tube with colloidal gold is used for comparison. These 11 tubes are allowed to stand in a dark place for 24 hours. Normally, colloidal gold solution is red-orange in color; this may change to various degrees of purple and blue to colorless in response to chemical reactions (decolorization) that ensue when an abnormal amount of globulin is present in the cerebrospinal fluid. These color changes are expressed numerically as follows:

| | |
|---|---|
| 0 | Red-orange, no change |
| 1 | Red-blue |
| 2 | Purple |
| 3 | Blue |
| 4 | Pale blue |
| 5 | Colorless |

There are 10 numbers to a report if 10 dilutions are used as described. A normal curve would be 0000000000, a pathological curve, 5555542100 (paretic); other variants are 0123320000 (tabetic) and 0011234531 (meningitic).

### Treatment and nursing intervention

Treatment is principally by the administration of procaine penicillin up to 10 or 15 million units.

Benzathine penicillin given in weekly doses of 3 million units with a total of 6 or 9 million units has become the preferred treatment of late syphilis. The cerebrospinal fluid should be examined at intervals of 6 months and more treatment given as indicated, depending on the number of cells in the fluid.

The client with general paresis presents a major problem in management and supervision because of personality changes and psychotic manifestations. He or she must be protected from self and others who may take advantage of the impaired judgment.

Many of these clients are so incapacitated by their cerebral dysfunction that they are committed to mental institutions for prolonged care. Their numbers have been decreasing as a result of improved antisyphilitic therapy and better public education.

If the client has tabes dorsalis, the nurse supervises activity to prevent falls and places side rails up at night to prevent injury when the client attempts to walk unaided in the dark. Treatment is directed toward relief of pain caused by dorsal root involvement. Nursing care is symptomatic according to individual needs.

**Expected outcomes**
1 Individual will be protected from inappropriate and unsafe acts that affect self or others.
2 Individual or family will describe general goals and medications involved in treatment.
3 Pain will be absent.

## BOTULISM

Botulism, caused by *Clostridium botulinum,* is a relatively rare bacterial intoxication that is often fatal. The spores produced by *C. botulinum* are harmless and can remain dormant in soil or food for years. In this state, before germination, they may be ingested with raw fruits and vegetables without ill effects. The spores require an airtight, oxygen-free, low-acid environment to germinate and produce botulin, a deadly poison. They do not germinate at low temperatures; consequently frozen foods properly stored are generally safe. The botulinum bacillus may be found in improperly processed food, especially nonacid types under anaerobic conditions. The toxin is destroyed by boiling; destruction of the spores requires higher temperatures. The mode of transmission is the ingestion of contaminated food from jars or cans inadequately processed during canning.

The symptoms generally appear within 12 to 36 hours after eating the contaminated food; usually the shorter the time after exposure, the more serious the reaction. The symptoms relate primarily to the central nervous system: weakness, dizziness, headache, difficulty in swallowing and speaking, paralysis, constipation or diarrhea, hoarseness, and vomiting. Oculomotor or other cranial nerve paralysis may occur. Convulsions, coma, and cardiac or respiratory failure may develop if treatment is delayed or unsuccessful.

Bacteriological and toxicological tests may identify the bacterium or its toxins in suspected food or stomach contents.

The immediate treatment consists of intravenous administration of botulinum antitoxin (available from the Center for Disease Control, U.S. Public Health Service, in Atlanta), stomach lavage, and artificial respiration as indicated by the severity of the symptoms.

This is a reportable disease. The inspection and regulation of the commercial processing of canned and preserved foods by the government (U.S. Food and Drug Administration) are the best controls to prevent botulism. The education of housewives who do home canning regarding the importance of maintaining certain standards of time, pressure, and temperature to ensure the destruction of spores and the boiling of home-canned vegetables for at least 3 minutes before serving also contribute to the rare incidence of this disease. According to the statistics, commercially processed canned food is much safer than home-canned food, which is reported to cause some botulism each year, with a mortality of about 30%.

The following precautions should be taken with canned food:

1. Do not use a can with a swollen end; this might be caused by harmless bacteria but could be the result of *C. botulinum* gases.
2. When you open a sealed container (can, glass jar, or plastic), if the food squirts out under pressure, throw it out *without* tasting it.
3. If a can is opened and the food looks or smells bad, do not eat it.
4. Use a steam pressure cooker for home canning; use only fresh food in good condition; be certain that the food, jars, and all utensils used while canning are clean; process foods according to standard directions; make sure jars are sealed airtight; and store in a cool, dry place.

If the contents of a can are suspicious, lye may be added and the can placed in a safe place for 24 hours. It should then be buried. In this way the bacteria and toxins, if present, are destroyed, and there is no danger of contaminating other food growing in the area.

**Expected outcomes**
1 Homemakers who do home canning will be instructed on safe procedures.
2 Consumers will avoid faulty cans in commercial foods.

## RABIES

Rabies, or hydrophobia, is an infectious disease of the brain caused by a specific virus that is generally fatal. It may occur in any warm-blooded animal, but it is relatively uncommon in man. It is considered primarily a disease of animals; dogs and cats as well as wild animals are susceptible. The saliva of a rabid animal is infectious. The mode of transmission to man is through a break in the skin caused by the bite of a rabid animal. Persons, especially children, should be warned not to handle dead or sick wild animals. Domestic animals should be immunized. If a domestic animal bites a person, the animal should be isolated, confined, and observed for 10 days. If during this time abnormal behavior is manifested, the animal should be killed and its brain examined.

The incubation period depends on the extent of the laceration and the site of the wound in relation to nervous tissue. It usually lasts from 4 to 6 weeks.

Prevention of rabies in a human being bitten by a rabid animal depends on the administration of five intramuscular doses of human diploid cell vaccine (HDCV) and rabies immunoglobulin. HDCV eliminates the discomfort and complications formerly associated with the duck embryo vaccine (DEV). HDCV may be given whenever the potential for rabies exists now that problems have been conquered. Serological testing is recommended for those with compromised immunity and for clients treated by DEV, but not for those treated with HDCV.

Preexposure vaccine is available for administration to individuals at high risk for rabies, such as dogcatchers. The local health department should be consulted for the specific regimen to be followed.

The symptoms may be preceded by apprehension and irritability. Malaise, headache, fever, anorexia, insomnia, restlessness, and local sensory changes (such as tingling, numbness, and pain at site of wound) may occur. During the initial 24 hours, mild spasms of the larynx and pharynx with the sensation of choking, difficulty in swallowing, and hoarseness may be manifested.

This disease is characterized by an *excitement stage* that may occur within 24 to 72 hours of the onset of symptoms. It may be characterized by extreme fear and suffering, excitement, violent spasms of the larynx increased by swallowing, and beginning hydrophobia. These symptoms increase progressively—spasms spread, convulsions follow, and then delirium occurs.

The *final stage* is characterized by paralysis of muscles, coma, and respiratory failure. The disease rarely lasts more than 5 days, and death is inevitable unless vigorous treatment is started early.

Negri bodies are present within the nerve cells, and lesions may be observed within the spinal sympathetic and cranial nerve ganglia. These are especially widespread in the medulla.

### Treatment and nursing intervention

The wound caused by a rabid animal should be thoroughly cleansed with soap or a detergent solution and left unsutured for several days. The individual must be isolated for the duration of the illness. All those in attendance should wear protective gowns and gloves and should be cautioned about contact with the contaminated saliva.

Apart from the administration of the rabies vaccine and rabies immunoglobulin, treatment and nursing care are directed toward prevention and treatment of complications, alleviation of discomfort, and the protection of others with vaccine and from the source of infection. Anticonvulsant medication, suctioning, tracheostomy, oxygen therapy, and mechanical ventilation may be administered.

On October 10, 1970, while asleep, Matthew Winkler, a 6-year-old boy living on a farm in Will-shire, Ohio, was bitten on the thumb by a rabid bat. Four days later, Matthew began receiving duck embryo vaccine. By November 3, his temperature rose to 104° F, and he complained of a stiff neck. He was admitted to St. Rita's Hospital in Lima, Ohio. Matthew improved during the ensuing week and then became increasingly lethargic. A lumbar puncture was done, and the cerebrospinal fluid showed white blood cell and protein changes. Although there was evidence of nervous system involvement, the physicians did not believe it was rabies. By November 14, Matthew's speech became garbled and unintelligible, and he became more somnolent. After consultation with experts at the U.S. Public Health Center for Disease Control in Atlanta, it was decided that the boy was too sick to transfer to another hospital. Dr. Michael Hattwick, considered the top rabies expert of the Communicable Disease Center, left at once for Ohio.

Meanwhile Matthew developed increasing difficulty in talking and breathing. A tracheostomy was performed and oxygen administered. With the onset of twitchings in his left upper extremity, anticonvulsant medication was started. Two weeks later his condition slowly improved. Physical and speech therapies were started. On January 27, 1971, he was discharged from the hospital to be followed up by his own pediatrician. According to Dr. Hattwick, Matthew Winkler is the first documented person to survive rabies.

**Expected outcomes**

1 Consumers will be taught to avoid handling sick or wild animals.
2 Pet owners will know the importance of immunizing pets.
3 Clients with the disease will be instructed on requisite health care.
4 Significant others and clients will be involved in planning, implementing, and evaluating care when rabies is actual or expected.
5 Health care providers will be informed about changes in caring for those who may be at risk for developing rabies because of the advent of human diploid cell vaccine.

## TETANUS

Tetanus, commonly called *lockjaw*, is an acute infectious disease caused by the toxin of the tetanus bacillus, *Clostridium tetani*, an anaerobic organism. It is introduced into the body through an open wound. This spore-forming bacillus is commonly found in earth and manure and is hard to destroy; the spores may live for months or years under suitable conditions.

The incubation period may extend from 2 days to 3 weeks, depending on the character, extent, and location of the wound. The toxin, tetanospasmin, is second in virulence to botulin and passes up the nerves to the spinal cord and brain. Minute hemorrhages, edema, and inflammatory changes may be found in the medulla.

Symptoms may initially involve the jaws, with difficulty in opening the mouth and tonic spasms of the masseter muscles. Headache, back pain, stiffness of the lower extremities, elevated temperature and pulse rate, and apathy may be manifested.

As increasing numbers of nerve cells are invaded by the tetanus toxin, their inhibitory control over muscle activity is lost. Spasms may spread to muscles of the back; the head is retracted, producing the opisthotonus position; spasms of the laryngeal and pharyngeal muscles cause difficulty in breathing and swallowing; slight stimulation can increase pain and spasms and produce convulsions. If the costal and diaphragmatic muscles are involved, respirations may be severely affected; dyspnea, cyanosis, and asphyxia may result.

Clients with tetanus may display a facial appearance characteristic of this disease: features are tense; face is immobile; forehead is wrinkled; eyes are sunken; corners of the mouth are drawn with the lips pouting in a fixed, ghastly smile *(risus sardonicus)*.

Deep reflexes become hyperactive; sweating may be profuse; urination is difficult. Complications of respiratory failure, nephritis, pneumonia, and fractures of the vertebrae may develop.

Death occurs in about 35% of individuals infected with tetanus.

This disease is relatively uncommon in the United States. Active immunization with tetanus toxoid gives protection. The initial inoculation is preferably given in infancy or early childhood with diphtheria toxoid and pertussis vaccine.

Routine tetanus immunization and the administration of a booster injection are given every 10 years in the absence of an injury. If an injury has occurred, the booster should be given every 5 years rather than after each injury. Active immunization against tetanus is recommended for international travelers.

This disease should be reported to the local health department.

## Treatment and nursing intervention

The specific treatment depends on whether the individual has previously had a course of active immunization. It may vary from a booster injection to a large dose of tetanus antitoxin intravenously or a complete active immunization series. Tetanus immune globulin (human) instead of the tetanus antitoxin is given intramuscularly to clients who have a history of horse-serum sensitivity or other allergies. Penicillin also may be administered in large doses intramuscularly. The wound should be cleansed meticulously, debrided, cauterized as necessary, and left open for a few days.

During the acute stages of the illness the client should be maintained in a quiet, semidark room with minimal external stimuli. If possible, staff should be assigned and not changed so that the optimal environment may be maintained. The seriously ill client should be cared for in an intensive care unit, if available, where changes in condition may be closely monitored. Tracheostomy, suctioning, and intermittent positive-pressure respiration may be necessary for several weeks. The client may require sedative and anticonvulsant medication and nasal or intravenous feedings. Chlorpromazine (Thorazine) has been found effective for relieving reflex muscle spasms.

The principles employed in the physical and psychological treatment of clients with acute central nervous system disease may be applied to the care of these clients.

The favorable prognosis for recovery from tetanus depends on the prompt administration of the specific antitoxin and the treatment and prevention of complications.

### Expected outcomes
1 The public will be informed about the need for tetanus immunizations.
2 Involved clients and significant others will be educated in disease process and health care management.
3 Clients and significant others will be involved in care planning, implementation, and evaluation.

## REFERENCES

Andruzzi, E.: The alcoholic patient with coexisting longterm illness, Nurs. Clin. North Am. **5:**35-45, March 1970.

Arehart-Treichel, J.: Slow agents of death, Nurs. Digest **2:**81, 1974.

Bennett, J.V., et al.: *Hemophilus influenzae* meningitis, Pediatrics **53:**951, 1974.

Bond, J.O.: St. Louis encephalitis, Nurs. Outlook **14:**26-27, Oct. 1966.

Borgeson, L.: How much danger in canned foods? Family Health, Nov. 1971.

Brachman, P.S.: The new NCDC isolation manuals, a brief review, Nurs. Clin. North Am. **5:**175-177, March 1970.

Cluff, L.E., and Johnson, J.E., III, editors: Clinical concepts in infectious disease, ed. 2, Baltimore, 1978, The Williams & Wilkins Co.

Eaglstein, W., Katz, R., and Brown, J.: The effects of corticosteroid therapy on the skin eruption and pain of herpes zoster. J.A.M.A. **211:**1681-1683, 1970.

Elgin, D.: Nursing care study: meningitis—a pediatric emergency, Nurs. Times **70:**541, 1974.

Ellenberg, M.: Current status of diabetic neuropathy, Metabolism **22:**658, May 1973.

Etsinger, J.: Medical miracle—age seven—plays in backyard, loves pizza, Manchester Evening Herald, March 9, 1971.

Faich, G.A., Graebner, R.W., and Sato, S.: Failure of guanidine therapy in botulism A, N. Engl. J. Med. **285:**773-776, 1971.

Fallon, R.J., et al.: Meningococcal disease, Br. Med. J. **2:**272, 1974.

Foote, F.M., commissioner: Botulism—a major concern in home canning, Connecticut State Department of Health, Weekly Health Bull. **53:**Sept. 20, 1971.

Francis, B.J.: Current concepts in immunization, Am. J. Nurs. **73:**646-649, 1973.

Franco, L.M.: Acute disseminated intravascular coagulation, Cardiovas. Nurs. **15:**22-27, Sept.-Oct. 1979.

Furr, S.C.: Subacute sclerosing panencephalitis—care of the child, Am. J. Nurs. **72:**93-95, Jan. 1972.

Garner, J.S., and Kaiser, A.B.: How often is isolation needed? Am. J. Nurs. **72:**733-737, 1972.

Glenn, J.D., and Karels, Sister R.G.: Pediatric paralysis in Botoga, Am. J. Nurs. **73:**299-301, 1973.

Howard, J.: Botulism, Life Magazine, pp. 29-31, Sept. 10, 1971.

Kaufman, D.M., et al.: Computed tomography in herpes simplex encephalitis, Neurology **29:**1392-1396, Oct. 1979.

Kealy, S.L.: Respiratory care in Guillain-Barré syndrome, Am. J. Nurs. **77:**58, Jan. 1977.

Lamas, E., and Lobato, R.D.: Intraventricular pressure and CSF dynamics in chronic adult hydrocephalus, Surg. Neurol. **12:**287-295, Oct. 1979.

Levitt, L.P., Lovejoy, F.H., and Daniels, J.B.: Eastern equine encephalitis in Massachusetts—first human case in 14 years, N. Engl. J. Med. **284:**540, 1971.

Manginello, F.P., et al.: Neonatal meningococcal meningitis and meningococcemia, Am. J. Dis. Child. **133:**651, June 1979.

Magnaes, B.: Communicating hydrocephalus in adults, Neurology **28:**478-484, May 1978.

Messert, B., and Wannamaker, B.B.: Reappraisal of the adult occult hydrocephalus syndrome, Neurology **24:**224, March 1974.

Morrison, S., and Arnold, C.: Patients with common communicable diseases, Nurs. Clin. North Am. **5:**143-155, March 1970.

Nankervis, G.A.: Bacterial meningitis, Med. Clin. North Am. **58:**581, 1974.

Petrlik, J.C.: Diabetic peripheral neuropathy, Am. J. Nurs. **76:**1794, Nov. 1976.

Rahal, J.J., Jr., et al.: Combined intrathecal and intramuscular gentamicin for gram-negative meningitis: pharmacologic study of 21 patients, N. Engl. J. Med. **290:**1394, 1974.

Recommendation of the Immunization Practices Advisory Committee: Supplementary statement on rabies vaccine serologic testing, Morbidity and Mortality Weekly Report, Communicable Disease Control Center, vol. 30, no. 42, Oct. 30, 1981.

Risk, W.S., and Haddad, F.S.: The variable natural history of subacute sclerosing panencephalitis, Arch. Neurol. **36:**610-614, Oct. 1979.

Rocklin, R., et al.: The Guillain-Barré syndrome and multiple sclerosis. In vitro cellular responses to nervous-tissue antigens, N. Engl. J. Med. **284:**803-808, 1971.

Rodman, M.J.: Drugs for treating tetanus, RN **34:**43-50, Dec. 1971.

Rosenthal, M.S.: Viral infections of the central nervous system, Med. Clin. North Am. **58:**593, 1974.

Scott, T.F.M., and Wanglee, P.: Treamtent of encephalitis, Hosp. Med. **6:**88-97, Feb. 1970.

Steigman, A.J.: Mumps vaccine, Lancet **2:**1276, 1974.

Stone, M.H.: Normal pressure hydrocephalus, Nurs. Clin. North Am. **9:**667, Dec. 1974.

Top, F., and Wehrle, P.F., editors: Communicable and infectious diseases: diagnosis, prevention, treatment, ed. 8, St. Louis, 1976, The C.V. Mosby Co.

Tweed, G.G., Coyle, N., and Miller, B.: Guillain-Barré syndrome, Am. J. Nurs. **66:**2222-2226, 1966.

Varki, A., and Puthuran, P.: Value of second lumbar puncture in confirming a diagnosis of aseptic meningitis, Arch. Neurol. **36:**581-585, Sept. 1979.

Victor, M.: Delirium, Hosp. Med. **6:**116-129, March 1970.

Williams, B.B., and Lerner, A.M.: Some previously unrecognized features of herpes simplex virus encephalitis, Neurology **28:**1193-1196, Nov. 1978.

Williams, J.D., et al.: Ampicillin-resistant *Haemophilus influenzae* meningitis, Lancet **1:**864, 1974.

# 21

# INTRACRANIAL SPACE-OCCUPYING LESIONS

Intracranial tumors are neoplasms that arise from any of the cells of the structures within the cranium. Thus it is possible to have tumors originating from the meninges, the blood vessels, the nerve cells or glia, the pituitary body, or the pineal gland. Metastatic tumors and those originating from the skull are also encountered. As with any neoplasm, these may be either benign or malignant, but because of their relationship to vital structures, histologically benign lesions may have malignant effects. By far the largest number of these tumors arise from the glia, supporting cells of the brain, and are called *gliomas*. These constitute almost 60% of all intracranial tumors. The *meningiomas,* benign tumors that arise from the meningeal coverings of the brain, amount to about 15%; the *metastatic tumors* account for 10%; and the remaining 15% include about 3% *pituitary adenomas,* 5% *acoustic neurofibromas,* and a scattering of others. Gliomas are not encapsulated, grow from the brain tissue itself, and invade its adjacent parts. Of these, 50% are *glioblastomas* and *medulloblastomas;* they grow relatively rapidly. The less active types, of which the *astrocytoma* is the most common, constitute the other 50%.

Brain tumors cause over 40% of the deaths (exclusive of strokes) resulting from diseases of the central nervous system. The peak incidence occurs in childhood and during the fifth decade of life, with a slightly higher incidence in males than in females.

## TUMOR CHARACTERISTICS

Tumors are characterized by a number of features. They may be single, multiple, multicentric, localized, or systemic. Also, the various tumors differ in their patterns of growth and may involve surrounding tissue through destruction, infiltration, or expansion. At times the individual may have more than one type of tumor simultaneously, such as when the individual with Recklinghausen's neurofibromatosis has meningiomas, neurinomas, and spongioblastomas simultaneously. When the tumor is evaluated in relation to its degree of malignancy, morphological and clinical features are considered in the effort to evaluate the total effect of the tumor. Thus if the same type of tumor is present in two different portions of the body, it may be considered to be benign at one site and malignant at the other. The following seven characteristics are commonly evaluated when one is estimating tumor malignancy:

1. Macroscopic and histological appearance
2. Tumor growth and volume
3. Effect on adjacent tissue
4. Structural alterations and displacements resulting from any increased intracranial pressure
5. Involvement of ventricular system in tumor growth
6. Encroachment of the growth on vital centers, including the hypothalamus and reticular formation
7. Vascular disturbances related to tumor growth

The signs and symptoms of intracranial tumors vary and may have as many presenting phenomena as there are functions in the brain. These signs may be the result of gradual or rapid loss of a particular function leading to failure of vision or loss of strength, sensation, speech, memory, or reason, or there may be manifestations of stimulation resulting in convulsions, hallucinations, pain, or paresthesias. These indications of dysfunction are the most important ones to recognize if an early diagnosis of intracranial tumor is to be made. Only infrequently does the early symptomatology include headache, vomiting, and failing vision, which until about 60 years ago were considered essential before entertaining a diagnosis of cerebral tumor. When these latter symptoms are present, intracranial pressure has already increased considerably. Even before this time the neurological examination may show beginning *papilledema,* which is one of the most important signs in the early differential diagnosis of brain tumor. No specific symptoms corresponding to the different types of neoplasms have been identified other than those associated with the pituitary tumors.

## DIAGNOSIS

Helpful information is gained from radiographic examination. The plain films may show unusual calcification, abnormal vascularity, and erosion or hyperostosis of bone. Radioisotope radiation (brain scanning) of brain tumors now approaches 95% accuracy. The lesion must be more than 2 cm in diameter for the scanning to be effective. If multiple lesions are suspected, this technique is most helpful in localizing them. If the lesion is lateralized, a carotid angiogram is made of the side of the tumor, but if there are no localizing indications, bilateral carotid angiograms may be made. If localization is not yet accomplished, pneumoencephalography is undertaken, and if filling of the ventricles is not attained with this procedure, ventriculography is performed as a last resort. Cerebral angiography has come to supplement air studies because this procedure generally gives more information by demonstrating the distortion or abnormality of the vascular pattern and in some instances foreshadows the histological diagnosis by revealing characteristic vascular architecture and circulation time for glioblastomas and meningiomas. Angiography is also helpful if the existence of more than one lesion is suspected (as in metastatic carcinoma). Computerized axial tomography is also valuable in localizing the lesion.

The diagnosis of an intracranial tumor is further supported by the persistent and increasingly severe physical signs and symptoms. Headache becomes generalized and progressively more troublesome. Readily recognizable deficits, such as hemiplegia and hemianesthesia, lateralize the *supratentorial* lesion. If the motor weakness or sensory impairment were limited to an upper or lower extremity or the face, the relative position of the tumor in the hemisphere would be obvious (near the longitudinal sinus if the foot were affected, nearer the fissure of Sylvius if the face were involved). Impairment of speech and homonymous hemianopia would point to the *temporal* lobe as the seat of the trouble. Loss of smell, loss of memory, or personality changes would direct the attention to a *frontal* lobe lesion.

If the signs and symptoms include principally incoordination in the use of the extremities and unsteadiness of gait with staggering, in addition to severe headache and disturbance of vision with obvious papilledema, the lesion is generally *infratentorial*. If associated unilateral disturbances of the cranial nerves are present, such as loss of hearing, facial paralysis, impaired sensation over the face, or difficulty in swallowing or phonating, the lesion in the posterior fossa can be lateralized to one or the other side.

Thus the diagnosis of intracranial tumors is differentiated into two categories for the purposes of diagnostic studies. In supratentorial tumors, papilledema is frequently the most prominent sign when symptoms of the tumor first become obvious, since the cranial vault is a fixed space after childhood. Radiographic studies often reveal convolutional markings on the skull. Both of these signs are caused by the generalized increases in intracranial pressure often obvious in supratentorial tumors. Pressure exerted at various points in the cerebrum may result in several problems, including sensorimotor disturbances and seizures. Electroencephalography (EEG) is valuable in localizing many of the cerebral tumors as well as the focal pattern of seizures. However, EEG is only a screening tool, since it does not reveal the presence of tumors in the brainstem, ventricles, or suprasellar region. EEG is often followed by radiographic films of the skull, which reveal such changes as the increased convolutional markings previously mentioned, changes in the sella turcica, erosion or hyperostoses of the skull, and sometimes tumor calcification in certain types of tumors.

When EEG and radiographic studies of the skull indicate a lesion, carotid angiography is performed. Cerebral tumors often displace blood vessels. If bony structures make visualization of small vessels difficult, results are computed by the process of electronic subtraction.

Scintigraphy is another diagnostic technique whereby the brain is studied by means of isotope scanning. In this technique the tumor picks up the labeled substance, whereas the substance does not penetrate normal tissue to a significant extent. Although the process of tumor affinity for the substance is not well understood, it is often explained in relation to the cerebral edema around the lesion, which results in increased concentrations of the substance in the interstitial spaces; to the increased blood flow to the tumor from increased vascularity in the lesion; and to the increased capillary permeability that results from the break in the blood-brain barrier. One feature of scintigraphy is that low-grade tumors (astrocytomas, oligodendrogliomas) pick up the substance poorly and may evade diagnosis by this method. However, the highly malignant tumors (meningiomas, glioblastomas, and metastases) pick up the substance readily. Thus diagnosticians rely on gamma scans and three-dimensional views of the lesion to gain more precise data on the location of the lesion.

Positron scanning is sometimes used in preference to gamma scanning because it provides a sharper image and is quick and uncomplicated. It is particularly valuable in indicating the presence of midline tumors and multiple metastases.

Another technique frequently utilized in detecting supratentorial masses is echoencephalography (ultrasonography). In this two-dimensional brain-scanning technique, which is safe and painless, a contrast is seen between normal and defective tissue. Because of its safety the technique may be done on a client repeatedly.

One of the greatest advances of our times is the widespread use of computerized axial tomography, also known as the CAT scan. In this technique, complete visualization of brain lesions in proper dimensions is available as the machine makes photographic impressions in a slice pattern all over the brain. The procedure may be either invasive, with the use of dye, or noninvasive.

Ventriculograms and CAT scans may be indicated to reveal the presence of midline tumors even at the earliest stages.

Although tumors of the infratentorial region are characterized by various symptoms according to location of the lesion and type of tumor, like supratentorial tumors, a few general statements may be made about the diagnosis of these tumors, which invade the posterior fossa.

Symptoms from tumors in the posterior fossa may include cerebellar signs, cervical signs (obligatory head position or neck pain), cranial nerve involvement, or long tract signs. In tumors of the brainstem, pyramidal tract signs are seen early in the disease course.

If the lesion in the posterior fossa does not involve the ventricular system, there are no signs of increased intracranial pressure. However, a lumbar puncture often suggests the presence of a tumor when it results in the presence of tumor cells, an increased cerebrospinal fluid pressure, elevated protein levels, and a normal glucose level and cell count. EEG is not particularly reliable in indicating the presence of a tumor in the posterior fossa. Radiographic studies of the skull frequently reveal changes in bony structure. Pneumoencephalograms are often utilized to detect these tumors, since many of them eventually result in involvement of the ventricular system. Sometimes the dye used in a ventriculogram obstructs the ventricular system and must then be immediately removed while the client undergoes surgical decompression. When a carotid angiogram indicates that a supratentorial space-occupying mass and internal hydrocephalus are lacking, but the practitioner realizes that the client has had subarachnoid hemorrhages, increased intracranial pressure from a lesion near the tentorium, or obstructions in the basilar or vertebral arteries, a vertebral angiogram may be indicated to gather more data. In vertebral angiography, cerebellar tumors are noted only at the end stages, but arteriovenous malformations are visualized early.

Dural sinus venography is the method utilized to indicate narrowing of sinuses and interferences with cranial drainage, which often occur in lesions of the posterior fossa. If the lesion involves the ventricular system, echoencephalography is valuable in indicating the lesion.

For some reason, brain scans show opposite results in the infratentorial area. Low-grade malignancies pick up the substance readily, whereas highly malignant tumors may evade detection through brain scanning.

A *pituitary tumor* manifests itself in various ways, depending on the age at which it first appears, the specific type of cell involved, and the ease with which it has extended up from the sella turcica to compress the optic chiasma or hypothalamus. There are three types of cells—eosinophilic, basophilic, and neutrophilic—in the pituitary body, and each gives rise to a specific type of tumor. The *eosinophilic tumor* may develop before the bones have ossified. Since these cells are responsible for growth, their overactivity causes *gigantism,* whereas if the tumor develops after the bones have ossified, there is an overgrowth of the bony prominences, and the resulting picture is *acromegaly.* These two conditions, gigantism and acromegaly, have an associated impaired tolerance for carbohydrates. The other two types of cells give rise to tumors that appear after maturity. The *basophilic adenoma* is a rare tumor and is usually minute, measuring only a few millimeters in size; nevertheless, it has extremely powerful effects and causes the typical picture of pituitary basophilism (Cushing's syndrome), which is characterized by a grotesque and painful obesity of the trunk with thin extremities, plethoric facies, hirsutism, large striae over the abdomen, arterial hypertension, and hyperglycemia. The neutrophilic cells may give rise to a *chromophobe adenoma*. Clients who have this tumor manifest sluggishness, a sallow appearance with fine skin and hair (which is also sparse), a tendency to a female habitus in the male, loss of libido, amenorrhea, increased glucose tolerance, and low basal metabolism. The characteristics described result from the effects of glandular dysfunction and are specific for this type of tumor. Other distinguishing manifestations, called *neighborhood* signs and symptoms, are caused by compression of adjacent structures by the expanding tumor (except the basophilic adenoma, which has never been known to reach a size capable of doing this). Vision may be impaired, the visual fields may demonstrate *bitemporal hemianopia,* and the fundi may demonstrate primary optic atrophy. Radiographic examination of the skull shows an enlargement and thinning of the walls of the sella turcica.

## TREATMENT AND NURSING INTERVENTION

The basophilic adenoma is treated with radiation. This is probably the only tumor of the nervous system that is thus treated before histological verification (biopsy). In this instance, if an adrenal neoplasm has been ruled out, the clinical picture is so distinctive that it constitutes virtual certainty of diagnosis. The eosinophilic (chromophilic) tumors and the neutrophilic (chromophobic) tumors should be removed surgically as completely as possible, and radiation therapy should then be given to obtain the maximum therapeutic effect.

The treatment of all other intracranial tumors is preceded by histological identification. Generally they are removed as completely as possible even if malignant. Radiation therapy may be given with temporary benefit to some of these, particularly the medulloblastomas. Tumors that arise from structures not primarily neurological (such as bone, meninges, and blood vessels) are removed with greater success, since they do not infiltrate the brain, as do the gliomas, and when completely extirpated do not recur.

Chemotherapy has recently been employed in an effort to combat the malignant glioma that to date has been unresponsive to standard forms of therapy, including surgery and radiation therapy. In some instances, these drugs have been therapeutically effective. Because of the continuous advances in treatment modalities, especially in relation to chemotherapy, it is not practical to quote specific regimens. To gather the latest data the nurse may utilize the following two resources: (1) communicate with or visit an oncological specialty unit connected with a national computerized program or (2) telephone the following:

Cancer Information Service (1-800-638-6694) or the Office of Cancer Information (1-301-496-5583)

for details on all aspects of cancer for either the layman or the health professional.

In Chapter 12 the most frequently used diagnostic tests and procedures are described. The responsibilites of the nurse in preparing the client and equipment, in assisting the physician, and in the aftercare of the client and equipment are given in detail. Criteria for indications and contraindications in the administration of these tests are also included.

To clarify and emphasize special points of nursing care, intracranial tumors are said to occur in the supratentorial or infratentorial region. *Supratentorial* lesions are all those located in the cerebrum or the anterior two thirds of the brain; *infratentorial* lesions occur in the cerebellum or brainstem, the posterior one third of the brain.

The nursing care of clients with intracranial lesions is based on the signs and symptoms of disturbed physiology and is directed toward the early recognition, prevention, and treatment of complications. The clinical signs, symptoms, and probable complications of specific localized tumors were discussed earlier in this chapter. The basic nursing care for clients with intracranial tumors before operation is the same for all, regardless of the pathological condition. Individual modifications are determined by the symptomatology and whether the lesion is above or below the tentorium. In addition, when planning the client's care, consideration is given to personality, reaction to the illness, fears, and emotional needs, as well as the physical manifestations of disease. To the extent possible the alert client is involved in developing and implementing the nursing care plan. Chapter 27 gives detailed suggestions that can be applied in the care of clients with intracranial lesions who are gravely, acutely, or chronically ill.

It is most important that nurses be familiar with the client's history, objective findings, subjective complaints, suspected diagnosis, and proposed treatment to plan and administer effective nursing care intelligently. Only by knowing these things can they evaluate the client's progress. They can thus note and report changes in condition to avert complications that may be fatal. Most neurologists and neurosurgeons with nurse specialists depend on them to a great extent for accurate observations of these clients. Nurses have the most frequent, the longest, and the most personal contacts with the clients in each 24-hour period. Observe clients with increased intracranial pressure closely and accurately, and report changes immediately to the physician. One cannot emphasize too strongly the importance of these observations in the management and treatment of clients with increased intracranial pressure.

## INCREASED INTRACRANIAL PRESSURE

The first step in the diagnosis of a brain tumor is to eliminate the possibility of any space-occupying lesion other than a neoplasm. A detailed history should assist in eliminating such problems as trauma that has resulted in a hematoma or inflammatory processes that may result in granulomas or abscesses.

Whenever a primary space-occupying lesion exists, several secondary processes may result, including the following:
1. Brain edema
2. Cerebrospinal fluid disturbances resulting from interferences in absorption, drainage, or overproduction
3. Interrupted blood flow caused by intracranial compression

An illustration of these generalized and specific effects of increased intracranial pressure is given in the boxed material on p. 538.

Brain edema may be either localized or diffuse. This edema may be primary or secondary. In primary lesions, edema occurs as a response to certain malignant brain tumors. In the secondary type of brain edema the problem is caused as the lesion impedes normal circulation by mechanical obstruction or disturbs the blood-brain barrier through hypoxia.

Local necrosis results as edema produces parenchymal lesions. Microscopic studies reveal an excess of fluid in the astrocytes of the gray matter and in the intercellular spaces of the white matter. Macroscopically, one notes flattening of gyri, narrowing sulci, and tissue displacement.

The flow of cerebrospinal fluid may be impaired by direct compression of the ventricular system or by indirect compression resulting from displacement of neighboring structures. Areas most frequently affected by mechanical compression include the foramina of Magendie, Luschka, and Monro and the aqueduct of Sylvius.

As intracranial pressure mounts, the immediate effects may include increased blood flow in response to vasomotor paralysis or venous conges-

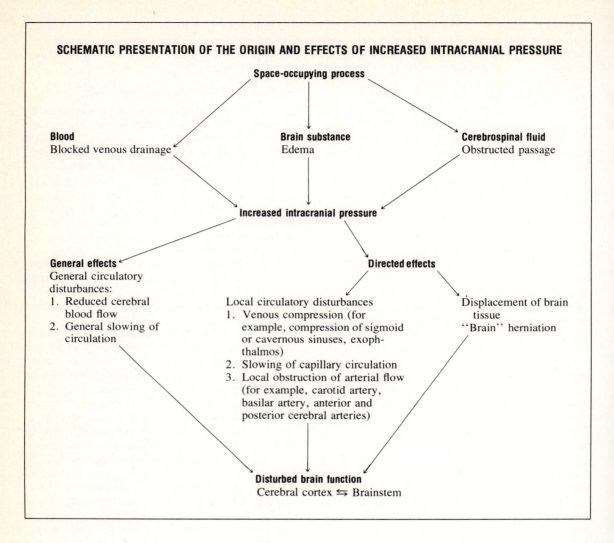

**SCHEMATIC PRESENTATION OF THE ORIGIN AND EFFECTS OF INCREASED INTRACRANIAL PRESSURE**

Space-occupying process

**Blood**
Blocked venous drainage

**Brain substance**
Edema

**Cerebrospinal fluid**
Obstructed passage

**Increased intracranial pressure**

**General effects**
General circulatory
disturbances:
1. Reduced cerebral
   blood flow
2. General slowing of
   circulation

**Directed effects**

Local circulatory disturbances
1. Venous compression (for
   example, compression of sigmoid
   or cavernous sinuses, exophthalmos)
2. Slowing of capillary circulation
3. Local obstruction of arterial flow
   (for example, carotid artery,
   basilar artery, anterior and
   posterior cerebral arteries)

Displacement of brain
tissue
"Brain" herniation

**Disturbed brain function**
Cerebral cortex ⇆ Brainstem

tion. As intracranial pressure remains elevated, compression interrupts blood flow to as much as half the normal capacity. Concurrently, oxygen supplies to the brain are deficient. Although brain tissue is perfused poorly, the actual amount of circulatory flow through the head may be increased in such vascular tumors as glioblastomas, arteriovenous shunts, and other vascular neoplasms. In these instances, increased blood supplies are utilized by the tumor itself, and surrounding brain tissue develops edema because of diminished oxygen supplies. The process of edema formation re-sults in ischemia and hypoxia cause tissue necrosis and damaged endothelium.

Blood flow may also be impaired at the point of exit from the cranial cavity if lesions in the posterior aspect of the cranium compress sigmoid and cavernous sinuses.

### Assessment

The following observations are made routinely by the nurse.

*State of consciousness.* The nurse observes the client's orientation as to person, place, and time;

alertness in verbal and physical response to the nurse's testing; and degree of lethargy, drowsiness, stupor, or coma. Variations in the quality of a client's response are monitored very closely and determined at specified intervals even if it is necessary to wake a sleeping client. A change in the level of consciousness may be one of the first signs of increasing intracranial pressure. The level of consciousness may be partially evaluated when one tests the pupillary reaction; generally if the client is comatose, the pupils are fixed bilaterally.

Refer to Chapter 9 for detailed information on the use of the Glasgow Coma Scale, a method of providing a rapid, standardized, thumbnail sketch of the client's status in terms of consciousness. Utilize the Glasgow Coma Scale in conjunction with thorough serial neurological assessments.

*Ocular signs.* Note the pupils' size, equality, and reaction to light. Normally, pupils are equal in size and react readily to light. An intracranial hemorrhage may cause the pupil on the affected side to become dilated and fixed, that is, it will not react when a beam of light is directed on the pupil. The client may have double vision or progressive failure of vision because of papilledema (choked disc).

*Vomiting.* Note characteristics and frequency of vomiting, whether or not it is projectile, and if it is accompanied by nausea or retching. If the client is conscious, caution him or her not to strain while vomiting or while using the bedpan because the intracranial pressure is thereby increased.

*Function.* Note motion and strength of facial muscles and extremities. If the client is conscious, ask him or her to show the teeth, smile, wrinkle the nose, close the eyelids tightly and resist attempts to open them, wrinkle the forehead, frown, raise the arms, grip the nurse's hands simultaneously, raise the legs singly and together, raise the knees, pull the feet up, and push the feet down against the resistance of the nurse's hands.

These tests of motor function are directed to the early recognition of *hemiparesis* (weakness on one side of the body) or *hemiplegia* (paralysis of one side of the body). These may occur on the side opposite the lesion in a client with increasing intracranial pressure and generally indicate the need for immediate treatment.

*Vital signs.* Pulse, respiration, and blood pressure are measured at the intervals ordered by the physician according to the needs of the individual client. If there is clinical evidence of increased intracranial pressure, it may be necessary to record them at 30-minute intervals. Rectal temperatures are taken every 2 to 4 hours. If the temperature is rising or if treatment has been instituted for hyperthermia, it should be taken every 15 to 30 minutes. Pulse and respiration should be measured for 1 full minute. Whenever possible, blood pressures should be determined on the same arm with the client in the same position for reliable interpretation. Changes in vital signs that indicate increasing or increased intracranial pressure are slowly falling pulse and respiration rate with an associated rise in blood pressure. If the client is untreated, lengthening periods of apnea follow, and respiration ceases.

*Pain.* Headache is an important symptom of increasing intracranial pressure. The nurse should note its location, duration, and severity. The position the client assumes for maximum comfort may be significant and should be recorded.

*Convulsions.* Convulsions may occur in clients with discrete lesions involving the frontal or parietal lobes or in clients with increased intracranial pressure. Accurate observation of a convulsive episode and in detailed charting of it may assist the physician in localizing the intracranial lesion. (For description, refer to Chapter 14.)

*Other considerations.* Increasing restlessness or the exaggeration of any symptom or sign may be slow in onset or dramatically sudden. Only early recognition of changes and immediate treatment can ensure the prolongation of the client's life. Many of these clients present diagnostic problems, in the solution of which the neurological nurse can assist the physician immeasurably by accurately recorded observations.

## Position

Unless contraindicated the client should be kept out of bed. If this is not feasible, elevate the head above the level of heart at a 30- to 40-degree angle and stabilize the head so that the chin does not compress any blood vessels in the neck or obstruct the airway. The upright position reduces venous congestion, improves drainage from the brain, may prevent a further increase in intracranial pressure, and makes the client a better surgical risk. Clients with brain tumors usually prefer this position, as it frequently relieves headache. If the client is confined to bed, a cradle and a footboard should be used, and the client should be postured as outlined in Chapter 9, with a change of position at least every 2 hours. Stuporous or unconscious clients should be supervised closely and positioned on alternate sides to prevent aspiration and help maintain an open airway. Weakened or paralyzed extremities require special attention and care to prevent footdrop and wristdrop, muscle stretching, joint contractures, decubitus ulcers, deformities, and burns. If the client has any changes in state of consciousness or if he or she is subject to seizures, use side rails when the individual is unattended to prevent falling out of bed and injury. Use subsequent restraints with great caution and only when necessary to keep the client in a particular position in bed. They generally defeat their purpose by further exciting the client. The evidence of irritation on wrists and ankles where they have been used improperly is a bad reflection on the nursing staff. More extreme circulatory disruption may have legal implications. For minimal local reaction and prevention of circulatory disturbance, it is suggested that the restraints be made of quilted muslin, approximately 3 inches wide for the wrist and ankle and 6 inches wide for the knee. Ideally, restless uncooperative clients should have someone in constant attendance. This opportunity may be utilized as an educational experience for the nursing student. It also may be possible to have a member of the family stay with the client for stated periods of time. The involvement of the family not only serves to supplement the nursing staff but also may calm the client and help the family through this period of stress.

## Nutrition

The diet should be well balanced and the meals supervised to ensure adequate nutrition. Supplementary feedings may be utilized as indicated. If possible, clients should be weighed once weekly. If vomiting is a problem, artificial feedings may have to be administered. If intracranial pressure is greatly increased, the fluid intake by mouth may be restricted to 1500 ml each 24 hours.

## Hygiene

If the client is confined to bed, the nurse should follow the suggestions outlined in Chapter 9 for detailed nursing care. Supervise the hygiene of ambulatory clients. Preoperative oral hygiene is most important in reducing the incidence of local postoperative complications.

## Elimination

The client with urinary retention or incontinence needs catheter drainage. The bowels should be kept open with mild cathartics, and enemas should be avoided. Caution the client against straining at stool because of the danger of compression of the midbrain or medulla oblongata, which can result in respiratory failure. If the client is stuporous or unconscious, a colon lavage is performed every 2 or 3 days to prevent the occurrence of involuntary defecations or impactions.

## Emotional needs

Independence should be encouraged. The nurse can help psychologically by anticipating the clients' wishes if the clients are aphasic, by avoiding situations with which they cannot cope, and by arranging trays and articles clockwise on the bedside table to aid those with rapidly failing vision. Avoid causing needless emotional trauma, and maintain a positive and optimistic attitude toward the client and his or her ultimate recovery.

After the diagnostic study is completed, the client needs diversional therapy, occupational and physical, according to individual needs and preferences. If the client has a disability, occupational therapy is directed toward its constructive amelioration if possible, that is, strengthening weakened extremities by activities such as weaving.

During the preoperative period the nurse makes every attempt to facilitate the client's adjustment to the illness, the hospital, and the staff. The approach will, through necessity, be modified for the individual client. The nature of the illness, ability to cooperate, personality, and intelligence must be considered. Too much emphasis cannot be placed on adequate psychological preparation of the client before a new diagnostic test, procedure, or treatment is instituted.

## Medications

Whenever the dose of a medication is stated in this text, it is the amount generally used for an adult. This may vary with the individual, and the nurse should not administer any medication without the written order of the physician.

*Analgesics.* Analgesics may be given for the relief of headache; aspirin, 0.6 gm, and caffeine citrate, 0.12 gm, are as efficacious as any.

*Anticonvulsants.* Phenobarbital, phenytoin (Dilantin), trimethadione (Tridione), and others may be used to control seizures. Chapter 14 discusses the treatment of paroxysmal disorders.

*Hypertonic solutions.* Urevert (30% solution), urea, and mannitol (50% solution) have been found extremely effective for the temporary reduction of increased intracranial pressure. However, mannitol is used less often now, since practitioners may not believe that it is beneficial to have a clinical picture of improvement while the intracranial mass keeps expanding, as in the case of intracranial bleeding. When the nature of the lesion is known, mannitol may still be utilized. Steroids are an important adjunct to the treatment of clients with cerebral edema (Chapters 23, 27, and 28).

*Narcotics.* Codeine has been used effectively to alleviate the headache associated with increased intracranial pressure. Morphine is contraindicated because of its depressing effect on the central nervous system and the possibility of obscuring clinical signs. In general, narcotics should be used with discretion in light of their addictive properties and their effect on the central nervous system.

*Cathartics.* If dehydration is desired, 30 ml of a saturated solution (50%) of magnesium sulfate is given before breakfast. Clients find this more palatable if a few drops of essence of peppermint are added and if it is served chilled. A slice of lemon or a piece of hard candy taken afterward helps remove the unpleasant taste. Milk of magnesia, 30 ml, given at bedtime may be effective in maintaining regular bowel elimination. If not successful, the addition of 4 ml of liquid extract of cascara sagrada should be effectual. Strong purgatives are contraindicated.

*Vitamins.* Supplementary vitamin therapy may be given orally if the client has anorexia (poor appetite) or intramuscularly if the client is vomiting.

## PREOPERATIVE NURSING INTERVENTIONS
### Preparation for operation

When surgical intervention has been decided on, an explanation is given to the client, family, or significant others by the physician. The extent of this depends on the individual client and the physical and psychological condition. Reassurance and reinforcement of details are given whenever necessary by the nurse.

Permission for operation is signed by the nearest relative after a detailed explanation by the physician. In some instances the client may be considered sufficiently competent to sign the permission; however, the nearest relative is also consulted. The practice varies in different institutions.

Orders are left in writing on the chart the afternoon before the scheduled operation.

If, up to this time, the client's elimination has been adequate, there should be no need for enemas before surgery. Since any rectal procedure may be uncomfortable and fatiguing, the routine use of enemas is discouraged.

Clients are usually questioned about their wishes concerning a visit from their respective clergy or other spiritual practices.

### Preparation of client

On the evening before surgery the client is given a bath to avoid becoming overtired in the morning. This also is the time to reinforce explanations given to the client regarding his or her operation by the various health team members.

On the morning of the operation, if the client is a man, shave his face. The procedure for clipping the hair and shaving the head is determined by institutional policy. It is generally done by the neurosurgeon after the client is anesthetized to reduce the trauma. The head is first shaved with electric clippers and then gone over again with a straight razor. It is important that the shaving be done by an experienced person to eliminate nicking or cutting the scalp, since this may increase the danger of infection. Shaving the head usually takes 30 to 45 mintues.

If possible, before the preoperative medication is given, the client ambulates to stimulate the circulation. The client receives morning care, including scrupulous oral hygiene. Dentures, unless otherwise ordered, are removed, placed in a labeled container, and put in the designated place. If the client is wearing a wedding ring, it is removed or secured with a piece of tape placed around the ring; other valuables are removed and stored in a safe place. A clean gown and emboli stockings are put on the client.

During preoperative preparation of the client the nurse can establish an expected client outcome on which to build the plan of care. These are arrived at after a thorough neurological assessment to identify base-line information. An example of an expected client outcome in the preoperative phase of hospitalization is as follows: The client will state his knowledge about his neurological condition. Other expected client outcomes that may be identified in reference to the neurological client will include the following areas:

1. Vital signs
   Temperature
   Pulse
   Respirations
   Blood pressure
2. Neurological signs
   Pupils and eye signs
   Motion and strength of extremities
   Mobility and symmetry of facial muscles
3. Orientation
   Person
   Place
   Time

Encourage the client to use the bedpan or urinal. During this preparation of the client for operation note subjective and objective reactions, reassure the client as necessary, and try to allay any apprehension. Usually, if it is not contraindicated, the client is permitted to see the immediate family before leaving for surgery. Generally, visitors are not permitted after the preoperative medication has been given.

Instruct the client's family regarding the possible duration of the operation; if they wish to remain in the hospital, direct them to a suitable waiting room. Cranial operations generally last 3 to 6 hours. This will be a very trying and anxious period for the family, and every attempt is made by the hospital staff to make it less so.

Someone is responsible for attending the family at intervals to inform them of the general progress being made in the operating room and to reassure them as necessary. It is important that the needs of relatives and friends are not overlooked and the opportunity to help them and to lay the foundation for involving them actively in the future care of the client is recognized. By developing good relations with the families of the clients from the time of admission to the hospital, the staff is doing a great deal to minimize the psychological trauma that is, of necessity, a part of every illness.

## POSTOPERATIVE NURSING CARE
### Preparation of postoperative environment

The client is placed in an intensive care unit until his or her condition is sufficiently stable for a safe return to the general unit. The bed is taken to the operating room so that the client can be moved directly from the operating table to the bed. This eliminates unnecessary jostling and moving and can be done under the supervision of the neurosurgeon to minimize the danger of trauma and hemorrhage.

### Preparation of bed

The bed is made with a draw sheet made from a large sheet folded lengthwise and then in half and placed across the bed to the top of the mattress. This will be used as a turning sheet and should support the head and entire back to be effective in preventing trauma when the client is turned. A large Pliofilm-covered pillow is placed on the bed to be used under the head of the client who has had a supratentorial operation; a small, firm, Pliofilm-covered pillow is used after an infratentorial operation or if the client is stuporous or unconscious. The cradle and extra equipment are left in the room and placed on the bed after the client's return. The remaining equipment is collected in the room or placed on the bedside table to expedite postoperative care. This eliminates needless trips, leaving the client alone or unprotected, and loss of time if an emergency occurs.

## POSTOPERATIVE INTERVENTIONS
### After supratentorial operation

If a large tumor is removed, leaving a large cavity, keep the client off the operative site. Elevate the head of the bed to a 45-degree angle, and turn the client every 2 hours. If the client is in shock, keep the head flat; elevation of the head is related to the amount of intracranial pressure present (position the client as suggested in Chapter 9).

Take temperature on return, then every hour for 4 hours, then every 2 hours for 24 hours, and then every 4 hours (may be ordered more or less frequently, depending on the site and extent of the lesion and the condition of the client).

Take pulse, respiration, and blood pressure on return, then every 30 minutes for 6 hours, then every hour for 18 hours, and then as needed by the individual client.

Limit fluids to 1500 ml in 24 hours. Measure output.

Give soft diet as tolerated. Administer prescribed pain medication as required for headache. Suction as necessary.

## After infratentorial operation

Keep the client off the back, position him or her flat on either side with a small head pillow, and turn every 1 to 2 hours (position the client as suggested in Chapter 9). Take the temperature routinely as after supratentorial operation. Vital signs should be checked at approximately the same intervals as after supratentorial operations.

Give nothing by mouth for 24 hours. Measure output.

Suction if necessary. Watch for respiratory difficulty because of surgical proximity to vital structures.

## Observations

Compare preoperative and postoperative observations and vital signs. General observations are also made regarding the condition, color, and warmth of the client's skin. The amount and color of any drainage on the dressing are noted.

## Position

Unless otherwise ordered, a client who has not recovered completely from anesthesia or one who is weak, stuporous, or unconscious is kept off the back and placed on the side. The position on the side facilitates breathing, prevents the tongue from falling back and obstructing the glottis, and ensures a better airway. If the client's head is so placed on a small, firm pillow that the mouth is dependent, the danger of aspiration of mucus or vomitus is lessened. In this position, secretions will drain freely from the mouth. Turning is done cautiously for the first 48 hours. The head of the bed should be labeled if the position is restricted.

After supratentorial surgery the client is kept in approximately the same position as during the operation. If this was upright, lowering the head will increase the blood supply to the brain and may start venous bleeding; therefore unless the client is in shock, it is contraindicated. If the blood pressure is dangerously low or symptoms of shock are present, the position is altered as necessary to treat shock. However, no nurse should assume responsibility for lowering the client's head without a written order from the resident or attending surgeon. Trendelenburg's position is generally contraindicated because the increased blood flow to the brain may precipitate a hemorrhage. For treatment of shock after intracranial surgery the optimum position of the client is flat on the side with the head on the same plane as the rest of the body.

After an infratentorial operation the client is kept flat on either side for the prevention of complications. The client is instructed regarding restrictions of position and activity. He or she is kept off the back for the first 24 to 48 hours because of the increased danger of aspiration caused by impaired swallowing and gag reflexes. On the third day the head of the bed is usually elevated 15 degrees and on the seventh day, 30 degrees. Thereafter it is raised progressively until the tenth day when, if all has gone well, the client usually sits up.

## Nutrition

After an operation on the anterior two thirds of the head (supratentorial region) the client generally tolerates fluids well. If residual symptoms of increased intracranial pressure are present and vomiting persists, it is advisable to stop everything by mouth for 24 hours because the associated straining may cause postoperative bleeding. Intravenous fluids are frequently used during this period. It is desirable that the intravenous fluids be controlled by an infusion device to ensure accuracy of the fluid delivery. When vomiting is not a problem, encourage the client to take a soft diet on the first and second postoperative days and a regular diet by the third day. After major intracranial surgery, all clients are assisted with feeding for approximately 48 hours to prevent unnecessary activity or fatigue and to ensure an adequate intake.

The client who has had an operation on the posterior one third of the brain (infratentorial region) is permitted nothing by mouth for 24 hours. Sometimes because of edema or trauma the functions of the glossopharyngeal and vagus nerves are disturbed, resulting in loss of the gag reflex and considerable difficulty in swallowing. After 24 hours, before the client is tried on fluids, test for gag and swallowing reflexes. If they are present, offer clear water through a straw, never by spoon or cup, since this may cause choking or aspiration. Once it is established that the client has no residual swallowing difficulties, fluids can be given freely unless limited. Soft food is given on the second day after operation, a regular diet on the fourth day.

If the client develops facial weakness or paralysis, fluids are taken through the opposite or unaffected side of the mouth to reduce drooling and other feeding difficulties. This can best be done while the client is on the side, with the paralyzed side uppermost. It is important to give careful mouth care after meals because of the likelihood of food being left in the mouth on the paralyzed side and acting as a focus for sordes and infection.

### Elimination

Unless the client becomes distended, uncomfortable, or restless because of a full bladder, he or she is usually so dehydrated that 12 hours or longer may safely separate voiding times. Usually the problem is one of incontinence rather than retention. If the client is stuporous, unconscious, or incontinent, catheter or condom drainage may be instituted to keep the individual dry, to prevent pressure sores, and to maintain bladder function. It is important to maintain intake and output records for 72 hours postoperatively.

A cathartic is given when indicated and unless contraindicated is followed by an enema the next day. (If the client is unable to retain an enema or if there is increased intracranial pressure, a colon lavage should be substituted.) Thereafter, cathartics and enemas are used as indicated to ensure adequate bowel evacuation every second or third day.

### Drug therapy

When doses are stated, they are to be used only for adults. This may vary with the individual, and the nurse should not administer any medication without the written order of the physician. On the other hand, it is important that the medications prescribed for the client are given as needed.

Four types of drugs are commonly used after the client has undergone cranial surgery. These four types are osmotic diuretics, steroids, anticonvulsants, and analgesics. Refer to Chapter 28 for specifics on each drug.

### Dressing

The dressing is checked frequently for drainage. If a drain has been left in, note the amount and color of the drainage. Any dressing with drainage should be changed immediately or reinforced with sterile sponges (4 by 8 inches); Surgiflex is placed around the head and anchored securely in place with adhesive tape. Check all dressings carefully and frequently for moisture or other evidence of leakage of cerebrospinal fluid. Report a wet, colorless drainage to the physician immediately, since this may be the result of wound rupture, requiring immediate repair to reduce the danger of wound contamination and infection. Disoriented or restless clients should be prevented from disarranging the dressing, putting the fingers underneath, or even removing it. Well-padded wrist restraints may be used with caution (on the physician's written order), provided that the client is not further excited by such a restraint. At times, it may be desirable and effective for an adult member of the family to remain with the individual.

If a drain has been used, it may be removed in 24, 36, or 48 hours, depending on the operative procedure and the wishes of the neurosurgeon. Expect drainage for the first 24 hours postoperatively if a drain has been put in place. The dressing may be draped with a sterile plastic covering when a drain is in so that it will not necessitate frequent dressing changes.

***Care of scalp after removal of dressings.*** Frequently, after the dressing is removed, the scalp is covered with crusts. The application of pHisoHex soaks will soften these crusts. They are readily removed when a cleansing shampoo is given. Most female clients are self-conscious about shaved heads and must be reassured frequently regarding their appearance. A nurse can help by screening the client before dressings are changed and other care is given. A pretty scarf helps the client's morale and is less conspicuous than, and is used instead of, a cap or towel. Although a wig may be an expensive item, its cosmetic and psychological effect may justify its purchase for some clients, and, when possible, this is done by the client or family before surgery. If bone has been removed, leaving a defect in the skull, the client is informed about this and prepared for the resulting change in appearance. If the neurosurgeon plans to insert a plate for protective and cosmetic reasons, the client is so informed. This will decrease the initial reaction to the defect.

## Activity

For the first 24 to 48 hours the client's activity is closely supervised, and he or she depends on the nurse for complete care. The position of the head is changed with caution to avoid jostling and jarring. The individual is turned with a sheet by two nurses. These restrictions are placed on the client to lessen the dangers of postoperative trauma and bleeding. By the third day, if the operation has been successful, most clients become progressively more independent and are able to turn with increasingly less aid and require less help with personal hygiene, feeding, and so forth. Establish normal routines as soon as possible. Some clients, depending on their personalities, will need more guidance, reeducation, and at times even more discipline than others. The client and family may need assistance in adjusting to problems and residual disabilities, if any. Implementing a comprehensive care plan can do much to prevent or ameliorate psychological sequelae after cranial surgery.

The client may be permitted out of bed the day after operation, depending on the condition. To reduce the possibility of untoward reaction, the head of the bed is gradually elevated to a high gatch; then, if no subjective or objective reaction occurs, the client dangles with the feet on a chair for 20 minutes under constant supervision with frequent checking for changes in pulse, color, and skin moisture. Avoid fatigue. If no adverse reaction occurs, 4 to 5 hours later the client is helped into an armchair at the bedside. Encourage the client to remain in the chair at least 30 minutes the first time, unless there are specific contraindications. The next day he or she should be up twice in a chair, the length of time as tolerated. This is increased progressively until he or she begins to ambulate. By the end of 2 weeks if all has gone well, the client is usually ready for convalescent or home care.

Physical therapy helps maintain muscular tone and stimulate circulation. It can be initiated in the form of massage and active and passive exercises to all extremities on the third postoperative day. If the client has no impairment of motor function, it can usually be discontinued when unassisted ambulation begins.

## POSTOPERATIVE COMPLICATIONS

The complications that may occur after intracranial surgery are presented in the following summary.

### Shock

The probable cause of shock is excessive loss of blood during or after operation.

*Signs and symptoms.* (1) Appearance of pallor. (2) occasionally slight cyanosis, (3) cold, moist, or sweaty skin, (4) rapid, thready pulse, (5) rapid, shallow respiration, (6) restlessness, (7) appearance of anxiety that may change to apathy, (8) thirst, (9) subnormal temperature, and (10) low and falling blood pressure.

*Prevention and nursing interventions.* During the preoperative period, adequate fluid should be given. Sedatives and reassurance as necessary allay anxiety and ensure a good night's sleep.

During operation, blood transfusions and other fluids are given intravenously as necessary.

Close observation of the client is made, with careful checking of the vital signs at frequent intervals. Strength is conserved when needs are anticipated and visitors are supervised and limited.

*Treatment.* Treatment includes the administration of blood plasma or other fluids intravenously, placement of the client in a horizontal position if intracranial bleeding is not a contraindication, and giving of stimulants for the circulatory and central nervous systems.

### Continued increased intracranial pressure

The probable causes of continued increased intracranial pressure are intracranial hemorrhage, cerebral edema, hematoma, or meningitis.

*Signs and symptoms.* (1) Changes in the level

of consciousness, with diminishing alertness, (2) increasing headache with or without vomiting, (3) restlessness, (4) irregular pupils (usually dilated on the side of the hemorrhage), (5) slowly falling respirations (may progress to periods of apnea), (6) falling pulse rate, (7) slowly rising blood pressure, (8) papilledema and visual disturbances, (9) elevation of the bone flap, (10) weakness or paralysis of one side of the body, (11) convulsions, and (12) increased cerebrospinal fluid pressure.

*Prevention and nursing interventions.* Observe the client closely, with careful checking of the vital signs at frequent intervals. Elevate the head. Limit fluids as ordered, and measure intake. Straining when vomiting or when at stool is minimized. Instruct the client regarding any restrictions and supervise him or her during activity. Refer to Chapter 27 intracranial pressure monitoring.

*Treatment.* Elevate the client's head to at least 30 degrees. Dehydration is the conservative treatment of increased intracranial pressure. The dehydration regimen includes hypertonic solutions intravenously; magnesium sulfate intramuscularly, by mouth, or by rectum; limited fluid intake; diuretic drugs; and ventricular or lumbar punctures for the removal of cerebrospinal fluid.

Steroids also have been effective in reducing the incidence and severity of postoperative edema and its associated complications.

If other measures are not effective, the client is returned to the operating room for further surgery.

### Hyperthermia

The probable causes of hyperthermia are disturbance of the heat-controlling mechanism in the hypothalamus and brainstem, local or general infection (especially wound, meningitic, respiratory, or urinary), pronounced dehydration, excessive blankets, and thrombophlebitis.

*Signs and symptoms.* Rising temperature.

*Prevention and nursing intervention.* The temperature is taken frequently. Fever in the first 24 to 48 hours postoperatively is common. If the temperature reaches 101° F, superfluous bedclothes are removed. Adequate fluid intake is maintained. Aseptic technique is used during dressings or catheterization. Change position frequently to prevent respiratory infections. Encourage deep breathing whenever the position is changed. Give aspirin or acetaminophen as ordered.

*Treatment.* Discover the cause, and treat symptomatically. Remove excess coverings. Give fluids, antipyretics, and sponge baths. For a sustained temperature of 101° F or above, a hypothermia unit is used. (Refer to Chapter 27.)

### Meningitis

The probable causes of meningitis are contamination at operation or wound infection.

*Signs and symptoms.* (1) Headache, (2) fever (frequently preceded by a chill), (3) increased sensitivity to light (photophobia), (4) hyperirritability, (5) slow pulse, (6) respiratory arrhythmia, (7) delirium, (8) nuchal rigidity, (9) soreness of skin and muscles, (10) focal or generalized convulsions, (11) increased white blood cells in the spinal fluid, and (12) Kernig and Brudzinski signs.

*Prevention and nursing intervention.* Maintain strict aseptic technique when doing dressings or lumbar punctures. Recognize and report early symptoms. Chart the vital signs carefully. Special nursing care is based on the presenting symptoms.

*Treatment.* Maintain adequate fluid intake. Avoid bright lights in the room. Keep noise and external stimuli to a minimum. Discover the cause, and treat symptomatically. Administer antibiotics as ordered. Lumbar punctures may be done to remove cerebrospinal fluid. Give anticonvulsants as ordered. Place side rails on the bed as necessary. Follow the regimen for the treatment of hyperthermia as indicated. (See Chapter 20.)

### Wound infection

The probable causes of wound infection are break in operative technique, rupture of the wound with leakage of cerebrospinal fluid, contamination of the wound by the client, or break in sterile technique during dressings.

*Signs and symptoms.* (1) Moist or saturated dressings without evidence of serosanguineous drainage (wound rupture), (2) clinical evidence of wound infection, and (3) fever.

*Prevention and nursing intervention.* Maintain strick aseptic technique during dressings. Report wet dressings immediately so that early treatment may be initiated. Report elevation of temperature. Staff members with colds must wear masks during dressings. Supervise the client closely to prevent removal of the dressing. Reinforce the dressing whenever necessary with a sterile towel.

*Treatment.* Before initiating antibiotic therapy, culture the wound. Special irrigations and medicated dressings may also be indicated.

## Headache

Headache is the rule rather than the exception for the initial 24 to 48 hours after intracranial surgery. At times, it is severe and may last for several days. The type of treatment depends on whether or not a lesion has been removed.

*Prevention and nursing intervention.* Avoid jostling the bed and jarring the client's head. Maintain the client's position with the head at a 45-degree elevation unless this is contraindicated. Administer analgesics as ordered. Maintain a quiet environment with restriction of visitors.

*Treatment.* Analgesics and dehydrating drugs may be given. If headache is caused by increased intracranial pressure, cerebrospinal fluid may be removed by ventricular or lumbar puncture. Fluid intake is limited.

## Vomiting

If vomiting becomes a problem, withhold oral feedings. It may be necessary to go to intravenous fluids. Administer antiemetics as ordered. If intracranial pressure is increased, it should be reduced, as discussed previously.

## Anorexia

Anorexia is usually an individual problem. Whenever possible, allow for the client's likes and dislikes. Serve smaller feedings frequently and as attractively as possible. At times, you may need to give supplementary vitamins or even to resort to total parenteral or enteral fluids to ensure an adequate caloric intake.

## Dysphagia

The probable cause of swallowing difficulties is injury to the glossopharyngeal and vagus nerves.

*Signs and symptoms.* (1) Inability to swallow food or fluids without regurgitating or choking, (2) increased drooling of saliva, and (3) diminished or absent swallowing and gag reflexes.

*Prevention and nursing intervention.* Give nothing by mouth for 24 hours after a suboccipital craniectomy. Test the gag and swallowing reflexes before initiating oral feedings. At the first indication of dysphagia the client should be closely supervised during the intake of food and fluid to prevent aspiration. It may be helpful to keep the client turned on the side with a low head gatch during feedings. If the problem is acute, stop oral feedings and institute tube feedings. These clients usually have increased secretion of mucus and phlegm that they cannot expectorate or swallow, thereby increasing the hazards of aspiration. Suction should be used only when necessary. Provide adequate mouth care.

## Aspiration

The probable causes of aspiration are a depressed level of consciousness, profound cachexia, difficulty in swallowing, improper technique in feeding the client before he or she has fully recovered from anesthesia, or the improper elimination of vomitus and mucus.

*Signs and symptoms.* (1) Choking on taking fluid, (2) cyanosis, and (3) respiratory difficulties.

*Prevention and nursing intervention.* The client must not be left alone while still under the effects of anesthesia. Keep a stuporous or unconscious client flat in bed and turned on the side with the mouth dependent to facilitate drainage of mucus. Suction is used whenever necessary to keep the passages open and clean. Oral feedings are withheld if difficulty in swallowing is encountered.

*Treatment.* If necessary, establish an adequate airway by removing the material aspirated, changing position, suctioning, or performing a bronchoscopy or tracheotomy.

## Respiratory complications

*Respiratory collapse* may result from compression of the respiratory center by herniation of the cerebellar tonsils in association with an infratentorial tumor or from edema of the medulla oblongata after operation in the posterior fossa. Early signs of respiratory involvement are manifested by the abnormal rate and depth of respirations; changes should be noted and reported immediately.

*Respiratory infections* are probably caused by

the aspiration of mucus, fluid, or vomitus; shallow breathing resulting in the poor exchange of oxygen; or prolonged lying on the back followed by inflammation of the dependent part of the lungs (hypostatic pneumonia). The manifestations are variable; they include cyanosis, dyspnea, chills, fever, cough, sharp pain in the side aggravated by deep inspiration, and abdominal distention. These manifestations can be prevented by good nursing care: Posture an anesthetized or unconscious client on the side with the mouth dependent to prevent aspiration, and support the uppermost arm to facilitate chest expansion. Check the airway frequently, and maintain its patency. Suction as indicated to remove mucus and phlegm. Turn the client at least every 2 hours to stimulate the circulation of oxygen throughout the lungs to prevent stasis. If the client is conscious, encourage deep breathing and coughing. Splinting of the chest with subsequent shallow, depressed respirations can be prevented when the client is given adequate medication at the first sign of chest pain. Maintain resistance to infection by adequate caloric intake.

*Treatment.* The treatment of respiratory collapse consists of the administration of oxygen and artificial respiration (manual or mechanical) supplemented by the use of decompressive and dehydrative measures. Early tracheostomy improves the client's chance of recovery. The prognosis is grave.

Treatment of respiratory infections requires good general nursing care that is directed toward maintaining a suitable, well-ventilated, quite environment and the physical and psychological comfort of the client and promoting relaxation and sleep; chemotherapy and oxygen are administered as necessary.

### Herpes, sordes, and parotitis

The probable causes of herpes, sordes, and parotitis are dehydration, fever, and inadequate oral hygiene.

*Signs and symptoms.* The eruption of vesicles primarily on the lips is a symptom of herpes. Sordes is a dark brown or blackish crustlike collection on the lips, teeth, or gums. Parotitis is characterized by inflammation, tenderness, and swelling of the parotid gland secondary to oral sepsis that has spread by way of Stenson's duct.

*Prevention and nursing intervention.* Provide

oral hygiene every 2 hours and after meals during acute febrile or postoperative periods. Encourage adequate fluid intake (3000 ml during febrile conditions unless contraindicated). The lips, tongue, and mucous membranes should be kept moist by frequent lubrication. Report tender or swollen cervical glands immediately.

*Treatment.* Oral hygiene is administered every hour. Thorough mastication of food is encouraged, and fluid intake is maintained. Chewing gum or sucking hard candy to stimulate salivation is helpful in preventing and treating parotitis. Radiation therapy to the parotid area may be indicated.

### Convulsions

For description, nursing care, and treatment of convulsions, refer to Chapter 14.

### Periocular edema

Puffing or swelling of the eyelids and surrounding tissue may follow head injury or intracranial surgery. Report the first sign of local swelling. The eyes and lids should be kept clean by irrigation whenever necessary. During the early stages of periocular edema, apply iced compresses or small ice bags. If bags are applied, they can be held in place by an eye patch. If edema is pronounced and the skin appears taut and thin, a coating of petrolatum jelly may be applied locally as a protective measure before the treatment is begun. If edema does not recede with cold applications, hot saline solution compresses should be applied 20 minutes on and 10 minutes off. Some physicians use hot and cold applications alternately. Early treatment hastens recovery and alleviates discomfort; periocular edema normally subsides within a 3- to 4-day period.

### Corneal ulceration

The probable cause of corneal ulceration is the neglect of eye care in clients who are unconscious or have corneal anesthesia or facial paralysis.

*Signs and symptoms.* With corneal anesthesia or facial paralysis, blinking of the eyelids is diminished with reduced secretion and increased dryness of the eye. Irritation of the cornea or conjunctiva, if untreated, will result in ulceration of the cornea and blindness.

*Prevention and nursing intervention.* Careful

frequent examination should be made of the eyes of a client with impaired or absent corneal reflexes. If a client is conscious, inform him or her of any disability and give instructions for preventing complications, for example, blinking frequently, refraining from rubbing the eyes, wearing protective glasses when outdoors, and using an eye cup at certain specified intervals during the day and immediately after being exposed to the wind. These are precautionary measures to prevent injury to the cornea. It should be pointed out that because of the loss of the corneal reflex, he or she cannot perceive foreign bodies that may become embedded in the eye and lead to a complication.

The nurse should irrigate the eyes of the unconscious client with saline solution every 2 hours and, if ordered, instill lubricant in the eyes twice daily. Early signs of irritation should be reported immediately so that specific treatment can be instituted. The application of a butterfly dressing serves to protect the cornea by keeping the eye closed. The gauze collodion butterfly dressing has many advantages over sutures. It is easily and painlessly removed, and the eye can be examined as desired to check improvement. A transparent eye shield made of clear radiographic film (Fig. 27-1) may also be used. This permits frequent inspection of the eye. The shield may be secured to the skin with cellophane tape. An eye patch may also be used, but it is generally less well tolerated, both physically and psychologically, by the client.

### Bladder complications

Bladder complications may be incontinence, retention, retention with overflow (dribbling small amounts of urine with a large residual), or cystitis. The causes are impairment of consciousness, mental and physical deterioration, and pathological or surgical involvement of the frontal lobes. These conditions prevent conscious control of the external sphincter muscle of the bladder.

*Signs and symptoms.* (1) Restlessness, (2) distention, (3) local discomfort, (4) inability to void, (5) inability to control urination, (6) incontinence, (7) dribbling with retention, and (8) loss of the awareness of bladder fullness and the need to urinate.

The following are symptoms of cystitis: (1)

burning or pain on urination, (2) urine usually grossly cloudy and full of sediment, (3) many white cells on microscopic examination, and (4) chills and fever.

*Prevention and nursing intervention.* To prevent cystitis, check frequently for bladder distention, and accurately measure intake and output to prevent overdistention and stretching of the bladder. Fluid intake to 3000 ml each 24 hours should be encouraged unless contraindicated. Encourage the client to use the bedpan or urinal at regular intervals under optimum conditions to stimulate voiding. Maintain strict aseptic technique for any catheterization. Avoid repeated catheterizations by utilizing catheter or condom drainage if the client is unable to void.

*Treatment.* The following measures are used to treat cystitis. The bladder is irrigated with solutions as ordered. Antibiotics may be ordered. Force fluids unless contraindicated. Measure intake and output. Treat chills and associated symptoms symptomatically. Examine urine daily to evaluate progress.

### Bowel complications

Bowel problems generally do not occur after intracranial surgery unless the level of consciousness is impaired.

Some of the complications of prolonged unconsciousness are constipation, impactions, and diarrhea. Prevention may be facilitated by careful use of cathartics and colon lavages and by modification of the feeding-tube mixture.

Abdominal distention, characterized by cramplike, colicky pains, and palpable distention of the rectum and lower bowel before operation, by guarding against the swallowing of air during the administration of anesthesia, by the restriction of ginger ale and orange juice in the immediate postoperative period, and by stimulating peristalsis and the normal expulsion of gas (the intake of solid food is generally effective).

*Treatment.* Turn the client from side to side frequently, and posture him or her on the abdomen unless contraindicated. A rectal tube is inserted. Neostigmine bromide (Prostigmin) or vasopressin (Pitressin) may be administered intramuscularly and a rectal tube inserted to stimulate the expulsion of flatus. Enemas or colon lavages may be helpful after the second postoperative day.

## Cranial nerve dysfunction

The cause of disturbed motor function is injury to the pyramidal tracts, the facial nerve, or other cranial nerves.

*Signs and symptoms.* (1) Diminished motion and strength of an extremity (paresis). (2) Complete inability to move an extremity (paralysis). (3) The loss of function may involve one extremity (monoplegia) or both extremities on the same side of the body (hemiplegia); the facial muscles may be involved. (4) Movements of the eyeballs (oculomotor, trochlear, and abducens nerves) and the muscles of chewing, swallowing, and talking (trigeminal, glossopharyngeal, and vagus nerves) also may be involved.

*Prevention and nursing intervention.* Prevention is directed toward the early recognition and treatment of presenting symptoms and toward preventing contractures, muscle stretching, footdrop, and wristdrop.

*Treatment.* If the upper extremity is affected, the forearm, wrist, and hand are supported in a sling to prevent muscle stretching, local discomfort, and wristdrop. If a sling cannot be used, the arm should be flexed slightly at the elbow and placed in a neutral position on the bed, with the wrist and hand supported on a small pillow. After the acute stage the client should frequently open and close the hand on a firm rubber ball to stimulate circulation and muscle tone. If the lower extremity is involved, the principles for positioning the client outlined in Chapter 22 should be applied to maintain maximum comfort and prevent additional complications. Physical therapy in the form of massage and exercise stimulates circulation and maintains muscle tone and the range of joint movements. If the paralysis is complete and permanent, reparative surgery may be necessary. The client is encouraged to eat and drink on the unaffected side. If the client has difficulty in swallowing, oral feedings may be omitted and tube feedings given.

## Decubitus ulcer

The cause of decubitus ulcer is pressure on the skin that interferes with the local blood supply. Prolonged rest or immobilization in one position (clients with hemiplegia or paraplegia may develop a pressure sore in a few hours), irritation of the skin by urinary or fecal incontinence, poor skin hygiene, debilitation, emaciation, and malnutrition may be contributing factors. The incidence of decubitus ulcers increases in individuals over 60 years of age. The loss of skin elasticity and subcutaneous fat, the decrease in glandular secretions, and the generalized skin atrophy characteristic of the aged increase the risk of skin breakdown.

*Signs and symptoms.* (1) Redness, (2) cyanosis, (3) induration, (4) necrosis, and (5) ulceration.

*Treatment and nursing intervention.* Refer to Chapter 25.

## Hiccup

The probable cause of hiccup is spasmodic contraction of the diaphragm accompanied by closure of the glottis caused by irritation of the respiratory center or phrenic nerve.

*Treatment.* Carbon dioxide and 10% oxygen are inhaled until mild hyperpnea results. As an alternate procedure, the client may keep breathing into a paper bag with a closed top until the carbon dioxide content is increased. This is repeated whenever necessary if the attack recurs. (The theory is that carbon dioxide may stimulate the respiratory center and cause regular contraction of the diaphragm instead of the irregular spasms that result in hiccups.) Atropine sulfate, 0.0008 gm intravenously (adult dosage), may be given. Thorazine also may be used with good effect. Procaine (Novocain) block or section or avulsion of the phrenic nerve may be done if other measures are ineffective.

## Visual disturbances

*Diplopia* (double vision) results from the dissociation of two images that would normally fuse into one and is caused by the involvement of the oculomotor, trochlear, or abducens nerves. The client is generally more comfortable if one eye is covered with an eye patch. If glasses are worn, one lens can be made opaque by being coated with Bon Ami. *Photophobia* (sensitivity to light) may be caused by meningeal irritation and may be alleviated when the room is darkened or dark glasses are worn. Progressive *loss of vision* may result from optic atrophy resulting from pressure on the optic nerves or may be secondary to papilledema.

*Nursing intervention.* The nurse can help the client adjust to the disability and the modified way of life. Assist with the activities of daily living as necessary, always encouraging the client to do as much as possible alone, thereby developing independence and self-confidence. He or she should be taught how to feed him- or herself by being oriented to the clock position of different foods on the plate and how to read braille as soon as the physician decides that blindness may result. Literature may be obtained from the local association for the blind to aid in rehabilitation of these clients.

## Speech disturbances

Speech disturbances include impairment of the comprehension, elaboration, and expression of ideas and result from a disturbance of the dominant hemisphere (the left side of the brain in right-handed persons). If the impairment is complete, it is called aphasia; if partial, it is called dysphasia. The types of speech disturbances are motor and sensory. The motor type is an inability to name common objects or to express simple ideas in words or writing; the sensory type is an inability to comprehend the written or spoken word.

Develop a simple way to communicate with the aphasic client. Reinforce the meaning of words with gestures, and encourage the client to respond in any way he or she is able.

Speech therapy, conducted over a period of time by a trained therapist, is directed toward helping the aphasic client learn how to express him- or herself and toward preventing further psychological disability and isolation from others. The nurse participates in the program planned by the therapist by providing the client with opportunities to practice, by spending time, and by listening.

*Nursing intervention.* Anticipate the client's needs to avoid undue frustration and anxiety. If the disturbance is motor in type, supply the client with a pad and pencil to express wants in writing if he or she is able. This will help minimize the emotional reaction to disability.

## Thrombophlebitis

Thrombophlebitis may be caused by immobility of the legs after surgical procedures, venous stasis, or the increased coagulability of the blood subsequent to dehydration.

*Signs and symptoms.* (1) Redness, (2) swelling, (3) tenderness, (4) pain in the leg, and (5) low-grade fever.

*Prevention and nursing intervention.* Prevent thrombophlebitis by maintaining adequate fluid in-take, encouraging deep breathing, frequently changing the position to facilitate venous drainage from the legs, and instituting special exercises while the client is on bed rest.

*Treatment.* Treatment of thrombophlebitis includes bed rest, elevation of the legs, antiemboli stockings, anticoagulants (heparin, dicumarol, coumarin), and ligation of the involved vein.

## Changes in personality and behavior

Personality and behavior changes may be the result of local disturbances of the frontal lobes or of diffuse disease of the brain.

*Signs and symptoms.* Any of the following manifestations may be present: (1) loss of memory, (2) defects in moral and ethical judgment, (3) euphoria, (4) untidiness, (5) apathy, (6) active or passive lack of cooperation, (7) irritability, antagonism, and hostility, (8) resistiveness, (9) assaultiveness and aggression, (10) incontinence of urine, and (11) regression to an earlier level of adjustment.

*Treatment and nursing intervention.* It is important to understand the cause of the client's behavior and to be objective in dealings. These clients cannot be held responsible for their actions, and the practitioner must develop skill and patience in caring for them. They must be supervised closely and, depending on their residual manifestations, may require a planned regimen of rehabilitation. If these clients become resistive or assaultive, sedatives or tranquilizers may be used.

Unless contraindicated, phenobarbital or ataractic drugs in small doses may help make them more tractable. Clients who regress to a childish level of mental functioning must be taught social behavior; their ability to function on an adult level, to reason, and to cooperate must be redeveloped. Operant conditioning or other behavior modification techniques may be used effectively. Changes in personality and behavior may be transient or may continue for several days, weeks, or months, depending on the underlying cause.

## Rehabilitation

If a neurological disability persists, the nurse can do a great deal by attitude and approach in helping the client to accept it and to make an optimal adjustment. Even clients with inoperable lesions and a life expectancy of 3 to 12 months should be kept as independent as possible, not only for their own morale, but also to decrease the burden of care imposed on their families when they are taken home. Institute occupational and diversional therapies as soon as possible, according to each client's needs and potentialities. Keep the client active and independent as long as possible. The family should participate in daily care and should be informed about any special problems or needs. When the client is discharged, a referral to the local public health nursing agency will ensure continuity of nursing services for the client and support and guidance for the family. Chapter 25 and discharge outcomes in Chapter 22, as appropriate, give further detail.

## REFERENCES

Bolin, K.L.: Assessing the status of the neurological patients, Am. J. Nurs. **77:**1478-1479, Sept. 1977.

Burrows, E.H., and Leeds, N.E.: Neuroradiology, Edinburgh, 1980, Churchill Livingstone, Medical division of Longman Group Ltd.

Cancer Nursing. Read this journal for valuable information about clients with oncological problems.

Carnevali, D.L.: Preoperative anxiety, Am. J. Nurs. **66:**1536-1538, 1966.

Cottrell, J.E., and Turndorf, H.: Anesthesia and neurosurgery, St. Louis, 1979, The C.V. Mosby Co.

Crosley, C.J., et al.: Central nervous system lesions in childhood leukemia, Neurology **28:**678-685, July 1978.

Cushing, H.: Intracranial tumours, Springfield, Ill., 1932, Charles C Thomas, Publisher.

Dandy, W.E.: Surgery of the brain, Hagerstown, Md., 1945, W.F. Prior Co., Inc.

Dean, J.C., et al.: The medical oncology nurse clinician, Ariz. Med. **32:**420, May 1975.

Duffy, P.E., editor: Tumors of the nervous system, Philadelphia, 1976, F.A. Davis Co.

Fankhauser, R., et al.: Tumours of the nervous system, Bull. WHO **50:**53, 1974.

Finlay, D.B., and Franklyn, P.: Changes in the skull in acute lymphoblastic leukemia of childhood, Clin. Radiol. **30:**431-433, 1979.

Hannan, J.F.: Talking is treatment too, Am. J. Nurs. **74:**1991, Nov. 1974.

Home Study program: The brain-damaged patient: approaches to assessment, care and rehabilitation, Am. J. Nurs. **79:**2117-2138, Dec. 1979.

Ingraham, F.D., and Matson, D.D.: Neurosurgery in infancy and childhood, ed. 2, Springfield, Ill., 1969, Charles C Thomas, Publisher.

Kistler, J.P., et al.: Computerized axial tomography: clinicopathologic correlation, Neurology **25:**201, March 1975.

Levin, A.B., et al.: Treatment of increased intracranial pressure: a comparison of different hyperosmotic agents and the use of thiopental, Neurosurgery **5:**570-575, 1979.

Lieberman, A., and Ransohoff, J.: Treatment of primary brain tumors, Med. Clin. North Am. **63:**835-848, July 1979.

Mahaley, M.S., Jr.: Experiences with antibody production from human glioma tissue, Prog. Exp. Tumor Res. **17:**31-39, 1972.

Mullan, S.: Current mortality of the surgical treatment of brain tumors, J.A.M.A. **182:**601-608, 1962.

O'Brien, M.: Pediatric neurological surgery, New York, 1980, Raven Press, Publishers.

Oerlemans, M.: Eli, Am. J. Nurs. **72:**1440-1441, 1972.

Newton, T.H.: Radiology of the skull and brain; vol. 5, Technical aspects of computed tomography, St. Louis, 1980, The C.V. Mosby Co.

Posner, J.B.: Diagnosis and treatment of metastases to the brain, Clin. Bull. **4:**47, 1974.

Rand, R.W.: Microneurosurgery, St. Louis, 1978, The C.V. Mosby Co.

Ransohoff, J.: Parasagittal meningiomas, J. Neurosurg. **37:**372-378, Sept. 1972.

Recent advances in the treatment of primary brain tumours, a seminar, Arch. Surg. **110:**696, June 1975.

Scogna, D.M., and Smalley, R.V.: Chemotherapy-induced nausea and vomiting, Am. J. Nurs. **79:**1562-1564, Sept. 1979.

Schneider, G.: Is it really better to have your brain lesion early? A revision of the "Kennard principle", Neuropsychologia **17:**557-583, 1979.

Schoenberg, B.S., et al.: The resolution of discrepancies in the reported incidence of primary brain tumors, Neurology **28:**817-823, Aug. 1978.

Shallice, T., and Evans, M.E.: The involvement of the frontal lobes in cognitive estimation, Cortex **14:**294-303, 1978.

Smith-Cowper, F.: Special nurses needed for very special nursing, Nurs. Times **75:**2168-2169, Dec. 13, 1979.

Smith, J., and Geist, B.L.: Evaluation and care of the acute craniotomy patient, J. Neurosurg. Nurs. **10:**102-111, Sept. 1979.

Smith, R.R.: Essentials of neurosurgery, Philadelphia, 1980, J.B. Lippincott & Co.

Taylor, J.R.: Headache: When should you suspect brain tumor? Med. Times **100:**65-75, Nov. 1972.

Wagner, F., editor: Neurosurgery of tumors, New York, 1980, Raven Press, Publishers.

Wheeler, P.: Care of a patient with a cerebellar tumor, Am. J. Nurs. **77:**264, Feb. 1977.

Yohn, D.S.: Oncogenic viruses: expectations and applications in neuropathology, Prog. Exp. Tumor Res. **17:**74-92, 1972.

# 22

# INTRAVERTEBRAL TUMORS

Intravertebral tumors occur much less frequently than intracranial tumors, and, although they are composed of similar pathological types, the incidence of the various kinds differs. Carcinoma metastasizes to the vertebrae much more frequently than to the bones of the skull. Hematoma and abscess are much more infrequent within the vertebrae than within the skull. The simplest classification depends on whether the tumor is extradural or intradural, and, of these, the *extradural* tumors constitute about 25%, most of which are of a malignant nature (metastatic). The *intradural* tumors, 75%, are subdivided into those originating from the meninges, blood vessels, or nerve roots (extramedullary), and those originating from the glial tissue of the spinal cord (intramedullary). The extramedullary tumors occur almost three times as frequently as the intramedullary and fortunately (since they are benign) constitute 50% of all intravertebral tumors. They are principally *meningiomas* and *neurofibromas* and may be completely removed by operation. The intramedullary tumors are almost all *gliomas*. More than half of them originate from the ependyma, which lines the central canal. Some can be excised surgically, but the rest infiltrate and are not removable without causing such damage to the spinal cord that complete loss of the sensory and motor function below the level of the lesion results.

*Abscesses* are mentioned here because they act as space-occupying lesions. They are extremely rare and may be either extradural or intradural. They occur secondary to infections elsewhere in the body. The onset is rapid, and the diagnosis and clinical picture are as mentioned under tumors. The treatment is decompression with drainage and the systemic and local administration of antibiotics to control the infection.

The signs and symptoms depend on the level and location of the tumor (in relation to the meninges and spinal cord). If the tumor develops adjacent to a nerve root, as happens most frequently with the extramedullary and occasionally with the extradural tumor, pain is the first symptom and may persist for months or years before there are manifestations of compression of the spinal cord itself. The metastatic tumors, epidural abscesses, and hematomas that usually occur in the thoracic spine cause a rapidly developing paraplegia. At first, this is flaccid in type with loss of all reflexes and sensation below the level of the lesion. It is accompanied by urinary retention. Later the extremities become spastic, the reflexes exaggerated, and the bladder hypertonic. Intramedullary tumors cause a painless, slowly developing paralysis of a spastic type with overactive reflexes, clonus, extensor plantar responses and loss of sensation below the level of the lesion. Intradural extramedullary tumors may manifest a similar picture, but as just mentioned, pain usually precedes the development of paralysis that may affect one leg before, or more seriously than, the other.

The diagnostic study of the client is first directed to establish whether a tumor is present. One determines this, after the history and examination have been obtained, by examining the spinal fluid, studying the radiographs, and doing a myelogram if necessary. Examination of the cerebrospinal fluid includes the determination of the total protein level, which is elevated considerably if a block exists, and determination of the number of cells, which are increased if an abscess or other infection exists. The cerebrospinal fluid Wassermann or Kahn reaction will be positive, and the colloidal gold curve will be abnormal in the presence of neurosyphilis. Spinal dynamics are tested to determine whether the cerebrospinal fluid circulation is obstructed. Radiographic examination of the spine may show destruction of bone, and a myelogram may reveal incomplete or no filling at a certain level because the mass prevents, in part or wholly, the passage of the opaque material. Myelography is especially helpful in localizing the exact level of the lesion if the spinal dynamics are normal. The site of the lesion is determined by the neurological examination if a sensory level is demonstrated. If the radiographic examination demonstrates changes in the bone that correspond to the clinical signs, the level of the pathological condition is verified. Tomograms of the vertebral column are especially valuable in demonstrating early changes suggestive of a primary intradural tumor. (Refer to Chapter 12.)

### Treatment and nursing intervention

Refer to Expected outcomes in Chapters 6, 17, 23, and 26.

The treatment is surgical; the purpose is to decompress the spinal cord that has been flattened by the tumor. This can be considered a palliative measure in the management of malignant and nonremovable lesions, with great care being taken that the spinal cord is not further injured during the procedure. The first step in operative treatment of a spinal cord disease is a laminectomy. This can be done at any level of the vertebral column and may be limited to one segment or extended over several vertebrae. (For some conditions a hemilaminectomy is preferable and consists of the removal of laminae on one side only.) After determination of the exact level of the lesion, a midline longitudinal incision several centimeters long is made down to the spinous processes of the vertebrae. The paravertebral muscles are dissected from the spinous processes and laminae and retracted to each side; thus the posterior aspect of the vertebral column is exposed. The spines and laminae are removed with rongeurs, and the dura is exposed. If the lesion is intradural, a longitudinal incision is made in the dura, which is retracted to either side with stay sutures. Thus the spinal cord is exposed and,

if possible, the tumor removed. The dura is closed with interrupted silk sutures. The defect left by the removal of bone is filled in by the paravertebral muscles and fasciae that are approximated carefully with interrupted silk sutures. The skin is closed in the same way, and a protective and supportive dressing is applied.

Radiographic therapy is helpful in the treatment of some of the intramedullary tumors that cannot be removed satisfactorily.

To be able to give effective nursing care to clients with disorders of the spinal cord, nurses should know its normal anatomy and physiology, including the tracts and blood supply. They have special responsibilities in caring for these clients, the performance of which will have considerable bearing on their ultimate progress. To plan nursing care intelligently, they should know and recognize the signs and symptoms of a disturbed condition. The early recognition and prevention of complications is, to a large extent, the responsibility of the nurses. However, they should recognize the importance of communicating with other team members, thus assuring their cooperation and collaboration in the provision of effective, comprehensive care for the client.

To be sure, all clients with spinal cord disease do not present the same challenge; this varies according to the degree of permanent disability the individual client must accept and to which he or she must adjust. Many clients have benign neoplasms of the spinal cord that are successfully removed, and they make remarkable recoveries. However, even their convalescence may be fraught with discomfort and be unnecessarily prolonged, depending on the caliber of nursing care given.

*Observation.* The following observations should be begun during the admission of the client.

GAIT. The client's gait should be noted to determine whether there is any impairment of function of the lower extremities. When out of bed, the client may require assistance.

FUNCTION. Motion and strength of all extremities should be tested grossly to enable the nurse to recognize subsequent changes.

SKIN. Examine the body for cleanliness, nutrition, dehydration, edema, rash, bruises, and decubitus ulcers. If the client is able to take a tub bath, the temperature of the water should be checked with a bath thermometer to avoid burning a client who has no perception of temperature.

ELIMINATION. Assess the client for evidence of bladder or bowel distention and question him or her about possible disturbances in bladder and bowel function, such as frequency, urgency, dribbling, incontinence, retention, constipation, or diarrhea. Determining the time of the last voiding and defecation is helpful in making the nursing care plan.

VITAL SIGNS. Temperature, pulse, respiration, blood pressure, height, and weight are measured.

During the admission procedure, note the client's general attitude, emotional reaction, and degree of acceptance, and help in the adjustment to the hospital environment. Refer to Chapters 6, 10 to 11, 15, and 17 for specific detail helpful in assessment, history-taking, and client communication. If the client is admitted to a ward or semiprivate room, introduce him or her to other clients and acquaint him or her with the facilities of the unit. Provide additional information concerning hospital regulation and routine according to needs. The client should also be informed of his or her rights and encouraged to ask questions and participate actively in the planning and implementations of care. Avoid tiring the client, but in the initial contact much can be done to provide reassurance and to develop a positive relationship that will result in a more comfortable, cooperative client. All pertinent information should be charted on the nurse's notes and relayed to the total health team for addition to the comprehension care plan.

*Diagnostic study of client.* The practitioner does a complete physical and neurological examination on every client, and a woman should be present to chaperone each female client. Client needs should be considered in relation to privacy, explanations, emotional support, and covering when the room is excessively cool. After the practitioner has completed the physical examination, tested the cranial nerves, and observed the client's gait, the client should be draped for the rest of the examination. This may be done with a draw sheet or a bath blanket in the following manner: Place a sheet or blanket next to the client; fanfold top bedclothes to the foot of the bed; remove the hospital shirt, cover the client's chest with the shirt, and tie sleeves across her back (the chest drape is usually omitted when a male client is examined); fold the sheet or blanket toward the center and place it between the extended legs. This serves to protect the client from exposure and facilitates the examination. When the examination of reflexes, special sensations, and musculature is completed in this position, the client is assisted onto the abdomen and draped in a similar fashion for further sensory examinations. At this point the various levels of sensory alteration are tested with a skin pencil or pen.

In addition to the blood tests generally ordered (complete blood count, blood Kahn, sedimentation rate, serum calcium, serum phosphate, alkaline phosphatase, urea nitrogen, and glucose), urinalysis and radiographic examinations of the chest and spine are made. Lumbar puncture and spinal dynamics are important aids in determining the absence or presence of an obstruction of the spinal canal. A Pantopaque myelogram and a CAT scan may be necessary before the lesion is localized. The nurse is responsible not only for preparing the equipment and assisting the physician with these special tests but also for understanding these procedures and any complications that may occur. Fortified with this knowledge, the nurse can do much to reassure an apprehensive client. This will also enable the nurse to obtain the client's maximum cooperation and to prepare for any possible ill effects. Depending on the nature of the client's illness and the condition, the diagnostic study may be completed within a 2- to 7-day period. Meanwhile the physician orders supportive and preventive care. When the diagnosis is well established, the decision is made as to whether surgical therapy is indicated.

*Position and activity.* Unless contraindicated, the client should be out of bed a few times each day, walking with assistance if necessary, or seated in a chair. If acutely ill or too disabled to be out of bed, the client should be postured at all times and turned at least every 2 hours. A bed cradle and footboard are used routinely. Posturing is directed toward the prevention of complications that may occur with any loss of motor function.

A large turning sheet placed under the client should extend from above the shoulders to below the hips to facilitate change of position without fatiguing the patient or nurse. Fracture boards, sectioned to permit elevation of the head gatch, may be placed under the mattress to prevent its sagging and to ensure equal distribution of body weight. The side-lying and back-lying positions are described in detail on pp. 560 to 562. Physical therapy in the form of massage and active and passive exercises may be given during the period when the client is being studied or treated in preparation for operation. If the client has weakness or paralysis of the extremities, physical therapy is particularly helpful in maintaining muscle tone, stimulating circulation, maintaining the normal range of movement of the joints, and preventing contractures. The client should be taught to do supplementary flexion and extension exercises of the extremities several times a day. The nurse, through teaching and guidance, can do much to enlist the client's cooperation and active participation in the regimen to prevent complications. The level of the client's cooperation depends to a large extent on the skill of the nurse, the client's recognition and understanding of the need, and the acceptance of the responsibility.

*Nutrition.* It is important that a well-balanced diet be given during this period. A high-protein, high-vitamin, high-calorie diet may be a vital factor in preventing the complications of decubitus ulcers, lowered bodily resistance with increased susceptibility to infections, and loss of morale. Anemia or other nutritional disturbances should be treated specifically and corrected before surgery. Fluids should be measured, and the client should be encouraged to take up to 3000 ml a day.

*Hygiene.* Daily cleansing baths are given, with frequent alcohol rubs. The use of powder is discouraged because of the danger of causing pressure sores when it is applied unevenly to damp skin. Meticulous attention is paid to all pressure areas, and the skin over these parts is examined closely every time the client's position is changed. If there is involvement of the anterolateral tracts with diminution or loss of temperature perception, caution should be used to prevent burning with hot bath water. Hot-water bags or electric pads should not be used. If a disturbance of the autonomic nervous system is present, the skin may be excessively dry and require frequent applications of lotions containing lanolin, mineral oil, or other emollient substance. The client should participate in the daily care according to ability and should

be encouraged to take an interest in his or her personal appearance.

*Client elimination.* Urinary output should be measured, and if the client has difficulty in voiding, utmost care is used to prevent cystitis. Repeated catheterizations for retention may be used or may be obviated by the use of a retention catheter and some type of drainage. Whether placed on catheter drainage or not, the client is checked frequently for distention to prevent stretching of the bladder. He or she may not experience any local discomfort yet may become overdistended and, as a result, because of the tearing of mucous membrane, may be more susceptible to urinary tract infection. Fluids are measured and given at regular intervals, and the client is encouraged to take up to 3000 ml a day. If the client is on complete bed rest and catheter drainage, the intake of milk and fruit juices is restricted because of the increased possibility of stones forming within the bladder and urinary tract.

These clients may have diminished intestinal tone, sluggish peristalsis, and relaxed anal sphincters. Involuntary stools or impactions may result unless proper elimination is maintained. Abdominal distention may be troublesome and should be treated symptomatically by colon lavage, rectal tube, and the intramuscular injection of neostigmine bromide (Prostigmin) or vasopressin (Pitressin). Sometimes posturing the client on the abdomen will suffice to relieve local distention by increasing the expulsion of flatus. If the client tends to be constipated, anticonstipation foods are included in the diet. Milk of magnesia and liquid aromatic cascara sagrada may be given the night before the colon lavage. This treatment is given until good results are obtained and the solution returns clear. Neostigmine or vasopressin, given 20 to 30 minutes before the colon lavage is begun, increases peristalsis; thus adequate cleansing of the bowels is accomplished more quickly. If the lavage is not effectual, an impaction should be considered and a rectal examination done. If an impaction is found and cannot be removed manually without discomfort to the client, hydrogen peroxide retention enemas should be given. If, because of existing contraindications, operation must be delayed indefinitely, one attempts to initiate evacuation by developing the conditioned bowel reflex. If the client cannot be taken to the bathroom for this purpose, an old-fashioned commode can be used at the bedside at regular intervals.

*Complications.* During the preoperative period, nursing is symptomatic and based on the manifestations of a disturbed function and the physical and emotional needs of the client. It is directed toward the treatment of existing complications and the early recognition and prevention of others, such as the following: (1) pressure sores, (2) contractures or other deformities, (3) footdrop and wristdrop, (4) bladder and bowel disturbances, (5) respiratory difficulties, and (6) psychological complications.

*Pressure sores* are caused by prolonged pressure on devitalized areas and may be prevented by rigid adherence to the following regimen: Change the client's position at least every 2 hours, and use correct anatomical posturing so that the weight is equally distributed over the body surface. Elevate the heels to avoid pressure. Doughnuts should not be used. A sponge rubber or air mattress may be used. Pliofilm instead of rubber sheeting should be used to protect the bed (eliminates coarse wrinkles and decreases warmth and excessive sweating). Bed linen should be free from wrinkles and crumbs.

The client should be kept dry. Meticulous hygiene is given to keep the skin clean and as free as possible from contaminating materials. Frequent alcohol rubs stimulate the circulation and toughen the skin. Powder should not be used. All pressure points are inspected frequently. (See Chapter 25.)

Body weight is maintained to ensure adequate padding over pressure points. Nutrition is maintained by a high-protein, high-vitamin, high-calorie diet. Adequate fluid intake prevents dehydration.

Urinary incontinence may be prevented by the use of some form of catheter drainage, and involuntary defecations may be prevented by the use of colon lavages as indicated. (Further detail is in Chapter 25.)

Daily massage and passive movements should be given to stimulate the circulation. The client should be ambulated if possible. The CircOlectric bed also may be helpful.

*Contractures* or *other deformities* should be prevented if possible. Physical therapy, especially passive exercises, maintains the normal range of joint movements. Massage maintains muscle tone.

The client is postured in such a way as to prevent stretching of weakened muscles. The position should be changed every 1 to 2 hours.

Hubbard baths or exercises under water, unless contraindicated, relieve muscle spasm and pain, stimulate circulation, and improve muscle tone. Muscle spasms may be relieved by medications such as neostigmine bromide (Prostigmin), mephenesin (Tolserol), methocarbamol (Robaxin), carisoprodol (Soma), or chlorzoxazone (Paraflex).

*Wristdrop* and *footdrop* inevitably follow paralysis of the upper or lower extremities if the following preventive measures are not applied: Continual support is given to a paretic or paralyzed extremity; the upper extremity is supported by the use of a sling when the client is out of bed, an aluminum cock-up splint when in bed. If a splint is not available, it can be easily improvised by use of basswood with cotton or sponge rubber and strips of adhesive tape; the hand end should have approximately a 2-inch elevation to ensure good support of the wrist; the fingers should be maintained in a functional position. Posterior molded casts may also be used to support the wrists when the client is in bed. If the client is cooperative, the wrists and adjacent parts may be postured on small pillows without other supportive devices. The lower extremities are postured so that the feet are always firmly supported to dorsiflexion at right angles to the legs. This support counteracts the pull of gravity on the weakened muscles and thus helps prevent footdrop.

*Bladder* and *bowel disturbances* should be anticipated. Bladder distention and incontinence may be prevented. Residual urine, which may cause cystitis, also should be prevented. Instructing the client how to use the Credé technique at specific intervals may be an effective means of emptying the bladder. Complications in the male client can be reduced by use of external condom drainage instead of a retention catheter. Strict aseptic technique is maintained, and the drainage apparatus is kept functioning efficiently when in use. Sufficient fluids are offered at regular intervals, and the intake as well as the output is measured.

The abdomen is checked frequently for distention. Dietary and fluid regimens are maintained as ordered. Neostigmine, vasopressin, cathartics, or suppositories may be administered as needed. Good elimination is ensured by means of a colon lavage every second or third day until bowel function can be reestablished through a reconditioning process.

*Respiratory difficulties* may become a problem. Deep breathing, sighing, and yawning should be encouraged. If the client has thoracic pain, adequate medication is given to control it to avoid splinting of the chest. (Procaine [Novocain] blocks may be used if medication is not effective.)

The client's position is changed every 2 hours. If the client is able, frequent ambulation is encouraged. Drafts or exposure to cold should be prevented. Systemic resistance is maintained and exposure to infection avoided. Early signs of respiratory involvement are reported.

*Psychological complications* may be manifested by anxiety, apprehension, fear, depression, irritability, withdrawal, or overdependence on the nurse. A positive and optimistic approach is used. The client should be encouraged to be as self-reliant as possible and taught to participate in the daily care and in the prevention of complications. Nutritional intake should be maintained at an optimal level.

Diversional and occupational therapy is provided according to the client's particular need and capacity. If the client is ambulatory or able to be in a wheelchair, he or she is encouraged to leave the room and join other clients in the lounge or television room. Frequently, being with other clients, talking, socializing, or playing various games will alleviate anxiety and reduce preoccupation with the physical condition. A positive attitude should be encouraged, and the cooperation of family and friends is enlisted in maintaining morale. Avoid overtiring the client.

Reassurance should be based on facts. The client is helped to accept and to adjust to any residual disability. The nurse should not belittle symptoms or, on the other hand, be oversympathetic. In the preoperative period the nurse can lay the psychological foundation for such rehabilitation as may be necessary after operation.

### Preoperative nursing intervention

*Preparation of client.* Permission for operation is obtained, and the family is notified of the hour of operation. A clergyman is notified if desired by the client.

Blood typing and Rh factor are checked, and blood units are reserved in the event they are necessary.

Local physical preparation usually is done by the nurse the night before the scheduled operation; if the client is unduly apprehensive, it may be delayed until the next morning. The procedure is explained to the client by the person doing it. For thoracic, lumbar, or cervical operation the area is scrubbed with Betadine soap and water, shaved, and cleansed with alcohol. A perineal preparation may be done on the female client with a sphincter disturbance to facilitate subsequent care. The procedure for clipping the hair varies according to institutional policy. For high cervical operations the area extending from the nape of the neck to the occipital protuberance is clipped with an electric clipper. A shampoo is then given. The area is scrubbed with soap and water, shaved with a straight razor, and cleansed with alcohol. Any evidence of dermatitis, seborrhea, or abrasions is reported immediately to the physician. (Skin lesions predispose to wound infection and, if severe, may be a contraindication to operation.)

A cleansing enema (a colon lavage is substituted if the client does not have sphincter control) is given the night before operation. (An effective and complete evacuation of the lower bowel will contribute materially to the client's comfort after operation and will lessen the possibility of abdominal distention.)

A shower or bed bath is generally given the night before the operation if the client is scheduled for operation before noon. (This eliminates needless rushing in the morning and prevents overtiring the client, which may predispose to postoperative shock.)

A sedative is generally ordered at bedtime.

On the morning of operation, care is given as necessary, and artificial dentures are removed; a hospital shirt and pajama trousers are put on the client.

The preceding meal is omitted.

Temperature, pulse, respiration, and blood pressure are taken and recorded on the chart.

Motion, strength, and sensation of the extremities are tested and the observations charted.

The client's mental attitude is noted and reassurance given as necessary.

The client is asked to void; the output is measured. If distended and unable to void, the client should be catheterized. (The bladder is emptied completely to prevent distention during the hours of operation.) If the client has been on catheter drainage, the set is temporarily disconnected, the catheter released, the bladder emptied, and the catheter secured with a rubber band. (Screw clamps should not be used for this purpose because of the possibility of causing trauma to the skin.)

Preoperative medication is given as ordered. The chart is completed with the detailed observation that have been made to facilitate evaluation of the client's condition after operation.

### Preparation for postoperative intervention

*Environment.* While the client is in the operating room, the postoperative bed and unit are prepared. Whenever possible, the client returns to a single or two-bed room. This ensures quiet and adequate rest for the client and, in the critically ill, reduces the possibility of inflicting emotional trauma on other clients. (This should be avoided if neurosurgical clients are not segregated and if other clients on the unit are being prepared psychologically and physically for similar surgical treatment.) After the postoperative bed has been made, the room is cleaned and well aired before the client returns. Whenever possible, the bed is elevated to expedite the administration of nursing care. Raising the bed to a higher level also protects the nurse by preventing unnecessary fatigue and muscle strain. The level of the mattress is then about the level of the nurse's waist and eliminates the need to bend or stoop when giving nursing care. An air flow mattress can be used to aid in preventing decubitus ulcers.

It is recommended that a fracture board be used. Fracture boards are used beneath the mattress to keep it from sagging and to ensure equal distribution of the weight of the body.

The use of a bed cradle is suggested because it does not interfere with the posturing of the client. It serves to elevate the bedclothes, thereby reducing the possibility of footdrop. A draw sheet is used to assist in moving the client.

The nurse checks the oxygen equipment and other equipment needed to restore the airway to ensure its availability in case of emergency. If the client is having a high cervical operation, the respirator is also checked for quick, efficient use in case of emergency. Nurses caring for such a client should be familiar with the operation of the respirator.

*Procedure for making the bed.* The mattress is folded, and fracture boards are placed on the spring. A large sheet is placed on the bed, and the corners are mitered and tucked in. A large sheet is folded lengthwise, and then in half and placed across the bed as a draw sheet. The height of the sheet on the bed depends on the level of the operative procedure. If the operation is to be in the cervical or high cervical area, the sheet is placed to the head of the bed to ensure firm support and good alignment of the operative area when the client is turned; if surgery is to be in the thoracic or lumbar area, the sheet is placed so that the entire back is well supported. By using this sheet the client can be turned in log-fashion easily and safely by two nurses. The cradle, footboard, bolsters, sandbags, and pillows should be arranged neatly and conveniently at the bedside.

### Postoperative nursing intervention

*Return to bed.* The head nurse on the floor is notified by the operating room nurse 10 to 15 minutes before the operation is completed. This enables the head nurse to send the postoperative bed to the operating room to receive the client directly so that unnecessary movement is eliminated. The nurse will require help to transfer the client from the operating table to the bed. The circulating nurse puts a dry, warm gown on the client and covers him or her with warm blankets before transferring to the bed. This initial change of position is most safely and effectively executed by four trained persons. The back is well supported and in good alignment at all times; care is exercised to avoid needless jarring, rough handling, or exposure of the client during transfer to the bed. He or she is then carefully transported to the recovery room and on to the unit by the physician, nurse, and assistant. The management and care of the client from this point on is directed toward the prevention of complications and toward maintaining comfort and morale.

*Position.* If the client is conscious, to ensure

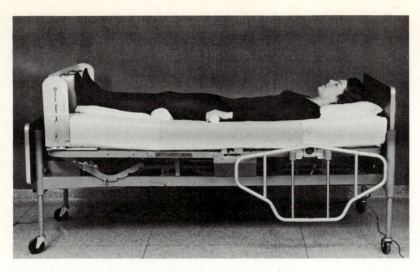

**FIG. 22-1.** Client postured on back showing good body alignment. Note use of footboard.

good hemostasis of the wound the physician generally orders that, depending on the extent of the laminectomy, the individual be kept flat on the back for 4 to 8 hours. The client should be postured as directed in previous chapters, with the body in good alignment, 10-degree flexion of the knees, calves supported, heels elevated from pressure of any kind, and feet maintained in firm dorsiflexion. The upper extremities are separated slightly from the sides and the wrists supported as indicated to prevent wristdrop (Fig. 22-1). Clients in the supine position who have had cervical or high cervical laminectomies do not have head pillows because of the increased danger of wound trauma. If indicated, the head and neck may be immobilized with sandbags and the client is instructed not to turn the head or flex the neck. Clients with laminectomies at other levels may have a head pillow, preferably a small, firm one for maximum support and comfort.

If the client has not recovered from anesthesia, he or she is postured on the side until completely conscious. During this critical period, this is the position of choice to prevent respiratory difficulties secondary to aspiration of mucus or vomitus and to ensure a better airway. The posture of the client in the lateral recumbent position has been described previously (Fig. 22-2). Adequate support is placed under the uppermost arm and leg to help maintain the alignment of the client's back and to facilitate expansion of the chest. The body weight is distributed equally over the shoulder, back, buttock, and lower extremity, which is slightly hyperextended on the bed. No back pillow is necessary if the client is postured correctly. Moreover, it is contraindicated because the client, feeling its support, tends to recline backward against it, thus throwing the body out of alignment and possibly causing injury to the wound. Feet are supported at right angles to the legs in firm dorsiflexion. A small, firm head pillow is used whenever the client is on the side. This helps prevent myositis of the neck muscles and is especially important in preventing trauma to the wound after high cervical laminectomies.

*Change of position.* As soon as the client is well oriented, explicit instructions are given on activity permitted. Depending on the individual's ability to understand, reasons are given for the necessary restrictions to ensure maximum cooperation. The individual is instructed to breathe deeply, sigh, and yawn for a few minutes at fre-

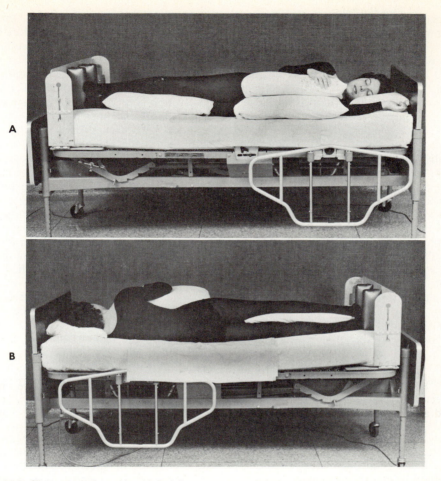

**FIG. 22-2.** Client postured on side with bed flat as recommended after surgery on spine. **A,** Anterior view. **B,** Posterior view. Side rails on bed should be used.

quent intervals to increase the intake of oxygen and thus expand the lungs.

The period during which the client is not permitted to turn alone is determined by the following: the site of operation, the extent of the laminectomy, the degree and extent of paralysis, the rate of healing of the wound, and the individual neurosurgeon's orders. This period may extend from 2 to 10 days or longer.

As soon as the physician permits, the client is turned by two nurses, using the turning sheet, to alternate positions at least every 2 hours. Some clients fatigue more quickly and may have to be turned every hour. Shorter intervals are not encouraged. After the third day, clients who have had thoracic or lumbar laminectomies may be postured in the prone position. If the client has paraplegia or is debilitated, this position is especially recommended as an alternate to the side and back positions in the regimen to prevent bedsores.

Turning the client with a sheet is directed toward preventing trauma to the wound, which may cause pain or rupture. This method of changing the position also lessens the likelihood of fatiguing the client and the nurses. The procedure for turning a client is as follows (Fig. 22-3): The client, with the arms folded across the chest, is positioned on the back in the middle of the bed on the turning sheet and is instructed to take no active part in the subsequent change of position. The turning sheet is rolled tightly from either side toward the client by the nurses, who are holding it firmly to afford maximum support to the entire back (Fig. 22-3). To turn the client onto the right side, the nurse on the client's left moves him or her to the edge of the bed by pulling the rolled sheet toward him or herself while the other nurse holds the sheet taut (Fig. 22-3). Then the nurse on the right unfolds the sheet, straightens it and removes any wrinkles. The nurse on the left, grasping the rolled sheet tightly, turns the client onto the right side, and straightens the sheet on the left side, checks the alignment of the client's back, and pulls out his or her right buttock to anchor in position (Fig. 22-3). A firm small pillow is placed under the head, and the supportive devices are put under the left arm and leg and against both feet.

To turn the client onto the back the posturing equipment is removed; the sheet is rolled toward the client from either side. The nurse on the left leaves enough sheet to cover the back. While the nurse on the client's right pulls the sheet up and toward him- or herself, the other nurse, supporting the client's back with the sheet by holding the rolled end securely, eases the client onto the back. This position is adjusted as necessary, the turning sheet is straightened, and the extremities are supported with the appropriate bolsters.

It is important for the client, if able, to maintain muscle tone and to stimulate circulation by doing regular exercises as instructed by the nurse, physical therapist, or physician. These usually begin on the second or third postoperative day and consist of hourly flexion and contraction of the voluntary muscles of the upper and lower extremities and abdomen. The exercises can be done safely without interfering with the client's alignment or position.

*Observations.* The observations detailed here should be made.

**GENERAL.** The color of the face, lips, and nail beds; warmth of the body and moisture of the skin; level of consciousness; and orientation should be noted.

**VITAL SIGNS.** Vital signs are checked at the intervals ordered and recorded on the chart and special observation sheet. Generally, temperature is ordered *immediately,* then every 2 hours for the first 24 hours, and then every 4 hours; respiration, pulse, and blood pressure are measured every 30 minutes for 6 hours, then every hour for 6 to 12 hours as indicated by the client's condition, and finally every 2 to 4 hours as the client convalesces. Generally, blood pressures are stabilized within 12 to 24 hours, and these measurements are discontinued. Temperature, measurements are continued until the client has been afebrile for 3 days. After the fourth postoperative day the temperature is taken at night only when ordered or after an elevation to 100° F or above. Changes in the vital signs should be reported because they may be the first warning of systemic shock, hemorrhage, or infection.

**FUNCTION.** The motion, strength, and sensation (light touch, pinprick, temperature, and position) of each extremity should be tested when the client has recovered fully to determine any change in the preoperative status. These observations are made every 2 to 4 hours during the first 48 hours after operation. This activity will afford the client some exercise and will stimulate the circulation. It will also enable the nurse to recognize the first symptoms of a disturbed function that may result from spinal cord edema, trauma, or hemorrhage. Change in function should be reported to the physician for further evaluation.

**DRESSING.** The dressing is examined for moisture and serosanguineous drainage each time the client's position is changed. A wet dressing suggests wound rupture with leakage of cerebrospinal fluid. If not immediately reported and treated, this may lead to wound infection. Generally a few skin sutures are inserted by the physician, and the wound is redressed. Drains are rarely used in spinal cord surgery. If serosanguineous drainage is present, sterile compresses are used to reinforce the dressing as necessary. If the dressing has become soiled or wet because of incontinence, the dressing may be changed and wound contamination prevented.

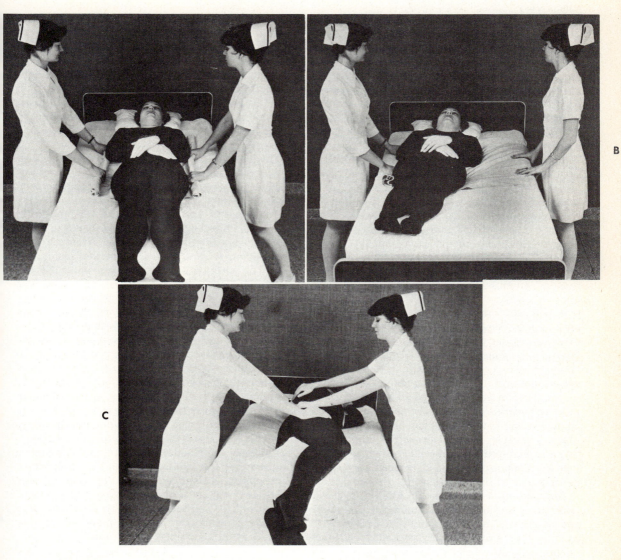

**FIG. 22-3.** Demonstration of procedure for turning client. **A,** Position preliminary to turning. **B,** Client has been moved to side of bed. **C,** Buttock pulled out to maintain alignment of client's back; client's back is supported while being turned to supine position.

**ABDOMEN.** The client is examined for evidence of bladder or bowel distention every 3 to 4 hours. The early recognition of distention will prevent unnecessary physical discomfort, and the response to therapy will be quicker and more satisfactory.

**SKIN.** The anterior surface of the client's body is examined on return from the operating room to note any reddened or excoriated areas. These may develop on the forehead, chin, iliac crests, and knees if the client has been kept in the prone position for the duration of the operative procedure. Every time the client is turned, vulnerable areas of the body should be examined meticulously for early evidence of breakdown of the skin.

*Nutrition.* After the client has reacted, encourage the use of fluids to 3000 ml each 24-hour period. The client is given solid food as early as possible to stimulate peristalsis and to lessen the occurrence of distention. After operation, some clients are able to eat and enjoy solid food the same evening. All clients are taught the importance of eating and are encouraged to increase their food intake gradually on the first postoperative day. If nausea or vomiting persist, dry melba toast or crackers may be well tolerated and retained. By the second postoperative day, most clients, unless complications are present, are able to eat a regular diet. All clients who have had laminectomies are fed during the initial 36 to 48 hours. By the third postoperative day, clients who are postured on their sides are able to feed themselves. Trays need to be prepared to facilitate this process; supervision is given as necessary; and the amount of the food eaten is carefully noted. If the client is paraplegic or quadriplegic, he or she is given a high-protein, high-vitamin, high-calorie diet to maintain weight and to help prevent the development of decubitus ulcers.

*Elimination.* Fluid intake to 3000 ml every 24 hours at regular intervals is encouraged, and intake and output are measured carefully. The client is examined for distention every time attended. Many clients with disturbed spinal cord function have sphincter and sensory disturbances. Because of this, urinary retention may result, and the bladder may become overdistended without causing discomfort. The nurse, by frequent observations, can detect and report early bladder distention before it is so severe that the mucous membrane may be torn and cystitis may develop. On the other hand, the client may void small amounts frequently without ever completely emptying the bladder. The residual urine that collects further increases the hazards of bladder infection. Therefore the amount and frequency of voiding are important determinants of bladder function and important guides toward the use of specific treatment. If frequent catheterizations are necessary because of retention, some form of bladder drainage with the insertion of a Foley catheter is recommended. Urinary antiseptics or antibiotics may be ordered to prevent or treat cystitis. Urinalysis is done as indicated in the care of the client.

Abdominal distention may occur as a result of gas formation. Peristalsis may be sluggish or impaired because of a pathological condition and may be further inhibited by the use of narcotics. Elimination of gas may be induced by the intramuscular injection of neostigmine or vasopressin and the insertion of a rectal tube. After the third postoperative day, unless contraindicated, the client is postured on the abdomen; the prone position frequently aids in the expulsion of gas. The intake of solid food as early as possible after operation is recommended to prevent the formation of gas. During the first 3 or 4 postoperative days, fruit juices and gas-forming foods are eliminated from the diet to lessen further the possiblity of distention.

Unless contraindicated, a cathartic is given the second postoperative night; if it is not effective, an enema is given the following morning. Enemas are given with great care to avoid overdistention of the intestines. If the client has impaired control of the anal sphincter and has difficulty in retaining or expelling the solution, a colon lavage should be substituted. This treatment is regulated so that measured amounts may be given and siphoned back with less danger of causing distention. It is less likely to fatigue the client, eliminates the use of a bedpan, which may cause further discomfort, and can be given until satisfactory results are obtained. The abdomen should be soft and the lower bowel empty at the completion of the procedure. If the client does not have a bowel movement regularly, a cathartic is given every second or third night followed by an enema in the morning as necessary. Mechanical interference with the passage of a rectal tube, the sensation of rectal full-ness or discomfort, or the involuntary seepage of fluid fecal matter suggests a fecal impaction. A rectal examination is done to determine whether there is an impaction, and, if one is present, man-ual removal should be attempted. If the impaction cannot be removed in this manner, retention ene-mas may be given.

After thoracic or lumbar laminectomy the cli-ent should not be placed on a bedpan while lying on the back. Elevation of the buttocks and hips so that the client can be placed on the bedpan will transfer the bulk of the weight to the operative area and may cause local trauma. Instead, turn the client onto the side by means of the turning sheet, place the bedpan in position, and, if the operation is at the lumbar area, place a small pad at the operative site for support. Roll the client back onto the bedpan. Elevate the head of the bed as per-mitted by the client's condition and need; place a bolster under the knees to support them and in-crease comfort. During the first 24 hours after operation, bedpans are used as seldom as possible. It is recommended that clients use fracture pans for voiding receptacles during this period.

As soon as the client is able to sit in a chair comfortably for at least 30 minutes, the reestab-lishment of regular bowel elimination is initiated. If the client is paraplegic, the regimen outlined in Chapter 17 is followed. If the client does not have any residual impairment of sensory or motor function, one may reestablish the previous pat-tern of bowel function by instituting a regular time for using the toilet, by including bulk-forming foods in the diet, by forcing fluids, by giving prune juice each morning as necessary, and by regular exercise.

*Hygiene.* Every attempt is made to keep the body as clean as possible. A daily bath is given. The nurse should avoid overtiring the client and should not be dogmatic as to the time the bath is given. Pain should be relieved before the client is subjected to any nursing care, or the therapeutic effect of such care will be greatly diminished. The bath affords an excellent opportunity for testing the client's sensory and motor functions. The client is generally able to help with the bath by the third postoperative day. The extent of the par-ticipation will depend on the level of operation,

the condition, and the progress of convalescence. The wrong kind of voluntary activity too soon may cause rupture of the wound or may increase local pain. If the client is too low in bed, he or she should be moved carefully to a higher level on the turning sheet by four nurses. A client with a thoracic laminectomy should never be hoisted by the armpits or shoulders because this may cause rupture of the wound.

Back rubs are given to the back and extremities, unless contraindicated, at least every 4 to 6 hours. Ideally the back and all possible pressure areas are rubbed with lotion every time the client is turned. The use of powder is discouraged because of the danger of its being applied unevenly to a damp surface, caking, and contributing to the de-velopment of a pressure sore.

Bed linen is changed as necessary. The draw sheet and bottom sheet should be tightened fre-quently to keep them free of wrinkles. The turning sheet should be dry and smooth at all times.

*Dressing.* The dressing is examined frequently for its condition and for signs of drainage. Gen-erally the first dressing is done on the third post-operative day, at which time the sutures are re-moved. A protective dressing is applied, and un-less complications occur, no other dressing is done until the time for its removal. This depends on the site of operation and the condition of the wound. Usually, high cervical dressings are re-moved on the tenth postoperative day and the thoracic and the lumbar dressings on the four-teenth day. Some neurosurgeons recommend the use of a Thomas collar for 3 to 5 days after high cervical operations. This collar is made of card-board cut to fit the individual client's neck and firmly covered with cotton and bandage. It is placed around the neck over the dressing and an-chored securely in back with a strip of 3-inch tape. This keeps the client from turning the head lat-erally and from flexing it anteriorly, thus protect-ing the wound. If continued support is advisable, this collar may also be used for the first few days after the client is permitted out of bed.

TECHNIQUE. If a dressing tray is used, petrolatum gauze, tincture of benzoin compound, and 3-inch tape are added to the routine setup and taken to the bedside. The client is screened as necessary. A bath blanket is placed over the client, and the top bedclothes are fanfolded to the foot of the bed. The client is then turned onto the abdomen and postured in a comfortable position. A firm pillow under the chest and one under the legs to elevate the toes from pressure will add to comfort. If the client has a cervical wound, a pillow may be placed under the forehead to keep the operative area in good alignment and to facilitate breathing. If the wound is at a lower level, the head may be turned to either side for comfort. Arms are straight at the sides. The client is covered with a bath blanket until the practitioner is ready to begin. A double sterile field is prepared on the bedside table previously cleared of all articles, and transferred to this field, by means of a sterile forceps, are sterile scissors, forceps, and a straight clamp, about six sponges 4 by 4 inches, six sponges 4 by 8 inches, two sterile towels for draping, and two 6-inch strips of sterile petrolatum gauze. The articles are then covered with a sterile towel.

The practitioner removes the outer dressing and discards it into the receptacle. He or she puts on sterile gloves and removes the rest of the dressing with forceps. Thimerosal (Merthiolate) or alcohol is sometimes used and should be available. Some practitioners believe that the application of either solution actually causes local discomfort, and therefore use no antiseptic before removing the sutures. After the removal of the sutures, petrolatum gauze may be placed over the incision; otherwise it is covered by large compresses (4 by 8 inches), the number depending on its site and extent. While the practitoner gently holds the dressing in place, the adhesive marks from the surrounding skin are removed with ether, alcohol is applied and the area is dried. Next a rolled sponge (4 by 8 inches) is saturated with tincture of benzoin and applied this to the area with patting motions. (This routine is beneficial in preventing irritation of the skin by the adhesive.) While the tincture of benzoin is drying, strips of tape are prepared, the number and length of which vary according to the size of the client and the site and extent of the wound. Usually four strips about 12 inches long suffice. These strips are then applied evenly over the dressing and back, the client is covered, supporting pillows are removed, and the individual is turned on the side and repostured. The bedclothes are rearranged, the bath blanket is removed, and the room temperature is adjusted to comfort.

During the entire procedure the client is kept informed. Questions are answered, and reassurance is given as necessary. Used articles are replaced and replenished as necessary. The bedside unit is left in order.

This routine will, of course, be modified if wound complications arise. These will require special dressings. Under such circumstances the nurse will be guided by the physician in preparing for the dressings.

*Medications.* After a laminectomy, most clients complain of pain in the operative area for the first 24 to 72 hours. They are kept as comfortable as possible, and medications should be given as ordered. (Morphine is never given to clients with high cervical lesions because of its depressant effect on the central nervous system and the increased danger of respiratory complications.) As the client convalesces, he or she requires progressively less medication. The severity of the pain is evaluated and medicine prescribed according to the individual client's needs. Especially after thoracic operations, clients are kept free from pain to prevent splinting of the chest and to facilitate free and deep respirations. Sedatives are given as necessary after the first postoperative night to ensure adequate rest and sleep. Refer to a pharmacology book for more detail.

*Convalescence.* The period of bed rest depends on the level and extent of the operative procedure and the presence or absence of complications or residual disabilities. Ambulation routines vary with the physician. Trends are toward earlier ambulation. If surgery is limited to disc removal, clients may ambulate within a day and be discharged within 3 days. Refer to surgical management of spinal trauma in Chapter 23. Clients who have an uneventful convalescence generally follow the routine described below in getting out of bed.

After a high cervical operation and after the seventh day the head of the bed is elevated progressively to a high gatch, and the client dangles the legs on the tenth day. He or she sits on the edge of the bed with adequate support and constant supervision for 10 to 20 minutes as tolerated. (The client is more comfortable if the feet are supported on a chair.) This is repeated in the afternoon if no adverse reaction occurred. The following day the client is helped into a chair at the bedside in the morning and again in the afternoon. Activity is increased according to capacity. If the bed is high and cannot be lowered, a stool should always be used by the client to get out of or into bed to avoid muscular strain. After thoracic operations, clients are more susceptible to wound trauma and therefore are kept in bed for 2 weeks or longer, depending on the extent of the laminectomy. Sometimes they are permitted out of bed only if they are wearing a brace for support. The routine for progressive ambulation is otherwise the same as that followed for other clients. After lumbar operation, clients usually ambulate, unless paraplegic, by the seventh day.

*Physical therapy.* Massage and active and passive exercises are begun on the third day for the purpose of stimulating circulation and maintaining the normal range of joint motion and muscular tone. Other forms of physical therapy are ordered according to the individual client's need. These may include rehabilitation exercises aimed at promoting ambulation with or without artificial devices and crutches, Hubbard baths to aid in establishing return of voluntary motor function, electrotherapy for stimulation or for relief of pain, or the use of a walker to help clients overcome residual gait disturbances.

If the client is quadriplegic, the tilt table may be used in the upright position daily for 1 hour to prevent osteoporosis. If the client is paraplegic and has been immobilized in a recumbent position for some time, the tilt table may be used to stabilize the circulation preliminary to the client's standing erect with the help of braces. Take the client's blood pressure before transferring to the tilt table. If the client does not become dizzy, tilt the head of the table to a 30-degree angle. Increase the elevation gradually each day until the client is maintained in the upright position without any ill effects. Thereafter, place the client on the tilt table in the upright position for 1 hour each day until fitted with braces.

The principles suggested earlier in this chapter are helpful in the approach to the client. Occupational therapy is used constructively for maintenance of morale, retraining and exercise of weakened muscles, development of work habits, evaluation of capacities and abilities, and formation of the foundation for vocational guidance if the client, because of residual disabilities, is not able to return to the former occupation.

*Postoperative complications.* The following complications may occur postoperatively: (1) respiratory failure or infection, (2) depression, (3) anxiety, (4) decubitus ulcer, (5) footdrop and wristdrop (6) contractures or other deformities, (7) bladder retention, distention, incontinence, or infection, (8) bowel distention, incontinence, constipation, diarrhea, or impaction, (9) muscular spasms, (10) wound rupture, (11) wound infection, (12) shock or hemorrhage (manifested by changes in the vital signs and in the general condition of the client) and (13) spinal cord edema or hemorrhage (manifested by changes in motor and sensory functions that are usually progressive).

The first eight complications were discussed in the first part of the chapter in the discussion on preoperative nursing care. The principles stressed for the early recognition, prevention, and treatment of complications should be applied during the postoperative period (Chapter 26).

Treatment for any of these complications is symptomatic. Most of them are more easily prevented than cured, and the responsibility for their prevention to a great extent rests on the nurse. Throughout the entire hospital stay the psychological and physical nursing care of these clients is most important and its successful and effective execution reduces the incidence of complications, helps the patient move toward recovery, expedites rehabilitation, and gives great satisfaction to the nurse.

### Expected outcomes

By the time that the client has been discharged from the hospital after surgery, the client and significant others can expect to:

1 Describe the pathological process and the anticipated results of the surgery performed.
2 Specify ways that the home environment may be modified to facilitate independence in the client.
3 Discuss the use and plans for acquiring any and all equipment needed by the client.
4 Identify specific resource people and agencies who may provide physical, psychosocial, economic, or vocational assistance in relation to expected deficits in functional capacities.
5 Identify specific ways that the activities of daily living will need to be modified to be appropriate to client activity restrictions.

**6** State rehabilitative measures and exercises that need to be done to improve function and prevent complications.

**7** Identify specific concerns and problems that require the attention of the physician.

**8** Explain the plan for all aspects of follow-up care at least up to the time of the next appointment with the physician and nurse.

## REFERENCES

Abbassioun, K.: Back pain and weakness in the lower limbs, Clin. Pediatr. **13**:992, Nov. 1974.

Brownlowe, M., Cohen, F., and Happich, W.: New washable woolskins, Am. J. Nurs. **70**:2368-2370, 1970.

Clark, C.L.: Catheter care in the home, Am. J. Nurs. **72**:922-924, 1972.

Elsberg, C.A.: Tumors of the spinal cord and the symptoms of irritation and compression of the spinal cord and nerve roots, New York, 1925, Paul B. Hoeber, Inc.

Elsberg, C.A.: Surgical diseases of the spinal cord, membranes, and nerve roots: symptoms, diagnosis, and treatment, New York, 1941, Paul B. Hoeber, Inc.

Epstein, B.S.: The vertebral column, Chicago, 1974, Year Book Medical Publishers, Inc.

Epstein, B.S., Epstein, J.A., and Postel, D.M.: Tumors of spinal cord simulating psychiatric disorders, Dis. Nerv. Syst. **32**:741-743, 1971.

Fager, C.A.: Indications for neurosurgical intervention in metastatic lesions of the central nervous system, Med. Clin. North Am. **59**:487, March 1975.

Giesy, J.D.: Incontinence: causes, diagnosis and treatment, Hosp. Care **3**:1-6, 15, Jan. 1972.

Harvin, J.S., and Hargest, T.S.: The air-fluidized bed: a new concept in the treatment of decubitus ulcers, Nurs. Clin. North Am. **5**:181-187, March 1970.

Javid, R., Belmusto, L., and Owens, G.: Results of surgical intervention for spinal cord compression due to metastatic tumors, N.Y. State J. Med. **65**:409-411, 1965.

Kelly, M.M.: Exercises for bedfast patients, Am. J. Nurs. **66**:2209-2213, 1966.

Kottke, F., and Blanchard, R.: Bedrest begets bedrest, Forum **3**(3):57-72, 1964.

Langford, T.L.: Nursing problem: bacteriuria and the indwelling catheter, Am. J. Nurs. **72**:113-115, Jan. 1972.

Lapides, J., et al.: Self-catheterization for urinary disease, Curr. Med. Dialog. **39**:826-831, 1972.

Linden, R.: Catheter care team heads off urinary infections, Hospitals **46**:86-95, May 16, 1972.

Marchant, M., et al.: Interdisciplinary learning on a neurological service, Am. J. Nurs. **72**:1638-1639, 1972.

May, C.M.: Wheelchair patient for a day, Am. J. Nurs. **73**:650-651, 1973.

McDermott, N.K.: The nursing role in a specialized infection control unit, Nurs. Clin. North Am. **5**:113-121, March 1970.

Nugent, G.R.: Expanding intraspinal lesions, Hosp. Med. **5**:31-44, Sept. 1969.

Olson, E.V.: The hazards of immobility—effects on psychosocial equilibrium, Am. J. Nurs. **67**:794-797, 1967.

Torelli, M.: Topical hyperbaric oxygen for decubitus ulcers, Am. J. Nurs. **73**:494-496, March 1973.

Vinken, P.J., and Bruyn, G.W., editors: Handbook of clinical neurology, tumors of the spine and spinal cord, New York, 1975, Elsevier Scientific Publishing Co.

# PART SEVEN

# DISORDERS RELATED TO EXTRANEUROLOGICAL PROCESSES

# 23

# NEUROLOGICAL TRAUMA

The ideal management of clients with major craniocerebral and spinal column injuries involves cooperative multidisciplinary approaches to diagnosis and health care delivery. Continuous assessment of neurological status, physiological extension of injury, and psychological adaptation must be provided, along with specialized support personnel, facilities, and equipment for continuous therapeutic care. The chance for successful neurologic recovery after major craniocerebral or spinal column trauma lies in early injury recognition at the scene of the accident, appropriate movement of the client, transportation, resuscitation, and management of acute care. With the increased availability of specialized mobile emergency care units, the improved standard of care for clients with neurological trauma continues to decrease overall morbidity and mortality, as well as the lifetime cost of injuries.

## PRINCIPLES OF NURSING INTERVENTION

Numerous management approaches exist for the therapeutic care of the client with neurological trauma. Each client is a mosaic of unique problems and needs that require the nurse to develop individualized therapeutic techniques, as well as adaptation plans for the client in self-care. Nursing skill, adaptability, and analytical powers of problem-solving are soundly tested in clients with neurological trauma, who can be totally dependent on the nurse for survival, communication, protection, and interpretation of needs.

### Expected outcomes
The care of clients with neurological trauma should include:
1 Restoration or maintenance of function of the body part or individual.

2 Prevention of complications of the injuries or therapeutic treatment.
3 Maintenance of the correction of any injuries by supportive care and client teaching.
4 Encouragement and development of the client's adaptive processes for self-care.

Treatments for neurological trauma may be classified as conservative, operative, and postoperative. Examples of conservative treatments would include casts, traction, and exercise. Operative and postoperative treatments would include laminectomy or spinal fusion, craniotomy or cranioplasty, ventriculostomy, intracranial pressure monitoring, special beds, and physical therapy. Nursing management for neurological trauma clients centers around assessment, planning, intervention, and evaluation of client outcomes. Parameters for the specific areas of acute, general, and rehabilitative care are based on neurological, physiological, and psychosocial assessment. The nursing assessment of neurological trauma clients is a continuous process in all phases of care, with the level of intervention and encouragement of self-care occurring throughout. Areas to be assessed in all phases of care are listed in Table 23-1.

Nursing management during the acute phase of neurological trauma to head or neck includes (1) airway, (2) bleeding, (3) neurological and vital signs, (4) constant reassessment of client status, (5) fluid and electrolyte balance, and (6) other injuries. Nursing management during general and rehabilitative care periods center on those specific nursing actions necessary to accomplish the previously mentioned nursing outcomes and client outcomes for self-care. The critical period for the establishment of a therapeutic relationship and re-

**TABLE 23-1.** Client areas to be assessed for neurological trauma

| Neurological | Physiological | Psychosocial |
|---|---|---|
| 1. Orientation | 1. Neurological and vital signs | 1. Cognitive ability |
| 2. General cerebral functioning | 2. Muscle tone and activity | 2. Emotional response |
| 3. Muscle strength | 3. Joint function | 3. Social environment |
| 4. Communication ability | 4. Nutrition | 4. Economic factors |
| 5. Visual fields | 5. Elimination | 5. Cultural influences |
| 6. Hearing | 6. Rest and sleep | 6. Health resources |
| 7. Balance, coordination, and gait | 7. Sexuality | 7. Family support |
| 8. Swallowing and respiratory function | 8. Body alignment and position sense | 8. Self-motivation |
| 9. Peripheral, cranial, and spinal nerve functioning | 9. Environmental safety | |
| 10. Reflexes | 10. Oxygenation | |
| 11. Sensation | 11. Circulation | |
| | 12. Comfort | |
| | 13. General physical condition | |

habilitation is the initial approach to the client. The nurse should approach the client and the family by using the following techniques and remembering that the client, the family, and nurse him- or herself will have varying degrees of shock and anxiety and that effective, serial intervention does make a critical difference in the care of the client.

1. Approach the client and family in a calm, matter-of-fact manner.
2. Assess the client's perception of the injury and the facts pertinent to the history.
3. Explain proposed treatments and procedures.
4. Answer questions honestly and accurately.
5. Give client and family the opportunity to ask questions.
6. Encourage client and family to verbalize feelings.
7. Help client to adapt self-image, self-care, and environment.
8. Praise client for efforts toward self-care and rehabilitation.
9. Encourage client and family participation in care to extent possible.
10. Involve client and family in the planning of care whenever possible.
11. Repeat this process until the client and family fully understand the situation and their role in treatment.

## HEAD INJURIES

Trauma to the head may cause fractures of the skull and injuries to soft tissue or skin such as contusions, edema, hemorrhage, or lacerations of varying degrees of severity just like trauma to any other body part. However, trauma to the head is generally cause for greater concern because of the hidden injuries that cannot be seen. The slightest bump can produce a concussion. Contusion and laceration of brain tissue require a more severe blow. Skull fractures are generally of little importance, unless the brain tissue is depressed or lacerated, or cerebrospinal fluid is leaking. The general effects of head injuries are (1) increased intracranial pressure, (2) cerebral edema, and (3) sensorimotor dysfunction. The most significant effect of head injury is loss of consciousness. The duration of unconsciousness often indicates the severity of the injury.

Craniocerebral trauma is a status condition pursuant to head injury. Once the injury has occurred, the subsequent dynamic process of brain damage can be prevented, controlled, or allowed to recur. The resultant cellular hypoxia and prolonged periods of increased intracranial pressure may produce more damage than the initial injury.

### Mechanics

The mechanics of head injury may be categorized into two types: direct and indirect (acceleration-deceleration). The pathological condition after cerebral trauma is variable in degree and location and depends on the character and situation of the cause. *Direct injury* to the head includes falls, assault, or striking one's head on a stationary object, as in an automobile accident, where over 70% of victims suffer head injuries. An *indirect* or acceleration-deceleration head injury is frequently seen in emergency rooms with simultaneous cervical spine injury. This injury results when an automobile collides with another object and the head is thrust forward and then backward with coincidental rotation of the head on its axis. Head injuries may also occur secondary to medical conditions such as diabetes, heart conditions, and epilepsy, which put the client at risk for falls.

The subsequent disorder and symptoms dictate the management of the head injury. A *cerebral concussion* may be characterized by shock of the brain's soft tissue without bruising or laceration. Momentary loss of consciousness and some post-traumatic amnesia can occur, but symptoms generally dissipate after 48 hours. Repeated concussions can have a cumulative effect of microscopic change and permanent neuronal damage. Pathological studies have demonstrated alterations in neurons (vacuolation and loss of Nissl substance) and shattering of myelin or rupture of axis cylinders on initial injuries.

A *cerebral contusion* is more serious than a concussion and is characterized by multiple bruising or laceration of brain tissue. When unconsciousness occurs, it may range from a stuporous state wherein the client will object to interference, or appear disoriented, aggressive, or agitated, to coma with decerebrate or decorticate posturing in response to stimuli; deep coma may also result in death.

If an alert, awake client has a recent memory loss persisting more than 24 hours, the concussion is termed severe even if the client never lost consciousness.

*Coup-contrecoup phenomenon.* Technically, the term "*coup-contrecoup phenomenon*" relates to direct head injury; however, the sequence of events after the initial impact of brain tissue within the skull is comparable to an acceleration-deceleration injury. Coup is the bruising of the brain tissue below the point of the injury. The re-

bound of the brain is directly proportional to the force of the blow, propelling the brain into the side opposite the injury, or contrecoup. Shearing forces stress nerve fibers, blood vessels, and tendons in the brainstem. Resultant effects of the coup-contrecoup phenomenon usually last 36 to 72 hours and can include tissue shock, laceration, hemorrhage, cerebral edema, increased cerebrospinal fluid production, increased intracranial pressure, and loss of sensorimotor function. An important aspect of maxillofacial, eye, and ear injuries is that coincidental head injury and the coup-contrecoup phenomenon usually are combined and contribute to a dynamic process after such injuries.

### Types of brain injury

Since the brain's encasement, the skull, is a nearly inexpansible container, the cranial contents—blood, brain, cerebrospinal fluid—have little room to expand when the volume of one of them increases. Such is the case when hemorrhage occurs after injury. The two common hematomas that arise from hemorrhage of cerebral tissue are located in the subdural and epidural spaces.

*Subdural hematoma.* Subdural hematoma results from an accumulation of blood from the cortical veins and arterioles and venules between the arachnoid and dura mater (Fig. 23-1). The bleeding characteristically is slow. Symptoms may not be apparent for weeks or months after injury. The clot, generally located over the frontal or temporal lobes, may be unilateral or bilateral, causing acute, subacute, or chronic symptomatic outcomes. Symptoms are usually preceded by a "symptomless period" followed sometime later by increasing drowsiness, headache, seizures, minimal unilateral dilatation of the pupil, increasing intracranial pressure or insidious coma. This hematoma is generally aspirated through burr holes or intracranial surgery.

*Epidural hematoma.* An epidural hematoma is a surgical emergency. The hematoma lies in the epidural space between the skull and dura mater (Fig. 23-2). The middle meningeal artery or the dural sinuses may have been traumatized, causing rapid formation of a large hematoma. A coincidental temporoparietal skull fracture is generally involved. Symptoms are preceded by a "lucid" interval of hours or a day after transient loss of

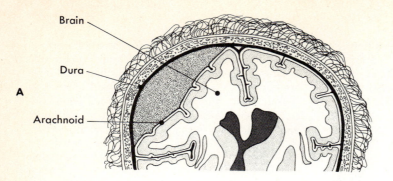

Brain

Dura

Arachnoid

A

FIG. 23-1. A, Subdural hematoma. B, Epidural hematoma.

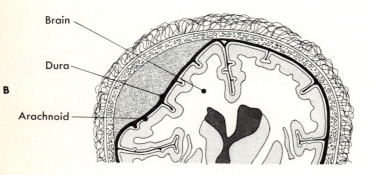

Brain

Dura

Arachnoid

B

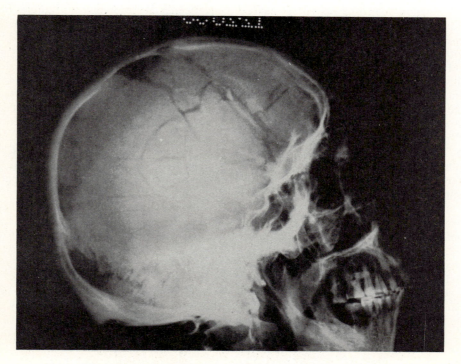

FIG. 23-2. Comminuted fracture of frontal and parietal bones of skull.

consciousness, and followed by rapidly developing signs of increased intracranial pressure and coma as the blood accumulates. The blood must be evacuated immediately through burr holes, and the client may possibly require large amounts of blood replacement, depending on the extent of the arterial hemorrhage, after appropriate coagulation and blood studies for type and cross-match are complete.

*Supratentorial herniation.* Supratentorial herniation may occur after severe head injury and coup-contrecoup phenomenon. The brainstem may have been the brunt of a direct blow to the head, causing severe damage to the vital functions regulated by the brainstem or a separation of the brainstem and cerebellum from the cerebral hemispheres and tentorium. Brain tissue herniates through the opening in the tentorium (tentorial hiatus) as a result of cerebral edema, hematoma enlargement, or severely high intracranial pressure with symptoms of rapidly deepening coma, sudden apnea, decerebrate or decorticate posture, and nuchal rigidity. Emergency measures include intravenous infusion of mannitol, as an osmotic dehydrating agent, and large doses of dexamethasone (Decadron) to act as an anti-inflammation agent. Appropriate neurosurgical procedures follow cerebral dehydration to preserve the client's life.

## Skull fractures

The diagnosis of head injury may be as simple as examining gross evidence of trauma and interpreting the extent of injury from the history of known mechanism of trauma or may require radiographic examination of the head to determine the extent of the injury. Skull fractures may be *linear,* a simple break in the continuity of the bone without alteration of the relationship of the fracture fragments; *comminuted,* a fragmented interruption of the skull from multiple linear fractures (Fig. 23-3); or *depressed,* the displacement of comminuted fragments (Fig. 23-4). A *compound* fracture may be linear, comminuted, or depressed and complicated by scalp, mucous membrane, paranasal sinus, eye, ear, or tympanic membrane lacerations. Symptoms of fracture in the anterior cranial fossa include periorbital ecchymosis ("raccoon eyes"), epistaxis, or cerebrospinal fluid rhinorrhea. In maxillofacial injuries, hyphema,

unilateral limitation of upward gaze (iridoplegia), lack of accommodative effort, and unilateral or bilateral anosmia may occur along with an anterior fossa fracture. Temporal area fractures generally produce a hemotympanum or cerebrospinal fluid otorrhea. Bleeding from the ear indicates obvious temporobasilar skull fractures with herniation of brain tissue through the middle ear space and enhanced possibility of rupture of the dural sinuses and posttraumatic meningitis. Sensorineural and conductive hearing loss and disturbances of balance, as well as nystagmus and facial nerve palsy, may be profound. Battle's sign, ecchymosis over the mastoid process, may be associated with temporobasilar fractures but does not develop for 24 to 36 hours after the injury and should be assessed accordingly by the nurse or family member and reported if found. Basilar skull fractures, posterior cranial fossa, are most easily diagnosed by the symptoms of brainstem herniation rather than radiographic examination.

## Diagnostic studies

A lumbar puncture may be performed to determine the character of the cerebrospinal fluid and its pressure, unless contraindicated by increased intracranial pressure. Bloody cerebrospinal fluid is frequently found in clients with severe head injuries. In itself, it does not warrant specific medical attention. Laboratory studies should include a complete blood count with differential, blood glucose, serum electrolytes, blood urea nitrogen, blood gases, and ethanol assessments when indicated. A chest roentgenogram is done to show possible aspirated material and injury to that area. A base-line ECG is also useful. An electroencephalogram is frequently performed, since it may be helpful in establishing a diagnosis, a comparison with subsequent extension of an injury, and a probable course. Changes in brain waves may be found as a result of cellular damage, or subdural or epidural hematomas. CAT scans are also frequently performed at various states of the treatment regime to obtain data predictive of outcome.

The management of a head-injured client is integrated into the daily care of each phase—acute, general, and rehabilitative—of the injury with client outcomes specific to the client's course. Clients with head injuries are treated conservatively,

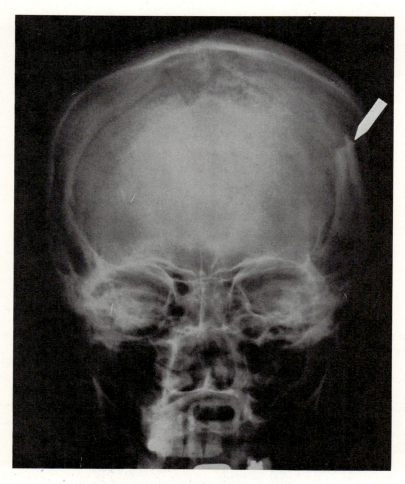

**FIG. 23-3.** *Arrow,* Depressed fracture of parietal bone.

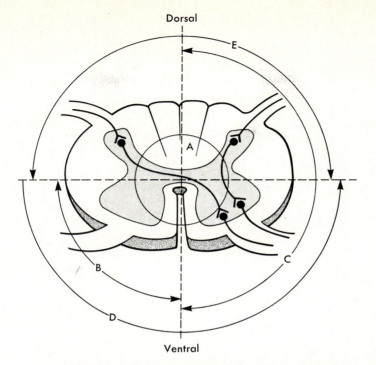

**FIG. 23-4.** Quadrants affected in cervical spine injury.

but aggressively, so that an accurate diagnosis and care appropriate to the extent of the injury are provided. The specific nursing approaches to, and outcomes for, head injuries have been discussed early in this chapter. Nursing management of head injuries is directed toward assessment, appropriate physician, dependent and independent intervention, and client teaching.

### Summary: head injury—critical care considerations (Tables 23-2 to 23-4)

1. In the first hours of treatment, skilled practitioners have a key role in decreasing secondary damage resulting from hypotension, hypoxemia, and anemia.

2. Stabilization of vital functions and resuscitation become the primary priority, whereas treatment of the head injury is secondary.

3. Treat all clients with head injuries as if they had a cervical cord injury, until you have proof to the contrary.

4. Begin treatment by establishing an adequate airway. Remove foreign matter and dentures. Place an oral airway into the unconscious client's mouth to prevent the tongue from moving back to occlude the oropharynx. Check for and remove contact lenses after the more critical maneuvers are accomplished.

5. When needed and when the practitioner is adequately prepared, a cuffed endotracheal tube may be introduced by the "blind" method so that a neck extension can be avoided. When clients with a diminished level of consciousness have normal gag responses, hyperventilate them before inserting the tube for better results. If they seem nauseated, depress the cricoid cartilage with your finger to decrease the urge to vomit.

6. Since intoxicated clients and awakening concussion victims may vomit, many practitioners elect to empty the gastric contents. If there is any possibility of introducing the nasogastric tube into the brain, because of the existence of an anterior

**TABLE 23-2.** Acute phase of head injuries

| Assessment | Intervention | Expected outcomes |
|---|---|---|
| **Neurological** (see Chapter 11) | Approach client in therapeutic manner. Inform client of the process of the neurological examination before initiating the exam. Explain the rationale for the various parts of the examination, regardless of level of consciousness. Observe and record all responses to the neurological examination. Answer questions honestly. Collaborate findings, if significant, with physician. Look for identification indicating special problems, that is, epilepsy, diabetes, hemophilia. Search accident scene for containers or substances, and take these to emergency room, when relevant. Question witnesses or significant others about the same information. Refer to Chapter 9 for detail on the care of the comatose client. | The client should: |
| 1. Orientation | | 1. Be informed of all aspects of neurological examination. |
| 2. General cerebral functioning | | 2. Be instructed in the rationale for the assessment procedures. |
| 3. Cranial, spinal, and peripheral nerve | | 3. Have continuous reassessment of injury status, regardless of extent. |
| 4. Sensation (Figs. 3-4 and 3-5) | | 4. Be provided privacy during examination. |
| 5. Reflexes | | 5. Have cervical spine injury ruled out by radiological examination. |
| 6. Visual fields (Fig. 11-13) | | 6. Have concurrent conditions identified, that is, substance ingestion, disease (diabetes). |
| 7. Pupil size, equality, and reaction to light | | |
| 8. Communication ability | | |
| 9. Muscle strength and motion | | |
| 10. Hearing | | |
| 11. Balance, coordination, and gait | | |
| 12. Respiratory function | | |
| **Physiological** | Establish all details of the accident or injury from the client, family members, or witnesses. Assess all physiological parameters and plan care appropriate to the findings. Answer all questions honestly and approach client therapeutically. Follow through on medical orders. As soon as the client's condition permits, cleanse all body surfaces, bandage appropriately, and provide change of clothes to provide reestablishment of self-image. Make observations at appropriate intervals. Record and report significant changes. Collaborate findings, if significant, with physician. Follow strict joint-ly prepared medical and nursing regimen for initial 24 to 48 hours after injury or until client is stable. Awaken client frequently to determine consciousness and general response. Monitor all indicators of progressive intracranial pressure or brainstem herniation. Narcotics should not be given for pain because of depression of physiological parameters and effect on pupils. | The client should: |
| 1. Neurological and vital signs | | 1. Be informed of the necessity for factual information regarding the injury. |
| 2. Headache, kind and site | | 2. Cooperate to best of ability for accurate information for evaluation of changes in care. |
| 3. Vomiting, if projectile, may indicate epidural hematoma | | 3. Have continuous reassessment of injury status, regardless of extent. |
| 4. Amount, color, and kind of drainage from any orifice | | 4. Be provided privacy during assessment. |
| 5. Muscle tone and activity | | |
| 6. Joint function | | |
| 7. Bladder or bowel distention or incontinence | | |
| 8. Detailed description of any convulsive phenomena or focal signs | | |
| 9. Unusual behavior—include medications, drugs, or alcoholic consumption | | |
| 10. Oxygenation and respiratory pattern | | |
| 11. Bleeding and circulation | | |
| 12. General physical condition or other injuries | | |

13. Nutrition
14. Elimination
15. Environmental and self-safety (include allergies)
16. Rest and sleep
17. Comfort
18. Sexuality

**Psychosocial**
1. Cognitive ability
2. Emotional response
3. Social environment surrounding injury or accident if pertinent
4. Cultural influences
5. Family support

Approach client and family therapeutically. Offer support appropriate to situation. Plan care, including socioeconomic and cultural influences of client. Record and report any significant changes in cognitive ability or emotional response.

The client should:
1. Receive treatment regardless of economic situation.
2. Have continuous reassessment as appropriate to determine extent of injury.
3. Cooperate with the gathering of factual information to plan care appropriate to psychosocioeconomic and cultural needs.
4. Have family supported by the nurse while diagnostic procedures or examinations are being conducted to determine extent of injury.

fossa fracture, utilize a laryngoscope to improve visualization during the procedure.

7. Since the passage of the nasogastric tube may induce vomiting even in the comatose client, it may be wise to intubate the client before insertion of the nasogastric tube.

8. When intubation is not possible, place the unconscious client in a semiprone position to decrease the possibility of aspiration. Use some type of bulky cervical collar to discourage neck movement. Avoid restraint of the extremities if the unconscious client is agitated.

9. Whether the client is aroused or not, the practitioner should use a soothing but firm voice and manner to give the client concrete directions, to let the client know that he or she is in good hands, and to try to diminish agitated or disorganized, panicked behavior. Avoid the tendency to arouse false hope or guarantee outcomes.

10. Because inadequate respiratory status may cause rapid deterioration in the neurological condition, it is vitally important for practitioners and their agencies to agree on procedural matters involving resuscitation. When abnormal respirations exist, many emergency practitioners have permission to administer oxygen after an airway is patent until blood gas determinations may be made. In some clients, intubation and assistive ventilation devices are required because of the extent of the injury. In general, the $Pco_2$ should not exceed 35 mm Hg and the $Po_2$ should remain above 80 mm Hg. (Refer to Chapter 9 for brain resuscitation therapy.)

11. The intricacies of circulation are beyond the scope of this text. The practitioner needs specific orders and training, since exact treatment modalities vary according to other systemic problems. Arterial hypotension must be treated. Overhydration may be a problem, however, when the client has cerebral edema or a convulsive disorder.

12. Because you need to monitor intake and output during the acute phases and because spinal injuries resulting in spinal shock cause the renal system to retain excessive fluid for the first 2 to 4 days of treatment, it is wise to insert an indwelling catheter through that time period. Specific gravities should be done on urine at specified intervals.

13. A quick head-to-toe assessment should be accomplished to locate other injuries. A few points

**TABLE 23-3.** General care phase of head injury

| Assessment | Intervention | Expected outcomes |
| --- | --- | --- |
| **Neurological**<br>Same as acute phase<br>**Physiological**<br>Same as acute phase | Same as acute phase<br><br>Assess all physiologic parameters and plan care appropriate to the extent of the injuries. Continue to approach client therapeutically and follow through on medical orders. Record and report any significant changes. Collaborate with the physician to move client on to self-care when appropriate. Observe at regular intervals and change intervals according to condition of client. Be alert for insidious changes or symptoms of subdural hematoma. Provide care based on specific needs. Encourage client to change positions or change position for him or her every 2 hours as indicated by individual limitations. Continue measuring intake and output with appropriate fluid encouragement. Diet should be given as tolerated. If client is comatose, follow prescribed nursing regimen as outlined in Chapter 9. If surgery has been indicated, follow prescribed postoperative routine and special observations (refer to Chapter 26). Increased intracranial pressure may be fluctuating; so be alert to significant changes and report accordingly (refer to Chapter 21). Intracranial pressure monitoring equipment may be utilized with the necessary care required, as outlined in Chapter 27. The nurse accepts considerable responsibility for maintenance of life supports and recognition of additional complications, in conjunction with the physician and other specialists on the health team. If decerebrate or decorticate posturing is present, ensure client safety and protection of all body parts and surfaces. Convulsions may occur as a posttraumatic phenomenon or other physiologic response, requiring seizure precautions and observation (refer to Chapter 14). The use of narcotics should still be contraindicated and analgesics or tranquilizers used only after complete assessment, before and after administration. Maintain appropriate cervical spine alignment even though injury has been ruled out. Be alert for delirium tremens or withdrawal symptoms of alcohol or drug abuse, as well as dynamic effect on physiological parameters in assessment. | Same as acute phase<br><br>The client should:<br>1. Have same outcomes as the acute phase satisfied.<br>2. Be included along with the family in care as appropriate.<br>3. Have continuous evaluation for cervical spine injury. |
| **Psychosocial**<br>1. Same as acute phase<br>2. Economic factors<br>3. Health resources<br>4. Self-motivation | Same as acute phase. Encourage self-motivation of client self-care as appropriate to the extent of the injury. Evaluate health care resources and economic factors to obtain appropriate community assistance. | The client should:<br>1. Have the same outcomes as the acute phase is accomplished.<br>2. Be encouraged in self-care within the extent of ability. |

**TABLE 23-4.** Rehabilitative phase of head injury

| Assessment | Intervention | Expected outcomes |
|---|---|---|
| **Neurological**<br>Same as previous phases | Same as previous phases | The client should:<br>1. Be informed of the need for continuous comparison with base line. |
| **Physiological**<br>Same as previous phases | Same as previous phases | The client should:<br>1. Be continuously encouraged to move toward self-care.<br>2. Receive honest answers regarding sexuality, economic independence, and limits of mobility. |
| **Psychosocial**<br>1. Same as previous phases<br>2. Establish learning needs | Include verbal teaching and written pamphlet on care for head injuries before discharge, if client is hospitalized. If not a hospitalized client, provide written and verbal instructions for home care. The usual pamphlet giving instructions for head injuries includes the following information:<br>1. In the event of any unusual change, contact your physician.<br>2. Limit activity for 24 hours.<br>3. Diet should include nonalcoholic liquids and foods as tolerated.<br>4. Bed or chair rest.<br>5. Unusual sleepiness or difficulty in awakening should be reported immediately. Check client every 2 hours.<br>6. Planned rest periods.<br>7. Possible residual effects such as dizziness, headache, and memory losses may persist for 3 to 4 months after trauma. Alert the physician to this complication for evaluation.<br>8. Care of abrasions and lacerations as indicated should be given to patient and family members.<br>9. The importance of ongoing outpatient care to physician and physical therapy as indicated to evaluate complications and progress.<br>10. Notify physician for unusual irritability, restlessness, vomiting, persistent headaches, vision changes or change in pupil size, dizziness, fluid coming from ears or nose, weakness or paralysis, seizures, change in respiratory patterns, difficulty with speech, unusual behavior, or loss of consciousness.<br>The nurse should stress that if the symptoms suddenly change, the client should be taken to the emergency room immediately. The nurse should also instruct family members and client in the importance of required medications, dosage, frequency of administration, purpose, adverse outcomes, and avoidance of over-the-counter medications unless approved by the physician. | The client should:<br>1. Be motivated to self-care. |

of interest for multiple injured clients would include the following:

*Scalp*—Palpate and look for any signs of fracture, bruises, deformity, and lacerations hidden by hair. Think about symptoms that occur with intracranial bleeding and blood clot formation.

*Ears*—Look for cerebrospinal fluid drainage.

*Face*—Facial lacerations look messy, but seldom involve bleeding significant to evoke shock. However, nosebleeds are a different matter, since they may continue or be associated with tissue swelling that could compromise the airway. If the eye orbit has endured a direct blow, you will usually notice subconjunctival hemorrhage and periorbital ecchymosis. You will observe the nostrils to detect any clear or bloody cerebrospinal fluid drainage. You will assess vision and eye movement when you assess the cranial nerves. Should you see that part of the face has been severed—ears, eyelid, tongue, or other body part—place that part in a bottle of Ringer's lactate that has been cooled in an ice container, so that surgeons may utilize that body part sometime during the day for reattachment to the victim.

*Thoracic area*—Note rib deformities, asymmetric chest movement, muscles used in respiration, and unusual breathing patterns.

*Abdomen*—Diagnosis may be facilitated as the practitioner considers the force and type (penetrating or nonpenetrating) injury that may have occurred. For example, if a lap belt is used with shoulder harnesses in a car, the victim may have abdominal, lumbar spine injuries, or fractures in the pelvis. Symptoms including nausea, vomiting, pain, tenderness, abdominal rigidity, distention, shock, and a lack of bowel sounds are all notable. Be specific in describing these items.

*Cervical injury*—If the client is conscious, palpate the spinous processes. When injured, they are tender and may be unusually spaced. Suspect cervical injury when the neck is held in a tilted manner or when voluntary movement is limited. Avoid flexion and extension of the neck during assessment. Additional signs that may be helpful in the less responsive client include evidence of facial or mandibular fractures (an indication that great force may have been applied, so that the probability of injury to the cervical area is greater), atonic anal sphincter, or diaphragmatic breathing.

*Musculoskeletal structure*—Check all extremities carefully for any injury. After the client is stable, immobilize affected extremities to prevent further injury.

*Focal signs*—Note any asymmetric signs of movement or paralysis.

*Seizures*—Note body movement, point of origin, body parts involved, transient paralysis after the seizure. Refer to Chapter 14 for details on client care during a seizure.

*Cranial nerves*—When evaluating the second and third cranial nerves (pupillary response to light), remember that the immediate dilatation and fixation of the pupil often occurs after a direct blow to the orbit or to the third cranial nerve. If a dilated, fixed pupil results later, think about the possibility of an intracranial hematoma. Always consider the possibility of substance abuse, use of eye medications, seizures, or congenital asymmetry. If the client is unconscious, qualified practitioners may assess some cranial nerves as follows: the third, fourth, and fifth are assessed when cold water is placed in the client's ear, so that eyes move to the stimulated side. Test the fifth and seventh by watching for a blink when a wisp of cotton is drawn across the cornea and by noting facial response to a slight pinprick to the internal nasal tissue. A gag response and normal verbalization (if possible) confirm the integrity of the ninth and tenth. Others cannot be tested.

*Increased intracranial pressure*—Refer to Chapters 21 and 27 for an explanation of the problem and of ways to avoid increasing the pressure.

*Motor*—Assess carefully as mentioned in Chapter 11 and in this chapter. Establish a base line early. Include the Glasgow Coma Scale in this process. Continue to perform serial evaluations. Report any trends in client progress to the physician in charge.

*Body temperature*—If spinal shock is present (refer to Chapter 15), normalize body temperature without burning the client. Watch for sudden changes in temperature in head-injured clients, as this is an indication of serious problems.

*Other considerations*—Be aware of the need to chart adequately, get appropriate permissions, report certain situations to legal officers, and transmit information only to those qualified to receive personal client data. Consider your preparation, your agency policy, and your state laws to determine what role you will play in prehospital care and emergency room services. Refer to section on spinal cord injury in this chapter.

## Complications

The complications of head injury are many and variable in degree. The least may result in only a prolonged or uncomfortable convalescence, whereas the most severe may culminate in death. The complications are as follows:

1. Shock
2. Increased intracranial pressure
3. Change in respiratory patterns
4. Hyperthermia
5. Vomiting
6. Wound infection, osteomyelitis, or meningitis
7. Epidural or subdural bleeding or hematomas
8. Electrolyte imbalances and metabolic disturbances
9. Emotional disturbances
10. Corneal ulceration
11. Convulsions
12. Bladder or bowel retention or incontinence
13. Sensory dysfunctions
14. Motor disabilities
15. Headache
16. Periocular edema
17. Delirium tremens
18. Drug abuse withdrawal
19. Brainstem herniation

## SPINAL INJURIES

Trauma to the vertebral column may include concurrent injuries to the head, thorax, and extremities. Spinal trauma with associated injury to nerves, soft tissue, bony canal, and intravertebral discs usually results in laceration and contusion of delicate tissues and surrounding membranes, fractures, dislocation, paralysis, paresthesia, spinal shock, loss of motor function, hidden injuries, or simply a strain of supporting musculoskeletal structure. Movement of the head or trunk in bending forward, backward, or sideways requires a mobile, uninjured vertebral column. Spinal trauma, regardless of severity, with resultant distortion and deformity, whether obvious or suspected, is a cause of great concern because of the possibility of an incomplete injury extending to a complete injury with motion of the head, neck, or extremities. The results of mismanagement of spinal injuries in clients who sustain spinal column trauma can be awesome and irrevocable.

As a result, since 1972 the National Institute of Neurologic Diseases and Stroke (NINDS), the Rehabilitation Services Administration of the Department of Health, Education, and Welfare, and the National Spinal Cord Data System have aided in the development of a responsible emergency care system designed to educate the public and professionals, evaluate the system itself, rehabilitate clients, and gather epidemiological statistics on spinal cord injury.

### Incidence

Spinal injuries are usually the result of vehicular accidents, gunshot wounds, falls or falling objects, water and sports accidents, or pedestrian traffic collisions, and can lead to very serious results or death. Less serious mishaps generally result from lifting heavy objects, minor falls, or improper posture weakening the spinal ligmentous musculoskeletal arrangement, ultimately leading to injury with exertion. Annually, 6000 to 9000 new cases of spinal cord injury occur in the United States, with incidence primarily confined to males between 18 and 25 years of age. There is no significant difference in the incidence of paraplegia as opposed to quadriplegia.

### Current concerns

The estimated cost of the initial injury is $25,000 to $50,000, with each subsequent hospital admission totaling $10,000. The approximate lifetime cost is $200,000 if the client is rehabilitated, and $600,000 if not. The costliness of long-term care for the client with a spinal cord injury has prompted efforts toward the improvement of diagnostic techniques and research studies on the chemical changes that take place after injury to the spinal cord. The aim is to find a method for early detection and pharmacological treatment during those most critical first 24 hours to prevent, arrest, or reverse the chemical changes that take place in the myelin after injury. Current research into enzymes and hyperbaric or high-concentration oxygen environments, nerve and bone stimulators, and nerve and bone grating techniques may in the future minimize some of the more disabling effects of injuries. As a result of surgical research, many long-term results of injuries such as dislocation of healed fractures or surgically stabilized spines have been approached anteriorly, as well as posteriorly (with laminectomy), giving added strength and stability to the vertebrae. Also, the application of the halo frame and body cast has aided both medical and nursing care by promoting early ambula-

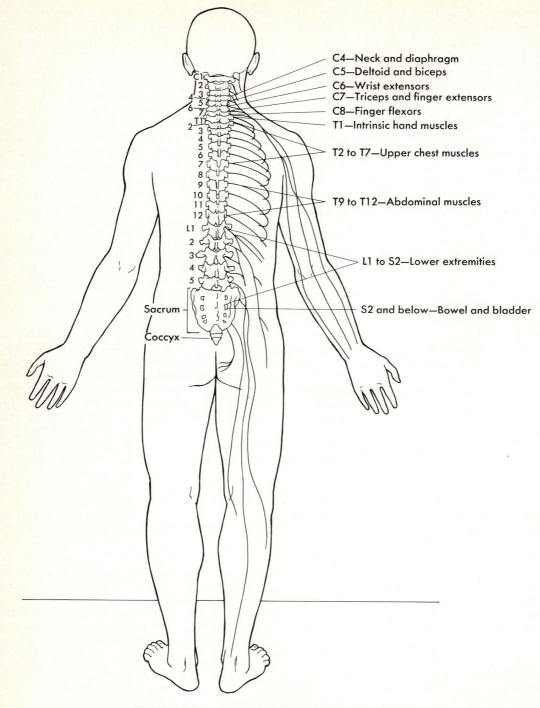

C4—Neck and diaphragm
C5—Deltoid and biceps
C6—Wrist extensors
C7—Triceps and finger extensors
C8—Finger flexors
T1—Intrinsic hand muscles

T2 to T7—Upper chest muscles

T9 to T12—Abdominal muscles

L1 to S2—Lower extremities

S2 and below—Bowel and bladder

Sacrum

Coccyx

**FIG. 23-5.** Relationship of spinal nerves to gross muscle functions.

tion, preventing complications of prolonged bed rest, and reducing hospital cost of the injury (Fig. 23-5).

## Types of injury

Injuries to the spinal cord can be categorized in a variety of ways and for each segment of the vertebral column. For practical purposes of discussion, trauma to the spinal cord is divided into specific types of spinal cord lesions and injuries, as shown in Table 23-5.

Spinal injuries are diagnosed by use of the history of the accident, results of the level of spinal cord injury from the neurological examination, and radiographic findings of the level of bony injury. Stability of the bony support is contingent on the integrity of the supraspinous ligament, intraspinous ligament, facet joint capsule, ligamentum flavum, and anterior and posterior longitudinal ligaments. If the ligamentous support remains intact, despite possible bony injury, the spine generally remains stable.

Crushing injury to one or more vertebral bodies is often associated with head injury, and damage to the intravertebral discs and spinal cord. Fractures may consist of (1) wedges or compression of the vertebral body, (2) dislocation of the pedicle with resultant intraspinous ligament damage, or (3) rupture of the intervertebral disc and dislocation of the vertebral body. Spinal injuries are grouped according to the mechanism of injury to the spinal column.

*Mechanisms. Flexion injuries* are classified as having a fracture present in the form of a wedge or compression of a vertebral body with or without dislocation of the vertebral alignment, a fracture of a pedicle with or without intraspinous ligament damage and dislocation, or fracture of the vertebral body and rupture of intervertebral disc. A flexion injury is generally the result of a force striking the posterior fossa and propelling the neck onto the chest. Other flexion injuries can occur by lateral exaggeration of the neck to one side or the other, usually resulting in a wedge fracture of the vertebral body. Rotation with flexion injury may occur as the head is twisted in one direction and the trunk in the opposite direction. Flexion injuries are common to the cervical and lumbar spine. If the force of injury does not interrupt the posterior ligmentous complex, the force is usually transmitted to the vertebral body, resulting in a wedge or burst fracture to the body. If the posterior ligament complex remains intact and the bone fragments are compact, the fracture is considered stable, generally fusing itself and making surgical fusion unnecessary.

*Rotational-flexional injuries* usually result in shearing of ligamentous support and dislocation of facet joints and distortion of vertebral alignment. This injury is common to the cervical spine and requires surgical stabilization and realignment with halo and body cast or skeletal traction. The aggressiveness of treatment depends on the client's age, social factors, and the significance of anterior dislocation or narrowing of the spinal canal. Cervical spine stability depending on ligamentous integrity

**TABLE 23-5.** Types of spinal cord trauma

| Types of spinal cord syndromes by affected areas | Categories of cord lesions by motor evaluation | Mechanism (types of spine injuries) |
|---|---|---|
| 1. Anterior<br>2. Posterior<br>3. Central<br>4. Brown-Sequard<br>5. Cervical root | 1. Complete at bony level<br>2. Graded complete<br>3. Partial with caudal gain or sparing<br>4. Partial with secondary incomplete or partial loss<br>5. Uniform partial lesion | 1. Flexion injury<br>  a. Wedge-burst fractures<br>  b. Fractures with dislocation of pedicles or vertebral body<br>  c. Lateral injury with fracture<br>  d. Rotational injury with spinal cord compression<br>2. Vertical compression injury with spinal cord compression<br>3. Hyperextension injury with compression of interspinous ligaments and ruptured intervertebral discs. |

and presence or absence of rupture of the facet capsule is cause for great concern during any stabilization and realignment procedure attributable to impending or hidden neurological deficit. The immediate goal is stability without deficit, while one tries to prevent complete cord lesion or potential instability of the spine.

*Vertical compression* injuries usually result from a force projected along an axis from the top of the head through the vertebral bodies to the level of the shoulders. In the case of the thoracolumbar spine, the force is usually projected caudally from the buttocks or feet, such as falling down a flight of stairs with both feet extended or jumping from a building roof. The vertebral body classically bursts with spinal cord compression. As long as the ligamentous support structures remain intact, the injury impacts itself, eliminating the need for surgical fusion. Bony fragments may, however, impinge on nerve roots or the spinal cord, necessitating surgical removal. Decompressive laminectomy may be indicated, if the intervertebral discs are ruptured and instability is suspected.

*Hyperextension injuries* occur because of a force such as sudden acceleration and deceleration experienced in many rear-end vehicular accidents, often causing compression of the intraspinous ligament, rupture of the intervertebral discs, disruption of the anterior longitudinal ligament, and fracture of the vertebral body or pedicle. This injury is most commonly associated with a "whiplash" or "hangman's injury" in automobile accidents, "clotheslining" in football, and diving injury in water sports. The history of this injury is most significant since radiographic examination often misses occult injuries. The spine, regardless of the extent of the injury, must be stabilized and aligned to prevent dislocation and neurological impairment. Decompression laminectomy with spinal fusion may be indicated for severe injuries. Cervical collars or braces may be used, if the spine is not malaligned and the ligamentous structures are stable. Bony malalignment and ligamentous instability necessitate skeletal traction by Crutchfield or Gardner-Wells tongs and, at a later point, halo frame and body cast.

Injury located in the thoracolumbar region is generally treated through open reduction with Harrington rod placement for posterior fixation. After myelography, decompressive laminectomy of the intravertebral discs or foraminotomy of nerve roots may be indicated to prevent neurological deficit.

***Categorization by affected cord area.*** After consideration of the type of spinal injury, attention is turned to injuries of spinal cord and category of cord lesions. Spinal cord lesions classically present neurological syndromes and correlate with the specific type of injury, as well as functional outcomes. The most common type of spinal cord syndrome is the *anterior cord syndrome* occurring after acute flexion injury of the cervical spine. Injury to the anterior spinal artery or ventral aspect of the spinal cord or both results in loss of upper and lower motor function; dorsal column sensation ("sacral sparing") and scattered peripheral sensation are usually preserved.

*Posterior cord syndrome* is rarely seen but is associated with cervical hyperextension injuries. The motor function of the extremities remains intact, but posterior dorsal column sensibility (light touch, proprioception) is lost.

*Central cord syndrome* is a frequent occurrence from hyperextension injuries in the elderly or flexion injuries with little evidence of displacement. It is the second most common spinal cord syndrome with the area of injury primarily located in the central gray matter. Neurological deficit results in mixed loss of upper and lower motor neuron lesions with flaccid paralysis related to the most traumatized area and spastic involvement (upper motor neuron) below the level of the lesion.

The *Brown-Sequard syndrome* can present variations in the acute phase after injury. This syndrome and associated spinal injury are usually manifested by rotation-flexion injury, where subluxation or dislocation of the fracture fragments occurs or by unilateral pedicle-laminar injuries. Neurologically, the client presents with motor weakness on the ipsilateral side of the injury and loss of sensation of pain and temperature on the contralateral side. An interesting phenomenon can occur with this particular syndrome in that significant neurological recovery often occurs and clients receive a false impression that total recovery may occur. Clients should be encouraged to work with the syndrome as recovery occurs, but care should be taken not to give false hope.

The *cervical root syndrome* may be associated

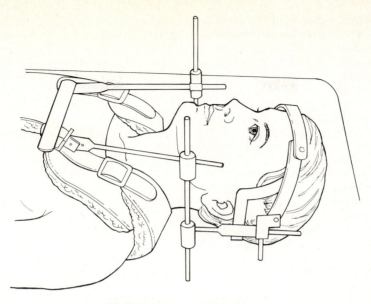

**FIG. 23-6.** Halo frame and body cast.

with flexion injuries followed by specific nerve root loss of function. This syndrome is common with ruptured intervertebral discs, with neuroforamina encroachment after injury, or as a sequela to degenerative arthritis (Fig. 23-6).

*Categorization by motor assessment.* Spinal cord lesions can also be categorized by motor evaluation for even better prognostic implications throughout all treatment periods. This categorization, based solely on motor function, seems to be more constant than one based on wide variation in presentation of sensory function. A *motor complete lesion* at the bony level generally results in total motor functional loss within two cord segments caudal to injury level. Vertebral-body malalignment necessitates the two-cord segment allowance for diagnostic purposes. A *graded complete lesion* occurs with caudal displacement of fracture fragments or vertebral bodies, creating complete loss of motor function between two to four segments beneath the point of impact of the bone.

*Partial motor loss at the level of injury with caudal gain or sparing* is the motor definition of the central cord syndrome wherein greater weakness occurs in the upper extremities as compared to the lower. A *partial motor loss* occurring at the level of injury with *partial or total secondary motor loss* at least four segments beneath the point of injury, signifies a poor prognostic implication. *Partial motor loss in a uniform pattern* corresponds to the root syndrome or multiple root deficits and can occur in cervical, thoracic, or lumbrosacral regions.

The spinal cord may be so damaged that function of the distal segment is permanently interrupted and integrated activity with the upper levels of the nervous system is impossible. Along with the motor loss, additional manifestations of spinal cord injuries are the immediate loss of sensory functions and reflexes below the level of the injury, urinary retention, bowel distention, priapism for a few hours, absence of perspiration in the paralyzed parts, neurogenic shock, need for respiratory assistance, vasomotor-system hypotension, dermal edema, and, in hot weather, faulty autoregulation of body temperature.

*Resulting damage.* The distinction between motor disturbances resulting from lesions of the voluntary motor pathways, whether lower or upper motor neuron in origin, can be made by observation of impaired muscle functioning or understanding of the interruption of impulses to the myoneural junction, peripheral nerves, or central nervous system. Lower motor neuron lesions interrupt essential motor cell activities from the corticospinal, rubrospinal, olivospinal, vestibulospinal, reticulospinal, and tectospinal tracts and from the intersegmental and intrasegmental reflex neurons through which neural impulses travel to skeletal muscle. Locations of the lesions may be the cell body or axons in the ventral gray column of the spinal cord or brainstem. Symptoms of lower motor neuron lesions include flaccid paralysis of involved muscles, muscle atrophy after degeneration of the muscle fibers, diminished or absent reflexes, or no pathological reflexes in the involved extremities. Upper motor neuron lesions affect the transfer of impulses from the motor strip of the cerebrum to the lower motor neurons through the corticobulbar or corticospinal tracts. Lesions located in the cerebral cortex, internal capsule, brainstem, or spinal cord may disrupt the impulses essential for voluntary muscle activity. Symptoms of an upper motor neuron lesion include spastic paralysis or paresis of involved muscles, little or no muscle atrophy, hyperactive deep tendon reflexes, pathological reflexes, and diminished or absent superficial reflexes. Either lesion can occur in a spinal cord injury, but the hallmark of which motor neuron will be affected lies solely on the location, the type of spinal injury and syndrome produced, and the category of spinal cord lesion. For a more detailed discussion of disturbances of motor function, refer to Chapter 15. Chapter 25 discusses rehabilitation of the disturbances.

### Cervical spine injury

If the cervical spine has been injured, the paralysis may include all or part of the four extremities and the trunk. The respiratory muscles also may be involved so that only the accessory muscles about the head (nose, mouth, and neck) carry on breathing, and respiratory failure may result.

### Thoracic spine injury

Fractures of the thoracic spine spare the upper extremities and respiratory mechanism, since the paralysis involves only the muscles of the lower extremities, bladder, and rectum. These muscles become spastic after the initial flaccidity recedes. The atonic bladder becomes hypertonic but with treatment may function automatically.

### Lumbar spine injury

Fractures of the lumbar spine cause injury to the *cauda equina* (lumbar and sacral spinal roots) and *conus medullaris*. The result is a persisting flaccid paralysis of the lower extremities, bladder, and rectum. Consequently, automatic urinary activity is never achieved. Refer to Chapter 25 for information on physiology and to Chapter 15 for motor disturbances.

### Autonomic hyperreflexia

An impending syndrome that may occur at any time after injury, with reports as long as 6 years after the initial insult, is *automatic hyperreflexia*. This syndrome is associated with a massive uncompensated cardiovascular response to stimulation of the sympathetic divisions of the autonomic nervous system. Those clients most likely to be affected have lesions at the T7 level or above. Autonomic hyperreflexia is characterized by paroxysmal hypertension, a pounding headache, sweating above the level of the lesion with flushing of the skin, cutis anserina below the level of the injury, nasal congestion, nausea, and bradycardia. The symptoms may develop singly or in combination and are generally associated with a distended bladder or instrumentation of the bladder, bowel distention, pressure on the glans penis or testicles (bulbocavernous reflex), or sharp stimuli to the genitoanal area. Any of the symptoms left untreated can lead to serious damage and even death.

### Summary

The management of a client with a spinal cord injury is integrated much the same as that for the client with a head injury and is generally divided into acute, general, and rehabilitative phases, with outcomes specific to the client's course of symptoms. Services of the spinal cord injury center should be utilized when possible. Specific nursing care outcomes for and approaches to clients with spinal cord injuries include the prevention of paralysis in those clients who have fractures and are not paralyzed, as well as the outcomes previously discussed for neurological trauma. Nursing management is again directed toward assessment, intervention, and client teaching in all phases of care.

*Prehospital intervention in spinal injuries.* The goals of early management are to (1) preserve life, (2) prevent further neurological deficit, (3) prevent deformity, and (4) prevent complications in other body systems. Some general signs that indicate spinal cord damage has occurred include numbness, tingling or sensory loss, loss of motor function, signs of spinal deformity, pain during spine motion, depressed or absent reflexes, and flaccidity when unconscious. Injury may be of a penetrating (knife wound or projectile) or of a nonpenetrating nature (falls, ejection, or trauma related to motor vehicles).

Four important facts need to be established during the initial assessment; they are (1) how the accident occurred, (2) the amount of force, (3) the extent and location of the injury, and (4) the sensorimotor and reflex capacities. Any motor or sensory sparing observed at this time is a good sign.

Refer to the critical care summary for head injuries in this chapter, to Chapter 9 on coma, to Chapter 21 on increased intracranial pressure, to Chapters 11 and 12 on assessment and diagnostic tools, and to Chapter 27 on adjunctive interventions for related information.

The priorities in prehospital care are outlined below:

1. The A, B, C's of resuscitation (airway, breathing, and circulation) are of primary importance.
2. Early edema of the cord may be relieved by a large intramuscular dose of dexamethasone (Decadron).
3. Utilize the appropriate board and an adequate number of trained personnel to free the victim from the accident and safely effect transport to the hospital.
4. Pad bony extremities to prevent skin breakdown.
5. An esophageal obturator airway may be used to provide an airway so that vomiting and aspiration are prevented.
6. Realize that involvement of the cord at C3 and C4 can cause rapid fatality whereas involvement at cord levels of C4 and C5 may

result in respiratory difficulty because of diaphragmatic involvement. Both of these types of injuries require assistive ventilatory support.
7. For thoracic and lumbar injuries
   a. Use a full board or a special scoop stretcher.
   b. Look for chest injuries when you find thoracic spine injuries because a great force is required to damage the barely mobile thoracic vertebrae.
   c. In lumbar injuries, look for abdominal injuries and pelvic fractures.
8. Emotion is first characterized by shock and disbelief and then by panic with thought disorganization and minimal comprehension during the first days of treatment.

If there are subjective or objective signs of injury to the cervical region, the position of the head should not be adjusted by anterior flexion on the chest or by elevation onto a support. These manipulations may result in increasing the degree of spinal cord damage and may even cause permanent loss of function. The individual with a possible cervical cord injury should be transported flat on the back without a head pillow on a wooden board (6 by 3 feet) (Fig. 23-7). It is generally wise to immobilize the neck and exert gentle traction by manual pressure on the occiput and mandible. This should only be done by the physician. The ambulance driver is cautioned to drive with the utmost care and to avoid abrupt stops. Reckless driving may so jar the client that further injury will result.

If the client has difficulty moving or lifting the legs, injury to the spinal cord at the thoracic or lumbar levels may be indicated. To avoid causing further local trauma, one should use great care in moving the client. Shoulders, back, and hips are kept in good alignment at all times. The position should not be changed without competent and sufficient help.

*At emergency room.* Perform a history and do a base-line assessment. Compare findings to those in the prehospital assessment. Leave the client on the transport board until injuries are confirmed and the presiding physician is present to supervise movement. Remove all clothing. Cut clothing if necessary. Look for other injuries. Utilize a soft

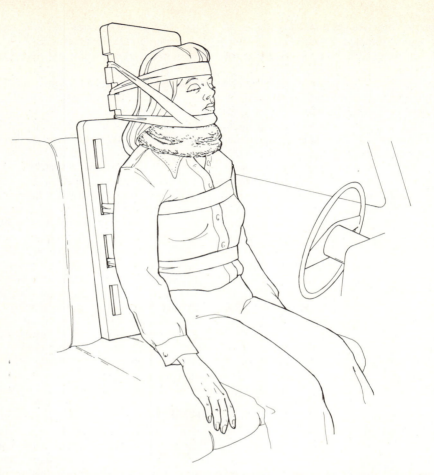

**FIG. 23-7.** First aid method of immobilization of spinal injury. Note use of a soft collar, which may be made from a heavy towel or other appropriate material.

collar and sandbags to discourage movement of the neck until the diagnostic evaluation is complete. Begin fluids and medications and give tetanus injection as necessary. Perform cultures before starting any antibiotics. Clean wounds and bandage. Avoid the use of iodine-containing solutions in areas prepared for radiographic study because iodine distorts x-rays. Stay with the client during the radiographic studies until spinal damage can be assessed. Monitor any client movement carefully. Provide skin care when the client is on a hard surface for a period of time. Continue serial assess-

ments. Motor integrity needs to be assessed only one segment above and below the established point of injury. Sensation should be marked on a diagrammatic chart (Figs. 3-4 and 3-5). If the client is in a coma, determine motor function by noting that there is no reflex activity below an injury involving spinal shock. (Refer to Chapter 9.) Internal and external stabilization of the spine is done so that the client may be mobilized early in the total treatment program. Continue with the acute phase at spinal injury (Table 23-6).

**TABLE 23-6.** Acute phase of spinal injury

| Assessment | Intervention | Expected outcomes |
|---|---|---|
| **Neurological** | Approach client in therapeutic manner, inform the client of the process of the neurological examination before initiating the exam. Explain the rationale for the various parts of the examination, regardless of consciousness. Observe and record all responses to the neurological examination. Answer questions honestly. Collaborate findings, if significant, with physician. | The client should: |
| 1. Orientation | | 1. Be informed of all aspects of the neurological examination. |
| 2. General cerebral functioning | | 2. Be instructed in the rationale for the assessment procedures. |
| 3. Cranial, spinal, and peripheral nerve functioning | | 3. Have continuous reassessment of injury status, regardless of extent. |
| 4. Sensation | | 4. Be provided privacy during examination. |
| 5. Reflexes | | 5. Have appropriate radiographic studies and repeat studies if necessary to diagnose injury. |
| 6. Respiratory function | | |
| 7. Muscle strength and motion | | |
| 8. Pupil size, equality, and reaction to light. | | |
| 9. Objective and subjective signs of head injury | | |
| 10. Communicative ability | | |
| 11. Visual fields | | |
| 12. Boundaries of functional loss of spinal integration | | |
| 13. Sacral sparing and anal wink | | |
| 14. Presence or absence of bulbocavernous reflex | | |
| 15. Balance, coordination, and gait, if client is ambulatory | | |

*Continued.*

**TABLE 23-6.** Acute phase of spinal injury—cont'd

| Assessment | Intervention | Expected outcomes |
|---|---|---|
| **Physiological—serial assessments** | Establish all details of the accident or injury from the client, family members, or witnesses. Assess all physiological parameters and plan care appropriate to the findings. Answer all questions honestly and approach client therapeutically. Follow through on medical orders. As soon as the client's condition permits, cleanse all body surfaces, bandage appropriately, and provide change of clothes. If client was admitted to the emergency room with spinal board in place or any other form of head and neck fixation device, *do not remove* or let anyone else remove the apparatus until instructed to do so by the physician in charge. Cut away clothing to avoid unnecessary movement. Try to pad and rub skin over bony prominences when board remains in place for more than 1 hour. Accompany client to radiology department to ensure proper movement and assessment of client during radiographic procedures. Before moving client, ensure safety by having ample numbers of trained personnel standing by to help move the client. Maintain strict body alignment at all times. Do not turn or move head at any time, and instruct client and family to do the same. Utilize semihard collar and sandbags lateral to head to discourage movement. Make observations at appropriate intervals. Collaborate significant findings immediately with physician. Maintain client airway. Have mechanical ventilator and tracheostomy tray available, especially when cervical injury is a problem. Take care when suctioning client not to traumatize gag reflex so that client will not have an urge to move the head. Use care when obtaining rectal temperature to | The client should: 1. Be informed of the necessity for factual information. 2. Cooperate to best of ability for accurate information to evaluate changes in care. 3. Have continuous reassessment of injury status, regardless of extent. 4. Be provided privacy during examination. |
| 1. Neurological and vital signs | | |
| 2. Pain at the level of injury | | |
| 3. Headache, kind, and site | | |
| 4. Oxygenation and respiratory pattern | | |
| 5. Muscle tone and activity | | |
| 6. General condition or other injuries | | |
| 7. Bleeding and circulatory status | | |
| 8. Amount, color, and kind of drainage from any orifice | | |
| 9. Joint function | | |
| 10. Bladder or bowel distention | | |
| 11. Description of any convulsive phenomena | | |
| 12. Nutritional, fluid, and electrolyte status | | |
| 13. Previous elimination pattern | | |
| 14. Loss of perspiration below a significant level | | |
| 15. Rest and sleep | | |
| 16. Comfort | | |
| 17. Environmental safety and self-safety | | |
| 18. Personal hygiene | | |
| 19. Details of accident | | |
| 20. Last ingestion of medication and what medication was necessary | | |

ly. Auscultate bowel sounds and breath sounds routinely. Cooperate in getting essential laboratory work done including complete blood count with differential, SMA-6, SMA-12, type and cross match, coagulation studies, and arterial blood gases. Administer medications only as ordered after complete assessment of the client. Morphine is generally contraindicated with spinal cord trauma, but analgesics, sedatives, and tranquilizers are also restricted until the rehabilitative phase. Injections should not be given below the level of the injury, unless no other route is available. Steroids may be given in large doses with routine precautions being taken. If a client requires surgery, his or her preparation and safety until received back in the room is the same as listed above. Posture the client correctly and maintain the position or positions appropriate to the injury. Understand the concepts and principles of neurogenic shock and the autonomic hyperreflexia syndrome so that nursing care plans can reflect precautions for these two specific syndromes (refer to Chapter 15). Use general nursing care management for head injuries as outlined previously in this chapter. Monitor all indicators of increased intracranial pressure (refer to Chapter 21). Support client and family by helping them verbalize feelings and fears during all phases of acute assessment and care.

## Psychosocial

1. Cognitive ability
2. Emotional response
3. Social environment surrounding injury or accident, if pertinent
4. Cultural influences
5. Family support

Approach client and family therapeutically. Offer support appropriate to situation. Plan care including psychosocioeconomic and cultural influences of client. Record and report any significant changes in cognitive ability or emotional response. Consider the necessity to provide repeated explanations due to shock, disbelief, fear of unknown, panic about situation/loss of functions during first days of treatment.

The client should:

1. Receive treatment regardless of economic situation.
2. Have continuous reassessment as appropriate to determine extent of injury.
3. Be informed of the necessity of factual information to plan care appropriate to psychosocioeconomic-cultural needs.
4. Have family supported by the nurse while diagnostic procedures or examinations are being conducted to determine extent of injury.

**TABLE 23-7.** General care phase of spinal injury

| Assessment | Intervention | Expected outcomes |
|---|---|---|
| **Neurological**<br>Same as acute phase | Same as acute phase. Modify neurological examination to client progress; spinal shock may last from 3 days to 3 months (see Chapter 15). | The client should:<br>Do same as acute phase. |
| **Physiological**<br>Same as acute phase | Treatment is the same as the acute phase with additional management required. Maintain parenteral fluid infusion with special attention to infusion sites, if below the level of the injury. Ensure sterility of urinary drainage system by appropriate indwelling catheter care and then intermittent catheterization, as discussed in Chapters 25 and 27. Accurate intake and output as ordered. Assess urine frequently for signs of renal sediment and be alert for possible renal calculi. Monitor bowel sounds and elimination frequently, giving enemas or suppositories as needed, usually every 3 days, for bowel training. Refer to Chapter 25 for further detail on bowel and bladder training. Perform range-of-motion exercises as ordered within limits of client tolerance. Encourage client to participate to functional limits in all aspects of care. Monitor all bony prominences every 2 hours and provide skin care as needed. Turn at least every 2 hours. Consult physical or occupational therapist for aids to prevent contractures, activities of daily living supplies, and effective exercise program for prevention of muscle-disuse atrophy. Maintain skeletal traction or halo frame alignment. Provide aseptic environment for pins in skull with skeletal traction. Know care of client with the identified neurological injury on special bed or frame. Take effective action to prevent the hazards of immobility, especially orthostatic hypotension, pneumonia, osteoporosis, and thrombophlebitis. Utilize diet modifications to ensure acid-ash diet to keep urine acidic. Force fluids to 3000 to 5000 ml per day. Provide emotional support, and instruct client in all aspects of care. Provide adequate rest periods between all activities to prevent frustration. Establish daily routines to facilitate client rehabilitation from the onset of injury. | The client should:<br>Do same as acute phase. |
| **Psychosocial**<br>1. Same as acute phase<br>2. Economic factors<br>3. Health resources<br>4. Self-motivation<br>5. Sexuality | Same as acute phase. Encourage self-motivation of client self-care appropriate to the extent of the injury. Evaluate health care resources and economic factors to obtain appropriate community services and rehabilitation center as indicated. Refer to Chapters 6 and 7. | The client should:<br>1. Do same as acute phase<br>2. Be encouraged in self-care within the extent of ability. |

**TABLE 23-8.** Rehabilitative phase of spinal injury

| Assessment | Intervention | Expected outcomes |
|---|---|---|
| **Neurological** Same as previous phases | Same as previous phases with modification according to client progress. | The client should: 1. Be informed of the need for continued comparison with base line. |
| **Physiological** Same as previous phases | Same as previous phases with progressive incorporation of client to self-care within functional limits. Plan daily care activities to include muscle-building activities in bed or wheelchair and during ambulation as able. Continue efforts at bowel and bladder training. Be alert for symptoms of autonomic hyperreflexia. Make contract for daily pattern of care and stick to it for client compliance during rehabilitation. Plan program for supportive, guidance, and client care supervision to include appropriate significant others. | The client should: 1. Be continuously encouraged to move to self-care. 2. Receive honest answers regarding sexuality (refer to Chapter 6). 3. Be accepted without judgment while coping with adjustments inherent in the physical condition. |
| **Psychosocial** 1. Same as previous phases 2. Establish learning needs | Include verbal instructions of self-care. Provide a written schedule of treatments as necessary, if client requires family-assisted care. Provide diversional activities that the client can complete. Give honest, appropriate praise for tasks completed. Give positive approval for any motivation toward self-care. Only give negative responses after collaboration with physician to prevent interference with motivation level. Deal with body image changes realistically and support client and family in their efforts to cope. Encourage verbalization of body changes, loss of function, and behavioral changes. Involve family at client's direction. Complete appropriate referrals to home-help agencies. Instruct client and family in: 1. Importance of keeping physician appointments for check-ups. 2. Need for continued rehabilitation. 3. Need for planned rest periods. 4. Medication administration. 5. Self-catheterization, rectal suppository, or enema instillation for bladder and bowel training. 6. Observation of bony prominences every 2 hours, and need for position change while client is sleeping. 7. Symptoms of autonomic hyperreflexia and how to combat symptoms; physician should be notified immediately. 8. Forcing of fluids and observation of urine for sediment. 9. Continuing of a nutritionally appropriate, acid-ash diet with foods to tolerance. | The client should: 1. Be motivated to self-care. 2. Receive discharge teaching for care. |

## Complications

The following complications may occur with spinal cord injury:

1. Systemic shock (considered the leading cause of death).
2. Respiratory failure (especially in cervical injuries).
3. Pneumonia (especially in thoracic injuries because respirations become shallow as a result of splinting of the chest when pain is not relieved).
4. Urinary tract infections (may be the cause of death within months to years after transection of the spinal cord).
5. Acute or chronic malnutrition.
6. Decubitus ulcers and burns.
7. Footdrop and wristdrop.
8. Muscle spasms and contractures.
9. Pain.
10. Anxiety and depression.
11. Autonomic hyperreflexia.
12. Paralysis.

Spasticity may occur from 2 weeks to several months after a spinal cord injury. Pain generally occurs later and is most likely to be in the lower extremities. Some paraplegic and quadriplegic clients complain of both pain and muscle spasms. Autonomic hyperreflexia can occur at any time during the client's recovery and after rehabilitation. See Tables 23-6 and 23-7.

## RUPTURE OF INTERVERTEBRAL DISC

Rupture of an intervertebral disc consists of the protrusion of a part of the *nucleus pulposus* posteriorly through a laceration of the *anulus fibrosus* and the posterior longitudinal ligament. The cause is a less violent degree of trauma than that which fractures the spine. This is usually caused when one lifts a heavy object or wrenches or falls on the back. The ligament and capsule of the disc are torn, and the fibrocartilaginous material squeezes out and pinches the adjacent nerve root by compressing it against the bone. More than 90% of these ruptures occur in the lower lumbar and lumbosacral regions. They are rare in the thoracic region and occur only occasionally in the cervical region.

The signs and symptoms associated with a ruptured lumbar disc are characterized by pain in the lower back with radiation down the back of one leg. Movement of the back is greatly restricted, and walking is painful. The discomfort is aggravated by coughing, sneezing, or straining. On examination, the back appears straight with loss of the lumbar curve; the paravertebral muscles are spastic; mobility of the spine is restricted; the affected leg cannot be straightened when the thigh is flexed; jugular compression aggravates the pain; the ipsilateral ankle jerk may be less active than the other; and sensation is impaired over the foot or leg, depending on the particular lumbar or sacral nerve root being compressed. Somewhat similar findings, stiffness of the neck and local pain radiating down the arm to the fingers, are noted when the herniation occurs in the cervical region.

The diagnosis is made on the basis of the clinical picture with doubtful situations clarified by myelography (Fig. 23-8).

### Treatment and nursing intervention

The treatment consists of neurosurgical operation to remove the damaged disc. This is performed through the small opening between the laminae of the vertebrae where the disc has been ruptured. Generally, little or no bone is removed, and the stability of the vertebral column is unaltered. Fusion of the spine is usually not indicated unless an associated congenital instability of the vertebral column is present. The fusion is then done by an orthopedic surgeon.

During the preoperative interval, treatment is systematic and directed toward the relief of pain. Fracture boards under the mattress may give some relief. The principles of nursing care are the same as those outlined earlier in this chapter. Conservative medical treatment consisting of prolonged bed rest, physical therapy, the wearing of a brace, or the use of some form of traction has been attempted with variable success.

The preoperative preparation of the client is for the most part similar to that outlined in Chapter 22. The principles of nursing care emphasized in Chapter 26 for the postoperative client are applied in the nursing care of the client after the removal of a disc. They are modified after the initial 24 hours, and these clients are permitted more spontaneous activity. They are turned and

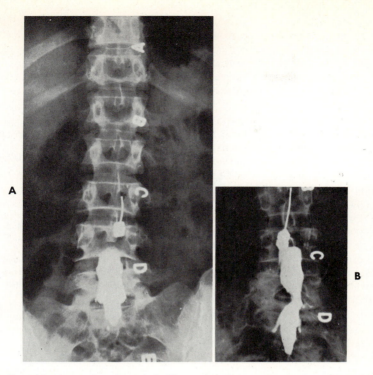

**FIG. 23-8. A,** Normal lumbosacral myelogram. **B,** Abnormal myelogram showing filling defect at lumbosacral level; spinal needle is in situ.

postured in the same way as long as they remain on absolute bed rest. The length of time in bed varies with the individual neurosurgeon and ranges from 1 to 5 days.

If a fusion is to be done, the client is measured for and fitted with a back brace before operation. (If this is not available, a circular cast may be substituted.) The brace is applied immediately after the completion of the surgical procedure and is not removed for the following 6 weeks. The client is not turned unless the brace is securely fastened in place; however, one may loosen it by opening the apron whenever necessary. Special instructions and demonstrations in adjusting, applying, and removing this brace should be given to the staff. The position of the client is changed every 2 hours by two nurses using the turning sheet. (The client is not permitted to turn him- or herself.) He or she is turned in log-fashion, as previously described, to reduce the danger of caus-

ing local pain and discomfort. The client should be postured at all times. During this initial 6-week period, the head is not elevated. At the end of this time, radiographic examination is made, and if bone union has progressed favorably, the client is gradually permitted out of bed. The brace is removed at night for the next week and then for increasing periods during the day until he or she is able to go without it. The time varies with the individual and is regulated according to the findings on radiographic examination. It may be 8 weeks or longer before the brace is finally removed.

## Conservative treatment

When myelography indicates a middle-grade protrusion of an involved disc, and all other conservative measures have been exhausted, physicians may inject the basic polypeptide aprotinin (Trasylol) into the affected intravertebral disc to diminish pressure associated with swelling and to thereby reduce associated nerve root compression. Further studies continue into client safety, results, and complications in this treatment method. Certainly, aprotinin represents an improvement over the chondrolytic agent chymopapain, a substance with very serious risks up to and including possible shock and paraplegia.

After surgery of the lumbar spine, there is the possibility that the removed nucleus pulposus will regenerate, or, if not, that the original problem and habits causing the first injury may result in trauma to the level about any spinal fusion. To avoid this event, the Low Back School was formed to (1) educate clients in anatomy, (2) assess habits, postures, and muscle strength, and (3) prescribe and instruct clients in corrective exercises and daily living habits. The acid test is the postinstruction negotiation of a deliberate obstacle course. Nurse specialists with appropriate education who are collaborating with physicians and physical therapists may wish to consider the possibilities of innovative practice opportunities herein (Attix and Tate, 1979).

## REFERENCES

Adelstein, W.: Brain stem injuries, J. Neurosurg. Nurs. **10:** 112-116, Sept. 1978.

Attix, E., and Tate, M.A.: Low Back School, J. Miss. State Med. Assoc. **20:**4-9, Jan. 1979.

Bailey, R.W.: The cervical spine, Philadelphia, 1974, Lea & Febiger.

Bakay, L., and Glasauer, F.: Head injury, Boston, 1980, Little, Brown & Co.

Benvenuti, C.S.: Independence for the quadriplegic: the Bantam Respirator, Am. J. Nurs. **79:**918-920, May 1979.

Birum, L.H., and Zimmerman, D.S.: Catheter plugs as a source of infection, Am. J. Nurs. **71:**2150-2152, 1971.

Braun, W.: Intradisc injection of Trasylol in lumbar intervertebral disc syndrome, Neurosurg. Rev. **1:**21-24, 1979.

Brower, P., and Hicks, D.: Maintaining muscle function in patients on bed rest, Am. J. Nurs. **72:**1250-1253, 1972.

Browse, N.L.: Physiology and pathology of bedrest, Springfield, Ill., 1965, Charles C Thomas, Publisher.

Burry, M.: The decerebrate patient, J. Neurosurg. Nurs. **11:** 6-9, March 1979.

Carol, M., et al.: Acute care of spinal cord injury: a challenge to the emergency medicine clinician, Crit. Care Q. **2:**7-21, 1979.

Christopherson, V.A.: Role modifications of the disabled male, Am. J. Nurs. **68:**290-293, 1968.

Clark, C.L.: Catheter care in the home, Am. J. Nurs. **72:**922-924, 1972.

Confirmation and cure of acute subdural hematoma, Nursing72 **2:**15, Feb. 1972.

Cooper, P.R., et al.: Serial computerized tomographic scanning and the prognosis of severe head injury, Neurosurgery **5:** 566-569, Nov. 1979.

Crewe, N.M., et al.: Spinal cord injury: a comparison of pre-injury and post-injury marriages, Arch. Phys. Med. Rehabil. **60:**252-256, June 1979.

Ducker, T.B., et al.: Emergency care of patients with cerebral injuries, Postgrad. Med. **55:**102, Jan. 1974.

El Ghatit, A.Z., and Haason, R.W.: Educational and training levels and employment of the spinal cord injured patient, Arch. Phys. Med. Rehabil. **60:**405-406, Sept. 1979.

Garrett, A.M.: Functional potential of patients with spinal cord injury, Clin. Orthop. Rel. Res. **112:**60-66, Oct. 1975.

Giesy, J.D.: Incontinence: causes, diagnosis and treatment, Hosp. Care **3:**1-6, 15, Jan. 1972.

Gifford, R., and Plaut, M.: Abnormal respiratory patterns in the comatose patient caused by intracranial dysfunction, J. Neurosurg. Nurs. **7:**57-61, July 1975.

Gudeman, S., et al.: The genesis and significance of delayed traumatic intracerebral hematoma, Neurosurgery **5:**309-313, Sept. 1979.

Hardy, A.G., and Elson, R.: Practical management of spinal injuries for nurses, ed. 2, New York, 1976, Longman, Inc.

Hardy, J.H., and Rossier, A.B.: Spinal cord injuries, Acton, Mass., 1975, Publishing Sciences Group, Inc.

Hargest, T.S., and Artz, C.P.: A new concept in patient care: the air-fluidized bed, AORN J. **10:**50-53, Sept. 1969.

Harvin, J.S., and Hargest, T.: The air-fluidized bed: a new concept in the treatment of decubitus ulcers, Nurs. Clin. North Am. **5:**181-187, March 1970.

Isler, C.: Decubitus/old truths, and some new ideas, RN **35:** 42-45, July 1972.

Jaffee, G.: Bob can walk again, Am. J. Nurs. **63:**85-86, July 1963.

Jamieson, K.G.: The traumatic intracerebral hematoma: report or 63 surgically treated cases, J. Neurosurg. **37:**528-532, 1972.

Jones, J.S.: Accept my disability? Never, Am. J. Nurs. **72:** 1983, Nov. 1972.

Kaplan, L.I., et al.: Pain and spasticity in patients with spinal cord dysfunction, J.A.M.A. **182:**918-925, 1962.

Kaste, M., et al.: Chronic bilateral subdural haematoma in adults, Acta Neurochir. **48:**231-236, 1979.

Katton, K.R.: Trauma and no trauma of the cervical spine, Springfield, Ill., 1975, Charles C Thomas, Publisher.

Keller, N.: Care without coordination: a true story, Nurs. Forum **6:**280-323, 1967.

Kottke, F., and Blanchard, R.: Bedrest begets bedrest, Forum **3**(3):56-72, 1964.

Kunkel, J., and Wiley, J.: Acute head injury, Nursing79 **9:** 22-23, March 1979.

Kurze, T., and Pitts, F.W.: Management of closed head injuries, Surg. Clin. North Am. **48:**1271-1278, 1968.

LaBaw, W.: Diary of a doctor's recovery from brain trauma, Resident Staff Physician **15:**61-67, Dec. 1969.

Landauer, A.A., Milner, G., and Patman, J.: Alcohol and amitriptyline effects on skills related to driving behavior, Science **163:**1467-1468, 1969.

Langford, T.L.: Nursing problem: bacteriuria and the indwelling catheter, Am. J. Nurs. **72:**113-115, Jan. 1972.

Lapides, J., et al.: Self-catheterization for urinary disease, Curr. Med. Dialog. **39**:826-831, 1972.

Larrabee, J.H.: Physical care during early recovery, Am. J. Nurs. **77**:1320-1329, Aug. 1977.

Lazure, L.: Defusing the dangers of autonomic dysreflexia, Nursing80 **10**:52-53, Sept. 1980.

Lindh, K., and Rickerson, G.: Spinal cord injury: you can make a difference, Nursing74 **4**:41, Feb. 1974.

McInerney, D.P., and Sage, M.R.: Computer-assisted tomography in the assessment of cervical spine trauma, Clin. Radiol. **30**:203-206, 1979.

Marshall, A.M.: The nurse and acute spinal injury, J. Neurosurg. Nurs. **7**:1-9, July 1975.

Martin, M.A.: Nursing care in cervical cord injury, Am. J. Nurs. **63**:60-66, March 1963.

May, C.M.: Wheelchair patient for a day, Am. J. Nurs. **73**: 650-651, 1973.

Merskey, H., and Woodforde, J.M.: Psychiatric sequelae of minor head injury, Brain **95**:521-528, 1972.

Meyd, C.: Acute brain trauma, Am. J. Nurs. **78**:40-44, Jan. 1978.

Morris, V., and Traber, W.: After the battle, Am. J. Nurs. **72**:97-99, Jan. 1972.

Nagler, B.: Psychiatric aspects of cord injury, Am. J. Psychiatry **107**:49-56, 1950.

Nayer, D.D.: They don't notice her wheelchair, Am. J. Nurs. **71**:1130-1133, 1971.

Nolan, J.: Who's afraid? Am. J. Nurs. **68**:1730-1731, 1968.

Norsworthy, E.: Nursing rehabilitation after severe head trauma, Am. J. Nurs. **74**:1246, July 1974.

Oldfield, R.C., and Williams, M.: Cerebral trauma in infancy and intellectual defect, J. Neurol. Neurosurg. Psychiatry **24**:32-36, Feb. 1961.

Olson, E.V.: The hazards of immobility, Am. J. Nurs. **67**:779-797, 1967.

Parkinson, J.: The spinal cord-injured patient autonomic hyperreflexia, J. Neurosurg. Nurs. **9**:1-4, March 1977.

Parsons, L.C.: Respiratory changes in head injury, Am. J. Nurs. **71**:2187-2191, 1971.

Pemberton, L.: Nursing on unconscious patient, Nurs. Mirror **149**:41-43, Sept. 13, 1979.

Pfaudler, M.: Care of patients with severe spinal cord injuries. In (Panel of authorities): Current practice in critical care, vol. 1, St. Louis, 1979, The C.V. Mosby Co.

Reeves, K.R.: Children's reactions to head injuries, Am. J. Nurs. **70**:108-111, Jan. 1970.

Rimel, R.W., et al.: Assessment of recovery following head trauma, Crit. Care Q. **2**:97-104, 1979.

Rimel, R.W., and Tyson, G.: The neurologic examination in patients with central nervous system trauma, J. Neurosurg. Nurs. **11**:148-155, Sept. 1979.

Roberson, F.C., et al.: The value of serial computerized tomography in the management of severe head injury, Surg. Neurol. **12**:161-167, Aug. 1979.

Romano, M.D.: Family response to traumatic head injury, Scand. J. Rehabil. Med. **6**:1, 1974.

Rusk, H.A. editor: Rehabilitation medicine, ed. 4, St. Louis, 1977, The C.V. Mosby Co.

Saxon, J.: Techniques for bowel and bladder training, Am. J. Nurs. **62**:69-71, Sept. 1962.

Schmorl, G., and Junghanns, H.: Human spine in health and disease, ed. 2 (E. Besemann, trans.), New York, 1971, Grune & Stratton, Inc.

Schutz, M.K.: Head trauma: what must be done when all else fails, RN **42**:52-54, May 1979.

Shea, J.D., et al.: Autonomic hyperreflexia in spinal cord injury, Southern Med. J. **66**:869-872, Aug. 1973.

Stauffu, E.S.: Diagnosis and prognosis of acute cervical spinal cord injury, Clin. Orthop. Rel. Res. **112**:9-16, Oct. 1975.

Steichen, F.M.: The emergency management of the severely injured, J. Trauma **12**:786-790, 1972.

Stevens, J.: Diagnosis of severe low-back pain, Hosp. Med. **6**:133-162, March 1970.

Sutton, N.G.: Injuries of the spinal cord: management of paraplegia and tetraplegia, London, 1973, Butterworth & Co. (Publishers), Ltd.

Suwanwela, C., Alexander, E., Jr., and Davis, C.H., Jr.: Prognosis in spinal cord injury with special reference to patients with motor paralysis and sensory preservation, J. Neurosurg. **19**:220-227, 1962.

Sverdlik, S.S., and Rusk, H.A.: Rehabilitation of the quadriplegic patient, J.A.M.A. **142**:321-324, 1950.

Swift, N.: Head injury: essentials of excellent care, Nursing74 **4**:27, Sept. 1974.

Tyson, G.W., et al.: Acute care of the head-injured patient. In Acute care of the head and spinal cord injured patient in the emergency department, Charlottesville, Va., 1978, Department of Neurosurgery, University of Virginia.

Tallalla, A., et al.: Subdural hematoma with long-term hemodialysis for chronic renal disease, J.A.M.A. **212**:1847-1849, 1970.

Torelli, M.: Topical hyperbaric oxygen for decubitus ulcers, Am. J. Nurs. **73**:494-496, 1973.

Trigiano, L.L.: Independence is possible in quadriplegia, Am. J. Nurs. **70**:2610-2613, 1970.

Tudor, L.L.: Bladder and bowel retraining, Am. J. Nurs. **70**: 2391-2393, 1970.

Verhonick, P., Lewis, D., and Goller, H.: Thermography in the study of decubitus ulcers, Nurs. Res. **21**:233-237, May-Feb. 1972.

Wahl, S.: Only a concussion, Nursing76 **6**:44-45, Aug. 1976.

Wiley, L., editor: Hazardous head injury, Nursing72 **2**:11, Feb, 1972.

Williams, A.: A study of factors contributing to skin breakdown, Nurs. Res. **21**:238-243, May-June 1972.

Wing, S.: Cervical spine injuries: treatment and related nursing care, J. Neurosurg. Nurs. **9**:138-140, Dec. 1979.

# 24

# CEREBROVASCULAR DISORDERS

Cerebrovascular disease encompasses topics such as hypertension, stroke, hemorrhage, transient ischemic attacks, pseudobulbar palsy, cerebral arteriosclerosis, subclavian steal syndrome, arteriovenous malformations, and peripheral vascular disease.

Hypertension is discussed first because the practitioner may intervene successfully in blood pressure control so that the incidence of stroke may be decreased.

## HYPERTENSION

Early disability, death, and illness are major problems in the almost 35 million Americans who currently have hypertension, and in the 25 million more who have borderline hypertension. Although hypertension increases the incidence of several serious problems, such as renal failure and congestive heart failure, it also puts the same 13% of the United States population in jeopardy of experiencing stroke.

Morbidity and mortality from disease processes related to hypertension can be effectively reduced as clients are diagnosed early and agree to comply with a program of long-range hypertension control.

Treatment requires a client. Unfortunately, the health education efforts impact personally on too few individuals. More vigorous efforts are needed to reach some 50% of the affected individuals who are informed of their problem. For those individuals who are informed of their hypertension, about half comply with the treatment regime adequately to control their high blood pressure. Borderline clients told to at least control high risk factors such as sodium intake may fail to recognize high sodi-

um foods without supervision. The high sodium content in some fast foods deceives a lot of people.

Although hypertension is most commonly seen in men over 35 years of age and in women over 45 years of age, it is also being detected in young populations up to and including the neonate. As more women enter the job market, statistics reveal increased problems in these women, who are subjected to increased stress from expanded roles. Although the problem is more serious in blacks than whites, it does not seem to leave any group of the population unaffected, regardless of age, education, geographic locale, or socioeconomic status.

### Understanding blood pressure

Blood pressure readings may vary. However, consistent elevations of blood pressure are abnormal. The normal blood pressure is maintained through an intricate physiological relationship among renal, endocrine, neurological, and cardiovascular processes. These body systems work to regulate heart rate, stroke volume, and total peripheral resistance. Five hemodynamic factors are expressed in any hypertensive reading; they are peripheral resistance, blood viscosity, elasticity of arterial walls, blood volume, and cardiac output.

The "normal" blood pressure has not been satisfactorily defined. However, many view an adult diastolic pressure of more than 90 as the point beyond which risks of increased morbidity are more prevalent.

### Determining elevations

Cause and severity are both considered when hypertension is defined. Many factors influence specific elevations in the diastolic and systolic blood pressure, including exercise, stress, age, and psychological events. One criterion for the determination of elevated blood pressure is related to age. In this instance a diastolic blood pressure greater than 90 mm Hg for individuals between the ages of 15 and 55 years of age and 100 mm Hg for those 55 years and older is considered to be an elevated blood pressure. However, the diagnosis of hypertension is not applied until a casual blood pressure taken without regard to particular preparation, time of day, or environment is elevated on three consecutive daily or weekly readings. Correct technique is essential so that the most accurate reading is possible. To review this technique, refer to an article entitled "Correcting Common Errors in Blood Pressure Measurement" (Agler and Malcolm, 1965). When serial determinations are needed for close comparison, the same cuff on the same arm is utilized. Additionally, basal blood pressure measurement, wherein the pressure is measured before activity as the client awakes from sleep, may be helpful.

### Physiological basis for elevations

The most common cause of elevated blood pressure is an increase in total peripheral resistance. This increase may be related to catecholamine secretion, pressoreceptor changes, or influences of the renin-angiotensin-aldosterone system.

*Catecholamine secretion.* Review the section on catecholamines in Chapter 4. The main chemical substances regulating sympathetic nervous system functions are norepinephrine and epinephrine. These substances have powerful vasoactive properties, which can increase blood pressure. Pheochromocytoma is one instance wherein abnormal amounts of mainly epinephrine are released.

*Pressoreceptor changes.* Pressoreceptors (or baroreceptors) situated in the carotid sinus function by maintaining normative blood pressure levels, unless they are "influenced" to maintain elevated blood pressure levels.

*Renin-angiotensin-aldosterone system.* As investigators continue to explore the precise mechanism for elevations of blood pressure, they are directing their research efforts toward the understanding of the renin-angiotensin-aldosterone (RAA) hormonal system, the complex wherein

blood pressure is controlled through adjustments in blood volume and vasoconstriction.

Renin, a proteolytic enzyme, releases angiotensin I from angiotensinogen, its liver substrate. Angiotensin I is quickly changed to angiotensin II, a potent pressor substance that can release the mineralocorticoid aldosterone, thereby augmenting sodium and water retention.

The RAA system is being extensively investigated. Current findings reveal important differences in clients with low, normal, and high renin activity. High-renin clients seem to experience an increased incidence in morbidity, mortality, and decreased intravascular volume, whereas low-renin clients tend to do the opposite. Research continues to assess the significance of renin activity.

### Vessel changes

Regardless of the cause, investigators have documented the fact that atherosclerotic changes in such organs as the heart, brain, kidneys, and retina are hastened by hypertension.

When vessels undergo excessive pressures, acceleration in the production of hyaline connective tissue and hyperplasia of the arterial media ensues. As pressures continue to mount, fibrinoid necrosis of the arterioles becomes evident. Since the arteries of the internal capsule of the brain are small and thin walled, microaneurysms may develop with these changes, so that the individual is at increased risk for thrombosis or cerebral hemorrhage.

### Hypertension categorized

According to contemporary terminology, hypertension is separated into four categories, including essential (primary), secondary, malignant, and labile. In *essential hypertension* the cause remains unknown, and the client may be asymptomatic in the early phases. *Secondary hypertension* is defined as elevated blood pressure related to a known organic disorder such as stricture of the renal artery or pheochromocytoma. In *malignant hypertension,* symptoms appear rapidly, and death often follows. *Labile hypertension* refers to the periodic increases in blood pressure than may eventually develop into essential hypertension. Within these categories, blood pressure elevations are further described as mild, moderately severe, or severe according to the following criteria:

Mild                     Diastolic blood pressure less than
                         120 mm Hg
Moderately severe        Diastolic blood pressure between
                         121 and 140 mm Hg
Severe                   Diastolic blood pressure over 140
                         mm Hg

These definitions are accepted by the American Medical Association.

Essential hypertension is by far the most prevalent type of hypertension, since it afflicts some 90% of the clients diagnosed with hypertension. In essential hypertension the diastolic blood pressure is the most accurate indicator of disease severity. Systolic elevations may develop secondary to diastolic elevations. The periodic increases in systolic blood pressure seen in labile hypertension may also result in essential hypertension.

Although the precise cause of essential hypertension is unknown, cardiac, hormonal, neurological, and renal mechanisms are all known to induce alterations in blood pressure readings.

Secondary causes of hypertension include diseases of the renal, endocrine, or neurological systems. Hypertension may also be substance related; that is, dependent on taking oral contraceptives or consuming excessive quantities of licorice.

Problems in maintaining normative pressures may occur at all ages. Thus it is important to establish base-line data at all ages from the newborn period until late maturity, especially for those with known disorders and for those at risk in the development of problems that affect blood pressure.

Practitioners interested in current information on treatment and points important in blood pressure control should write for the free 1980 Report of the Joint National Committee on Detection, Evaluation, and Treatment of High Blood Pressure (HBPIC, Box JNC 5. 120/80, National Institutes of Health, Bethesda, MD 20205).

## Nursing intervention

The assessment is usually an outpatient process geared toward these explicit objectives:
1. Identify hypertension and confirm its presence.
2. Evaluate the degree of hypertension and the integrity of target organs.
3. Assess coexisting disorders and risk factors that may affect therapeutic intervention and outcomes.
4. Specify individual client habits that are positive or negative in blood pressure control.
5. Identify motivating factors that will assist the client in compliance with a therapeutic program for blood pressure control.
6. Prevent complications.

The nurse is in an ideal position to detect individuals who are at increased risk for developing elevated blood pressures. In eliciting the blood pressure reading the nurse notes readings that are at the high end of the normal range for the age group, records periodic elevations of blood pressure, and evaluates individuals with tachycardia for their greater tendency to develop essential hypertension. In considering racial and sexual differences the practitioner is aware that blacks have essential hypertension more often and with greater severity than whites, that men are more likely to develop hypertension than women until after menopause, and that women with elevations in blood pressure while pregnant or taking birth control pills have a greater tendency to develop essential hypertension. Other factors that may predispose an individual to essential hypertension include a positive family history, obesity, or the existence of a concurrent medical condition such as diabetes mellitus.

In the United States, approximately 20% of the population over 50 years of age have hypertension. This may exist by itself or may be associated with conditions such as cerebral arteriosclerosis, hemorrhage, or thrombosis. The development of these complications can be prevented or at least arrested by suitable treatment. A more vigorous therapeutic regimen has been developed in the past decade with the administration of ataractic drugs, adrenergic inhibitors, vascular smooth muscle dilators, and diuretics.

Arterial hypertension generally occurs in individuals between 35 and 55 years of age. Heredity is considered a major factor in the development of essential hypertension. Although both the systolic and diastolic blood pressures tend to increase with age, the systolic pressure shows a greater increase. Generally for individuals less than 45 years of age the upper normal blood pressure is 135/90 mm Hg; for those more than 45 years of age, the upper normal blood pressure is considered to be 150/100 mm Hg.

If hypertension is discovered in a person less than 35 years old without a family history of hypertension, he or she should have an intensive evaluation to determine the cause. If there is a sudden onset of hypertension after the age of 50 years, investigative study should be directed toward determining the primary cause.

### Presence of hypertension

Serial blood pressure determinations, evaluations of retinal integrity, and a thorough general history and physical examination assist the physician in diagnosing the client as a hypertensive.

Various standardized blood pressure tests are utilized to determine the type of hypertension and the response to postural changes and sedation. Generally the blood pressure is taken three times: after the client has been resting in the supine position 10 to 15 minutes, then after sitting, and then after standing. Some physicians average the three readings; others use only the third reading. Unless severe hypertension is present or target-organ damage has occurred, the physician generally determines a client's blood pressure by obtaining blood pressure determinations on at least three separate visits. For borderline cases even more measurements may be needed before the diagnosis of hypertension is established. Some physicians further recommend that clients take their own pressure at home daily, and record the readings for two to three weeks. The excitement of seeing the physician is known to raise the pressure in some individuals. If hypertension is suspected in a hospitalized client, many physicians prefer to avoid treating the milder cases until ambulatory status is resumed and pressures change to approximate more typical conditions.

### Assessing hypertension

Some physicians recommend that the initial evaluation be geared toward the severity of the hypertensive condition. In general, younger clients require the most intensive workup since their hypertension tends to be more severe and less responsive to treatment. A thorough history and physical examination is vital. Although the automated chemistry profile may be ordered to reduce client costs, the minimum testing if ordered indi-

vidually should include a complete blood count with hematocrit to determine general health, serum creatinine or BUN, serum potassium, serum uric acid, blood glucose, serum cholesterol, and serum triglycerides in clients younger than 60 years. Additionally the client should have a urinalysis, wherein protein, blood, and glucose are assessed. When individually warranted, the urine examination should include microscopic analysis. A chest roentgenogram and an electrocardiogram are also advisable. Other tests such as plasma renin activity, urine aldosterone, renal function studies, and so on should be reserved for situations where they are required to identify a primary cause for hypertension.

### Integrity of target organs

Target organs prone to complications affecting prognostic and therapeutic outcomes for the hypertensive client include the brain, eyes, heart, and kidneys.

***Brain.*** The practitioner should elicit a thorough history, particularly in relation to any prior neurological conditions such as stroke or transient ischemic attacks. A careful physical assessment should reveal any neurological deficits, systolic or both systolic and diastolic bruits over the carotid artery, and retinal changes. When cerebrovascular disorders are apparent, further testing such as carotid or vertebral angiography and ophthalmodynamometry are indicated.

Arterial hypertension may result in cerebral disturbances.

The signs and symptoms of the cerebral disturbance caused by arterial hypertension occur most frequently in middle-aged individuals but may be seen in young adults. These include headache, vertigo, tinnitus, syncope, irritability, difficulty in concentration with errors in judgment, and fatigue. Some of these symptoms may be caused by the anxiety that hypertensive individuals frequently manifest rather than by a cerebral disorder. However, complaints of severe frontal headache on arising in the morning may be serious and demand prompt treatment. At times, there are acute episodes, associated with a rapid rise of blood pressure to a high level, that are characterized by intense headache, vomiting, drowsiness, and possibly unconsciousness. One side of the body may show weakness, and convulsions may occur. The reflexes are pathological, and papilledema, with narrowing of the retinal arteries and small hemorrhages, may be seen with the ophthalmoscope. The arterial pressure may rise to 250 mm Hg, and the cerebrospinal fluid pressure may also be elevated. These manifestations are transitory, and recovery usually takes place within a week. Recovery becomes less likely with subsequent attacks. The diagnosis of this condition is facilitated by a previous history of hypertension, but on occasion it may be difficult to distinguish between it and intracranial tumor. Continued observation over a period of 1 or 2 weeks will demonstrate progression if the disease is neoplastic.

*Eyes.* An expert assessment of the retinas is extremely important. The data gleaned are as follows:

1. The severity of spasms in retinal arterioles can be directly correlated with the diastolic blood pressure level.
2. The duration of hypertension is assessed by determination of the heightened light reflex and arteriovenous nicking collectively termed "sclerosis."
3. When retinal hemorrhages and exudate are present in the absence of papilledema, prompt medical attention is warranted.
4. If retinal hemorrhages, exudate, and papilledema are evident, the condition is termed "malignant hypertension," a medical emergency.

*Heart.* The history of the client who has had cardiac problems may include angina pectoris, myocardial infarction, or chronic congestive heart failure. Physical findings may include the addition of third or fourth heart sounds, cardiac enlargement, or sustained apex impulse. The electrocardiogram indicates appropriate findings. Radiographic chest films reveal any left ventricular enlargement.

*Kidneys.* Negative findings on urinalysis with microscope assay reveal normal renal status in most cases. Primary renal disease with resulting secondary hypertension is the case when proteinuria is found before the appearance of elevated blood pressure. Renal disease is secondary if hypertension is noted before the finding of an abnormal urinalysis. If renal disease is suspected, appropriate studies may include intravenous pyelo-gram, CAT scans, retrograde pyelography, and others.

## Coexisting disorders and risk factors

In the zeal to treat hypertension, the practitioner should not overlook concurrent illness or fail to place blood pressure control in its proper perspective in relation to the client's total health status.

Compliance with the hypertensive treatment regime effectively reduces complications of all disorders except coronary atherosclerosis. Other risk factors, in addition to hypertension, must be regulated to diminish the morbidity and mortality currently associated with coronary disease.

After hypertension has been diagnosed the goal of therapy is to avoid acceleration of the atherosclerotic process in an attempt to reduce the possibility of such disorders as stroke, heart attack, cardiac failure, and renal disease. Along with regulation on a pharmacological management program the client is encouraged to avoid or minimize conditions that augment atherosclerotic changes such as obesity, hypercholesterolemia, hypertriglyceridemia, consumption of excessive amounts of sodium, cigarette smoking, or regular involvement in activities that negate the opportunity for exercise or result in stressful life situations or patterns.

Diagnostic consideration should be given to possible causes of secondary hypertension when the history and physical indicate the existence of renal vascular hypertension, primary aldosteronism, Cushing's syndrome, coarctation of the aorta, and pheochromocytoma. Although these conditions are rare, when they are found medical treatment can resolve all these problems except pheochromocytoma. Surgical management provides at least temporary relief from primary aldosteronism and atherosclerotic renovascular disease. Finally, since the use of oral contraceptives accounts for the main type of reversible hypertension in women during the childbearing years, this fact should be elicited and evaluated during the history process.

## Nursing assessment

Refer to Chapters 5, 6, and 11 for information related to the assessment process. Suffice it to say that the nursing assessment compiles a unique combination of data not only on body systems, but also on activities of daily living and relevant psychosocioeconomic factors. These data are crucial to the development of treatment individually tailored to accomplish the objectives listed as 4 and 5 (p. 602), wherein positive and negative client habits and motivating factors that may assist the client in treatment compliance are identified.

## Complications

The most serious complications that may occur with untreated hypertension are congestive heart failure; myocardial infarction; cerebrovascular disease, especially stroke; and progressive renal failure.

## Treatment and nursing intervention

Treatment may utilize some or all of the following suggestions: physical rest, including 9 hours of sleep at night and a rest period of 1 to 1½ hours' duration during the middle of the day; daily exercise; frequent vacations; reduction of nervous stress and strain, with the development of a calm, realistic outlook on life; practice of relaxation techniques; psychotherapy; sedatives or medications to reduce symptoms of nervousness, irritability, and high blood pressure; renal extract; restrictive diet if obesity, kidney, or heart complications coexist; and the avoidance of any excess (such as alcohol, tobacco, coffee, strenuous physical activity, hot and cold baths, emotional stress, violent coughing, vomiting, abdominal straining, food, or sexual activity) that may be a precipitating factor in causing a cerebral hemorrhage. Some physicians advocate that pork and all pork products and other grossly salty foods be eliminated from the diet and that the salt intake be restricted to 3 to 5 gm a day. Some physicians prohibit smoking. If economically and personally possible, the client may be advised to move to a rural area, preferably in a tropical climate, and he or she should be given help in adjusting physically and psychologically to advancing years.

Drug therapy for hypertension is indicated for many clients. Although medication needs may be expressed in general terms, each client's need for amounts and types of medications and the response to pharmacological agents vary greatly. The antihypertensive drug chosen for the individual depends on the degree of hypertension, age, general health, adequacy of renal function, and reaction to and tolerance of the drug.

Many physicians prescribe thiazide diuretics as a solitary medication. If more medication is required, one goes to "step 2," which involves the selection and addition of a sympathetic blocking agent. After reasons for failure of treatment are exhausted, the client may honestly require additional medication. "Step 3" is the addition of a peripheral vasodilator, such as hydralazine.

Most clients are usually controlled at the "step 2" phase of treatment. Guanethidine, the "step 4" addition, is now restricted to those with severe hypertension, because the discovery of new agents has expanded treatment alternatives. Refer to Chapter 28 for a list of medications used to treat hypertension. Both the client and family should be familiar with the side effects and reportable symptoms that may occur.

In general, treatment is palliative and directed toward relief of subjective symptoms and prevention of complications. The client is instructed about the complications that may occur in hypertension and impressed that hypertension is a chronic disease that will worsen unless the medical regime is fully instituted. Each client will react differently and all discussions should be related to particular needs. Many clients are helped by participating in group therapy with other hypertensive persons. It may also be helpful for a family member to be trained in taking the blood pressure at home so that the client can identify the activities that increase blood pressure. Treatment is successful only to the extent and ability of the client to cooperate and to pursue a rigidly moderate and modified way of life.

The nursing care of the client with high blood pressure is directed toward enlisting the client's cooperation in following the routine prescribed by the physician, educating the client and family to appreciate and understand the need for certain modifications in life-styles, assisting the physician and client with the diagnostic tests and therapeutic procedures, and controlling the psychological and physical environment of the client to facilitate the amelioration of symptoms and to retard the progress of disease. These clients are usually ambulatory and require no special nursing care other than that just implied, which consists primarily of instructing, supervising, encouraging, guiding, and reassuring. The nurse can help the client plan a new way of life within the restrictions imposed by the disease.

## Nursing intervention to decrease noncompliance

Poor compliance with treatment, especially in the mild hypertensive client who is asymptomatic, is a great problem. Since most hypertensive clients are treated on an outpatient basis, a nurse specialist in cooperation with the physician can set up a program to (1) make appointment times convenient, (2) keep waiting room time short and productive because planned educational efforts with audiovisual aids make self-learning possible, (3) ensure personalized, frequent follow-up and communication with the client and family, (4) utilize principles of relaxation therapy and behavior modification to instruct the client in essential life-style changes, (5) organize group sessions for the acquisition of factual information and the sharing of feelings, (6) serially measure objective data such as weight, blood pressure, home charts of blood pressure, and the presence or absence of stressors as individually established, and (7) reinforce all aspects of learning regarding treatment compliance in relation to life-style, diet, excesses, personal habits, smoking, weight, medication, and blood pressure measurement. The nurse can also provide specific individual and group training in relaxation therapy.

Cost containment is possible when the physician and the nurse cooperate to streamline treatment to what is individually appropriate for each individual. Client follow-up when carefully planned can also be individualized so that the least number of drugs, at the lowest possible cost, with the fewest side effects, can be prescribed. All these efforts improve client compliance. When the client has been through a well-organized, comprehensive educational program, and a personalized care approach, the following outcomes are possible:

### Expected outcomes
The client will:

1 Describe all items prescribed in hypertensive control and how they can be utilized and accomplished effectively and efficiently.
2 Explain the importance of treatment compliance.
3 Identify all prescribed medications in terms of dosage, special instructions for use, storage, minor side effects that must be tolerated, expected benefits from medication, and adverse outcomes or intolerable side effects that need to be reported to the physician.
4 Explain the relationship and problems that may be encountered when alcohol and over-the-counter drugs are consumed simultaneously with prescriptive medication and the need to notify the physician before one ingests these substances
5 Demonstrate that an available significant other can and does take the blood pressure correctly and records it at specified intervals.
6 Identify blood pressure readings that are normal and abnormal for him- or herself and discuss the relationship of elevated blood pressure to pathophysiological outcomes.
7 Explain exact ways that the daily routine, monetary budget, and schedule have been modified to accommodate the required blood pressure treatment.
8 Discuss typical daily habits with which exercise, relaxation techniques, medication, and other prescriptive items have been consistently associated and accomplished, such as toothbrushing, mealtime, or a certain time of day.
9 Have a blood pressure within the normal range.
10 Show steady progress toward achieving the ideal weight.
11 Decrease tobacco use by at least 50%.
12 Take all prescribed medications unless otherwise indicated by the physician.
13 Keep all appointments with the physician and nurse.

## CEREBRAL ARTERIOSCLEROSIS

Cerebral arteriosclerosis may be a part of a generalized arteriosclerosis or may occur independently of vascular changes in the extracranial circulation. The clinical picture results from inadequate nourishment of the nerve cells and the development of cerebral atrophy. It can be confused with presenile and senile dementia, which may occur without arteriosclerosis. It is normally considered to be a concomitant of old age, but it may appear as early as 50 years of age.

The symptoms include headache, dizziness, irritability, and difficulty in sleeping, concentrating, and remembering. Frequently the condition may be mistaken for a psychoneurosis, but as the disease progresses, the diagnosis becomes clear. Memory for recent events is lost, and the client may become disoriented and have delusions and hallucinations. Mental faculties deteriorate to such an extent that the client does not recognize even family members, and he or she becomes very untidy about personal appearance. This person's behavior may be obnoxious to those around, especially if they believe the acts are deliberate or if they do not understand the nature of this illness.

### Treatment and nursing intervention

Treatment and nursing care are dictated by the physical, emotional, and mental manifestations of the disease. The prevention of complications is emphasized. The regimen of medical therapy outlined for the care of the hypertensive client is recommended with some modifications in the care of these clients, since they usually belong to a much older age group and have more notable and characteristic personality changes. To facilitate adjustment to the client, the nurse should clearly understand the reason for the behavior, mood swings, and uncooperativeness. This will also be a guide in helping the family to understand the physical and mental changes taking place in the client so that they can better adjust to them and plan more intelligently for subsequent care.

Clients with cerebral arteriosclerosis are chronically ill with various degrees of disability. Because they are often irritable, unreasonable, suspicious, forgetful, difficult to get along with, and unpleasant, the nurse and the client's family must develop great patience and tact in all their contacts. These clients may show signs of deterioration, becoming slovenly and untidy in their personal appearance and eating habits. In the hospital the nurse can cope with these traits by adequate supervision of hygiene and matter-of-factly screening the client at mealtime to avoid upsetting the other clients. If it is undesirable for the client to share the family mealtime because of the presence of young children at home, he or she should be given a tray and have needs attended to before the rest of the family eat. This must be done tactfully to avoid making the client feel rejected and unwanted.

These clients are encouraged to be as independent and as active as possible. Since they are frequently preoccupied with their bodily discomforts, a definite attempt is made to divert them and to keep them interested in other things. They are permitted to work and go out as they desire unless the disease has progressed to the point where they are no longer responsible. Aged persons should be permitted to follow their established way of life if possible. This disease may last 10 years or more; for most of this time the client will be cared for at home. The members of the family should so understand and adjust to the client's illness that they can continue living their own lives without being adversely affected by the restrictions imposed on them. It is particularly important that children in the family should not be deprived or neglected because of the vagaries, whims, and needs of such a client. An objective attitude will indirectly have a good influence on this person also. As the disease progresses, the client becomes more of a behavioral problem and may have to be institutionalized.

If there is an acute episode secondary to a cerebral thrombosis, bed rest is indicated. The time in bed depends on the severity of the attack and its objective signs and symptoms. Most practitioners believe, because of the age of these clients and their predisposition to complete invalidism, that the shorter the period in bed the better.

### TRANSIENT ISCHEMIC ATTACKS

In the United States, atherosclerosis is the most prevalent cause of ischemic cerebrovascular disease. The presence of a transient ischemic attack (TIA) is indicative of an impending stroke in about 25% to 35% of the affected clients. However, no definitive method has yet been devised to detect which individuals will go on to have a stroke when proper intervention is lacking. TIA differs from stroke in that ischemic focal cerebral processes last for less than 24 hours with no continuing neurological impairment. Many individuals experience transient episodes of slurred speech and paralysis on one side and fail to seek medical attention because symptoms disappear without intervention. However, intervention at this point may be one of the most important steps in stroke prevention for the individual prone to stroke (Fig. 24-1).

TIA results when a temporary decrease or interruption of the blood supply occurs because of a partial or complete obstruction within the carotid or vertebrobasilar system or possibly as the result of a radical fall in blood pressure. Common sources of obstruction are related to emboli from atheromatous extracranial arterial plaques that may originate in the cervical carotid artery, a prosthetic heart valve, or an abnormal heart valve during a period of auricular fibrillation. Although the role

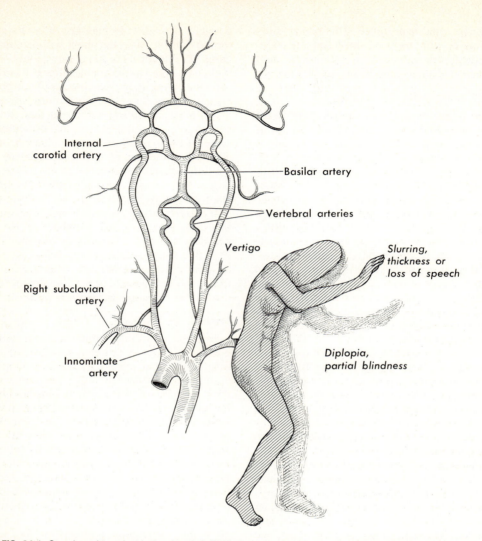

**FIG. 24-1.** Overview of transient ischemic attack (TIA) showing carotid and vertebrobasilar arteries as most common points of obstruction.

of hypotension in relation to the cause of TIA remains in dispute, sudden hypotension in a client with inadequate cerebral circulation resulting from generalized cerebrovascular disease is believed to be a factor in inducing ischemic attacks. In all these instances, microemboli disintegrate so that normal blood supply is reestablished within 24 hours without neurological deficit.

The diagnosis is established when no apparent cause is found for the following symptoms, which dissipate within 24 hours: (1) Double vision. (2) Unilateral blindness. (3) Staggering or uncoordinated gait. (4) Precipitous falls from weakness in the legs. (5) Numbness or weakness in one side of the body. (6) Speech impairments, that is, loss, thickness, or slurring.

Since symptoms may be gone before the individual is examined, the physical assessment may not be exceedingly helpful in confirming the diagnosis. However, the neurological examination may be valuable in localizing problems that could contribute to TIA. Sources of the emboli are sought. The atheromatous plaque may be in a major vessel if cholesterol or platelet fibrin emboli are visualized in retinal arterioles. Other common origins of TIA include embolus movement after auricular fibrillation, stenosis of the mitral valve or a prosthetic heart valve. Narrowing or the existence of an ulcerated plaque in the carotid artery is indicated by the presence of a pronounced bruit in the neck.

Further findings in the client who has experienced a TIA and who may be a candidate for stroke include elevations in fasting blood glucose levels; in blood pressure; and, in clients younger than 50 years of age, in serum cholesterol levels. An angiogram frequently reveals areas of stenosis or atheromatous plaques. The electrocardiogram may demonstrate an abnormal Q wave or ST segment. The neurological examination may be essentially normal between attacks except for the carotid bruits and the unequal superficial artery pulses in patients with atherosclerotic disease.

To differentiate TIA from other neurological problems such as stroke, space-occupying lesions, or multiple sclerosis, the practitioner reviews the history, physical assessment and additional data gleaned from the angiogram, brain or CAT scan, and lumbar puncture. Paroxysmal disorders should be ruled out as the causative problem. Additional diagnostic studies may be indicated by other symptoms that may be present in an individual. In general, most neurological abnormalities that mimic TIA are differentiated by their presence at a previous time, their longer onset, or their tendency to cause neurological problems that persist beyond 24 hours.

Two major courses of treatment are available for the client who has experienced TIA, including vascular surgery and anticoagulant therapy. *Vascular surgery* is designed to remove the genesis of the problem, thereby reducing the frequency of TIA and the danger of impending stroke. Endarterectomy is a procedure wherein plaques are removed from the arch of the aorta or the cervical carotid artery. Vein grafts or Dacron prostheses may be utilized to bypass constricted vessel segments. When the client does not have a problem remedied by or accessible to surgery, or when the client is a poor candidate for surgery because of concurrent physical problems, *anticoagulant therapy* in the form of heparin, warfarin (Coumadin), or aspirin, is utilized. Problems that preclude the use of anticoagulants include lack of client consent and adherence to therapy, lack of essential laboratory facilities, ulcers in the gastric mucosa or urinary bladder, and hypertension. In addition, treatment is given to clients with such underlying pathological processes as obesity, arrhythmias, hypertension, polycythemia, leukemia, thrombocytosis, and migraine attacks. Research continues into the complete role of aspirin in reducing TIA.

The most significant role of the nurse in relation to TIA is one of early identification and referral of individuals who report such transient symptoms. Beyond this primary role in prevention the nurse continues to support and educate the client and family through the process of diagnostic studies and surgery. When started on anticoagulant therapy, the client needs to be educated as to the effect of other medications in prolonging bleeding time (aspirin), the need for periodic checks on clotting time, the need for regular administration of medication, the problems that may result from interferences with clotting in injury, and the greater tendency to bruise. A Medic Alert tag and billfold identification are important for these clients because medical practitioners require these data to treat traumatic injuries during emergencies. Activities of daily living should be reviewed to point out possible situations that may augment the chance of injury.

## STROKE

"Stroke" is a term used to describe a cataclysmic, pathological vascular event that involves brain tissue and results in permanent neurological deficits. Stroke does not give a definitive picture of the underlying problem, but it does describe accurately the sudden dramatic impact of the event. The phrase "cerebrovascular accident" often used interchangeably to describe the event is inaccurate because stroke is not an accident. Rather, stroke has pathological antecedents, within or outside the cerebral circulation, that often give warning symptoms in transient ischemic attacks or small strokes. A transient ischemic attack can last for several minutes to several hours, but the individual has no lasting neurological deficits. Signs may be of visual changes; sensory, speech, and behavioral changes; and paresis to paralysis.

## Pathophysiology

A review of earlier chapters of anatomy and physiology of the brain will provide some understanding of the great variation in strokes because of the specific functions of each area of the brain. Stroke can be a quick devastating event because of the brain's circulatory and metabolic needs for survival. The brain uses some 15% of the cardiac output and consumes 20% of the oxygen supply available to the entire body. Brain metabolism does not occur without oxygen and depends totally on glucose to supply its operational needs. When an interruption to the cranial blood supply persists for 4 to 8 minutes, permanent brain damage occurs. Permanent brain damage occurs quickly because the neurons of the central nervous system cannot regenerate. However, when the blood supply is interrupted gradually, collateral circulation can develop to meet the needs of the brain tissue. The neurological deficits that persist after a stroke are thus directly related to the extent of central nervous system neuronal death. Functional return for a stroke client is in turn related to the resumption of circulation to allow viable neurons to resume function.

## Extent of problem

The true status of stroke as a national and worldwide health problem is difficult to ascertain because stroke is not a reportable disease as are infectious diseases. Stroke can be used as a catchall when multiple disorders are present. Stroke is listed as the third cause of death in the United States. It is also the second cause of chronic illness and disability, with approximately 1,820,000 people being disabled to some extent by the residual effects (*Heart Facts,* 1980). Figures from a 1980 study give the incidence of stroke as 196 per 100,000 of population. Other studies give figures between 177 to 200 per 100,000. Under 35 the incidence is approximately 4.1 per 100,000, but from age 35 upward the incidence increases rapid-

ly to 2737 at 85 and beyond. The greatest increase in incidence occurs between 75 and 85 (*National Survey of Stroke,* 1980). Stroke can be considered primarily a problem of the aged with men having a higher incidence than women at all ages. However, one out of seven strokes do occur under 65 years of age.

## Types

The pathological causes of stroke relate to three processes: hemorrhage, thrombosis, and emboli. Hemorrhage may be subarachnoid (5.9%) or intraparenchymal because of aneurysms or arteriovenous malformations (6.3%). Embolic infarctions (5.4%) occur from valvular cardiac disorders, tumors, or released plaques of the cerebral vessels. The greatest percentage of strokes, however, occur from thrombotic infarctions (82.4%) of the basis of atherosclerosis (*National Survey of Stroke,* 1980). The thrombic areas for infarction are related to mechanical narrowing and obstruction of intracranial and extracranial vessels. Such obstructions usually occur at bifurcations of arteries where circulation is slowed and turbulence occurs, such as the bifurcation of the common carotid artery.

## Risk factors

Certain risk factors obtain to all cardiovascular diseases, but the chief risk factor in stroke is hypertension. Studies show that 34,290,000 have high blood pressure and black Americans are almost 50% more likely to have hypertension than whites (*Heart Facts,* 1980). The risk factors of high serum cholesterol, diabetes, hypertension, and cardiac disease show some familial tendencies. The risk factors of obesity, cigarette smoking, and stress are essentially controlled by the individual. The use of oral contraceptives, particularly with an estrogen content over 0.05 mg in women 40 years of age and less has increased the incidence of cerebroarterial thrombosis three to nine times in this age group (Bickerstaff, 1975). Multiple combinations of risk factors put the individual at greater risk; two factors, three times the risk; and three factors, five times the risk (*Heart Facts,* 1980). Essentially the best treatment for stroke is prevention through early detection and treatment of risk factors. The media have contributed greatly in placing the facts before the public, but education remains the domain and responsibility of health care providers.

## Morbidity and mortality

The mortality trend for stroke has shown a decline since 1914, but a much greater rate of decline in 1969 and 1972, as did all the cardiovascular diseases. Death rates from cardiovascular diseases are influenced by cycles of epidemic respiratory infections. A compromised respiratory tree will place added stress on the cardiovascular system, which may result in congestive heart failure or related cardiovascular problems, such as stroke. After the severe epidemic of 1968 the mortality for pneumonia and influenza fell considerably. Stroke rates declined proportionately. Overall mortality in 1975 was 156.8 per 100,000, down from 259.5 per 100,000 in 1960. The decline in mortality for black Americans exceeded the decline for whites overall (Soltero et al., 1978). The many reasons for decline are not clear. It can only be assumed that control of infections and control of risk factors, hypertension in particular, play a significant part. The part microsurgical procedures plays in eliminating problems of aneurysms and cerebral artery bypass grafts that better vascularize the brain has yet to be determined because the procedures are relatively new (McDowell, 1977).

Different geographic areas of the United States and other parts of the world show variations in incidence. For example, in 1975 the highest mortality in the United States appeared in Savannah, Georgia, and the lowest in both Hagerstown, Maryland, and Pueblo, Colorado (Stolley et al., 1977). These variations relate to the ethnic groups as well as to population life-styles. With standard methods of data collection that are being adopted worldwide a better picture of stroke should soon be available.

## Nursing intervention

Each stroke is unique because of the underlying causes and the multiple sites where the brain may be damaged. Consequently, nursing care must be based both on the underlying pathological process and on a detailed assessment of resulting deficits and maintained abilities of the client. Nursing goals must contain the elements of prevention, support, and restoration to provide comprehensive care these clients and families deserve.

## Assessment

A thorough history and physical assessment of the stroke client is a vital adjunct to the data gathered in special diagnostic techniques. When complete, the compilation of this data provides a definitive picture of the client's problem and an adequate basis for a comprehensive plan of care. Chapters 11 and 12 give general parameters of neurological assessment and information as to the availability of diagnostic tests.

In relation to strokes the practitioner needs to gather additional specific data beyond the basic information gleaned from the general neurological assessment. A stroke profile is shown here for your consideration.

### PROFILE FOR STROKE*

High blood pressure
History of brief, transient stroke episodes
Atherosclerosis, especially in the heart, neck, and legs
Diabetes
Elevated blood cholesterol and fat levels
Gout and high red blood cell level possibly significant
Heavy smoking believed to be significant

*According to the American Heart Association Council on Stroke.

Particular attention is directed to the following questions during the client interview because they assist in identifying the genesis of the problem:
- Preexisting disease
- Associated laboratory findings
- Precipitating factors
- Mode of onset
- Residual impairments
- Alterations in cognitive or behavioral capacities, including memory

In general, when neurological capacities return to normal after the event, the episode is termed a transient ischemic attack. When the client reports a headache as part of the event, the problem is usually related to hemorrhage rather than ischemia. If the onset is rapid and sudden, the event is usually caused by embolism or hemorrhage. When the progression of symptoms has a more gradual or intermittent pattern, it is more often the result of ischemia. Events associated with hemorrhage or emboli are most frequently described in connection with waking activity, whereas those related to infarctions or ischemia frequently have their onset during sleep or rest. Alterations in cognitive and behavioral processes are most often related to multiple microembolic events or generalized ischemia.

Significant others who have close contact with the client may provide valuable data about the client in general and in relation to events seen during or after an episode. Their observations frequently clarify changes in the client, which the affected individual may be unable to relate because of lack of awareness, aphasia, or denial.

The past history also contains valuable information that may give the practitioner insights into the cause of the abnormal event. Generalized arteriosclerotic disease may be suspected when the past history is earmarked by hypertension, diabetes mellitus, or ischemic heart disease. Focal neurological disorders and localized headaches point to the possibility of an aneurysm or an arteriovenous malformation. Embolic processes are suggested when the past history includes valvular heart disease, cardiac arrhythmias, or sclerosing subacute bacterial endocarditis (SSBE).

After gleaning data from the history the practitioner continues the assessment through physical examination. A thorough examination is indicated. Points of emphasis listed herein relate specifically to findings that earmark entities related to cerebrovascular disease or stroke.

As a part of the neurological assessment, the practitioner evaluates extracranial arteries by palpation and auscultation. In assessment of the extracranial arteries the following findings are significant. A thrill in any extracranial artery reveals the presence of a pathological lesion at that point. Occlusion of the ipsilateral carotid artery may be detected as the practitioner notes a lack of pulsations when the finger is positioned over the internal artery or the tonsillar fossa. Ipsilateral disease in the external (common carotid) artery is suspected when palpation reveals decreased pulsation in one occipital or superficial temporal artery. The subclavian steal syndrome is often indicated when there are irregularities in pulse arrival to the radial arteries.

Auscultation of the orbit and major arterial courses—carotid, vertebral and subclavian—is especially helpful in detecting bruits. The points of bifurcation deserve special attention in auscultation. Although bruits may be present in normal individuals and absent in some with extreme interferences in extracranial circulation, the identification of a bruit is a frequent finding at the point where blood flow becomes turbulent to bypass an atherosclerotic plaque.

Thermographic examination is often done to assess the circulatory integrity of the carotid system. Since the skin of the medial forehead is supplied by the ophthalmic artery, uneven temperatures may signal the possibility of occlusive processes on the side with reduced temperature.

Doppler ultrasonography is a technique utilized to indicate the direction and velocity of blood flow and the amplitude of the arterial pulse in the orbit and at the point of carotid bifurcation. A reversal of blood flow occurs when the internal carotid artery becomes occluded.

Abnormalities in blood pressure are indicative of more problems than hypertension in relation to cerebrovascular disease. Comparison of pressures in both arms is an important means of determining subclavian steal syndrome. Circulatory insufficiency may also be elicited and monitored as blood pressure measurements are performed during the Valsalva maneuver.

When qualified personnel, monitoring equipment, and resuscitative support are available, hypersensitivity to carotid sinus reflexes may be assessed through carotid artery massage and compression. Dangers inherent in this assessment technique include resulting extreme cerebrovascular insufficiency and potential problems related to dislodging an embolus from an atherosclerotic plaque.

Ophthalmoscopic examination is also an integral part of neurovascular assessment. Indications of increased intracranial pressure, as well as hypertension and atherosclerotic changes in the retinal arteries, are apparent as the retinas are visualized. Ophthalmodynamometry may also be a valuable diagnostic aid, since pressures in the ophthalmic artery, the first major branch off the internal carotid artery, indicate the general status of carotid artery system pressures. When discrepancies in pressure exist, the side with lower pressure may be obstructed by an occlusive lesion.

The diagnostic study in suspected cerebrovascular disease continues with an electrocardiogram, an electroencephalogram, radiographic examination of the skull and chest, a lumbar puncture, an angiogram, and varied blood studies. Radioisotopic brain scanning and computerized axial tomography may also be used to rule out a space-occupying lesion.

The cerebrospinal fluid is usually bloody after a cerebral hemorrhage; it remains normal in appearance after a cerebral thrombosis or embolus. The skull radiograph may reveal a pineal shift as the result of cerebral edema (cerebral thrombosis) or intracerebral hemorrhage. The angiogram may differentiate further between cerebrovascular diseases by revealing specific abnormalities: narrow or obstructed vessels (such as found in thrombosis and embolism) or an avascular area with displacement and stretching of surrounding arteries and veins (pathognomonic of hemorrhage). The electroencephalogram also may help localize the area of involvement.

Extradural and subdural hematomas may produce similar signs and symptoms and should be ruled out as diagnostic possibilities. A history of head injury is generally sufficient to establish a differential diagnosis.

## Hemorrhagic stroke

Hemorrhagic stroke resulting from hypertension, ruptured aneurysms, ruptured arteriovenous malformations, trauma, and hemorrhagic diseases has a high mortality, 50% to 75% (Taylor and Ballenger, 1980), especially with early development of coma. If there has been only a small amount of bleeding and the client survives, recovery can be complete. This type of stroke is likely to occur during active hours, suddenly, with or without headache with accompanying hypertension. It presents certain signs depending on the location. If in the basal ganglia, early hemiparesis progresses to hemiplegia and hemianesthesia, and stupor and coma quickly occur, depending on the extent of the bleeding. If in the cerebellum, symptoms include vomiting, vertigo, ataxia, occipital headache, eye deviation, possible paralysis, ipsilateral facial weakness, stupor, and coma later. If in the

pons there is early coma, quadriplegia, external and internal ophthalmoplegia, and decerebrate rigidity. Medical management is conservative and supportive of vital systems (see Chapter 9 for care of the comatose client) and may include reduction of increased intracranial pressure, seizure control, blood pressure stabilization, and continuity of adequate ventilation.

*Nursing intervention.* Nursing intervention for an intercerebral hemorrhagic stroke entails close monitoring for extension of the process and for prevention of complications related to bed rest. These are the complications of respiratory infection, urinary tract infection, pressure sores, thrombophlebitis, and contractures. (See Chapter 25 for specific preventive practices for positioning, pressure sores, and range-of-motion exercises.) Full-length support hose are routine for prevention of phlebitis. When the client has stabilized and the condition causing the hemorrhage is under control, the client is allowed to resume activities gradually. The danger of bleeding in the same area is unlikely. The special problems of swallowing and handling of secretions require careful supervision. A fluoroscopic examination of swallowing may be necessary to determine aspiration with swallowing when the pons and cerebellum are involved. Nasogastric feeding or surgical gastrostomy may be necessary for feeding until sufficient cough and swallowing reflexes return. The best foods to use with swallowing problems are semisolids, the consistency of mashed potatoes, because they stimulate the swallowing reflex better than fluids do. Nasogastric, gastrostomy, and oral feedings may be combined for a period of time until the client can swallow sufficient food without danger of aspiration.

## Hemorrhage from cerebral aneurysm

Hemorrhage from a cerebral aneurysm occurs in the subarachnoid space, whereas hemorrhage from an arteriovenous malformation can be both subarachnoid and intercerebral. Cerebral aneurysm problems occur most frequently in middle age as do weakened vessel aneurysms of other sites in the normal process of aging (Fig. 24-2). Arteriovenous malformation hemorrhage can occur at any age, but it usually occurs in the young adult. Aneurysms are usually asymptomatic until the time of

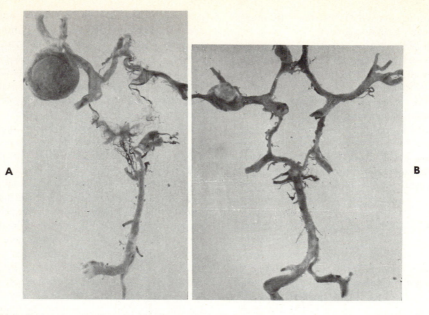

**FIG. 24-2.** Postmortem specimens of basilar cerebral arteries. **A,** Large aneurysm of middle cerebral artery. **B,** Two aneurysms (middle and anterior cerebral arteries).

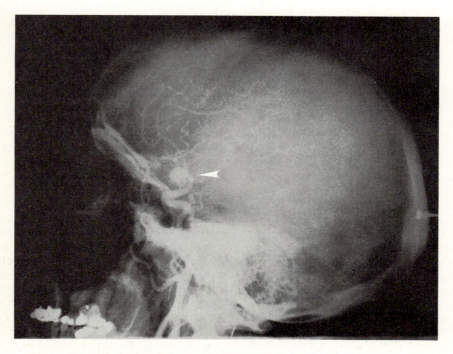

**FIG. 24-3.** Cerebral angiogram showing aneurysm. *Arrow,* Lateral view.

rupture when a severe headache occurs (Fig. 24-3). The rupture is often related to very great physical activity. The person may be hypertensive at the time of the insult but is not necessarily hypertensive. He may become unconscious or have transient periods of consciousness and unresponsiveness. Signs of meningeal irritation are evident when there is bleeding into the subarachnoid space. Those in whom unresponsiveness and coma persist have a poor prognosis. Mental confusion, drowsiness, speech disturbances, numbness, paresis, and paralysis may occur. Seizures may be present also, especially in arteriovenous malformations (Jones et al., 1978). Neurological deficits tend to clear as does mental cloudiness, but aneurysms have a tendency to bleed within 6 to 8 weeks. Bleeding after 2 weeks is usually fatal (Sahs, 1975).

*Treatment and nursing intervention.* Early awareness of renewed bleeding is an important goal in management during the acute phase of care. Serial assessments at regular, frequent intervals and additional evaluations as indicated by client status are imperative in detecting early clinical signs of bleeding. As explained in Chapter 9 alterations in the level of consciousness are frequently the first indications of increasing intracranial pressure.

Widespread use of aminocaproic acid (Amicar) in the contemporary management of subarachnoid hemorrhage reduces the incidence of recurrent bleeding by inhibition of clot lysis throughout the body. Fibrinolytic activity is eliminated in the cerebrospinal fluid as aminocaproic acid crosses the blood-brain barrier. It is interesting to note that recanalization of thrombi in blood vessels occurs in about 10 to 14 days, the period when the greatest number of clients experience a return of bleeding. Fibrinolytic resolution of the thrombus in the aneurysm is believed to be a possible cause of recurrent bleeding. Nausea and diarrhea are two common symptoms associated with the administration of aminocaproic acid and are managed symptomatically when they occur. When individuals have a history of renal insufficiency, pulmonary embolism, or ischemic heart disease, aminocaproic acid is contraindicated.

TREATMENT. Medical treatment of aneurysms and arteriovenous malformations initially is conservative, with treatment of symptoms and maintenance of vital functions. At a later time when the client's condition is stable, surgical intervention to prevent recurrence of bleeding is desired. These procedures may consist of a metal clip to occlude the aneurysm, wrapping it with material to prevent another break, ligating it proximally and distally, embolizing it, or gradually occluding the common carotid with a Selverstone clamp when the aneurysm is inaccessible surgically. Arteriovenous malformations are best treated by excision when not in a motor area, but ligation, radiation, or embolization may be used.

Embolization is a procedure done in the operating room with the client under general anesthesia. The client is prepared and draped as for a carotid endarterectomy with a radiographic cassette in lateral projection under the client's head and shoulders. The common carotid artery and its bifurcation are exposed. A Silastic catheter is passed into the artery and sutured to the arterial wall.

The emboli are then placed in the end of the catheter. These emboli are Silastic spheres impregnated with barium sulfate. They are then flushed into the artery, and the catheter is clamped. Radiographic films are taken to check the placement of the emboli. It is desirable to place them proximally to the feeding arteries at the origin of the arteriovenous malformation. As soon as this is accomplished, the catheter is withdrawn and the artery closed.

It may be several days or weeks before surgery can be done, if at all, so that symptomatic medical treatment and preventive nursing measures are crucial to the outcome of the client.

ENVIRONMENTAL CONTROL. Hemorrhage is controlled initially by complete bed rest with the head of the bed elevated 15 to 20 degrees. Any discomfort the client with hemorrhage experiences must be controlled so that he or she will remain quiet and not initiate further bleeding. Careful assessment for headache and agitation is imperative to give adequate amounts of analgesia. Phenobarbital and meperidine hydrochloride (Demerol) are the usual drugs if the client is alert. Phenytoin (Dilantin) or codeine are given when the client is confused. These drugs must be evaluated as to their effects on seizures, blood pressure, and level of consciousness, all in relation to further bleeding. External stimuli are kept to a minimum by limitation of visitors, no radio or television, and assurrance of quiet with a closed door. Photophobia may be present; so lighting is limited. Accordingly, the client's level of consciousness is evaluated carefully, with consideration for all the measures that reduce responses to stimuli to be sure that no other disorder is occurring. The client may require orientation at regular intervals when he or she wakes up. The client may also need light restraints when confused.

ELIMINATION. Bowel and bladder status are evaluated for continence, cerebral control, and changes in elimination. An indwelling catheter may be necessary when the client is incontinent and there is great danger of skin breakdown or if there is an obstruction in the urethra. External collecting devices, however, are preferred because of the almost certain danger of urinary tract infection from an indwelling catheter. Stool softeners, bulk agents, and cathartics should be employed early to prevent Valsalva maneuvers with straining at stool. This maneuver could precipitate further bleeding. Enemas or other rectal stimuli such as a thermometer are contraindicated. These stimuli, such as bowel straining, could provoke a Valsalva maneuver.

LONG-RANGE PLANS. Because of prolonged bed rest and the guarded prognosis of bleeding, there is much anxiety for the family and client, increasingly so as the client becomes more alert. The client and family must be apprised of tests, procedures, and any changes to alleviate their fears. Concerns should be explored and encouragement given to clients and their families to ventilate feelings. The early explanations around treatment must be continued so that all new activities for the client and family can be approached with confidence and understanding. They may need considerable help in planning the future because the client's life-style may undergo great change as a result of the residual impairments from the stroke.

## Embolic stroke

Embolic stroke is sudden in onset because of the short time it takes for the embolus to travel from the heart to a cerebral vessel and is not related to activity. There may be a fleeting warning of headache before consciousness is lost. It occurs in people with known heart disease, and with arterial fibrillation, the risk of stroke rises to 50%.

The embolus may cause neurological deficits initially, and then as it travels or disintegrates into smaller segments and reaches smaller vessels, symptoms disappear. The middle cerebral artery, the vertebrobasilar system, and the inferior cerebellar arteries are the usual sites for emboli to lodge. The person's future with this type of stroke will depend on the source of the emboli, the potential for further emboli release, and his cardiac capacity to take on an extra work load with paresis or paralysis.

## Thrombotic stroke

Thrombotic stroke usually occurs at rest and may develop over a period of hours. The person often has had one or more transient ischemic attacks. Ideally the person who sustains a transient ischemic attack will seek medical evaluation immediately. That individual may be a candidate for surgery for removal of plaques, endarterectomy, or a cerebral bypass graft. Surgery has proved effective in warding off major strokes. Thrombotic stroke can occur at any age, but it usually occurs in middle age or older. However, the use of estrogen birth control pills has greatly increased the incidence of thrombotic stroke in young women. The person who sustains a thrombotic stroke often can lay claim to one or more risk factors—hypertension, diabetes mellitus, smoking, and hyperlipemia. The basic cause of thrombotic stroke is atherosclerosis, which may or may not be present also as coronary artery disease or peripheral vascular disease. Trauma and infections, most commonly facial, sinus, and middle ear, may precipitate the stroke.

*Symptoms.* Thrombotic stroke attacks the major vascular systems serving the brain, the carotid system, and the vertebrobasilar system. The carotid system occlusion is recognized by monoparesis to contralateral hemiplegia, sensory deficits, visual deficits in monocular blindness or homonymous hemianopia, speech and language problems, opposite-side neglect, confusion, and bruits over the involved artery and at times the opposite artery. The vertebrobasilar system occlusion manifests in any limb-weakness combination, unilateral or bilateral hemianopia, paralysis of eye muscles with rotational and pupil abnormalities, nystagmus, diplopia, numbness in varying degrees, dysarthria, dysphagia, ataxia, and cranial nerve palsies (Marshall, 1972).

On regaining consciousness from a stroke, the client has a characteristic picture of hemiplegia with or without speech disturbance, depending on the side of the brain affected, and the affected side becomes spastic, with exaggerated tendon jerks, clonus, and an extensor plantar response. Convulsions are frequently associated with cerebral hemorrhage, rarely with cerebral thrombosis or embolism. Nuchal rigidity is generally present after a hemorrhage but is absent after a thrombosis or embolism. The client may be incontinent of urine and may develop fecal impactions. If he or she is unable to communicate because of aphasia, the client will be easily frustrated and may be depressed and afraid of dying. Even though sensorimotor speech areas are not affected, the individual may manifest impaired intellectual function, poor judgment, memory lapses, poor concentration with short attention span, and little initiative. The client may be overly dependent, demanding and irritable, or apathetic and withdrawn. Because of age, he or she may be upset by hospital practices and may have difficulty in adjusting to the new routines. As the client improves, he or she may become preoccupied with somatic complaints and be privately concerned about the impact of disease on sexuality, family-social relationships, body image, and life-style (Chapter 6).

*Treatment and nursing interventions.* Initial treatment for completed thrombotic strokes is conservative in maintaining vital systems and preventing secondary complications, particularly with coma. Deep coma in basilar infarctions usually means death in a few days. Preventive nursing care during the unstable period is first-stage rehabilitation as is the nursing for other types of stroke. Clients with thrombotic stroke can be involved in a rehabilitation program as their vital systems become stable. These people can be mobilized early, whereas people with hemorrhage and emboli are kept quiet and uninvolved. Careful assessment of abilities and deficits is to be made early by nursing as well as other disciplines. Nursing capitalizes on the client's abilities regardless of how few, so that he or she can experience success from efforts and not be overcome by losses. Activities must be tempered also by other concurrent diseases or normal aging, such as chronic obstructive pulmonary disease, coronary artery disease, angina, and arthritis.

## Outcomes in stroke

Each type of stroke has its own rate of survival and potential for independent functions. The survival rate overall for strokes is approximately 75% after 3 weeks. Chances for survival increase with each day according to studies, one of which gives the following figures: 90% for 24 hours, 84% for 72 hours, 81% for 7 days, 76% for 2 weeks, and 74% after 3 weeks (Herman et al., 1980). In long-term survival, there is a 35% to 45% mortality up to 5 years, but after 5 years, stroke effect on mortality is lost (Hutchinson, 1975). Survival rates for hemorrhagic stroke are between 25% and 50%, but chances for independent function after the early months of bed rest are very high. Functional capacity for persons sustaining embolic strokes will depend on the underlying cause, cardiac in nature usually, and consequently the capacity may be limited. The thrombotic stroke presents the greatest challenge both in numbers and potential for rehabilitation. Although the nature of brain damage in stroke indicates there should be a leveling off of improvement after 6 months, many people continue to show gains for several years. To date, studies have not given a clear picture of the pathological process occurring with brain tissue during the circulatory interruption at the time of stroke, but there appears to be some evidence of greater neuron recuperation (Ginsberg and Reivich, 1975). This may account in part for improved function for an extended period of time. Physical conditioning and long-term support of families and professionals can also account for some of the steady improvement. Each stroke client should have, as his right in long-term follow-up, regular assessments of his abilities with therapies added to improve his capabilities.

*Right-sided brain strokes.* Although each stroke is a unique entity, there are certain problems related to sites of brain damage that require consideration and management. Right-sided brain strokes have a special set of problems as do left-sided brain and brainstem strokes. Right-sided brain damage will have spatial and balance problems often along with field cuts as homonymous hemianopia. Consequently these people do not recognize potentially dangerous situations and overestimate their capacities. Sensory losses and agnosia compound their problems. They learn best by verbal instructions and require strict supervision. (See Chapter 25 for techniques of ambulation and instruction in self-care.) In addition, the original flaccid paralysis usually becomes spastic paralysis, along with flexion contractures to further compound problems. Flexion contractures result quickly if range-of-motion exercises are not continued. Nursing and all disciplines need to emphasize the importance of keeping joints mobile. This can be a problem when the individual with stroke considers function as his or her only goal.

*Left-sided brain strokes.* Those with left-sided brain strokes primarily have speech and language problems that lead families and friends to believe they are demented. Communication problems are the greatest blocks to acceptance. (See Chapter 25 for speech and language.) Self-care and mobility skills, however, are readily learned because of the intact right side of the brain.

*Additional problems.* Vertebrobasilar strokes with cerebellar, pons, and cranial nerve involvement can present even greater frustration for the person with this type of stroke. Balance, monoparesis to quadriplegia, depressed gag and swallowing reflexes, and dysarthria can cause the person to give up if he or she does not have reassurance in explanations and encouragement to persevere.

## Pseudobulbar palsy

Pseudobulbar palsy is caused by bilateral thromboses or hemorrhages in the internal capsule. It occurs in the late decades of life (55 to 80 years of age) and is usually preceded by one or more minor strokes. Characteristic manifestations of pseudobulbar palsy include the following: excessive crying and laughing without adequate provocation and with little affect, exaggeration of facial expressions, inability to swallow without choking, increasing difficulty in chewing and talking, abnormal salivation and drooling, impairment of intellectual functions (failure of memory, diminished interest in life, and irritability), and increasing difficulty in walking. These disabilities are the result of degeneration of the pyramidal tracts about the bulb (medulla oblongata) rather than degeneration of the nuclei of the bulb, hence the name "pseudobulbar palsy."

Examination also discloses hypertension with associated vascular changes in the fundi and peripheral arteries.

*Treatment and nursing intervention.* Treatment and nursing care are supportive and symptomatic. The prevention of complications is of vital importance and the basis of medical and nursing care. Because of general inanition the client is very susceptible to intercurrent infection. Maintenance of adequate nutrition poses a serious problem because of the great difficulty in chewing and swallowing. Food must be strained or blended in an electric blender and all oral intake carefully supervised. *Aspiration pneumonia* occurs frequently, and the nurse has a tremendous responsibility in preventing this. Suction equipment should be kept at the bedside and used as indicated. Meticulous mouth care is also important.

If the client has weakness of the extremities, he or she should be postured correctly at all times and turned at frequent intervals. Allowances must be made for emotional and intellectual impairment, and the staff must exercise considerable tact and patience as well as vigilance in their care.

The principles of nursing care are to alleviate the emotional and physical distress and to sustain him or her and the family during any crisis that may be precipitated by this illness.

## Rebuilding life

Stroke leaves its mark on people. The self-image is attacked. Frustration and depression may remove the veneer of manners to reveal the person's worst personality traits in some people and the best traits in others. Personality changes are based on organic brain disease, which may be concurrent, but not the stroke. Trying to rebuild a life is not easy because this group, like any other group with obvious physical disability, is shunned. It is difficult to get back into the community. For this reason special groups, stroke clubs, for stroke clients and their families have been organized to aid in socialization and sharing of experiences that make life more tolerable. The American Heart Association has supported and given direction for development of these resocialization groups. Information is available from the American Heart Association.

"Resocializing Through a Stroke Club" (O'Connor, 1976) is an interesting article that describes the positive aspects of group encounters.

All families do not react in the same way to the crisis situation that is created when one of its members has a stroke. Some are immobilized and unable to accept any responsibility; others are supportive to the client and eager to help in any way possible. Their involvement and interaction with the client should be encouraged. Although the physician bears the primary responsibility for explaining to the family the nature of the client's illness, condition, prognosis, and plan of treatment, the nurse can reinforce and clarify the physician's explanations, provide opportunities for the family to talk about the client, and listen and involve them in daily care. The nurse can answer their questions, help them understand the particular problems presented by the client, and teach them how to approach solving them. The family, especially a spouse, needs the opportunity to verbalize and explore feelings regarding alterations in the client and their life-style.

When the client has recovered from the effects of the stroke and is ready for convalescent or home care, he or she and the family are instructed in what to do and what not to do in order to prevent a second attack.

Although about 90% of the clients who survive strokes can be taught how to ambulate and care for their own needs, they may manifest changes in personality and behavior and have difficulty in adjusting to the home setting. The family may also need help in reintegrating the client into the family unit and in aiding him or her to learn to accept disabilities and develop abilities. Referrals may be made to the public health nurse, who will visit the client at home and help the individual and the family by making changes in the physical environment to facilitate ambulation and self-care activities, by contacting other community agencies for help with special economic or social problems, by stimulating new interests and activities, and by strengthening family relationships and clarifying problems as they occur.

A number of films have been produced over the years to educate professionals and the public. Two of the best are *The Inner World of Aphasia* and *I Had a Stroke*. The personal experiences of the people in the films show clearly the conflicts and frustrations of both the people with strokes and their families. The approaches the people have made in the films can give guidance to professionals and reassurance to those with strokes and their families.

Stroke as a national health problem should decrease in importance with better control of risk factors and new improved surgical interventions. But to date, the greatest hope for clients who have had a stroke is in skilled long-term preventive and supportive care by all professionals.

### Expected outcomes

By the time that the client is discharged from the hospital after a stroke, the following outcomes may be expected.
The client will:

1 Identify limitations and methods of increasing personal independence in relation to activities of daily living, such as eating, mobility, toileting, bathing, and grooming.

2 Describe the safe use of appliances required to achieve independence in activities of daily living.

3 Describe safety measures and specific ways to compensate for any loss—sensory, perceptual, or motor—in functional capacities.

4 Detail all aspects of therapy and medication use required in the home setting with the inclusion of significant others as necessary.

5 With the assistance of significant others demonstrate any specific speech or physical exercise to be practiced at home.

6 With the assistance of significant others, show the method by which prescribed therapy will be integrated into the daily routine at home.

7 Have a written reminder of return visits with the physician and other therapists. A reminder telephone call will be made to the client to verify this appointment after discharge.

8 Be able to state realistic short-term goals for therapy that are reevaluated and revised at each visit after hospitalization.

9 Receive emotional support from others as an outcome of the thorough psychosocioeconomic support provided in the assessment and intervention by the health team for and with significant others.

10 With the aid of significant others identify all changes that need to be made at home to remove architectural barriers, secure needed financial resources, and obtain assistive devices.

11 Develop the type of therapeutic relationship with the nurse and physician wherein any problem, such as physical functions, employment, sexuality, emotional outbursts, and communication problems, may be openly and freely discussed.

## SUBCLAVIAN STEAL SYNDROME

When impairments occur in pressure gradients within the vascular system, blood destined for the anastomotic arteries of the circle of Willis is rerouted to other areas. This phenomenon is termed the subclavian steal syndrome.

The arteriovenous malformation is the most common intracerebral abnormality resulting in this event. In arteriovenous malformations, dilated arteries often decrease resistance to blood flow, and blood is thus directed away from normal vessels into the malformation. Once shunted into the malformation, it is unable to supply brain tissue, since the malformation lacks capillaries. Instead, blood moves directly on to become part of the venous system.

Several extracranial syndromes are cited as processes that "steal" blood destined for the brain. Points of obstruction include the left subclavian artery near the origin of the left vertebral artery, the brachiocephalic artery near the origin of the right common carotid artery, and the coarctation of the aortic arch near the origin of the left and right common carotid arteries. At these points, blood flow is reversed and is able to reach other vessels as alternative routes of flow are established. However, the most common example of the steal syndrome in ordinary practice is the subclavian steal syndrome.

In the subclavian steal syndrome an obstruction occurs proximal to the origin of the vertebral arteries, which results in reversed blood flow in the vertebral artery. The cause of this obstruction is most commonly atherosclerosis, though it may result from congenital atresia, coarctation of the aorta, dissecting hematoma, trauma, and Takayasu's disease. Blood flow that becomes reversed at the point of obstruction returns to the heart and upper extremities before supplying the brain.

The severity of symptoms is directly related to the functional capacity of the collateral circulation. The client experiences symptoms when the collateral circulation is unable to compensate for the excessive blood flow directed to the involved arm. When the client engages the upper extremities in activity, vertebrobasilar insufficiency may occur because the increased metabolic demands of the arms require increased blood supplies.

Symptoms of vertebrobasilar insufficiency are varied and depend on which artery or arteries experience a break in circulation. Symptoms are specific to the structure or structures involved in interrupted blood supplies. Carotid insufficiency is not commonly associated with the subclavian steal syndrome.

In the affected arm, exercises or elevation may result in tingling, numbness, and claudication.

A difference in radial pulses and a delay in pulse-arrival time, as determined by plethysmography, are common features of the subclavian steal syndrome. On measurement an inequality of as much as 20 mm Hg between the two arms is common, with greater differences occurring as elevation of the arms or exercise aggravates the problem. After the problem is suspected an angiography is performed to localize the causative lesion and often more clearly delineates the problem when exercise is employed during the procedure. After the angiogram, surgery is often performed in symptomatic clients. Surgical procedures include endarterectomy and bypass grafting. Chapter 26 gives further detail on surgical procedures.

Nursing intervention is related to identification of potential cases, careful determinations of pulses and blood pressure, and education and psychosocial support inherent in the process of diagnostic procedures and surgical intervention. Management of vertebrobasilar insufficiency closely parallels the care given to the stroke client even though these episodes are usually of a transient nature.

## PERIPHERAL VASCULAR DISEASE

*Raynaud's disease* is a vasomotor disorder of unknown cause and attributable to intermittent spasms of small cutaneous arteries or arterioles that interfere with the circulation of blood to the extremities; it is characterized by attacks of impaired sensation and numbness and tingling, especially in the tips of the fingers, toes, ears, and nose. These parts are pale and cold, and severe pain, which is caused by vascular spasm, may accompany the local pallor. After minutes or hours the skin becomes deeply cyanotic. This stage of cyanosis may last from a few seconds to several minutes, and occasionally the skin may become black and gangrenous. There is no impairment of the general circulation, as in thromboangiitis obliterans or arteriosclerosis.

About 75% of the clients with Raynaud's disease are women, and the onset of symptoms usually occurs before the age of 40 years. Symptoms are usually precipitated by exposure to cold; emotional stress may be a precipitating factor in 20% of those afflicted. If the local sensory, color, and temperature changes are not secondary to some other disease, the course of the disorder is relatively benign and rarely incapacitating.

## Treatment and nursing intervention

If possible, a person with Raynaud's disease should live in a warm climate. Exposure to extremes of temperature should be avoided. Treatment is palliative and preventive, and the following principles of care are recommended: keep the client's body warm, protect the extremities from exposure to chemical, mechanical, and thermal trauma, have him or her abstain from smoking, instruct the client in the importance of meticulous hygienic care of the involved areas, and provide specific treatment for associated conditions. Eliminate all drugs that stimulate vasoconstriction, and if the client is obese, prescribe a low-calorie diet, If warming the hands does not give relief during an attack, alcohol taken by mouth or papaverine hydrochloride given intravenously may relieve the symptoms. Nicotinic acid, phenoxybenzamine hydrochloride, cyclandelate, azapetine phosphate, tolazoline hydrochloride, and neostigmine bromide (Prostigmin) have also been used with good results. Paravertebral blocks may be administered with good therapeutic effect. Various ganglionic and adrenergic drugs may be tried if other treatment is ineffective in relieving pain and preventing necrosis of the tissue. The client should wear gloves when touching cold objects. This is especially important when refrigerated or frozen foods are handled.

Surgical treatment is indicated if the circulation is seriously affected or if the pain is severe and is not alleviated by medical treatment. Sympathectomy (lumbar or thoracic) is done to relieve pain caused by vasoconstriction of the peripheral arteries and to improve the circulation. This procedure decreases the client's disability during cold weather and prevents the development of ulcers. Nursing care is symptomatic and depends on the site of the operation and the client's general condition.

Other peripheral vascular diseases, thromboangiitis obliterans (Buerger's), arteriosclerosis, and thrombophlebitis, which most commonly affect the lower extremities, especially numbness and tingling, may be treated by vasodilating drugs, a low-fat diet, and regular exercise. Meticulous foot care and the prohibition of smoking also should be emphasized. Refer to Chapter 16 for a discussion of the peripheral vascular diseases in relation to trophic changes.

## REFERENCES

Agler, B., and Malcolm, B.: Correcting common errors in blood pressure measurement, Am. J. Nurs. **65:**133-164, Oct. 1965.

Agranowitz, A., and McKeown, M.: Aphasia handbook for adults and children, Springfield, Ill., 1975, Charles C Thomas, Publisher.

Amacher, N.J.: Touch is a way of caring, Am. J. Nurs. **73:** 852-854, 1973.

American Heart Association: Heart Facts, Dallas, Texas, 1980, The Association.

Barton, J.: To help a hemiplegic, you have to know how it feels to be one, nurses learn, Mod. Nurs. Home **24:**37-38, April 1970.

Bickerstaff, E.R.: Neurological complications of oral contraceptives, New York, 1975, Oxford University Press, Inc.

Booth, K.: Subclavian steal syndrome: treatment with proximal vertebral to common carotid artery transposition, J. Neurosurg. Nurs. **12:**28-31, March 1980.

Brower, P., and Hicks, D.: Maintaining muscle function in patients on bed rest, Am. J. Nurs. **72:**1250-1253, 1972.

Browse, N.L.: Physiology and pathology of bed rest, Springfield, Ill., 1965, Charles C Thomas, Publisher.

Buck, M.: Dysphasia: the patient, his family, and the nurse, Cardiovasc. Nurs. **6:**51-56, Sept. Oct. 1970.

Buell, U., et al.: Sensitivity of computed tomography and serial scintigraphy in cerebrovascular disease, Radiology **131:**393-398, May 1979.

Burnside, I.M.: Clocks and calendars, Am. J. Nurs. **70:**117-119, Jan. 1970.

Burnside, I.M., editor: Psychosocial nursing; care of the aged, ed. 2, New York, 1980, McGraw-Hill Book Co.

Burt, M.M.: Perceptual deficits in hemiplegia, Am. J. Nurs. **70:**1026-1029, 1970.

Caplan, L.R., and Mohr, J.P.: Harvard stroke registry: make-up and purpose, Neurology **29:**755, May 1979.

Caplan, L.R.: Vertebrobasilar disease: time for a new strategy, Curr. Concepts Cerebrovasc. Dis. **15:**11, July-Aug. 1980, American Heart Association.

Carlson, C.E., coordinator: Behavioral concepts and nursing intervention, ed. 2, Philadelphia, 1978, J.B. Lippincott Co.

Chater, N., et al.: The spectrum of cerebrovascular occlusive disease suitable for microvascular bypass surgery, Angiology **26:**235, March 1975.

Chiu, L.C., et al.: Computed tomography and brain scintigraphy in ischemic stroke, Am. J. Roentgenol. **127**:481, Sept. 1976.

Dandy, W.E.: Intracranial arterial aneurysms, Ithaca, N.Y., 1944, Comstock Publishing Associates.

Daniels, L.M., and Kochar, M.S.: Monitoring and facilitating adherence to hypertension therapeutic regimens, Cardio-Vasc. Nursing **16**:7, March-April 1980, American Heart Association.

Drummond, E.E.: Communication and comfort for the dying patient, Nurs. Clin. North Am. **5**:54-63, March 1970.

Feigenson, J.S.: Stroke rehabilitation, Curr. Concepts Cerebrovasc. Dis. **15**:21, Nov.-Dec. 1980, American Heart Association.

Fields, W.S.: Stroke diagnosis and management, current procedures and equipment, St. Louis, 1973, Warren H. Green, Inc.

Fowler, R.S., and Fordyce, W.: Adapting care for the brain-damaged patient, Am. J. Nurs. **72**:2056-2059, 1972.

Fox, J.L.: Vascular clips for the microsurgical treatment of stroke, Stroke **7**:489, Sept.-Oct. 1976.

Fox, M.J.: Talking with patients who can't answer, Am. J. Nurs. **71**:1146-1149, 1971.

Freese, A.S.: Stroke: the new help and the new life, New York, 1980, Random House, Inc.

Fujishima, M., et al.: Prognosis of occlusive cerebrovascular diseases in normotensive and hypertensive subjects, Stroke **7**:472, Sept.-Oct. 1976.

Galloway, D.B., et al.: Propranolol in hypertension: a dose-response study, Br. Med. J. **2**:140, July 17, l976.

Gaspard, N.J.: The family of the patient with long-term illness, Nurs. Clin. North Am. **5**:77-84, March 1970.

Gaul, A., Thompson, R., and Hart, G.: Hyperbaric oxygen therapy, Am. J. Nurs. **72**:892-896, 1972.

Gerdes, L.: The confused or delirious patient, Am. J. Nurs. **68**:1228-1233, 1968.

Geschwind, N.: Aphasia, N. Engl. J. Med. **284**:654-656, 1971.

Gifford, R.W.: Raynaud's disease, Hosp. Med. **6**:37-53, March 1970.

Ginsberg, M.D., and Reivich, M.: Cerebral vascular pathophysiology. In Towers, D.B., editor: The nervous system: Vol. II, The clinical neurosciences, New York, 1975, Raven Press, Publishers.

Glaser, B.G., and Strauss, A.L.: Time for dying, Chicago, 1968, Aldine Publishing Co.

Goda, S.: Communicating with the aphasic or dysarthric patient, Am. J. Nurs. **63**:80-84, July 1963.

Griffith, E., and Madero, B.: Primary hypertension—patient's learning needs, Am. J. Nurs. **73**:624-627, 1973.

Groteboer, J.: Stroke, carotid endarterectomy, and the neurosurgeon, J. Neurosurg. Nurs. **10**:52-62, June 1978.

Hachinski, V., et al.: Symptomatic intracranial steal, Arch. Neurol. **34**:149, March 1977.

Harvey, W.P., editor: Desk reference issue on hypertension, Med. Times, **106**(5): entire issue, May 1978.

Hatano, S., et al., editor: Hypertension and stroke control in the community, Geneva, 1976, World Health Organization.

Herman, B., Schulte, B.P., van Luijk, J.H., et al.: Epidemiology of stroke in Tilburg, The Netherlands, Stroke **11**(2): 162-169, March-April 1980.

Hill, M.: Helping the hypertensive patient control sodium intake, Am. J. Nurs. **79**(5):906, May 1979.

Hoffman, E.: Don't give up on me! Am. J. Nurs. **71**:60-62, Jan. 1971.

Hulicka, I.: Fostering self-respect in aged patients, Am. J. Nurs. **64**:84-89, May 1964.

Huston, J.C.: Overcoming the learning disabilities of stroke, Nursing75 **5**:66, Sept. 1975.

Hutchinson, E.C., and Acheson, E.J.: Strokes: natural history, pathology and surgical treatment, Philadelphia, 1975, W.B. Saunders Co.

Irey, N.S., et al.: Oral contraceptives and stroke in young women: a clinicopathologic correlation, Neurology **28**:1216-1219, Dec. 1978.

Jackson, B.S.: Chronic peripheral arterial disease, Am. J. Nurs. **72**:928-934, 1972.

Johnstone, M.: Home care for the stroke patient, New York, 1980, Churchill Livingstone, Medical Division of Longman, Inc.

Jones, D., Dunbar, C.F., and Jirovec, M.M.: Medical surgical nursing: a conceptual approach, New York, 1978, McGraw-Hill Book Co.

Kahn, R.: Stroke rehabilitation in general hospitals, Hospitals **45**:47-50, Nov. 1, 1971.

Katz, D.M.: Doppler sonography diagnosis of cerebrovascular diseases, Stroke **7**:439, Sept.-Oct. 1976.

Keller, H.M.: Noninvasive angiography for the diagnosis of vertebral artery disease using Doppler ultrasound, Stroke **7**:364, July-Aug. 1976.

Kerber, C.: Use of balloon catheters in the treatment of cranial arterial abnormalities, Curr. Concepts Cerebrovasc. Dis., vol. 14, July-Aug. 1979, American Heart Association.

Kinkel, W.R., and Jacobs, L.: Computerized axial transverse tomography in cerebrovascular disease, Neurology **26**:924, Oct. 1976.

Kricheff, I., et al.: Simplified solid-particle embolization with a new introducer, Radiology **131**:794-795, June 1979.

Kübler-Ross, E.: On death and dying, New York, 1969, Macmillan Publishing Co., Inc.

Kübler-Ross, E.: What is it like to be dying? Am. J. Nurs. **71**: 54-61, Jan. 1971.

Librach, I.M.: Subarachnoid hemorrhage, some pitfalls, Br. J. Clin. Pract. **29**:43, 1975.

Licht, S., editor: Stroke and its rehabilitation, Baltimore, 1975, The Williams & Wilkins Co.

Marchant, M., et al.: Interdisciplinary learning on a neurological service, Am. J. Nurs. **72**:1638-1639, 1972.

Marshall, J.: A survey of occlusive disease of the vertebro-basilar arterial system. In Vinken, P.J., and Bruyn, G.W., editors: Handbook of clinical neurology: Vol. XII, Part 2, Vascular diseases of the nervous system, New York, 1972, American Elsevier Publishing Co.

McCaig, C.: Embolization of cerebral arteriovenous malformations, AORN J. **28**:232-239, Aug. 1978.

McCombs, J., et al.: Critical patient behaviors in high blood pressure control, Cardio-Vasc. Nursing **16**:19, July-August, 1980, American Heart Association.

McCormick, G.P., and Williams, M.: Stroke: the double crisis, Am. J. Nurs. **79:**1410, Aug. 1979.

McDowell, F.H., et al.: Treatment of impending stroke, Stroke **11**(1):1, Jan.-Feb. 1980.

McDowell, F.H.: The extracranial/intracranial bypass study, Stroke **8**(5):546, Sept.-Oct. 1977.

McHenry, L.: Cerebral circulation and stroke, St. Louis, 1978, Warren H. Green, Inc.

Medical highlights: Asymptomatic bruits in cervical arteries, Am. J. Nurs. **80:**1357, July 1980.

Mervin, F.: The plight of dying patients in hospitals, Am. J. Nurs. **71:**1988-1990, 1971.

Morris, M., and Rhodes, M.: Guidelines for the care of confused patients, Am. J. Nurs. **72:**1630-1633, 1972.

Mullan, S.: Conservative management of the recently ruptured aneurysm, Surg. Neurol. **3:**27, Jan. 1975.

National High Blood Pressure Coordinating Committee: The 1980 Report of the Joint National Committee on Detection, Evaluation, and Treatment of High Blood Pressure, U.S. Department of Health and Human Services, 120/80 National Institutes of Health, Bethesda, Md.

O'Brien, M.T., and Pallett, P.J.: Total care of the stroke patient, Boston, 1978, Little, Brown & Co.

O'Connor, A.B., compiler: Nursing in neurological disorders, Contemporary Nursing Series, New York, 1976, American Journal of Nursing Co.

Olson, E.V., et al.: The hazards of immobility—effects on psychosocial equilibrium, Am. J. Nurs. **67:**794-797, 1967.

Peripheral vascular disease, a diagnostic guide, Emergency Med. **9:**127, Jan. 1977.

Perkins, W.H.: Speech pathology, an applied behavioral science, ed. 2, St. Louis, 1977, The C.V. Mosby Co.

Petrie, J.C., et al.: Methyldopa and propranolol or practolol in moderate hypertension, Br. Med. J. **2:**137, July 17, 1976.

Phillips, P.: Nursing care study—subarachnoid hemorrhage caused by a ruptured aneurysm, Nurs. Times **72:**1270, Aug. 19, 1976.

Powell, B.R., et al.: Rehabilitation, performance and adjustment in stroke patients: a study of social class factors, Genet. Psychol. Monogr. **93:**287, May 1976.

Reinmuth, O.M.: Intracranial bypass surgery for cerebral arterial disease and the responsibility of the practicing physician, Stroke **10**(3):344-347, May-June 1979.

Research News: Treatment reduces deaths from hypertension, Science, vol. 206, Dec. 1979.

Robertson, J.T.: Cerebral arterial spasm, Clin. Neurosurg. **21:**100, 1974.

Rodman, M.J.: Drugs used in cardiovascular disease. 2. Treating hypertension, RN **36:**41-54, April 1973.

Ross-Russell, R.W.: Cerebral arterial disease, New York, 1976, Longman, Inc.

Rusk, H.A., editor: Rehabilitation medicine, ed. 4, St. Louis, 1977, The C.V. Mosby Co.

Sahs, A.L.: Medical management of vascular diseases of the brain. In Towers, D.B., editor: The nervous system: Vol. II, The clinical neurosciences, New York, 1975, Raven Press, Publishers.

Salazar, J.L., et al.: Intracranial neurosurgical treatment of occlusive cerebrovascular disease, Stroke **7:**348, July-Aug. 1976.

Sarno, J.E., and Sarno, M.T.: Stroke: a guide for patients and their families, New York, 1979, McGraw-Hill Book Co.

Schmeidek, P., editor: Microsurgery for stroke, New York, 1978, Springer-Verlag New York, Inc.

Siev, E., and Freishtat, B.: Perceptual, dysfunction in the adult stroke patient, Thorofare, N.J., 1976, Charles B. Slack, Inc.

Smith, G.W.: Care of the patient with a stroke, ed. 2, New York, 1976, Springer Publishing Co., Inc.

Soltero, I., et al.: Trends in mortality from cerebrovascular diseases in the United States, 1960 to 1975, Stroke **9**(6):549-555, Nov.-Dec. 1978.

Steinberg, F.U., editor: Cowdry's the care of the geriatric patient, ed. 5, St. Louis, 1976, The C.V. Mosby Co.

Stolley, P.D., Kuller, L.H., Nefzger, M.D., Tonascia, S., Lilienfeld, A.M., Miller, G.D., and Diamond, E.L.: Three-area epidemiological study of geographic differences in stroke mortality. II. Results, Stroke **8**(5):551-557, Sept.-Oct. 1977.

Stryker, S.: Speech after stroke, Springfield, Ill., 1978, Charles C Thomas, Publisher.

Taylor, J.W., and Ballenger, S.: Neurological dysfunctions and nursing interventions, New York, 1980, McGraw-Hill Book Co.

Troost, B.T.: Dizziness and vertigo in vertebrobasilar disease, Stroke **11**(3):301-303, May-June 1980.

Ward, G.W., et al.: Treating and counseling the hypertensive patient, Am. J. Nurs. **78**(5):824-828, May 1978.

Webb, P.H.: Neurological deficit after carotid endarterectomy, Am. J. Nurs. **79**(4):654-658, April 1979.

Weinberg, J., et al.: Training sensory awareness and spatial organization in people with right brain damage, Arch. Phys. Med. Rehabil. **60**(11):491-496, Nov. 1979.

Wende, S., et al.: Cerebral magnification angiography: physical basis and clinical results, New York, 1974, Springer-Verlag New York, Inc.

WHO Meeting, Tokoyo, March 11-13, 1974: Hypertension and stroke control in the community. In Hatano, S., et al., editors: Proceedings, Geneva, 1976, World Health Organization.

Wingquist, D.: Of life's span the final stages, Nurs. Homes **22:**32-34, March 1973.

Wyka, C.A., et al.: Group education for the hypertensive, Cardio-Vasc. Nurs. **16:**1, Jan.-Feb. 1980, American Heart Association.

Yarnell, P., et al.: Aphasia outcome in strokes: a clinical neuroradiologic correlation, Stroke **7:**516, Sept.-Oct. 1976.

Yaşargil, M.G., et al.: Arteriovenous malformations of vein of Galen: microsurgical treatment, Surg. Neurol. **3:**195, Sept. 1976.

# PART EIGHT

# ASSISTIVE INTERVENTION

# 25
# REHABILITATION

## CONCEPTS AND PRACTICES

The phrase "rehabilitation involving all the areas of nursing practice" expresses best the philosophy of the nursing profession. When there are major interferences in life-style caused by disease or injury, there are requirements for adaptations of the physical body and coping by the emotional makeup. The process of rehabilitation addresses itself to the extensive changes physically and emotionally that leave permanent handicaps. Rehabilitation endeavors to assist and support the individual in returning to the previous life-style, however it has changed.

Fordyce states, "Rehabilitation is concerned typically with people who have disabilities with enduring and pervasive effects. The essence of the rehabilitation process is recognition that what happened to the client affects, and will continue to affect, many aspects of his life extending beyond the limits of bodily function" (Krusen et al., 1971). Families, not the individual alone, are affected and become involved in the rehabilitation process. Rehabilitation endeavors to preserve spared abilities and discover new talents within the individual to help him or her function in society on the same level and with the same opportunities as neighbors.

Nursing, as philosophically stated by Henderson (Harmer and Henderson, 1955), is rehabilitation. "Nursing is primarily assisting the individual (sick or well) in the performance of those activities contributing to health or its recovery or to a peaceful death, that he would perform unaided if he had the necessary strength, will or knowledge. It is likewise the unique contribution of nursing to help the individual to be independent of such assistance as soon as possible."

Nursing in rehabilitation is client and family centered because of the many adjustments that the patient alone cannot handle. Many disciplines, as well as medical specialists, are involved in the adjustment process, and they enhance and reinforce each other in helping the client change to a new way of life. This change must be a "creative procedure," as stated by Krusen (Krusen et al., 1971).

Neurological problems, medical or surgical, by their very nature imply changes in function and deficits. Nursing, as well as the other disciplines involved, has developed and is seeking constantly better methods to prevent, limit, or control these inherent problems. Because neurological problems are almost always lasting, there is great need for client and family education. Nursing plays a large part in this educational process. Rehabilitation requires a thorough assessment of the client and family for physical and psychosocial strengths as well as weaknesses to devise a plan of attack for the problems involved. This chapter will consider problems or potential problems with current nursing practice that promote rehabilitation.

## PERCEPTION: INTEGRATION OF ENVIRONMENTAL STIMULI

How each person views the environment and responds to it involves a multitude of circuits in one of the most complex computers ever developed: the cerebrum. Experiences and patterns of responses to different types of stimuli are recorded over a period of time in a memory bank for quick recall and responses to similar experiences. This is learning. Particular areas of the cerebrum are responsible for the interpretation of certain types of stimuli, and through many cross tracts, as yet not fully understood, integration to a larger experience occurs. Breaks in the receiving organs or in the integration process present special problems. Professionals must be alert for problems when any insult occurs in the nervous system and must work with clients to help them compensate for deficits or distortions in perception.

## Visual disturbances

Visual disturbances present special problems for function. Causes of visual disturbance can be in the eye, in the optic radiation, or in the optic cortex. Cataracts, refraction problems, and glaucoma may have been present long before a neurological insult occurred in an elderly individual (Mossman, 1976). Visual field restrictions (Fig. 11-13) are common with head trauma, tumors, and strokes. Cortical blindness can occur from head injuries and stroke with posterior cerebral artery involvement.

The larger component of visual disturbance, however, lies in the realm of special perception and reasoning. The right cerebral hemisphere has been recognized as dominant for visual-spatial perception, reasoning, and the concept of time. The left hemisphere is dominant for speech and language skills. The hemispheres, however, are not independent but are linked together by cross tracts of the corpus callosum, which allows each hemisphere to assert some degree of control over the other. The process of special perception consists of the interpretation of multiple stimuli to form a conscious or an unconscious idea, which in turn forms a concept. The function of the parietal lobes is to synthesize stimuli into perceptions, impressions that form ideas. This is called *morphosynthesis*. Denny-Brown states that although this process is bilateral, it is more developed in the hemisphere corresponding to the preferred hand. Others see morphosynthesis primarily in the nondominating parietal lobe, usually the right parietal lobe (Mossman, 1976). Several tests have been developed to measure perceptual deficiencies. One example is the Bender-Gestalt Visual Motor Test, consisting of meaningless geometric designs the individual is

asked to copy. Another test frequently used is the Wechsler Adult Intelligence Scale (WAIS) of assembly and completion tasks of varying levels of perception and analysis (Mossman, 1976). The Raven Coloured Matrices Test asks the person to match geometric designs and is useful in detecting field defects as well as perception problems (Raven, 1962). Before working with a client who has sustained cerebral injury, one should make a careful visual assessment, looking for perceptual overlays of the right hemisphere.

A client who had a stroke with right middle cerebral artery involvement in addition to perceptual problems often has left homonymous hemianopia (Fig. 11-13). This person may neglect food on the left side of the tray, misinterpret what he or she has read because of starting in the middle of the page, and frequently bump into objects on the left (Figs. 25-1 and 25-2). This person must be taught to compensate by looking to the left to scan the environment and increase the visual field. There is usually a lack of depth perception also. It is important to place frequently used objects within easy reach and within the right visual field to prevent falls. Approach these individuals on their right side so as not to startle them. Otherwise they may move quickly and lose balance. Place this client so that the visual field is toward the center of activity in a room; in this way, he or she receives maximum stimulation from the environment and does not feel isolated (Fig. 25-3). Perceptual problems will be considered further in the discussion of mobility.

## Reasoning deficits

The other large problem related to perceptual deficits has to do with reasoning and judgment and is usually observed as impulsiveness. This quality, as Mossman states, defies measurement and can be the saboteur of independence in self-care and mobility. The difficulty is a phenomenon of cortical disinhibition, with the inability to withhold a response even without a proper stimulus. Inaccurate perceptual input coupled with cognitive deficiencies results in poor judgment and lack of reliability. Premorbid personality traits, poor memory, or denial mechanisms will enhance the problem. This person, usually with right parietal lobe involvement, will attempt to walk when the

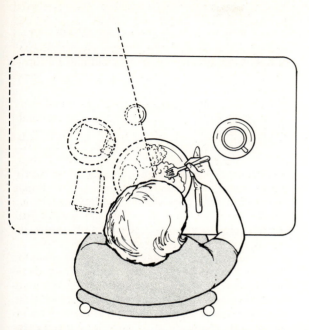

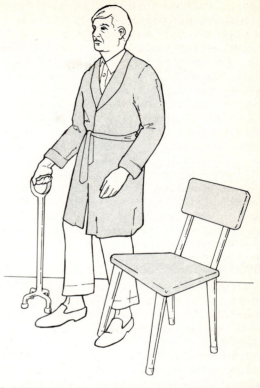

**FIG. 25-1.** Dinner for left hemiplegic with field cut. Person may not be able to find bread and butter, napkin, or milk.

**FIG. 25-2.** Left hemiplegic with field cut is unaware of furniture on left and bumps into it.

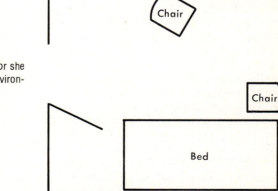

**FIG. 25-3.** Place person with field cut in room so that he or she may see who is approaching as well as other parts of environment.

leg cannot support him or her, touch a hot stove, or leave the refrigerator door open. The relationship between cause and effect or the ability to plan ahead and anticipate consequences is lost, introducing a myriad of hazards into the person's life (Mossman, 1976).

The person with judgment problems, or loss of "quality controls," will require close supervision for all activities. This person often talks as if understanding the hazards, but behavior does not bear this out. The person may be able to relearn through great diligence personally and on the part of professionals step-by-step safe behavior. However, he or she may also be easily distracted and forget safe patterns. These persons frequently do better in a familiar environment with stimuli they understand, where they need not develop new environmental perceptions.

## SPEECH AND LANGUAGE

Language may be one of man's greatest accomplishments. It has allowed through symbols and sound the reconstruction of the past, description of the present, and hypotheses about the future (Krusen et al., 1971). Language and speech also may be considered another aspect of how man receives and responds to the environment. In language, man receives environmental information through sense organs and analyzes it on the basis of part experiences to form a symbol or idea. Linguistic ability allows the formulation of responses in language symbols and the initiation of a plan of action, including word choice and grammar for the motor cortex (Speech Department, Strong Memorial Hospital, The University of Rochester). The motor cortex carries through the response to the environment in speech or other actions. A break any place in the circuitry shown above will disrupt language and speech.

Disruption in language communication makes rehabilitation extremely difficult. It is important to determine the extent of the disruption early and to discover the best methods of communicating. A careful evaluation will reduce frustration on the part of the person who has sustained the loss as well as those helping.

Aphasia, apraxia, and dysarthria relate chiefly to disruption of the language model. These problems are usually seen in stroke and head injury victims

## LANGUAGE MODEL

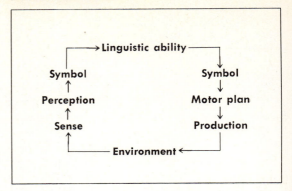

with left cerebral damage. Aphasia, "the disturbance or loss of ability to comprehend, elaborate or express speech concepts" (Miller and Keane, 1972), has many shadings. They are usually classified under receptive aphasia and expressive aphasia.

*Receptive aphasia* may exist first in distorted auditory images, wherein the sounds of speech do not correspond to the sounds the person knew before brain injury. Words may sound like gibberish, and the person appears hard of hearing. Fortunately, this distortion of sound is most often intermittent. The person may or may not have speech.

Another deviation is poor auditory comprehension of words. These persons can repeat words, but the words have no meaning, similar to a foreign language. These persons may make association-comprehension errors such as *table* for *chair* or *fork* for *knife*. Some may understand concrete terms but not concepts. In addition, there is usually a reduced ability to retain what has been said ranging from only one to two words to as much as one sentence.

Along with auditory receptive problems of language there usually exist some visual receptive language problems. The person may be able to read but does not understand what is read. Alternatively, he or she may not be able to read aloud but can read silently with fairly good comprehension, though rate and accuracy are likely to be reduced. Reading impairment may be compounded by visual-field restrictions. Individuals with right-field restrictions are more likely to compensate than those with left-field restrictions. Poor visual-spatial perception of right-sided brain damage may interfere with reading because the person has problems following one line and moving to the next line. It must be remembered that although only one hemisphere seems to be damaged, some subtle changes may exist in the other to compound the problem.

*Expressive aphasia* is more obvious, as the listener hears the speech errors. It must be remembered that an inappropriate response may be made because the person did not understand the question on the basis of auditory difficulties. Also the person may understand the question but cannot formulate an answer because of a break in motor speech production. A person with speech production difficulties often has problems in ''word finding''—knowing what he or she wants to say but not being able to find the word. The individual may substitute several words for one word *(circumlocution)* if the problem is mild. He or she may make substitution errors, such as ''I write with a watch.'' Some persons use only nouns or verbs and have a telegraph style of speech. The mildly impaired individual may make grammatical errors as to verb tenses, word order, or plurals. One may assume that some individuals have language problems when the problem is really in the speech organs of teeth and tongue. The speech is slurred, but there are no grammatical problems *(dysarthria)*.

Some individuals may have no voluntary speech, but old patterns of association may be initiated in counting, naming the days of the week or months of the year, or swearing. This speech is referred to as ''automatic speech'' and can be used socially in giving the name or singing. Often a concerned relative mistakes this for linguistic ability. This situation, wherein the person is unable to initiate voluntary speech but has the motor ability, may be referred to as *speech apraxia*. Apraxia occurs in other situations where the person cannot initiate an action but may perform automatically. For example, when the person is asked to comb the hair, the person will not comply. If however, the comb is placed in the hand, he or she will comb the hair. Limited but appropriate automatic answers of yes or no can be very useful, and the person becomes much more socially acceptable. Certain per-

sons use only jargon, but with changes in voice inflection there is no question of meaning. In like manner, gestures, and facial expressions are often quite adequate for communication and should be utilized when voluntary speech is limited or lacking.

Writing is on a higher symbolic level than speaking and requires the additional processes of visual configuration of letters. Writing may be the best method of communicating when there is interruption of motor speech. Other conceptual problems of arithmetic may be affected and show up better when writing is attempted (Mossman, 1976).

## Evaluation

Because speech and language are made up of many parts, suspected language impairment must be evaluated systematically. The following screening form will give the nurse a base line quickly and help establish a reasonable method of communication.

**Speech and language screening***

1 *Auditory comprehension: receptive aphasia*
Close your eyes.
Touch your right ear.
Point to the pencil, key, nickel, cut, etc.
Which one do we spend, drink, write with?
Put the nickel beside the pencil.
Put the comb between the pencil and the key.

2 *Speech: expressive aphasia*
What is this? (Examiner holds up or points to object—pen, cup, watch, etc.)
Definitions: What does robin mean? Island? Bargain?
Use the interpretation of proverbs for high-level training.

3 *Reading comprehension: receptive aphasia*
Match the following words to the objects (print each work on separate strips of paper): pencil, key, nickel, cup.
Have the client read the following sentences and mark, point to, or say yes or no (print sentences far apart, one at a time, using large, clear letters):
Are there 7 days in a week?   Yes   No
Is Christmas in June?   Yes   No
Does the sun rise in the east?   Yes   No
Do you tell time with a watch?   Yes   No

4 *Writing: expressive aphasia*
Have the client copy these shapes: ○ + □
Ask the client to write his or her name.

---

*From Speech Department, Strong Memorial Hospital, The University of Rochester.

Have the client copy simple words. (Examiner writes them first, one at a time.)

Have the client write words from dictation: man, rain, watch, information.

5 *Speech production: dysarthria or apraxia*

Have the client imitate tongue protrusion, elevation, depression, movement laterally. (Note drooling or swallowing difficulty.)

Have the client repeat rapidly ta-ta-ta-ta-ta-ta-ta, etc.

Have the client say the following words, either by reading them or repeating them after the examiner: cross, seven, Massachusetts, Methodist Episcopal.

Speech pathologists have a number of tests to measure speech deficits. These tests are used on a regular basis to give measurable indications of improvement. Some of the tests used frequently are the Minnesota Test for Differential Diagnosis of Aphasia (Schuell, 1965), Porch Index of Communication Ability (Porch, 1967), and Functional Communication Profile (Sarno, 1965).

## Intervention

When working with an individual who has speech and language problems, the following list should be used as a guide to reduce anxiety and frustration and to promote success:

1. Be calm and objective.
2. Use a normal tone of voice.
3. Proceed slowly; do not hurry.
4. Choose a setting with few or no outside distractions.
5. Avoid confrontation with new or strange situations.
6. Treat the person as an adult.
7. Allow for emotional behavior and uncontrollable lability.
8. Avoid interruption; allow the person to finish whatever he or she is attempting.
9. Watch for fatigue, limit attempts.
10. Do not discuss unpleasant news.
11. Encourage every attempt at language.
12. Focus on progress.
13. Encourage self-help.
14. Use short, simple directions.
15. Give one direction at a time.
16. Substitute one word for another when the person has difficulty understanding.

When teaching new skills to an individual who has severe receptive problems, it may prove less frustrating to use gesture only. Speech only distracts and confuses the individual performing the job at hand.

## Summary

Speech and language skills set man apart from other species, and when these skills are limited or lost, the person may feel less than human; others often treat him or her so. It is extremely important, therefore, for professionals to help the person so afflicted and the family to find and employ a satisfactory form of communication.

## DECUBITUS ULCERS

Any break in the neurological monitoring system of the peripheral nerves, the spinal and thalamic tracts, or the cognitive higher functions may quickly lead to decubitus ulcers. The ulcers, better considered pressure sores, result when cell metabolism is impaired. Impaired blood circulation, limiting vital nutrients, is the ultimate cause of pressure sore formation, but the loss of the warning signs of pressure and pain is the basic problem. It would follow that clients in coma, clients with neuropathies, and clients with spinal cord injuries are prime candidates for pressure sores. On a circulatory basis, clients with arteriosclerosis, metabolic disorders, and general aging are also ultimately candidates for pressure sores. These clients usually have sensory deficits also.

Guttmann in 1955 identified the intrinsic and extrinsic factors associated with clients with spinal cord injuries that lead to decubitus ulcer formation. He stated first that the most important intrinsic factor is lowered tissue resistance to pressure caused by the interruption of spinal vasomotor pathways, with loss of control of skeletal muscles as well as skin and mucosal muscles. The lack of muscle tone and control in the vascular bed allows pressure that would not normally block blood vessels to occlude these vessels and results in ischemia of the body part, usually the lower extremities, where blood flow pressure is normally less than in the upper extremities. Second, loss of sensation is a causal factor. Normally, discomfort, the first symptom of impaired circulation, does not come into play to prompt movement and relieve pressure. Exton-Smith in 1961 found that the number of pressure areas an elderly population of 50 persons developed was directly related to the number of spontaneous movements they had during sleep. The third intrinsic factor is the anatomical arrangement of certain body parts, namely, the distance of bony weight-bearing prominences from the skin and the thicknesses of padding of muscle and fat between bone and skin. Fourth, spasticity of the lower limbs, especially adductor spasm, causes shearing stress on the skin to produce ulcers on the inner surface of the knees and ankles (Guttmann, 1973).

Three extrinsic factors are identified as pressure, maceration from exposing the skin to moisture (urine, fecal incontinence, and perspiration), and cold. The work of Kosiak in 1958 on pressure-time studies with dogs demonstrated an inverse relation in the formation of ulcers. The greater the pressure, the less was the time required to produce an ulcer. At 600 mm Hg an ulcer will develop in slightly under 2 hours, whereas 11 hours were required for an ulcer to form at 150 mm Hg. Mechanically the studies demonstrated that pressure is exerted both internally from bones and externally from the force applied (Krusen et al., 1971).

Other candidates for pressure sores with limited circulation and metabolic disturbances will have part or all of the foregoing factors contributing to their ulcers. The elderly, with all systems slowing and reaction times increased, become candidates. Any person who has a tight appliance such as a bandage or cast can readily develop pressure sores. Edema, because of constriction, will aggravate the situation. Decreased movement of a body part, increased or decreased sensation, and change in skin color indicate circulatory impairment that can damage all tissues. Diabetics are a population characterized for ulcer formation because of their easily disrupted metabolic balance and early development of atherosclerosis and neuropathies.

Several scales have been developed to indicate quickly those persons who will develop pressure sores. A scale developed by Gosnell (1973) rates mental status, continence, mobility, activity, and nutrition. According to this scale, when the total score dropped to 11, the candidate was in jeopardy. Factors of temperature elevation and poor nutrition appeared critical in precipitating ulcers (Table 25-1) (Gosnell, 1973).

Pressure sores are usually described as to the stage of development, which in turn indicates the extent of treatment required. Campbell in 1959 classified them according to the tissue layers involved (Table 25-2), as follows:

*Stage I:* Redness of area (epidermis) that will blanch and subside if pressure is removed, and no tissue damage will ensue.

*Stage II:* Redness, swelling, induration, occasional blistering, and desquamation of epidermis. This situation may be reversible with relief of pressure and increased circulation.

*Stage III:* Necrosis of skin with exposure of fat. The area may heal spontaneously if it is small.

*Stage IV:* Skin and fat necrosis extending to muscle. This stage must have intervention, specifically débridement, and may require surgery.

*Stage V:* Skin, fat, and muscle necrosis. Débridement and surgical closure are required in most cases.

*Stage VI:* Bone involvement or periostitis, ostitis, or osteomyelitis. Surgical intervention is necessary.

*Stage VII:* Osteomyelitis, septic arthritis, possible pathological fracture, and septicemia. This stage may precipitate a cancerous process. Surgical treatment may involve amputations of mutilation.

**TABLE 25-1.** Rating scale for decubitus ulcer formation

| Mental status | Continence | Mobility | Activity | Nutrition | Score | |
|---|---|---|---|---|---|---|
| 5 Alert | 4 Fully controlled | 4 Full | 4 Ambulatory | 3 Good | Mental status | _____ |
| 4 Apathetic | 3 Usually controlled | 3 Slightly limited | 3 Walks with assistance | 2 Fair | Continence | _____ |
| 3 Confused | 2 Minimally controlled | 2 Very limited | 2 Chairfast | 1 Poor | Mobility | _____ |
| 2 Stuporous | 1 Absence of control | 1 Immobile | 1 Bedfast | | Activity | _____ |
| 1 Unconscious | | | | | Nutrition | _____ |
| Date | | | | | TOTAL | _____ |

**TABLE 25-2.** Decubitus ulcers: stages and treatment

| Stage | Physical signs | Treatment | Prognosis | Nursing orders and modalities |
|---|---|---|---|---|
| 1 | Redness over pressure area, no induration <br><br> ———————— Epidermis | Relieve pressure increase circulation | Will subside if pressure is relieved | 1. Do not position on affected area. <br> 2. Turn at least every 2 hours. <br> 3. Give exquisite skin care. <br> 4. Mobilize. <br> Alternating pressure mattress, sheepskin boots, and so on <br> Massage, cold, and heat treatment |
| 2 | Redness, swelling, induration, occasional blistering, and desquamation of epidermis <br><br> Skin <br> Sub. areolar tissue <br> Muscle | Relieve pressure <br> Increase circulation <br> Prevent secondary infection <br> Improve nutrition | May be reversible with pressure relief and increased circulation | 1. Do not position on affected area. <br> 2. Turn at least every 2 hours. <br> 3. Give exquisite skin care. <br> 4. Protect any broken areas. <br> 5. Mobilize. <br> Massage, cold, and heat treatment <br> Ultraviolet treatment |
| 3 | Necrosis of skin with exposure of fat <br><br> Fat layer | Relieve pressure <br> Increase circulation <br> Prevent and treat secondary infection <br> Improve nutrition | May heal spontaneously if small | 1. Do not position on affected area. <br> 2. Follow regular turning schedule. <br> 3. Mobilize. <br> 4. Give high-protein, high–vitamin C diet. <br> 5. Institute exercise and recreational programs. <br> Alternating pressure mattress <br> Massage <br> Ultraviolet treatments <br> Débridement <br> Debrisan (dextranomer) <br> Hydrotherapy <br> Surgical intervention |
| 4 | Skin and fat necrosis extending to muscle <br><br> Skin <br> Fat | Relieve pressure <br> Increase circulation <br> Prevent and treat secondary infection <br> Improve nutrition | Must have intervention <br> Débridement <br> Trial of conservative therapy <br> Surgery if indicated | 1. Do not position on affected area. <br> 2. Follow regular turning schedule. <br> 3. Give high-protein diet. <br> 4. Institute exercise and recreational programs. <br> Alternating pressure mattress <br> Débridement <br> Topical antibiotics <br> Debrisan <br> Surgical intervention |
| 5 | Skin, fat, and muscle necrosis <br><br> Skin <br> Fat <br> Muscle <br> Bone | Relieve pressure <br> Increase circulation <br> Remove necrotic tissue <br> Prevent and treat secondary infection <br> Improve nutrition <br> Relieve anemia | Requires surgery in most cases | 1. Do not position on affected area. <br> 2. Follow regular turning schedule. <br> 3. Give high-protein diet. <br> 4. Institute exercise and recreational programs. <br> Alternating pressure mattress <br> Other areas: use Stryker, Foster, or flotation devices <br> Débridement <br> Debrisan <br> Surgery |

**TABLE 25-2.** Decubitus ulcers: stages and treatment—cont'd

| Stage | Physical signs | Treatment | Prognosis | Nursing orders and modalities |
|---|---|---|---|---|
| 6 | Bone involvement (periostitis, ostitis, osteomyelitis) <br> Skin / Fat / Muscle / Bone | Relieve pressure <br> Increase circulation <br> Remove necrotic tissue <br> Treat secondary infection <br> Improve nutrition <br> Relieve anemia | Requires surgery <br> Little hope of spontaneous healing | 1. Do not position on affected area. <br> 2. Give high-protein diet and supplementary feedings. <br> 3. Institute exercise and recreational programs. <br> Alternating pressure mattress <br> Use Stryker, Foster, or flotation devices <br> Secondary infection treated topically or systemically <br> Surgical débridement |
| 7 | Osteomyelitis, septic arthritis, possible pathological fracture, septicemia | Remove necrotic tissue <br> Control infection <br> Improve nutrition <br> Relieve anemia | Problem almost insurmountable by any means <br> May be candidate for mutilation surgery | 1. Do not position on affected area. <br> 2. Give high-protein diet and supplementary feedings. <br> 3. Institute exercise in affected limbs. <br> Alternating pressure mattress <br> Use Stryker, Foster, or flotation devices <br> Surgical intervention |

It is, however, difficult to determine the extent of skin and underlying tissues involved with present tools. Vrebonic et al. (1972) are researching heat as a measure of tissue involvement, seeking hard data for application in the clinical setting.

Only gross estimates can be made about tissue involvement with induration. Induration is best considered an iceberg with the surface indicating only a small fraction of tissue damage.

## Prevention

The best treatment for pressure sores has been and remains prevention. This means a careful assessment and monitoring by those involved in care. One should use a guide that incorporates a scale similar to Gosnell's and those neurological and metabolic diseases that make clients subject to pressure sores.

The most common sites for pressure have been identified and pressure readings on different surfaces taken. The average capillary pressure at heart level is usually considered to be 25 to 30 mm Hg, and this should be used as a base for all pressure readings (Guyton, 1976). The usual sites identified are occiput, scapula, sacrum, heel, shoulder, elbow, trochanter, knee, malleolus, and ischium. One unpublished study reported readings taken with the person supine on a standard hospi-

tal mattress to be $174 \pm 20$ mm Hg at the occiput, $46 \pm 5$ mm Hg at the sacrum, and $150 \pm 32$ at the heel (Jones, 1973). A study done in England with five subjects reports three types of beds that exert pressures less than capillary pressure on crucial sites. They were the LAL (mobile air support system or air jet support system) bed, feather pillows or foam, and a water bed (Redfern et al., 1973). These systems often prove cumbersome as well as expensive, the LAL bed in particular. Consequently, they are not in wide use; however, more consideration should be made of them as treatment modalities.

Alternating pressure devices will leave areas free of pressure periods of time, but pressure periods always exceed safe readings. They are an adjunct, not an answer, and the practice of positioning for total relief of pressuring is a must. Alternating pressure devices may even cause ulcers in debilitated individuals. It should be remembered that once tissue injury has occurred, it requires less insult for a second injury. The usual length of time considered safe for one position is 2 hours.

Other common surfaces that reduce pressure are foam and synthetic acrylic "sheep skin." Small, spot type of "water mattresses" often prove effective.

Other preventive measures include diet, cleanliness, and control of moisture. A well-balanced diet with supplements, depending on the client's state of nutrition, is essential. Skin lubrication to prevent skin breaks is as important as eliminating excesp moisture to prevent maceration.

## Treatment

Many treatments and special devices have evolved to treat pressure sores. What these treatments and devices contribute is regular observation with a change of position to relieve pressure. A study by Fernie (1975) in Toronto with a bogus "light machine" proved nursing attention alone made the difference in decubitus ulcers. When tissue damage has occurred, the dead tissue must be removed by the body scavenger system or external débridement before healing can take place. Débridement may be achieved by the physician surgically, by enzymes such as collagenase and protolytic enzyme ointment (Travase), by hydrogen peroxide, by dextranomer (Debrisan) by Whirlpool baths, or a system of dressing changing from wet to dry. (The wet dressing loosens or macerates dead tissue. As the dressing dries out, the dead tissue becomes imbedded in the gauze dressing and can be removed with the dressing.) Combinations of these are often prescribed by the physician. Secondary infection may be limited by use of a solution with a pH around 5 (Leveen, 1973). Betadine is one example of a solution with this pH.

Large areas close slowly by granulation; this tissue is delicate and breaks down readily with limited stress. Therefore full-thickness flap grafts are frequently employed over areas such as the ischium, sacrum, and trochanter. (A plastic surgery text is recommended for greater detail.)

## Summary

Pressure sores can be an extremely expensive addition to a rehabilitation program both in terms of money and time. A decubitus ulcer will curtail all other activities. With the imposed bed rest, strength and endurance are greatly reduced. A dollar figure for each decubitus ulcer was calculated in 1975 to be from $10,000 to $15,000 (Fernie, 1975). The cost of lost productivity is incalculable. Above all, nursing must be aggressive in teaching clients and familes to recognize the signs of pressure sores and in ingraining a systematic method of

checking potential sites for ulcer formation. Clients and families must be helped to learn tolerances for bed surfaces and time schedules for moving that eliminate signs of pressure. The water bed, which is growing in popularity for the able bodied, might be the best investment over time for the decubitus ulcer–prone individual.

## BOWEL RETRAINING

Involve the client, physician, and nursing staff on all shifts in the initial observation and development of the plan.

Review all data pertinent to bowel habits before the present illness and the current pattern of elimination.

Determine the time of day that seems most typical of the client's pattern.

Encourage the client to be as active as possible, to develop the tone and strength of the muscles that he or she can use, and to assume the sitting position frequently.

Explain the proposed program to the client, and enlist active participation.

Arrange for the client to have the necessary food and fluids.

Insert a bisacodyl (Dulcolax) suppository high into the rectum against the rectal wall about 15 minutes before the client is scheduled to use the toilet.

Substitute a glycerin suppository as soon as effective results are achieved with Dulcolax. As the client progresses, the suppository should be discontinued.

Assist the client as necessary to use the toilet at the specified time each day.

Control the consistency of the stool with prune juice, diet, fluid intake, Colace, Metamucil, or Serutan.

If the client does not have a bowel movement, give an enema of a prepared solution of sodium phosphate, 120 ml, in a disposable plastic container with an attached rectal nozzle (Travad, Clyserol, Fleet).

## BOWEL AND BLADDER PROBLEMS

Western culture normally is repelled by human wastes, more often on an aesthetic than on a health sanitation basis. Therefore in the rehabilitation process, bowel and bladder management has a high priority. To the professional, loss of control also means a chance for skin breakdown and decubitus ulcer formation.

### Defecation

Management of the bowels of individuals who have lost certain neurological controls is based on "habits" that so-called normal persons find effective. However, the "habits" are normal physiological occurrences in the normal defecation process. Defecation is a reflex that occurs when feces enter the rectum and distend the rectal wall, initiating afferent signals that spread through the myenteric plexus. A reflex peristaltic wave is thus initiated in the descending and sigmoid colon and travels toward the anus. As the peristaltic wave approaches the anus, the internal anal sphincter closure is inhibited by the phenomenon of "receptive relaxation."

Most physiologists believe the directional movement of the bowel occurs because of a special organization of the intramural nerve plexus that preferentially allows analward movement signals. When stimulated electrically, the bowel contracts above and relaxes below. This is the receptive relaxation that gives propulsion to the entire gut. If the external anal sphincter is relaxed, defecation will occur. The reflex itself is weak and must be fortified by another reflex in the sacral segments of the spinal cord. When the afferent fibers in the rectum are stimulated, signals are sent to the spinal cord and then reflexly back to the descending and sigmoid colon, rectum, and anus via parasympathetic fibers that greatly intensify the peristaltic waves and convert the weak movement to a powerful process of defecation, which may empty the bowel all the way from the splenic flexure to the anus.

Additionally, these afferent signals initiate taking a deep breath, closing the glottis, and contracting the abdominal muscles to push down on the contents of the colon. At the same time the pelvic floor is contracted to push feces downward. Normally an individual will prevent defecation until in a socially acceptable position. This is controlled voluntarily by the external sphincter, a skeletal muscle. If the external sphincter is kept contracted, the reflex ceases after a few minutes and does not return for several hours. Persons who inhibit the normal reflexes too often can become severely constipated (Guyton, 1976).

The defecation reflex can be stimulated by the intake of food. Mass movement of the colon is caused principally by the duodenocolic reflex. This results as filling of the duodenum initiates a reflex from the duodenum to the colon and increases the activity of the entire colon. This mass movement reflex can be stimulated only a few times a day

and usually occurs most abundantly for about 10 minutes during the first hour after breakfast (Guyton, 1972). This is the reflex individuals so often attribute to their morning coffee, morning hot water, or some other special food.

The neurologically impaired individual usually has problems with voluntary control, so that the normal reflex must be used more effectively with regard to timing and management. To aid in management the consistency of stool must be considered first. The desired consistency is a formed semisolid. This can be achieved through a balanced diet containing adequate roughage and at least 2000 ml of fluid daily. Drugs to soften the stool, for example, dioctyl sodium sulfosuccinate (Colace), or drugs to add bulk, for example, psyllium hydrophilic mucilloid (Metamucil), will help to bring about the desired consistency. The defecation reflex can be assisted by suppositories, which stimulate the reflex arc. These may be of glycerin, quite gentle, or bisacodyl (Ducolax), more irritating and stimulating. Digital stimulation may be sufficient for some individuals.

In setting up a bowel program, it is best to obtain a bowel history to discover what measures the person has found to be effective in the past. This is particularly true for the elderly. But it must be remembered also that in the elderly more stimulation may be necessary because muscle tone in general has decreased. Individuals with spinal cord injuries can no longer depend on old patterns but must develop a new conditioning program.

The following schedule often proves effective for individuals with stroke and spinal cord injuries after dietary, fluid, and drug measures for stool consistency have been initiated, and the desired stool has resulted. This regimen will not work if the person is constipated or obstipated.

1. Give a suppository (start with bisacodyl) approximately ½ to 1 hour before breakfast.
2. Eat breakfast.
3. Sit on the toilet or commode immediately after breakfast.
4. The young child may be instructed to use a potty chair so that his or her feet may be firmly planted on the floor.
5. Games such as bubble or balloon blowing may be used to instruct the young child in successful bowel evacuation.

Thus the normal function is being used to the fullest. This procedure is usually carried out every other or every third day, if this works out better for the person. Some individuals may find themselves too rushed in the morning and convert to the evening hour. Using the abdominal muscles and closing the glottis may be brought into play deliberately at the evening hour. This type of program helps to maintain and increase muscle tone. Large enemas that decrease bowel tone should be a practice of the past. Until a person with a spinal cord injury is able to manage on a toilet or commode, it is best to allow him or her to defecate in bed, while protecting the bedding with waterproof pads. The pressure of a bedpan for the amount of time that may be required could produce a decubitus ulcer.

## Urinary tract management

Management of the urinary tract for infections is a more critical issue than continence. Urinary tract infections, especially in individuals with spinal cord injuries, are one of three causes of death, with decubitus ulcers and respiratory infections being the other two. Urinary tract infections with progressive kidney damage hold the same place for degenerative neurological diseases such as multiple sclerosis and amyotrophic lateral sclerosis.

Catheters have provided a means of keeping the person dry, keeping the urinary tract open, and allowing free drainage. However, they have also proved a source of infection despite adherence to strict aseptic technique. Attention has been focused on how to eliminate catheters, how to cut down on infections, and how to keep the person free from soiling. Different methods have been practiced to trigger the micturition reflex to achieve a management similar to that of the bowel. The micturition reflex is initiated by stretch receptors in the bladder wall as it fills. Impulses are carried to the sacral segments of the cord through the pelvic nerves and then back again to the bladder through the parasympathetic nerves of the pelvic plexus. Once the reflex begins, it is self-regulating; that is, the initial contraction of the bladder causes a further increase in the afferent impulses from the bladder, which causes a further increase in reflex contraction of the bladder. The cycle repeats itself

again and again until the bladder has reached a strong degree of contraction. Once the micturition reflex has occurred, the sacral portion of the spinal cord usually remains in an inhibited state for at least a few minutes or sometimes up to an hour or more. However, as the bladder fills more, the reflexes become more powerful and more frequent. The desire to empty the bladder usually occurs when the pressure rises to about 12 to 15 mm $H_2O$. This is the voiding pattern of infants or young children who have not learned voluntary control.

The voiding reflex also can be facilitated or inhibited by centers in the brain. There is a strong facilatory center in the upper pons, a strong facilatory center in the hypothalamus, a moderately strong inhibitory center in the midbrain at approximately the level of the superior colliculus, and several centers in the cerebral cortex that are chiefly inhibitory. When it is time to urinate, the cortical centers can facilitate activation of the sacral micturition centers to initiate a micturition reflex and inhibit response of the external urinal sphincter so that urination can occur (Guyton, 1972).

Any interruption in the fiber tracts from the brain to the bladder, the tracts as yet unknown, will interfere with continence and the type of voiding. The micturition reflex also can be weakened when a catheter is left in place for a long period of time. The reflex is not called into play, and the bladder loses tone. Individuals suffering brain injury caused by trauma, tumors, or stroke frequently lack control immediately after injury. These persons must respond quickly to the urge to void. If the person is unaware of voiding, he or she voids automatically. A toileting schedule of every 1 to 2 hours may help the individual develop the ability to recognize bladder filling and emptying. When relearning does not occur, it is a sign of extensive brain damage.

Frequency and urgency of voiding may occur when a urinary tract infection is present and may interfere with controls. Urine must be checked regularly for color, odor, particles, pH, and microorganisms to discover and treat infections early. Infection will interfere with learning control and will damage the kidneys. This is especially true if the person has had a catheter in for any length of time. Urinary tract infections can occur within 24 hours after a catheter has been inserted.

The individual with a spinal cord injury presently has no voluntary control and will have either an automatically emptying bladder, if the reflex arc is intact (injury above the sacral segment), or potentially a flaccid, nonemptying bladder, if all fibers of the sacral segments are damaged. Fortunately in most instances, sufficient sacral fibers remain intact for there to be a reflex. However, with certain practices the individual can become catheter free and eliminate a major source of infection. Management depends on a sufficient micturition reflex that will empty the bladder, leaving less than a 100 ml residual.

This management has been achieved through intermittent catheterization and drugs. Intermittent catheterization allows the bladder to fill and respond to reflexes that are intact. Catheters suppress this filling stimulus. Guttmann and Frankel in 1966 reported the results of an 11-year study of intermittent catheterization in the early management of traumatic paraplegia and quadriplegia. Of 409 men treated, 80.7% were discharged with sterile urine; additionally, 67 women had sterile urine, a rate of 59.7%. Those clients treated with only intermittent catheterizations had a 7% infection rate, whereas those treated originally with Foley catheters had a 61% infection rate in men and 20% in women (Guttmann, 1966).

In 1974 Lapidis et al. theorized that "most cases of urinary tract infection are caused by some structural or functional abnormality of the urogenital tract which leads to decreased resistance of tissue and to bacterial invasion. . . . Maintenance of a good blood supply to the bladder by avoiding high intravesical pressures and overdistention is the key to prevention of urinary tract infection. Residual urine in itself and the bacterial flora in the urethra and vagina are of little import in the genesis of urinary infection." On this theory, Lapidis began clean, intermittent self-catheterization. Results of 100 clients after 4 years showed 65% had completely negative urine and 41% had no antibacterial medication after initial treatment (Lapidis et al., 1974).

A regimen that has proved effective at the Medical Center of the University of Rochester is the following (Gibson, 1977):

1. Limit the fluids to 1500 mg/day so that the bladder will not become overdistended.
2. Catheterize every 6 hours until the client voids spontaneously.
3. Catheterize every 8 hours if he or she consistently voids 300 to 400 ml or if he or she has 200 to 300 ml of residual urine after voiding (catheterizing immediately after voiding).
4. When the residual postvoided urine falls to 100 to 150 ml or less, catheterize every 3 to 4 days.
5. Then check the client weekly as a precaution.
6. Appropriate modification can be made in this plan when the client is a child.

The micturition reflex may require extra stimulation; it is assisted by the drug bethanechol chloride (Urocholine), which acts on the parasympathetic fibers in the bladder. An overactive reflex may be reduced by methantheline (Banthine) or oxybutynin (Ditropan).

Male clients use external collecting devices such as condoms, a DuVaul external urinal, or a McGuire urinal. These devices are attached to leg bags when the person is mobile and to straight drainage when in bed. Female clients may wear a protective pad for stress incontinence during physical conditioning activities.

The individual and family members are taught how to perform sterile catheterizations. This technique is to be used as long as the person is hospitalized. Paraplegic and occasionally quadriplegic female clients (level of lesion C6 or C7) learn self-catheterization first in bed by using a mirror. Paraplegic female clients whose injury is to the lower cord may need to continue this practice for several months after discharge; so they are taught to do this procedure while sitting on a toilet.

Clean catheterizations are done with the person cleaning the meatus with soap and water only. Catheters for clean self-catheterization are boiled for 20 minutes and kept in a clean container, for example, a fruit jar. When the client returns to work, various clean containers can be used, for example, compacts or cosmetic bags for women and Dopp kits for men. Some clients, such as children with spina bifida, may use the same catheter several times, washing it only with soap and water between catheterizations.

Female quadriplegics will require catheters if they cannot transfer to a toilet for voiding. It is too much of a hardship for someone else to keep these women dry when they cannot care for themselves. The catheter is changed weekly, with no irrigations between changes to introduce organisms. The person is also required to have a fluid intake of 2500 to 3000 ml daily to keep the urinary tract flushed. The overall objective is to keep the individual with impaired bladder function, if at all possible, free of an indwelling catheter and free of infection.

### Associated problems

One problem that may occur in the client with a spinal cord injury during bladder conditioning (or later if some obstruction occurs in the urethra or bladder neck) is autonomic dysreflexia or hyperreflexia. This is characterized by exaggerated autonomic responses to stimuli. Individuals who have cervical lesions or high thoracic lesions are at greatest risk because the normal controls of the hypothalamus and brainstem autonomic areas no longer function. In these high lesions a stimulus such as a distended bladder or distended bowel will initiate excessive sympathetic or parasympathetic discharges. The result is severe hypertension of the exaggerated reflex, which can be a crisis for the person with a spinal cord injury. The hypertension results when stimuli arising in the bladder travel cephalad through the pelvic nerves to the spinal cord and ascend by way of the spinothalamic tracts and posterior columns to the level of the spinal cord injury. These impulses then complete the reflex through autonomic outflow of neurons in the lateral horns to cause spasm of the pelvic viscera, arteriolar spasm in the splanchnic vessels, pilomotor erection, and sweating. Splanchnic vasoconstriction can cause elevated blood pressure, stimulating receptors in the aortic arch and carotid sinus to send impulses to the vagus and glossopharyngeal nerves and to the vasomotor regulatory centers in the medulla. The vagus nerve transmits impulses to the heart, resulting in bradycardia. The high blood pressure with the bradycardia results in a pounding headache. The blood pressure may rise to 300/160 mm Hg.

Superficial vasodilatation can occur in areas above the cord injury, resulting in flushing of the face and neck, engorgement of the large temporal and neck vessels, and nasal congestion. Seizures may follow. The danger of this dysreflexia is in its relationship to acute myocardial failure and intracranial or retinal hemorrhage.

Nurses must always be alert for signs of bradycardia, flushing, and headache in clients with high cord injuries. If the client is supine, he or she should be placed in the sitting position immediately, because this normally reduces the blood pressure significantly. The physician must be called immediately to aid in the management of this crisis. The blood pressure must be checked every 3 to 5 minutes. The source of stimuli must be investigated immediately. A distended bladder or bowel is the usual cause. The bladder requires immediate emptying and follow-up as to cause. If the source is a distended rectum, it should not be evacuated until the blood pressure subsides. Dibucaine (Nupercaine) ointment should be placed in the rectum 10 minutes before one attempts evacuation (Taylor, 1974). The physician may use phentolamine (Regitine) to control the elevated blood pressure. To control frequent episodes of autonomic dysreflexia, oral ganglionic blocking agents such as pentolinium (Ansolysen) or mecamylamine (Inversine) may be used.

### Summary

Bladder and bowel management has posed many problems, but with the engagement of the normal physiological processes and regulation with certain drugs, acceptable patterns can be established to allow persons to move freely in society.

## PARALYSIS, PARESIS, AND WEAKNESS

Paralysis, paresis, and generalized weakness can result in deforming contractures unless preventive practices of positioning and exercise are started when these conditions first appear. Preventive practices also must be continued as long as the conditions exist.

Paralysis is defined as the loss or impairment of the ability to move parts of the body. It is a symptom of a variety of physical and emotional disorders (Miller and Keane, 1972). The most frequent types of paralysis dealt with in rehabilitation are flaccid and spastic paralysis. *Flaccid paralysis* results when lower motor neurons are affected. These neurons consist of cell bodies located in the anterior gray column of the spinal cord or brainstem and an axon passing by way of the peripheral nerves to the motor end plates of the muscles. These are the essential motor cells for motor activities. Lesions result from trauma, toxins, infections, vascular disorders, degenerative processes, neoplasms, and congenital malformations (Krusen et al., 1971). Poliomyelitis, a viral infection, was an all-too-often example until the Salk vaccine. Guillain-Barré syndrome is a more common example of an infectious process at the present time.

Contractures develop in flaccid paralysis because of the nature of the loose connective tissue around body joints. Normally, loose connective tissue develops between organs and other structures, such as joint capsules, fasciae, intermuscular layers, and subcutaneous tissues, where movement occurs continually. This tissue will elongate under prolonged tension or shorten where there is no motion. When a body part is immobilized, the collagenous and reticular networks become contracted, so that the tissue becomes dense and hard and loses the suppleness of normal aerolar tissue (Chusid, 1979).

*Spastic paralysis* involves the upper motor neurons, which convey impulses from the motor area of the cerebrum and which are essential for voluntary muscular activity. The processes of the nerve cells of the motor cortex pass through the internal capsule, brainstem, and spinal cord by way of the corticobulbar or corticospinal tracts to the lower motor neurons (Chusid, 1979). The reflex arcs of the lower motor neurons are intact, and the interaction results in spasticity.

Contractures develop in spastic paralysis in the same manner as in flaccid paralysis. The abnormal tightness and shortening of joints cause the areolar tissue to change to a dense meshwork of tissue and tight bands. This change in connective tissue can occur within 1 week of immobility or, with trauma, in as short a time as 3 days. The tension of the shortened connective tissue has been measured as 14 kg/cm² of cross section, a considerable force. Contractures caused by spasticity may develop in any joint, but those that affect walking, bathing, and dressing are most disabling. Hip, knee, ankle, and toe contractures will disturb posture and bal-

ance, limiting or making walking impossible. These leg contractures, as well as shoulder, elbow, and wrist contractures, make dressing difficult and often painful.

Spasticity is defined as a lower threshold to the stretch reflex, an enlarged area from which the reflex may be obtained and an exaggeration of the stretch reflex associated with a tendency to develop contractures in the antigravity muscles. Reviewing the anatomy and physiology of the muscle spindle and neuroinnervation may clarify how and why spasticity occurs (Fig. 25-4). Muscle contains two types of fibers: short round (intrafusal) fibers and long cylindrical (extrafusal) fibers. Two types of sensory impulses originate within these muscle spindles: a larger rapidly conducting, monosynaptic afferent fiber originating in the smaller muscle spindle (gamma efferent), and a higher threshold, polysynaptic, conducting fiber originating in the longer muscle spindle bodies in the anterior horn of the spinal cord (alpha efferent). The polysynaptic afferent fibers of the long muscle fibers synapse with motor fibers of the short muscle fibers in the ventral horn to form a loop. Stretch or movement of the long muscle fibers stimulates the sensory endings within the short muscle fibers (Mossman, 1976). Thus the reflex arc is set in motion.

The motor nuclei in the anterior horn are under constant influences of supraspinal facilitation and inhibition through the descending tracts of the spinal cord. The cerebellum also is involved, as it controls the rate of motor fiber discharge and modifies the afferent discharges from the muscle spindle. The cerebellum coordinates motor and sensory activity in a smooth-running servomechanism. Constant muscle activity through the muscle sensors is called *muscle tone*. The exaggerated, uncontrolled muscle activity is spasticity. Spasticity develops when there is a disruption of the extrapyramidal motor system, the servomechanism. Lesions may be located in the cerebral cortex, internal capsule, cerebral peduncles, brainstem, or spinal cord (Mossman, 1976). Spasticity is increased further with emotional upset and any infection. Clients with spinal cord injuries can often judge the extent of their urinary tract or pressure sore infections by the increase in spasticity.

Problems attendant with spasticity relate to mobility and self-care. Clonus, a reverberating self-

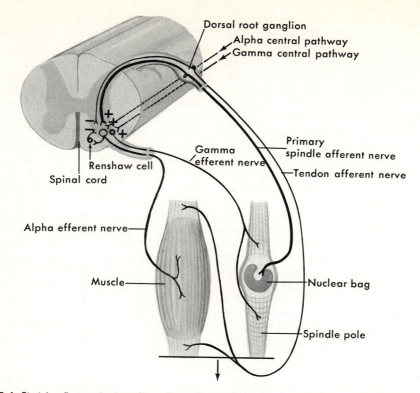

**FIG. 25-4.** Stretch reflex mechanism. (From Schottelius, B.A., and Schottelius, D.D.: Textbook of physiology, ed. 18, St. Louis, 1978, The C.V. Mosby Co.)

perpetuating segmental stretch reflex, may be triggered in the affected leg of a stroke client when the foot first hits the ground. Full weight bearing does suppress the reflex, but walking may be difficult, and the client feels insecure. Bracing resolves some of the problems. A spastic arm and shoulder make dressing difficult and more so if there is pain from a subluxated shoulder. The corticospinal control disruption in cerebral palsy presents the same type self-care and ambulatory problems. Clients with spinal cord injuries may have such severe reflexes that they can be thrown out of a wheelchair or bed. Restraining straps are needed for the wheelchair and sheet restraints for the bed. Clients may have the strength to perform self-care activities, but spasms may prevent these activities. Certain paraplegic and quadriplegic clients, however, can learn to trigger extensor spasms to allow

them to stand and do bed and even car transfers with minimal or no assistance.

Spasticity is treated medically by drugs, nerve injection, and occasionally surgery. Surgery is not used so frequently as in the past, since it was found that the interruption of one reflex pattern allowed other reflexes to come into play that often were as debilitating as the eliminated spastic pattern. Phenol nerve block, chemical neurolysis, is used instead, primarily for the lower legs and forearms. A phenol block may last up to 6 months and may be repeated. This treatment is less risky than surgery.

Drugs used to relieve spasticity include diazepam (Valium), which works on the polysynaptic pathways, and more recently dantrolene (Dantrium), which acts on the muscle body. Those two drugs may be used in combination, since diazepam in doses to depress spasm often makes the person very drowsy, too drowsy to engage in any meaningful activity.

Paresis is defined as incomplete paralysis, which is a common symptom of degenerative diseases such as multiple sclerosis and tertiary syphilis. Debilitating but reversible situations such as severe trauma may leave individuals extremely weak with poor muscle tone and limited endurance. These persons with weakness or paresis can develop contractures in the same manner as those with flaccid paralysis.

If an individual who has developed paralysis, paresis, or weakness is expected to be mobile in the future, the skeletal system must be maintained to assume the functional upright position for walking, that is, of a plumb line dropping from the ear to the shoulder, to the hip, to the knee, to the ankle. This position distributes the body weight for easily maintained balance. It also allows for good aeration of the lungs. One of the positions for a bed client must be this flat aligned position (see boxed material on p. 644). Other bed positions must allow for good lung aeration as well as prevention of contractures. Splints may be used to help maintain functional positions of hands and feet, especially with spastic paralysis. Light splints can be molded from Duraplast.* This material can be remolded quickly to relieve a pressure point or to improve the functional position of an extremity. Velcro straps are used to keep the splints in position. Anyone wearing a splint, especially someone with spasticity, must have the skin checked carefully and regularly for pressure. If a splint fits well, it is more readily tolerated.

## Exercise

Exercise is one of the most important parts of any rehabilitation program. It maintains the existing functional capabilities of the individual and upgrades or retrains other capacities. An exercise program is a type of athletic training program from a medical prescription. A program may have one or several components. A range-of-motion program for freely moving joints is essential for independent or assisted mobility. Other exercises provide for developing strength, endurance, and coordination. Exercises are also classified as active (the individual performs the exercise), passive (the person is exercised), and active assistive (the person exercising is given physical assistance as necessary). Passive exercise will maintain range of motion, increase blood flow, and give a sense of well-being, but it will not build muscle strength or endurance.

The normal activity of a healthy individual gives full range of motion many times a day to all parts of the body, including joint capsules, muscles, subcutaneous tissue, and ligaments. With restriction of the range of motion for any reason, tightness occurs. To maintain full joint range of motion, one should carry all joints through a full range three times twice daily (Krusen et al., 1971). The reader is referred to a standard text on physical medicine for exact joint ranges. The individual should carry out the exercises as much as possible after being instructed. When the individual is being exercised by a therapist, nurse, or family member, the following measures will facilitate the program:

1. Stabilize the joints above and below the joint being exercised.
2. Support the stabilized joints by the palms of the hands, not grasping tightly. Do not give support at the muscle belly, especially when inflammation or pain is present.
3. Move the joint smoothly and at a slow even rhythm.
4. Exercise the individual when he or she is warm and relaxed.

Exercises to stretch, that is, increase the range of motion, should be done under the supervision of a physician. As a rule, tight muscles can be stretched vigorously unless there is inflammation. This stretching should be done beyond the point of pain, but there should be no residual pain. With persons who have had prolonged disuse, paralysis, or anesthesia, caution must be used because of osteoporosis with the danger of fractures (Krusen et al., 1971). For increasing various joint ranges by stretching, refer to a text on physical medicine.

Exercises to develop strength and endurance make it possible to carry on useful activities, in particular, the activities of daily living. *Strength* can be defined as the maximal tension that can be

---

*Johnson & Johnson, Health Care Division, New Brunswick, N.J.

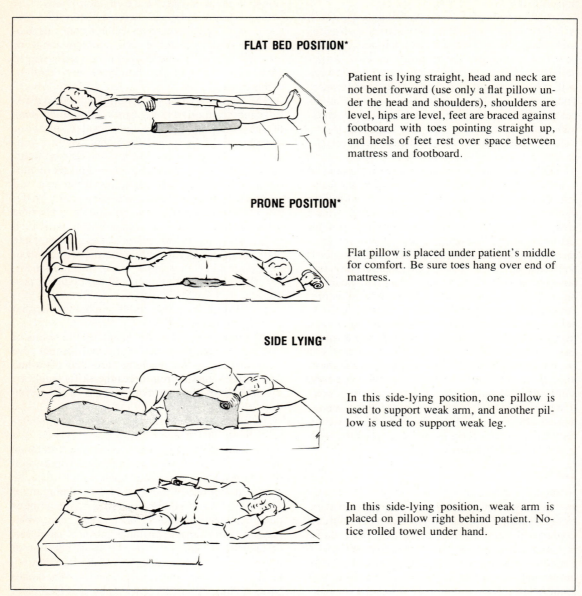

**FLAT BED POSITION***

Patient is lying straight, head and neck are not bent forward (use only a flat pillow under the head and shoulders), shoulders are level, hips are level, feet are braced against footboard with toes pointing straight up, and heels of feet rest over space between mattress and footboard.

**PRONE POSITION***

Flat pillow is placed under patient's middle for comfort. Be sure toes hang over end of mattress.

**SIDE LYING***

In this side-lying position, one pillow is used to support weak arm, and another pillow is used to support weak leg.

In this side-lying position, weak arm is placed on pillow right behind patient. Notice rolled towel under hand.

*Reprinted with permission of the American Heart Association.

exerted by a muscle during a contraction. *Endurance* is the ability of a muscle to contract and exert tension over a prolonged period of time (Krusen et al., 1971). To accomplish a task, the individual requires strength (force) sufficient to move (distance) a body part. In mechanical terms, this is called *work*. A better measure of the person's ability to function is how many times he or she can perform this task per unit of time or how much power he or she has. The use of maximal strength gives rapid muscle fatigue, but this is rarely required for functional activities. Repetitive activities at less than maximal strength produce fatigue at a slower rate (Krusen et al., 1971).

Increasing tension on a muscle, according to several studies, is the method by which muscle strength is increased. This can be done through isometric exercise, tensing but not shortening muscles, or concentric exercise, shortening muscles. One study reported that regularly recurring exercise in which tension exceeded 35% of the muscle strength resulted in an increase of muscle strength. Tension fo 20% to 35% maintained strength, and less than 20% did not maintain strength. De Lorme developed a series of progressive resistive exercises in 1945 to increase strength, to increase use of more muscle units, and to withstand the discomfort of heavy exercise (Krusen et al., 1971). (Refer to a text on physical medicine for the method.) These and similar exercises are used as a basis for building strength.

Exercises for endurance are designed around factors of muscle strength, circulation, and muscle metabolism. As a muscle becomes stronger, work against a constant load requires proportionately less of the muscle to be contracting at any instant and leaves a greater recovery period for muscle fibers after contracting. During muscle activity, motor units contract, but they contract intermittently. Tension is sustained through the irregular contractions and relaxations of many motor units. If the rest period between muscle contractions is not long enough for metabolic recovery, the muscle becomes fatigued. It takes 20 times longer for metabolic muscle recovery than for a contraction. Metabolites developed in a muscle during work serve as stimuli to increase local circulation, cardiac work, and respiration. A decrease in the blood pH caused by muscular metabolites will dilate the arterioles, capillaries, and veins within the muscles. Repeated and prolonged exercise may increase the number of capillaries by 40% (Krusen et al., 1971).

Exercises for developing endurance consist of low resistance and high repetition. The exercises need to be repeated hundreds of times each day and should result in muscle fatigue at the end of an exercise period. The resistance on the muscle should be between 15% and 40%. The greater the resistance, the more quickly fatigue will result. Boredom can be the greatest problem with this type of exercise (Krusen et al., 1971). Occupational therapy plays an important part in adapting crafts of interest to the individual to those muscle groups that need to regain strength and endurance.

Exercise for coordination requires careful analysis of the task to be accomplished to determine the muscles used and the exact sequence in which the task is to be performed. The person learning the task must be rational, old enough to comprehend and follow instructions, and able to cooperate and concentrate on the muscular task during the exercise period. The person must have intact proprioception to monitor activity. When the person becomes fatigued or inattentive, the activity should be ended (Krusen et al., 1971). (The reader is referred to a standard text on physical medicine for exact techniques for teaching particular coordination skills.) Nursing reinforces the skills taught by the disciplines of physical or occupational therapy. The teaching and learning involved follow the same principles for learning any new skill. Because fewer ways are available for learning, it is important for the person not to expend energy on habits he or she must unlearn.

In any exercise to develop strength and endurance the cardiac and respiratory systems require observation. The Committee on Exercise of the American Heart Association in 1972 published guidelines for training healthy individuals. Heart rate was indicated as a good measure to use in regulating or prescribing intensity of exercise. Heart rate studies from Scandinavia, other European countries, and the United States established safe maximal heart rates for specific decades of life in healthy individuals. One method of calculating maximum safe rate for endurance exercises is to take 75% of the age-corrected predicted maximum heart rate. For example, at age 50 years, the maximum rate for an untrained person is 187; multipled by 75%, this equals 138. This rate can be established only after cardiac examination.

It must be remembered that with illness and deconditioning, cardiac output will decrease, and maximal heart rate may actually increase slightly. When starting exercise for strength and endurance, the goal of pulse rate may be set at 40% over the resting pulse. For example, a resting pulse of 72 plus 40%, or 28, equals 100. With any existing cardiac problems, full-scale cardiac testing is required. The exercise program is then set up by the cardiologist, with guidelines for monitoring. With any conditioning program, muscle power is developed slowly at a submaximal level.

## MOBILITY

A number of elements are necessary for safe mobility activities. First, there must be voluntarily controlled muscle power sufficient to push or pull the individual's body weight. This power will differ for various activities, from rolling in bed, to sitting up, to walking. Weight will be borne according to the strength of the supporting limbs. The more equal the weight distribution, the less energy is used. The better functioning muscles must expend more energy to support the total body weight when one or two extremities are weak and the individual fatigues quickly. Conditioning exercises for strength and endurance are preparatory. External bracing may be prescribed by the physician to compensate for limited muscle strength. The brace will slow down the fatigue rate of the weak muscles and increase endurance.

Second, the person must have adequate balance. This requires proprioception, a knowledge of where the body is in space, muscle power, and muscle control to keep the body upright. Persons with right parietal lobe damage usually have balance problems.

Third, the person must have judgment about abilities and limitations in order to recognize potential danger. Again, this is related to the right parietal lobe. Visual field restrictions will also impair judgment. Without adequate balance and judgment the individual cannot become as mobile as the muscle power would indicate. The func-

tional level must be kept lower to prevent bodily injury. When an individual is being mobilized, he or she must be taken through the developmental motor patterns to an upright standing position. Bringing a person to the feet and expecting him or her to walk after being cared for in bed for several days will most likely end in failure. Such an experience could delay involvement in mobility activities. First teach the person to roll from side to side in bed while he or she grips the mattress. Assist with only enough force to make up for any lack of power (see boxed material opposite). The second stage is sitting (see boxed material on pp. 648 and 649 for the steps a client who had a stroke would use). Assistance must be given for placing the legs, rolling to the strong side, and rising when the person begins this maneuver. As he or she gains strength and balance, help is withdrawn to only standby assistance. Individuals with quadriplegia and paraplegia may be lifted and placed in chairs long before they are capable of assisting themselves to a sitting position. For principles of lifting and moving, refer to *Lifting, Moving and Transferring Patients* (Rantz and Courtial, 1977).

The next step of mobilization is moving from bed to chair, a transfer (see boxed material on p. 650 for the steps a stroke client would use). Special slings or trapezes will be used by quadriplegics and paraplegics before they acquire sufficient power to lift themselves from bed to chair (Rantz and Courtial, 1977). It is important that the person lift to cut down on the friction of sliding from one surface to another. Sliding can result in friction burns. Lifting also prevents bruises from protruding parts of furniture.

Ambulation may require assistive devices such as canes or walkers, depending on the limbs affected (see boxed material on pp. 650 and 651 for the limited assistance devices a client who had a stroke would use). For special ambulation training, refer to standard texts on physical medicine and rehabilitation (for example, *Physical Medicine* [Rusk, 1977]).

In summary, there are certain rules to follow for each of the mobility activities:

1. Start movements from the strong side of the body.

*Text continued on p. 654.*

## ROLLING OVER IN BED*

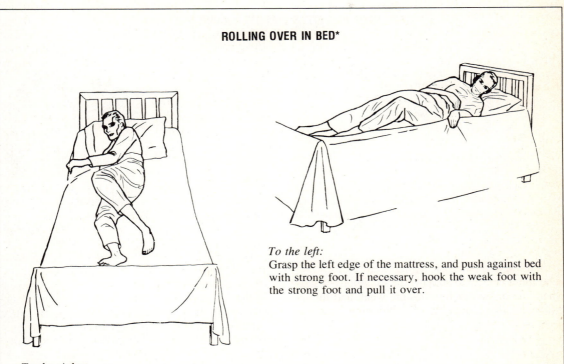

*To the left:*
Grasp the left edge of the mattress, and push against bed with strong foot. If necessary, hook the weak foot with the strong foot and pull it over.

*To the right:*
Grasp the right edge of the mattress, pull with strong arm, and push against bed with strong foot.

*Reprinted with permission of the American Heart Association.

**GETTING UP AND SITTING ON THE SIDE OF THE BED***

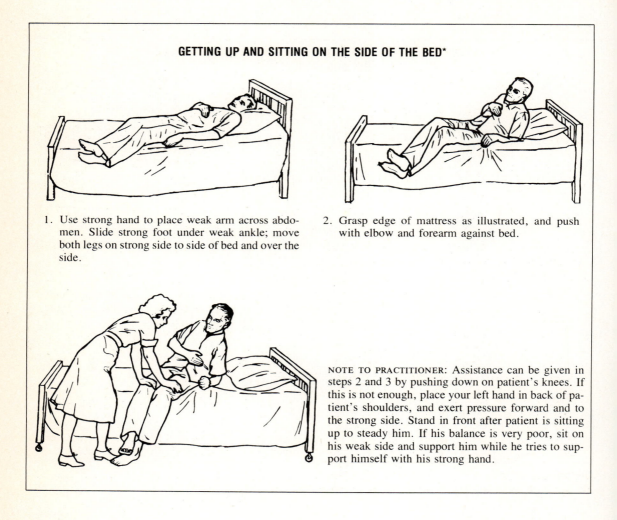

1. Use strong hand to place weak arm across abdomen. Slide strong foot under weak ankle; move both legs on strong side to side of bed and over the side.

2. Grasp edge of mattress as illustrated, and push with elbow and forearm against bed.

NOTE TO PRACTITIONER: Assistance can be given in steps 2 and 3 by pushing down on patient's knees. If this is not enough, place your left hand in back of patient's shoulders, and exert pressure forward and to the strong side. Stand in front after patient is sitting up to steady him. If his balance is very poor, sit on his weak side and support him while he tries to support himself with his strong hand.

**GETTING UP AND SITTING ON THE SIDE OF THE BED —cont'd**

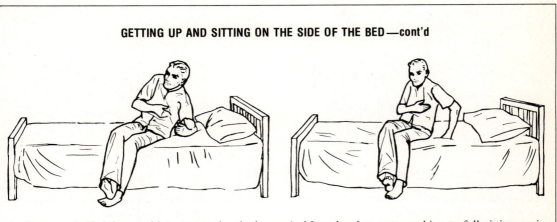

3. Come to half-sitting position, supporting body weight on strong forearm.

4. Move hand to rear, pushing to full sitting position.

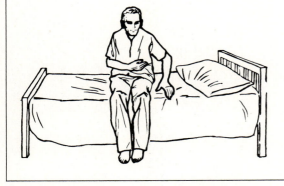

5. Move around until sitting securely on side of bed; uncross legs.

CAUTION: If patient feels dizzy when he first sits up, stand in front of him and give support if needed.

*Reprinted with permission of the American Heart Association.

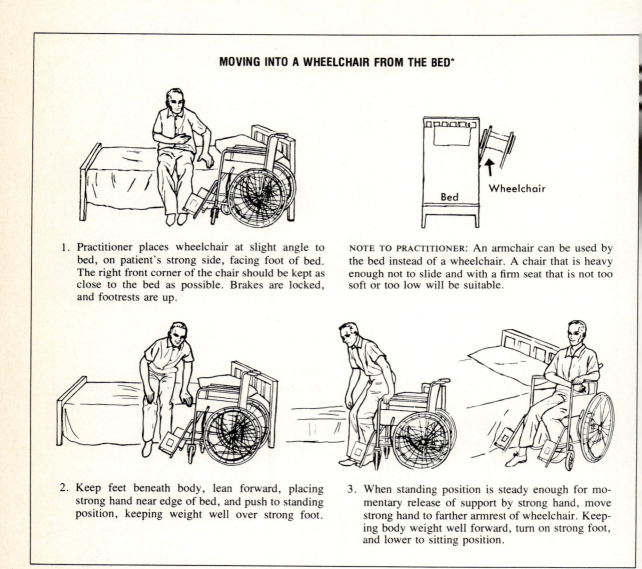

## MOVING INTO A WHEELCHAIR FROM THE BED*

1. Practitioner places wheelchair at slight angle to bed, on patient's strong side, facing foot of bed. The right front corner of the chair should be kept as close to the bed as possible. Brakes are locked, and footrests are up.

NOTE TO PRACTITIONER: An armchair can be used by the bed instead of a wheelchair. A chair that is heavy enough not to slide and with a firm seat that is not too soft or too low will be suitable.

2. Keep feet beneath body, lean forward, placing strong hand near edge of bed, and push to standing position, keeping weight well over strong foot.

3. When standing position is steady enough for momentary release of support by strong hand, move strong hand to farther armrest of wheelchair. Keeping body weight well forward, turn on strong foot, and lower to sitting position.

*Reprinted with permission of the American Heart Association.

## WALKING WITH SUPPORT*

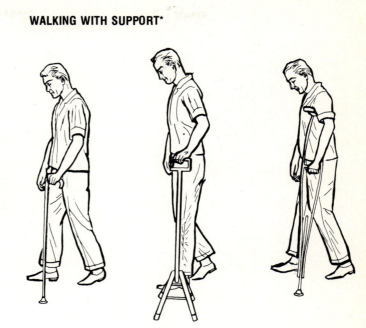

NOTE TO PRACTITIONER: Proper height of cane and crutch hand support. The height, when the support is placed on the floor, should allow patient's elbow to be bent slightly, as illustrated.

CAUTION: Do not let weak foot get ahead of cane or crutch.

### Cane

Place cane ahead of strong foot and slightly out to side. Step ahead with weak foot, placing it opposite cane. Take all of body weight on weak leg and the cane, and step ahead with strong foot. Repeat steps.

*or*

Start with both feet and cane in line, all slightly separated. Step ahead with cane and weak foot at the same time. Then taking body weight on weak leg and cane, step ahead with strong foot. Repeat steps.

### Crutch for support

Be sure there is space under the arm between top of crutch and underarm. Be sure crutch has ''Safe-T-Tip.'' Directions for walking with crutch are the same as for cane.

### Wide-base cane

Place cane a few inches ahead of strong foot, then bring weak foot forward and place it opposite cane. Shift body weight to weak leg and cane, and step ahead with strong foot. Repeat steps.

NOTE TO PRACTITIONER: Usually short steps are easier than long steps. Try to keep the patient's steps uniform in size. Be sure cane is equipped with ''Safe-T-Tip.''

*Reprinted with permission of the American Heart Association.

## CLIMBING STAIRS*

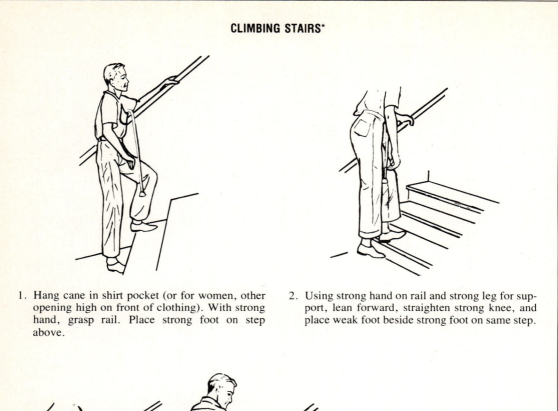

1. Hang cane in shirt pocket (or for women, other opening high on front of clothing). With strong hand, grasp rail. Place strong foot on step above.

2. Using strong hand on rail and strong leg for support, lean forward, straighten strong knee, and place weak foot beside strong foot on same step.

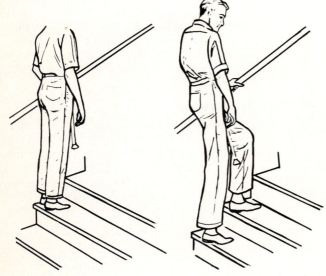

RULE: Go up with strong foot first. Bring weak foot to same step.

NOTE TO PRACTITIONER: It is not advisable for patient to go up and down stairs without a handrail unless he has nearly normal strength and balance. There should be a handrail down the center of the steps or one along each side. Going up and down stairs using a handrail can be done by a patient with a very weak leg provided he places his feet carefully and his weak knee is straight when he takes his weight on it.

3. Repeat steps 1 and 2, climbing one step at a time.

*Reprinted with permission of the American Heart Association.

# DESCENDING STAIRS*

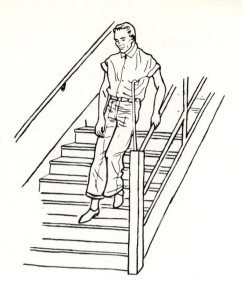

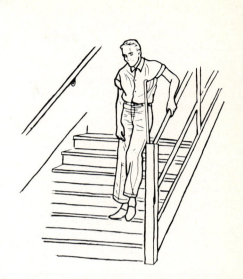

1. Make sure toes of strong foot overlap edge of step before starting down. Grasp handrail with strong hand. Place weak foot on next step below, bending strong knee as weak foot goes down.

2. When weak foot is firmly placed with knee straight and leg is able to support body weight, step down to same step with strong foot.

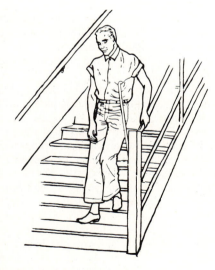

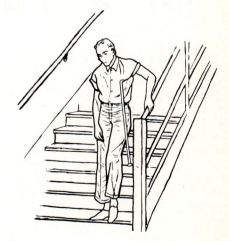

3. Repeat steps 1 and 2.

RULE: Go down stairs with weak foot first. Bring strong foot down to the same step.

*Reprinted with permission of the American Heart Association.

2. Achieve balance at each step of a maneuver before starting the next.
3. Stop before becoming overfatigued.
4. Be patient; accept small gains.

## DRESSING

The principles that apply to mobility practices apply to the skills of dressing. The same problem of perception, balance, and dexterity apply. Upper extremity mobility is even more important for this task. Certain guidelines follow, exemplified well with stroke clients (see also boxed material on pp. 655 and 656):

1. Start dressing the extremity on the affected side first.
2. Maintain balance at every stage.
3. Teach the individual with perceptual problems using verbal instructions.
4. Color code parts of clothing for identification for the perceptually impaired, for example, use colored thread on the collar of the shirt to indicate which side of the garment is right as well as the neck opening.
5. Instruct individuals with damage to the left side of their brain by showing. Do not confuse them with verbal instructions.

## ADJUSTMENT TO DISABILITY

Rehabilitation for the neurologically impaired individual requires an extended time in soul-searching for adjustment. Each person adjusts according to past experiences and previous methods of coping.

The value that the disabled individual places on him- or herself may appear to change the personality, especially since negative values are placed on a disability. Society and culture determine human values, with youth and the body beautiful ranking high in Western culture.

Besides evoking a negative response for its presence, the disability has so powerful a stimulus that it causes a spread-of-effect phenomenon. This means that persons seeing the disabled individual assume he or she cannot perform certain tasks associated with the disability as well as others completely unrelated. As an example, if a person is blind, persons speak loudly to him or her, as if the hearing ability was impaired. This same spread-of-effect phenomenon is often displayed by the disabled in overgeneralizing the effects of their dis-

abilities. This is not unexpected because of the amount of negative feedback the person receives from friends (Krusen et al., 1971). He or she becomes a member of another minority group.

The negative aspects of the disability must be put into perspective with the total assets the person possesses. The individual must think positively about what he or she can do compared with others rather than what he or she cannot do. The value system of the general public must be shifted to an asset value system of present and potential abilities. All treatments and techniques in rehabilitation must be directed toward helping the disabled make this shift.

In making the value shift, the adjustment to a disablity, there are certain stages an individual goes through to make peace with the "new person" who has evolved. This process is essentially the process of grief and grieving over a loved one, the person before the disability. Fink in 1967 developed a model of the "psychological phases of crises," which identifies the stages of shock (stress), defensive retreat, acknowledgement (renewed stress), and, finally, adaptation and change. There is no time framework. Each person must go at an individual pace, which may be a few months to many years for the final resolution.

In the initial stage of shock the person feels panic, anxiety, and helplessness, with no ability to plan, reason, or understand what is happening. Professionals must give information but not expect the person to internalize the meaning. This is also the time dominated by the acute medical problem of the trauma.

As the person enters the stage of defensive retreat, he or she may appear euphoric except when challenged; then the result may be anger. The individual avoids reality through wishful thinking. This may be seen in a champion skier who has a cervical spine injury and says he or she will be back on the slopes next winter. This person is resisting change, although the physical condition is beginning to indicate the degree of functional ability. Professionals must work with the person to help him or her realize remaining abilities and not to allow him or her to avoid a program because of a belief in ultimate recovery. Professionals do not destroy these fantasies but hope the client will recognize the reality of the situation.

When the person acknowledges what has hap-

## PUTTING ON A SHIRT OR DRESS*

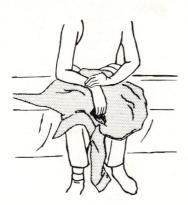

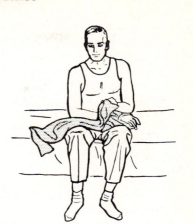

1. Spread shirt on lap inside up and collar away from body.

2. Using strong hand, place weak hand in right armhole and pull sleeve up weak arm.

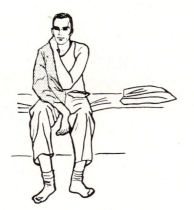

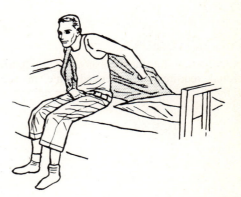

3. Throw rest of garment behind body, and pull right sleeve all the way up.

4. Reach behind with strong hand, and place it in left armhole. Work sleeve into position.

NOTE TO PRACTITIONER: Dressing while sitting on side of bed is easier than in wheelchair if balance is good. If balance is poor, have patient sit in wheelchair or heavy armchair to dress.

An open-down-the-front dress, sweater, or coat is put on the same way as a shirt, but it is necessary to stand up and straighten the skirt before it can be fastened.

Large buttons are easier to fasten than snaps.

*Reprinted with permission of the American Heart Association.

## PUTTING ON TROUSERS*

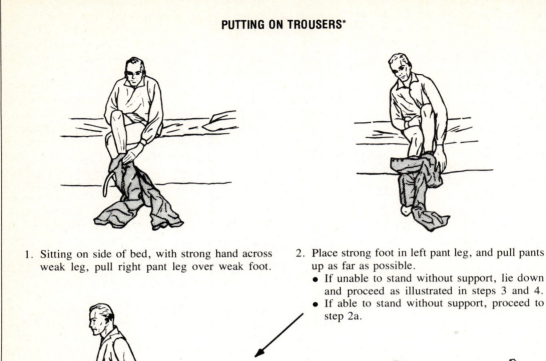

1. Sitting on side of bed, with strong hand across weak leg, pull right pant leg over weak foot.

2. Place strong foot in left pant leg, and pull pants up as far as possible.
   - If unable to stand without support, lie down and proceed as illustrated in steps 3 and 4.
   - If able to stand without support, proceed to step 2a.

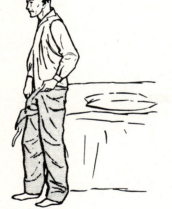

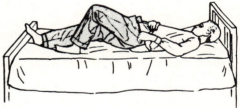

3. Lie down; bend strong knee and hip, pushing strong foot against bed to raise hips. Pull pants up over hips.

2a. If standing balance against bed without support of strong hand is possible, stand leaning against bed for support and pull pants up with strong hand.

NOTE TO PRACTITIONER: If patient cannot cross legs, he can rest his weak foot on a small stool to assist in this activity.

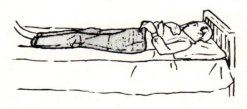

4. Fasten front of pants.

*Reprinted with permission of the American Heart Association.

pened, one observes great depression, apathy, and even a desire for suicide if the reality is too overwhelming. Physically the person may have reached a plateau, and the goal of being completely well is shattered. The depression and grief should be considered a favorable sign that the person is grappling with reality. Without this mourning state the person can never resolve the feeling of loss. Professionals must keep the person involved in a program for small gains but never give false hope. They must listen to the client, allow the expression of despair, and allow crying.

As the person adapts, he or she begins to feel satisfaction in attainments and to recognize abilities. The individual needs opportunities to test the new person in reality situations, to go out in public with friends, and to visit old and new places for pleasure. This is a time to develop new skills and areas where he or she can excel. Sports such as the Paraolympics, started by Guttmann in England, have opened up new vistas for persons who had written themselves off. This is also the time the individual recognizes the date he or she became a different person. Many celebrate the date over the years as a second birthday.

Families go through the same phases of adaptation as the person who has sustained the trauma. Professionals must listen and counsel them as well as the victims. Depending on their coping abilities and the significance of the trauma, families may not progress through the stages as quickly as the victims. Professionals may need to give the disabled person the support the family cannot. The person with the disability may be the one to support the family through this grief and grieving process. Some disabled persons may plateau on a lower level of function, preferring to retain the sick role. It may allow the person to withdraw from a reality that was difficult to handle before the injury or illness. He or she may have received so much satisfaction while in the sick role at an earlier time that a return is welcomed. Alternatively, the family may prefer him or her in a dependent, passive role, and they will condition him or her accordingly.

The professional, regardless of discipline, must assist the person to shift values and to look to assets. This requires careful assessment in all areas of function and coping on a regular basis, weekly being a good general time frame. Long-term goals can be projected early, with short-term goals based on the steps required to reach the long-term goals. The disabled person must be involved in setting goals. A contract of sorts for teaching and learning is required between the professionals and the person or family.

When the illness or injury is self-limiting, goals may be projected for months or years. Time tables can be adjusted according to progress. When the underlying disease process is progressively degenerative, goals will become lower, and the time table is controlled by the progression of the disease. Multiple sclerosis and amyotrophic lateral sclerosis are common examples of this progressive type of disease. Goal setting and contract formation must continue regardless of the disease course. Goals may eventually consist of preventing complications or maintaining the status quo. If these goals keep the person comfortable and allow the use of abilities, they are most acceptable. Goal setting and contracts must always be individual.

Adaptation is perhaps the most difficult part of a rehabilitation program, but the knowledge and the skill that professionals can impart to the disabled person will make it possible for him or her to become a contributing member of society, with the same rights and privileges as any other member of society.

## REFERENCES

Campbell, R.M.: The surgical management of pressure sores, Surg. Clin. North Am. **39**:509, 1959.

Chusid, J.G., Correlative neuroanatomy and functional neurology, ed. 17, Los Altos, Calif. 1979, Lange Medical Publications.

American Heart Association, Committee on Exercise: Exercise testing and training of apparently healthy individuals: a handbook for physicians, Dallas, 1972, American Heart Association.

Di Mascio, S.: Debrisan for decubitus ulcers, Am. J. Nurs. **79**(4):684-685, April 1979.

Fernie: Phoney treatment shows nurses how to prevent bedsores, The Toronto Star, Nov. 3, 1975, p. A3.

Fink, S.L.: Crisis and motivation: a theoretical model, Arch. Phys. Med. Rehabil. **48**:593, 1967.

Gibson, C.H.: Personal communication, 1977.

Gosnell, D.J.: An assessment tool to identify pressure forces, Nurs. Res. **22**:55-59, Jan.-Feb. 1973.

Guttmann, L.: Spinal cord injuries, comprehensive management and research, Oxford, 1973, Blackwell Scientific Publications, Ltd.

Guttmann, L., and Frankel, H.: The value of intermittent catheterization in the early management of traumatic paraplegia and tetraplegia, Paraplegia **4:**63-81, Aug. 1966.

Guyton, A.C.: Textbook of medical physiology, ed. 5, Philadelphia, 1976, W.B. Saunders Co.

Henderson, V., and Nite, G.: Principles and practices of nursing, ed. 6, New York, 1978, Macmillan Publishing Co.

Jones, R.H.: Personal communication, 1973, Rochester, N.Y.

Krusen, F.H., Kottke, F.J., and Elwood, P.M., Jr.: Handbook of physical medicine and rehabilitation, ed. 2, Philadelphia, 1971, W.B. Saunders Co.

Lapidis, J., et al.: Follow-up on unsterile, intermittent self-catheterization, J. Urol. **3:**184-187, Feb. 1974.

Leveen, H., et al.: Chemical acidification of wounds, an adjuvant to healing and the unfavorable action of alkalinity and ammonia, Ann. Surg. **178:**745-753, Jan. 16, 1973.

Miller, B.F., and Keane, C.B.: Encyclopedia and dictionary of medicine and nursing, Philadlephia, 1972, W.B. Saunders Co.

Mossman, P.L.: A problem oriented approach to stroke rehabilitation, Springfield, Ill., 1976, Charles C Thomas, Publisher.

Porch, B.E.: Porch Index of Communication Ability, Palo Alto, Calif., 1967, Consulting Psychologist Press.

Rantz, M.J., and Courtial, D.: Lifting, moving and transferring patients: a manual, St. Louis, 1977, The C.V. Mosby Co.

Raven, J.C.: Coloured Progressive Matrices, London, 1962, E.T. Heron & Co., Ltd.

Redfern, S.J., et al.: Local pressures with ten types of patient support systems, Lancet **2:**277-280, Aug. 11, 1973.

Sarno, M.T.: Functional Communication Profile, New York, 1965, Institute of Rehabilitation Medicine, New York University Medical Center.

Schuell, H.: Minnesota Test for Differential Diagnosis of Aphasia, Minneapolis, 1965, University of Minnesota Press.

Taylor, A.G.: Autonomic dysreflexia in spinal cord injury, Nurs. Clin. North Am. **9:**717-725, Dec. 1974.

Verbonic, P.J., Lewis, D., and Goller, H.: Thermography in the study of decubitus ulcers, preliminary report, Nurs. Res. **21:**233-237, May-June 1972.

# 26

# SURGICAL TECHNIQUES AND NURSING INTERVENTION

Surgical intervention is an important aspect of treatment for the neurological client. It is usually not the first choice of treatment; however, at times it can be the only choice of treatment. This chapter deals with the three phases of the surgical experience and the operating room nurse's role in each phase. Also, basic neurosurgical procedures are described and illustrated.

The operating room nurse plays a vital role with the neurosurgical client in the preoperative, operative, and postoperative phases of the surgical experience. He or she provides the client with continuity of care throughout the phases.

## PREOPERATIVE PHASE

In the preoperative phase the operating room nurse assesses the client's physiological, psychological, and sociocultural status and begins by reviewing the client's chart. The nurse notes the client's vital signs, medications currently being taken, and allergies and checks the operative permit. Additionally the nurse reviews the client's medical history, looking specifically for the presence of chronic diseases and the history of the reason the client is to undergo surgery. The operating room nurse confers with the floor nurses to obtain information about the client's reaction to the hospitalization and diagnosis.

Next the operating room nurse visits the client and family in the room, beginning by introducing him- or herself and stating the reason for the visit.

In assessing the neurosurgical client the nurse may want to use an assessment tool, such as the one shown on pp. 660 to 664. This provides a systematic way in which to collect the record data. Particular to the neurosurgical client the nurse notes the client's level of consciousness, affect, speech, reflexes, motor ability, and pupils. The data collected from this visit are used to develop a plan of care for the operative phase. This increases the efficiency and effectiveness of the care given to the client in both the operating room and the recovery room.

Another objective of the preoperative visit is to provide the neurosurgical client with information about the upcoming surgery. The operating room nurse can give the client the time of surgery, approximately how long it will last, and how long he or she will be in the recovery room. The nurse can utilize this time to explain the dressing, intravenous tube, urinary catheter, heart monitor, and other equipment specific to the surgery scheduled. The family is included in the teaching and is given information about the time they should arrive the morning of surgery and where they can wait while the client is in surgery. The client receives basic preoperative teaching concerning postoperative recovery, such as turning, coughing, deep breathing, and leg exercising. The operating room nurse also includes information about postoperative pain. The client is told to expect pain and reassured that adequate pain medication will be available. This information-giving period is followed by a session in

*Text continued on p. 664.*

**Preoperative assessment tool for use by the operating room nurse***

## PREOPERATIVE ASSESSMENT TOOL

Name _____ Age _____

### SUBJECTIVE DATA†
### Current medical/surgical history
*(to elicit the client's knowledge about the hospitalization and establish
a base line for preoperative teaching)*

1. What brought you to the hospital? _____

2. What type of surgery are you going to have? _____

3. What has the doctor told you about your surgery? _____

   _____

4. What has the nurse told you about your surgery? _____

   _____

5. What do you want the surgery to do for you? _____

   _____

6. How long do you expect to be in the hospital? _____

### Past medical/surgical history
*(to determine any factors that might influence the client's present hospitalization
and reaction to surgery and recovery)*

1. Have you been in the hospital before? _____

   | REASON | WHEN |
   |--------|------|
   | a. _____ | _____ |
   | b. _____ | _____ |
   | c. _____ | _____ |

   Did you have any problems during any of those hospitalizations? _____

   If so, what? _____

2. Have you ever had surgery before? _____

   | REASON | WHEN |
   |--------|------|
   | a. _____ | _____ |
   | b. _____ | _____ |
   | c. _____ | _____ |

   Did you have any problems after your surgery? _____

   If so, what? _____

3. Did you have pain when you were hospitalized before? _____

   Describe this pain: Location _____ Quality _____

   Quantity _____

   Did pain medication relieve the pain? _____

*Previously unpublished tool of Rebecca Smith.
†Subjective data are anything the client states.

## PREOPERATIVE ASSESSMENT TOOL—cont'd

How long did you take the pain medication? _____

What was the name of the pain medication? _____

Are you in pain now? _____ If so, describe the pain: _____

Location _____ Quality _____ Quantity _____

Chronology _____ Setting _____

Associated manifestations _____

Alleviating factors _____

4. Are you allergic to any medications? _____

   WHAT

   a. _____

   b. _____

   c. _____

   How do you react to it? _____

5. Were you taking any medication(s) at home? _____

   | WHAT | HOW OFTEN |
   |------|-----------|
   | a. _____ | _____ |
   | b. _____ | _____ |
   | c. _____ | _____ |

   LAST DOSE

   a. _____

   b. _____

   c. _____

6. Do you have any other health problems you have not mentioned (emphysema, diabetes, tuberculosis, arthritis, epilepsy, heart disease, cancer, hypertension)? _____

## OBJECTIVE DATA‡
### Current medical/surgical history

1. What is the operation proposed for the client? _____

2. Is the client currently taking medication? (Include especially those drugs that might affect the client's reaction to anesthesia: antihypertensives, antidepressants, monoamine oxidase inhibitors, steroids.)

   _____

‡Objective data are anything the nurse observes or takes from the chart.                    *Continued.*

## Preoperative assessment tool for use by the operating room nurse—cont'd

### PREOPERATIVE ASSESSMENT TOOL—cont'd

WHAT                                                                           HOW OFTEN

a. _____          _____

b. _____          _____

c. _____          _____

### Level of consciousness

1. Is the client oriented to time, person, and place? _____

2. Is the client confused? _____ Explain: _____

3. Is the client semicomatose? _____ Explain: _____

4. Is the client comatose? _____ Explain: _____

### Level of anxiety

1. Is the client anxious about the impending surgery? _____

2. Describe the client's behavior (like wringing hands, restlessness): _____

### Patterns of coping/adaptation (check one):

Excessive laughing _____ Crying _____ Changing the subject _____ Developing tension head-

ache _____ Denying need for surgery _____ Having transient rash _____ Displaying anger _____

Exhibiting muscle tightness _____

### Body image

1. To what degree will the client's physical appearance be altered by the surgery? _____

2. Does the client talk about the affected part or avoid the subject?_____

3. Does the client take an interest in his or her physical appearance (like wearing makeup, combing hair)?

_____

4. Does the surgery affect the masculine or feminine image? _____

5. Is the client able to acknowledge the upcoming loss? _____

### Skin color

1. Is the client's skin pale, cyanotic, yellowish, pink, or ashen? _____

2. If none of these, describe: _____

### Skin temperature

1. Is the skin warm, hot, cool, or cold to touch? _____

### Skin integrity

1. Is there a rash present? _____ Describe: _____

2. Are there any abrasions? _____ Describe: _____

3. Is there any unusual skin condition? _____ Describe: _____

## PREOPERATIVE ASSESSMENT TOOL—cont'd

### Body structure and size

1. Describe briefly the size and general appearance of the client (include things like catheter, Levine tube): _____

2. Does the client have any physical limitations or prostheses? _____ Describe: _____

3. Does the client have any sensory impairment? _____

   Eyes _____ Speech _____

   Ears _____ Touch _____

### Laboratory data

1. Base-line vital signs: Temperature _____ Pulse _____ Respiration _____ Blood pressure _____

2. Are there any unusual results of the diagnostic studies? _____

   Study _____ Results _____

3. Complete blood count: White blood cells _____ Red blood cells _____ Hematocrit _____

   Hemoglobin _____

4. Blood type: _____ Cross match: _____

5. Urinalysis (anything abnormal): _____

6. Chest radiograph results: _____

7. Electrocardiogram results: _____

8. SMA-12 (anything abnormal): _____

### Nursing summary of objective data

*Continued.*

## Preoperative assessment tool for use by the operating room nurse—cont'd

### PREOPERATIVE TEACHING CHECKLIST

1. Turn, cough, and deep breathe
   a. Explained _____
   b. Practiced _____
   c. Returned _____
2. Leg exercises
   a. Explained _____
   b. Practiced _____
   c. Returned _____
3. Intravenous fluids
   a. Explained the purpose and approximate time of continuance _____
4. Postoperative pain
   a. Explained approximate length of time to expect pain and gave information about pain medication _
5. Blood pressure, pulse, and temperature
   a. Explained frequency of taking these and why _____
6. Preoperative preparation
   a. Explained about the enema, skin preparation, signing the surgical consent, nothing to eat or drink
      after midnight, and why _____
7. Urinary catheter
   a. Explained reasons for having one and approximate length of time having the catheter _____
8. Heart monitor
   a. Explained that it is placed on in surgery and why _____
9. Recovery room
   a. Explained procedures that will take place and approximate time would be there _____
10. Premedication
    a. Explained when it will be given and why _____
11. Family members
    a. Explained when to be there and where to wait _____

which the client has the opportunity to ask questions about the surgery. Specific questions about the surgical procedure and anesthesia is referred to the surgeon and anesthesiologist.

A final objective of the preoperative visit is to help allay some of the client's anxiety about sur-gery. One can accomplish this by providing the client with adequate information, as discussed previously. Also, simply being a familiar face in the operating room helps to comfort the client.

During the preoperative visit, the operating room nurse can establish expected client outcomes for the three phases of the client's surgical experience. Once they are identified, an individualized nursing care plan can be developed.

**Expected outcomes**
**Preoperative:**
1 The client states his or her knowledge of the upcoming operative procedure.
2 The client states his or her knowledge of the events before surgery.
3 The client demonstrates turning, coughing, and deep breathing.
**Operative:**
1 The client will remain in a safe environment.
**Postoperative:**
1 The client is able to turn, cough, and breathe deeply.
2 The client will demonstrate improved neurological function.

These expected outcomes should be based on the institution's standards of care. Using this as the base, the operating room nurse can audit his or her care at appropriate intervals. The results of this evaluative process lead to improvements in client care delivery. This is an integral part of a quality-assurance program in the operating room.

In summary, the preoperative visit is an important function of the operating room nurse to assess the client and plan care accordingly. A visit from the nurse complements that of the surgeon and anesthesiologist. Most important, the client is provided with continuity of care.

## OPERATIVE PHASE

Despite improved neurosurgical techniques and therapeutic results, the majority of individuals continue to react with fear and awe when the question of neurosurgery arises. This is especially true when brain surgery is contemplated; many believe that if the client survives at all, he or she will be retarded, paralyzed, blind, or so helpless as to require care like a child. In competent hands the hazards associated with surgery on the nervous system are no greater than major surgery elsewhere in the body.

Morally, neurosurgical treatment is justified when the expected beneficial effects outweigh any possible harmful ones. However, when surgery of the frontal lobe is contemplated for the treatment of clients with intractable disease (mental or physical), the moral implications of the procedure should be carefully considered for the individual client.

The scope of neurological surgery is broad. In addition to diseases of the nervous system, many general medical conditions are treated neurosurgically. This is done by the interruption of neurophysiological pathways.

## GENERAL NURSING CONSIDERATIONS

The following are considerations for the neurosurgical client beginning the operative phase. They are discussed sequentially as the client would experience them.

As the neurosurgical client arrives in the surgical suite, he or she is greeted by the operating room nurse, who checks the identification band, operative permit, and chart record. At the same time the operating room nurse reassesses the client's physiological and psychological status.

The next consideration is the anesthetizing of the client. The first step in the anesthetic process is starting the intravenous drip, which is done by the operating room nurse. Various types of anesthesia are used, depending on the physical and emotional condition of the client and the preference of the individual neurosurgeon and anesthesiologist. Anesthesia is administered by one or more of the following methods: intravenous route, inhalation, endotracheal route, spinal injection, or local infiltration.

The neurosurgical client, when under general anesthesia, is likely to experience depressed respiration and circulatory function. For this reason, it is important to note that a patent airway is maintained: hypothermia or induced hypotension can be used; extreme muscle relaxation is not necessary; and return of consciousness and reflexes as soon as possible is preferred.

If ordered by the neurosurgeon or anesthesiologist, the operating room nurse assists with the attachment of the heart monitor, application of the Doppler device, insertion of the central venous pressure line, placement of the nerve stimulator, insertion of a urinary catheter, application of the cautery ground pad, and insertion of a nasogastric tube.

The position of the client for neurosurgery is determined by the site of operation. The operating room nurse assists the surgeon and anesthesiologist in achieving the position of choice. Throughout the surgical procedure the nurse is responsible for maintaining the client's position (Fig. 26-1). This includes checking for pressure points, preventing pressure on nerves and blood vessels, protecting the client from metal surfaces (burn hazard), and checking the patency of tubes.

After being positioned, the neurosurgical client is ready to be prepared. The extent of the preparation is determined by the operative procedure to be done. The preparation consists in shaving the hair and then scrubbing the area with a bactericidal antiseptic such as Betadine. In most cranial surgeries the client's hair is removed after the client comes to the surgical suite and is anesthetized. This helps reduce the preoperative anxiety associated with body-image change for the client. The actual shaving of the hair is usually done by the neurosurgeon, who knows how much is necessary to be removed for the incision. Fig. 26-2 illustrates

the usual extent of a cranial preparation. The hair removed is sealed in an envelope and attached securely to the client's chart or returned to the unit.

The operative setup required for neurosurgical procedures is quite extensive. This includes preparation of the surgical suite as well as instrumentation. (See the boxed material on p. 674.)

As the techniques of modern neurosurgery have progressed, they have necessitated continued refinement and development of specialized equipment and instrumentation. The neurosurgical and microneurosurgical instruments are shown in Fig. 26-3, *A* and *B*, respectively.

The last nursing consideration of the neurosurgical client before the operative phase is completed is that of the cranial dressing. It includes the entire head. The exact type of dressing will vary according to the neurosurgeon's preference. The dressing must be sterile and thick to protect the incision site (Fig. 26-4).

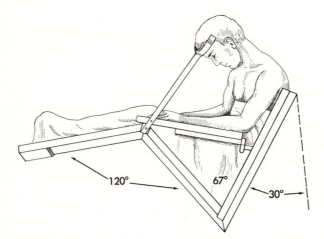

**FIG. 26-1.** Client prepared for suboccipital craniotomy is positioned on operating room table in semi-Fowler's position with attached headrest immobilizing head.

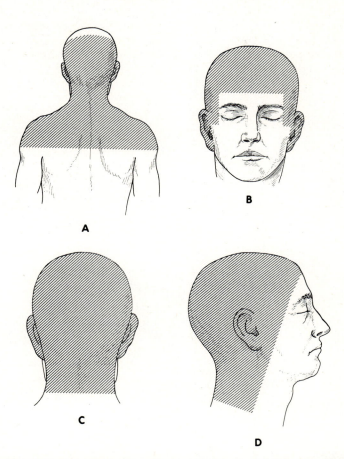

**FIG. 26-2.** *Shading,* Areas to be prepared for different types of craniotomies. **A,** For posterior craniotomy. **B** and **C,** For craniotomy, frontal tumor excision. **D,** For major scalp surgery. (From Pate, M.O.: The preparation manual, Long Island City, N.Y., 1963, Edward Weck & Co., Inc.)

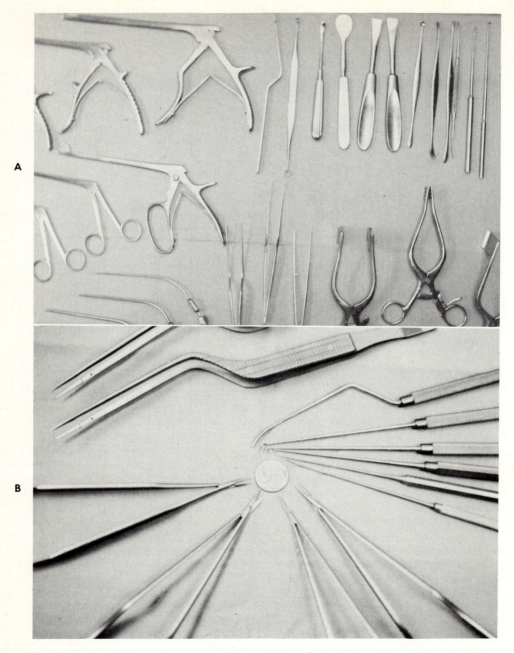

**FIG. 26-3. A,** Neurosurgical instruments. **B,** Special microneurosurgical instruments used for procedures requiring great precision.

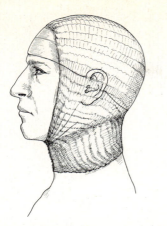

**FIG. 26-4.** Typical head dressing used after neurosurgery.

## NEUROSURGICAL PROCEDURES

Neurosurgical procedures may be classified, according to the part of the nervous system that is involved, in four major groups, as follows:

**I** Brain and cranial nerves
**II** Spinal cord and nerve roots
**III** Peripheral nerves
**IV** Autonomic nervous system

### Brain and cranial nerves (group I)

To approach the brain and cranial nerves, one must make an opening in the skull. The location and dimension of the opening must be determined carefully, since these restrict the accessibility to the area concerned. (Intracranial surgery does not allow the introduction of a hand, as is possible in abdominal surgery.) The exposure is accomplished by the removal of bone (craniectomy) or by the turning of an osteoplastic bone flap (craniotomy).

*Craniectomy.* A craniectomy may be small or large (1 to 5 cm), depending on the suspected pathological condition. It may be only a burr hole, such as is made when one performs a ventriculography or explores for a hematoma. It also is possible through such an opening to aspirate cerebrospinal fluid, blood, or pus or to biopsy a lesion. For other procedures one enlarges the original burr hole by nibbling away additional bone with a rongeur to permit greater exposure. This is done in the approach to the trigeminal nerve in the temporal fossa (Fig. 26-5), to the cranial nerves (fifth, eighth, ninth, and tenth) in the posterior fossa, and for space-occupying lesions in the brainstem or cerebellum (suboccipital craniectomy). The posterior root of the trigeminal nerve is divided, manipulated, or decompressed in the treatment of trigeminal neuralgia.

There are two approaches in treating trigeminal neuralgia. The first is extracranial. The procedures include resection or avulsion of the peripheral branches of the fifth cranial nerve. One noninvasive procedure is the alcohol injection that offers relief for up to 12 months, the average being 4 to 9 months. An inherent danger in this procedure is the possibility that the alcohol will diffuse into the cranial cavity, with damage resulting to the brain and cranial nerves.

The second approach is the intracranial. One procedure involves exposing and sectioning by temporal craniotomy for the retrogasserian ganglion in the middle cranial fossa. A second procedure is the suboccipital craniectomy, in which the sensory root in the posterior fossa is sectioned. After the rhizotomy the client will experience permanent numbness on the affected side of the face.

Recent research is determining if the retrogasserian rhizotomy is effective in alleviating symptoms of epilepsy, cerebral palsy, and spasticity caused by other diseases. This treatment mode is still in the experimental stages.

*Craniotomy.* A series of burr holes (three to six) is made as a preliminary step in the craniotomy operation. The bone between the holes is cut with the Stryker pneumatic drill (Fig. 26-6). The bone remains attached to the muscle, which acts as a hinge when the flap is turned. (This may be compared to a door that may be opened or closed.) The dura is then incised following the outline of the bone flap but opening in the opposite direction so that its base (hinge) is near the midline (Fig. 26-7). This procedure is used for the removal of supratentorial tumors, abscesses, and chronic subdural hematomas; the excision of specific cortical areas for the relief of seizures, focal pain, tremors, and mental disease; and the treatment of aneurysms and other vascular anomalies. If the tumor cannot

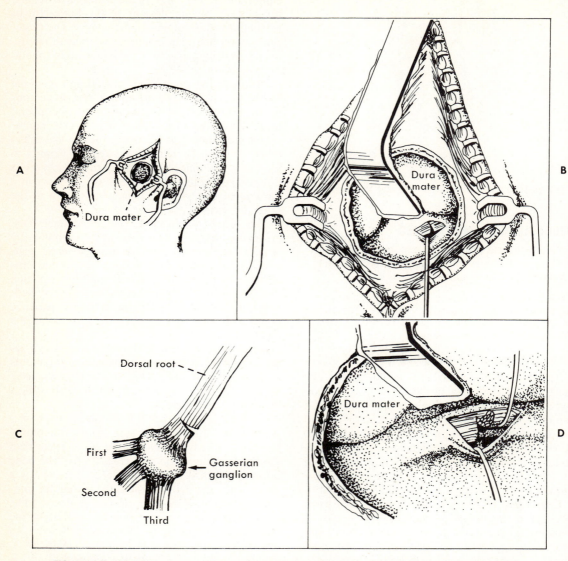

**FIG. 26-5.** Partial section of posterior root of trigeminal nerve. **A,** Skin retracted, bone removed, and dura mater exposed. **B,** Dura mater incised, posterior root exposed and partially cut. **C,** Trigeminal nerve showing three divisions, gasserian ganglion, and sectioned root. **D,** Close-up view of sectioned posterior root.

**FIG. 26-6.** Pneumatic craniotomy drill with three different headpieces.

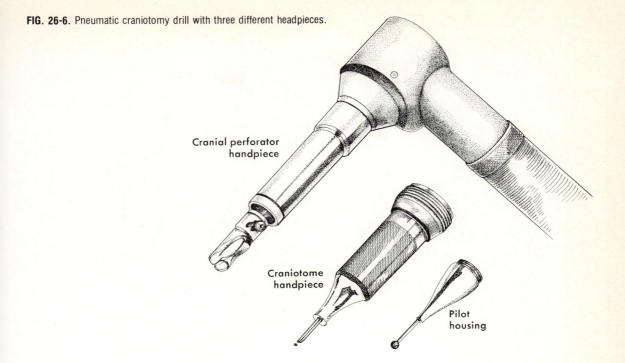

Cranial perforator
handpiece

Craniotome
handpiece

Pilot
housing

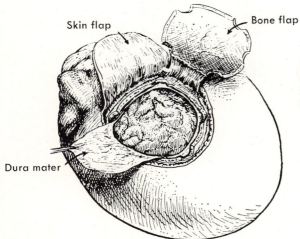

Skin flap

Bone flap

Dura mater

**FIG. 26-7.** Demonstrating relationships of scalp, bone, and dural flaps in craniotomy. (From Sachs, E.: Diagnosis and treatment of brain tumors and care of the neurosurgical patient, ed. 2, St. Louis, 1949, The C.V. Mosby Co.)

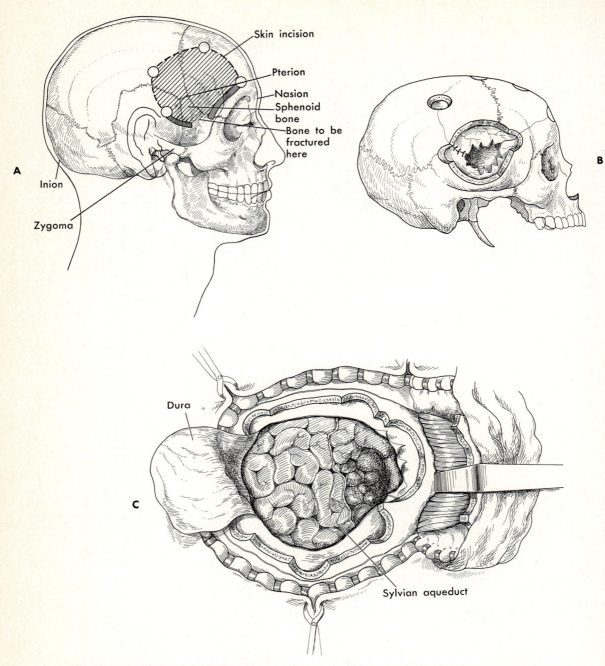

**FIG. 26-8.** Craniotomy with subtemporal decompression. **A,** Skin incision and placement of burr holes for frontotemporal craniotomy. **B,** Bony defect. **C,** Malignant cerebral tumor exposed.

be removed because of its position or nature, the neurosurgeon makes a subtemporal decompression by leaving an opening in the dura and overlying skull (Fig. 26-8). After the purpose of the procedure is accomplished, the closure is done in layers (dura, muscles, fasciae, galea, and scalp) with interrupted silk sutures. Some neurosurgeons suture the bone flap to the skull with interrupted silk or wire sutures; others secure the bone flap by suturing the pericranium. The most important step in the closure is the careful suturing of the galea. This prevents disruption of the wound and promotes maximum wound healing. These same fundamentals are applicable to the closure of all cranial procedures. Dressings are applied as described in Chapter 21.

A cerebral aneurysm, if its size and location permit, is exposed when an osteoplastic flap is made. The frontotemporal flap is frequently used to approach all anterior circulation aneurysms, including internal carotid, middle cerebral, posterior

communicating, anterior communicating, carotid bifurcation, and anterior cerebral aneurysms. Posterior circulating aneurysms are exposed through a posterotemporal flap or suboccipital flap, depending on their location. The brain must be extremely relaxed for a subtemporal and transtentorial approach to the brainstem. This is the reason clients are not operated on in acute conditions. Spinal drainage, dexamethasone (Decadron), and mannitol are used for brain relaxation.

The artery is occluded with Yaşargil or Heifetz aneurysm clips or ligatures on either side of the aneurysm. If the aneurysm cannot be clipped, it can be wrapped with fine mesh gauze and coated with Biobond acrylic. In this way the circulation to the weakened, dilated area is interrupted, and the danger of rupture is eliminated. If the lesion cannot be handled in this direct way, a more remote approach, ligation of the common carotid artery in the neck, is performed on the appropriate side in an attempt to reduce the arterial pressure

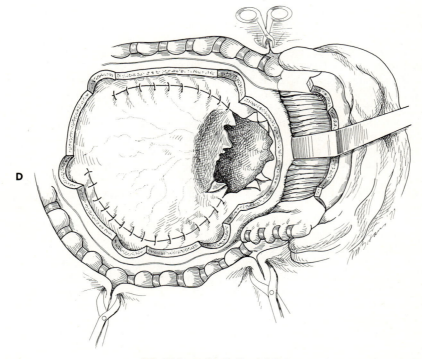

**FIG. 26-8, cont'd. D,** Dural defect.

## Operating room setup for neurosurgery

| BASIC ROOM SETUP | | ANESTHESIOLOGIST |
|---|---|---|
| Microscope | Oversized Mayo stand | Blood gas analyzer |
| Fiberoptic light source | Surgical steps | Central venous pressure setup |
| Headlight | Stools | Doppler device |
| | | Blood warmer |
| Hypothermia unit | Foley catheter set | |
| Air tanks | Clippers | Heart monitor and defibrillator |
| Gomco suction unit | Razor | Electroencephalograph unit |
| Intravenous poles | Spinal tray | |
| Radiographs | Dressing chart | Spinal drainage |
| Backup suction unit | | Arterial line |
| | Mayfield headrest | Nerve stimulator |
| Electrosurgical unit | Bath blankets for padding | |
| Malis bipolar coagulation unit | Arm rests | |
| Cryosurgical probe | Laminectomy frame | |

at the weak spot; thus the likelihood of rupture is diminished. Hypothermia can be used during cerebral aneurysm surgery to decrease cerebral blood flow.

Microneurosurgery techniques are frequently employed in aneurysm surgery because of the critical location and delicate nature of some aneurysms. This consists of using the microscope and microneurosurgical instruments (Fig. 26-3, *B*).

Another procedure involving cerebral circulation is cerebral artery bypass. Microvascular technique makes the treatment of clients who have had a cerebrovascular accident possible. The procedure consists of a bypass where the superficial temporal artery is anastomosed to a branch of the middle cerebral artery.

During the procedure, monitoring of cortical oxidative metabolism is growing in popularity. This involves a Teflon-coated platinum electrode inserted into the cortex near the site of the anastomosis. This catheter is attached to a blood flowmeter, which, as the blood moves through the constant-area cross section of the magnetic field, reflects a voltage that is directly proportional to the rate of the blood flow. These measurements are taken before and after the anastomosis.

Another procedure concerning the cerebral cir-

culation, though not directly involving the brain and cranial nerves, is carotid endarterectomy. This consists in exposing the carotid arteries in the neck at the site of occlusion, incising the vessel or vessels, and removing the clot and associated sclerotic tissues.

Depressed skull fractures are generally treated surgically. If simple, they may be treated without operation at the discretion of the neurosurgeon; if compound or comminuted, they should be operated on immediately so that the incidence of infection is reduced and further damage to the brain is prevented. If bone fragments are fixed, a burr hole is made in an adjacent nonfractured area to facilitate their elevation. Foreign bodies and loose comminuted pieces of bone are removed. Lacerations of the dura are repaired as necessary. After the depressed fragments have been realigned, the scalp is sutured.

*Cranioplasty.* Bone defects may result from extensively comminuted fractures, or osteomyelitis of the skull, or after the removal of tumors involving the skull (meningioma). Depending on the size and location of the defect, a cranioplasty (Fig. 26-9) may be indicated. This consists of the insertion of a substitute (such as bone, tantalum, Vitallium, or plastic) previously prepared in size and shape to

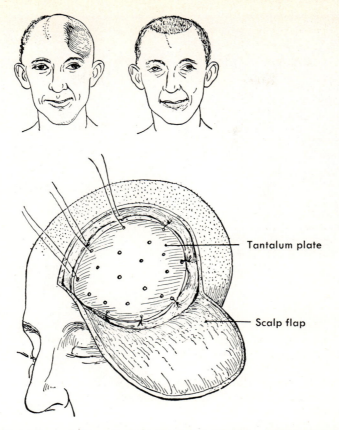

**FIG. 26-9.** Client before and after cranioplasty. Defect of skull has been repaired with tantalum plate.

fit into the defective area. This is indicated in supratentorial defects for protection of the brain and for its cosmetic effect. This problem is not present in defects of the infratentorial region because this area is adequately protected by the neck muscles (trapezius, sternocleidomastoid, splenius capitis, and semispinalis capitis).

Large dural defects are encountered with some extensive skull fractures and after the removal of certain meningeal tumors. They are corrected by the use of fascia (previously removed from the client's thigh or temple), fibrin film, or polyethylene film. The material is sutured to the remaining dura.

***Stereotactic surgery*** (Fig. 26-10). Beginning with Cooper's observation that the choroidal artery supplies the basilar ganglion region, techniques for the treatment of Parkinson's syndrome have rapidly developed. Spiegel and Wycis, Cooper, and numerous others have contributed considerable data derived from their treatment of large numbers of clients by the production of lesions in selected areas of the thalamus.

Using internal landmarks, coagulating electrodes, cryosurgical probes, wire loops, and other lesion-producing devices have been inserted stereotactically into preselected sites with great accuracy.

The cryosurgical technique appears most effective, since in the process of freezing brain tissue selectively, functional changes that may occur are reversible with rewarming before permanent dam-

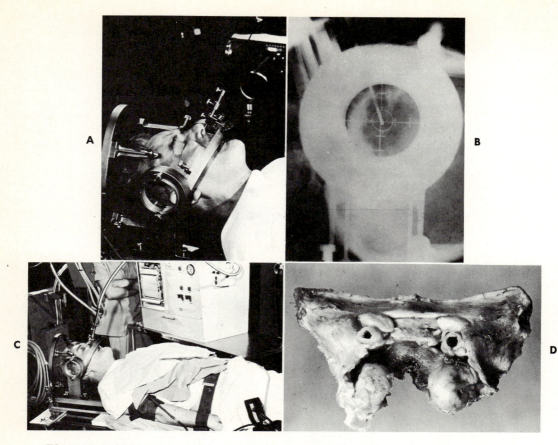

**FIG. 26-10. A,** Client's head is fixed to stereotactic unit. Twist drill is inserted into anterior wall of sphenoid sinus by way of left nostril into nasopharynx. **B,** Lateral radiographic film demonstrating freezing unit properly placed in target area (pituitary gland). Circle and cross hairs are positioned at target point before insertion of cannula. **C,** Cannula in client's left nostril is attached to freezing unit on table. Radiographic equipment is seen in upper left background. Since procedure is performed with client under local anesthesia, body straps are used to immobilize client. **D,** A sella turcica viewed from above, demonstrating bone perforation at base through which cannula was inserted. To either side of sella, internal carotid arteries are seen (below, siphon; above, with open lumen, cranial extensions). Above sectioned arteries, optic nerves are seen passing into orbits.

age is produced. This technique permits moment-to-moment neurological assessment of the client during the production of the lesion.

*Psychosurgery.* Psychosurgical procedures of numerous types have been employed in the past for the treatment of intractable mental disease. Some of these have been modified and utilized to alleviate severe systemic pain after other therapeutic and remedial measures have been unsuccessful. These operations, for the most part, have been performed through small craniectomies in the frontal regions. They consist of the interruption of the connections between the frontal lobes and the thalamus and hypothalamus. The original bilateral frontal leukotomies, though therapeutically effective, had undesirable associated phenomena (physical, intellectual, and social deterioration). The attempt to eliminate the resulting disabilities led to several variations in the technique. These included unilateral as well as partial bilateral leukotomies, resection of specific cortical areas (gyrectomy), and thalamotomy.

**LEUKOTOMY.** The classic *frontal leukotomy* is performed by incision of the cortex and, under direct vision, division of the frontal white matter in a plane anterior to the lateral ventricle. Modifications of this procedure have consisted of fractional division of the frontal white matter. Through selective elimination, it has been learned that the greatest therapeutic benefit is achieved simultaneously with the least regression when the medial third of the frontal white matter is interrupted bilaterally. Another variant of frontal leukotomy is called *transorbital leukotomy.* A sharp, pointed instrument (transorbital leukotome) is introduced into the conjunctival sac between the eyeball and upper lid. When the orbital plate is reached, the leukotome is directed parallel to the nose and tapped with a hammer to pierce the bone. It is inserted into the frontal white matter and moved to the right and left, thus dividing the thalamofrontal radiation. The maximum depth of penetration into the brain is 5 cm.

**RESECTION OF SPECIFIC CORTICAL AREAS.** Resection of specific cortical areas (gyrectomy, topectomy) has been performed. The most satisfactory results have followed the removal of areas 9 and 10 (Fig. 3-12). *Cingulectomy,* the resection of the gyrus cinguli on the medial aspect of the frontal lobe, has been mainly effective in the treatment of clients with obsessional neuroses.

**THALAMOTOMY.** A more direct anatomical approach to the origin of the thalamofrontal pathways, the dorsal medial nucleus of the thalamus, has been accomplished through stereotactic surgery, thalamotomy. This involves the application of a mechanical device to the skull, with the help of which electrodes are introduced to specific nuclei in otherwise inaccessible parts of the brain. Radiographic examinations of the skull are made before and during the operation to verify the position of the electrodes. The dorsal medial nucleus of the thalamus is destroyed by electrocoagulation, freezing, or ultrasound or with a radioactive substance; thus the physiological pathways to the frontal lobe are interrupted.

A similar technique is applied to destroy the ventrolateral nucleus of the thalamus for the relief of parkinsonism.

***Treatment of nonobstructive and obstructive hydrocephalus.*** Specific procedures for the treatment of nonobstructive (communicating) hydrocephalus are choroid plexectomy (Dandy), lumbar subarachnoid ureterostomy (Heile), and lumbar subarachnoid peritoneostomy. Specific procedures for the treatment of obstructive hydrocephalus are third ventriculostomy (Dandy), ventriculocisternostomy (Torkildsen), auriculoventriculostomy, ventriculoureterostomy (Matson), and ventriculoperitoneostomy (Cone).

**CHOROID PLEXECTOMY.** Choroid plexectomy is accomplished through bilateral craniectomies in the parietal regions. Transcortical incisions are made to permit access to the choroid plexuses of the lateral ventricles; these are excised. Some neurosurgeons prefer to coagulate rather than to excise the choroid plexus. This operation is directed toward curtailing the production of cerebrospinal fluid; thus the total amount within the ventricular system is reduced. All the other operations are designed to direct the cerebrospinal fluid into channels that will facilitate its circulation or elimination.

**LUMBAR SUBARACHNOID URETEROSTOMY.** The lumbar subarachnoid ureterostomy permits the disposal of excessive cerebrospinal fluid (nonobstructive hydrocephalus) through the ureter to the bladder. The operation consists of a laminectomy of the second and third lumbar vertebrae and a nephrectomy. One end of a polyethylene tube is inserted into the lumbar subarachnoid space and sutured to the dura mater. The other end is passed through an opening in the psoas muscle along with spinal column into the retroperitoneal space and inserted a distance of 4 to 6 cm into the ureter of the resected kidney.

**LUMBAR SUBARACHNOID PERITONEOSTOMY.** The lumbar subarachnoid peritoneostomy is another attempt to accomplish the elimination of excessive cerebrospinal fluid. It consists of a lumbar laminectomy and a lateral abdominal incision extending into the peritoneum. One end of a polyethylene tube is inserted into the subarachnoid space as previously described, and the other is carried subcutaneously around the flank into the peritoneal cavity, where it is sutured in place. (This procedure is not always effective.)

**THIRD VENTRICULOSTOMY.** The third ventriculostomy is performed after a unilateral frontal crani-

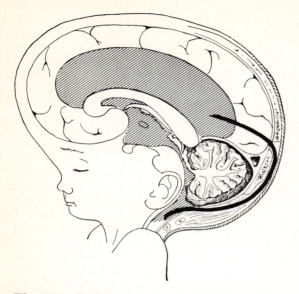

**FIG. 26-11.** Torkildsen operation, ventriculocisternostomy, showing catheter in place: one end in occipital horn of lateral ventricle, other in cisterna magna.

otomy by elevation of the frontal lobe and opening of the anterior wall of the floor of the third ventricle. This allows the cerebrospinal fluid to drain into the cisterna chiasmatis of the subarachnoid space.

**VENTRICULOCISTERNOSTOMY.** The ventriculocisternostomy (Fig. 26-11) consists in making a burr hole in either occipital region and a midline suboccipital craniectomy. A rubber catheter (No. 10 or 12 French) or polyethylene tube is passed beneath the scalp between the two openings. Incision are then made in the dura mater over the cisterna magna and the occipital lobe. One end of the catheter is inserted 4 to 5 cm into the occipital horn of the lateral ventricle, and the dura is sutured around it. The rest of the catheter is laid over the dura toward the cisterna magna to determine the length required. The surplus is cut off, and the tip of the free end is introduced into the cistern. The dura is sutured around the catheter to secure it in place.

**AURICULOVENTRICULOSTOMY.** The auriculoventriculostomy consists of the insertion of a Silastic catheter into a lateral ventricle; the other end of the catheter is passed through the jugular vein into the right auricle. This system maintains normal ventricular pressure by channeling the excess cerebrospinal fluid through the auricle into the general circulation. This has become the treatment of choice for hydrocephalus.

**VENTRICULOURETEROSTOMY.** The ventriculoureterostomy is an operation in which a shunt is effected between the occipital horn of a lateral ventricle and a ureter. A burr hole is made in one occipital area, and the dura and cortex are incised. A nephrectomy is performed. A subcutaneous tunnel is prepared to join the occipital and renal areas. The polyethylene tube is placed over the proposed course, and the appropriate length is cut and passed through the tunnel. The ends are inserted into the ventricle and ureter as previously described.

**VENTRICULOPERITONEOSTOMY.** Ventriculoperitoneostomy is another shunt procedure devised to bypass an obstruction between the third and fourth ventricles. This is accomplished when a tube is passed subcutaneously, with one end being inserted into the lateral ventricle and the other into the peritoneal cavity as just described. (See Table 13-2.)

*Treatment of craniosynostosis.* Craniosynostosis, premature closure of the cranial sutures, is treated by various methods directed toward enlarging the cranial cavity and permitting the brain to develop. The most commonly applied procedure is the resection of the suture or sutures involved. To prevent reunion, pieces of polyethylene film are used to cover the free margins of bone. Other attempts to correct the deformity are bilateral *craniectomies* or *morcellation* of the entire skull. The latter consists of cutting the skull into small pieces, approximately 3 to 5 cm in size. These are laid over the dura in a pattern to conform to their original position. The interruption of the continuity of the skull allows the intracranial contents to expand; thus the bony fragments are kept apart until the brain reaches its maximum growth (Chapter 13).

*Treatment of encephaloceles.* Encephaloceles are treated by the removal of the bulging deformity to prevent infection, to expedite physical care, and to correct the cosmetic defect. Any neurological deficit already present is not improved by the procedure. The protrusion is dissected down to the point where it comes through the defect in the skull. The sac is opened, and any cerebral ele-

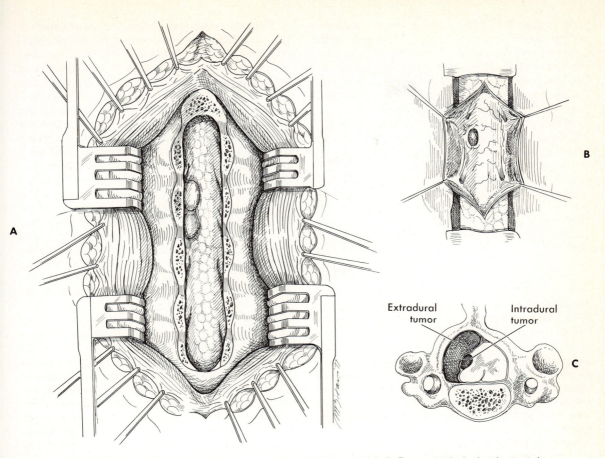

**FIG. 26-12. A,** Laminectomy completed, dura mater and tumor exposed. **B,** Dura mater incised and retracted, revealing pia-arachnoid membrane over spinal cord and part of tumor. **C,** Diagram showing cross section of tumor site and location of extradural and intradural disorder.

ments within it are freed and replaced in the cranial cavity. The sac is amputated at its base, and the defect is covered as necessary with pericranium (Chapter 13).

## Spinal cord and nerve roots (group II)

*Treatment of meningoceles.* Meningoceles are treated by excision. An elliptical incision (generally horizontal for lumbar lesions and vertical for thoracic and cervical defects) is made around the protrusion, and dissection is carried down to the bone, where the neck of the sac is isolated. The sac is opened, and if any nerve elements are contained within it, they are dissected free and re-

placed as possible within the dura mater. The sac is amputated near its base, and the dural opening is closed tightly with sutures. No attempt is made to repair the bony defect or to approximate the paraspinal muscles and fascia. A flap of fascia is elevated and reflected to the other side to cover the bony defect. The skin is closed very carefully in two layers. A sterile dressing is applied and sealed with Elastoplast. Pliofilm or other waterproof material is secured over the dressing to prevent contamination by excreta.

*Laminectomy.* To approach the spinal cord and its nerve roots, one must first carry out a laminectomy (Fig. 26-12). This consists in making a midline incision in the back over the spinous processes of the vertebrae to be exposed. The extent of the incision will depend on the number of laminae to be removed. It is continued down through the fascia; the paraspinal muscles are dissected from both sides of the spinous processes and the laminae of the vertebrae to be exposed. The spinous processes and laminae are cut off with rongeurs. The dura is thus exposed and then incised longitudinally in the midline. The pia-arachnoid is incised as necessary to accomplish the purpose of the procedure. The operation is completed by closing of the dura with interrupted silk sutures; the muscles and fascia are approximated in separate layers and sutures with interrupted silk or wire. The skin is closed with interrupted silk sutures, and a sterile dressing is applied and secured with strips of adhesive tape or Elastoplast. The spinal cord is adequately protected by the layers of muscles and fascia; therefore the bony defect that occurs after a laminectomy need not be repaired.

A laminectomy is performed for the removal of neoplasms, abscesses, ruptured cervical intervertebral discs, bony fragments, and foreign bodies, whether they are extradural or intradural. It is also a preliminary step in operations for the relief of pain and involuntary spasmodic movements. In some circumstances, when the purpose of the operation can be accomplished through a unilateral approach, *hemilaminectomy,* it is not necessary to do a complete laminectomy.

*Chordotomy.* A chordotomy consists in division of the anterolateral tracts (pain-conducting pathways) in the spinal cord at the appropriate level on the side opposite to the site of the pain. On occasion, it may be necessary to do it bilaterally. After the spinal cord has been exposed, the dentate ligament at the level selected for the chordotomy is divided. A clamp is applied to the ligament, and it is drawn posteriorly toward the midline to expose the anterolateral part of the cord. A chordotomy knife is introduced into the spinal cord immediately anterior to the dentate ligament and directed toward the anaterior spinal artery. The tissue anterior to this line is divided with the knife. This procedure is generally indicated in the treatment of diffuse pain caused by malignant disease.

During the past several years a new technique, the *high cervical percutaneous chordotomy,* has

permitted nonsurgical stereotactic destruction of the anterolateral spinothalamic tracts. By the method developed by Mullan and his associates and perfected by Rosomoff and his group a new era in the control of pain experienced by cancer clients has been made possible.

This technique permits the destruction of the spinothalamic tract simply by the stereotactic insertion of a spinal needle laterally between C1 and C2. A wire electrode is then inserted into the anterior quadrant, and by use of a radiofrequency generator, a lesion is made and the sensory fibers are destroyed. Rather exact control of the size of the lesion allows the neurosurgeon to follow stepwise the anesthetic level as it develops. This procedure can be carried out in terminal cancer clients with minimal morbidity. Bilateral procedures may be performed without any bladder dysfunction being caused. If the level of anesthesia falls or if the perception of pain recurs, the percutaneous chordotomy may be repeated.

*Rhizotomy.* A rhizotomy consists in the division of one or more spinal nerve roots (anterior or posterior). After laminectomy the root or roots to be divided are identified either anatomically or with the help of electrical stimulation. They are picked up individually with a nerve hook and cut. The anterior roots are divided to stop the involuntary spasmodic movements associated with paraplegia or torticollis. The posterior roots are divided to eliminate pain in a restricted area (involvement of specific nerves by compression, inflammation, or irremovable neoplasm) (Fig. 26-13).

*Treatment of ruptured lumbar intervertebral discs.* Ruptured lumbar intervertebral discs (Fig. 26-14, *A*) are usually removed through a unilateral interlaminar approach. This consists in making a midline incision, 6 to 8 cm long, over the level of the lesion. The lumbar fascia is incised, and the paraspinal muscles are dissected from the spinous processes and laminae above and below the herniated disc. The ligamentum flavum between the selected laminae is excised to expose the spinal dura and compressed root. In some instances one must enlarge the natural opening between the laminae by rongeuring 1 to 2 mm of the adjacent laminae. The compressed nerve root is retracted away from the ruptured material, which is then removed (Fig. 26-14, *B* to *D*). The defect that re-

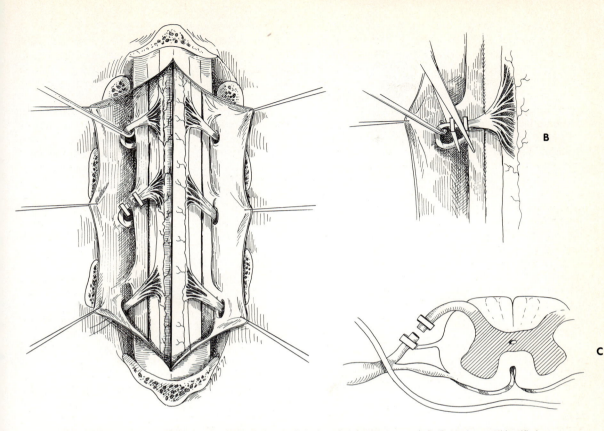

**FIG. 26-13.** Posterior rhizotomy after laminectomy. **A,** Spinal cord and roots exposed. **B,** Posterior root identified. **C,** Diagram showing cross section of spinal cord and divided posterior root.

sults from the removal of the intervertebral disc is negligible. The lateral vertebral joints prevent close contact of the anterior bodies. A fusion is indicated when there is unusual instability of the lower spine.

*Skeletal traction.* Skeletal traction is the treatment of choice for fracture-dislocations of the cervical spine. This is accomplished by the application of Crutchfield or halo tongs to the skull. To eliminate the possibility of further injury to the spinal cord, these procedures are sometimes carried out with the client in a specially prepared bed (see discussion of fracture bed, Chapter 27). The head of the client, by being at a suitable elevation, is accessible for the operative procedure. The scalp over the vertex in the parietal regions is prepared over an area 15 cm in size, as described in the next section.

**CRUTCHFIELD TONGS.** The two sites for the insertion of the tongs are selected over the lateral parietal eminences (about midway from the top of the ear to the midline bilaterally). A local anesthetic is injected into the scalp, a stab wound is made down to the skull, and a drill hole (3 mm, children; 4 mm, adults) is made in the outer table of the skull. The points of the tongs are inserted into these openings, and the tongs are tightened to secure them in place. Small sterile dressings are applied with collodion over the wounds and around the inserted points. Traction is applied with weights.

**HALO TONGS.** Application of halo tongs is similar

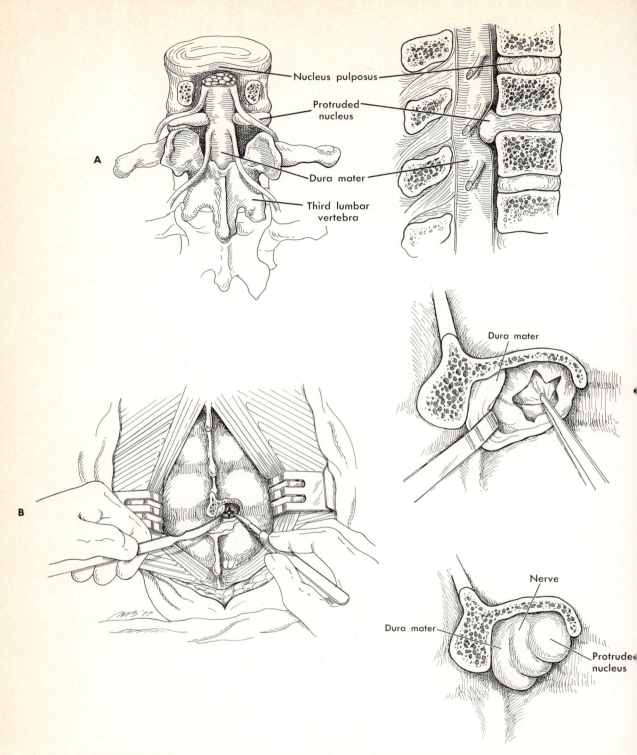

Nucleus pulposus

Protruded nucleus

Dura mater

Third lumbar vertebra

A

B

Dura mater

Nerve

Dura mater

Protruded nucleus

**FIG. 26-14. A,** Herniation of lumbar intervertebral disc. **B,** Interlaminal removal of herniated disc, removal of part of lamina, exposing nucleus pulposus. **C,** Observe relationship of dura mater, nerve, and protruded nucleus. **D,** Removing extruded disc.

to that of Crutchfield tongs. Insertion of the tongs is in four sites, two anterior and two posterior. With these tongs the client can be put into traction similar to that used with Crutchfield tongs. Another alternative is to apply a spica cast with additional halo attachments that immobilize the cervical area. This allows the client to be ambulatory without damage to the cervical fracture.

## Peripheral nerves (group III)

Peripheral nerve surgery is done for the removal of tumors (neurofibromas) of the peripheral nerves, the repair of divided nerves, and the alleviation of pain. The operations included in this field are neurotomy, neurectomy, neurexeresis, neurotripsy, neurolysis, neurorrhapy, nerve anas-

tomosis, and the excision of tumors. A *neurotomy,* the division of a nerve, is performed to relieve localized peripheral pain. *Neurectomy,* the excision of a nerve, and *neurexeresis,* the avulsion of a nerve, are also applied in the treatment of local pain. *Neurotripsy,* the crushing of a nerve, is performed to accomplish temporary (a matter of months) interruption of function. Its most common application is to the phrenic nerve in the treatment of pulmonary tuberculosis. (This results in a paralysis of the diaphragm and limits the activity of the lung.) *Neurolysis,* the freeing of a nerve from adhesions or callus about a fractured bone, is applied for the relief of pain and to promote the recovery of nerve function. *Neurorrhaphy,* the suture of a divided nerve (Fig. 26-15), is done in the repair of

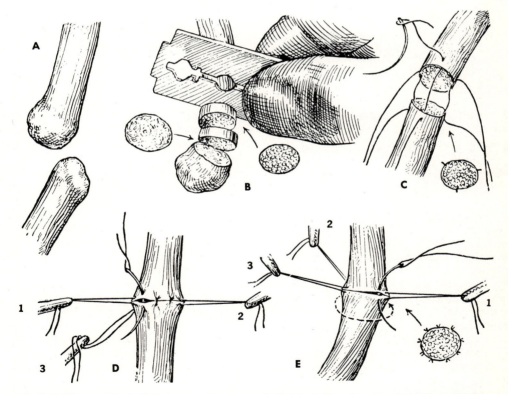

**FIG. 26-15.** Nerve repair. **A,** Divided nerve with neuroma. **B,** Serial resection of neuroma to healthy nerve fibers. **C,** Placement of sutures in perineurium. **D** and **E,** Approximation and tying of sutures. (From Sachs, E.: Diagnosis and treatment of brain tumors and care of the neurosurgical patient, ed. 2, St. Louis, 1949, The C.V. Mosby Co.)

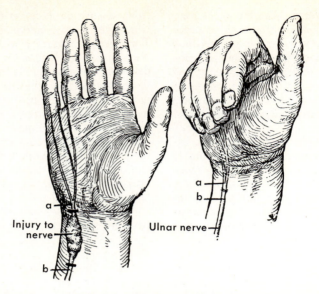

**FIG. 26-16.** Traumatic neuroma of ulnar nerve; note limits of excision of lesion and sutured nerve ends, as identified by points *a* and *b*. (From Sachs, E.: Diagnosis and treatment of brain tumors and care of the neuro-surgical patient, ed. 2, St. Louis, 1949, The C.V. Mosby Co.)

injuries of nerves, in the approximation of nerve ends after the removal of a tumor of the nerve, and in nerve anastomoses.

The length of the skin incision depends on the location and nature of the lesion. The management of a neoplasm or of a traumatic neuroma is the same as just described in that after resection of the mass the two ends of the nerve must be approximated and sutured meticulously with interrupted fine silk sutures in the perineurium (Fig. 26-16). The same type of approximation is used in the anastomosis of a healthy nerve with one whose function has been destroyed as in facial paralysis (hypoglossal-facial; spinal accessory–facial). Since the removal of the lesion shortens the nerve, it is sometimes necessary to flex the limb to approximate the nerve ends. This flexion must be maintained so that there is no chance that the nerve sutures are pulled out. Therefore after the application of a sterile dressing a plaster cast is used to maintain the desired position for at least 6 weeks. This gives the nerve a chance to regenerate.

The brachial plexus may be compressed by a su-pernumerary (cervical) rib, bands between rudimentary and normal ribs, an aberrant artery, a subclavian artery, or the anterior scalene muscle. The symptoms (pain in the shoulder and arm with paresthesias) associated with these conditions are caused by compression of the brachial plexus. A skin incision, 8 to 10 cm, is made just above the medial third of the clavicle, and the dissection is carried down to the anterior scalene muscle, which is then divided. The brachial plexus is inspected for any constricting elements (bands, aberrant artery, fibers of scalenus medius muscle), and these are resected. If a cervical rib is present, it is excised.

## Autonomic nervous system (group IV)

Surgery of the autonomic nervous system is performed for the treatment of circulatory disturbances (Raynaud's phenomenon, thromboangiitis obliterans, peripheral arteriosclerosis, essential hypertension, angina pectoris, and frostbite) and for relief of intractable pain (in causalgia, biliary and pancreatic diseases, idiopathic dysmenorrhea, and renal and ureteral disorders). The therapeutic effect in the management of vascular disease is accomplished by elimination of vasospasm and improvement of the peripheral blood supply. The relief of pain in the conditions mentioned is achieved by the interruption of afferent pathways in the sympathetic division. This surgery (sympathetic ganglionectomy, splanchnicectomy, and presacral neurectomy) consists in performing various procedures on the sympathetic division of the autonomic nervous system and entails the removal of one or more ganglia with their intervening sympathetic chain in the thoracic and lumbar regions.

*Thoracic sympathectomy.* Thoracic sympathectomy (sympathetic ganglionectomy) is accomplished through a paravertebral incision over the transverse processes of the thoracic vertebrae at the desired level. The paravertebral muscles are incised and retracted to expose the transverse processes of the vertebrae and the adjacent segments of ribs. These are resected; the retropleural space is exposed with the sympathetic chain as it lies along the side of the vertebral bodies. An upper thoracic sympathectomy (second through fifth thoracic nerves) is performed for the relief of causalgia, angina pectoris, and Raynaud's phenomenon involving the upper extremities. A lower thoracic sympathectomy (sixth through twelfth thoracic nerves) and the interruption of the splanchnic nerves (sympathetic ganglionectomy–splanchnicectomy) is done in the treatment of biliary and pancreatic diseases.

*Lumbar sympathectomy.* Lumbar sympathectomy (sympathetic ganglionectomy) is most commonly done through an anterior abdominal muscle–splitting incision to the retroperitoneal space. The peritoneum and abdominal contents are retracted medially to expose the sympathetic chain that lies between the psoas muscle and the vertegral column. Two or more ganglia and the intervening chain are resected. This is done to treat circulatory disorders of the lower extremities (thromboangiitis obliterans, frostbite, and peripheral arteriosclerosis) and causalgia.

*Thoracolumbar sympathectomy.* Thoracolumbar sympathectomy (ganglionectomy and splanchnicectomy), sixth through twelfth thoracic and first through third lumbar nerves, is performed through a hockey-stick incision parallel to and 3 inches from the spine. The thorax is entered after removal of a segment of one or two of the adjacent ribs. The pleura is separated from the posterior thoracic wall so that the sympathetic chain and ganglia are disclosed. The lower half (sixth through twelfth thoracic nerves) of the thoracic sympathetic chain with the ganglia and splanchnic nerves are removed. The lumbar chain (first through third lumbar nerves) is then removed through a retroperitoneal approach into the flank. The procedure must be done bilaterally, and approximately a week should intervene between the two stages. This operation is performed in the treatment of essential hypertension.

*Presacral neurectomy.* Presacral neurectomy is performed through a left paramedian abdominal incision. The intestines are retracted into the upper abdominal cavity; the posterior peritoneum is incised over the bifurcation of the aorta, and the superior hypogastric plexus is resected. This is done for the relief of idiopathic intractable dysmenorrhea.

## POSTOPERATIVE PHASE

The postoperative follow-up is the final aspect of the operating room nurse's role. The nurse may visit one or more times, depending on the institution's policy. The objectives of the postoperative visit are to continue to give support to the client, to evaluate the nursing care given to the client in the operative phase, and to plan for and implement alternative nursing actions, if necessary.

The operating room nurse continues to give information to the client during the postoperative phase and observes the client turning, coughing, deep breathing, and leg exercising to reinforce this teaching. The operating room nurse can answer questions pertaining to the equipment, such as dressings, intravenous lines, and any drains.

The operating room nurse utilizes this time to evaluate nursing care given in the operative phase, checking the client's vital signs, level of consciousness, affect, speech, reflexes, motor ability, and pupils to compare with the preoperative assessment. Any signs of postoperative complications are also noted by the nurse. He or she assesses the data and determines if the complication relates to the nursing care given in the operating room.

Finally, alternate nursing actions are planned for the institution, if necessary. If a postoperative complication is possibly related to nursing care given in the operating room, a new procedure may need to be developed.

## SUMMARY

The neurosurgical client requires comprehensive care from the preoperative to the postoperative aspect of the surgical experience. The operating room nurse plays an important role in helping to provide continuity of care for the client. The members of the surgical team must work together to maintain excellent client care.

### REFERENCES

Alexander, C., Schrader, E., and Kneedler, J.: Preoperative visits: the operating room nurse unmasks, AORN J. **19:**401, Feb. 1974.

Alksne, J.F.: Stereotactic thrombosis of intracranial aneurysms, N. Engl. J. Med. **284:**171-174, Jan. 28, 1971.

Allwood, A., and Lundy, C.: Cerebral artery bypass surgery, Am. J. Nurs. **80:**1284-1287, July 1980.

Ammerman, B.J., and Smith, D.R.: Giant fusiform middle cerebral aneurysm: successful treatment utilizing microvascular bypass, Surg. Neurol. **7:**255, May 1977.

Anchie, T.I.: Acoustic neuroma: a benign tumor, J. Neurosurg. Nurs. **12:**11-17, March 1980.

AORN Convention 1976: Changing face of operating room nursing, Paper presented by J. Persson et al., Miami Beach, Fla., March 1976.*

AORN Convention 1977: Care of patients having local anesthetics, Paper presented by J. Dahle et al., Anaheim, Calif., March 1977.*

AORN Convention 1980: New JCAH standards impact on quality assurance, Paper presented by J. Affeldt et al., Atlanta, Ga., March 1980.*

Ayers, C., and Walton, L.: A guide for the preoperative visit, AORN J. **19:**413, Feb. 1974.

Backlund, E.O., et al.: Controlled subtotal evacuation of intracerebral hematomas by stereotactic technique, Surg. Neurol. **9:**99-101, Feb. 1978.

Bader, D.: Micro-surgical treatment of intracranial aneurysms, J. Neurosurg. Nurs. **7:**25, July 1975.

Bader, D.: Microtechnical nursing in neurosurgery, J. Neurosurg. Nurs. **7:**22, July 1975.

Beckford, A.R., and Teter, A.: A study of three patients with "Y" shunts, J. Neurosurg. Nurs. **9:**128-132, Sept. 1977.

Behrends, E.A.: Intraoperative monitoring of cortical oxidative metabolism, J. Neurosurg. Nurs. **12:**22-27, March 1980.

Bucy, P.C.: Intracranial tumors: where we have been and where we are going, Clin. Neurosurg. **25:**305-309, 1978.

Butterworth, G.A.: Interfascicular autologous nerve grafts in the microsurgical repair of peripheral nerves, J. Neurosurg. Nurs. **9:**63-66, June 1977.

Cassidy, F.M.: Adult hydrocephalus, Am. J. Nurs. **72:**494-499, 1972.

Coleman, P.: The problem of spasticity in the management of the spinal cord–injured patient and its treatment with special reference to percutaneous radiofrequency thermal selective sensory rhizotomy, J. Neurosurg. Nurs. **8:**97, Dec. 1976.

Connolly, E.S., deLima, A.M., and Rowland, M.L.: Operating room inservice on microneurosurgery, AORN J. **20:**452, Sept. 1974.

Dooley, D.M.: Spinal cord stimulation, AORN J. **23:**1209, June 1976.

Dye, W.S., and Brown, C.M.: Surgical correction of carotid and vertebral artery stenosis, Surg. Clin. North Am. **53:**241, Feb. 1973.

Ehni, G.: The surgical nurse and neurological surgery, J. Neurosurg. Nurs. **6:**7, July 1974.

Fedun, P.C.: Preoperative evaluation of patients undergoing microanastomosis for brain ischemia, J. Neurosurg. Nurs. **12:**46-53, March 1980.

Garrido, E., and Stein, B.: Microsurgical removal of intramedullary spinal cord tumors, Surg. Neurol. **7:**215, April 1977.

Grabow, J.D., et al.: Cerebellar stimulation for the control of seizures, Mayo Clin. Proc. **49:**759, Oct. 1974.

Greenwood, J.: The evolution of neurosurgery and the neurosurgical nurse, J. Neurosurg. Nurs. **5:**39, Dec. 1973.

Harris, L.O.: The specialized role of the neurosurgical operating room nurse, J. Neurosurg. Nurs. **12:**128-133, Sept. 1980.

Hartley, M.B.: Hypothermia, AORN J. **24:**764, Oct. 1976.

Healey, K.M.: Does preoperative instruction make a difference? Am. J. Nurs. **68:**62, Jan. 1968.

Heimburger, R.F.: Early repair of myelomeningocele (spina bifida cystica), J. Neurosurg. **37:**594-600, Nov. 1972.

Hoffman, J.: Arterial blood gas analysis as a basic criterion for the management of the neurosurgical patient, J. Neurosurg. Nurs. **9:**29, March 1977.

Jacobs, G.B., Rubin, R.C., and Wille, R.: The treatment of intracranial aneurysms, J. Neurosurg. Nurs. **8:**149, Dec. 1976.

Kay, E., and Boone, E.: Stereotactic surgery for Parkinson's disease, Am. J. Nurs. **72:**2200-2205, 1972.

Kellogg, M.: Update: operating room nursing, AORN film, March 1977 (AORN convention), Davis & Geck Co.

Kelly, D., et al.: Modified leucotomy assessed clinically, physiologically and psychologically at six weeks and eighteen months, Br. J. Psychiatry **120:**19-29, Jan. 1972.

Kline, D.G.: Tensions of aneurysm surgery, AORN J. **20:**385, Sept. 1974.

Koons, D.D.: Local hypothermia in the treatment of spinal cord injuries. Report of seven cases, Cleve. Clin. Q. **39:**109-117, Fall 1972.

*For cassettes of these programs contact the Association of Operating Room Nurses, Inc., 10170 East Mississippi Ave., Denver, CO 80231.

Lamb, S.: Interstitial radiation for the treatment of brain tumors using the stereotactic method, J. Neurosurg. Nurs. **12:**138-144, Sept. 1980.

Lee, R.M., and Madeja, C.: Neurosurgical clinician provides continuity of care, AORN J. **20:**426, Sept. 1974.

Lindeman, C.: Study evaluates effects of preoperative visits, AORN J. **19:**427, Feb. 1974.

Lindeman, C.A., and Stetzer, S.L.: Effect of preoperative visits by operating room nurses, Nurs. Res. **22:**4, Jan.-Feb. 1973.

Loetterle, B.C., et al.: Cerebellar stimulation: pacing the brain, Am. J. Nurs. **75:**958, June 1975.

Madeja, C., Plank, N., and Reuta, R.: The neurosurgical nurse as a departmental assistant, J. Neurosurg. Nurs. **7:**99, Dec. 1975.

McCaig, C.: Review: positioning for neurosurgery, AORN J. **28:**1053-1060, Dec. 1978.

McConnell, E.A.: After surgery: how you can avert the obvious hazards . . . and the not-so-obvious ones, Nursing77 **7:**32, March 1977.

McKenzie, S.: Stereotaxic radiofrequency coagulation: a treatment for trigeminal neuralgia, J. Neurosurg. Nurs. **4:**75, July 1972.

Morgan, M.E.: Surgical nurse clinical specialist, AORN J. **23:**638, March 1976.

Murphy, M.: Preoperative teaching, integration of nursing and social work services, J. Neurosurg. Nurs. **9:**5, March 1977.

Nevins, S.K.: Pre- and postoperative care of patients undergoing transsphenoidal pituitary surgery, J. Neurosurg. Nurs. **8:**45, July 1976.

Ostrow, L.: New hope for patients with trigeminal neuralgias, Am. J. Nurs. **76:**1301, Aug. 1976.

Poole, M.V.: Percutaneous electrocoagulation for tic douloureux, AORN J. **24:**887, Nov. 1976.

Rand, R.W.: Microneurosurgery, St. Louis, 1969, The C.V. Mosby Co.

Ridgeway, M.: Preop interviews assure quality care, AORN J. **24:**1083, Dec. 1976.

Rimel, R.W.: Nurse practitioners and neurosurgical manpower, Surg. Neurol. **7:**19, Jan. 1977.

Rutecki, B., and Seligson, D.: Caring for the patient in a halo apparatus, Nursing80 **10:**73-77, Oct. 1980.

Sachs, E.: Diagnosis and treatment of brain tumors and care of the neurosurgical patient, ed. 2, St. Louis, 1949, The C.V. Mosby Co.

Salmon, J.H.: Adult hydrocephalus, evaluation of shunt therapy in 80 patients, J. Neurosurg. **37:**423-428, 1972.

Sele, S.C.: The treatment of tic douloureux by vascular decompression of the trigeminal nerve, J. Neurosurg. Nurs. **9:**19, March 1977.

Shields, C.B.: Cerebral revascularization, AORN J. **27:**905-924, April 1978.

Slocombe, I.: Posterior cervical stabilization with anterior cervical fusion: an alternative approach to cervical fractures, J. Neurosurg. Nurs. **11:**34-36, March 1979.

Smith, R.A.: Preoperative assessment by the operating room nurse, Unpublished paper, University of Evansville, Evansville, Ind., Nov. 1976.

Smith, R.B., Petruscak, J., and Solosko, D.: In a recovery room, Am. J. Nurs. **73:**70-73, 1973.

Spiegel, E.A., and Wycis, H.T.: Stereoencephalotomy, New York, 1952, Grune & Stratton, Inc.

Stetzer, S.: Preoperative visits meet patient's tangible needs, AORN J. **19:**441, Feb. 1974.

Stibitz, M.A.: Intraoperative care during spinal cord stimulation, AORN J. **23:**1213, June 1976.

Stowe, S.M.: Hypophysectomy for diabetic retinopathy, Am. J. Nurs. **73:**632-637, 1973.

Sundaresan, N., et al.: Transaxillary transthoracic sympathectomy, Surg. Neurol. **7:**149, March 1977.

Wille, R.L.: Neurosurgical nursing: past, present, and future, Heart Lung **8:**891-895, Sept.-Oct. 1979.

Wille, R.: The nurse's role in the specialty of neurological surgery, J. Neurosurg. Nurs. **8:**77, Dec. 1976.

Winslow, E.H., and Fuhs, M.F.: Preoperative assessment for postoperative evaluation, Am. J. Nurs. **73:**1372, Aug. 1973.

Wren, L.: Nursing care of a craniotomy patient in the operating room, J. Neurosurg. Nurs. **10:**49-51, June 1978.

Yura, H., and Walsh, M.B.: The nursing process: assessing, planning, implementing, evaluation, New York, 1973, Appleton-Century-Crofts.

# 27

# ADJUNCTIVE INTERVENTION

To initiate effective nursing intervention based on medical therapy, accurate assessments of all neurological deficits and disorders must be made. Such assessments are made by physical examination, neurological assessment, neurological diagnostic testing, radiological studies, and, when indicated, surgical procedures. History taking of illnesses and accidents are an integral part of planning nursing care. The essence of nursing intervention is based on the development of a therapeutic relationship with the client and family; the client's cooperation and acceptance of those actions necessary to accomplish physical and psychosocial care; and continuity, consistency and excellence in those interventions necessary to return the client to a functional level of performance or to comfort the client and family when death is imminent. Specific nursing interventions are discussed in this chapter with the emphasis on assessment as outlined in previous chapters, intervention, and the need for client and family teaching throughout hospitalization, rehabilitation, and discharge.

## INTERVENTION FOR HYPERTHERMIA

Remove blankets, gown, and other excess clothing if the client's temperature reaches 101° F. Maintain room temperature at 70° F. Use a standing electric fan at the bedside of the client to aid in cooling the body. (Be certain it is positioned so the client cannot reach it and accidentally cause injury.) Antipyretics may or may not be given. These drugs are little to no value in hyperthermias that result from injured thermoregulatory centers (stroke, cerebral tumor, or intracranial surgery, or after head injuries) but are effective in treatment of temperature elevations from pyrogens. Unless contraindicated, increase fluid intake to 3000 ml every 24 hours.

If hyperthermia has a specific cause, such as wound infection, meningitis, cystitis, pneumonia, or phlebitis, treat symptomatically and systemically. If the temperature continues to rise and reaches 103° F or above, a tepid sponge bath is administered. Intravenous dantrolene sodium has been approved by the Federal Drug Administration for the treatment of malignant hypertension (*FDA Bulletin,* p. 27, Nov. 1979).

If the temperature does not fall with these treatments, cool to ice-cold colon lavages may be given. An oxygen tent may be used to supplement the regimen by providing added cool moisture.

If hyperthermia is believed to be caused by damage to the hypothalamus (edema, hemorrhage, or trauma), the most effective method of reducing and controlling the body temperature is with a hypothermic machine. Rectal temperatures are taken frequently until the temperatures lower to a reduced, safer level.

Comfort measures for clients with an elevated temperature should include keeping the skin dry and clean, frequent mouth care, frequent positional changes and skin care over bony prominences, and emotional support for the client and family when the client is irritable or stuporous.

The client should have an explanation of why the temperature must be lowered and receive physical and emotional support during discomfort.

# HYPOTHERMIA

*Definition.* Hypothermia is the controlled reduction and maintenance of body temperature 10° to 15° below normal as an adjunct to the medical or surgical treatment of selected clients. It also may be used to treat clients with elevated temperatures.

The physiological response to hypothermia is related directly to the degree of temperature achieved. As the temperature falls, the rate of metabolism decreases; as metabolism slows, glandular, liver, and kidney functions decrease; as the neuromuscular tissue in the heart (pacemaker) becomes more affected by the cold, the circulation slows; as plasma pools in the peripheral capillary beds, the volume of blood in the circulation diminishes. Since the metabolic activity of the body is reduced in proportion to the fall of temperature, previously jeopardized tissues need less blood and have a better chance to survive.

With a temperature of 86° F (30° C) the metabolism of the body is reduced by almost 50%; with a temperature of 68° F (20° C) the metabolism is reduced to 25% of the normal rate. Although it has been reported that a child survived a temperature of 60.8° F (16° C), it is generally recommended that induced hypothermia be maintained above 82° F (27.8° C) to prevent irreversible complications. The optimal level of hypothermia is related directly to the reason it is being used and to the reaction of the particular client. The critical temperature below which myocardial irritability is altered with resulting arrhythmia varies with the individual, depending on age, physical condition, and the type of anesthetic used, if any.

The physiologic effects of cold on the human being are described in Table 27-1.

With hypothermia, oxygen consumption is reduced; pulse, respiration, and blood pressure fall, cerebral function diminishes; brain bulk is reduced; the venous and cerebrospinal fluid pressures decrease; and cerebral blood flow is reduced about 6% for every degree the centigrade temperature is reduced below normal.

Various methods for lowering the temperature of the human body have been developed. They may be classified in four groups: (1) *external cooling* by immersion of the body in ice water, by forcing cold air around the client in a tight enclosure, by wrapping with electrically refrigerating blankets, or by the application of cracked ice, sponges, or ice bags; (2) *internal surface cooling* by ice-water enemas, by cold saline solutions poured into the thoracic or abdominal cavities, or by the circulation of ice water in a balloon placed in the stomach; (3) *internal vascular cooling* by removing venous blood, cooling it, and returning it to the circulation; and (4) *ventricular cooling* by introducing a hypothermic physiological solution into a ventricle through an indwelling catheter.

The procedure of caring for the client with a hypothermia electronic machine includes principles of care and observation, which may be followed when other methods are used to induce hypothermia.

*Purposes.* (1) To reduce metabolic activity so that oxygen requirements are decreased, (2) to prevent, to control, or to combat dangerously high temperatures, (3) to control cerebral edema, (4) to

**TABLE 27-1.** Physiologic effects of cold on the human being

| Temperature | | Comments |
|---|---|---|
| 98.6° F | 37.0° C | Normal body temperature; normal metabolism |
| 96.0° F | 35.5° C | Heart and respiration slow; rate of metabolism decreases |
| 92.0° F | 33.3° C | Higher mental processes impaired; difficulty in performing complex physical acts; responds to verbal commands |
| 90.0° F | 32.2° C | Diminished response to external stimuli; becomes stuporous |
| 86.0° F | 30.0° C | Generally becomes unconscious; rate of metabolism 50% of normal (heart action apparently not disturbed) |
| 82.0° F | 27.8° C | Pupillary reaction to light absent; corneal and gag reflexes absent; blood pressure, pulse, and respiration continue to fall; ventricular fibrillation may develop |
| 68.0° F | 20.0° C | Rate of metabolism only 25% of normal; human being in grave jeopardy; death may occur suddenly |

facilitate certain surgical procedures by reducing blood flow, (5) to reduce intracranial pressure, (6) to decrease circulation time, (7) to reduce the amount of anesthetic given during surgery, (8) to reduce operative risk in debilitated clients, and (9) to relieve intractable pain.

*Indications.* (1) Vascular surgery, (2) cardiac surgery, (3) cardiac arrest, (4) prolonged neuro-surgical procedures on the brain, (5) amputations, (6) shock, (7) hyperthermia, (8) surgery on ''poor-risk'' clients, and (9) terminal cancer with intract-able pain.

*Preparation of equipment.* Assemble all equipment. Utilize the manual of operating instructions distributed with each machine to ensure its safe and effective use.

*Preparation of client.* If the client is conscious, the physician explains the procedure to him or her. A permit for the treatment is obtained from the client if possible, or from a responsible relative.

If the client is not in a single room, draw curtains to provide privacy and sufficient space for equipment and staff.

Place a draw sheet over the client and remove the top bedclothes. Remove pajamas.

Turn the client on the side, and place the bath blanket on the bed. Turn the client on the other side, and pull it through, making certain that it is free of wrinkles. Position the client on the back.

Take and record pulse, respiration, and blood pressure; note and record the level of consciousness and strength of extremities.

Open the cut-down tray and assist the physician as necessary in preparing for the administration of intravenous solutions. (Oral intake may be unsafe if gag reflexes and other reflexes are depressed.)

Catheterize the client with a Foley catheter, inflate the Foley balloon, and leave it in place. Empty the bladder, and attach the connection tip and drainage tube to the catheter. Place the end of the tube in the drainage bottle, place in holder, and attach to frame of bed. Record the amount of urine, and check its specific gravity carefully since urinary output may be decreased with lowered body temperature.

Utilize a cardiac monitor to facilitate the detection of cardiac arrhythmias caused by lowered body temperature.

*Procedure.* Turn the client on the side; place a vinyl pad on the bed and cover with draw sheet. Turn client and pull through the pad and sheet. Place client on the back. Place second vinyl pad over client, leaving the sheet next to the body.

Insert the temperature probe into the rectum, and place its plug in the jack in the electronic control box.

Approximate the holes on the two vinyl pads, and tie with tape or bandage. Repeat on the other side. The bath blanket, previously placed on the bottom draw sheet, may be wrapped around the pads that now enclose the client. (This helps to maintain the desired temperature.)

Remove protective caps from male couplings on the machine, and connect tubes attached to vinyl pads.

Check level of solution, and add more if it is not above the minimum mark.

Turn on the machine, and set the dial for the desired temperature (initially this may be done by the physician).

Read temperature meter, and record every 3 to 5 minutes until the desired body temperature is reached. (This takes from 2 to 4 hours, depending on the level desired and the client's temperature at the beginning of the treatment.)

*Intervention during hypothermia.* Read and record temperature meter every 15 minutes after the desired temperature is reached.

Measure and record pulse, respiration, and blood pressure every 5 minutes until the client's temperature is stabilized and then every 15 to 30 minutes, depending on the client's condition.

Note size and reaction of pupils, and check level of consciousness each time the vital signs are taken.

Check color of lips and nail beds frequently.

Check for and report immediately any skin discoloration, induration, or edema.

Measure intake and output accurately. Check specific gravity of urine as ordered.

Change the position of the client at least every 2 hours unless contraindicated.

If the client is unconscious, apply the principles of mouth, eye, and skin care as outlined in this chapter and in Chapter 9.

Use suction as necessary to maintain an open airway. If the client is conscious, encourage coughing and deep breathing.

If the temperature goes below 90° F (32.2° C), test the gag reflex before giving any food or fluid by mouth.

Report any changes in the client's condition.

Watch for complications: changes in vital signs not in ratio to the fall or rise of temperature, increased intracranial pressure, respiratory obstruction, respiratory arrest, cardiac arrest, oliguria, anuria, frostbite.

Although shivering is a normal response to cold and the body's attempt to maintain its heat, it increases venous and cerebrospinal fluid pressure and oxygen requirements and must be controlled if treatment is to be effective. (Curare, succinylcholine, and chlorpromazine are a few of the drugs that may be used for this purpose.)

Remember that the signs of infection or inflammation may be masked during the course of treatment.

Noted that, in general, the effect of drugs is reduced with hypothermia, and so higher doses may be required for therapeutic results.

*Specific cautions.* The manufacturer states that the electrical equipment is not explosion proof, and the extension legs of the cart should be used to elevate the unit to the 5-foot level if explosive gases are in its vicinity. Keep the unit at least 3 feet away from any oxygen equipment.

Be certain that the ground wire is connected and the machine grounded before starting the treatment. Utilize safe practice geared toward the use of an electrical machine.

Make certain that the unit is on the open frame of the cart so that air circulates around the base of its compressor to prevent overheating.

Use the correct solution, and check the level frequently.

*Intervention after hypothermic treatment.* The machine is usually turned off when the temperature is recorded at 94° to 96° F. This allows for the tendency of the temperature to drift downward. The tapes securing the vinyl pads are untied, and the pads are removed.

Cover the client with a warm blanket. Remove the sheets on top of and under the client; remove the blanket from beneath the client.

Assist the client into pajamas.

Replace top bedclothes.

Measure temperature, pulse, respiration, and blood pressure every 30 minutes until they are stabilized and then every 4 hours unless otherwise ordered.

Continue observations on level of consciousness, size and reaction of pupils, motion and strength of extremities, and color and condition of skin.

Check dressings frequently (as temperature rises, bleeding may occur).

Measure intake and output.

Encourage the client to move, to breathe deeply, and to cough.

Continue special nursing care as indicated.

Remember that a hypothermic reaction may occur several days after treatment has been discontinued.

If the Aquamatic Thermia machine is used to raise the client's temperature to normal after several hours or days of hypothermia, the same meticulous observations should be made and special nursing care continued.

### CHARTING

Note time treatment was begun and discontinued.
Describe client's condition and reaction to treatment.
Record intake and output.

## Iced alcohol sponge (rarely used)

*Purpose.* To reduce body temperature by increasing surface evaporation of heat from the body after the application of alcohol and ice.

*Contraindications.* (1) Severe cachexia or debility, (2) very aged or very young clients, (3) systemic shock, (4) chills, and (5) convulsions.

### EQUIPMENT

2 large round basins
Large pitcher
Cracked ice (large pieces)
6 bath towels
4 ice bags and covers
6-foot rubber sheet
2 bath blankets
Alcohol, 70%
Rubber gloves
Electric fan (optional)
Rectal thermometer
Lubricant
Watch
Sphygmomanometer and stethoscope

*Preparation of client.* If the client is conscious, explain the nature of the treatment and the reason for applying the ice and alcohol. Prepare him or her for a possible unpleasant reaction to the cold applications, and try to elicit cooperation before beginning the procedure.

Draw curtains around the unit. Place bath blanket over the client, remove the top bedclothes, fold them neatly, and place them on a chair.

Turn the client on the side and place a rubber sheet covered with a bath blanket on the bed. Turn the client on opposite side and pull through the rubber sheet and blanket. Posture the client on this side. Make sure the leg and arm bolsters are well protected with rubber sheeting.

Measure the rectal temperature, pulse, respiration, and blood pressure. Record with the time on the observation sheet.

*Procedure.* Put on rubber gloves to protect the hands from the cold solution. Wring out each towel individually and apply to the body in the following order: towel 1 to the back, towel 2 to the uppermost arm, towel 3 to the lower extremity on the bed, towel 4 to the uppermost lower extremity, and towel 5 to the chest, abdomen, and other arm.

Remove the bath blanket as soon as the towels are applied. Place ice bags in the axillary and popliteal regions. Change towels continually, one by one, following the same order, always keeping one towel submerged in the basin.

Measure temperature, pulse, and respiration every 10 minutes and record on vital sign sheet. Check blood pressure every 30 minutes unless indicated more frequently.

Continue treatment until temperature falls to 100° F unless any of the following occur: severe chill, symptoms of shock, or severe emotional reaction. If the temperature does not fall within the first 20 minutes of treatment, start the electric fan.

Change the client's position to alternate sides every hour. Change the bottom blanket as necessary. Keep the client as dry as possible.

Cover the client with a bath blanket. Remove towels, ice bags, rubber sheet, and blanket. Change bed linen as necessary.

Posture the client in a comfortable position. Cover the patient with a sheet and remove the bath blanket. Remove curtains.

Measure the client's temperature, pulse, respiration, and blood pressure, and record. Continue these observations every 30 to 60 minutes as indicated by the client's condition until they are stabilized.

## CHARTING

**Nurse's notes**
Procedure, date, and time begun and ended
Significant reactions
Aftercare

# INTERVENTION FOR NUTRITION AND FLUID BALANCE

Neurological clients who have a depressed or absent gag reflex as a result of intracranial surgery, neurological disorders, spinal cord or head injuries, general debilitation, or unconsciousness are not given food or fluids orally to prevent aspiration. Therefore nutritional, fluid, and electrolyte needs are met through nasal gastric feedings and intravenous infusions. Both short- and long-term nutritional, fluid, and electrolyte needs can be balanced through physiological feedings proportioned to meet the body's daily requirements and prevent a negative nitrogen balance.

**Expected outcome**
The client should be informed of the need to reestablish nutritional balance and to cooperate in the placement of the nasal gastric tube.

## TUBE FEEDING

*Definition.* The insertion of a small Levin tube through the nostril into the stomach when the client is unable or refuses to take adequate nourishment by mouth. This tube may be left in for several days but should be changed at least every 5 days. The nostrils should be alternated to prevent irritation of the mucous membrane.

*Contraindication.* Bilateral nasal obstruction or disease.

## EQUIPMENT

Tray
Polyethylene nasal tube
2-ounce funnel
Lubricant, water-soluble

500 ml graduate
200 ml cup
20 ml syringe
3 towels
Emesis basin
Unsterile sponges (3 by 3 inches)
Roll of ¼-inch adhesive tape
Tongue depressors
Flashlight
Rubber band or plastic clamp
Nutrient solution
Water

*Preparation of equipment.* Place towel on tray. Arrange the rest of the equipment neatly on the tray. Fill cup with water (room temperature). Fill graduate with fruit juice or tube feeding mixture. Cover tray and carry to client's bedside.

*Preparation of client.* Explain the procedure to the client. Tell him or her how to swallow the tube and how to relieve the feelings of distress by breathing through the mouth. For the unconscious client, still explain the procedure as usual, but proceed with great care because of inability to swallow or breath through mouth or on mechanical ventilator. Remove artificial dentures. Raise the head of the bed to approximately a 45-degree angle. Screen the client.

*Procedure.* Put a protective pad on the client with its surplus over the top bedclothes to protect them. Tuck a towel under the client's chin, and secure it under the neck of the pad.

Squeeze lubricant on a sponge, and apply to the first 6 inches of the tube. (Because of the danger of droplets being aspirated, no oily solution should be used to lubricate the tube.) The nurse gives final instructions to the client and then inserts the tube into the nostril, through the esophagus, and into the stomach (22 to 30 inches in an adult).

Using a flashlight and tongue depressor, the position of the tube in the pharynx is checked during the procedure to determine whether it is going into the esophagus or lies curled in the mouth. If the client has difficulty in swallowing the tube, sips of water or cracked ice may assist the process. The position of the tube may be tested when its end is inverted into a glass of water. If air bubbles appear, the tube may be in the trachea or the lung; if so, remove and reinsert the tube.

After testing for the tube placement in the stomach, attach the 20 ml syringe to the tube and aspirate, measure, and return stomach contents. Attach a funnel to the tube, pour in about 50 ml of water to clear the tube of mucus. Follow this with 100 to 200 ml of fruit juice or tube feeding mixture. (Commercially prepared solutions providing the daily required nutrients including vitamins and minerals are available. Generally these solutions are high in protein and calories and low in bulk.) The total amount of each feeding must be determined by the needs, age, and stomach capacity of the individual client. The average adult tolerates feedings of 200 ml every 2 to 3 hours. Follow each feeding with approximately 30 ml of water to clear the tube and to prevent blockage.

Secure the tube to the nose with a narrow 2-inch strip of adhesive tape, bifurcated through its center for 1 inch. Place the undivided end across the nose, and wind the divided ends alternately around the tube. This serves to keep the tube in place and prevents distortion of the nares. The rest of the tube should be brought across the cheek, behind the ear, and anchored on the forehead with a second strip of adhesive tape. Fold the end of the tube on itself, and secure with a rubber band or plastic clamp.

Remove superfluous equipment, and leave remainder on the tray on the bedside table.

*Nursing intervention with retention nasal tube.* Lubricate the nares frequently to prevent formation of crusts. Give mouth care as indicated. Aspirate a few milliliters of stomach contents before each feeding and allow to return to stomach. If greater than 50 ml of stomach contents is aspirated, hold the feeding and return the aspirate. Turn client to the right side to facilitate drainage from the stomach. Follow each feeding with 30 ml of water to keep the tube open. Follow each feeding by a short rest period to reduce the possibility of regurgitation of stomach contents. If vomiting occurs, it may be caused by the consistency or content of the tube feeding mixture, increased gastric motility, decreased gastrointestinal absorption, or the method of administration. Administer specific feedings as ordered, usually with high-vitamin, high-calorie, or high-protein content. (Gastrointestinal complications have been reduced appreciably by substitution of a well-balanced soft diet that has been prepared in an electric food blender for the traditional tube feeding mixture. Some clients can be given a blended meal three times a day rather than smaller amounts every 2 or 3 hours.) Supplementary vitamins may be given as necessary.

Measure intake.

Crush all tablet medication, and thoroughly dissolve in 15 to 30 ml of water before administering through the tube.

Watch for lesions of the nose, mouth, tongue, and gums.

Watch for symptoms of dehydration, alkalosis, and acidosis.

Clamp tube before removal to prevent aspiration.

*Warning.* If the client is suspected to have an aneurysm, high blood pressure, or severe arteriosclerosis, he or she should be cautioned against retching and vomiting.

*Complication.* When the client being tube fed also has a tracheostomy or endotracheal tube, it should be noted that the prolonged pressure on the walls of the esophagus and trachea produced by the nasogastric, endotracheal, or tracheostomy tubes may produce a tracheoesophageal fistula. This is manifested by the appearance of gastric contents in the tracheal excretions and demands immediate intervention.

### CHARTING

**Nurse's notes**
Date and time nasal tube is inserted
Significant reactions
Total intake at end of each 8-hour period

## INTERVENTION FOR ORAL HYGIENE

**Expected outcome**
The client should be able to explain the procedure and rationale for the need for continued oral hygiene.

## MOUTH CARE ROUTINE

*Purposes.* (1) Maintenance of good oral hygiene, and (2) prevention of complications: herpes, sordes, parotitis, aspiration, and respiratory infection.

*Indications.* (1) All seriously ill clients, (2) all stuporous or comatose clients, (3) all febrile clients, (4) all clients with trigeminal neuralgia, (5) all clients with facial or bulbar paralysis, and (6) all clients with intracranial surgery.

### EQUIPMENT

Small tray with 2-inch rim (individual setup)
Wide-mouthed, covered jar containing Cook's mouth ointment*
  or glyoxide solution
4-ounce bottle of mouthwash
Gauze sponges (4 by 4 inches)
Tongue depressors
Toothbrush
Emesis basin
Small rubber sheet and towel
Suction machine

*Preparation of client.* Position on side. If client has facial paralysis, have the affected side uppermost. Cover rubber sheet with towel, and place under client's chin and over bedclothes. Place emesis basin at angle of jaw.

*Procedure.* Cleanse mouth with antiseptic solution, if the client is conscious and able to expectorate. Use suction as necessary to remove excess secretions. Brush the teeth. Apply Cook's ointment or glyoxide to the tongue, gums, and mucous membrane of the mouth. This can be done with a toothbrush or gauze squares. Gums are massaged briskly. This is done until tongue and mouth are clean. A padded tongue depressor is used to separate the teeth when indicated to prevent accidental biting of the nurse's fingers. Apply ointment to lips to prevent drying and herpes. Remove basin and protective covering. Repeat procedure every 2 hours or more often if indicated.

*Supplementary care to ensure good oral hygiene.* Maintain adequate fluid intake. Use suction as necessary to keep mouth and throat free of mucus. Posture the unconscious client on the side to facilitate drainage from the mouth.

### CHARTING

**Nurse's notes**
Procedure and time
Condition of client's mouth

---

*Ingredients for Cook's mouth ointment are boric acid, 22.50 gm; menthol, 0.09 gm. mineral oil, 60.00 gm; white petroleum jelly, 60.00 gm; and oil of nutmeg, 0.45 gm.

# INTERVENTION FOR OPHTHALMIC PROTECTION

### Expected outcome

The client should be able to detail the need for protection of the eyes and cooperate in the application of treatments.

## EYE CARE ROUTINE

*Purposes.* (1) To keep the eye clean, (2) to lubricate the eye, and (3) to prevent complications secondary to corneal anesthesia or facial paralysis.

*Indications.* (1) All unconscious clients, (2) all clients with corneal anesthesia, (3) all clients after section of the fifth cranial nerve, and (4) all clients with facial paralysis.

### EQUIPMENT

Small tray with 2-inch rim (individual setup)
Special glass solution container with dropper and bulb attachment
Cotton balls
Normal saline solution
Homeostatic eye drops or methylcellulose
Emesis basin
Small plastic sheet and towel
Eye cup

*Preparation of client.* Adjust position as necessary so that the head is turned to the right when the right eye is being treated and to the left when the left eye is being treated. If the client is sitting in a chair, tilt his or her head back and turn to the side as indicated.

*Procedure.* Place protective plastic sheet and towel at the angle of the client's jaw and over the shoulder. Adjust emesis basin at the outer corner of the eye. Use ophthalmic saline solution and, while holding the eye open, irrigate from the inner to the outer canthus. (A saturated cotton ball may also be needed.) Repeat this procedure until all exudate has been removed and the eye is clean. Dry eyelids gently with cotton. Insert one or two drops of homeostatic ophthalmic drops or a lubricant such as methylcellulose into lower sac of eye (never onto eyeball directly) to prevent drying of the cornea. Remove basin and protective drape. Repeat procedure with other eye as indicated. Eye care is administered at least every 4 hours and more frequently if indicated.

If the client is conscious, he or she is given the following instructions with additional explanation as necessary: never rub the affected eye, blink the eye at frequent intervals, avoid irritation of the cornea by contact with the pillow, wear protective glasses whenever outside, and irrigate eye at regular intervals and on returning indoors. The conscious, cooperative client is taught the use of the eye cup, and the procedure is supervised as indicated by the individual client's need.

Eyes are inspected for early signs of inflammation and irritation at frequent, regular intervals. The physician is notified at the first sign of inflammation or irritation.

If indicated, an eye shield may be made of transparent radiographic film. To make such a shield, cut a circle 9 cm in diameter. Make two 3 cm slits opposite each other. Close these openings by overlapping the adjacent material and securing it with hypoallergenic tape so that a cone-shaped shield results. Place this over the affected eye, and fix its rim to the skin with hypoallergenic tape (Fig. 27-1). This shield not only protects the eye but also is comfortable and does not interfere with vision.

As an alternate for this shield, a butterfly dressing may be applied as a preventive measure to close the eyelids of an uncooperative client. The

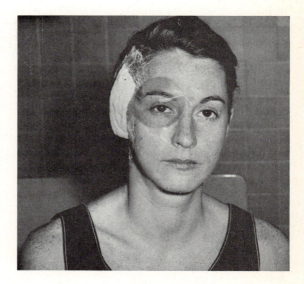

**FIG. 27-1.** Transparent eye shield in place. Note collodion dressing.

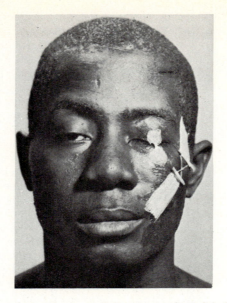

**FIG. 27-2.** Nonsurgical closure of eye with gauze-collodion dressing (butterfly). Anterior view of facial sling is also shown.

butterfly dressing is made as follows: Cut a 1-inch length of 1-inch bandage in half, and discard one piece. Twist the center tightly until a bow effect results. Close the eye and place the upper part of the bow in the center of the upper eyelid. Moisten well with collodion on a cotton applicator. Exert gentle pressure on the lid to keep it lowered until the collodion is dry and the upper part of the bow is anchored securely. With the eye closed, exert slight traction (eyelashes should be on a level with the twisted center), place the lower part of the bow on the skin of the infraorbital region, and check to see if the eye is well closed. Moisten well with collodion and hold in place until dry (Fig. 27-2).

### Treatment for periocular edema

*Definition.* Swelling of the eyelids and the surrounding tissues caused by trauma.

*Purposes.* (1) To relieve local edema by prolonged cold application and (2) to check the progress of periocular edema.

*Indications.* At the first sign of periocular edema after head injury or cranial surgery.

**EQUIPMENT**

Pliofilm
Hypoallergenic tape (1-inch width) or 4 paper clips
Cracked ice
Eye patch with tapes long enough to encircle the head
Petroleum jelly

*Procedure for making Pliofilm container.* Cut a piece of Pliofilm 9 inches square. Place small, flat pieces of ice in its center. Fold in half. Roll the three open edges tightly to prevent leakage of fluid as the ice melts. Secure with paper clips placed at each corner or with long strips of hypoallergenic tape.

*Procedure for application of Pliofilm ice bag to eye.* Protect the upper eyelid and surrounding tissue with a thin coating of petroleum jelly. Apply Pliofilm ice bag. Apply eye patch, and tie tapes around the head.

*Nursing intervention.* Observe for possible leakage of fluid from the bag. Refill with ice as necessary. Examine the lids for early signs of burning.

Administer eye care at frequent intervals to prevent collection of mucus or formation of crusts on lids.

# INTERVENTION FOR MAXILLOFACIAL OR EYE ORBIT INJURIES

### Expected outcome
The client should have the procedure explained and need for cooperation in the application of the facial sling emphasized.

## FACIAL SLING

*Definition.* The application of a gauze collodion sling to weakened facial musculature.

*Purposes.* (1) To prevent stretching of weakened or paralyzed facial muscles, (2) to facilitate eating and drinking by achieving better lip alignment, (3) to lessen the danger of biting the mucous membrane of the cheek on the affected side, and (4) for cosmetic effect.

*Indication.* Clients with facial paralysis.

### EQUIPMENT

2 strips of 1-inch bandage (4 inches long—the length may vary, depending on the client's age, sex, and facial structure)
2 cotton applicators
Plain applicator
Collodion
Medium rubber band
Electric hair dryer

*Preparation of client.* Explain treatment and its purpose to the client. Have him or her sit in a comfortable position in a chair or in bed.

*Preparation of equipment.* Collect all equipment, and take to the bedside. Cut two 1-inch lengths from a wooden applicator. Connect dryer.

*Procedure.* Place the 1-inch piece of wood across the center of the first 4-inch length of bandage and fold lengthwise, making a 2-inch strip. Repeat the same procedure with the second lenth of bandage. Open a bottle of collodion, and insert a cotton-tipped applicator.

Place the open, double end of folded bandage on the forehead in line with the eyebrow, the applicator end slightly slanted toward the nose. Moisten the entire strip with collodion. Hold securely in place, and turn on the dryer until the dressing is completely dry.

Place the open, double end of the second bandage strip so that traction will be exerted on the upper lip and the lower part of the cheek. The folded end with stick is in line with the upper part of the sling and separated from its by a distance of approximately 1 inch. Moisten the entire strip with collodion, hold, and use the dryer as necessary.

Place a rubber band under the stick edges of the upper end of the lower strip, twist once, and anchor on the stick of the upper strip. For greater traction, the rubber band can be twisted around the sticks.

Check the position of the client's lips, and adjust the sling for maximum alignment. (A strip of hypoallergenic tape, which is inconspicuous but less durable, may be used instead of collodion gauze.)

*Nursing intervention.* Check the sling for efficient functioning. Adjust the rubber band traction as necessary. To remove, cover the eye and dissolve collodion with acetone applied with a sponge.

# INTERVENTION FOR BOWEL ELIMINATION

### Expected outcome
The client should have all procedures explained as well as the need for continued bowel elimination.

## RECTAL TREATMENTS

The detailed procedure for administering retention enemas has been purposely omitted. Only the differences from accepted practices have been outlined. Preparation and position of client, preparation and aftercare of equipment, and charting should be carried out as the nurse has been previously taught.

### Medicated retention enema for removal of fecal impaction
#### INGREDIENTS

Hydrogen peroxide, 30 ml
Sodium bicarbonate, 8 ml
Water to make a total of 240 ml

*Procedure.* Give 60 ml with a small enema bucket or gavage bag. Repeat at hourly intervals until all solution has been given. Follow the next morning by a soapsuds enema or colon lavage.

## Colon lavage

*Definition.* The filling of the lower bowel with a specific solution under low pressure and emptying by gravity flow. This is repeated until adequate fecal material has been removed and the solution siphoned back is clear.

*Indications.* (1) When the client has diminished sphincter control, is unable to retain solution, or becomes overdistended because of an inability to expel the solution. (2) Clients with increased intracranial pressure who, while trying to expel an enema, may strain and cause a secondary rise in intracranial pressure. (Straining may even cause displacement of a posterior fossa tumor and may result in respiratory collapse.)

This method is advocated to prevent fluid absorption, to regulate the amount of solution given, and to evaluate the amount siphoned off.

### EQUIPMENT

Enema bucket
Plastic protective sheet
Large pitcher
Lubricant
Toilet tissue
Bedpan
Bedpan cover
Emesis basin
Bath blanket
Solution as ordered (soapsuds, tap water, saline solution, sodium bicarbonate, dilute hydrogen peroxide)
Bath thermometer
Tray

*Preparation of equipment.* Arrange necessary equipment on the bedside tray (emesis basin, enema bucket, lubricant, tissue). Prepare solution in pitcher at required temperature. Collect all remaining equipment and carry to the bedside.

*Preparation of client.* Draw curtains around the bed. Cover the client with a bath blanket and fanfold top bedclothes to the foot of the bed. Turn the client onto the side and posture comfortably. Place plastic sheets under the client's buttocks. Explain the treatment to the client before proceeding.

*Procedure.* Place bedpan next to the client on the bed. Lubricate catheter. Fill enema bucket, flush solution through tube to remove air, bend on itself, insert it into the rectum, straighten tube, and allow contents to flow into rectum under low pressure. Then lower enema bucket below level of mattress until colonic contents begin to appear in tube. If the client complains of distress before the bucket is empty, lower it and begin to siphon back the solution. If the client expels the solution around the tube, the bucket is lowered immediately. Have client use the bedpan frequently to evacuate fecal material and retained solution.

Repeat the procedure until the return is satisfactory and the lower bowel and rectum seem empty. Move the tube to various levels in the rectum to ensure complete evacuation of the solution and thus prevent subsequent involuntary defecation. If the colon lavage is correctly done, even though it may take 1 hour, the client is not fatigued by the procedure and suffers no ill effects. Abdominal massage during the period of siphonage of the fluid sometimes increases the return. The abdomen is soft and flat at the end of the procedure.

*Nursing intervention.* Remove the bedpan, emesis basin, and plastic sheets. Cleanse client with soap and water, and dry. Change linen as necessary. Turn client and posture him or her in a comfortable position. Rearrange bedclothes and remove bath blanket. Remove the curtains and dispose or cleanse the equipment appropriately.

### CHARTING

**Nurse's notes**
Procedure, date, and time begun and ended
Solution used and amount
Results
Significant reactions

# INTERVENTION FOR PAIN

### Expected outcome
The client should have relief from pain or discomfort.

Paravertebral block and alcohol injections are not nursing interventions but may be part of a pain-relief program that the nurse may be involved in by intervening with client teaching for the procedure. (Refer to Chapter 10 for further detail on pain.)

## PARAVERTEBRAL BLOCK

*Definition.* Infiltration of the sympathetic rami and ganglia with an anesthetic solution.

***Purposes.*** (1) To alleviate pain in specific areas of the body, (2) to determine probable reaction to sympathectomy in the treatment of peripheral vascular disease of the extremities, (3) to dilate blood vessels to cause local pooling of the blood, and (4) to counteract cerebrovascular spasm or thrombosis.

***Contraindication.*** The use of procaine hydrochloride (Novocain) or its derivatives is contraindicated if sensitivity is known or suspected.

***Dangers.*** (1) Puncture of a blood vessel, (2) puncture of the pleura, causing pneumothorax, and (3) pulmonary puncture.

## EQUIPMENT

**Sterile**
10 ml syringe
2 ml syringe
2 No. 25 needles
4 No. 20 needles (8 to 10 cm long)
6 sponges (3 by 3 inches)
4 applicators
2 towels
Gloves

**Other**
Procaine (Novocain), 2%, 30 ml ampule
Epinephrine, 1 ml ampule
Thimerosal (Merthiolate) or Betadine
Alcohol, 70%
File

***Preparation of client.*** An explanation of the test is given, and the treatment permit is signed. No preliminary medication is given unless the client is apprehensive. The therapeutic results are evaluated more accurately if the block is done when the client has pain.

***Procedure.*** The position depends on the site of injection; it may be prone, supine, or lateral recumbent.

For a thoracic block the client lies prone with the chest elevated on a large pillow, arms above the head in a comfortable position, forehead or chin on a sandbag to facilitate breathing, or supine with the head rotated to the side opposite the proposed site of injection.

For a lumbar block the client lies in the prone position with a pillow under the abdomen, head turned to the side, and arms in a comfortable position.

If the blocks are done with the client in the lateral recumbent position, he or she should lie on the unaffected side with the knees and hips flexed.

The area is exposed, and the client is covered with a bath blanket.

The physician palpates the client to determine the site for injection and then puts on sterile gloves and prepares the area with thimerosal or Betadine.

Sterile drapes are applied.

The physician draws procaine into the syringe and injects it superficially into the skin where the block is to be done (3 to 6 cm from the midline).

Long needles are inserted at the proper level through the skin wheals; 5 to 6 ml or procaine is injected through each needle. The needles are removed, the area is cleansed and dried, and a protective dressing is applied. (The local anesthetic effect will last about 1 hour.)

***Nursing management.*** The client's position is changed as necessary to make him or her comfortable. He or she is examined by the physician to evaluate the success of the procedure. The previous routine is then resumed.

## CHARTING

**Nurse's notes**
Procedure, physician, date, and time
Significant reactions
Site of puncture and number of injections
Solution and amount used
Significant reactions

## ACUPUNCTURE

The practice of acupuncture apparently began in China more than 5000 years ago. It reached its peak by the middle of the nineteenth century; thereafter its use steadily declined. Although modern physicians in China forbade the practice of acupuncture in the more advanced city hospitals, the practitioners of folk medicine continued to use it.

In 1958, because of the lack of conventional anesthetics in the People's Republic of China, Chairman Mao Tse-tung ordered his physicians to try acupuncture as an anesthetic. He is credited with the modern revival of acupuncture. Extensive research has been conducted in China on acupuncture for more than 15 years. It has been used widely as an anesthetic agent and for its analgesic action. About 95% of the clients in Friendship Hospital in Peking choose acupuncture rather than any other anesthetic. It has been used effectively in both minor and major surgical procedures. Its greatest advocates admit that they do not know how or why acupuncture works as an analgesic or an anesthetic; all they know is that it does.

During the early 1970s, several American physicians visited China. Although they were impressed by the level and quality of Chinese medical practice, most of them were excited by the application of acupuncture for the control of pain and as an anesthetic. Dr. Wu, the vice-president of the Beijing (Peking) Academy of Medical Sciences, states that acupuncture has two disadvantages as an anesthetic: (1) it does not relax skeletal muscles and (2) it is not effective in open heart surgery when a heart-lung machine is used. While in China, Dr. Tkach interviewed surgeons, acupuncturists (qualified physicians), and nurses at Friendship Hospital and was impressed by their candor and belief in acupuncture.

The following procedure for performing acupuncture is based on reports of current practice in a teaching hospital in Beijing.

*Definition.* The insertion of one or more special, sterile, wire-thin stainless steel needles with a twirling motion into soft tissue of various parts of the body (number of identified acupuncture points ranges from 600 to 1000). The rotation of the needle or needles is continued manually or automatically with low-voltage electric current.

*Purposes.* (1) To produce an anesthetic effect and (2) to alleviate pain.

*Indications.* According to Chinese surgeons, it is used effectively in most surgical procedures and in most medical conditions accompanied by pain.

*Preparation of client.* According to Dr. Wu, patients being prepared for acupuncture anesthesia at Friendship Hospital in Beijing are admitted 2 days before surgery is scheduled. Two surgeons, who are to perform the surgery, are assigned to the client on admission. They take the history, examine the client, and explain in detail what will happen. (If the procedure is in the United States the doctor must obtain written permission.) The client is then taken to the operating room, where the surgeons describe the surgical procedure, what the acupuncturist will do, the insertion of the nee-

dles, and their effect. The client is then encouraged to talk with other clients who have had the same procedure. Finally, if the client wishes, the surgeons provide him or her with an acupuncture needle with which to experiment on him- or herself. Generally, fluids are not withheld before surgery.

One can hypothesize that this sustained personal contact with the surgeons would have a profound psychological effect on the client, instill confidence, and alleviate anxiety or apprehension about the surgery.

*Procedure.* After the client, clad in pajamas, is assisted onto the operating table, the acupuncturist scrubs the selected site or sites (ears, nose, hands, head, upper arms, torso, thighs, and so on), inserts the special needle or needles (varying in length from ½ inch to several inches), and with a twirling motion penetrates the soft tissue. He or she then attaches electrodes to the needle or needles. The electrodes connect to a 9-volt battery capable of generating a pulsing current of 60 to 120 surges per minute. (The rotation of the needles may also be continued manually.) Local anesthesia is accomplished in about 20 minutes. Pulse, respiration, and blood pressure are taken by the acupuncturist periodically during the surgery.

After the operation is completed, the client is assisted off the table and walked out of the surgical suite.

*Advantages.* Since the client remains conscious throughout the procedure and is active immediately after its completion and since no systemic reactions occur with acupuncture, the possibility of complications is greatly reduced. There is no nausea or vomiting. Generally, fluids are administered during surgery, and dehydration is not a problem. Respiratory complications do not occur. There is no pain during the immediate postoperative period. Because the client is ambulatory, the danger of clotting is greatly reduced. No deaths have been reported after the use of acupuncture as an anesthetic agent. Psychologically the client seems not only to tolerate the surgical procedure very well but also to enjoy it. He or she is aware of what is happening and able to cooperate and follow any of the surgeons' requests.

No special observations or nursing care is required after acupuncture. Postoperative nursing care is planned according to the nature of the operation and the client's condition and special needs.

*Other considerations.* When acupuncture is employed for the relief of pain, the technique of insertion and rotation of the special needles is as just described. The number and length of needles may vary, as well as the points of insertion. For additional information, see Chapter 10.

## ALCOHOL INJECTION

*Definition.* Injection of alcohol by the introduction of a long slender needle into the peripheral branches of nerves for the interruption of sensory fibers.

*Purpose.* To secure relief from severe and uncontrollable pain, especially that caused by disease of the fifth cranial nerve. (If successful, the client may be free from pain for 6 to 18 months. If the nerve regenerates, the pain returns.)

*Indications.* (1) Clients who refuse operative treatment and (2) old or debilitated clients who are poor operative risks.

*Contraindications.* (1) Diffuse painful conditions of the face when functional disease is suspected and (2) infection at the site of injection.

### EQUIPMENT

**Sterile** (on tray)
5 ml syringe
2 ml syringe
2 No. 25 needles
1 No. 22 needle
2 medicine glasses
6 sponges (3 by 3 inches)
Cotton balls
Fenestrated sheet
2 pairs of gloves
2 trigeminal needles—long and slender with rubber markers to designate the maximum depth of insertion

**Other**
Procaine (Novocain), 2%
Alcohol (for injection), 95%
Betadine
Skull and applicator
Chair (dental or barber)
Plastic sheet
Head towel and safety pins

*Preparation of client.* After describing the treatment and its possible effects, the physician obtains written permission from the client or the nearest relative.

Administer preliminary medication as ordered. Explain procedure to the client, discussing what may be expected and how he or she can best cooperate to ensure a successful result. Reassure as necessary before and during the procedure. Have the client wear pajamas and robe, and place a towel around the head in turban fashion and fasten with pins. Take the client to the treatment room in a wheelchair; wrap in a blanket for warmth if necessary. Assist him or her into the special chair.

*Procedure.* The nurse adjusts the dressing rubber sheet and towel around the client's shoulders. The physician, after checking the landmarks and depth on the skull, locates the area for injection on the client's cheek. The client is asked to tell the physician when and where a sharp pain is felt during the treatment. The physician puts on gloves. The nurse uncovers the sterile equipment and stands beside the client to offer reassurance as necessary, to prevent contamination of the area by the client, and to observe reactions.

Hand restraints may be required to prevent contamination of the surgical field by the client during the procedure.

The physician prepares the skin in routine fashion and then drapes the area with a fenestrated sheet. Procaine is injected for superficial anesthesia. From 1 to 3 ml of 95% alcohol is drawn into the 5 ml syringe. The trigeminal needle is adjusted.

Alcohol is not injected until the physician is reasonably certain of being in the right location. The technique for introduction of the needle can be found in textbooks on minor surgery and anesthesia. The client usually has a characteristic paroxysm of pain when the nerve has been reached by the needle. After the injection is completed, the needle is removed and the area cleansed. A small piece of cotton with collodion is applied to the puncture wound.

*Nursing intervention.* Remove the drapes and protective plastic sheet. Return the client to bed. After a rest period, its length depending on the client's needs, he or she may resume the usual routine.

The physician does a sensory examination to determine the area of anesthesia and the success of the treatment. If there is corneal anesthesia, the nurse instructs the client to blink the affected eye frequently and not to rub it. The nurse should examine the eye at stated intervals for signs of irritation and administer irrigations or oil instillations as ordered.

*Complications.* (1) If the needle is advanced too far, the brain may be penetrated. (2) An artery may be punctured and bleeding result. (3) Corneal irritation, keratitis, and loss of vision in the affected eye. (4) Local edema and ecchymosis. (5) Transient herpes may occur in the area of distribution of the nerve.

### CHARTING

**Nurse's notes**
Procedure, physician, date, and time
Significant reactions
Site of injection
Solution and amount used

## INTERVENTION FOR RESPIRATORY SUPPORT IN FAILURE

### Expected outcome
The client should have relief from impaired respirations and decreased apprehension from need for respiratory support.

### RESPIRATOR

Both negative- and positive-pressure respirators are manufactured for use in the sitting or recumbent position in the hospital, office, or at home. These machines may be used with the application of a face mask, a mouthpiece, or an adapter to a tracheostomy tube. A micronebulizer is available for the relief of spasms and edema. The nebulizer moistens and mobilizes tenacious secretions, restores the cleansing action of the cilia, and facilitates the excretion of mucus and purulent material from the bronchial tree.

The Monaghan Ventalung* may be used by the attachment of a face mask, mouthpiece, or tracheostomy adapter. With this machine, intermittent positive-pressure breathing may be instituted to wash out carbon dioxide, to remove deep secre-

tions, and to improve alveolar ventilation. It may also be used as a resuscitator to prevent hypoventilation and to maintain respiratory function.

A portable respirator with a thoracoabdominal shell that permits complete chest expansion is also available.* This high-dome plastic shell with its inflatable foam-rubber seal comes in 34 different sizes, fits over the client's chest and upper abdomen, and adjusts to the configuration of the body. It is kept in place by two nylon straps that are secured firmly across the thoracic and lumbar regions. Because the client's arms and legs are free, the position can be changed, and the administration of medical treatment and nursing care is facilitated. This respirator can be operated with alternating and direct electric current in an automobile, airplane, or ship, as well as in the hospital or home. It also can be run on its battery for as long as 4 hours.

The Mueller-Mörch piston respirator† is designed to maintain prolonged artificial respiration for clients with respiratory failure associated with disease of the central nervous system (poliomyelitis, Guillain-Barré syndrome, tetanus, and barbiturate poisoning), postoperative depression, or crushing injuries of the chest. This compact respirator is portable and operates on alternating current. In case of failure of electrical power or while the client is being transported, operation of a hand crank permits uninterrupted breathing. It differs from most other respirators because it operates on an open, "leaky" system and is most effective when used with an uncuffed endotracheal tube or tracheostomy tube. This respirator aids in expelling secretions, prevents excessive inflation of the lungs, and allows the client with a tracheostomy to phonate. This respirator occupies little space (37 inches by 30 inches by 9 inches) and, when in use, can be placed under most hospital beds. The position of the client is not restricted, and since no part of the body is encased, treatment and care are not complicated.

*Definition.* An apparatus designed to maintain respiratory activity by changing the pressure within an airtight chamber by means of mechanical suc-

---

*Monaghan, 500 Alcott St., Denver, CO 80204

---

*Monaghan, 500 Alcott St., Denver, CO 80204.
†Mueller & Co., Chicago, Ill.

tion, thereby causing the thorax alternately to expand and relax when voluntary respiratory movements are impaired or absent.

*Purposes.* (1) To maintain an adequate exchange of oxygen and carbon dioxide within the alveoli of the lungs, (2) to relieve anoxia, (3) to restore alveolar ventilation, (4) to prevent respiratory acidosis, (5) to rest weakened muscles, and (6) to support inadequate respiratory activity in debilitated or elderly clients.

*Indications.* (1) Respiratory failure caused by intracranial or other lesions of the nervous system. (2) Poliomyelitis, the spinal type with involvement of the diaphragm or intercostal muscles. (The respirator has been used indiscriminately for all respiratory dysfunction, including that resulting from involvement of the bulbar respiratory centers, but the value of its use under these circumstances is doubtful.) (3) In the presence of low vital capacity (less than 250 cc of air); increased, shallow respirations with the first signs of dyspnea or cyanosis, increased restlessness, and apprehension.

Although most hospitals now have inhalation therapy units with staff specially trained in the use of respirators, the nurse remains responsible for the total care of the client and assists the inhalation unit's staff as necessary. The nurse supports the client psychologically and instructs and supervises as necessary.

Adequate ventilation of the lungs can be accomplished most effectively with a mechanical respirator connected to the client's endotracheal tube (cuffed) or to a tracheostomy tube. The latter is preferred if the respirator is to be used for a long period of time.

Several types of pressure-cycled and volume respirators are employed. Regardless of the type in use, the nurse monitors the client's progress at frequent intervals, noting the level of consciousness, pupillary reaction, color, motion and strength of extremities, vital signs, laboratory data, intake and urinary output, character and amount of secretions, edema, and reaction to respirator. Nursing care is administered according to the condition and special needs of the client. *Respiratory Nursing Care: Physiology and Technique* (Wade, 1981) and *Respiratory Care of Patients with Neuromuscular Disease* (Lavigne, 1979) give further detail.

# INTERVENTION FOR THROMBOEMBOLISM

### Expected outcome

The client should have effective thromboembolism-prevention measures instituted to provide adequate circulation.

## ANTIEMBOLISM STOCKINGS

*Purpose.* (1) Promote circulatory flow for clients during neurosurgical procedures and (2) prevent circulatory stasis as a complication of prolonged bedrest.

*Indications.* (1) All stuporous and unconscious clients, (2) all clients with spinal cord injuries, (3) surgical clients for neurosurgical procedures that may be positioned in a circulatory compromised posture, (4) all clients with a prior history of circulatory problems, and (5) all debilitated, elderly, or neuromuscular impaired clients who may not have the strength to ambulate or exercise their extremities.

Antiembolism stockings are indicated for those clients who are at risk for the development of circulatory stasis and possible thromboembolism. Neurosurgical clients who will be confined to bed for a prolonged period of time, the neurosurgical client who may be undergoing a long procedure or will be positioned in a circulatory compromising posture, or the traumatized and debilitated clients routinely should be assessed and fitted for antiembolism stockings. Numerous stockings are available. The most recent advancement in antiembolism stockings has been made by the Patient Care System Division of Zimmer USA.* The PCS† antiembolism stocking is being preferred over other antiembolism stockings because of its unique construction. This stocking has a clear-view window located over the toes to allow observation of the toes, a low-pressure designed heel, popliteal and femoral compliance zones to allow for improved circulatory flow, and special construction for easier application and comfort.

Antiembolism stockings are not by any means the sole intervention available for thromboembolism prevention. Clients should move their legs as frequently as possible, ambulate early during the course of hospitalization, have the legs exercised

---

*Zimmer USA, Warsaw, Indiana 46580.
†Pressure Controlled Stockings.

by the nurse if they require assistance, or have tilt-table exercise or movement on special beds to prevent thromboembolism.

## INTERVENTION FOR SPINAL CORD INJURY

### Expected outcome

The client should have the need for special beds and treatments explained so that cooperation during hospitalization and rehabilitation may lead to functional recovery.

### FRACTURE BED

*Definition.* A specially arranged bed for the treatment of injuries of the spine by hyperextension (Figs. 27-3 and 27-4).

*Purpose.* To reduce incomplete vertebral fracture-dislocations or compression fractures of the spine without resorting to the use of manipulation or traction.

### EQUIPMENT

Hospital bed (3-gatch Decker bed if available)
Fracture boards
2 6-inch shock blocks
2 firm mattresses
Sponge rubber or air mattress
2 to 6 bath blankets (number depends on the degree of hyperextension desired by the physician and the thickness of the blankets)
4 large sheets
Footboard
Cradle
Knee bolster
Calf bolster
4 sandbags ⎫
Roll of 4-inch
   adhesive tape ⎬ only for cervical injury
4 tongue depressors
4 safety pins ⎭
3 draw sheets
Blanket (depending on weather)
Spread
Adjustable supports for prevention of wristdrop as indicated by the level of the lesion

*Preparation of equipment.* Cover the footboard neatly with draw sheet, and pin it. Fold bath blanket so that, when placed across the bed, it completely covers the width of the mattress. Roll tight-

ly and without wrinkles. If the roll is not large enough, add another similarly folded blanket and roll. Repeat this with subsequent blankets until the roll is large enough to produce the amount of hyperextension desired by the physician. Secure the roll with a bandage, and cover neatly with the draw sheet. (If a Decker bed is used and the gatch is jointed at the fracture level, the blanket roll is unnecessary.)

Turn the bed around so that the foot becomes the head (particularly important with cervical injuries because it expedites nursing care and the use of traction). Remove wheels from the foot of the bed (now the head of the bed), and elevate on shock blocks.

*Preparation of client.* Posture the client comfortably on a stretcher, and do not move him or her until the bed foundation is completed. Explain the purpose of the bed to the client. Explain restriction of motion and change of position to ensure the client's cooperation in maintaining the best position for maximum reduction and alignment of the fracture.

*Method of making fracture bed.* Place the fracture boards on bedspring. Add the two mattresses. Cover the mattresses with a large sheet, miter corners, and tuck in. Place sponge rubber mattress with flotation pad or inflated air mattress on top of other mattresses. Cover with a large sheet, miter corners, and tuck in. The sheet must be taut and free of wrinkles.

Place the blanket roll at the designated level for hyperextension: shoulder level for cervical lesions and at the site of fracture for others. (The blanket roll is placed between the two upper mattresses.) Add draw sheet, tighten sheets, and tuck them in. Fold third large sheet lengthwise and then in half, and place crosswise on the bed according to the level of the lesion. If the lesion is in the cervical region, the sheet extends to the end of the mattress; if in the thoracic or lumbar areas, it extends above the level of the shoulders and below the level of the buttocks. (This sheet is used to adjust the client's alignment and to facilitate moving to the side of the bed or to a higher or a lower position in bed.)

If the client has an injury of the cervical spine, form a trough by applying broad strips of adhesive tape to the middle 8 to 10 inches of the top mat-

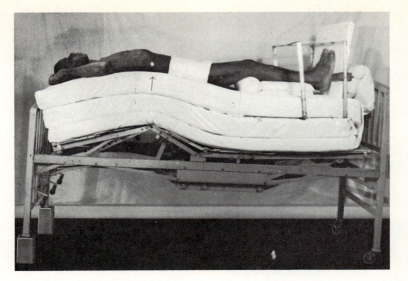

**FIG. 27-3.** Decker bed with elevation of gatch at thoracic level for hyperextension of client with fracture at that point. *Arrows,* Apex of break should be aligned with level of fracture. Lower extremities should be supported and postured at all times.

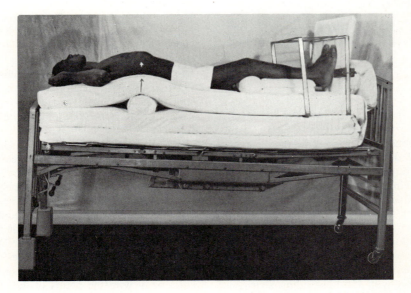

**FIG. 27-4.** Hyperextension fracture bed made by using blanket roll when Decker bed is not available or not suitable for treating fracture.

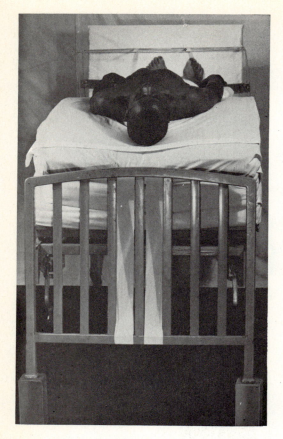

**FIG. 27-5.** Hypertension fracture bed demonstrating head trough for treatment of client with injury of cervical spine.

tress. These strips start at the level of the blanket roll and extend over the mattress, which is firmly depressed to obtain the desired degree of hyperextension, and down to the bottom of the bed frame, where they are securely fastened (Fig. 27-5). (The following method of securing the strips to the bed frame to prevent slipping has been found successful: extend strips along the mattresses on the inner surface of the bed frame, secure to the bottom of the frame, and extend up over the anterior part of the frame; place tongue depressors across ascending adhesive strips at the level of junction with the descending strips and bring the two surfaces together. Insert safety pins through both strips of adhesive tape above the

tongue depressors to prevent their slipping.) The tape must be kept taut at all times to maintain the desired hyperextension. It should be checked at frequent intervals and adjusted as necessary. The foundation of the fracture bed is now ready for the client.

*Transfer of client with spinal injury from stretcher to bed.* Six people, including two physicians, are required for the safe transfer of the client. They should be assigned to definite positions and should have a good understanding of what is to be done.

Place the stretcher beside the bed. If the turning sheet is not under the client, the sheet on which the client is lying should be loosened and rolled tightly on each side to the outer limits of the client's body.

If a cervical injury is suspected, a physician stands at the client's head, which is maintained in slight hyperextension when the physician applies manual traction. If the injury is at a lower level, a nurse is assigned to the head position to support the client's head in good alignment with the rest of the spinal column. If a thoracic or lumbar injury is suspected, the greatest support is maintained at the fracture level. A physician and a nurse are stationed alongside the stretcher with their adjacent hands close to the fracture site and holding the rolled sheet tightly. Their other hands are at a distance that will give maximum support to the client's trunk. Directly opposite them and on the far side of the bed the second physician and another nurse stand on foot benches in a similar position. The sixth attendant is delegated to the foot of the stretcher, where he or she is responsible for moving the client's lower extremities onto the bed.

As soon as each person has assumed the designated position, the leader of the team counts aloud to three. At the count of "three" the client is moved into the bed. With the sheet still being used, the client is positioned in the center of the bed at the optimum level to effect adequate hyperextension. This sheet is then slowly and gradually removed in the following manner: Two physicians, facing each other at opposite sides of the bed, simultaneously depress the mattress under the client's body with the palms of their hands. At the same time, two nurses in similar positions gently pull the sheet from the head of the bed down toward the foot. This should be done piecemeal to avoid jarring the client. The team may have to repeat the procedure three to four times at different levels of the client's body before the sheet can be removed safely.

After the sheet is removed, the alignment of the client's body is rechecked and adjusted as necessary. A small bolster is placed under the knees, a square bolster is placed under the calves, and the feet are placed in firm dorsiflexion against the footboard. A cradle is placed over the bed. The top of the bed is made in the usual manner.

The client remains on the back until good union of the fracture line is assured. Every precaution is taken to prevent the complications of decubitus ulcers, contractures, footdrop, wristdrop, and hypostatic pneumonia.

### Stryker frame (Fig. 27-6)

*Definition.* The Stryker frame was designed in 1937 by Dr. Homer Stryker of the University of Michigan Hospital orthopedic staff. It is a modified form of a Bradford frame and consists of two metal frames with canvas covers and thin protective padding. The frames are supported on a movable cart fitted with a special pivot device at each end. This permits easy change of the client's position from the prone to the supine and vice versa.

*Purposes.* (1) To facilitate the administration of nursing care to clients with spinal cord injury: (a) to change the client's position effectively without causing further trauma to the spinal cord by maintaining necessary alignment and immobilization; (b) to avoid causing the client additional discomfort, pain, or fatigue; (c) to enable the client, while lying on the anterior frame, to feed him- or herself, to read, or to perform light occupational therapy in a safe and comfortable position; (d) to protect the nurse from fatigue and muscle strain in handling the client; and (e) to eliminate the need for more than one nurse in turning a client.

(2) To facilitate the administration of the necessary nursing care with greater ease and less danger of complications after fusion of the spine: (a) to prevent local trauma, which may be caused by inexpert moving of the client or by the voluntary activity of an uncooperative client; (b) to prevent the occurrence of pressure areas and decubitus ulcers during the first 48-hour postoperative period when the client may be kept flat on the back; (c) to enable the nurse to give effective back care; (d) to permit changing the client's position every 2 hours, thus eliminating complications, discomfort, and fatigue caused by prolonged immobilization in one position; and (e) to facilitate elimination and expedite the administration of rectal treatments.

(3) To facilitate the administration of care and treatment of the chronically ill, disabled bed client: (a) to maintain good alignment of the client's body by application of the principles of good posture; (b) to maintain the client's morale through the movability of the frame, which permits change of environment and a greater range of social activity; (c) to reduce the incidence of complications such as pneumonia, depression, anorexia, decubitus ulcers, footdrop, wristdrop, contractures, and muscle stretching; and (d) to prevent overdependence on the nurse by enabling the client in the prone position to wash the face and hands, to feed him- or herself, to read, and to develop independent activity.

*Contraindications.* (1) Cervical cord injuries treated by immobilization and hyperextension without the use of Crutchfield tongs. (2) Compression fractures of the thoracic or lumbar spine that are reduced by hyperextension. (3) When a client's position in bed is not restricted and allows posturing on the sides as well as on the face and back. (4) When a client is over 6 feet tall, weighs over 200 pounds, or the physical structure is such that it prevents one from assuming a safe and comfortable position between the two frames before the turning process. (5) When a client is broader than the external limits of the frame. This results in local pressure and discomfort and precipitates the occurrence rather than the reduction of complications. (6) When the client may become disturbed emotionally and cannot adjust to the turning mechanism of the Stryker frame.

### EQUIPMENT

Movable cart with overhead frame and underlying tray
Anterior and posterior frames covered with canvas securely fastened and continuously kept taut
Headpiece
Arm supports
Foot support

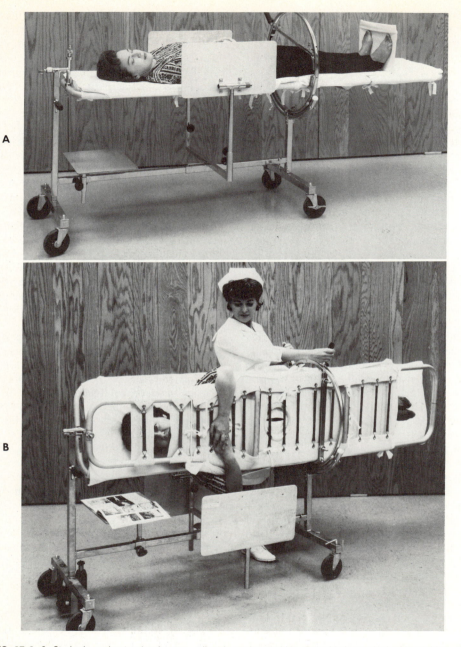

**FIG. 27-6. A,** Stryker's wedge turning frames—client in supine position. For added security in this position, arm boards may be turned up as side boards and ring closed over client. **B,** One nurse using turning handles to turn client. Arm boards have been lowered, and ring is closed over client. (Courtesy Stryker Corporation, Kalamazoo, Mich. In Larson, C.B., and Gould, M.: Orthopedic nursing, ed. 9, St. Louis, 1978, The C.V. Mosby Co.)

Muslin covers with tapes, made to specifications, to cover both frames (anterior covers in one piece with perineal opening, posterior covers cut in three pieces to match the canvas supports)

The preceding pieces of equipment are available commercially. The following equipment can be added to the Stryker frame as special needs suggested modifications:

Foam rubber mattress (1 to 2 inches thick) long enough to cover the anterior frame with a cross slit to parallel the perineal opening in the canvas support

Foam rubber mattress (1 to 2 inches thick) sectioned to cover the three canvas supports of the posterior frame

Muslin cover for foot support

Small head pillow and case for use by client when on the posterior frame

Foam rubber pads (1 inch thick), same size as the arm supports, with pillowcases to be placed on the arm supports for greater comfort

Small bolster with cover to be used under knees to maintain 10 degrees of flexion

Square firm bolster, size and thickness depending on the size of the client, to support calves and elevate heels

The square bolster for supporting the calves extends from the knee bolster to approximately 3 inches above the heels. Posturing the lower extremities in such a way will aid in the prevention of muscle strain, stretching, and contractures. The maintenance of the feet in firm dorsiflexion by means of the foot support will elevate the heels from pressure and thus prevent the development of pressure sores in this area. Footdrop will also be prevented.

It has been our practice to put the hospital shirt on the client on the anterior frame with the opening to the front. The open sides of the shirt in the prone or supine position are never left beneath the client because of the danger of wrinkles resulting in the formation of pressure areas. The top bedclothes are modified according to the needs of the individual client and the environment.

*Preparation of equipment.* Assemble the parts of the frame as directed by the printed instructions on the arm supports. After the posterior frame has been placed on the cart, add foam rubber mattress sections, and cover with muslin covers. Tie all tapes securely. Place the anterior frame on a stretcher or other suitable surface, and add foam rubber mattress and muslin covers. Tie all tapes securely. Lock wheels of cart.

Prepare the remainder of the equipment, and arrange neatly and conveniently for its subsequent use.

*Preparation of client.* Explain the working mechanisms of the frame to the client. Elaborate on the reasons for its use in his or her care. Demonstrate to the client the turning of the frame with its resulting change of position. (Use ambulatory client or member of the staff as a model.)

*Transfer of client to Stryker frame*

FROM BED. With six persons, follow the technique described in moving a client with a spinal cord injury onto a fracture bed. If the level of the bed is much higher than the posterior frame, move the client to the far side of the bed, place the posterior frame in good position on the bed, and then transfer as directed. Two orderlies can then replace the frame on the cart and secure it in place.

FROM STRETCHER. Place the posterior frame on a second stretcher, and proceed as just described.

Check the client's position to be sure the body is in correct alignment and centered in the middle of the frame. Be certain that no part of the body is resting on the metal supports.

Posture the lower extremities as previously suggested. Place a small pillow under the head unless contraindicated. Place arm supports in holes in the metal frames. Add covered foam rubber pillows, and posture the client's upper extremities in a comfortable, neutral position. If weakness or paralysis exists, place additional support under wrists and hands to prevent wristdrop.

*Turning of client.* Cover the client with a draw sheet. Remove top bedclothes, head pillow, and the client's gown. Remove the arm boards, and slide under the frame. Remove the foot support and bolsters. Place the anterior frame over the client with the face support over the face. Press the ends of the frame down over the bolts and screw on the wing nuts. The client fits snugly between the frames.

Fold a large sheet lengthwise and fasten it around the two frames to prevent the legs being dislodged during the turning process. Instruct the client to fold the arms around the anterior frame, and tell him or her in which direction the frame will be turned. Two persons should turn the client. One goes to each end of the frame and grasps a turning handle. The locking device is pressed to release the wedge lock, and the client is turned over quickly.

After turning, rock the frame gently to be sure it has locked automatically into place. Remove the restraining sheet and posterior frame.

Adjust the face mask and the client's position as necessary. Put shirt on backwards. Replace the top bedclothes, and remove the draping sheet. Add arm boards if the client is to be at rest. Otherwise, adjust platform tray for reading, eating, or occupational therapy activities.

Change the position of the client at least every 2 hours during the daytime and every 4 hours at night, unless indicated more frequently for the prevention of complications. Special nursing care, depending on the client's condition, must be administered for the prevention of complications.

During the convalescent period the client is taught rehabilitative exercises and the use of the longitudinal overhead bar to improve the muscle tone of the upper extremities. Whenever possible and if the weather permits, the client is wheeled outdoors on the roof or in the yard.

## CircOlectric Universal Hospital Bed (Stryker)*

The manufacturer of the Stryker frame has designed the CircOlectric bed (Fig. 27-7), which embodies, improves, and extends the principles of the Stryker frame. An illustrated manual of instruction for the operation of the CircOlectric bed is provided.

This bed is operated electrically. If the use of electricity is contraindicated because the client on the CircOlectric bed is in the operating room or receiving oxygen, or if there is a failure of electric power, it may be operated manually with a hand crank.

Whereas the Stryker frame permits only two positions, prone and supine, the CircOlectric bed allows a variety of positions: horizontal, vertical, and sitting. Instead of turning the client in a horizontal plane from the prone to the supine position, or vice versa, the change of position is accomplished in a vertical direction. The turning of the client can be interrupted at any level and a particular position maintained without jeopardizing

the alignment of the client's body. Levers are provided for head and knee gatches. This bed may be used as a tilt board to prevent osteoporosis, and circulation can be stimulated by several changes of position. Hypotensive reactions, experienced by clients when elevated to a sitting or standing position after prolonged horizontal immobilization, can be eliminated.

Equipment for cervical, pelvic, and Buck's traction is available. A transfer sling, side rails, and other special accessories may be purchased from the manufacturer.

Nursing intervention of the client on the CircOlectric bed is directed toward the prevention of complications, the promotion and restoration of health, and the achievement of physical, emotional, social, and spiritual well-being. The principles of care should be modified or elaborated according to the individual needs of the client and the particular problems created by the illness. When it is utilized for a client with a fractured spine, be certain that the frame position places the spinal column in correct alignment for appropriate healing.

Thoracic and lumbar injuries are immobilized early on either a Stryker or a Foster frame, not on a CircOlectric bed because the CircOlectric bed places extra stress on the injury from the axial loading of the spine that occurs during the vertical turning posture.

## Skeletal traction

*Definition.* The application of traction with weights to the vertebral column by means of tongs (halo, Gardner, or Crutchfield) or piano wire (Hoen), which is fixed to the skull.

*Purpose.* To reduce fractures or fracture-dislocations of the cervical spine. (This facilitates nursing care, since it permits moving the client without causing more injury.)

### EQUIPMENT

The following equipment is needed in addition to the instruments required in the operating room:

Special tongs or piano wire
Bar
Pulley
Rope
Weights

---

*Orthopedic Frame Co., Kalamazoo, Mich.

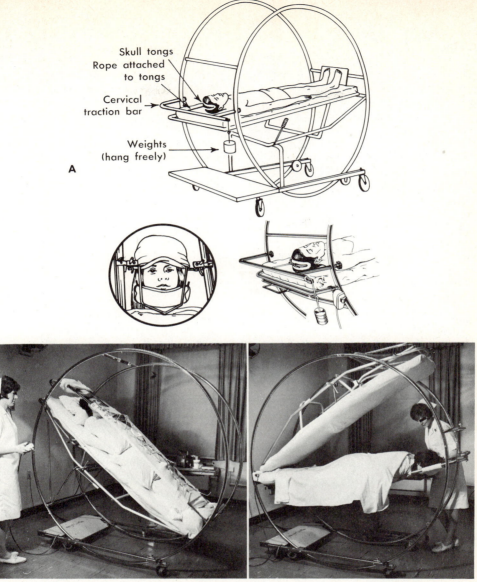

Skull tongs
Rope attached
to tongs

Cervical
traction bar

Weights
(hang freely)

**A**

**B**

**C**

**FIG. 27-7.** CircOlectric bed consists of an anterior and a posterior frame and provides for vertical turning as opposed to lateral turning of client. Thus, standing, Trendelenburg, and sitting positions also may be utilized. Since bed is operated with electric motor, even a very helpless client may be able to adjust his position and assume a greater degree of independence. The many benefits (physiological and psychological) derived from frequent position changes and from self-dependence may be augmented with use of this bed. In addition to hospital use. CircOlectric bed can be used advantageously in the home to facilitate care of disabled person. **A,** Use of CircOlectric bed for client with skull tongs (cervical traction). Arrangement of traction apparatus provides for maintenance of continuous traction as client is turned vertically from supine to prone position or vice versa. Note close view of adjustable facepiece. Support for head in either prone or supine position is an important factor in maintaining desired position of cervical vertebrae. **B,** Anterior frame has been put in position, and turning of client is started. **C,** Prone position, with posterior frame in elevated position. (**A,** From Orthopedic nursing procedure manual, University of Iowa Hospitals and Clinics, The University of Iowa, Iowa City, Iowa. In Larson, C.B., and Gould, M.: Orthopedic nursing, ed. 9, St. Louis, 1978, The C.V. Mosby Co.)

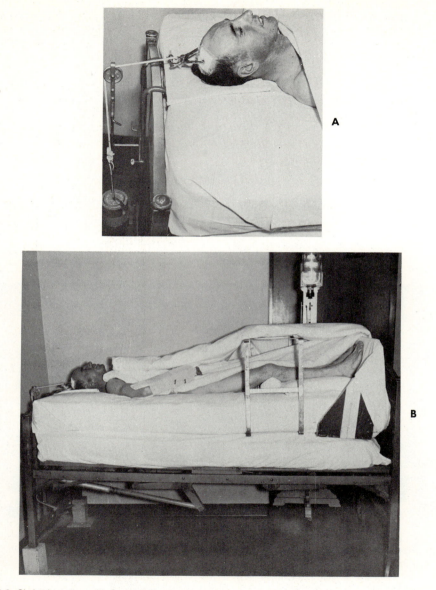

**FIG. 27-8.** Skeletal traction with Crutchfield tongs for treating clients with fracture-dislocation of cervical spine.

*Preparation of client.* The physician explains the procedure to the client and obtains permission. The hair is cut and the scalp shaved as necessary.

*Procedure.* Follow the principles to maintain the necessary alignment and traction of the neck, thus preventing additional spinal cord injury while the client is transferred to the operating table.

Using aseptic technique and a local anesthetic, the physician makes a small incision in each parietal region, perforates the outer table of the skull with a small drill, and inserts the points of the Crutchfield tongs. Sterile dressings are applied. (If piano wire is used, two lengths are inserted through two burr holes in each parietal region.) The client is transferred to the bed with the head at the foot end of the bed to which the pulley has already been attached. The physician connects the rope to the tongs and applies weights (10 to 20 pounds) to the other end (Figs. 27-8 and 27-9).

## Halo frame

*Definition.* The application of halo tongs to the skull and body cast combined to form a frame. (Refer to Fig. 23-1.)

*Purpose.* To stabilize the cervical spine after cervical spine fusion or cervical spine injuries.

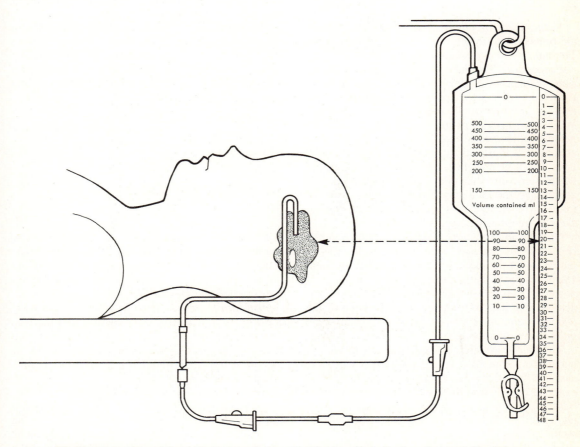

**FIG. 27-9.** Holter External Ventricular Drainage System. (Modified from illustration from Codman & Shurtleff, Inc., Randolph, Massachusetts.)

(This permits moving the client and early ambulation after cervical spine injury without causing more injury.)

### EQUIPMENT

The following equipment is needed in addition to the instruments in the operating room:

Halo tongs
Four posters for upright frame to tong attachment
Plaster
Heavy felt padding
Stockinet large enough to encircle body
Sheet cotton (Sofroll)
Bucket of warm water
Instruments to trim cast
Fracture table

*Preparation of client.* The physician explains the procedure to the client and obtains permission. The hair is cut and scalp shaved as necessary.

*Procedure.* The halo tongs are placed in the same manner as Gardner or Crutchfield tongs with the exception that four pins are inserted. The halo ring is approximated around the client's head. With the assistance of the operating room personnel the stockinet, felt padding, and sheet cotton are applied. Plaster is then rolled to form the body cast. The four upright posters are attached during the plaster-rolling technique. The posters are then attached to the halo ring and adjustment with the torque wrench renders the appropriate amount of skeletal traction (Chapter 23).

*Nursing intervention.* One prepares the client's bed by obtaining two three-fourths mattresses to put on top of the regular mattress and placing them 18 inches from the head of the bed. The client is positioned on the mattresses such that the shoulders should be 2 to 4 inches from the edge of the two additional three-fourths mattresses. Additional pillows are required to support the head.

The halo frame facilitates the turning of the client to the prone and lateral positions to dry the cast and for skin care. Turning the client at least every 2 hours is advised with the assessment of bony prominences and edges of the cast. The client should be cautioned against poking any instruments or implements down the cast. This may weaken the cast or injure the skin. Routine cast and pin care are required at least daily.

When the client ambulates, two persons should stand at either side. The client will have difficulty with maneuvering and planting the feet because of inability of bending the neck. When the client is dismissed from the hospital, he or she should be given instructions on cast and pin care.

### Pelvic traction

*Definition.* The application of a special belt around the waist and pelvis of the client attaching its two lateral strips of webbing to a spreader with a cord, pulley, and weights so that traction is exerted at the lumbosacral articulation and along the lower spine.

*Purposes.* (1) Relief of low back pain caused by injury or disease and (2) relaxation and decompression of tissues of the lumbar area.

*Advantages.* (1) Permits change of position without interruption of traction, (2) does not restrict movement of the lower extremities, (3) eliminates some adverse reactions to leg traction (local swelling, skin irritation, and phlebitis), and (4) facilitates nursing care.

### EQUIPMENT

Pelvic traction belt (size varies with each client)
Spreader, cord, and pulley
Weights (10 to 25 pounds)
Frame
2 shock blocks (10 to 12 inches high)
Foot cradle

*Preparation of client.* The physician explains the purpose of the traction to the client and determines the size of the belt by placing a tape measure around the client at a level 2 inches below the anterosuperior part of the spine.

*Procedure.* Screen the client. After removing the wheels, place the shock blocks under the legs of the foot of the bed. Place sheet over client, and remove top bedclothes. Remove nightgown or pajama bottoms. Help client into hospital gown if a pajama top is not available.

Attach frame to foot of bed. Fold sheet to waist. Place the pelvic belt under the client and around the waist and pelvis, and fasten the straps. (If the belt has been fitted correctly, the lateral soft hoods cap the iliac crests; there is a 2-inch spread at the buckle line; the row of buckles are straight down from the umbilicus.) Insert the two straps of webbing through the slip buckles and the Dee rings. Adjust so that the apex of each V-strap will be at the level of the knees. Secure the lateral straps to the spreader and adjust so that they are the same length. Attach cord pulley to the center of the spreader, and adjust over frame so that the spreader is from 6 to 12 inches above the toes.

Place weights on pulley, and increase the amount until the client feels the pull in the paravertebral area. William's position may be ordered to create further pull on the spine and lessen pull on hips and abdomen.

Instruct the client about the optimal position of the spreader, the activity permitted, and restrictions, if any.

Place foot cradle over knees of client (so that view of feet is not obstructed). Replace bedclothes over the cradle and drape over the legs, leaving the feet and traction apparatus uncovered. If desired, put socks on the client's feet.

*Nursing intervention.* Check for maximum comfort. (The upper strap is as tight as possible without causing any discomfort; the second and third straps are firmly secured but not tight; the bottom strap is loose enough to permit flexion of the hips.)

Change the client's position as necessary, always keeping the spreader straight. Check position of spreader, and enlist the client's help in maintaining its position. (At rest, the spreader is close to the feet but at least 6 inches above the toes.) If the spreader touches the foot of the bed or the pulley, instruct the client to pull him- or herself up in bed; if he or she cannot, have the client call the nurse to change position.

Encourage the client to move the legs, bend the knees, and flex and extend the feet at frequent intervals. If the client is permitted to be out of bed periodically, supervise him or her, as necessary, in the removal of the belt and its replacement.

## CHARTING

Note client's reaction to traction, time initiated, and intervals when traction is interrupted.

Note skin condition and local pressure during and after application of traction.

# INTERVENTION FOR INCREASED INTRACRANIAL PRESSURE

Increased intracranial pressure can result from brain tumors, inflammatory processes, or trauma. Brain tumors result in pressure on the surrounding tissues, leading to cerebral edema and possible necrosis of the tissue if treatment is not instituted. The same is true of an inflammation process and trauma. Both cause tissue damage with corresponding cerebral edema. In many cases, surgery is required; however, a conservative regimen may be instituted first.

### Expected outcome

The client should be able to explain the procedures for decreasing intracranial pressure, including safe and rapid control of the intracranial pressure.

### DEHYDRATION REGIMEN (CONSERVATIVE TREATMENT OF PATIENT WITH INCREASED INTRACRANIAL PRESSURE)

One or more of the following measures may be used to reduce increased intracranial pressure. The dosage given is that recommended for an adult.

1. Limited fluid intake: 800 to 1200 ml each 24 hours.

2. Magnesium sulfate: 30 ml saturated solution by mouth before breakfast daily or every other day. If the client is unable to retain medication by mouth, give as retention enema (60 ml slowly with a No. 24 catheter).

3. Hypertonic solutions intravenously: 250 ml of 25% glucose; 50 ml of 50% glucose; concentrated proteins (serum albumen and plasma); urea or mannitol, 50% (Chapter 21). Corticosteroids, though slow in action, also reduce cerebral edema. If mannitol is utilized, heed contraindications for use and risk of masking an expanding intracranial mass. Catheterize client simultaneously or as soon as feasible. After the hypertonic solution is administered for a rapid reduction of pressure, corticosteroids may be given to maintain the therapeutic effect. Decadron is often the medication of choice.

4. Removal of cerebrospinal fluid by lumbar or ventricular puncture: reduce pressure by one half the initial pressure or to 100 mm, whichever is lower (may be modified for the individual client).

5. Continuous ventricular drainage.

An important adjunct to this regimen is elevation of the head 30 to 45 degrees. This increases venous drainage from the brain.

## CONTINUOUS VENTRICULAR DRAINAGE

*Definition.* The automatic withdrawal of ventricular fluid by means of a special device that maintains intracranial pressure at any desired level.

*Purposes.* (1) To reduce increased intracranial pressure preoperatively or postoperatively, (2) to eliminate intermittent, repeated ventricular or lumbar punctures, and (3) to facilitate frequent recording of the intraventricular pressure.

*Contraindications.* None.

*Complications.* (1) Excessive subcutaneous loss of cerebrospinal fluid, (2) infection at the site of catheter or reservoir insertion, (3) air bubbles in the flush system, (4) break in sterility of the collection system, (5) overzealous drainage of cerebrospinal fluid causing subdural hematoma, (6) overhydration, (7) ventricular catheter obstruction, and (8) hemorrhage and neurological sequelae.

## EXTERNAL DRAIN UNIT

*Definition.* The stabilization of cerebrospinal fluid pressure within the ventricular system by means of an indwelling catheter and an external reservoir.

*Purposes.* (1) To regulate cerebrospinal fluid pressure and (2) to permit automatic drainage of cerebrospinal fluid by a closed sterile system when insertion of permanent shunt is contraindicated.

### EQUIPMENT*

38 cm radiopaque silicone rubber catheter
40.6 cm stylet for catheter placement
Subgaleal trocar
One-way valve
183 cm polyvinylchloride tubing with two clamps
Syringe for irrigation and priming of system
Latex injection and sampling site
Stainless steel tubing connector
Plastic collection bag with 50 cm pressure measuring tape and latex drain with clamp

### Other
Sterile gauze dressings and hypoallergenic tape

*Procedure.* The site of catheter insertion varies depending on the client's pathological condition

*Holter External Ventricular Drainage System; used with permission of Codman & Shurtleff, Inc., Randolph, Mass.

and the neurosurgeon's judgment. In the operating room the perforated catheter and stylet are introduced into the selected ventricle. The system is checked for the free flow of cerebrospinal fluid. The catheter is sewn into position on the skin at the exit site. Sterile dressings are applied. The external drain unit is clamped and prepared for connection to the catheter. The collection bag is temporarily suspended with the exit clamp closed while the tubing clamps are opened. The valve is flushed with 10 ml of sterile normal saline solution from a syringe and connected between the collection bag and distal clamp. The syringe is refilled with sterile normal saline, and the entire collection unit is flushed. The collection bag is positioned such that the corresponding centimeter marking on the measuring tape is in a horizontal line with a central line to the head. The placement of the central head line in relationship to the centimeter measuring tape will maintain the intracranial pressure at a corresponding millimeter of water pressure. For example, if the central head line is placed at the 20 cm mark, the intracranial pressure will be maintained at the 200 mm $H_2O$ mark (Fig. 27-9).

The advantage of this closed system is that the bag is permeable to gases; thus fluid collection is possible without a vent, and sterility is maintained. Cerebrospinal fluid for examination also may be removed through the stopcock without interrupting the system. Thus the need for repeated needle punctures is eliminated. The extralow pressure value prevents reflux of cerebrospinal fluid into the system. Because the system is disposable, the risks of infection and cross-contamination are reduced. Injection of drugs is by the easy access and fluid-sampling sites.

Nursing management of the client with an external drain unit has been greatly simplified by recent improvements in such units. Nursing responsibilities for these clients are centered around maintenance of a sterile collection system, a collection bag of appropriate height in relationship to the intracranial pressure for adequate drainage of the cerebrospinal fluid, and prevention of infection of the exit site of the catheter. Cautious monitoring of the intracranial pressure and client in regard to clinical status are required for effective nursing management in continuous ventricular drainage.

## SUBARACHNOID SCREW

The subarachnoid screw is a device for direct measurement of increased intracranial pressure. It is a hollow cylinder with a standard Luerlock on the external end. The subarachnoid screw can be inserted under local anesthesia in the operating room. The usual site of placement is in the frontal area of the skull and just behind the hairline. An incision exposes the dura mater, and the screw is locked into place with a wrench into the subarachnoid space. A sterile dressing or collodion is then applied at the site of insertion. A three-way stopcock is then put on the pressure screw to allow drainage of the cerebrospinal fluid and measurement of intracranial pressure.

The subarachnoid screw is hooked to a transducer that converts the cerebrospinal fluid pressure into an electric current that can then be monitored. A heparinized solution of 500 ml of normal saline solution and usually 1000 units of heparin are used as a basic flush for the intravenous tubing to prevent clotting of the system. High-pressure tubing and manometer are utilized to measure the intracranial pressure. The advantage of the subarachnoid screw over the traditional measurement of intracranial pressure is that changes in the pressure are detectable much sooner than physical signs. The pressure is measured with the same principle as that in central venous pressure, with zero millimeters of water pressure as a normal valve reading. Progressive rise or abrupt increases indicate developing intracranial pressure.

The nurse must know several things about the subarachnoid screw. It is a closed system and must be kept that way. It is easily removed when monitoring is no longer necessary, and it results in no permanent damage. The major risk of this system is the potential for infection. Aseptic technique is essential when changing dressings around the insertion site. All portions of the setup should be changed daily. Obtain random cultures and sensitivities if infection is suspected.

## INTRACRANIAL PRESSURE MONITORING

Compensatory mechanism and other parameters of intracranial dynamics can be evaluated by intracranial pressure monitoring. Since intracranial pressure monitoring is still a relatively recent advancement, variations in procedure from institution to institution are dependent on the monitoring technique and expertise of the neurosurgical staff. Ventriculostomy reservoirs, transducers, and electronic oscilloscopes are generally complemented by intra-arterial pressure monitors, electroencephalographs, electrocardiographs, and automated blood pressure analyzers. Intracranial pressure dynamics can thus be evaluated in terms of volume-pressure relationships, pressure waves, and cerebral perfusion pressures.

Normally, intracranial pressure ranges from 4 to 15 mm Hg or 50 to 200 mm $H_2O$. In Fig. 27-10, *A,* normal intracranial pressure is depicted. Subsequent increases in intracranial pressure are shown in Fig. 27-10, *B,* which demonstrates a curve with compensatory mechanisms beginning to be exhausted over time. Fig. 27-10, *C,* demonstrates the exhausted compensatory mechanisms, and sharp elevations of intracranial pressure. Usually if the intracranial pressure rises this rapidly, decompensation in neuronal tissue, client status, and death results when the intracranial pressure increase is left untreated.

Intracranial wave formations are generally based on fluctuations of pressure noted on the oscilloscope. Fig. 27-11, *A,* depicts possible formations of pressure waves in normal intracranial pressure. Elevated portions (Fig. 27-11, *B)* with sustained plateau waves indicates rises in intracranial pressure and the effect of compensatory mechanisms on lowering the pressure to a homeostatic level. Rapid, large wave fluctuations from the base line (Fig. 27-11, *C)* indicate failure of compensatory mechanisms and malignant increases of intracranial pressure.

*Nursing intervention.* The use of intracranial pressure monitoring is appropriate and pertinent only to a well-trained nursing staff. The interpretation of data and coordination of other equipment designed to evaluate the client's status such as intra-arterial line pressures, ECG, and EEG need to be evaluated carefully against the client's clinical picture. The nurse's role basically should encompass the activities that seek to prevent infection at the exit site, monitor cerebrospinal fluid leakage and pressure level, observe hematoma formation, and prepare the client's family for the sophisticated equipment they might find in use for the client. Also, supportive care to prevent complications of

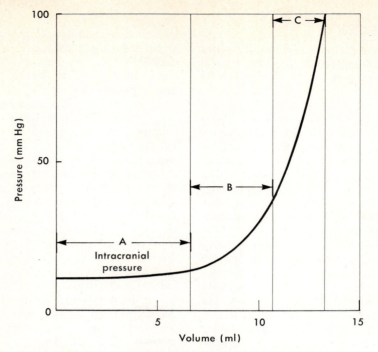

**FIG. 27-10.** Volume-pressure relationship in intracranial pressure monitoring.

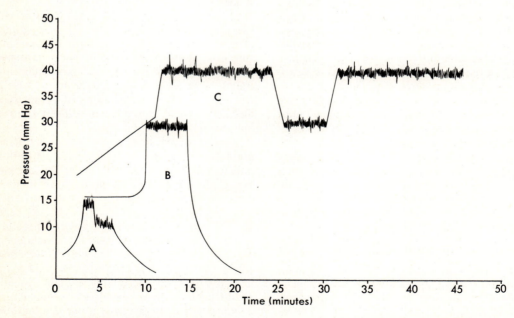

**FIG. 27-11.** Pressure-wave form relationship of increased intracranial pressure. *A,* In early stages, as volume increases, intracranial pressure is normal. *B,* When small margin of compensation is exhausted, intracranial pressure begins to rise. *C,* With intracranial pressure already raised, minor increase in volume causes major rise in pressure.

bed rest, hypoventilation or hyperventilation, and hypothermia are necessary to ensure the integrity of bodily functions, while decompensation is being prevented.

## RADIOTHERAPY

X-ray therapy, or radiotherapy, consists in the administration of roentgen rays to the neoplastic area. The treatment is given under standard conditions in a special environment. The dosage (duration and strength) and frequency of administration are controlled carefully. After the diagnosis has been determined histologically, treatment is given to clients with the following types of tumors: medulloblastoma, glioblastoma, and pituitary adenoma. The benefits to be derived from x-ray treatment of other tumors of the nervous system, including the malignant types, are questionable, but the psychological effect may warrant its continued use. Clients with syringomyelia are helped appreciably by radiation.

Before proceeding with the treatment, permission is obtained and the client told of the possible sequelae (loss of hair, superficial skin reactions, gastrointestinal disturbances, headache). These associated discomforts may result from the absorption of the products of protein breakdown and may be prevented or alleviated when the client fasts for the 2- or 3-hour period preceding the treatment. Nicotinic acid or chlorpromazine (Thorazine) may be given during the series of treatments to obviate nausea and vomiting. Marijuana is being used experimentally in treating nausea and vomiting. Appropriate detail on radiotherapy is available in the references. Cola syrup over cracked ice also may be effective in alleviating these symptoms.

The client is observed for signs and symptoms of increasing intracranial pressure during the course of treatment.

## REFERENCES

Alexander, E., Jr., Davis, C.H., Jr., and Kester, N.C.: Intracranial aneurysms: methods of treatment; value of hypothermia in the surgical approach, Arch. Neurol. Psychiatry **81:**684-692, 1959.

Benzinger, T.H.: The human thermostat, Sci. Am. **204:**134-147, Jan. 1961.

Bettice, D.: The cause of vomiting of tube feedings by neurosurgical patients, J. Neurosurg. Nurs. **3:**93-112, Dec. 1971.

Botterell, E.H., et al.: Hypothermia and interruption of carotid,

or carotid and vertebral circulation, in the surgical management of intracranial aneurysms, J. Neurosurg. **13:**1-42, Jan. 1956.

Bozza, M.L., and Rossanda, M.: A simplified method for safe and controllable hypothermia in neurosurgery, Acta Neurochir. **10:**153-161, Feb. 16, 1961.

Brunner, L.S.: The Lippincott manual of nursing practice, ed. 2, Philadelphia, 1978, J.B. Lippincott Co.

Chesney, D., and Chesney, M.O.: Care of the patient in diagnostic radiography, ed. 5, Philadelphia, 1978, J.B. Lippincott Co.

Collins, V.J.: Principles of anesthesiology, ed. 2, Philadelphia, 1976, Lea & Febiger.

Conner, G.H., et al.: Tracheostomy—when it is needed, Am. J. Nurs. **72:**68-74, Jan. 1972.

Cottrell, J.E., and Turndorf, H.: Anesthesia and neurosurgery, St. Louis, 1979, The C.V. Mosby Co.

Crutchfield, W.G.: Fracture-dislocations of the cervical spine, Am. J. Surg. **38:**592-598, 1937.

Devney, A.M., and Kingsburg, B.A.: Hypothermia in fact and fantasy, Am. J. Nurs. **72:**1424-1425, 1972.

Dison, N.: Clinical nursing techniques, ed. 4, St. Louis, 1979, The C.V. Mosby Co.

Downs, H.S.: The control of vomiting, Am. J. Nurs. **66:**76-82, Jan. 1966.

Eiseman, B., and Spencer, F.: Tracheostomy: an underrated surgical procedure, J.A.M.A. **184:**684-687, 1963.

Geffin, B., and Pontoppidan, H.: Reduction of tracheal damage by the prestretching of inflatable cuffs, Anesthesiology **31:**462-463, 1969.

Goloskov, J., and LeRoy, P.: A new method for managing extracellular fluid accumulations in central nervous system disorders, J. Neurosurg. Nurs. **8:**53-57, 1976.

Gurevich, I.: Some new concepts in tracheostomy suctioning, RN **35:**52-55, Sept. 1972.

Hanlon, K.: Description and uses of intracranial pressure monitoring, Heart Lung **5:**277-282, March-April 1976.

Helfet, A.J., and Lee, D.M.: Disorders of the lumbar spine, Philadelphia, 1978, J.B. Lippincott Co.

Hoen, T.I.: A method of skeletal traction for treatment of fracture dislocation of cervical vertebrae, Arch. Neurol. Psychiatr. **36:**158-161, July 1936.

Hope-Stone, H.F.: Radiotherapy in modern clinical practice, St. Louis, 1976, The C.V. Mosby Co.

Howe, J.R.: Patient care in neurosurgery, Boston, 1977, Little, Brown & Co.

Hrobsky, A.: The patient on a CircOlectric bed, Am. J. Nurs. **71:**2352-2353, 1971.

Jacquette, G.: To reduce hazards of tracheal suctioning, Am. J. Nurs. **71:**2362-2364, 1971.

Jones, A.: Nursing implications in the administration of urea, J. Neurosurg. Nurs. **7:**37-41, 1975.

King, E.M., et al.: Illustrated manual of nursing techniques, New York, 1977, J.B. Lippincott Co.

Krayenbuehl, H., et al.: Advances and technical standards in neurosurgery, vol. 6, Berlin, 1978, Springer Verlag.

Lavigne, J.M.: Respiratory care of patients with neuromuscular disease, Nurs. Clin. North Am. **14:**133-143, March 1979.

Leahy, I.M., et al.: The nurse and radiotherapy: a manual for daily care, St. Louis, 1978, The C.V. Mosby Co.

Mitchell, P., and Mauss, N.: Relationship of patient-nurse activity to intracranial pressure variations, Nurs. Res. **27:**4-10, Jan.-Feb. 1978.

Morley, T.P., editor: Current controversies in neurosurgery, Philadelphia, 1976, W.B. Saunders Co.

Nikas, D., and Konkoly, R.: Nursing responsibilities in arterial and intracranial pressure monitoring, J. Neurosurg. Nurs. **7:**116-122, Dec. 1977.

Ozuna, J.M., and Foster, C.: Hypothermia and the surgical patient, Am. J. Nurs. **79:**646-648, April 1979.

Pfaudler, M.: Care of patients with severe spinal cord injuries. In (Panel of authorities): Current practice in critical care, vol. 1, St. Louis, 1979, The C.V. Mosby Co.

Robinson, F.: An apparatus for continuous ventricular drainage and intraventricular therapy, J. Neurosurg. **5:**320-323, 1948.

Rosomoff, H.L., and Holaday, D.A.: Cerebral blood flow and cerebral oxygen consumption during hypothermia, Am. J. Physiol. **179:**85-88, Oct. 1954.

Ruge, D, and Wiltse, L.L., editors: Spinal disorders: diagnosis and treatment, Philadelphia, 1977, Lea & Febiger.

Sackett, J.F., and Strother, C.M., editors: New techniques in myelography, New York, 1979, Harper & Row, Inc.

Saunders, R., and Lyons, T.: External ventricular drainage, Crit. Care Med. **7:**556-558, Dec. 1979.

Smith, E.W.: *Pseudomonas,* the ever present menace, RN **35:**63-70, Feb. 1972.

Tilbury, M.S.: The intracranial pressure screw, Nurs. Clin. North Am. **9:**641, Dec. 1974.

Tillery, B., and Bates, B.: Enemas, Am. J. Nurs. **66:**534-537, 1966.

Tysinger, D.S.: Common misconceptions in inhalation therapy, J.A.M.A. (Alabama) **40:**1-7, Jan. 1971.

Uihlein, A., Terry, H.R., Jr., and Martin, J.T.: Induced hypothermia in neurologic conditions, Med. Clin. North Am. **44:**1079-1100, 1960.

Wade, J.F.: Comprehensive respiratory nursing care: physiology and technique, ed. 3, St. Louis, 1981, The C.V. Mosby Co.

Welsh, M.S.: Comfort measures during radiation therapy, Am. J. Nurs. **67:**1880-1882, 1967.

White, H.A.: Tracheostomy: care with a cuffed tube, Am. J. Nurs. **72:**75-77, Jan. 1972.

Wollman, H., and Larson, C.: Anesthesiology, Philadelphia, 1978, J.B. Lippincott Co.

Yashon, D.: Spinal injury, New York, 1978, Appleton-Century-Crofts.

Zimmer USA: Patient care systems package insert, PCS anti-embolism stockings, March 1979, Warsaw, Ind.

# 28
# MEDICATIONS IN COMMON USE

A complete discussion of medications utilized in neurological nursing is beyond the spatial limits of this book. As an alternative to avoiding the topic, this chapter has been written as an outline of major pharmacological agents in each classification. One example of each category has been expanded to include a brief tabular listing of trade and generic names, other agents and general action of the group, specific mechanism of the drug's action, adverse outcomes, drug interaction, nursing assessment, nursing management, and client outcomes.

When a nurse utilizes pharmacological agents in the care of neurological clients, it is important to use this as a general discussion requiring more specific information from the latest references. For further reading see the bibliography to this chapter.

For most of these drugs effects on pregnant women, newborns, and even young children may be indefinite. Adverse outcomes and drug interactions mentioned include the most probable situations, but are not totally inclusive of all possibilities. Because of variations in dosage that occur in different clients who may be utilizing medication for a classic or other therapeutic action, who vary in personal reactions and physical condition, and who exhibit age-related responses, no attempt has been made to suggest dosages.

Adverse outcomes tend to be more commonly apparent in debilitated clients, those at either age extreme, and clients on concomitant pharmacological therapy.

The nurse is responsible for all aspects of client safety regarding medication administration, drug actions (both desired and adverse), and possibilities for interaction with other substances. The nurse uses his or her knowledge to interpret orders and seek clarification as necessary before administration of prescribed medications. After assessment of the client's condition, need, and potential for drug effectiveness and interaction and administration of the drug, the outcome of and change in client condition is reported to the physician. The physician orders necessary laboratory and radiological studies to document, modify, or discontinue the drug when indicated.

Both the physician and the nurse should know what drugs are included in the Controlled Substances Act of 1970 and should comply with the state and federal laws regulating the use of these drugs.

**Expected outcomes**
The client who is taking medications will:
1 Identify prescribed medication name, use, and rationale for taking each drug.
2 Explain any special directions and precautions in taking the drug, in health care measures necessary while on the drug, and in any special storage instructions.
3 Recognize adverse outcomes and state what side effects can occur while the medication is making the client improve in health status. Report these to the physician.
4 State the desired outcome from the use of the medication or medications.
5 Describe the possible interaction between drug and alcohol ingestion, over-the-counter drugs, and interactions among other prescribed medications.
6 Explain all aspects inherent in self-administration of medications.
7 Before discharge, be assessed for previous history of drug compliance and receive written and verbal instructions or printed material outlining the above points, observations of specific outcomes, and when and what to report to the physician.

## ANTICONVULSANTS

| Classification | Drug | Mechanism of action | Adverse outcome |
|---|---|---|---|
| Hydantoins<br>Stabilize membrane ion movement to decrease grand mal, focal, and psychomotor seizures. | Phenytoin sodium (Dilantin Sodium)<br><br>*Other drugs:*<br>Mephenytoin (Mesantoin)<br>Ethotoin (Peganone) | Motor cortex. May promote efflux of sodium from neurons, which stabilizes the threshold against hyperexcitability caused by excess stimulation or environmental change that reduces membrane sodium gradient, which prevents cortical seizure foci from stimulating adjacent cortical areas sensitive to seizure activity. Reduces events in brainstem centers responsible for tonic phase of grand mal seizure. | Slurred speech, nystagmus, mental confusion, nausea, blurred or double vision, dizziness, constipation, fever, vomiting, skin eruptions, staggering gait, gingival hyperplasia, thrombocytopenia, and leukopenia. Rapid intravenous administration can depress atrial and ventricular conduction and induce ventricular fibrillation, osteomalacia, and hyperglycemia from inhibition of insulin release. Depression in protein-bound iodine. Toxic hepatitis, liver damage; unknown effects in pregnancy and nursing infants; phenytoin metabolism may be greatly altered when used in combination with other drugs; abrupt cessation of phenytoin use may result in status epilepticus. |
| Barbiturates<br>Nonspecific central nervous system depressants to decrease grand mal, focal, and psychomotor seizures. | Phenobarbital (Luminal Sodium)<br><br>*Other drugs:*<br>Amobarbital sodium (Amytal Sodium)<br>Aprobarbital (Alurate)<br>Butabarbital sodium (Butisol Sodium)<br>Metharbital (Gemonil)<br>Mephobarbital (Mebaral)<br>Pentobarbital sodium (Nembutal)<br>Secobarbital sodium (Seconal Sodium)<br>Primidone (Mysoline) Congener of phenobarbital | General CNS depressant that depresses the activity of nerve and skeletal, smooth, and cardiac muscles with reduction of oxygen consumption in selected tissues. Depression occurs through reduction in both excitatory and inhibitory postsynaptic potential of acetylcholine by presynaptic blockage of ganglionic cells. The basic antiepileptic action is unknown. | Respiratory depression, hypersensitivity reactions in clients with asthma, uticaria, or angioneurotic edema. Laryngospasm, hypotension with rapid intravenous infusion. Should not be used in clients with history of sensitivity to barbiturates, porphyria, or chronic pulmonary disease. Ataxia, vertigo, drowsiness, sexual impotence, megaloblastic anemia, nausea, anorexia, and vomiting. |

| Drug interaction | Nursing assessment | Nursing intervention | Expected outcomes |
|---|---|---|---|
| Barbiturates enhance the rate of metabolism of phenytoin. Dicumarol inhibits the metabolism of phenytoin in the liver. Coumarin anticoagulants increase serum levels of phenytoin. Isoniazide and chloramphenicol inhibit the metabolism of phenytoin resulting in phenytoin intoxication. Tricyclic antidepressants in high doses can precipitate seizures. Phenytoin increases metabolism of vitamin D with resultant effect on serum calcium. | *Assess client for:* Constipation, fluid, or electrolyte imbalance from nausea and vomiting, skin condition, rashes, bruising, shortness of breath, tiredness, bleeding tendencies (especially the mouth and gingiva), nystagmus, ataxia, slurred speech, dizziness, insomnia, mental confusion, motor twitching, and vital sign changes (especially pulse), blood glucose, data related to liver function. Effectiveness of seizure control. | *Nurse should:* Give laxatives as needed. Monitor lab data of electrolytes, hematocrit, hemoglobin, differential, platelets, and blood glucose, studies indicating liver function. Give soft foods to prevent severe gingival bleeding. Frequently brush teeth and massage gums. Use seizure precautions if status epilepticus is known from history. Make frequent neurological checks when dosages are changed. Give drug with or at meal completion. | *Client should have:* Reduction of grand mal seizure activity, seizure foci of status epilepticus, and psychomotor seizure activity. *Serum level:* 10 to 20 $\mu$g/ml. |
| Barbiturates inhibit the action of antihistamines or other drugs that have an enzymatic effect. Barbiturates serve as antagonists for CNS stimulants. Alkaline antacids inhibit absorption of some barbiturates. Barbiturates in certain dosages depress protein-bound iron. Phenobarbital inhibits hypnotics and increases the metabolism of vitamin D with resultant effect on serum calcium. | *Assess client for:* Respiratory depression and hypotension on intravenous infusion. Always assess for past reaction to barbiturates or client history of porphyria or chronic pulmonary disease, fluid and electrolyte imbalances, bruising, tiredness, drowsiness, and staggering gait. Effectiveness of seizure control. | *Nurse should:* Monitor respiratory rate and blood pressure during drug adjustments or intravenous infusion. Monitor lab data of hemoglobin, hematocrit, platelets, and differential. Use seizure precautions. Make frequent neurological checks during dose changes. Caution clients not to drive or operate mechanical or electrical equipment when they are drowsy. Give folic acid if megaloblastic anemia occurs. Monitor drug-usage patterns and responses. Observe client for withdrawal, if drug is suddenly discontinued; observe and report unusual behaviors to physician. | *Client should have:* Reduction of grand mal, psychomotor, and focal epileptic seizure activity when used in large dosages or in combination with other anticonvulsant drugs. |

*Continued.*

## ANTICONVULSANTS—cont'd

| Classification | Drug | Mechanism of action | Adverse outcome |
|---|---|---|---|
| Diones<br>   Useful in petit mal seizures and convulsions from picrotoxin, strychnine, and procaine. | Trimethadione (Tridione)<br><br>*Other drugs:*<br>Paramethadione (Paradione)<br>Primidone (Mysoline) | Elevate the threshold for synaptic potentials by prolonging synaptic recovery time and passively contributing to sodium efflux by reducing membrane sodium gradient, preventing central excitation, and enhancing CNS depression. | Because of adverse outcomes, it is used only when response to other drugs is inadequate. Skin rash, leukopenia, neutropenia, sore throat, epistaxis, hepatitis, jaundice, albuminuria, hemeralopia, lupus-like syndrome and myasthenia gravis–like syndrome, nausea, gastric pain, vomiting, vertigo, drowsiness, fatigue, personality changes, hiccups. Possible birth defects when used during pregnancy. Blood dyscrasias. Fatal aplastic anemia may precipitate grand mal seizures. |
| Succinimides (suximides)<br>   Utilized to decrease petit mal seizures. | Ethosuximide (Zarontin)<br><br>*Other drugs:*<br>Methsuximide (Celontin)<br>Phensuximide (Milontin) | Depression of motor cortex through elevation of threshold of synaptic potentials by prolonging synaptic recovery time and passively contributing to sodium efflux by reducing membrane sodium gradient, preventing central excitation, and enhancing CNS depression. The exact antiepileptic mechanism is unknown. | Nausea, vomiting, gastric upsets and pain, leukopenia, aplastic anemia, drowsiness, dizziness, hiccups, personality changes, sleep disturbances, skin rash, ataxia, lupus-like syndrome, bleeding tendencies, blood dyscrasias, gum hypertrophy. Should not be used in clients with history of hypersensitivity to succinimides. Abrupt withdrawal may cause petit mal status epilepticus. |

| Drug interaction | Nursing assessment | Nursing intervention | Expected outcome |
|---|---|---|---|
| Diones when given in combination with phenytoins elevate blood dione levels and may create overdosage. Paradione increases the metabolism of vitamin D with resultant effect on serum calcium. Aspirin potentiates effects of anticonvulsants by decreasing metabolism of anticonvulsants. | *Assess client for:* Skin condition, bleeding gums, epistaxis, vaginal bleeding and bruising tendencies, fluid and electrolyte imbalance from nausea and vomiting, staggering gait, drowsiness, shortness of breath, fatigue or difficulty arousing from sleep, any unusual or unexpected behavior patterns or reactions to verbal responses or physical treatments. Effectiveness of seizure control. | *Nurse should:* Monitor bleeding episodes for frequency and amount. Use seizure precautions if past history of grand mal seizures. Monitor lab data (especially hemoglobin, hematocrit, white cell count differential, platelets, bilirubin, liver function studies, electrolytes, and albumin in urinalysis) and report abnormalities to physician. Caution clients not to drive car or operate mechanical or electrical equipment when drowsy. Evaluate progress of unusual skin rashes or petechia. Report skin rashes immediately so that drug may be stopped. Use tridione as a last resort in pregnant women. Explain treatment regime to client and family. | *Client should have:* Reduction of petit mal seizure activity. The client may have a tendency toward grand mal seizure activity.<br><br>*Plasma level:* 40 to 100 $\mu$g/ml. |
| Zarontin when combined with other anticonvulsants can increase libido. Aspirin potentiates anticonvulsant effect by decreasing metabolism of anticonvulsants. | *Assess client for:* Fluid and electrolyte imbalance caused by nausea and vomiting, epigastric or abdominal pain, or vague gastrointestinal complaints, bruising or bleeding tendencies, fatigue or drowsiness, any unusual or unexpected behavior changes or reactions to verbal responses or physical treatments, skin condition, and gum condition. Effectiveness of seizure control. | *Nurse should:* Monitor lab data for hemoglobin, hematocrit, electrolytes, white cell count differential, and platelets. Note frequency and intensity of gastrointestinal complaints. Monitor bleeding or bruising for frequency and amount. Caution clients not to drive or operate mechanical or electrical equipment when drowsy. Report unusual or unexpected behavior or sleep disorders. Evaluate progress of skin conditions. | *Client should have:* Reduction of petit mal seizure activity. |

*Continued.*

## ANTICONVULSANTS—cont'd

| Classification | Drug | Mechanism of action | Adverse outcome |
|---|---|---|---|
| Miscellaneous anticonvulsants<br>Possess anticonvulsant properties or are used concomitantly with other agents for seizure control. | Valproic acid (the sodium salt is Depakene)<br><br>*Other drugs used as anticonvulsants:*<br>Carbamazepine (Tegretol)<br>Paraldehyde<br>Diazepam (Valium)<br>Meprobamate (Miltown)<br>Thiopental sodium (Pentothal Sodium) | Mechanism of action uncertain. Suggested mode of action is through increased brain GABA levels. No known effects on neuronal membrane potentials to date. | Hepatic failure, nausea, vomiting, gastrointestinal disturbances, abdominal cramps, bleeding tendencies, behavioral change, ataxia, nystagmus, weakness, dizziness, incoordination, transient alopecia, petechiae, diplopia, thrombocytopenia. Effects during lactation and pregnancy unknown. |

| Drug interaction | Nursing assessment | Nursing intervention | Expected outcome |
|---|---|---|---|
| Depakene is partially metabolized into ketones and is partially eliminated in the urine, leading to falsely positive urine ketone tests. Potentiates CNS depression activity of alcohol. An increase in serum barbiturate levels can lead to CNS toxicity. Potentiates the effects of anticoagulants. Concurrent use of valproic acid and clonazepam may result in petit mal status epilepticus. | *Assess clients for:* Jaundice, delirium, abdominal cramps, bleeding, history of alcohol abuse, behavioral change or unexpected response to verbal commands or physical treatments, nystagmus, staggering gait, alopecia, poor eye-to-hand coordination, fluid and electrolyte imbalances from nausea and vomiting, drowsiness. Monitor serum barbiturate levels and concurrently administered phenytoin levels. Evaluate effectiveness of seizure control. | *Nurse should:* Monitor lab data for hemoglobin, hematocrit, platelets, differential, partial thromboplastin time, bilirubin, prothrombin time, electrolytes. Monitor the frequency and intensity of bruising or bleeding. Use seizure precautions if history of multiple types of seizures. Institute safety measures for problems related to behavior, balance, and mobility. Report unusual behavioral changes. Caution clients not to operate automobile, or mechanical or electrical machinery when dizzy. Monitor and report anticonvulsant blood levels. Intake and output until effect on gastrointestinal system and weight control is established. Treat bowel abnormalities symptomatically. | *Client should have:* Reduction of petit mal seizure activity or reduction in multiple seizure types of complex origins. *Plasma levels:* 0.5 to 25 $\mu$g/ml. |

## DEPRESSANTS

| Classification | Drug | Mechanism of action | Adverse outcome |
|---|---|---|---|
| Analgesics<br>  Decrease presynaptic transmission of acetylcholine at neuronal junction in CNS in route to efferent tracts.<br>  Opiate derivatives (narcotics) | Morphine<br><br>*Other drugs:*<br>Codeine<br>Hydromorphone hydrochloride (Dilaudid)<br>Hydrochlorides of opium alkaloids (Pantopon) | Exact mechanism is unknown, but there are effects that decrease various neurotransmitter release at the neuronal junction in CNS and peripheral nerves. | Respiratory depression, pupil constriction, nausea, vomiting, hypermotility in stomach and small intestine with considerable decrease in peristalsis in large intestine, increase in smooth muscle tone in bladder and ureter, decreasing urine flow. Increase in biliary tract spasm. Altered emotional pain perception potentially creating habitual abuse. |
| Synthetic narcotics | Meperidine hydrochloride (Demerol Hydrochloride)<br><br>*Other drugs:*<br>Alphaprodine hydrochloride (Nisentil Hydrochloride)<br>Anileridine (Leritene)<br>Oxycodone (Percodan)<br>Methadone hydrochloride (Dolophine Hydrochloride) | Same as narcotic analgesics, but pharmaceutical structure is different. | Drowsiness, slight dilatation of pupils, respiratory depression, nausea, vomiting, decreased urinary output, constipation. |
| Synthetic nonnarcotics | Pentazocine (Talwin)<br>*Other drugs:*<br>Propoxyphene napsylate monohydrate (Darvon-N)<br>Levallorphan tartrate (Lorfan)<br>Naloxone hydrochloride (Narcan) | Similar to narcotic and synthetic narcotic analgesics | Similar to narcotic analgesics, but to milder degree. Transitory hallucinations, physical and psychological dependence; may precipitate seizures, increases sedation with concomitant CNS depressants; respiratory depression occurs to a lesser degree than with narcotic and synthetic narcotic analgesics. |

| Drug interaction | Nursing assessment | Nursing intervention | Expected outcome* |
|---|---|---|---|
| Alcohol, antihistamines, barbiturates, phenothiazides, benzodiazepines, tricyclic antidepressants enhance CNS depression. MAO inhibitors can give severe reactions of rigidity, excitation, sweating, and hypertension. | *Assess client for:* History of taking narcotic analgesics, pain history, review pain experience, vital signs, neurological checks, previous respiratory patterns of narcotic administration, depressed cough reflex, intake and output, bowel patterns, level of consciousness, age, debilitation, concomitant medications before administration, concurrent problems and disease conditions, psychosocial history. Evaluate effectiveness of pain relief. | *Nurse should:* Monitor client experience with narcotic analgesics. Evaluate pain and narcotic tolerance. Frequently check client's respiratory rate and pattern, neurological check and level of consciousness. Use with extreme caution in elderly, debilitated, severely traumatized, or CNS-depressed clients. | *Client should have:* Reduction in pain, relaxation, sedation. |
| Same as for narcotic analgesics. | *Assess client for:* Same as narcotic analgesics, plus drowsiness. Evaluate effectiveness in pain relief. | *Nurse should:* Same as narcotic analgesics. If client is taking orally, caution against driving automobile and operating machinery. | *Client should have:* Reduction in pain, relaxation, sedation, some drying of secretions when given as presurgery medication. |
| Same as narcotic and synthetic narcotic analgesics. | *Assess client for:* Same as other narcotic and synthetic narcotic analgesics. Evaluate effectiveness in pain relief. | *Nurse should:* Same as narcotic and synthetic narcotic analgesics. Use with extreme caution in above clients plus pregnant women, children, clients with myocardial infarct, and in those with diminished renal, respiratory, or hepatic functions. | *Client should have:* Same as synthetic narcotic analgesics. |

*Naloxone hydrochloride (Narcan), an effective antagonist, administered for overdosage.          *Continued.*

**DEPRESSANTS—cont'd**

| Classification | Drug | Mechanism of action | Adverse outcome |
|---|---|---|---|
| Hypnotics/sedatives Barbiturates | Secobarbital sodium (Seconal sodium) Refer to barbiturate listing under Anticonvulsants. | See barbiturates. | See barbiturates. |
| Nonbarbiturates | *Other drugs in classification of barbiturates* Ethclorvynol (Placidyl) *Other drugs:* Glutethimide (Doriden) Methyprylon (Noludar) Flurazepam dihydrochloride (Dalmane) Chloral hydrate (Noctec) Methaqualone (Quaalude) | Same as barbiturates, but with less excitation and do not suppress rapid-eye-movement sleep. | Should be used only with great caution in clients with porphyria, suicidal tendencies, or depression or in those with a history of prior drug dependence. Not recommended during first and second trimesters of pregnancy; safety during lactation and in children unknown. Use smallest possible dosage in elderly, debilitated, or those who might become dependent on drug. |
| Alcohol Primary and continuous CNS depressant | Ethanol (ethyl alcohol, anhydrous alcohol) | Depresses CNS integrating activity between reticular activating system and cerebral cortex. | Effects directly proportional to the blood concentration and of chronic use. Use with caution in clients with respiratory diseases. Should not be used by those with renal or hepatic diseases, or epileptics. Read *FDA Drug Bull.* **9**(2):June 1979 for important information on alcohol and drug interactions. Read *Loosening the Grip,* a good book on the topic (published by The C.V. Mosby Co.) |

| Drug interaction | Nursing assessment | Nursing intervention | Expected outcome |
|---|---|---|---|
| See barbiturates. | *Assess client for:* Same as barbiturates. | *Nurse should:* Same as barbiturates. | *Client should have:* Reduction in pain, relaxation, sedation. May be used as presurgery medication. |
| May cause a decrease in prothrombin time. When used with amitriptyline, may cause transient delirium. Barbiturates, CNS depressants, alcohol, or MAO inhibitors used simultaneously may increase depressive responses. | *Assess client for:* Same as barbiturates. | *Nurse should:* Same as barbiturates. | *Client should have:* Relief of insomnia or may have a reduction in seizure activity when used in combination with other anticonvulsants. |
| Same as barbiturates, narcotic and synthetic narcotic analgesics. May cause vasodilatation when combined with antihypertensive nitroglycerin. May cause hypoglycemia when used with insulin, sulfonylureas. Gastrointestinal bleeding with aspirin use. May increase or decrease prothrombin time with anticoagulants. May precipitate seizures with phenytoin use. *Alcohol antagonist:* Disulfiram (Antabuse) | *Assess client for:* History of alcohol use (frequency and amount), general history including concomitant medications, psychosocial history of abuse, medical or surgical conditions that may worsen if alcohol withdrawn, pain history, fever, and sleep disturbances. | *Nurse should:* Monitor all drug and alcohol ingestion. Seek psychological aid for appropriate clients and families in cases of alcohol abuse or pain. Monitor all clients' temperatures after alcohol baths for fever, and report abberations. Evaluate effects of alcohol and resolution of sleep disturbances. Caution clients not to operate vehicles or machinery if medication is taken with alcohol or after consumption of large quantities of alcohol. | *Client should have:* Reduction of fever through skin evaporation when used externally. However, ethanol is more commonly taken internally. When taken internally in proper proportions, should have improved appetite and digestion, relief from insomnia. |

## STIMULANTS

| Classification | Drug | Mechanism of action | Adverse outcome |
|---|---|---|---|
| Xanthines | Anhydrous theophylline (Theophyl)<br><br>*Other drugs:*<br>Caffeine<br>Theobromine<br>Aminophylline | May be mediated through inhibition of phosphodiesterase, resulting in an increase in intracellular cyclic AMP. Provides smooth muscle relaxation and increased oxygen supply to tissues. General CNS, cortical, medullary, and spinal cord stimulation and synaptic excitation. | Nausea, epigastric discomfort, headaches, insomnia, reflex hyperexcitability, tachycardia, flushing, hypotension, diuresis. Increased dosages are required for clients with history of tobacco abuse and may exceed toxic dose level (20 $\mu$g/ml) for therapeutic effect. |
| Amphetamines | Dextroamphetamine sulfate (Dexedrine Sulfate)<br><br>*Other drugs:*<br>Ephedrine<br>Amphetamine sulfate (Benzedrine Sulfate) | CNS stimulation may be mediated through sympathomimetic agent excitation of cortex, medulla, and spinal cord through depolarization of neuronal cells and stimulation of norepinephrine. | Same as for xanthines. Also apprehension, insomnia, increased libido, hallucinations, tremor when attempting fine coordinated muscle movements, increased suicidal and homicidal tendencies. |
| Nonamphetamine stimulants | Methylphenidate hydrochloride (Ritalin Hydrochloride)<br><br>*Other drugs:*<br>Phenmetrazine (Preludin)<br>Pemoline (Cylert)<br>Picrotoxin<br>Carbon dioxide<br>Pentylenetetrazole (Metrazole) | Similar action to amphetamines; more effective than caffeine, but less effective than amphetamines. | Nervousness, insomnia, headache, tachycardia, nausea, weight loss. |

| Drug interaction | Nursing assessment | Nursing intervention | Expected outcome |
|---|---|---|---|
| Toxic synergism with ephedrine. Combined with reserpine, precipitates tachycardia. Antagonizes propranolol. Combined with furosemide, increases diuresis. | *Assess client for:* Physiological and psychosocial manifestations of mental cloudiness, drowsiness, respiratory depression, CNS toxicity of morphine or other CNS depressants, tobacco abuse and tolerance to drug dosage, environment and family support system. | *Nurse should:* Monitor respiration and changes in level of consciousness. Provide support for client and family, as mental alertness changes. Involve family in activities with client to provide mechanism for ventilation of feelings and improvement of self-esteem. Support client and family during drug withdrawal periods. | *Client should have:* Relaxation of bronchial airway and smooth muscles, clearer flow of thought and ideas, allayed fatigue and drowsiness with improved motor activity (however, fine muscle coordination and timing may be adversely affected). Reversal of morphine intoxication. |
| Antagonizes adrenergic neuron blockade of guanethidine. Combined with MAO inhibitors causes headache, hypertensive crisis, cerebral hemorrhage. Used with sodium bicarbonate, enhances effects of amphetamine. | *Assess client for:* Same as for xanthines. Also assess for symptoms of drug abuse, insomnia, irritability, misperceptions, meal patterns, and nutritional preferences with continued anorexia. | *Nurse should:* Same as for xanthine. Also should provide small, frequent meals with caloric balance and improved nutrition during anorectic periods. | *Client should have:* Same as for xanthine. Should also have relief of inappropriate narcolepsy symptoms. |
| Same as amphetamines. Can inhibit metabolism of phenytoin. | *Assess client for:* Same as amphetamines. | *Nurse should:* Same as amphetamines. Drug should be taken early in morning or late afternoon to prevent insomnia. | *Client should have:* Same as amphetamines. Also, relief of inappropriate symptoms of minimal brain dysfunction, hyperkinetic child syndrome with improved attention span, emotional ability and mental alertness, improved respiratory ventilation. May be used to combat CNS depression with overdose of barbiturates. |

## PSYCHOTROPICS

| Classification | Drug | Mechanism of action | Adverse outcome |
|---|---|---|---|
| **Antipsychotics**<br>Phenothiazides | Chlorpromazine hydrochloride (Thorazine)<br><br>*Other drugs:*<br>Triflupromazine hydrochloride (Vesprin)<br>Thioridazine (Mellaril)<br>Perphenazine (Trilafon)<br>Prochlorperazine dimaleate (Compazine)<br>Trifluoperazine dihydrochloride (Stelazine) | Precise mechanism is unknown. Exerts strong antiadrenergic but weaker peripheral anticholinergic actions with little ganglionic blocking properties. Reportedly increased threshold levels in the cortex by blocking postsynaptic dopamine receptors in the brain. Subcortical action has been demonstrated, but is not well defined. | Drowsiness, jaundice, agranulocytosis, extrapyramidal parkinsonian reactions with motor restlessness in higher dosages. May lead to tardive dyskinesia, breast enlargement, false pregnancy tests, skin pigmentation, lupus-like syndrome, weight gain, constipation, decreased libido, urinary retention. Secondary extrapyramidal symptoms can occur and can mimic or lead to a missed diagnosis of primary CNS diseaes complicated by vomiting such as Reye's syndrome or encephalopathy. |
| **Antidepressants**<br>Tricyclics | Amitriptyline hydrochloride (Elavil)<br><br>*Other drugs:*<br>Imipramine hydrochloride (Tofranil)<br>Nortriptyline (Aventyl)<br>Doxepin hydrochloride (Sinequan)<br>Desipramine hydrochloride (Norpramin) | Precise mechanism is unknown. Believed that there may be enhanced activity of norepinephrine by blockage of the reuptake at storage granules in the nerve endings or potentiation of serotonin blockade by prevention of reuptake or its metabolism. | Seizures, hallucinations, insomnia, incoordination, inappropriate antidiuretic hormone syndrome, tachycardia and prolongation of conduction time, palpitations, skin rash, photosensitization, edema of face and tongue, dry mouth and mucous membranes, slurred speech, blurred vision, increased intraocular pressure, constipation, decreased libido, or impaired ejaculation. Use amitriptyline (Elavil) cautiously when the possibility of suicide exists. |
| **Monoamine oxidase (MAO) inhibitors** | Phenelzine sulfate (Nardil Sulfate)<br><br>*Other drugs:*<br>Isocarboxazid (Marplan)<br>Pargyline hydrochloride (Eutonyl)<br>Tranylcypromine sulfate (Parnate) | Not completely known, demonstrates blockade of the enzymatic deamination of serotonin and other biogenic amines and reuptake of monoamine oxidase for oxidative deamination intracellularly. | Hypertensive crisis related to foods high in tyramine because of inhibition of tyramine metabolism; agitation, hallucinations, hyperreflexia, hyperpyrexia, convulsions, tremors, inhibition of ejaculation, hyperhidrosis, mania, orthostatic hypotension, dry mouth. Electroconvulsive therapy is contraindicated. |

| Drug interaction | Nursing assessment | Nursing intervention | Expected outcome |
|---|---|---|---|
| Alcohol, benzodiaze-pines, CNS depressants result in additive CNS depression. Antacids inhibit absorption and should be given at a spaced interval from phenothiazides. When given with guanethidine, antagonizes antihypertensive effects. Combined with quinidine, increases cardiac depression. | *Assess client for:* Level of consciousness and mental status, bleeding tendencies, motor restlessness or tremors, history of seizure disorders, bowel and bladder regularity, fluid and electrolyte imbalances from nausea and vomiting, pain tolerance and frequency, skin condition or changing pigmentation. Prior ingestion of alcohol, barbiturates, analgesics, history of chronic respiratory disorders or acute respiratory depression. Effectiveness of thorazine in alleviating undesirable behavioral symptoms. | *Nurse should:* Provide emotional support for client and family during medication and potential psychotherapy. Use seizure precautions of known past history of epilepsy or seizure activity. Initiate bowel and bladder training program as indicated. Caution clients not to drive car or operate machinery when drowsy, and to wear protective clothing when exposed to intense sunlight or ultraviolet rays. In elderly clients, a lower than usual dose is recommended because of greater tendency for hypotension and neuromuscular dysfunction. | *Client should have:* Relief of excessive anxiety, tension, agitation, delirium tremors, pain, nausea, vomiting, and relaxation when used as a presurgery medication. |
| Potentiates effects of alcohol, amphetamines, antihistamines, MAO inhibitors, narcotic analgesics, sympathomimetic amines. May produce seizure activity in epileptic client on anticonvulsants. Long-term use with corticosteroids increases intraocular pressure. Impairs metabolism of oral anticoagulants. May cause antihypertensive blockade when combined with guanethidine. | *Assess client for:* Same as antipsychotics. | *Nurse should:* Same as for antipsychotics. Assist client in environmental and interpersonal behavior modification to decrease stress factors. | *Client should have:* Relief of symptoms associated with depression, phobia anxiety, and enuresis. |
| Potentiates effects of alcohol, amphetamines, anticholinergics, antihistamines, benzodiazepines, narcotics, antipsychotics, and tricyclic antidepressants. Contraindicated with propranolol. Enhances hypoglycemic effect of insulin. | | *Assess client for:* Nutritional and alcohol use history, history of concomitant and over-the-counter drugs, environmental stress factors and family unit, behavioral changes and mood swings, abnormal lab tests, especially liver function and electrolytes. Cumulative or toxic effects to liver or CNS. Ability to verbalize any sexual dysfunction. | |

*Continued.*

## PSYCHOTROPICS—cont'd

| Classification | Drug | Mechanism of action | Adverse outcome |
|---|---|---|---|
| Amphetamines<br>Refer to listing under Stimulants. | | | |
| Antianxiety drugs<br>Benzodiazepines | Diazepam (Valium)<br><br>*Other drugs:*<br>Chlordiazepoxide hydrochloride (Librium)<br>Chlorazepate dipotassium (Tranxene)<br>Oxazepam (Serax) | Precise mechanism unknown. Possible effects are concentrated in the vacillation of gamma-aminobutyric acid transmission in gray matter. | Contraindicated in clients with glaucoma. Drowsiness, ataxia, mental confusion, fatigue, nausea, constipation, urinary retention, hypotension, behavioral changes, or physical dependence can occur when combined with sedatives. Minor low-voltage, fast-activity EEG changes of little clinical correlation. May increase seizure activity when used as adjunct therapy for grand mal seizures requiring increased doses of anticonvulsants. Tapering of doses should be used when one withdraws the drug to prevent temporary increase in seizure activity. |
| Miscellaneous | Hydroxyzine pamoate (Vistaril)<br><br>*Other drug:*<br>Hydroxyzine hydrochloride (Atarax) | Specific mechanism unknown. Believed to inhibit action of acetylcholine in subcortical brain areas and antagonize the action of histamine at neuronal receptors. | Drowsiness, muscle tremor in higher dosages, dry mouth. |
| Propanediol carbamates | Meprobamate (Miltown, Equanil)<br><br>*Other drug:*<br>Tybamate (Solacen) | Specific CNS focus has not been identified. Inhibits electrical aftercharges in the limbic system and variety of responses from the hypothalamus and polysynaptic responses in the spinal cord. | Drowsiness, ataxia, anxiety or depression on arising from "hangover" feeling. Hypotension in elderly clients, abrupt withdrawal may precipitate seizures in higher dose ranges. |

| Drug interaction | Nursing assessment | Nursing intervention | Expected outcome |
|---|---|---|---|
| | | *Nurse should:* Teach client to avoid foods high in tyramine and alcoholic beverages. Use only medication prescribed specifically for the client. Teach client to modify environment to decrease stress factors. Enlist family in client care for support and verbalization of feelings. | *Client should have:* Same as for tricyclic antidepressants. |
| Potentiates effects of alcohol, narcotic analgesics, barbiturates, MAO inhibitors, CNS depressants, antihistamines. | *Assess client for:* Pathophysiological effects, history of glaucoma or progressive development of cataracts, level of consciousness and mood alterations, fluid and electrolyte imbalances for nausea and urinary retention, bowel and bladder habits, history of drug and alcohol abuse, previous seizure activity. | *Nurse should:* Help client to modify environment and stress factors. Incorporate family for support and verbalization of feelings. Initiate bowel and bladder training program. Caution client not to drive or operate machinery when drowsy. Use seizure precautions as indicated. Caution client against concomitant alcohol and CNS depressant use with diazepam. | *Client should have:* Relief of anxiety and tension. Reduction in seizure activity when combined with anticonvulsant. Reduction in rigid muscle spasticity, acute relief of agitation, and tremor with impending delirium tremens. |
| Potentiates effects of CNS depressants, alcohol, antihistamines, barbiturates, tricyclic antidepressants, and narcotics. Antagonizes effects of anticholinesterase. | *Assess client for:* Same as benzodiazepines. | *Nurse should:* Same as benzodiazepines. | *Client should have:* Relief of psychomotor agitation, anxiety, hyperkinetic symptoms in children with out mental impairment. Relaxation when used as presurgery medication. |
| Same as diphenylmethane antihistamines, that is, hydroxyzine pamoate and hydroxyzine hydrochloride | *Assess client for:* Pain tolerance and frequency, behavioral manifestations of anxiety and depression upon arising, incoordination, drowsiness. | *Nurse should:* Same as benzodiazepines. Monitor client in arising for "hangover" feeling after dosing. Monitor client for pathophysiological symptoms, rapid-eye-movement sleep deprivation. | *Client should have:* Relief of anxiety. Relaxation. Relief of musculoskeletal pain. Relief of seizure activity when combined with anticonvulsants. |

## SKELETAL MUSCLE RELAXANTS AND ANTAGONISTS

| Classification | Drug | Mechanism of action | Adverse outcome |
|---|---|---|---|
| Neuromuscular blocking agents<br>Nondepolarizing | Pancuronium bromide (Pavulon)<br><br>*Other drugs:*<br>Tubocurarine chloride (Tubarine)<br>Gallamine triethiodide (Flaxedil)<br>Alcuronium dichloride (Alloferin) | Act peripherally to antagonize neuromuscular receptor agents with resultant nondepolarization blockage by competition with acetylcholine at cholinergic receptor sites between the motor end plate and striated muscle. | Prolonged or profound muscle relaxation, skeletal muscle weakness, respiratory insufficiency, increased pulse, increased salivation if no anticholinergic agent is administered before light anesthesia for surgical procedures. Should not be given unless mechanical ventilator equipment and reversal agents are readily accessible and an experienced physician is supervising drug administration. |
| Depolarizing | Succinylcholine chloride (Anectine Chloride)<br><br>*Other drugs:*<br>Decamethonium bromide (Syncurine) | Antagonize and block sustained depolarization between the motor end plate and striated muscle. Compete with acetylcholine at cholinergic receptor sites producing rapid, initial muscle contraction and visible muscle fasciculations followed by inhibition of neuromuscular activity. | Profound and prolonged muscle relaxation, arrhythmias, cardiac depression, respiratory depression, dyspnea, excessive salivation, increased intraocular pressure. Should not be given unless experienced physician is available with resources to intubate and adequately ventilate the client. |
| Centrally acting muscle relaxants | Chlorphenesin carbamate (Maolate)<br><br>*Other drugs:*<br>Carisoprodol (Soma)<br>Methocarbamol (Robaxin)<br>Cyclobenzaprine hydrochloride (Flexeril)<br>Meprobamate (Equanil)<br>Chlorzoxazone (Paraflex) | Depress transmission of spinal and supraspinal polysynaptic response fibers. Acts selectively in CNS to produce sedative effect without loss of consciousness while relaxing skeletal muscle. | Drowsiness, sedation, nausea, vertigo, headache, skin rash, abnormal liver function studies. Diarrhea or severe weakness signal need to decrease dose. |

| Drug interaction | Nursing assessment | Nursing intervention | Expected outcome |
|---|---|---|---|
| Action is reversed by anesthetics, quinine, magnesium salts, neomycin, streptomycin, and gentamicin. Is not affected by narcotics or barbiturates. Aberrant metabolism may cause malignant hyperthermia. Neostigmine or atropine used to reverse drug effect. | *Assess client for:* Signs of fluid and electrolyte imbalances, asthma, myasthenia gravis, renal impairment, acid-base imbalance because of alteration in drug action. Adverse reactions to anesthesia, prolonged muscle relaxation, symptoms of malignant hyperthermia in immediate postanesthesia period. Monitor client for ventilatory and circulatory adequacy. | *Nurse should:* Observe clients with myasthenia gravis carefully for drug overdosages during crisis. Administer drug with extreme care and know precautions for client care after administration. Monitor mechanical ventilation of client and report changes in pathophysiological response of drug versus ventilation to physician. Support client's family by explaining drug therapy versus mechanical ventilation. | *Client should have:* (1) Neuromuscular blockade within 45 seconds of intravenous administration to facilitate mechanical ventilation of clients or adjunct for general anesthesia. (2) Decrease violent activity occurring in electroshock therapy. (3) Relieve spasms of tetanus. |
| Should not be mixed with barbiturates in the same syringe or administered through the same needle simultaneously. Neostigmine or procaine should not be given intravenously concurrently with succinylcholine; should be used to counteract overdose. Aberrant metabolism may cause malignant hyperthermia. | *Assess client for:* Prolonged muscle relaxation in clients with cirrhosis, severe anemias, malnutrition, fever, dehydration, antimalarial drugs. Symptoms of malignant hyperthermia immediately postoperatively. Vital signs, apnea, or arrhythmias. See nonpolarizing neuromuscular blocking agents. | *Nurse should:* Observe client postoperatively for aberrant metabolism of anesthetics. Know that intense muscle fasciculations in the immediate postanesthetic period may be attributable to drug metabolism and plane of anesthesia, not to the client's being cold. Be prepared to provide necessary ventilating support. | *Client should have:* Muscle relaxation (flaccid paralysis) within 2 minutes after intravenous administration with paralysis dissipated in 8 to 10 minutes. |
| When combined, MAO inhibitors, alcohol, and CNS depressants enhance sedative effects. Barbiturates and diphenhydramine, through enzyme induction inhibits chlorphenesin carbamate. Cross sensitization may occur with meprobamate. Phenothiazines may potentiate muscle relaxants. | *Assess client for:* Level of consciousness and neurological checks, paresthesia or tingling in fingers and toes, use of body mechanics, previous history of musculoskeletal trauma or surgery, alcohol abuse, family-support system, and history of pain location, description and pattern of occurrence. | *Nurse should:* Caution client not to drive or operate machinery when drowsy. Instruct client and family members in proper body mechanics. Instruct client in self-care for musculoskeletal trauma. Report any paresthesia or tingling if not present before medical and drug therapy is initiated. Caution clients against ingesting excess amounts of alcohol with drug therapy. Support client and family to verbalize feelings if repeated injury occurs to low back area. | *Client should have:* Relief from muscle spasm, skeletal-muscle pain, fibrositis, myositis, bursitis, or low back pain, or after trauma. |

*Continued.*

## SKELETAL MUSCLE RELAXANTS AND ANTAGONISTS—cont'd

| Classification | Drug | Mechanism of action | Adverse outcome |
| --- | --- | --- | --- |
| Direct-acting relaxant | Dantrolene sodium (Dantrium) | Depresses muscular contractile power without CNS or spinal cord selectivity. Muscular relaxation occurs postsynaptically from the myoneural junction by interfering with $Ca^{++}$ release from sarcoplasmic reticulum. | Muscle weakness, drowsiness, light-headedness, nausea, fatigue, malaise, diarrhea, excessive tearing, mental depression, speech disturbances, visual disturbances, photosensitivity, enuresis. Extreme weakness or diarrhea signals need for dosage reduction. |
| Antiparkinsonian agent | Carbidopa with levodopa (Sinemet) *Other drugs:* Levodopa (Dopar) Ethopropazine hydrochloride (Parsidol) Amantadine hydrochloride (Symmetrel) Biperiden hydrochloride (Akineton) Carbidopa (Lodosyn) | Improves dopamine action and inhibits decarboxylation of peripheral or CNS levodopa. When combined with levodopa, carbidopa increases levodopa available to brain tissue (corpus striation) to coordinate muscle movement. | Choreiform, dystonic movements, paranoid ideation, depression, possible suicidal tendencies, seizures, bradykinetic "on-off" phenomenon, anorexia, dysphagia, dry mouth, blepharospasm, urinary retention, dark urine, hoarseness, oculogyric crisis, insomnia. |

| Drug interaction | Nursing assessment | Nursing intervention | Expected outcome |
|---|---|---|---|
| Should be used cautiously in women over 35 years of age with concomitant estrogen therapy. Potentiated by CNS depressants. | *Assess client for:* Degree and specific origin of spasticity, cooperation of client in rehabilitation, history of liver or pulmonary disease, lab data (especially SGOT, SGPT, alkaline phosphatase, complete blood count, platelets, and bilirubin), hepatitis symptoms, exposure to direct sunlight or ultraviolet light, history and pathogenesis of spasticity or previous adverse reactions to general anesthesia, speech or visual disturbances. | *Nurse should:* Carefully observe clients who have severe pulmonary disease. Monitor liver function tests for hepatotoxity. Report all abnormal liver function studies. Caution clients not to drive or operate machinery when drowsy. Caution clients on exposure to high amounts of ultraviolet light. Monitor all pathophysiological and behavioral changes at peak dose levels. Monitor all postoperative clients for aberrant metabolism during anesthesia for need to institute dantrolene therapy in malignant hyperthermia crisis. | *Client should have:* Reduction of spasticity from stroke, spinal injuries, multiple sclerosis or cerebral palsy; beneficial effects after 1 week of therapy when drug is at peak dose. Reduction in skeletal muscle metabolism in malignant hyperthermia. |
| May cause increased intraocular pressure. Potentiates hypotensive effect of antihypertensives. Carbidopa-levodopa combination is recommended instead of levodopa alone to prevent vitamin $B_6$ interference with increased dopamine formation. Phenothiazides and diazepam may cause a deterioration in disease process. Anticholinergics decrease amount of available levodopa because of poor absorption from gastric mucosa with delayed emptying. | *Assess client for:* Orthostatic hypotension on arising, nutritional and fluid history, dysphagia, behavioral changes, lab data (especially BUN, SGOT, SGPT, lactic dehydrogenase, bilirubin, protein-bound iodine, alkaline phosphatase, and Coombs' test), pathophysiological progress of disease, family support system, seizure activity, intake and output, vital signs, and neurological checks. | *Nurse should:* Give medication after meals to prevent gastric irritation, anorexia, and dry mouth during meals. Instruct client to decrease high-protein foods in diet to stabilize dyskinesias. Vitamin $B_6$ need not be limited if the client receives carbidopa and levodopa in combination. Support client and family by providing knowledge about Parkinson's disease process and drug therapy. Exercise all extremities. Use support hose or anti-embolism stockings on client when getting client to standing or sitting position. (Refer to Chapter 27.) | *Client should have:* Reduction of muscular rigidity and tremor, but effects may not be apparent for 2 to 6 months. |

*Continued.*

**SKELETAL MUSCLE RELAXANTS AND ANTAGONISTS—cont'd**

| Classification | Drug | Mechanism of action | Adverse outcome |
|---|---|---|---|
| GABA (gamma-aminobutyric acid, gaba) analog | Baclofen (Lioresal) | Precise action not known. Possibly acts through inhibition of monosynaptic and polysynaptic reflexes at the spinal cord level through hyperpolarization of afferent terminals to mimic the effect of GABA on regulation of muscle tone at the myoneural junction. | Sedation, somnolence, ataxia, respiratory and cardiovascular depression, hallucinations (with abrupt withdrawal), constipation, nausea, urinary frequency, skin rash. Vertigo, mental confusion; contraindicated in epileptic clients. |

| Drug interaction | Nursing assessment | Nursing intervention | Expected outcome |
| --- | --- | --- | --- |
| Respiratory stimulants are contraindicated in the presence of respiratory depression. Alcohol and CNS depressants potentiate baclofen. | *Assess client for:* Locomotion status, vital signs, neurological checks (especially level of consciousness, respirations, and pulse), seizure activity, behavioral changes during dose titrations, bowel and bladder habit changes, lab data (especially serum and urine creatinine, electrolytes, urine protein, and albumin), ability for self-care, family support system. | *Nurse should:* Monitor spasticity level in clients who require some degree of spasticity for upright posture and balance for locomotion such that drug therapy is not preventing motion. Caution clients about operating an automobile or machinery when drowsy. Use seizure precautions when drug therapy is in upper dosage limits. Support client and family system for verbalization of feelings. Instruct client in self-care aspects of daily living. | *Client should have:* Muscle relaxation with spasticity from multiple sclerosis (especially the flexor spasms). Reduction of pain, clonus, and muscular rigidity. |

## AUTONOMIC AGENTS

| Classification | Drug | Mechanism of action | Adverse outcome |
| --- | --- | --- | --- |
| Parasympathetic stimulants—direct acting | Bethanechol chloride (Urecholine Chloride)<br><br>*Other drugs:*<br>Carbachol (carbamylcholine chloride)<br>Pilocarpine hydrochloride (Pilocar)<br>Pilocarpine nitrate with phenylephrine hydrochloride in polyvinyl alcohol (Pilofrin Liquifilm Ophthalmic) | Mimic stimulation of the parasympathetic nervous system by activating muscarinic receptors of effector cells in the detrusor urinal muscle, smooth muscles in the gastrointestinal tract, and ganglionic cells of CNS. | Flushing of skin, malaise, headache, hypotension, asthmatic attacks, nausea, diarrhea, abdominal cramps, borborygmi. Contraindicated in clients with epilepsy, Parkinson's disease, peptic ulcer, latent or bronchial asthma, pregnancy, coronary artery disease, bradycardia, hyperthyroidism. Infection, anatomic disorders, or recent surgery in the gastrointestinal or urinary systems require assessment before any administration of the drug. Injectable type may only be used subcutaneously. Otherwise pronounced symptoms of cholinergic excessive stimulation are evident. |
| Cholinesterase inhibitors | Pyridostigmine bromide (Mestinon Bromide)<br><br>*Other drugs:*<br>Ambenonium chloride (Mytelase)<br>Demecarium bromide (Humorsol)<br>Edrophonium bromide (Tensilon)<br>Echothiophate iodide (Phospholine Iodide)<br>Neostigmine bromide (Prostigmin Bromide) | Inhibit the destruction of acetylcholine by acetylcholinesterase liberating myoneural transmission of impulse movement across the neuromuscular junction. | Miosis, nausea, increased peristalsis, abdominal cramps, vomiting, increased salivation, diarrhea, muscle cramps, fasciculations, increased bronchial secretions, diaphoresis. Contraindicated for clients with obstructive intestinal or urinary system disorders. Administer cautiously to those with bronchial asthma. |

| Drug interaction | Nursing assessment | Nursing intervention | Expected outcome |
|---|---|---|---|
| Combined with ganglionic blocking agents causes hypotension. Atropine is specific antidote that blocks muscarinic action. | *Assess client for:* History of epilepsy or Parkinson's disease, history of urinary retention, neurogenic bladder atony or postoperative abdominal distention, fluid intake and nutritional patterns, length of time since surgical procedure, ability to ambulate, blood pressure, concurrent medications. | *Nurse should:* Have an ampule of atropine or Bristoject syringe of atropine at the bedside for treatment of toxicity when bethanechol is given subcutaneously. Monitor intake and output, bowel and bladder patterns, and diet. Provide client with adequate amounts of fluid for hydration. Try all methods of instituting micturition without catheterization. Use rectal tube for gas relief before drug administration. Ambulate clients as soon as possible postoperatively. | *Client should have:* Initiation of micturition and emptying of the bladder and increases in gastric motility, peristalsis, and tone. Relief of abdominal distention. |
| Quinidine, procainamide, and hydroxyzine antagonize drug effects because of their relative anticholinergic activity. Atropine is a specific antidote. Neomycin, gentamicin, bacitracin, and morphine may block acetylcholine release inhibiting action of pyridostigmine bromide. | *Assess client for:* History of myasthenia gravis pattern, client's ability to perform activities of daily living, respiratory difficulty or possibility of aspiration, especially while eating or drinking, family adjustment to the disease, pathophysiological progress of disease. (Refer to Chapter 17.) | *Nurse should:* Monitor client for symptoms of cholinergic crisis, primarily weakness in muscles (especially the respiratory musculature leading to respiratory areas). Teach client specifics about disease process and drug therapy. Do not instill false hope that during a remission the disease process is gone. Support family and help them understand disease process and management of client as disease progresses. Teach family member how to recognize early crisis symptoms and to give parenteral medications to prevent respiratory collapse until emergency help arrives. Encourage family and client to seek professional guidance in dealing with disease process as necessary. Set pattern of activities of daily living around symptoms utilizing rest periods and an alarm clock for medication administration to prevent crisis. | *Client should have:* Progressive muscle strength, ability to swallow and breathe with less effort. Less fatigue. |

*Continued.*

**AUTONOMIC AGENTS—cont'd**

| Classification | Drug | Mechanism of action | Adverse outcome |
|---|---|---|---|
| Antiparkinsonian-anti-cholinergic agents | Benztropine mesylate (Cogentin Methane-sulfonate)<br><br>*Other drugs:*<br>Procyclidine hydrochloride (Kemadrin)<br>Trihexyphenidyl hydrochloride (Artane) | Selectively block neuromuscular acetylcholine release preventing hyperexcitability and rapid metabolism of dopamine. Antihistaminic properties are not well defined in Parkinson's disease. | Dry mouth, anhidrosis, vomiting, nervousness, blurred vision, anorexia, constipation, listlessness, depression, nausea, numb fingers. Not recommended for young children or those with drug hypersensitivity. Unknown safety in pregnancy. |
| Beta adrenergic receptor antagonists | Isoproterenol hydrochloride (Isuprel)<br><br>*Other drugs:*<br>Isoproterenol sulfate (Norisodrine Sulfate)<br>Isoxsuprine hydrochloride (Vasodilan)<br>Nylidrin hydrochloride (Arlidin) | Synthetic sympathomimetic amines that affect the $beta_2$ receptor in the bronchial musculature stimulating relaxation of bronchi and trachea. Affect the cardiovascular system by lowering peripheral resistance, increasing cardiac output, and forcing contraction and oxygen consumption. Relax skeletal muscle by decreasing calcium levels needed for muscle contraction, resulting in increased blood flow through alteration of cyclic AMP; also, relax the alimentary tract. | Increased myocardial work and oxygen consumption, flushing of face, sore throat when inhaled in respiratory therapy because of alcohol content of mixture, sweating, nervousness, tremors, angina-like pain, nausea, vomiting, weakness. Contraindicated in clients with cardiac disorders; that is, arrhythmias with tachycardia or coronary insufficiency *may* be problematic to those with a sensitivity to sympathomimetic amines. Hazards unknown in pregnancy. |

| Drug interaction | Nursing assessment | Nursing intervention | Expected outcome |
|---|---|---|---|
| Combined with antihistamine increases anticholinergic effects in glaucoma. May decrease available levodopa absorption by delaying gastric emptying. MAO inhibitors and tricyclic antidepressants potentiate action of benztropine mesylate. When administered with anticholinergic drugs or phenothiazines, may result in paralytic ileus. | *Assess client for:* Degree of bradykinesic tremor, rigidity, and ability to perform activities of daily living, history of disease progress, pathophysiological disease progress, emotional status, nutritional and fluid patterns and preferences, bowel and bladder habits, ability to sweat and body temperature during warm weather, evidence of tardive dyskinesia, benztropine mesylate dosage. | Caution client not to drive or operate machinery when drowsy. Encourage client and family to interact and verbalize feelings. Drug should be taken after meals to prevent gastrointestinal irritation. Limit concentrated protein intake. Educate the client and family in disease process, drug therapy, and diagnostic procedures. Encourage exercise, posture control, and proper position to prevent contractures. Warn client to avoid extreme exertion during warm weather. | *Client should have:* Reduction in muscle rigidity, akinesia, and tremor. Drug effectiveness within 2 to 6 months. |
| Epinephrine and isoproterenol should not be administered simultaneously because of arrhythmogenic potential. Guanethidine antagonizes antihypertensive effect. Concomitant use with tricyclic antidepressants may enhance either the antidepressant or isoproterenol. | *Assess client for:* Vital signs (especially pulse, and blood pressure); neurological checks; pathophysiological conditions that may precipitate acute situation; client or family history of cardiopulmonary or renal disease, hyperthyroidism, diabetes, or hypertension; any infiltration at intravenous site or tissue necrosis. | Monitor all neurological signs and rapidly changing physical parameters of pulse, blood pressure, respirations for respiratory insufficiency, arrhythmias, or hypotension. Monitor all intravenous infusions, especially rate fluctuations. If client takes isoproterenol sublingually, should not swallow saliva after pill is dissolved. Caution clients to move to the upright position slowly to avoid effects of orthostatic hypotension. Teach client and family to self-administer drug and caution them against use of inhalants concurrently or excessive drug use. | *Client should have:* Bronchodilatation and breathe better with less effort, relaxation of skeletal muscles and alimentary tract, improved cardiac output, reduction in cerebral vasospasm after subarachnoid hemorrhage when combined with aminophylline. |

*Continued.*

## AUTONOMIC AGENTS—cont'd

| Classification | Drug | Mechanism of action | Adverse outcome |
|---|---|---|---|
| Adrenergic blocking agents | | | |
| Alpha adrenergic blockers | Ergotamine tartrate and caffeine (Cafergot)<br><br>*Other drugs:*<br>Ergotamine tartrate (Gynergen)<br>Ergotamine tartrate, caffeine, belladonna alkaloids, and phenacetin (Wigraine)<br>Phenoxybenzamine hydrochloride (Dibenzyline Hydrochloride)<br>Phentolamine hydrochloride (Regitine Hydrochloride)<br>Hydrogenated ergot alkaloids (dihydroergotoxine mesylate, Hydergine)<br>Methysergide dimaleate (Sansert Dimaleate) | Block sympathetic nerve activity by directly stimulating or blocking intimal alpha-adrenergic receptors in smooth muscle of peripheral and cranial blood vessels, also depressing central vasomotor center to effect selective vasoconstriction with concomitant decrease in pulsations of blood vessels. May also antagonize serotonin mechanism effects on cranial blood vessels. | Orthostatic hypotension, drowsiness, stuffy nose, nausea, vomiting, numbness, tingling, muscle pain, leg weakness, angina-like pain, localized pain and itching, temporary bradycardia or tachycardia. |
| Beta adrenergic blockers | Propranolol hydrochloride (Inderal)<br><br>*Other drugs:*<br>Metoprolol tartrate (Lopressor) | See Antihypertensives and diuretics. | See Antihypertensives and diuretics. |
| Adrenergic neuron blockers | Methyldopa (Aldomet)<br>Methyldopa and chlorothiazide (Aldoclor)<br>Guanethidine sulfate (Ismelin)<br>Reserpine (Serpasil) | See Antihypertensives and diuretics. | See Antihypertensives and diuretics. |

| Drug interaction | Nursing assessment | Nursing intervention | Expected outcome |
|---|---|---|---|
| Troleandomycin (TAO) may inhibit metabolism of ergotamine. Use with caution to guard against severe vasoconstriction when propranolol is given concomitantly. Sympathomimetic agents may cause extreme elevation in blood pressure. | *Assess client for:* History of pain or headaches, infection, pathophysiological responses to drug therapy, progress of headache-tension mechanism, support processes of family, self-motivation to modify environmental stress factors and for self-administration of drugs. | *Nurse should:* Caution client against using any more than the prescribed number of tablets in a 24-hour period because of possibility of CNS toxicity. Teach client proper use of sublingual tablets and self-administration. Support client and family to verbalize their feelings during drug therapy, diagnostic procedures, and identification of stress factors in environment. Advise client to seek professional counseling if necessary to verbalize feelings. Maintain quiet, calm, dark environment during attack. Provide comfort measures to prevent tension or stress in the client. (Refer to Chapter 14.) | *Client should have:* Temporary relief of vascular headaches that may be complicated by tension medication; may abort vascular headache, if administered in time. Relief of histamine cephalgia. |
| See Antihypertensives and diuretics. | See Antihypertensives and diuretics. | *Nurse should:* See Antihypertensives and diuretics | *Client should have:* See Antihypertensives and diuretics. |
| See Antihypertensives and diuretics. | *Assess client for:* See Antihypertensives and diuretics | *Nurse should:* See Antihypertensives and diuretics. | *Client should have:* See Antihypertensives and diuretics. |

## ANTIHYPERTENSIVES AND DIURETICS

| Classification | Drug | Mechanism of action | Adverse outcome |
|---|---|---|---|
| Thiazide diuretics | Chlorothiazide (Diuril) <br><br> *Other drugs:* <br> Hydrochlorothiazide (Hydro-Diuril) <br> Triamterene and hydrochlorothiazide (Dyazide) <br> Hydrochlorothiazide (Esidrix) <br> Methyclothiazide (Enduron) <br> Trichlormethiazide (Naqua) <br> Chlorthalidone (Hygroton) | Activate renal cortical tubule mechanisms by increasing sodium and chloride excretion (diuresis) by inhibiting absorption from the proximal and early distal tubules with resultant loss of potassium and bicarbonate. The mechanism of antihypertensive control is undetermined. | Anorexia, nausea, dizziness, vertigo, headache, thrombocytopenia, orthostatic hypotension, skin rash, muscle spasm, photosensitivity, hyperglycemia, glycosuria, hyperuricemia, acute gout, hypercalcemia. Contraindicated in those who are anuric and those with hypersensitivities to sulfonamide derivatives. |
| Loop diuretics | Furosemide (Lasix) <br><br> *Other drugs:* <br> Ethacrynic acid (Edecrin) | Inhibit sodium and chloride reabsorption in the proximal and distal tubules and loop of Henle. | Same as thiazide diuretics. |

| Drug interaction | Nursing assessment | Nursing intervention | Expected outcome |
|---|---|---|---|
| When used with cardiac glycosides, may cause digitalis, toxicity, and decrease in potassium. Antagonize hypoglycemic effect of insulin and oral hypoglycemic agents. Combined with corticosteroids, increase potassium loss. Antagonize oral anticoagulants by concentrating clotting factors. Increase BUN when combined with tetracyclines and doxycycline antimicrobials. May change response to tubocurarine and norepinephrine. | *Assess client for:* Presence and severity of hypertension. Identify coexisting disease processes that may alter approach to hypertension. Identify risk factors and environmental stressors, family and social history, vital signs and neurological checks (especially level of consciousness, blood pressure, and intake and output), retinal changes, lab data (especially BUN, hemoglobin, hematocrit, serum creatinine and electrolytes), diet history (especially ethnic influences), medication history and compliance, family support system. | *Nurse should:* Monitor all pathophysiological responses to therapy, diet, and intake and output. Monitor all lab data for signs of renal, electrolytic, or cardiac impairment. Teach client about all aspects of treatment, risk factors, taking own blood pressure, and importance of compliance to medical and drug regimen. Assist client and family in supportive therapy and verbalization of feelings. (Refer to Chapter 24.) | *Client should have:* Diuresis and reduction in blood pressure. A commonly selected drug for long-term hypertensive therapy. |
| Same as thiazides. Combined with aminoglycoside antimicrobial results in additive toxicity to auditory structures. Added to cephalosporin therapy may result in nephrotoxicity. Lithium toxicity may result when added to lithium carbonate therapy. When given simultaneously with indomethacin, diuresis and antihypertensive outcomes may be altered. When given with salicylates, toxic level may be lower. When administered with alcohol, narcotics, or barbiturates, the incidence of orthostatic hypotension increases. | | *Nurse should:* Same as thiazide diuretics. | *Client should have:* Same as thiazide diuretics. |

*Continued.*

## ANTIHYPERTENSIVES AND DIURETICS—cont'd

| Classification | Drug | Mechanism of action | Adverse outcome |
|---|---|---|---|
| Hypertonic osmotic diuretics | Urea (Ureaphil) Urea and invert sugar (Urevert) *Other drugs:* Mannitol (Osmitrol) Glycerol (glycerin) Glycerol in flavored water (Osmoglyn) | Interfere with sodium and water reabsorption and reduce intraocular and intracranial pressure by altering serum osmolarity. Shifting of aqueous humor occurs to the plasma in the anterior chamber of the eye and from intracerebral tissue to plasma in the skull by increasing renal blood flow and decreasing vascular resistance. During the infusion, sodium reabsorption is depressed in the proximal tubules and loop of Henle with increased water excretion from the distal tubule such that more water is excreted than sodium. | Hyponatremia, hypokalemia, circulatory overload, dizziness, headache, nausea, vomiting, fever, skin rash. Rapid infusion may result in congestive heart failure. Should be used with extreme caution in clients with impaired renal hepatic or cardiac conditions. |
| Hormonal antidiuretic | Vasopressin tannate (Pitressin Tannate) | A posterior-pituitary extract that acts through a cyclic AMP–mediated mechanism of influencing the distal tubules through altered permeability of water and urea to increase water reabsorption. Also stimulates alimentary tract and constricts smooth muscle. | Tremor, uterine cramps, angina, nausea, bronchial constriction, drowsiness, listlessness, headaches, circumoral pallor, anaphylaxis, cardiac arrest, shock. |

| Drug interaction | Nursing assessment | Nursing intervention | Expected outcome |
|---|---|---|---|
| Lithium carbonate should be utilized with caution and be closely monitored for clients on diuretics to avoid lithium toxicity. | *Assess client for:* Daily body weight, vital signs (especially blood pressure), at least hourly urinary output, intravenous site for signs of infiltration, signs or symptoms of cardiac arrest, congestive heart failure, pulmonary edema or circulatory collapse, lab data (especially serum and urine osmolarity, electrolytes, and hematocrit), ECG changes, level of consciousness and behavioral changes in postoperative period, anxiety, intravenous infusion rate (constantly monitored), obvious signs of fluid and electrolyte imbalance. Monitor client for evidence of increasing intracranial mass, whose symptoms are being minimized by the drug, especially in cases of trauma. | *Nurse should:* Make sure all crystals in solution are dissolved before administration. Use a warmed solution to mix crystals. Use filter or blood-warming coil with warm solution to ensure that all of drug dissolved. Administer through Angiocath or Intracath in a large vein. Monitor blood pressure *frequently*. Keep pace with urinary output by intravenous replacement. Monitor urine output at least hourly during acute administration (catheterization is necessary for accurate output). Have crash cart available at all times as well as plasma expander to avoid drastic fluid changes. Monitor all lab data. Allay client and family anxiety through emotional support. | *Client should have:* Diuresis. Reduction in intracranial and intraocular pressure. Decrease in cerebral tissue mass during neurosurgery. |
| Vasopressin is inactivated by trypsin and cannot be given orally. Acetaminophen, anesthetics, oral hypoglycemics, and neostigmine potentiate effects of vasopressin. Sensitivity to vasopressin is increased when vasopressin is combined with ganglionic blocking agents. Alcohol blocks action of vasopressin. | *Assess client for:* Weight, vital signs (especially blood pressure), history of cardiac or renal disease, history of polyuria and polydipsia, previous fluid intake and urinary output, signs of fluid and electrolyte imbalance, bowel pattern, measurement of abdomen (if used for ascites), ECG changes, lab data (especially serum and urine creatinine, hematocrit, serum and urine osmolarity, and electrolytes), check level of consciousness and neurological status. | *Nurse should:* Inform client of possible pain at injection site. Monitor frequent weight and vital sign checks. Auscultate bowel sounds. Keep strict and frequent intake and output. Monitor level of consciousness and neurological status. Monitor cardiorenal complications of drug therapy. Monitor bowel elimination and use rectal tube if necessary for gaseous distinction in ascites. Monitor ECG and lab data for drastic changes. Teach family to administer at home as necessary. Give emotional support and integrate family into care plan. Have crash cart available at all times. | *Client should have:* Increased ability to concentrate and a return of normal thirst and urine patterns. Increase in peristalsis with ability to expel gas. |

*Continued.*

## ANTIHYPERTENSIVES AND DIURETICS—cont'd

| Classification | Drug | Mechanism of action | Adverse outcome |
|---|---|---|---|
| Beta-adrenergic blocking agents | Propranolol hydrochloride (Inderal)<br><br>*Other drug:*<br>Metroprolol tartrate (Lopressor) | Compete with both beta$_1$ and beta$_2$ adrenergic receptors resulting in decreased heart rate and force of contraction, decreased renin-angiotensin feedback loop and vasodilatation responses. The antihypertensive and antimigraine effects have not been established. | Bradycardia, increase in atrioventricular block, hypotension, lightheadedness, behavioral changes, fatigue, nausea, epigastric distress, skin rash, respiratory distress, purpura, unknown safety in pregnancy, causes changes in some lab values. |
| Ganglionic blocking agents | Pentolinium tartrate (Ansolysen)<br><br>*Other drugs:*<br>Mecamylamine hydrochloride (Inversine)<br>Trimethaphan camsylate (Arfonad) | Combine with nicotinic receptors in ganglia by blocking myoneural acetylcholine release from preganglionic neurons. | Orthostatic hypotension, dilatation of pupils, blurred vision, dry mouth, constipation, blockage of sweat secretion. |

| Drug interaction | Nursing assessment | Nursing intervention | Expected outcome |
|---|---|---|---|
| May enhance hypoglycemic effects when combined with insulin and oral hypoglycemic agents. Enhances effects of tricyclic antidepressants. Concomitant use of propranolol with MAO inhibitors is contraindicated. Used with procainamide, increases cardiac depression. Must be withdrawn 48 hours before surgery or reversed by drug administration of isoproterenol or levarterenol. | *Assess client for:* History of cardiopulmonary and diabetic disease, vital signs and neurological checks (especially blood pressure and level of consciousness), pain history (especially frequency and location if migraine suspected), hyperthyroidism, skin condition, behavioral changes, tolerance to activity and foods, respiratory problems distress, risk and stress factors in environment, lab data (for renal or liver impairment), medication history and compliance, and family-support system. Refer to Chapters 5, 10, 11, and 24 for further information. | *Nurse should:* Teach client to take pulse and blood pressure and to call doctor if pulse drops below 50 and to hold the dose until doctor approves client to take same. Monitor all pathological responses to drug therapy, diet, and intake and output. Monitor lab data (especially BUN, SGOT, alkaline phosphatase). Teach client about all aspects of treatment and importance of compliance to medical and drug regimen. Assist client and family in supportive therapy and verbalization of feeling. | *Client should have:* Reduction in blood pressure, decrease in tonic sympathetic nerve responses from CNS vasomotor centers and inhibition of renin release from kidneys. A common choice for an ancillary agent in the long-term control of hypertension. |
| Cholinesterase inhibitors antagonize ganglionic blocking agents. | *Assess client for:* Vital signs (especially blood pressure), bowel and bladder habits, intake and output, autonomic dysreflexia in clients with spinal cord injuries, neurological checks (especially pupil dilatation), potentiated effects of drug if client on low-sodium diet or has hypertensive encephalopathy, history of smoking. Refer to Chapter 24 for general care of the hypertensive client before the crisis situation that necessitates the use of ganglionic blocking agents. | *Nurse should:* Caution client against standing in one place too long. If they have to, instruct to wiggle toes and move ankles, knees, and legs. Caution clients against getting heat exhaustion because of decreased sweating. Give laxatives for constipation, and oral hygiene for dry mucous membranes in mouth. Clients should be cautioned to avoid tobacco use during drug therapy or just before surgery. | *Client should have:* Controlled hypotension during emergency treatment of hypertensive crisis. Decreased blood flow through brain during neurosurgical procedures with trimethaphan. Reduction of autonomic dysreflexia in clients with spinal cord injuries. |

*Continued.*

## ANTIHYPERTENSIVES AND DIURETICS—cont'd

| Classification | Drug | Mechanism of action | Adverse outcome |
|---|---|---|---|
| Sympatholytic agents | Methyldopa (Aldomet)<br><br>*Other drugs:*<br>Methydopa and chloro-<br>   thiazide (Aldoclor)<br>Reserpine (Serpasil)<br>Guanethidine sulfate<br>   (Ismelin) | Not clearly known but has antihypertensive effect. Probably caused by metabolism of methyldopa to alpha-methylnorepineph-rine, which decreases arterial blood pressure through stimulation of alpha-adrenergic receptors, a false neurotransmitter, or decrease in plasma renin activity. | Sedation, weakness, extrapyramidal ataxia and tremor, headache, dizziness, dry mouth, depression, behavioral changes, orthostatic hypotension, bradycardia, angina, nausea, dry mouth, "black-tongue," abnormal liver function tests, direct positive Coombs' test, cramps, constipation, increased BUN, lupus-like syndrome, sexual disturbance in males. |
| Vasodilators | Hydralazine<br>   (Apresoline)<br><br>*Other drugs:*<br>Prazosin hydrochloride<br>   (Minipress)<br>Diazoxide (Hyperstat)<br>Sodium nitroprusside<br>   (sodium nitroferricya-<br>   nide, Nipride)<br><br>*Other drugs in category:*<br>Histamine<br>Nicotinic acid (niacin) | Direct effect on precapillary arterioles resulting in vascular dilatation and decreased peripheral resistance to blood flow. The most effective response is achieved when a drug such as propranolol is used simultaneously to reduce cardiac output and heart rate. | Headache, palpitations, nausea, tachycardia, angina, nasal congestion, flushing, constipation, lupus-like syndrome, orthostatic hypotension, peripheral neuritis. |

| Drug interaction | Nursing assessment | Nursing intervention | Expected outcome |
|---|---|---|---|
| May cause hypotension when combined with levophen, levodopa, MAO inhibitors, phenothiazides, procainamide, propranolol, and other vasodilators. Combined with sympathomimetic amines may result in hypertension, tachycardia, or cardiac arrhythmias. | *Assess client for:* Same as thiazide and loop diuretics. Also, assess lab data, especially BUN, Coombs' test, SGOT. Evaluate weight gain and edema. | Same as thiazide and loop diuretics. Caution clients to avoid driving or operating machinery when drowsy. | *Client should have:* Same as thiazide and loop diuretics. |
| May potentiate effects of MAO inhibitors. Antagonizes sympathomimetic amines. | *Assess client for:* Same as thiazide. Also, assess lab data (especially complete blood count, lupus erythematosus preparation, and antinuclear antibody titers). Monitor pulse and anginal symptoms. | Same as thiazide diuretics. Also monitor lab data for decreasing blood counts and continued positive lupus erythematosus preparation and antinuclear antibody titers, especially if lupus-like symptoms develop. | *Client should have:* Reduction in blood pressure with improved renal blood flow. |

# ANTIMICROBIALS

| Classification | Drug | Mechanism of action | Adverse outcome |
|---|---|---|---|
| Cell wall selectivity | Carbenicillin disodium (Geopen)<br><br>*Other drugs in classification:*<br>Ampicillin trihydrate (Amcill)<br>Procaine penicillin G (Duracillin)<br>Amoxicillin trihydrate (Larotid)<br>Cephalothin sodium (Keflin)<br>Cefazolin sodium (Kefzol)<br>Cephalexin monohydrate (Keflex)<br>Cefamandole nafate (Mandol) | Primary bactericidal action by interfering with bacterial cell wall synthesis of mucopeptides. Acts during miosis to increase intracellular osmotic pressure resulting in cell rupture and degradation. | Hypersensitivity reactions, non-specific increases in SGOT and SGPT, nausea, false-positive Clinitest results, emergence of resistant organism, neuro-muscular rigidity or convulsions. When dosage range approaches maximum recommended limits, look for blood dyscrasias, bleeding problems in clients with bleeding disorders. |
| Ribosome selectivity | Gentamicin sulfate (Garamycin)<br><br>*Other drugs:*<br>Erythromycin ethylsuccinate (EES, Pediamycin)<br>Erythromycin estolate (Ilosone)<br>Doxycycline hyclate (Vibramycin Hyclate)<br>Chloramphenicol (Chloromycetin) | Primary bactericidal action by inhibiting protein synthesis on the intracellular ribosome subunit in susceptible organisms. | Cross-resistance to other aminoglycosides. Ototoxicity and nephrotoxicity, hearing abnormalities, vertigo, numbness, skin paresthesia, muscle twitching, respiratory depression, nausea. |
| Transcription-mechanism selectivity | Nitrofurantoin (Furadantin)<br><br>*Other drugs:*<br>Sulfisoxazole (Gantrisin)<br>Nalidixic acid (NegGram)<br>Nitrofurantoin macro-crystals (Macrodantin) | Primary bactericidal action by interference with and prevention of the transcription process of bacterial strand replication of DNA. Breaks down the DNA strand before transcription or by mutation of replicating RNA strands by the introduction of incorrect components. | Fever, chills, chest pain, pulmonnary infiltration, eosinophilia, dyspnea, hepatotoxicity, headache, and vertigo. Should not be used in clients with anuria, oliguria, or significant renal impairment. |

| Drug interaction | Nursing assessment | Nursing intervention | Expected outcome |
|---|---|---|---|
| Are incompatible in solutions with multivitamins, heparin, polymyxin, tetracyclines, alkaline or acid pH, mycin antibiotics, calcium gluconate, carbohydrate solutions with alkaline pH. | *Assess client for:* Meningeal irritation, hypersensitivity reactions after infusion, infiltration, and irritation at intravenous site, history of previous antibiotic therapies, time of last series of antimicrobial therapy, lab data on reduction of white blood cell count or elevation of SGOT and SGPT, wound or incisions, neurological and vital signs. | Mix powdered solution with sterile bacteriostatic solutions when multiple doses are to be extracted from the vial, or may use sterile water for injection when one time only mixture required. Monitor client for hypersensitivity. Monitor lab work for evidence of antimicrobial activity or impaired renal or hepatic function. Note any pain or discharge from wounds or incisions, level of consciousness, muscle rigidity, vomiting, or increased intracranial pressure. Isolate client as indicated. Instruct client to avoid acidic foods. | *Client should have:* Relief of systemic infective symptoms and normothermia, general sense of movement to well-being. Improvement in objective lab data, such as the white blood cell count. |
| When two or more aminoglycosides are combined, severe ototoxicity and nephrotoxicity can result. Possible superinfection when combined with corticosteroids. May produce neuromuscular blockade with muscle relaxants. Decreases gut vitamin K production and prolongs prothrombin times. Combined with either furosemide or ethacrynic acid results in additive ototoxicity. | *Assess client for:* Signs or symptoms of ototoxicity, renal impairment, hypersensitivity with known history of aminoglycoside therapy, vital signs (especially for decreased respirations caused by respiratory muscle paralysis, muscle spasms or rigidity caused by neuromuscular blockade), lab data for reduction of white blood cell count, BUN, proteinuria, SGOT, SGPT, and serum creatinine. Monitor wounds and injuries, neurological and vital signs, and level of consciousness. | Same as cell-wall antimicrobials with the exception of acidic-food avoidance. | *Client should have:* Same as for cell wall antimicrobials. |
| Alcohol inhibits oxidation of medication. Alkalizing agents, antacids, nalidixic acid, and phenobarbital inhibit nitrofurantoin. Probenecid potentiates nitrofurantoin toxicity | *Assess client for:* Indications of hepatic or renal impairment and toxicity. Evaluate lab data for reduction of white blood cell count, increased SGOT, SGPT, BUN, proteinuria, and serum creatinine. Assess for drug hypersensitivity, history of microbial therapy, vital signs with emphasis on respiratory functions, and neurological checks. | *Nurse should:* Mix with water, milk, fruit juice, or infant formula as necessary to ensure client compliance. Provide client with acid-ash diet to acidify urine to potentiate effect of drug. Monitor physiological status of client, especially the cardiopulmonary areas. Monitor for hypersensitivity reaction. Monitor lab data for objective changes in client status. | *Client should have:* Same as cell wall and ribosome antimicrobials. |

## MISCELLANEOUS MEDICATIONS

| Classification | Drug | Mechanism of action | Adverse outcome |
|---|---|---|---|
| Anti-inflammatory agents | | | Psychosis, superinfection, peptic ulceration, fluid retention, increased intraocular and intracranial pressure, impaired wound healing, headache, nausea, decreased carbohydrate tolerance, moon face, vertigo, growth suppression, negative nitrogen balance, osteoporosis, changes in skin test reactions, muscle wasting, buffalo hump obesity, activation of latent amebiasis, menstrual disturbances, weight gain, malaise. |
| Corticosteroids | Dexamethasone (Decadron) | Physiologically synthetic adrenocortical steroid that exert biological inhibition against agents producing inflammation. Also influences carbohydrate, lipid, and protein metabolisms and fluid and electrolyte balances (thus homeostasis). | |
| | *Other drugs:* Methylprednisolone (Medrol) Prednisone (Deltasone) Hydrocortisone (Cortef) Betamethasone (Celestone) | | |
| | *Other drugs in category:* Acetylsalicylic acid (aspirin) Indomethacin (Indocin) Phenylbutazone (Butazolidin) Ibuprofen (Motrin) Naproxen (Naprosyn) Fenoprofen calcium dihydrate (Nalfon) | | |

| Drug interaction | Nursing assessment | Nursing intervention | Expected outcome |
|---|---|---|---|
| Combined with oral anticoagulants may antagonize and produce hypercoagulability. Combined with insulin and oral hypoglycemic agents may cause hyperglycemia. Phenytoin decreases activity of dexamethasone. Vitamin A could inhibit anti-inflammatory effect. Combined with furosemide, ethacrynic acid, or thiazide diuretics enhances potassium loss. | *Assess client for:* Symptoms of inflammatory process, physiological effects of drug therapy, nutritional and fluid history, intake and output, weight, vital signs, and neurological checks (especially pulse, blood pressure, and level of consciousness). Determine simultaneous medications and disease processes and assess them in relation to dexamethasone. | Monitor all objective complaints of gastrointestinal upset after drug ingestion. Monitor all lab data, especially complete blood count with differential urinalysis, and serum glucose. Observe clients on long-term steroid therapy for bruising or abnormal bleeding tendencies. Monitor objective signs of edema and note progress. Observe for subjective signs of increased intraocular and intracranial pressure. Weigh client daily. Ensure client safety during ambulation to prevent falls and pathological fracture. Encourage exercise to prevent muscle atrophy. Give medication with food, milk, or bread products. Caution clients not to take medication on an empty stomach. Ensure balanced diet within tolerance to include adequate quantities of vitamins A, C, and D. For clients who are taking oral hypoglycemics or insulin, or those with diabetic tendencies, test urine for glucose spillage and observe for symptoms of hyperglycemia. If diuretics are concurrently administered, observe for hypokalemia symptoms. Strictly monitor intake and output, and correlate with weight and edema findings. Enforce fluid restrictions if indicated. Monitor all wounds or injuries for signs of superinfection. Support client and family through all aspects of care and tests. Help client and family verbalize their feelings about the administration and side effects of the drug therapy. | *Client should have:* Reduction in inflammatory process. |

*Continued.*

## MISCELLANEOUS MEDICATIONS—cont'd

| Classification | Drug | Mechanism of action | Adverse outcome |
|---|---|---|---|
| Antineuralgia and anti-convulsant agent | Tegretol (Carbamazepine) | Mechanism of action is unknown, recent data show that carbamazepine may affect the spinal trigeminal nucleus, preventing potentiation of repetitive stimuli from hyperexcitability. | Drowsiness, dizziness, aplastic anemia, thrombocytopenia, agranulocytosis, jaundice, leukopenia, fever, sore throat, peripheral neuritis, nystagmus, ulcerations in the mouth, incoordination, agitation, speech disturbances, epigastric distress, purpura, impotence, abnormal liver function tests. |
| Antivertigo and anti-histamine agents | Meclizine hydrochloride (Antivert, Bonine, Vertrol)<br><br>*Other drugs:*<br>Dimenhydrinate (Dramamine) | Basic mechanism unknown. Potentiate effect on vasodepressor blocking response to histamine but exhibit weak blocking responses to acetylcholine. | Dry mouth, blurred vision, drowsiness. |
| Antiemetic, anticho-linergic, and antihis-taminic agents | Benzquinamide (Emete-Con)<br><br>*Other drugs in category:*<br>Prochlorperazine dimaleate (Compazine)<br>Promethazine hydrochloride (Phenergan)<br>Trimethobenzamide hydrochloride (Tigan) | Mechanism in humans unknown. | Drowsiness, hiccups, dry mouth, blood pressure changes, dizziness, increased blood pressure, blurred vision, allergic skin response, fatigue, nervousness. |

| Drug interaction | Nursing assessment | Nursing intervention | Client outcome |
|---|---|---|---|
| May stimulate metabolism of doxycycline. Potentially dangerous when combined with MAO inhibitors. Decreases activity of oral anticholinergics. Decreases seizure control when used as an anticonvulsant in combination with tricyclic antidepressants. | *Assess client for:* Pain history, previous medication, nutritional history, history of seizure activity, lab data (especially complete blood count, platelets, serum iron, SGOT, SGPT, alkaline phosphatase, and BUN), plasma blood levels for drug, pathophysiological responses to drug therapy, support systems during tests, procedures and surgery, vital signs, neurological checks, intake and output, peripheral bruising or bleeding tendencies, gingival mucosa bleeding with dental care, concurrent drug therapy, pregnancy. | *Nurse should:* Monitor all lab data and plasma drug levels. Report any drug level approaching toxic levels immediately. Report any pain or seizure activity. Support client and family through all aspects of medical and surgical care and tests. Help client and family to verbalize their feelings. Teach client and family about all aspects of care. Caution client about driving or operating machinery when drowsy. Caution client to use care when ambulating to prevent bumping into objects and watching step to avoid falls because of potentiation of bruising and bleeding. Use caution during dental care to prevent gingival bleeding. | *Client should have:* Reduction in seizure activity, reduction in pain if drug used for trigeminal neuralgia; plasma blood level of 0.5 to 25 $\mu$g/ml. |
| Use judiciously with combinations of depressants, barbiturates, hypnotics, muscle relaxers, and alcohol, which may potentiate depressant effect. | *Assess client for:* Drowsiness, vertigo, condition of mouth and mucous membranes, history of motion sickness and methods of relieving it, patterns of vertigo attacks, past history of viral infections or ear infections, tinnitus, loss of hearing, and vomiting with vertigo. | Caution client not to drive or operate machinery when drowsy. Teach client to take safety precautions to prevent falls when having vertigo attack. Help client verbalize feelings. Help client and family develop support system during diagnostic testing and drug therapy. Instruct client to strictly curtail alcohol use while on drug therapy. | *Client should have:* Relief from motion sickness or vertigo associated with inner ear disorders. |
| Same as above | *Assess client for:* Obscured signs of overdosage of drugs or toxicity and signs to diagnose intestinal obstruction or increased brain tissue mass or pressure, drowsiness, nausea, or vomiting after hiccups. Changed blood pressure and vital signs. | *Nurse should:* Monitor all clients for postoperative potentiated sedative effect of drug-combined anesthesia and respiratory depression, and pathophysiological responses masked by drug therapy. Monitor clients in postoperative period for aspiration of vomitus. Caution clients not to drive or operate machinery when drowsy. | *Client should have:* Reduction in nausea and vomiting postoperatively or after anesthesia. |

*Continued.*

**MISCELLANEOUS MEDICATIONS—cont'd**

| Classification | Drug | Mechanism of action | Adverse outcome |
|---|---|---|---|
| Antiviral agent with antitranscription ability | Vidarabine (Vira-A) | Inhibits viral DNA synthesis and replication. Exact antiviral mechanism is unknown. | Diarrhea, anorexia, vomiting, psychosis, hallucinations, ataxia. Changes in lab data. |
| Antifibrinolytic agent | Aminocaproic acid (Amicar) | Inhibits fibrinolysis by inhibition of fibrinogen and plasmin activity in blood and tissue for competition against fibrinolysis of blood clots. | Nausea, diarrhea, malaise, nasal stuffiness, conjunctival suffusion, headache, skin rash. |

| Drug interaction | Nursing assessment | Nursing intervention | Expected outcome |
|---|---|---|---|
| Corticosteroids, ophthalmic preparations are contraindicated with vidarabine ophthalmic preparations. | *Assess client for:* acute fever, disordered mentation, altered level of consciousness, focal seizures, lab data (especially complete blood count, bilirubin, and SGOT), fluid and electrolyte imbalances, appetite and dietary pattern, intake and output, vital signs and neurological checks, and family support system. | *Nurse should:* Monitor client frequently for pathophysiological signs of drug therapy or extension of encephalitis. Support client and family in verbalization of feelings. Teach client regarding possible brain biopsy in surgery to confirm diagnosis or lumbar puncture, brain or CAT scan, EEG. Monitor clients with renal impairment or increased intracranial pressure very carefully for fluid overload. Once vial is mixed, should be used within 48 hours. | *Client should have:* Reduction of risk of mortality from herpes simplex virus, indirect encephalitis. |
| Antagonizes anticoagulants because of antifibrinolytic activity by decreasing prothrombin time. Can cause increased blood clotting when used with oral contraceptives. | *Assess client for:* Integrity of intravenous site, adverse effects of drug, neurological and vital signs, hypotension or bradycardia if intravenous rate fluctuates, intravenous site for any sign of infiltration, anorexia or nausea, signs of emboli in extremities (and Homan's sign), intake and output, respiratory difficulties, skin breakdown, bowel and bladder pattern, family support system. | *Nurse should:* Give drug diluted in 50 to 100 ml of solution and run over an hour. Do not give in same line as hyperalimentation or sodium lactate solutions. Use an intravenous control devise to ensure safe infusion. Support client and family by educating them regarding treatment and progress. Give fluids and foods that the client can tolerate within the restricted amount. Apply antiembolism stockings. Monitor sputum for change in color and signs of pulmonary emboli. Massage all reddened areas and monitor all broken areas with treatment appropriate to level of breakdown. Check for constipation or urinary distention while immobilized. Assist family through grief process if death is imminent. | *Client should have:* Fibrinolytic inhibition of the aneurysmal blood clot to prevent subarachnoid rebleeding. No development of complications associated with immobilization during therapy. |

## BIBLIOGRAPHY

Alcohol-drug interactions, FDA Bull., vol. 9, June 1979.

Baldessarini, R., and Stephens, J.: Lithium carbonate for affective disorders, Arch. Gen. Psychiatry **22:**72-77, Jan. 1970.

Beecher, H.: The powerful placebo, J.A.M.A. **159:**1602-1606, 1955.

Bergersen, B.S., and Goth, A.: Pharmacology in nursing, ed. 14, St. Louis, 1978, The C.V. Mosby Co.

Boyd, E.M.: The safety and toxicity of aspirin, Am. J. Nurs. **71:**964-966, 1971.

Bruni, J., and Wilder, B.J.: Valproic acid, Arch. Neurol. **36:** 393-398, July 1979.

Cooper, C.R.: Anticonvulsant drugs and the epileptic's dilemma, Nursing76 **6:**45-50, Jan. 1976.

Coulam, C.B., and Annegers, J.F.: Do anticonvulsants reduce the efficacy of oral contraceptives? Epilepsia **20:**519-524, 1979.

Di Mascio, S.: Debrisan for decubitus ulcers, Am. J. Nurs. **79:**684-685, 1979.

Dover, D., et al.: Treatment of acute intermittent porphyria with large doses of propranolol, J.A.M.A. **240:**766-768, 1978.

Evaluations of drug interactions, ed. 2, Washington, D.C., 1976, American Pharmaceutical Association Publishers.

Forsythe, W.I., et al.: Phenytoin serum levels in children with epilepsy: a microimmuno-assay technique, Dev. Med. Child Neurol. **21:**448-454, Aug. 1979.

Galloway, D.B., et al.: Propranolol in hypertension: a dose-response study, Br. Med. J. **2:**140, July 17, 1976.

Geigy Symposia Series: The addictive personality: treatment and prevention, Hartford, Conn., Nov., 1972, Ardsley, N.Y., 1973, Geigy Pharmaceuticals.

Gifford, R.W.: Clinical application of new antihypertensive drugs, Cleve. Clin. Q. **42:**255, Fall 1975.

Goodman, L., and Gilman, A., editors: The pharmacological basis of therapeutics, ed. 4, New York, 1970, Macmillan Publishing Co., Inc.

Hawken, M., and Ozuna, J.: Practical aspects of anticonvulsant therapy, Am. J. Nurs. **79:**1062-1068, June 1979.

Hollister, L.E.: Mental disorders—antianxiety and antidepressant drugs, N. Engl. J. Med. **286:**1195-1198, 1972.

Jackson, B.S.: Chronic peripheral arterial disease, Am. J. Nurs. **79:**928-934, 1972.

James, J., et al.: A guide to drug interactions, New York, 1978, McGraw-Hill Book Co.

Joynt, R.L.: Dantrolene sodium: long-term effects in patients with muscle spasticity, Arch. Phys. Med. Rehabil. **57:**212, May 1976.

Katz, D.L.: Sedatives and tranquilizers, N. Engl. J. Med. **286:** 757-760, 1972.

Kinney, J., and Leaton, G.: Loosening the grip: a handbook of alcohol information, St. Louis, 1978, The C.V. Mosby Co.

Kline, N.S., and Davis, J.M.: Psychotropic drugs, Am. J. Nurs. **73:**54-62, Jan. 1973.

Langan, R.J., and Cotzias, G.C.: Do's and don'ts for the patient on levodopa therapy, Am. J. Nurs. **76:**917, June 1976.

Laverty, R.: The mechanisms of action of some antihypertensive drugs, Br. Med. Bull. **29:**152, 1973.

Martin, E.W., et al.: Hazards of medications: a manual on drug interactions, Philadelphia, 1978, J.B. Lippincott Co.

Merck Sharp and Dohme: Product information summary, Sinemet (a combination of carbidopa and levodopa), West Point, Pa., 1975.

Modell, W., editor: Drugs of choice 1978-1979, St. Louis, 1978, The C.V. Mosby Co.

Mohney, S.: Some important clues to adverse drug reactions, RN **36:**48-49, 88-93, March 1973.

Monster, A.W., Herman, R., and Meeks, S., et al.: Cooperative study for assessing effects of pharmacological agents on spasticity, Am. J. Phys. Med. **52:**163, 1973.

Petrie, J.C., et al.: Methyldopa and propranolol or practolol in moderate hypertension, Br. Med. J. **2:**137, July 17, 1976.

Physicians' desk reference to pharmaceutical specialties and biologicals, ed. 34, Oradell, N.J., 1980, Medical Economics Co.

Ralston, S.E., and Hale, M.: Review and application of clinical pharmacology, Philadelphia, 1977, J.B. Lippincott Co.

Robinson, D.S.: Pharmacokinetic mechanisms of drug interactions, Postgrad. Med. **57:**55, Feb. 1975.

Robinson, M.B.: Levodopa and parkinsonism, Am. J. Nurs. **74:**656, April 1974.

Rodman, M.J.: Drugs for treating epilepsy, RN **35:**63-78, Sept. 1972.

Rosenberg, J.M.: Prescriber's guide to drug interactions, Oradell, N.J., 1978, Medical Economics.

Rusk, H.A.: Rehabilitation medicine, ed. 4, St. Louis, 1977, The C.V. Mosby Co.

Silverman, J.J., et al.: Clinical significance of tricyclic antidepressant plasma levels, Psychosomatics **20:**736-746, Nov. 1979.

Waddington, J.L., and Cross, A.L.: Pharmacology of (+) and (−) baclofen: GABA-dependent rotational behavior and [$^3$H]GABA receptor binding, Neuroscience Letters **14:**123-127, 1979.

Shank, L.F., and Ludewig, J.: Hypertension, Nurs. Clin. North Am. **9:**677, Dec. 1974.

Tsairis, P., and McDowell, F.H.: Drugs for skeletal muscle disturbances. In Modell, W., editor: Drugs of choice 1978-1979, St. Louis, 1978, The C.V. Mosby Co.

# APPENDIX

# AUDIOVISUAL RESOURCE LIST

Utilize this list to order audiovisual materials on neurological topics. Items with an *asterisk* are recommended but usually have some type of weakness that needs to be overlooked or supplemented. Items with a *dagger* are excellent in quality. The capital letter following the citation refers to the name of the source as listed in the *Key,* which follows.

KEY

*A* = American Academy of Pediatrics, 1801 Hinman Ave., Evanston, IL 60611

*B* = American Journal of Nursing Co., Educational Services, 555 West 57th St., New York, NY 10019

*C* = American Medical Association, Division of Continuing Medical Studies, 535 N. Dearborn, Chicago, IL 60610

*D* = Concept Media, P.O. Box 19542, Irvine, CA 92714

*E* = Conrad Berens International, Eye Film Library, 246 Danforth Ave., Jersey City, NJ 07305

$E^2$ = Crisis Communications Corporation, Ltd., 7215 Garden Grove Blvd., Suite J, Garden Grove, CA 92641

$E^3$ = Ear Research Institute, 256 South Lake St., Los Angeles, CA 90057

*F* = F.A. Davis, 1915 Arch St., Philadelphia, PA 19103

*G* = J.B. Lippincott, E. Washington Sq., Philadelphia, PA 19105

*H* = Martha Stuart Communications, Inc., 66 Bank St., New York, NY 10014

*I* = Medcom, Inc., 1633 Broadway, New York, NY 10019

*J* = Medical University of South Carolina, Division of Continuing Education, 171 Ashley Ave., Charleston, SC 29401

*K* = Michigan State University–East Lansing, College of Human Medicine, B 139 Life Sciences, East Lansing, MI 488401

*L* = Motorola Teleprograms Inc., Suite 23, 4825 N. Scott St., Schiller Park, IL 60176

*M* = Multimedia Educational Programs, % Medical Publications Center, McGraw-Hill Publishing Co., 4530 W. 77th St., Minneapolis, MN 55435

*N* = National Audiovisual Center, National Archives and Records Service, General Services Administration, Washington, DC 20409

$N^2$ = Nuclear Associates, 100 Voice Rd., Carle Place, NY 11514

*O* = Pennsylvania State University Audiovisual Services, 17 Willard Bldg., University Park, PA 16802

*P* = Robt. J. Brady Co., Rt. 197, Bowie, MD 20715

*Q* = Sister Kenny Insitution, Research and Education, 811 E. 27th St., Minneapolis, MN 55407

*R* = Trainex Corp., P.O. Box 116, Garden Grove, CA 92542

*S* = University of Arizona, Health Sciences Center, Division of Biomedical Communications, Tucson, AZ 85724

*T* = University of California–San Francisco, Educational TV Division, 431 North Bldg., San Francisco CA 94143

*U* = University of California–Los Angeles, Behavioral Sciences Media Lab, 760 Westward Plaza, Los Angeles CA 90024

*V* = University of Kansas, Division of Continuing Education Film Services, 746 Massachusetts St., Lawrence, KS 66044

*W* = University of Michigan, Medical Center,

Towsley Center for Continuing Medical Education, Box 57, Ann Arbor, MI 48109

*X* = University of Washington Press, Seattle, WA 98195

*Y* = University of Wisconsin Extension, Bureau of Audiovisual Instruction, 427 Lorch Ct., Rm. 106, Madison WI 53706

*Z* = Wayne State University Systems, Distribution and Utilization, 5448 Cass Ave., Detroit MI 48202

## Abuse

\*A different kind of hurt (child abuse), 16 mm, 18 min., sound, color, loan from V, cit. no. 8000102A

†Ordinary people: child abuse and neglect, 16 mm, 25 min., sound, color, guide, loan, and sale from L, cit. no. 8000577A

†Visual diagnosis of non-accidental trauma and failure to thrive, slides, 2 × 2, with cassette and guide, color, sale from A.

## Aging

†Aging: Who is listening? ¾-inch videocassette, 30 min., guide, sound, color, loan or sale, from B, cit. no. 7901283A

## Coma

†The comatose patient, two ¾-inch cassettes with guide, sound, color, 98 min., loan or sale from C.

†The comatose patient, 10 filmstrips with audiocassettes, color, sale from E².

## Coping

†Family stress in critical illness, slides or cassette with filmstrip, sale from P, cit. no. 7901487A

†The nature and management of stress, slides or cassette, guide, color, sound, sale from S, cit. no. 8000359A

\*Stress in critical care nursing practice, slides, filmstrip, or cassette from P, cit. no. 7901517A

## Dying

†American attitudes toward death and dying, filmstrip with cassette and guide, color, sale from D, cit. no. 7601368

†Viewpoint: the dying patient, filmstrip, cassette, and manual, color, sale from D, cit. no. 7601304

†The nurse and the grieving process, 16 mm, 45 min., sound, black and white, loan from T, cit. no. 7601338

†Guidelines for interacting with the dying patient, filmstrip, cassette, and manual, color, sale from D, cit. no. 7601414

†Nurse and the grieving process, 16 mm, 45 min., sound, black and white, loan from T, cit. no. 7601338

†Until I die, 16 mm, 30 min., sound, color, loan or sale from B

## Headache

\*Headache, ¾-inch videocassette, color, sound, 46 min., guide, loan or sale from C

## Hypertension

†Introduction to hypertension, ¾-inch videocassette, 26 min., sound, color, loan or sale from J

## Disorders in infants and young children

†Jean, The Bennetts, Dr. Voss, and Mrs. McGill: Sympathy; the Schuster family; How do you tell the parents? 16 mm with guide, 45 min., sound, color, loan or sale from Y, cit. no. 8000697A

†The neurologically suspect infant, 2 × 2 slides with 30 min. cassette, color, sale from N, cit. no. 7601617

‡Neurological disorders of the newborn, 2 × 2 slides with guide, loan free from K, cit. no. 7602114.

## Examination: underlying anatomy and physiology

†Autonomic nervous system, ¾-inch videocassette, sound, color, 29 min., loan free or sale from N, cit. no. 7600053

\*Cranial nerves: normal and abnormal signs, 16 mm, 27 min., sound, color, loan or sale from Z, cit. no. 7600120

†Denver Developmental Screening Test, ¾-inch cassettes, sound, color, 60 min. total, also available in 16 mm, sale from N, cit. no. 8000261A

†Exploring the human nervous system, 16 mm, 23 min., sound, color, loan free from N, cit. no. 7600194

†Indirect ophthalmoscopy of the peripheral retina, 16 mm, 45 min., sound, color, loan from E, cit. no. 7600260

†The neurological examination of infants, 16 mm, 26 min., sound, color, loan or sale from Q, cit. no. 7511145

†The neurological examination (pediatric), ¾-inch videocassette, 40 min., sound, color, guide, write J.B. Lippincott Co., Philadelphia.

\*Neuromuscular: physical appraisal of the adult in nursing practice, ¾-inch videocassettes, 50 min. total, sound, color, guide, contact W.

†Proprioception, vibratory, tactile, pain and temperature pathways, ¾-inch videocassette, 36 min., sound, color, loan free or sale from N, cit. no. 7600473

\*Spinal cord and its relations, 16 mm, sound, color, loan free or sale from N, cit. no. 7600524

### Infection

*Infections of the nervous system,* slides and sound, sale from F, cit. no. 7901223A

### Language disorders

†*Language disorders (aphasia),* filmstrip with cassette and guide, sale from D.

### Neurosis

*The neurotic child,* 28 min., sound, black and white, 16 mm, loan or sale from O, cit. no. 7600748

### Pain

†*The lower back pain syndrome,* 2 × 2 slides, guide, color, contact I, cit. no. 7601963

†*Neurophysiology of pain,* slides, cassette, or filmstrip, sale from P, cit. no. 7901502

†*Pain management,* ¾-inch videocassette with manual, black and white, 37 min., sound, sale from X, cit. no. 7602120

### Neurosurgery

†*Pathophysiology of neurosurgery,* 62 slides (2 × 2), color or black and white, guide, loan or sale from W, cit. no. 7901114A

### Seizures

†*The absence seizure,* 16 mm, 29 min., sound, black and white, free from N, cit. no. 7500005

†*Introduction to seizure disorders,* ¾-inch videocassette or filmstrip with cassette, sale from R, cit. no. 7601252

†*Children with seizures,* 2 × 2 slides with cassette and guide, sale from W.

*Neuroleptics and adjunctive medications,* two ¾-inch videocassettes, sound, 52 min. total, color, guide, loan or sale from X.

†*Nursing care in seizure disorders,* ¾-inch videocassette or filmstrip with cassette, sale from R, cit. no. 7601267.

*People who have epilepsy,* ¾-inch videocassette, sound, color, 29 min. loan or sale from H, cit. no. 7901059A

*Seizure disorders in children,* ¾-inch videocassette, 29 min., sound, color, loan or sale from O, cit. no. 7900845A

### Sleep

†*The nature of sleep,* filmstrip with 22 min. cassette, contact D, cit. no. 7602068

### Specific disorders; disabling conditions

†*Disabling and deforming conditions,* filmstrip with 32 min. cassette and manual, sale from D, cit. no. 7602098

†*Cerebrovascular disorders,* slides with cassette and test book, sale from N[2]

†*Gilles de la Tourette's disease,* 45 min., 16 mm, sound, color, loan or sale from U, cit. no. 7900818A

*Multiple sclerosis,* 16 mm, 26 min., sound, color, loan free from N, cit. no. 7500141

*Multiple dystrophy and related conditions,* 16 mm, sound, color, 32 min, loan free from N.

†*Stretching and mobilization for the Parkinson patient,* 16 mm, sound, color, 7 min., loan free from N, cit. no. 7600822

†*Mobilization of the stroke patient,* 2 × 2 slides with cassette, color, sale from W, cit. no. 7601833

*The diagnosis and treatment of trigeminal neuralgia,* ¾-inch videocassette, sound, color, 29 min., contact O, cit. no. 7901615A

### Sexuality

†*Medical conditions (i.e., hypertension) impact on sexuality (human sexuality and nursing practice: Program 3),* Filmstrip with cassette and manual, sale from D, cit. no. 7602111

†*Sexuality: a nursing concern,* filmstrip with cassette and manual, sale from D, cit. no. 7602136

### Trauma

*Head injuries,* ¾- or ½-inch cassette, 22 min., sound, color, loan or sale from M, cit. no. 8000318A

†*The multiply-traumatized patient,* ¾-inch videocassettes, 55 min. total, sound, color, guide, loan or sale from C, cit. no. 7901638A

†*Vestibular and non-vestibular nystagmus,* ¾-inch videocassette, 47 min., sound, color, contact E[3]

†*Dizziness of unknown origin,* ¾-inch cassette, 58 min., sound, color, loan or sale from E[3], cit. no. 8000346A

# INDEX

Encephaloceles, 14-15, 353
 differential diagnosis, 15
 surgical treatment of, 678-679
Encephalopathy, 172
 common findings in, 517-519
 metabolic, and coma, 201
 in niacin deficiency, 433
Endoneurium, 48
Endarterectomy, 609
Endorphins, 77, 234, 242-243
Endotracheal tube, insertion of, in comatose client, 577
Endurance, exercises for, 645
Enduron; *see* Methyclothiazide
Enema, medicated retention, for fecal impaction, 697
Engel's theory of pain, 217
Enkephalins, 77
Enophthalmos, 123
Enteric cytopathogenic human orphan virus, 511
Enteric viruses, differentiating, 511
Environment
 for client with multiple sclerosis, 454
 for client with Sydenham's chorea, 522
 enrichment of, 147-148
 after hemorrhagic stroke, 615-616
 for infant with hydrocephalus, 371
 intrauterine, 257
 after intravertebral tumor surgery, 559
 postoperative, preparation of, 542
 for unconscious client, 208
Environmental influences on development, 7-10
Enzyme multiple immunoassay technique, 402
Eosinophilic tumor, 536
Ependyma, 45
Ependymal layer of neural tube, 18, 20, 21
Ephedrine, 119
 properties of, 732-733
Epicritic sensation, 85
Epidemic meningitis, 503
Epidermoids, 354
Epidural hematoma, 573-575
Epigenesis theory of development, 4
Epilepsy, 165
 categorization, 384-385
 childbearing and, 408
 and differentiation from coma, 202
 EEG to detect, 304-305, 307
 factors involved in, 385-388
 general evaluation for, 388
 incidence, 385
 laws affecting epileptics, 408
 medical management of, 401-408
 medications for, 408-409
 multifactorial classification
  abdominal epilepsy, 395
  centrencephalic seizures, 392-394
  complex partial seizures, 392
  focal seizures, 389-392
  miscellaneous mixed convulsive problems, 394-395
 pathogenesis of, 385
 related problems, 395-401
 resources, 409

Epinephrine
 and blood pressure
  role in pupillary response, 123
 secretion of, 43
 to stimulate sympathetic division, 119
Epineurium, 48
Epithalamus; *see* Pineal body
EPSP; *see* Excitatory postsynaptic potential fibers
Equanil; *see* Meprobamate
Equipment for neurological assessment, 249-250
Erb's dystrophy, 463
Erection, physiology of, 156
Ergonovine, 119
Ergotamine tartrate, 411
 properties of, 748-749
Erythromycin, 511
 properties of, 758-759
*Escherichia coli,* 352, 510
Eserine, 59
Eskabarb, 398
Essential hypertension, 601, 602
Estriol levels in maternal urine, 259
Ethacrynic acid, 750
Ethanol, 730
Ethclorvynol, 730
Ethopropazine, 740
Ethosuximide, 392
 properties of, 724-725
Ethotoin, 722
Eutonyl; *see* Pargyline
Evaluation of speech and language, 631-632
Excitability, 71
Excitatory postsynaptic potential fibers, 73, 102, 106
Excitement phase of sexual arousal, 156
Exencephaly, 14, 353
Exercise for spastic clients, 643-646
Experimental situations, response to pain in, 220-221
Expressive aphasia, 631
Extension paraplegia, 447
External cooling, 689
Exteroceptors, 77, 78
Extradural tumors, 553
Extrapyramidal disorders, 472-486
Extrapyramidal tracts
 functions of, 102-105, 106
 influences of motor command centers on, 105
 interruptions in, 106-107
Extremities of neonate, assessment of, 271
Eye care
 routine for, 695-697
 for unconscious client, 208, 549
Eye orbit injuries, interventions for, 697
Eye shield, 695
Eyes, integrity of, in hypertension, 604

**F**

Facial nerve, 24, 25, 36, 38
 anatomy of, 58
 assessment of 291-292
Facial paralysis, 493-494
Facial sling, 697